Principles of Critical Care

To

Vera and my children, for the love and happiness we share;

my parents, for showing me the way;

my house-staff and nursing staff, for their unstinted support.

Preface to the Second Edition

It has been gratifying to observe that this book has become the standard text of critical care medicine in India. Love's labour has been rewarded and has indeed borne fruit. My hope that this work would be worthy of acceptance by intensivists, anaesthesiologists, colleagues practising other specialities, by residents, students and senior nursing staff has been realized. In a small way the book has perhaps helped critical care in India to strike deeper roots, to spread and to flourish.

I have succumbed to the pressure of producing a second edition. It has been a difficult and onerous task. I discovered that it is easier to write afresh, than to delete, modify, prune and add to what has already been written. Yet it was imperative that this task be undertaken, so as to keep reasonably abreast with the advances in this speciality. The new edition has been extensively revised; it incorporates several changes and several current trends in almost every chapter of the book. Because of popular demand, a new section has been devoted to Critical Care During Pregnancy.

The management of critically ill patients with different emergent problems has been increasingly influenced by set protocols, algorithms, and guidelines based whenever possible on scientific evidence. These have been included in various sections of the present edition. The concept of disease and its management based on scientific proof or evidence is unquestionably preferred to that based on 'opinions' or 'impressions', provided the scientific evidence is both trustworthy and strong. However, there are limits to science today and in the foreseeable future. There are many areas in critical care and emergency medicine where science has as yet to shed its light. Where science ends, empiricism whether we like it or not, begins. The same disease producing a critical illness is almost never exactly similar in any two patients, with regard to clinical presentation, natural history or management. These are modified not only by each patient's individual physiological adaptations to disease, but also by several protean factors, which we do not understand. Clinical judgment in the recognition and treatment of a critical illness therefore remains of supreme importance. Clinicians and intensivists should be aware of guidelines and other aids borne out of scientific study and evidence. But these should not strait-jacket thinking and lead to a tunnel-vision of what is very often a complex problem. In the management of every single critically ill individual, well designed protocols and guidelines should supplement and not supplant or usurp clinical judgement.

I very sincerely acknowledge my thanks to my distinguished contributors who have once again kindly and willingly contributed in an honorary capacity to this edition, thereby enhancing its prestige. I would like to express my deep gratitude to Dr Sumit Raisinghaney and Mr Neeraj Chawan, my research assistants, for their dedication, their perseverance and for their unstinted help and support. I would also like to thank the publishers and authors who have granted me permission to reproduce some figures and tables from their books/journals. Although every effort has been made to trace copyright holders of material printed in this book, in some cases, the copyright holders are yet to respond. The publishers will be glad to hear from them.

My gratitude above all to my wife Vera for correcting the page-proofs and for her forbearance and care during the many days and nights spent on this work. Finally, my sincere thanks to the Oxford University Press in Delhi and Bombay.

Preface

Critical care in India and other developing countries is nascent and needs to strike deeper roots if it is to flourish and prosper. The history of critical care in this country started in the late sixties and early seventies with the establishment of coronary care units in Bombay and in a few other big cities of India. These units though centralized, were designed and equipped chiefly to offer intensive care to patients with acute myocardial infarction. They had a poor concept of overall critical care, or of intensive respiratory care. Mechanical ventilator support was primitive, its use being mostly restricted to a token gesture of grace offered to a patient about to depart from this world. In the mid and late sixties, my medical unit at the Breach Candy Hospital, Bombay, started offering overall critical care, intensive respiratory care and successful ventilator support in critical illnesses due to a wide spectrum of disease. Intensive care in my unit, to start with, lacked good monitoring facilities and was initially offered in a few separate rooms within a general ward of the hospital. These were perhaps the first stirrings of critical care as we know it today in the city of Bombay, and perhaps in this country. However the real impetus to organized, centralized, overall critical care arose when, in early 1970, a 34-year old, 6-month pregnant lady was hospitalized in my unit at the Breach Candy Hospital for increasing breathlessness. She was dubbed as functional by the duty officer, when in fact she had acute poliomyelitis presenting with intercostal muscle weakness. She evolved over 24 hours because of bulbar and spinal involvement into an acutely ill, totally paralytic state which needed intensive care of multiple organ systems, together with prolonged ventilator support. We used a pressure-cycled Bird's ventilator, and with the able assistance of an anaesthetist colleague, Dr A. B. Bhatia, struggled and succeeded against great odds in keeping her alive. Successful ventilator support was continued for many months, and she was delivered by Caesarean section of a healthy baby at full term, whilst on ventilator support. About six weeks after initiating ventilator support we fortuitously acquired a Radiometer through the patient's brother who was a paediatric cardiac surgeon in Los Angeles, enabling us thereby for the first time to monitor arterial pH and blood gases by the Astrup technique. This was indeed the first blood gas analysis machine used for intensive patient care in this country. Unwittingly, the illness of this dear lady (who is still well), became an important landmark in the history of critical care both in this city and in this country. Starting in 1971, from a 2-bedded, centralized, reasonably well-equipped, multidisciplinary all-purpose intensive care unit, we graduated to a newly constructed 8-bedded well-designed and fully equipped unit which admitted critical problems in all branches of medicine and surgery. This unit over many years continues to have a medical audit as good as any unit in the West. It has also served to train numerous house physicians and registrars who have carried the message of critical care to other hospitals of this city and to many hospitals in other parts of the country. The concept of critical care has now been increasingly accepted and followed in most large hospitals of the big cities of this country.

Some of my colleagues, particularly those engaged in community medicine, preventive and social medicine, are of the opinion that in a poor large country like India, the encouragement of critical care is a misdirected effort. It is indeed true that increasing the number of critical care units in the country will not inflict even a small dent in the overwhelming health problems this country has to cope with. Should then the speciality of critical care be fostered and encouraged? The answer on principle is unquestionably yes. It is the physician's duty to care for the ill, and the more critically ill a patient, the more intensive the care a patient needs for survival. We however need to do this in all poor countries with a logical perspective. It would be unrealistic, futile and morally wrong to dot this huge country with numerous critical care units when even basic primary health care is lacking, and when ordinary hospital facilities in most parts of the country are hopelessly inadequate. Reason demands that well-equipped critical care units should in the forseeable future be confined to medium and large hospitals which have the infrastructure to support such units. It would also be wiser and profitable to organize general all-purpose intensive care units rather than copy the West and establish critical care units in different specialities and subspecialities. A multidisciplinary intensive care unit permits concentration of meagre resources with regard to staffing, equipment and technical expertise. Above all it encourages a more holistic approach, so that problems in the critically ill are considered in an overall perspective rather than in terms of disease afflicting isolated organ systems. There is also a crying need to formulate laws and regulations (non-existent at the present time) that govern the establishment and functioning of critical care units in developing countries. Financial lucre will otherwise continue to allow the mushrooming of so-called intensive care units which are veritable death traps for unwary, unsuspecting patients.

Efficiently functioning critical care units in the forseeable future will be largely confined to the big cities of this country. Should we not promote a modicum of better care for critical illnesses in the huge population of over 650,000,000 that resides outside these cities? This can for the present only be achieved by providing a better staffed and better equipped high-dependency ward in every district hospital of this subcontinent. These wards would not qualify by Western standards as critical care units, but in our experience could offer better care, with improved results, at a smaller cost.

This book is largely based on my numerous jottings and notes embodying my experience of problems in the diagnosis and management of critically ill patients over the last 30 years. A book of this magnitude, authored in the main by a single individual helped by just a few distinguished contributors, may seem audacious, but has the intrinsic advantage of presenting the uniform view of one who for many years has had to grapple with a wide spectrum of critical illnesses. It in no way detracts from the fact that for a successful outcome, critical care often needs team effort involving many specialities in medicine, surgery, and their allied branches. The emphasis in this book is on fundamentals that form the basis of care and on important problems that find their way to a busy unit. The book also includes in most chapters an insight into the nature of derangement of altered functions in a critical illness. Good management can then be better understood and need not be ritualized or didactic.

Critical care in developing countries encompasses both diseases prevalent in the West, as also special problems chiefly encountered in poor countries such as India. These problems particularly in relation to important fulminant tropical infections have been given due emphasis in this book. We also have to necessarily contend with lack of sophisticated gadgetry and equipment in many of our units. The successful management of many life-threatening problems under these circumstances and restraints is difficult but still possible, and has been discussed in relevant chapters.

It is essential to stress that the principles of good critical care are the principles of good medicine and surgery. Improvement in critical care can therefore only flow from improved standards in general medicine and surgery. A careful history, a good physical examination, and the evaluation of relevant laboratory and imaging data will always form the bedrock for correct diagnosis and management of life-threatening problems. Improved technology and invasive gadgetry can be of help, but they can never be a substitute for sound clinical acumen and experience gathered over years of trial and tribulation. The use of machines and in particular of invasive techniques, should never be an end in itself, but always a means to the solution of difficult problems. To feed a machine in a critical care unit just because it is there, is to court medical nemesis.

The speciality of critical care by its very nature often incites the caring physician to prompt or hurried action. Admittedly, there are a few emergencies which do demand immediate measures if life is to be salvaged. But in most critical situations there will be time to stand and wait, to think and deliberate—

> 'And time for all the works and days of hands
> That lift and drop a question on your plate.'

The physician must take time to muster the clinical discipline that allows a focused view on an emergent threatening problem, yet not lose an overall perspective of the patient. The initiate in critical care medicine should first and foremost be reminded ever so often of the Hippocratic dictum, *Primum Non Nocere*—first of all, do no harm. He should therefore be encouraged to think (without falling asleep) over a problem before jumping into action, else he may well become the prime iatrogenic hazard in the unit.

In the final analysis, critical care is care that aids and improves patient survival. It is doctors and nurses who care for patients and not machines. We should take comfort in the fact that there is no substitute for human ingenuity, endeavour and resources. Motivation and dedication towards providing better patient care can indeed compensate significantly in our part of the world for the lack of sophisticated technology and technical expertise.

I very sincerely acknowledge my thanks to all my extremely distinguished contributors who are all well-known specialists in their own fields, and who have so kindly and willingly contributed in an honorary capacity to this book. They have immeasurably enhanced the prestige of this book by their valuable contributors. I would like to acknowledge my immense gratitude most of all to Dr Ruby Jal Kharas, my research assistant, who has made this book her special baby. She has been of immense help in every single aspect of this book, and this book would have had to wait for many more months to see the light of day, if it had not been for her dedication and perseverance. I also owe an immense debt of gratitude to Mr S. M. Datta, Chairman of Hindustan Lever Ltd., India, who on behalf of his company has been kind enough to give a very generous subsidy towards the publication of this magnum opus. The price of this work has thereby been substantially reduced so that the book is now within reach of all students and all my medical colleagues. Dr Ramnik Parikh and Dr T. Rajgopal were instrumental in arranging for this munificent subsidy, and to them I express my sincere gratitude. I would also like to thank the publishers and authors who have granted me permission to reproduce some figures and tables from their books/journals. Although every effort has been made to trace copyright holders of material printed in this book, in some cases this has not proved possible. In a few cases, the copyright holders are yet to respond. The publishers will be glad to hear from them.

I would also like to thank Dr Shilpa Bhojraj for her assistance with the chapter on Control of Pain and Anxiety and the Use of Muscle Relaxants in the Critically Ill. My special thanks are due to Mrs Lavanya Ray and to Ms Rivka Israel for their excellent editorial advice and assistance. I am grateful to Mr Abe Aboody and Mr P. Balagangadharan of Alliance Phototypesetters for their kind cooperation and excellent work. I am also grateful to Mr V. Pradhan and Mr R. Prabhu for the good art work and X-ray plates. I also offer my thanks to Ms Katy F. Irani who has helped with the typing of this manuscript and with the Index. My gratitude to my wife, Vera, for having helped to correct the page proofs and for her extra forbearance and care during the many days and nights spent on this work. Finally, my sincere thanks to the Oxford University Press in Bombay and Delhi for their unstinted help and cooperation in publishing this work.

Contents

Preface to the Second Edition   vii

Preface   viii

1   An Introduction to Critical Care   1
- Overview   3
- Principles, Philosophy and Ethnics of Critical Care   4
- Organization of an Intensive Care Unit   8
- Critical Care Scoring   14

2   Cardiopulmonary Resuscitation and Cerebral Preservation in Adults   19

3   Basic Cardiorespiratory Physiology in the Intensive Care Unit   33

4   Procedures and Monitoring in the Intensive Care Unit   45
- Procedures in the Intensive Care Unit
  by Dr J.D. Sunavala   47
- Cardiac Monitoring in Adults
  by Dr J.D. Sunavala   59
- Respiratory Monitoring in Adults   77

5   Imaging in the Critical Care Unit   85
- Introduction   87
- Imaging Techniques in the Chest
  by Dr Anirudh Kohli   88
- Imaging Techniques in the Abdomen
  by Dr Anirudh Kohli   96
- Neuroimaging Techniques
  by Dr Anirudh Kohli   106

6   Clinical Shock Syndromes   113
- Overview of Shock Syndromes   115
- Hypovolaemic and Haemorrhagic Shock   120
- Cardiogenic Shock   128
- Sepsis and Septic Shock   141
- Cardiac Compressive Shock   155
- Anaphylactic Shock   159

7   Cardiovascular Problems Requiring Critical Care   161
- Acute Coronary Syndromes   163
- Unstable Angina   165
- Acute Myocardial Infarction   171
- Acute Left Ventricular Failure with Pulmonary Oedema   183
- Tachyarrhythmias in the Intensive Care Unit   190
- Bradyrhythms and Heart Blocks in the ICU   202
- Antiarrhythmic Drugs Used in the ICU   205
- Hypertensive Crisis and Aortic Dissection in the ICU   213
- Pulmonary Embolism   220

8   Respiratory Problems Requiring Critical Care   229
- Acute Respiratory Failure in Adults   231
- Oxygen Therapy   245
- Airway Management   255
- Acute Respiratory Crisis in Chronic Obstructive Pulmonary Disease (COPD)   267
- Acute Lung Injury (ARDS)
  by Dr F.E. Udwadia with Dr Z.F. Udwadia   274
- Acute Severe Asthma
  by Dr Zarir F. Udwadia   288
- Community-acquired Pneumonias Requiring Critical care
  by Dr Zarir F. Udwadia   295
- Massive Haemoptysis   301

9   Mechanical Ventilation in the Critically Ill   309

10   Fluid and Electrolyte Disturbances in the Critically Ill   339

11   Acid-Base Disturbances in the Critically Ill   359

12   Nutritional Support in the Critically Ill Adult   373

13   Fever and Acute Infections in a Critical Care Setting   389
- General Consideration and Non-Infective Causes of Fever in the ICU   391
- Nosocomial Infections   394
- Community-acquired Fulminant Infections Requiring Critical Care   413
- Use of Antibiotics in the ICU   431
- Treatment of Fungal infection in Critically Ill Patients   440

14 Surgical Infections in the Intensive Care Unit 445
    – Post-Operative Wound Infections 447
    – Nectrotizing Fasciitis and Clostridial
      Myonecrosis 450
    – Intra-abdominal Sepsis 453

15 Organ System Dysfunction Requiring
    Critical Care 463
    – Multiple Organ Dysfunction Syndrome (MODS) 465
    – Renal Dysfunction in the Critically Ill 479
    – Critical Care in Fulminant Hepatitis 491
    – Acute (Fulminant) Necrotizing Pancreatitis 503
    – Acute Gastrointestinal Bleeds Requiring
      Critical Care 510
    – Haemorrhagic Disorders in the ICU 520
    – Transfusion (Blood Product) Therapy 530
    – Endocrine Dysfunction in the Critically Ill 535
    – Diabetes Mellitus in the Critically Ill Patient 543
    – Neurological Disorders Requiring Critical Care 550
      A. Increased Intracranial Pressure
          by Dr Sarosh M. Katrak and
          Dr Noshir H. Wadia 550
      B. Cranial Trauma
          by Dr Sohrab K. Bhabha 557
      C. Acute Stroke
          by Dr Sarosh M. Katrak and
          Dr Noshir H. Wadia 562
      D. Fulminant Neurological infections
          by Dr Sohrab K. Bhabha 571
      E. Status Epilepticus
          by Dr Sarosh M. Katrak and
          Dr Noshir H. Wadia 577
      F. Peri-Operative Neurosurgical Care
          by Dr Sohrab K. Bhabha 584

16 Critical Care After Open Heart Surgery 589

17 The Immunocompromised Patient 603

18 Physical Injuries Requiring Critical Care 621
    – Intensive Care Management of Polytrauma
      by Dr N.S. Laud 623
    – Management of Critically Ill Burns Patients
      by Dr S.M. Keswani with
      Dr F.E. Udwadia 630
    – Critical Care in Poisonings 640
    – Envenomation in the ICU 653

19 Critical Care of the Cancer Patient 659

20 Control of Pain and Anxiety and the Use of
    Muscle Relaxants in the Critically Ill 667

21 Critical Care of the Transplant Patient 679

22 Critical Care in Pregnancy 687
    – Introduction 689
    – Critical Illness Not Specific to Pregnancy 691
    – Critical Illness Specific to Pregnancy 694

23 The Critically Ill Child 701
    – Cardiopulmonary Resuscitation in Infants
      and Children
      by Dr Y.K. Amdekar 703
    – Respiratory and Haemodynamic Monitoring
      of the Critically Ill Child
      by Dr Joseph Britto and
      by Dr P. Ramnarayan 705
    – Approach to Shock in the Paediatric Intensive
      Care Unit
      by Dr Y.K. Amdekar 715
    – Hypertensive Emergencies in Paediatrics
      by Dr Y.K. Amdekar 718
    – Heart Failure in Neonates and Children
      by Dr Y.K. Amdekar 719
    – Acute Respiratory Failure in Children and
      Hyaline Membrane Disease
      by Dr Y.K. Amdekar 721
    – Fluid and Electrolyte Disturbances in the
      Critically Ill Child
      by Dr Y.K. Amdekar 726
    – Nutritional Support in the Paediatric
      Intensive Care Unit
      by Dr Y. K. Amdekar 728
    – Paediatric Life-Threatening Infections Requiring
      Critical care
      by Dr Y. K. Amdekar 729
    – Acute Renal Failure in Infants and Children
      by Dr B. V. Gandhi 733

Appendix 737

Index 743

SECTION 1

An Introduction to Critical Care

1.1 Overview
1.2 Principles, Philosophy and Ethics of Critical Care
1.3 Organization of an Intensive Care Unit
1.4 Critical Care Scoring

CHAPTER 1.1
Overview

Critical care is the care of seriously ill patients with life-threatening illnesses or trauma, as also of patients who have the potential to develop life-threatening complications from their disease. Critical care should, correctly speaking, be reserved for patients with severe but potentially reversible problems. Patients with chronic terminal illnesses, with the end close at hand should be given every care at home or in the ward of a hospital, but not in critical care units.

The origin of the present day intensive care unit started with the use of the post-operative recovery room for immediate special post-operative care. This concept was given a further impetus during the poliomyelitis epidemic in the early 1950s when the use of mechanical ventilation salvaged many paralysed patients. Present day intensive care is however far more meaningful than mere post-operative care and ventilatory support. It incorporates the knowledge and experience of numerous specialities that have blossomed over nearly four decades from 1960 onwards. Pulmonary medicine with the concept of respiratory care, cardiology with the concept of the coronary care unit, and advances in anaesthesiology have all contributed greatly to the evolution of the modern day critical care unit. While specialities in medicine or surgery are sharply focused on a single organ system within the body, a general medical or surgical critical care unit is devoted to the patient as a whole, recognizing the overwhelming fact that there is a tremendous interdependence and interrelationship between various organ systems, so that a serious involvement of one strongly jeopardizes the function of others. The approach to critical care medicine is thus simultaneously holistic, viewing the patient in an overall perspective, and yet focused on one or more problems that constitute an immediate threat to life.

It was obvious from the 1960s onwards that critically ill patients are best and ideally cared for in special units which centralize equipment, staff and facilities, so necessary for the care of life-threatening problems. Intensive or critical care has blossomed into a speciality with special training and certification in the West, and also in many developed or quickly developing East Asian countries. The speciality is a young but growing one in our country. Doctors practising critical care medicine are often called 'Intensivists'— semantically speaking an inappropriate and rather unaesthetic term. Many such practitioners of critical care medicine are specialists in cardiology, pulmonary medicine, anaesthesiology, or in critical care itself. However the principles of critical care are the principles of general medicine and general surgery, rather than the principles applicable to any particular speciality. In my opinion the general physician or surgeon with a wide experience of medicine or surgery, and suitable training and exposure to acute medical or surgical problems, has the best aptitude and philosophy for organizing and directing a critical care unit.

It is important particularly in a poor country like ours, that the few good critical care units we have, admit patients who truly need appropriate care. It is sad to see critical care units cluttered with patients who are unquestionably better looked after in the wards, or at home. A critical care unit has its advantages and disadvantages. The chief advantage is that it provides better and more organized care. The main disadvantage is of a hostile environment contributing to anxiety, emotional stress, loneliness, fear, and a greater risk of developing nosocomial infections.

The following conditions require intensive or critical care:

(i) Acute life-threatening illnesses which are potentially reversible.

(ii) Acute illnesses with potential and likely to occur life-threatening complications.

(iii) Monitoring of vital parameters of patients with symptoms and/or signs that suggest the possibility of an evolving life-threatening illness.

(iv) Acute or immediate life-threatening crisis or complications in a chronic illness, even when the latter by itself is almost certain to cause death within a matter of months. An example of this is a patient with cancer at a stage when his life expectancy is 3–6 months. An acute complicating pneumonia in such a patient is a life-threatening emergency, which is treatable, curable and may well necessitate critical care.

A critical care unit as already mentioned should not be used for terminal cases where the end is close at hand. The tendency to use a critical care unit as the last halt or 'stopping station' before an expected departure from this world, should be strongly deprecated.

This section first deals with the principles and philosophy of critical care. This is followed by a short discussion on ethical principles governing critical care, on ethical issues in terminal illness, and on euthanasia. The section then discusses the organization of a critical care unit and ends with a description of current critical care scoring systems.

Principles, Philosophy and Ethics of Critical Care

The principles of critical care are in quintessence the same as those underlying good medicine and surgery. They include:

(i) Early Diagnosis and Identification of the Problem

The doctor in the critical care unit often deals with life-threatening illnesses with serious dysfunction involving one or more organ systems. The early diagnosis and identification of the problem is imperative for correct management. This is a basic dictum for all fields of medicine and surgery, but is indeed a matter of urgency in critical care medicine.

(ii) Anticipation of Possible Events and Complications

I consider this the very essence of good critical care. The treating doctor must have a firm grip on what is happening to a patient, and must acutely anticipate possible events and complications in the immediate future. This he can only do if he has the knowledge, wisdom and experience of judging the possible evolution of a life-threatening illness in a given patient. To be 'one step ahead in one's mind' with reference to an acutely evolving disease, is an important tactical advantage that often leads to victory for the patient and his doctor.

(iii) The Holistic Approach to a Critical Illness

The holistic approach has already been mentioned earlier. It cannot be overstressed that the patient must be viewed in an overall perspective with interrelated functions of interrelated organ systems. This is not to decry team effort involving various specialists in the management of a critical illness. Team effort is indeed crucial for success, as there is no single physician or surgeon who can know everything there is to know about the multiple facets of medicine and surgery. Yet team effort must needs be conducted and carefully orchestrated by a single individual, if it is to prove successful. Too many specialists and superspecialists individually looking after a critically ill patient, more often than not hasten his departure from this world. Their over-enthusiastic and often over-focused attention on the organ system of their choice, needs to be tempered and viewed with reference to the patient as a whole. The many problems in such patients should be considered in their overall perspective, priority being assigned to those needing immediate attention. Yet it must always be asked as to how best one can engage an emergent problem without seriously jeopardizing the function of other organ systems. A management decision in a not so critically ill patient is often easy and straightforward; a similar decision in a critically ill individual is beset with complex difficulties. The hazards involved in implementing a therapeutic procedure should always be balanced against the possible benefits. There are no clear-cut guidelines in many decisions that need to be made in the care of critically ill individuals. It is a question of experience, wisdom, and at times an intuitive feel of what is probably right or wrong in a given situation.

(iv) The Considered Use of Technology

The patient is to be cared for by the doctor and the nurses and not by machines. Machines and sophisticated gadgets are an adjunct to the doctor's skill and care; they cannot replace them. Merely because machines have been provided is no reason to use them. Invasive procedures and invasive gadgetry have an inherent risk even in the best of hands; they pose grave hazards in inexperienced or poorly trained hands. Invasive diagnostic procedures may help to fine-tune management in individual patients, but their overall influence on reducing morbidity and improving mortality in critically ill patients is debatable. It is remarkable how with increasing experience the use of invasive monitoring is significantly reduced. Again this is not to decry the use of sophisticated technology in the intensive care unit. It is merely to restress that in the final analysis good care rests with doctors and nurses, and not with machines.

(v) Primum non nocere

'First of all, do no harm'. This is an ancient Hippocratic tenet. Do not subject the patient to procedures and investigations which add to pain and suffering, when one is certain or almost certain that these can lead to no extra benefit. The risk-benefit ratio should always be kept in mind in all management decisions in the ICU.

(vi) The Practice of Evidence Based Medicine

Evidence based medicine is the rallying cry of modern medicine, a shining banner held aloft by the profession for all to view, a promised trail for a better future in health care. It is unquestionably important to judge the clinical effectiveness or otherwise of treatment options through scientifically accumulated evidence. It is even more important to gather evidence to ensure that a treatment option is not injurious to patients. I am all in support of evidence based medicine, but only up to a point. In critical care medicine, it may be impossibly difficult and even unethical to furnish scientific evidence as to the optimal approach to acutely emergent problems occurring in very critically ill patients with many variables. Evidence based medicine is merely one aspect of medicine. Medicine has several other aspects—social, cultural, economic, psychological, philosophical, religious, genetic, and the other nebulous aspects that characterize a trusting, caring doctor-patient relationship. Again, evidence can be imperfect, can change and is not sacrosanct. If it were, medicine would be static, whereas history teaches us that it is ever-changing, dynamic. It is also possible that the conclusions drawn from evidence based medicine in the Western world may not always apply to the rest. A study of the influence of racial and genetic factors may well alter present day evidence in relation to the management of different medical problems.

Finally, medicine is a science and art, in equal measure. Evidence based medicine ignores the art in medicine. It is the art in medicine that translates the application of its science to the care of an individual patient. I came across this ancient description of a good physician and I feel it has a timeless relevance.

'It was his part to learn the practice of medicines and the practice of healing, and careless of fame, to exercise that quiet art'.

(vii) Recognition of the Limits of Critical Care

Physicians involved with critical care must recognize the limits of such care. Critical illnesses are necessarily associated with a high morbidity and mortality, and quite often this morbidity and mortality cannot be improved despite all the care available in present times. The discerning physician learns to recognize the limits of care, knows when to draw the line, and recognizes the futility, and often the cruelty of aggressive management in patients who are well past the point of no return. Learning the limits of care is not easy; it is fraught with doubts, difficulties and danger. A working guideline is to struggle unto life or death in a young individual with a potentially reversible life-threatening illness, and to remember not to play *God* in the ICU. Yet in the old and feeble, in patients who are clearly dying, and in those with serious background illnesses, one must learn through wisdom and experience to temper care with reason.

Ethical Principles Governing Critical Care

The principles of ethics are rooted in religious, philosophical and sociocultural traditions. These vary in different cultures and countries, but the absolute values of good and evil, right and wrong, and the sanctity of human life, are remarkably similar in all civilized societies.

There are three basic ethical principles derived from these absolute values which govern the art and science of all medicine, and in particular of critical care medicine. The first is beneficence, and its companion-in-arms, non-maleficence. Beneficence is an all-important ethical principle and duty of the physician, which has been emphasized in ancient Ayurvedic texts, as also by Hippocrates. Beneficence directs the physician to do good by relieving suffering and restoring good health. Beneficence does not merely involve technical expertise and medical skill; it equally involves human qualities particularly in the care of critical illnesses. It is these human qualities which tend to be unfortunately forgotten or pushed into the background, by the frontiers of advancing technology in medicine. The chief of these human qualities expressed in a single word is 'humanity'. Humanity can be defined as the sensibility which enables a physician to feel for the distress and suffering of a patient, prompting him to relieve them. True humanity in a physician is the fount of sympathy and care for a critically ill patient. A critically ill but conscious patient in my opinion, has special antennae (very like what the child has for the mother), which enable him to promptly recognize, reach out, and clasp to his heart a physician who truly cares. This often makes the difference between life and death in a critical illness. In a similar manner, a critically ill individual often recognizes the pseudosympathy exhibited by some physicians, however brilliant and technologically well-equipped they may be. Knowledge and experience when linked to humanity, make a great physician and indeed a great man.

Non-maleficence is the companion-in-arms of beneficence. It reminds the physician that above all, he should do no harm. Beneficence and non-maleficence may at times in a critical care setting be in apparent conflict. Thus the use of a narcotic to relieve pain is beneficence in a dying patient, yet this may hasten death by depressing respiration, thus violating the tenet of non-maleficence. This conflict, as explained later is apparent and not real.

The second basic ethical principle governing decision-making and management in critical care medicine, is patient autonomy. This is the patient's right to self-determination—the right after being properly informed, to accept or refuse medical treatment offered to him including life support measures like mechanical ventilation. It is indeed the proper interpretation of the balance between the principles of beneficence and the principles of patient autonomy, that governs decision-making and management in critical care medicine. This balance is indeed difficult, and not easy to strike in a critical care setting. This is because patients who are seriously ill may be unable to make proper decisions about their own care. In fact they may often make the wrong decisions under the physical and emotional stress of their illness. In these circumstances, the physician must lean towards the principle of beneficence, and take management decisions which he genuinely believes are in the best interests of the patient. It is important to illustrate this point with true-to-life examples. A patient was brought in nearly dead after a sedative poisoning, with a note informing the physician that it was her express wish not to be resuscitated and treated. The directive was ignored; the patient was resuscitated and discharged in good health. She was forever grateful for being restored to life.

A patient with quickly progressive respiratory muscle weakness, in his extreme fright, agitation, anxiety and distress, refused intubation and mechanical ventilator support. The request was ignored, appropriate management decisions taken, and the patient was again ever grateful to the doctor for having ignored his directive.

There are many factors which distort, prejudice or interfere with autonomous decisions of patients in critical care medicine. These include fear, anxiety, depression, panic, lack of information, and abhorrence of invasive modalities of treatment which prompt them to decide (often wrongly) to 'die with dignity'. The working ethical principle is that in acute medicine, when confronted with a potentially reversible life-threatening illness, beneficence prevails over patient autonomy.

The third and final ethical principle is justice—to distinguish in patient care, the right from the wrong. If at times this is difficult or impossible to determine in absolute terms, one should determine what is more right or less wrong. In developing countries where resources are limited, justice dictates that treatment is administered to patients who are more likely to benefit from them. This often produces an ethical quandary. Witness for example a situation where there are three ventilators in an 8-bedded tetanus ward, and all 8 patients have severe tetanus requiring mechanical ventilation. Physicians should unquestionably be involved in the ethics of resource distribution that provide equitable medical care to the society in which they live and work. Yet ethical arguments limiting care because of limited resources, should not in my opinion be applicable to an individual patient already under intensive care. Wisdom however dictates that in all situations requiring protracted intensive care, the burden-benefit relationship should be carefully considered, and care be tempered with reason, when judged to be an exercise in futility.

Ethical Issues in Terminal Illness

A terminal illness is one that leads to death in the immediate future, so that the physician concentrates not on cure, but on relief of symptoms and on moral support to the patient and his family.

At times a patient with terminal cancer or terminal advanced organ system failure, is unwittingly admitted to a critical care unit. It is important to try and avoid such admissions to the best of one's ability. If such an admission does occur, one should explain the futility and the crippling expense likely to be incurred, to the patient and his family. Treatment in a ward or at home is invariably possible, if time is taken to explain the exact situation to the relatives.

What is more relevant in a critical care setting is the worsening of a patient with an acute but potentially reversible life-threatening illness, to a stage where death becomes inevitable in the immediate future. An all-important proviso in relation to a terminal illness in critical care medicine, is to constantly review the word 'terminal'. Knaus et al. (1, 2)* consider that patients with three or more organ system failure for more than 3–4 days have a 98 per cent mortality. It is basically bad judgment (for several reasons) to go by statistics in the management of an individual patient, as it breeds a nihilistic attitude to patient care. Interestingly enough, in our experience, severe multiple organ dysfunction due to tropical problems like tetanus or fulminant Pl. falciparum malaria, has a far better prognosis with a good survival rate.

Yet on a number of occasions in a critical care setting, the discerning physician can see the inevitability of death. The severe resource crunch in our poor countries should prompt the physician in such a situation, to refrain from using medical technology and skill that merely prolong death, or that make death excessively lonely, gruesome, dehumanised, perhaps even obscene, and ruinous to the patient and his family.

It is important in an acute illness which in spite of all efforts appears to progress to an inexorable fatal outcome, to ascertain the wishes of the patient and his relatives. There is no such legal document as a Living Will in our country, as there exists in many Western countries. Nevertheless, there is still a very strong bond in our part of the world between the physician and the patient and his relatives. The patient invariably follows his physician's advice, and the relatives are also similarly influenced. This is indeed an added and extremely heavy responsibility on the physician, because poor judgement can unnecessarily prolong the act of dying, and can also in the bargain, financially cripple the patient's family. Better judgement could have prevented both these calamities. Judgement is terribly difficult in some young patients. Alas! It is not always that a Daniel comes to judgement!

Management in an acute illness which is finally found to be terminal is further helped by the following principles:

(i) The proper training of residents and nurses in the medical management of a terminal illness. In this connection, a quote from a judgement delivered in the United Kingdom by Judge Delvin, is indeed of unsurpassed guidance and relevance—'the proper medical treatment that is administered and that has an incidental effect in determining the exact moment of death, is not the cause of death in any sensible use of the term' (3).

(ii) The offering of true compassion to the patient—a quality which cannot be bought, but which should come naturally to all trained staff in a critical care unit.

Withholding Life Support and Withdrawal of Life Support in the Critically Ill

It is comparatively easy to withhold life support in a patient who will inevitably die in a short or small time span of a few hours, or even a few days. It may be difficult however to withhold support when the time span of a terminal illness is more prolonged.

A problem often arises in withdrawing life support in hopeless situations, if this life support was already started at an earlier point in time, when the life-threatening acute illness seemed potentially reversible. Unfortunately, till recently brain death was not recognized in our country. At last the authorities that be, have passed an act in parliament recognizing brain death, and thereby permitting the withdrawal of life support in patients who are brain dead. Recognition of brain death and the sanction to remove life support in these patients has ended an agonizing era of utter helplessness and mental agony and torture for both relatives and staff in critical care units. There is some controversy as to whether one is justified in stopping nasogastric feeds in terminally ill patients. This question hardly ever arises in a critical care setting, as terminally ill patients devoid of life support quickly die, irrespective of whether one gives feeds as a token gesture or not. We certainly stop all parenteral feeds, not only because of their utter futility, but also because of the expense entailed.

Euthanasia

No discussion of ethics in relation to modern day medicine, including critical care medicine, can be complete without a short discussion on euthanasia.

Euthanasia includes:

(i) Voluntary euthanasia or intentional killing of patients who express a competent, freely made wish to die, because of the pain or suffering they experience.

(ii) Medically assisted suicide, at the patient's insistence and wish.

(iii) Homicide following a surrogate decision on a crippled or handicapped patient, or in a patient with a poor or hopeless quality of life. In this case, the patient is not involved in the decision.

Advocates of euthanasia remarkably enough invoke the ethical principles of beneficence, stating that the act is morally justified because it is 'doing good to the patient', and is in 'his or her best interest'. In my opinion, this act is wrong, unjustifiable, and violates the sanctity of life, as it is perpetrated with known intent to kill. Yet it must be clearly understood that withholding or withdrawing treatment, when it is certain that such treatment will be of no benefit and when death is inevitable, does not constitute euthanasia (even though some prefer to call this 'passive euthanasia'), because the intent is not to kill but to prevent prolongation of the act of dying.

I gather from discussions with my colleagues in the West, that a significant number of acutely ill patients who are about to die, as also patients with chronic but terminal disease, express a desire to be killed or to be medically assisted in suicide. It is amazing that in my long association of over 45 years with so many critically ill patients in their terminal state, there has not been a single individual who has persistently wished for euthanasia. There have been a few who have expressed a fleeting wish, but talking to them, and gently explaining measures to relieve their symptoms, have led to a resigned and comparatively unanguished acceptance of their destiny. Why is there this difference between the East and the West? I think it is basically related to sociocultural and religious differences. A patient's, and for that matter a physician's attitude to suffering, pain, impending death, and death itself, is conditioned by these sociocultural and religious factors. Most people in our part of the world and in the Far East believe that life cannot be divorced from pain and suffering, that we live in the midst of pain and suffering, and that each one in this world is apportioned one's share of pain and suffering. This is the law of 'Karma'—a belief that one reaps in the present life what one has sown in previous lives, and that one will reap in future existences what one sows in the present.

In our experience, suffering in a terminal illness (whether this is a sequel to an acute or chronic problem), almost always can be relieved by appropriate medication and compassion. This brings us to the question of whether it is imperative to tell the patient the exact truth, that his terminal illness will inevitably end fatally. Here again, East and West may differ. The relatives have a right to know the whole truth, and it is the moral obligation of the physician to appraise them of this truth. Many terminally ill patients either in critical care units or outside, know and feel that their illness is terminal, but barring rare exceptions, they do not wish to discuss death or dying with the physician. In fact, they will if possible, in no uncertain terms stop the physician from broaching the issue. I would agree that the ethical principle of patient autonomy includes the patient's right to know and understand the nature of his illness, so that an informed consent or dissent regarding management decisions is possible. Yet a patient also has a right to choose exactly how much he wants to know. If the physician is to exert beneficence, he must respect that right. Perhaps the patient's disinclination to discuss the end is due to a faint glimmer of hope that life will extend longer than what the physician feels, or what medical science expects. I am of the opinion that under these circumstances, a physician has no right to systematically destroy that glimmer of hope which keeps the patient more happy and peaceful towards the end of his life.

To die with dignity and to legalize euthanasia are slogans often linked together, as if one needs the latter to achieve the former. Legalizing euthanasia in our country, even in the most diluted form, could well open the floodgates to murder. Euthanasia however, under strict clauses and safeguards, has already been legalized in Holland. Perhaps in time to come, it may be similarly legalized in other Western countries as well. I am in no position to comment on the Western world, but for all the safeguards and guarantees against misuse that the Dutch for example have, is it not possible that a patient would want to end his 'suffering' as a matter of a cult, or even as a matter of duty that needs to be performed in time to come? Is it ever possible to quantify suffering? Is not suffering often a state of the mind? And cannot a state of the mind be subject to changing social pressures and social mores? Can most doctors claim to have the knowledge, experience, the Ostlerian wisdom and perspective to be truly able to enlist themselves to the cause of euthanasia in a patient who states, 'I cannot bear the suffering I am going through'? These are pertinent questions which are difficult to answer. Finally when one legalizes a solution to a problem like euthanasia, would the good that accrues clearly outbalance the evil or harm that could possibly result from this legal sanction? This again is a question that physicians all over the world should seriously consider.

REFERENCES

1. Knaus WA, Draper EA, Wagner DP et al. (1985). Prognosis in acute organ-system failure. Ann Surg. 202, 685.

2. Knaus WA, Wagner DP. (1989). Multiple organ system failure: Epidemiology and prognosis. Crit Care Clin. 5, 221.

3. Delvin P. (1985). Easing the Passing. The Trail of Dr. John Bodkin Adams. p 171. The Bodley Head, London.

Organization of an Intensive Care Unit

Critical care is ideally given in a centralized unit by trained medical and nursing staff using centralized equipment. A good unit necessarily uses the infrastructure of a well-equipped general hospital, and has therefore the back-up and support of sophisticated investigations, imaging techniques, physiotherapists, specialists and superspecialists in different fields of medicine and surgery. Such a critical care unit is possible only in large or medium sized general hospitals in the metropolitan cities of this country. In the Western world, particularly in the United States, most large institutions have special ICUs for different specialities and subspecialities. Thus besides a medical and surgical ICU, an institution may have separate critical care units for trauma, burns, cardiac surgery, general surgery, respiratory care, coronary care, neurosurgery and other specialities. In our part of the world, general all-purpose units are to be preferred. This allows for concentration of rather meagre resources with regard to staffing, equipment and technical expertise. Again, critical care basically necessitates a holistic approach to the ravages of a life-threatening disease. Physicians and surgeons in all-purpose critical care units are more appropriately trained to fulfil this purpose, as compared to their colleagues working in speciality care units. In our hospital except for a separate neonatal unit and a dialysis unit, there is one 8-bedded general medical intensive care unit, a new 4-bedded general medical and surgical intensive care unit, and one separate 12-bedded surgical care unit. The former admits all critically ill patients including any overflow from the surgical ICU. The surgical ICU chiefly caters to post-operative open-heart surgery; it also caters to general surgery, and handles any overflow from the medical ICU. The total number of ICU beds constitutes about 12 per cent of the total bed strength of the hospital. Our hospital ICUs are tertiary referral centres handling patients referred not only from other city and suburban hospitals, but also patients transferred from hospitals and ICUs all over the country, and also occasionally patients transferred from Middle Eastern countries.

Perfect facilities as those existing in ICUs of well known institutes in the West, can only be afforded by a handful of units in poor and developing countries. Distances in our subcontinent are vast, transport poor and at times medieval, so that it is imperative that critical care reaches out to the smaller hospitals in smaller towns and their surrounding districts. It is suggested that every medium sized hospital should organize and maintain a high dependency unit or ward which allows better nursing, better monitoring and observation, and more efficient handling of patients by a well trained medical staff, of problems related to acute medicine. The operational requisites of such a unit are discussed later. What needs to be deprecated, condemned and abolished are the small cubby holes attached to small 'nursing homes' in different cities of this country, whose sole claim to critical care is merely a name board with 'ICU' written above the entry door. These are death traps for the unwary, and do far more harm than good.

ICU Location

The ICU should as far as possible be in close relation to the operation theatre and the recovery room. This allows easy transport of critically ill patients from the ICU to the theatre and vice versa. This is specially important for the surgical ICU, or for a general intensive care unit which admits a high proportion of post-operative cases. If for some reason this has not been implemented, or is not possible, then the hospital should ensure rapid vertical transport through fast moving, promptly available elevators—a basic tenet which architects in this country often ignore. Doors and corridors used for this transfer should be spacious, and help and not hinder transport. It should never be forgotten that critically ill patients are at risk when moved from one department of the hospital to another. The ICU also has a special and close relationship with the casualty and emergency ward, with the laboratory, with the radiology-cum-imaging department, and with the physiotherapy department (which includes respiratory therapy) (Fig 1.3.1). If the hospital has a step-down or a high-dependency unit or ward, it needs must have a close relation with such a ward. The importance of a fairly large high-dependency ward of about 14 beds does not seem to be realized in our part of the world. Every good ICU should be closely associated with a high-dependency ward. Such a combination enables the ICU to be reserved exclusively for patients who truly deserve critical care. It also enables a quicker turnover and therefore a more economic, efficient and correct use of critical care. It reduces morbidity and

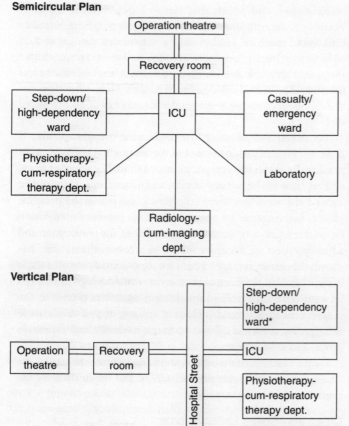

Fig. 1.3.1. Relationship between the ICU and other departments.

mortality in patients recovering from critical illnesses, as these patients on transfer from the ICU are often poorly observed and attended to in the general ward of a hospital. If a medical ICU has a high proportion of patients with ischaemic heart disease, it would be ideal to have the cardiac catheter laboratory in close relation to it, on the same floor. When multiple ICUs subserving different specialities are located in an institution, the interrelationship between the ICUs is of greater importance than the interrelationship between the ICU and the operation theatre or the recovery room. Even with multiple ICUs, the ancillary departments should be common to all units. Some large units may choose to decentralize their ICUs in order to enhance the functioning and integrity of a special service. Thus a coronary care or cardiac ICU may be adjacent to the cardiology unit, the cardiovascular surgery unit, and the cardiac catheter laboratory. Similarly a neurological ICU should be adjacent to the neurosurgery theatre and the neurology wards and department.

Design of the ICU

The design of the unit should take into consideration the integration and smooth functioning of three areas of importance and activity: (i) the Patient Area; (ii) the Staff Area chiefly for nurses and doctors, and (iii) the Support Area.

The design of an ICU should meet four basic requirements (1): (a) direct observation of the patient by the nursing and medical staff; (b) surveillance of physiologic monitoring; (c) provision and efficient use of routine and emergency diagnostic procedures and therapeutic interventions; (d) recording and maintenance of patient information.

A critical care unit should preferably be spacious so that movement of staff and equipment is easy, free and uncramped. This may be possible in a new construction. In a renovated unit however, the configuration of the existing room or wing determines and often restricts the design of the unit. A square-shaped wing is usually preferable to a rectangular one. In general, the ratio of the total unit footage per bed should range from 350–500 sq. feet/bed. A diagrammatic design of an ICU is given in **Fig. 1.3.2.**

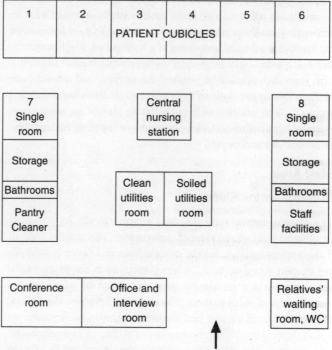

Fig. 1.3.2. Diagrammatic design of an ideal ICU.

Patient Bed Area

Each patient bed area should have a minimum floor space of 200 sq. feet. This applies to an open bay design in which curtains partition each bed area. If each bed area is separated from the adjacent bed by an actual partition, a larger floor space area/bed is necessary (250–350 sq. feet). The partitioning between beds in our unit extends from the ceiling downwards; in the upper 3/4 is transparent glass, and the lower 1/4 consists of a tiled wall which starts from the floor, and extends upwards to meet the glass partition. Thus a patient lying in bed has no view of the adjacent room. Each room has a sliding glass door; each room also has curtains which can if necessary be drawn across the partitions, as also across the entrance door.

The open bay design has one important advantage—the ability to encroach on the floor space of an adjacent bed, when there is shortage of space for equipment required for a patient. The major advantage of partitioned cubicles (with partitions designed as stated above) with sliding doors, is that it allows privacy, and yet provides easy access to the patient. Dying, death or an acute crisis in a unit can remain more isolated, and not affect the emotional and physical well-being of other critically ill individuals.

Each patient's bed area must necessarily be supplied by an oxygen outlet attached to a flow meter, by a central suction outlet, and by suitable power outlets. Each patient bed area should have large windows that allow natural light. Windowless ICUs are a feature of poor design, and are important contributors to patient disorientation and stress. As far as possible, oxygen outlets, suction lines and monitoring equipment should be wall-mounted. This saves space and allows more easy movement. Ideally there should be one wash basin to two beds; each wash basin must have an antiseptic solution bottle mounted on, or next to it (in our unit we use Sterillium solution containing 45 g 2-propanol, 30 g 1-propanol, and 0.2 g ethyl-hexadecyl-dimethylammonium-ethylsulphate). The soap dish should be washed frequently, and should have perforations at the bottom to prevent water from accumulating within it. The practice of hand washing should be assiduously followed both before and after examining or handling each patient, by all doctors and nurses.

Staff Area

Nursing Central Station

The nursing central station should be strategically located so as to allow an unhindered view of each patient. This may be difficult if the patient beds are in one straight line, and easier if the beds are shaped along an arch. When patient beds are in a straight line, two nursing stations may be necessary for unobstructed observation of each patient. The distance between the central station and each patient bed should be conveniently short, yet not so short as to obstruct movement of traffic, of equipment and of personnel. The station should have adequate room for storage of records, forms, charts and supplies. It should provide seating arrangements for 2 nurses and 1 doctor. A telephone hook-up with the central exchange of the hospital, and with other departments within the hospital, should be located in the central station. In our unit we have an alarm button which is activated whenever there is a cardiac arrest or any dire emergency in the ICU. This sounds a bell in the residents' quarters so that help from other senior residents is promptly available.

The space between the nursing station and the patient beds should be totally uncluttered and clean. The only piece of furniture permissible in this floor area is a mobile emergency trolley which carries all emergency drugs required for cardiopulmonary resuscitation, and which also carries a defibrillator monitor. Portable X-ray equipment, portable image intensifiers, portable ultrasound machine, equipment for respiratory therapy should all be kept in the equipment storeroom, and should never clutter the patient area of a unit. Ideally each bed requires a ventilator and this should be at the bedside of each patient. More often than not in developing countries, even good units may not be able to afford this luxury.

For constraints of space, the medication preparation area is generally located within the area of the nursing station. Whenever possible the medication preparation area should be separate from, and yet close to the nursing station and patient area. It should be located at a site where there is no visual observation by patients, and no interruption by phone calls. This prevents medication errors due to haste or disturbance. A study of the preparation and administration of drugs by nurses in a conventional unit, has shown that on an average 18 per cent, or one medication in six, is in error (2). The incidence of these errors could perhaps be reduced by a separate undisturbed medication area. Equipment in the medication area should include a counter-top, a medication refrigerator, a locked cabinet to house narcotics and expensive drugs, and a wash basin.

Acute emergencies would however necessitate the use of the emergency trolley with preparation of the medication in the central station or patient area.

Clean and Soiled Utility Rooms

Clean and soiled utility items should be housed separately. The clean utility room should contain procedure trays, bandages, pads, linen and intravenous solutions.

A soiled utility room must be accessible to but separate from other work areas. Waste material (suitably collected), disposables, soiled usable material awaiting transfer to central supply, and soiled linen are all housed in this room. The room should have a sink and a toilet where used bedpans can be flushed.

Storage Room

It is imperative to have a large storage area which houses equipment, stretchers, ECG machines, and numerous items of storage. A storage area should preferably consist of 20–25 per cent of patient and central station areas. A storage room must not be a dump. Each storage item should be kept in its appointed place. The room and all that it contains, should be kept scrupulously clean.

A sufficient sized, well-appointed storage area could also include a laboratory bench where basic ICU investigations like CBC, Hb, PCV, serum electrolytes, and estimation of blood gases can be done. If limited finance makes this impossible, the ICU must necessarily avail of the services of the central hospital laboratory for investigations.

Equipment

The level of equipment will depend on the type of ICU. A 2-channel monitor will suffice for an ICU in a small hospital in the city or at the district level. A tertiary (often called a Level III) unit in a teaching hospital, or in a hospital reputed for critical care, should be equipped with monitors that can display at least four physiological parameters. Equipment should be chosen by experienced physicians and surgeons. It is a sad commentary that in large teaching hospitals of poor countries, expensive and inappropriate equipment often lies unused, in a state of disrepair and decay.

A list of equipments desirable for a tertiary unit is tabled below (**Table 1.3.1**).

Table 1.3.1. Equipment desirable for a tertiary unit

1. Monitoring Equipment
   * Bedside and central monitors
   * 12-lead ECG recorder
   * Intravascular pressure monitoring devices
   * Cardiac output computer
   * Pulse oximeters
   * Expired CO_2 analyzers
   * Spirometers and peak flow meters
   * EEG monitor
   * Temperature monitors
   * Enzymatic blood glucose meters

2. Cardiovascular Therapy
   * CPR trolley
   * Defibrillators
   * Temporary transvenous pacemakers
   * Intra-aortic balloon pump
   * Infusion pumps and syringes

3. Respiratory Therapy
   * Ventilators—volume cycled, allowing different modes of ventilation
   * Humidifiers
   * Oxygen therapy devices and airway circuits
   * Nebulizers
   * Intubation/Tracheostomy trolley
   * AMBU bag
   * Fiberoptic bronchoscope

4. Dialysis Equipment—for haemodialysis, peritoneal dialysis, continuous arteriovenous haemofiltration

5. Radiological Equipment
   * Portable X-ray machine
   * X-ray view box
   * Image intensifier

6. Laboratory Equipment—not absolutely necessary within an ICU; central laboratory facilities may be utilized
   * Blood gas analyzer
   * Selective ion (electrolyte) electrode analyzers
   * Haematocrit centrifuge
   * Microscope
   * Osmometer

7. Miscellaneous Equipment
   * Dressing trolleys
   * Drip stands
   * Heating/cooling blankets
   * Bed restraints
   * Pressure distribution mattresses
   * Sterilizing equipment (e.g. autoclave)
   * Refrigerator

Kitchen and Nourishment Area

A kitchen or nourishment area is the space devoted for patient (and staff) nourishment. If possible, it should have a separate refrigerator, a wash basin, a gas stove, and a few storage cabinets.

Special Procedure/Treatment Room

It is preferable to do all diagnostic and therapeutic procedures as far as possible in the ICU patient room, so that patient transport and the hassles associated with this, are reduced to a bare minimum. A special room is used in some units, but this is a luxury that few units in developing countries can afford. In our opinion, it offers no specific advantage.

Medical Staff

Critical care is a multidisciplinary approach. Even so, there should always be one individual in charge, who directs and orchestrates this multidisciplinary approach. Too many superspecialists, each in sole charge of one organ system in a critically ill patient, can do more harm than good. In countries where critical care medicine has developed as a separate speciality (with separate formalized training requirements, and separate certification), the overall head is usually such a trained specialist—unfortunately and inappropriately termed an 'intensivist'. In India, critical care as a separate speciality is in the nascent phase; critical care training and certification are in the process of evolution. Intensivists who are both adequately trained and have acquired sufficient experience are for a large country such as India, relatively few in number. Till such time as training, certification and experience are all forthcoming, a physician with a wide background of experience (which necessarily involves critical care) should preferably head and direct such a unit.

The unit should also be staffed by two other trained doctors (for a 10–12 bedded unit) who have the experience to handle all emergency situations. Junior doctors in training should also rotate through a critical care unit, and should be encouraged to manage patients under close supervision of the better trained medical staff.

Nursing Staff

In my opinion, a well trained nursing staff is the central core of a well functioning unit. It is amazing as to how efficiently trained nursing staff can take quick management decisions in critically ill individuals. They can only do this if responsibility is not only given to them, but is forced upon them. To have junior, untrained or poorly trained resident doctors doing an 8 hour round-the-clock duty in an ICU in developing countries is extremely expensive, and has the following disadvantages:

(i) Till recently, almost all in-coming resident doctors to our unit had little or no training in critical care. They generally stayed for six months to a year and moved on to other jobs in other hospitals. This meant that by the time that they had gathered a modicum of experience and training, they left and one had to again cope with a fresh, untrained batch.

(ii) The practice of an '8 hour on-duty resident' system (with poorly trained residents) within a unit somehow lowers nursing standards in our part of the world. The nurses take no decisions and no responsibility because they feel that it is for the doctor on duty in the ICU to do so. In most units, the doctor has had little or no exposure to critical care, and is generally insufficiently trained to do what exacting standards demand. A laissez-faire attitude and a decline within the unit is observed.

We therefore devised a system over the years whereby a central core of very well-trained and dedicated nurses, together with two highly trained dedicated doctors look after the unit, all being strictly supervised by the physician in charge of the unit. The ratio of nurses to patients is invariably 1:1, and never less than 1:2. Of the 8 nurses on duty at any one time in the 8-bedded general ICU in our unit, 4 are very well trained, and 4 are trainees. We often lose the trainees to the Middle East, or to the United States, where nurses are far better paid. Even so we are fortunate to have a central core of nurses, headed and actively supervised by a dedicated Sister-in-Charge, who looks after the department.

The two well trained doctors are ably assisted by 3–4 senior residents who also manage the general wards of the hospital. Doctors are always present in the unit when needed, and can appear at a moment's notice when called. They do not necessarily have to be within the unit on an 8 or 12 hour rota. This method is money saving in poor countries, allows for excellent nursing which continues to improve, and breeds a healthy respect and rapport between doctors and nurses. Results (as judged by a medical audit) are good and perfectly comparable with any good unit in the West, proving that this system of management in poor countries does exceedingly well.

It is only over the last two years that we have had the luxury of obtaining reasonably trained residents in our unit. We have therefore now adopted the rota system of 8 hourly shifts of duty. Though this offers medicolegal protection in difficult times, we sincerely hope it does not lead to lowered nursing standards and enhances overall patient care and efficiency of the unit.

Support Services

A major ICU should have a 24 hour access to physiotherapy, radiography, imaging and laboratory services. Physiotherapists in our country double up as respiratory therapists as well. This is advantageous and again economical. An in-house system which provides trained technicians to maintain equipment and repair breakdowns in equipment is of vital importance. This is the support facility which is abysmally lacking or poor in all developing countries. It should be given top priority, else efficiency will always remain below par.

Any medium to large hospital housing an ICU must necessarily have its own generator which permits functioning of electrical equipment, even if the central power trips, or for some reason is interrupted. This is not uncommon in poor developing countries, and occasionally happens even in the city of Mumbai. The hospital generator should be triggered into action within a few seconds of failure of the main electrical supply.

Importance of Cleanliness

The importance of cleanliness cannot be overemphasized in poor tropical countries where there is a great deal of dust. The floor should be swabbed 8 hourly or even more frequently with an antiseptic solution. This cleaning procedure should always be done after visiting hours. It is absurd to see units insisting on having doctors and relatives change shoes on entering a unit which is basically unclean. We do not think that changing footwear before entering a unit is at all necessary; this procedure (particularly the way in which it is practised), probably introduces rather than prevents infection.

The patient bed area must be kept scrupulously clean, the side table bare and uncluttered; the windows and their frames should be spotless, and the curtains should be periodically washed and cleaned. It is sad but true that most units in the city and in this country lack the elementary aesthetic sense of cleanliness so necessary for good results. It is advisable that giving of bedpans, commodes and the washing of patients after the use of these should be done only by nurses, and not by separate staff who in many hospitals in poor countries are employed solely for this purpose. Non-nursing staff in developing countries lack knowledge regarding the basic principles of hygiene—principles which are so important for reducing the incidence of nosocomial infections in critical care units.

Swabs (at weekly intervals) should be taken from the ICU and its immediate environment and sent for cultures to the microbiology department. These include swabs from fixtures in the unit, from bedside tables, walls, curtains, antiseptic solutions in use, water humidifiers and other respiratory equipment. An awareness of the microbiological profile in an ICU helps in the control of nosocomial infection.

Continuing Education and Research

Continuing education for both doctors and nurses is absolutely essential. Junior and senior doctors should be involved in training programmes for nurses. Teaching at the bedside during clinical rounds is invaluable, and seems to be a forgotten art. Research should be encouraged, records kept, and an audit of performance within the ICU periodically performed and discussed.

Clinical Audit

A regular audit of ICU data must be performed to document ICU statistics. Such audits also help to point to aspects of critical care in an ICU which could be improved upon.

Operational Principles of a High-Dependency Ward

Critical care is nascent in developing countries like India where 75 per cent of its one billion people still live in rural areas with meagre medical facilities. District hospitals which drain small towns and adjoining rural areas should preferably have large (10–14 bedded) high-dependency wards offering as much critical care as possible, rather than small 2-bedded or 4-bedded ICUs which more often than not are ICUs in name, rather than in deed. A high-dependency ward should have an open bay design.

Basic Operational Requisites

The basic requisites are a highly motivated nursing and medical staff. No machines or instruments can match or replace human dedication, motivation and resources. The results in morbidity and mortality may not be as good as those observed in an excellent critical care unit described in the previous pages. They are however far superior to the results obtained from looking after very ill patients in a general ward, or from managing critically ill patients in poorly run ICUs in large general hospitals.

This was proven to the hilt in the 1980s, when the tetanus ward in one of the large teaching hospitals was converted into a high-dependency ward. The basic equipment of this high-dependency ward comprised of 3 outlets for central oxygen supply, 2 electrically operated suction machines, volume-cycled ventilators (starting with one and finally increasing to three), an ECG machine, and a defibrillator (which incidentally was a later acquisition). Equipment for prompt intubation or tracheostomy, AMBU bags, oxygen cylinders, and an emergency trolley completed the requirements of this ward. There were no monitors, yet the mortality of fulminant tetanus which was horrendous (well over 80 per cent, and often close to 100 per cent) was reduced to about 20 per cent. The overall mortality in tetanus in this high-dependency ward, was reduced from 30 per cent to about 12 per cent (3, 4).

There were just 2 nurses in this 9-bedded ward, and the house staff looking after this ward consisted of 2 registrars, 2 house physicians, and 2 interns. This staff also looked after a very busy male ward and female ward in general medicine. The above approach to the delivery of critical care in district hospitals and in large public hospitals in cities of developing countries has much

to commend itself. Even teaching hospitals in large metropolitan cities have intensive care units with beds far too meagre for the overall bed-strength of the hospital. Should not one deliver better care to the so many critically ill patients in the general wards of these hospitals? The creation of a couple of large high-dependency wards in big general hospitals could prove to be of great use, and is strongly recommended. If this proves difficult because of restrictions in finance or space, then each large medical and surgical ward should have one volume cycled ventilator, an emergency trolley for cardiopulmonary resuscitation, and one monitor-cum-defibrillator. There are many philanthropic donors and charitable trusts who would help in reorganizing wards for better patient care, provided bureaucratic obstacles are withdrawn.

REFERENCES

1. Hudson LD. (1985). Design of the intensive care unit form a monitoring point of view. Respir Care. 30.549.
2. Hill DW. (1983). Monitoring equipment and unit design. In: Care of the critically ill patients. (Eds. Tinker J, Rapin M). Springer-Verlag. New York.
3. Udwadia FE, Lall A, Udwadia ZF et al. (1987). Tetanus and its complications: Intensive care and management experience in 150 Indian patients. Epidem Inf. 99, 675–684.
4. Udwadia FE. (1994). In: Tetanus. Oxford University Press. Bombay, Delhi, Calcutta.

CHAPTER 1.4
Critical Care Scoring

Optimized distribution of medical and financial resources is of crucial importance in the delivery of health care, particularly in the poor developing countries of the world. To this end the critical care physician often has to make decisions about which patients are likely to derive the maximum benefit from admission to a critical care unit.

Illness scoring systems have been introduced in the past three decades to formulate some degree of priority for ICU admissions in patients with acute illness or trauma. These scoring systems are useful for medical audit purposes and for comparison of therapy and results in groups of patients who roughly have the same degree of physiological derangements produced by critical illnesses. However scoring systems have strong limitations, and critical care of individual patients should not be influenced by scoring protocols.

The commonly used trauma and critical care scores are briefly discussed below.

Glasgow Coma Score (GCS)

The Glasgow Coma Score judges the extent of coma in patients with head injury. It is useful for pre-hospital trauma triage as also for patient assessment after hospitalization. The scale is based on eye opening, motor response and verbal response (**Table 1.4.1**), and can be tested and scored by the physician within a couple of minutes. The total score is the sum of each response and varies from a minimum of 3 to a maximum of 15. The lower the score, the greater the severity of head injury in relation to CNS function.

Table 1.4.1. The Glasgow Coma Scale

Eye opening	Motor response	Verbal response
4 = Spontaneous	6 = Obedient	5 = Oriented
3 = To voice	5 = Purposeful	4 = Confused
2 = To pain	4 = Withdrawal	3 = Inappropriate
1 = None	3 = Flexion	2 = Incomprehensible
	2 = Extension	1 = None
	1 = None	

Trauma Score and Revised Trauma Score

These are useful for patients with trauma. The Trauma Score is based on the state of the cardiovascular and respiratory systems and on the Glasgow Coma Score (**Table 1.4.2**). Values are given to each parameter and these are added to give the total trauma

Table 1.4.2. Trauma Score

A. Systolic BP		B. Respiratory rate		C. Respiratory effort		D. Capillary refill	
> 90	4	10–24	4	Normal	1	Normal	2
70–90	3	25–35	3	Shallow or		Delay	1
50–69	2	> 35	2	retractions	0	None	0
< 50	1	< 10	1				
0	0	0	0				

E. GCS points

1. Eye opening		2. Motor response		3. Verbal response		(1 + 2 + 3)	
Spontaneous	4	Obedient	6	Oriented	5	14–15	5
To voice	3	Purposeful	5	Confused	4	11–13	4
To pain	2	Withdrawal	4	Inappropriate	3	8–10	3
None	1	Flexion	3	Incomprehensible	2	5–7	2
		Extension	2	None	1	3–4	1
		None	1				

TRAUMA SCORE (A + B + C + D + E) _____

score which ranges from 1–16. The lower the score the greater the risk for mortality.

The Trauma Score was found to underestimate the prognostic significance of head injuries. This led to the development of the Revised Trauma Score which is now widely used to assess the severity of trauma. The Revised Trauma Score is based on the Glasgow Coma Scale, the systolic blood pressure and the respiratory rate. Coded values are given for the above parameters and summed up (**Table 1.4.3**). Higher values have a better prognosis and lower values a poor prognosis.

Table 1.4.3. Revised Trauma Score *

Glasgow Coma Scale (GCS)	Systolic Blood Pressure (SBP) (mm Hg)	Respiratory Rate (RR) (Breaths/min)	Coded Value
13–15	> 89	10–29	4
9–12	76–89	> 29	3
6–8	50–75	6–9	2
4–5	1–49	1–5	1
3	0	0	0

*RTS = 0.9368 GCSc + 0.7326 SBPc + 0.2908 RRc, where the subscript c refers to coded value.

CRAMS Scale

The circulation, respiration, abdomen, motor, speech (CRAMS) scale is another trauma triage scale frequently used to decide which patients require urgent admission to a trauma unit (**Table 1.4.4**). Patients with a low CRAMS Score need urgent critical care.

Table 1.4.4. The CRAMS Scale*

Circulation	
Normal capillary refill and BP > 100 mm Hg	2
Delay capillary refill or 85 < BP < 100 mm Hg	1
No capillary refill or BP < 85 mm Hg	0
Respiration	
Normal	2
Abnormal (laboured or shallow)	1
Absent	0
Abdomen	
Abdomen and thorax non-tender	2
Abdomen and thorax tender	1
Abdomen rigid or flail chest	0
Motor	
Normal	2
Response to pain (other than decerebrate)	1
No response (or decerebrate)	0
Speech	
Normal	2
Confused	1
No intelligible words	0

*Score ≤ 8 indicates major trauma; Score ≥ 9 indicates minor trauma.

Injury Severity Score

This system assigns numerical scores to different body regions that may be injured. A manual of codes provides information on the scoring of each injury. The worst injury in each region is given a numerical value. This is squared and added to numerical values from each of the other anatomical regions. The total score ranges from 1–75 and co-relates with the mortality risk. The Injury Severity Score has some important limitations. It considers only the highest score from each body region, and considers injuries with equal scores to be of equal importance irrespective of the anatomical region injured. The ISS is frequently used as a measure of overall trauma, and forms a rough guide to mortality risk in the injured patient.

Acute Physiology, Age, Chronic Health Evaluation (APACHE)

The APACHE II Score is one of the most frequently used critical scales in critical illnesses. It is used in order to stratify prognosis and outcome in groups of patients, and to determine success of different forms of treatment (1–6). The APACHE II Score uses 12 easily measured variables (APS) and takes into consideration background disease or premorbid health (**Table 1.4.5**). The worst scores in the first 24 hours following ICU admissions are used. The 12 parameters considered are:

(i) Temperature (°C)
(ii) Mean Arterial Pressure (mm Hg)
(iii) Heart Rate (beats/min)
(iv) Respiratory Rate (breaths/min)
(v) Alveolar-Arterial Oxygen Gradient (A-aDO$_2$) if fractional inspired oxygen (FIO$_2$) is 0.5 or greater, or PaO$_2$ if FIO$_2$ < 0.5.
(vi) Arterial pH
(vii) Serum Sodium (mmol/l)
(viii) Serum Potassium (mmol/l)
(ix) Serum Creatinine (mg/dl)
(x) Haematocrit (%)
(xi) Leucocyte Count (cells/mm^3)
(xii) Glasgow Coma Score (GCS).

Depending on the degree of derangement, a weighted score is given to each parameter. Sedated, ventilated patients are given a GCS of 15 when neurological problems seem unlikely.

Scores are also assigned for increasing age, emergency post-operative or non-operative admission, and for the presence of background diseases resulting in pre-existing organ dysfunction. Double weighting is assigned to derangements of serum creatinine in the setting of acute renal failure, due to marked increase in mortality in critically ill patients with acute renal failure. The maximum possible APACHE II Score is 71. Increasing scores correlate with increasing mortality at each 5 point increment across a wide range of diseases.

The APACHE II scoring system is a useful scale in critical care medicine. Nevertheless it is wrong to allow APACHE II Scores to influence management in individual patients. A high initial APACHE II Score in post-operative coronary artery bypass surgery is not necessarily associated with a high mortality (6). It is also shown later in this book (see Chapter on Multiple Organ Dysfunction Syndrome) that tropical problems may be associated with severe multiple organ dysfunction (and high APACHE II Scores), and yet do not have the grim prognosis forecast by the APACHE II Score. A critique of these scoring systems is given in the Chapter on Multiple Organ Dysfunction Syndrome.

Table 1.4.5. APACHE II points (A + B + C below)

A. Acute Physiology Score (APS)

Points	High Abnormal			Normal			Low Abnormal		
	+ 4	+ 3	+2	+ 1	0	+1	+ 2	+ 3	+ 4
Temperature (rectal) °C	≥ 41	39–40.9		38.2–38.9	36–38.4	34–35.9	32–33.9	30–31.9	≤ 29.9
Mean BP mm Hg	≥160	130–159	110–129		70–109		50–69		≤ 49
Heart rate beats/min	≥180	140–179	110–139		70–109		55–69	40–54	≤ 39
Respiratory rate breaths/min	≥ 50	35–49		25–34	12–24	10–11	6–9		≤ 5
A-a DO₂ mm Hg if FIO₂ ≥ 0.5	≥ 500	350–499	200–349		< 200				
PaO₂ (FIO₂ < 0.5)					>70	61–70		55–60	< 55
Arterial pH	≥ 7.7	7.6–7.69		7.5–7.59	7.33–7.49		7.25–7.32	7.15–7.24	< 7.15
Serum Sodium mmol/l	≥180	160–179	155–159	150–154	130–149		120–129	111–119	≤ 110
Serum Potassium mmol/l	≥ 7	6–6.9		5.5–5.9	3.5–5.4	3–3.4	2.5–2.9		< 2.5
Serum Creatinine mmol/l (points are doubled in acute renal failure)	≥300	171–299	121–170		50–120		< 50		
Haematocrit %	≥ 60		50–59.9	46–49.9	30–45.9		20–29.9		< 20
Leucocytes cell/mm³	≥ 40		20–39.9	15–19.9	3–14.9		1–2.9		< 1
Neurological Points = (15 – actual Glasgow Coma Score)									

B. Age Points

Years	≤ 44		45–54		55–64		65–74		≥ 75
Points	0		2		3		5		6

C. Chronic Health Points

2   points for elective post-operative admissions, or
5   points if emergency operation or non-operative admission, if patient has significant chronic liver, cardiovascular, respiratory, or renal disease or is immunocompromised

Several variants of the APACHE II Scoring systems have been devised. These include Bion's 'Sickness Score' (**7, 8**), Mortality Prediction Models (**9–11**) and the Therapeutic Intervention Scoring System (**12, 13**).

None of these scoring systems have any significant advantage over the more frequently used APACHE II Score, and none of these should significantly influence decision making in individual patients. There is also little or no difference in the predictive ability of each of these systems over a wide range of scores (**11**).

The APACHE II scoring system (and its modifications) was not designed to judge individual patient outcomes. A new scoring system (the APACHE III score) has been introduced to objectively assess patient risk for death and other important outcomes related to patient stratification. This new system aims to provide—(i) An APACHE III score; (ii) a series of predictive equations that help to predict individual patient mortality at different times during the patient's stay in the ICU.

The APACHE III system is based on 17 physiological variables or parameters, and includes within its ambit a coma scale, age,

and pre-existing co-morbid conditions (**14**). The APACHE III Score is calculated by adding the coded variables for each category. A 5 point increase in the APACHE III score (range 0–299) is associated with increased risk of death. Further use and evaluation of this scoring system is necessary before it can be used routinely for triage decisions in critical care.

Other Important Scoring Systems in Critical Care

In the 1990s three other important scoring systems were devised to predict the outcome in critically ill patients. These were the Sequential Organ Function Assessment score (SOFA), the Multiple Organ Dysfunction Score and the Simplified Acute Physiological Score (SAPS I); this was further modified to SAPS II. Unlike the APACHE II scoring system which is used only on admission of the patient to the ICU, the SOFA Score, Multiple Organ Function Score and SAPS II Score are determined daily in a critically ill patient till either recovery or death occurs. These scoring systems take into consideration two obvious facts—(a) organ dysfunction is a continuum, varying from very mild at one end of the spectrum to hopelessly severe at the other end; (b) organ dysfunction is a dynamic process and the degree of dysfunction or failure could vary with time.

SOFA Score

The SOFA score is made up of scores from six organ systems graded from 0 to 4, depending upon the degree of dysfunction (15). A SOFA score > 15 is associated with a mortality > 80 per cent (16). We use this scoring system in our unit and find it valuable. However, as explained in the Chapter on Multiple Organ Dysfunction Syndrome, we have noted that in fulminant tropical infections (e.g. falciparum malaria), high SOFA scores do not necessarily predict death. The recovery rate in these infections is significantly higher than that predicted by the SOFA score (see Chapter on Multiple Organ Dysfunction Syndrome). **Table 1.4.6**

gives the details of organ function assessment through the SOFA system.

Multiple Organ Dysfunction Score

The Multiple Organ Dysfunction Score was devised because of the direct relationship between the number of organs that fail to mortality in ICU patients (17). The 'score' for each patient is assessed daily, allowing a better prediction of morbidity and mortality. (**Table 1.4.7**)

Simplified Acute Physiology Score (SAPS)

The SAPS I score was developed from a small database of about 700 patients in France, as a simplification of the APACHE scoring system (18). The SAPS I score had a range from 0 to 56 and was based on physiological parameters, age and invasive or

Table 1.4.6. The Sequential Organ Failure Assessment (SOFA) score

	SOFA Score				
	0	1	2	3	4
Respiration					
PaO_2/FIO_2	> 400	≤ 400	≤ 300	≤ 200 With respiratory support	≤ 100 With respiratory support
Coagulation					
Platelets ($\times 10^3$ /mm^3)	> 150	≤ 150	≤ 100	≤ 50	≤ 20
Liver					
Bilirubin (mg/dl)	< 1.2	1.2–1.9	2.0–5.9	6.0–11.9	> 12.0
(μmol/l)	< 20	20–32	33–101	102–204	> 204
Cardiovascular					
Hypotension	No hypotension	MAP < 70 mm Hg	Dopamine ≤ 5 or dobutamine (any dose)*	Dopamine > 5 or epi ≤ 0.1 or norepi ≤ 0.1*	Dopamine > 15 or epi > 0.1 or norepi > 0.1*
Central Nervous System					
Glasgow Coma Score	15	13–14	10–12	6–9	< 6
Renal					
Creatinine (mg/dl)	< 1.2	1.2–1.9	2.0–3.4	3.5–4.9	> 5
(μmol/l) or urine output	< 110	110–170	171–299	300–440 or < 500 ml/day	> 440 or < 200 ml/day

epi - epinephrine; norepi - norepinephrine.
*Adrenergic agents administered for at least 1 hour (doses given are in μg/kg/min).

Table 1.4.7. The Multiple Organ Dysfunction Score

	Points				
Parameter	0	1	2	3	4
PaO_2/FIO_2	> 300	226–300	151–225	76–150	≤ 75
Serum creatinine (μmol/l)	≤ 100	101–200	201–350	351–500	≥ 500
Serum bilirubin (μmol/l)	≤ 20	21–60	61–120	121–240	> 240
Pulse-adjusted heart rate*	≤ 10	10.1–15	15.1–20	20.1–30	> 30
Platelet count (x 10^3/dl)	> 120	81–120	51–80	21–50	≤ 20
Glasgow Coma Score+	15	13–14	10–12	7–9	≤ 6

*PAR = HR X (RAP / MAP); HR = heart rate, RAP = right atrial pressure,
MAP = mean arterial pressure.
+The best estimate in the absence of sedation.

Scoring method:
The most abnormal value for each parameter over a 24-hour period is selected for scoring purposes. The addition of scores of all six parameters gives the final score. It has been observed that scores between 13–16 carry a 50% mortality, scores between 17–20 a 75% mortality and scores >20 a 100% mortality.

non-invasive ventilation. Predictive results using the SAPS I were found to be comparable to those using the APACHE I score. The main drawback of the SAPS I as an outcome prediction tool was that it did not take into consideration the specific diagnosis and background diseases or chronic health status of the individual.

About a decade later, the updated SAPS II score was developed from a large database of more than 13,000 patients from ICUs across Europe and North America (19). The SAPS II score is calculated using 17 variables—12 physiological parameters, age, type of admission (emergency/elective), presence of AIDS, metastatic cancer or haematologic malignancy. The main outcome measure predicted by the SAPS II is vital status at hospital discharge. It has been found to perform better than SAPS I and its performance is comparable to that of the APACHE II. Modifications of the SAPS II have been used to make it more applicable at local ICU levels and also for clinical trials in specific diseases and conditions such as sepsis.

The SAPS III is currently being developed by the European Society of Intensive Care Medicine. The database for this score is expected to be very large, collected from ICUs all over the world. The SAPS III will consist of 4 modules—a basic evaluation module, an extended outcomes module, an infection module and a resources module. Along with predictive models for patient outcomes, the score is also expected to provide a reliable tool for evaluation of individual ICUs with a special emphasis on infection rates and cost-benefit ratios of investigations and therapies.

Critical Care Scoring in the Future

The evolution and practice of better future scoring systems need to take into account (a) factors which predict patient outcome; (b) effectiveness of therapy or management; (c) efficiency of delivered care.

Critical care is however a complex process. Patients receiving critical care constitute many variables related to different disease processes. The problem is further compounded by the fact that delivery of critical care in different parts of the world is influenced by cultural, social and economic factors. For these reasons it is difficult to quantify critical care with measurable values and compare these values with different institutions in different countries of the world.

Present scoring systems are a valuable guide to patient outcome and indirectly on how management can affect outcome. Yet it is our opinion that 'scores' should not influence management decisions in individual patients. Clinical judgement should never be replaced by any scoring system or scale.

REFERENCES

1. Knaus WA, Zimmerman JE, Wagner DP et al. (1981). APACHE—acute physiology and chronic health evaluation: a physiologically based classification system. Crit Care Med. 9, 591–597.

2. Scheffler RM, Knaus WA, Wagner DP et al. (1982). Severity of illness and the relationship between intensive care and survival. Am J Public Health. 72, 449–454.

3. Knaus WA, Draper EA, Wagner DP et al. (1982). Evaluating outcome from intensive care: A preliminary multihospital comparison. Crit Care Med. 10, 491–496.

4. Knaus WA, Le Gall JR, Wagner DP et al. (1982). A comparison of intensive care in the USA and France. Lancet. 2, 642–646.

5. Wagner DP, Knaus WA, Draper EA. (1986). Physiologic abnormalities and outcome from acute disease: evidence for a predictable relationship. Arch Intern Med. 146, 1389–1396.

6. Knaus WA, Draper EA, Wagner DP, Zimmerman JE. (1985). APACHE II: a severity of disease classification system. Crit Care Med. 13, 818–829.

7. Bion JF, Edlin SA, Ramsay G et al. (1985). Validation of a prognostic score in critically ill patients undergoing transport. Br Med J. 291, 432–434.

8. Bion JF, Aitchison TC, Edlin SA, Ledingham IMcA. (1988). Sickness scoring and response to treatment as predictors of outcome from critical illness. Intens Care Med. 14, 167–171.

9. Lemeshow S, Teres D, Pastides H et al. (1985). A method for predicting survival and mortality of ICU patients using objectively derived weights. Crit Care Med. 13, 519–525.

10. Lemeshow S, Teres D, Avrunin JS, Gage RW. (1988). Refining intensive care unit outcome prediction by using changing probabilities of mortality. Crit Care Med. 16, 470–477.

11. Lemeshow S, Teres D, Avrunin JS, Pastides H. (1987). A comparison of methods to predict mortality of intensive care unit patients. Crit Care Med. 15, 715–722.

12. Keene AR, Cullen DJ. (1983). Therapeutic intervention scoring system: Update. Crit Care Med. 11, 1–3.

13. Cullen DJ, Civetta JM, Briggs BA et al. (1974). Therapeutic intervention score system: a method for quantitative comparison of patient care. Crit Care Med. 2, 57–60.

14. Knaus WA et al. (1991). The APACHE III prognostic system: Risk prediction of hospital mortality for critically ill hospitalized adults. Chest. 100, 1619–1636.

15. Vincent JL, Moreno R, Takala J, et al. (1996). The SOFA (Sepsis-related Organ Failure Assessment) score to describe organ dysfunction/failure. Intensive Care Med. 22, 707–710.

16. Vincent JL, de Mendonca A, Moreno R et al. on behalf of the working group on 'sepsis-related problems' of the European Society of Intensive Care Medicine (1998). Use of the SOFA score to assess the incidence of organ dysfunction/failure in intensive care units: Results of a multicenter, prospective study. Crit Care Med. 26, 1793–1800.

17. Marshall JC, Cook DJ, Christou NV et al. (1995). Multiple Organ Dysfunction Score : A reliable descriptor of a complex clinical syndrome. Crit Care Med. 23, 1638–1652.

18. Le Gall JR, Loirat P, Alperovitch A, et al. (1984). A simplified acute physiology score for ICU patients. Crit Care Med. 12, 975.

19. Le Gall, Lemeshow S, Saulnier F. (1993). A new simplified acute physiology score (SAPS II) based on a European/North American multicenter study. JAMA. 270, 2957.

SECTION 2
Cardiopulmonary Resuscitation and Cerebral Preservation in Adults

Cardiopulmonary Resuscitation and Cerebral Preservation in Adults

A sudden unexpected cessation of effective cardiac pump function or beating of the heart is termed cardiac arrest. This may be reversible if promptly managed, but otherwise invariably leads to death. Cardiac arrest quickly results in a respiratory arrest and resuscitation therefore involves establishing an effective stable circulation as well as maintaining effective ventilation. Cessation of effective cardiac pump function results in an inadequate blood supply to all vital organs of the body, particularly to the brain and also to the heart muscle itself. Hypoxic brain damage and death always result if resuscitation is delayed, is not implemented, or is unsuccessful. In fact, even if the cardiorespiratory system is resuscitated and stabilized, hypoxic brain damage and death may result, if during resuscitation, or prior to it, the cerebral circulation has been compromised, leading to irreversible damage and death of nerve cells within the brain.

It is not the purpose of this chapter to enumerate the numerous causes of sudden cardiac arrest or cardiac death. Ischaemic heart disease remains the commonest cause in Western countries as also in India. In the sixties, 12 per cent of all natural deaths in the United States of America were sudden, and 88 per cent of all sudden natural deaths were due to cardiac causes (1). A prospective study in the same country demonstrated that 50 per cent of all coronary heart disease deaths are sudden and unexpected, and occur within one hour of the onset of symptoms (2). Cardiac arrest is a dreaded complication during surgery and anaesthesia; it can also complicate investigational procedures—pleural, peritoneal or pericardial paracentesis, intravenous pyelography, cardiac catheterization and coronary or cerebral angiography. It can occur as a consequence of electrolyte and metabolic abnormalities, or may be caused by drugs—particularly antiarrhythmic drugs like quinidine, procainamide and digitalis. It is an important cause of death following trauma, blood loss, asphyxia (due to drowning, carbon monoxide poisoning, inhalation of food or vomit), sudden large airways obstruction by a foreign body, and electrocution either by electric shock or lightning.

Basic Mechanisms

The mechanisms underlying cessation of effective cardiac pump function which if uncorrected lead to rapid loss of consciousness and death, are:

(i) Ventricular fibrillation (VF).

(ii) Ventricular tachycardia (VT) resulting in pulselessness and an unconscious state.

(iii) Cardiac standstill or asystole—a markedly severe brady-rhythm has well-nigh the same effect as an asystole or standstill.

(iv) Pulseless electrical activity (PEA)—here though the ECG or cardiac monitor show a normal or satisfactory electrical activity, the mechanical pumping action of the heart is either feeble or absent.

Management

A little over four decades ago, cardiac arrest of any aetiology, even if it occurred in a hospital setting, was invariably fatal. However, with the advent of coronary care units with good monitoring facilities, the use of newer antiarrhythmic drugs, and the electrical management of bradyrhythms, and ventricular tachyrhythms, there has been a dramatic reduction in the immediate hospital mortality rates in patients with potentially lethal arrhythmias. This is particularly so in patients with ischaemic heart disease. It has however been a worldwide observation that sudden deaths due to cardiac arrest occur far more frequently at home or during transport to a hospital soon after a major coronary event, rather than in a hospital. This led to the concept of mobile coronary care units equipped with CPR monitoring and defibrillators to provide intensive care facilities during the high-risk phase of acute myocardial infarction. In India, the funds for such mobile units are meagre. Even so, the city of Mumbai has several such mobile coronary care units in the form of well-equipped ambulances. These mobile units can unfortunately only make a minor dent in the incidence of deaths due to cardiac arrest amongst the 14 million inhabitants of the city. An effective set-up would require a controlling central station, a number of well-equipped ambulances with qualified doctors and paramedical staff, and a quick response to emergency calls. The latter is often an impossibility during the chaotic traffic jams witnessed in the city during peak working hours.

The principles of basic life support if propagated and taught to the lay public could also perhaps make a small dent in the incidence of deaths from cardiac arrest, specially in out-of hospital settings. This is being attempted rather indifferently in the larger cities of the country, and there is no statistical data on its efficacy in ultimate patient survival. In the final analysis an overall improvement in survival rates following cardiac arrest can only be expected if improvements in both pre-hospital (i.e. outside hospital) and in-hospital care are forthcoming. Since unquestionably more arrests occur outside rather than in an in-hospital setting, the importance of pre-hospital care needs to be repeatedly emphasised. Perhaps the most important factor in pre-hospital care is the use of immediate defibrillation by emergency rescue personnel at the scene of the cardiac arrest. Eisenberg and co-workers (3) showed that standard CPR used in the pre-hospital stage resulted in only 23 per cent of the patients reaching the hospital alive, and only 7 per cent being discharged alive. In contrast, immediate defibrillation at the scene of arrest resulted in 53 per cent of patients arriving alive at the hospital, and 23 per cent being discharged alive. Subsequent data support the basic concept that early defibrillation leads to improved survival rates (4–6). Another factor contributing to improved survival is the key role played by CPR administered by lay bystanders whilst awaiting the arrival of the rescue team or ambulance. It was observed that almost twice as many pre-hospital cardiac arrest victims were ultimately discharged alive when they had received bystander CPR (43 per cent), than when such basic life support was not provided (22 per cent).

Objectives and Principles of Management

(i) The chief objective is to restore and maintain stable, effective cardiopulmonary function resulting in effective transport of oxygen to the tissues of the body.

(ii) Since irreversible brain injury or death can occur within 4–6 minutes of the onset of arrest, immediate treatment is mandatory. Time is of essence, and every single second counts.

(iii) A pre-planned, well-organized management protocol is essential. Initially, it aims at Basic Life Support; in a hospital, particularly in an ICU setting, this graduates almost *pari passu* to Advanced Life Support, as detailed below.

(iv) There is a window of approximately 4 minutes from the cessation of effective cardiac function (with absence of major pulses) and of respiration, after which hypoxic injury to the brain progresses rapidly, leading to irreversible death. Resuscitation attempts after 10–15 minutes of arrest have rarely been found to be successful, and most doctors hesitate to resuscitate when more than 10 minutes have elapsed after an unattended cardiac arrest. Permanent brain damage and a vegetative state are the sequelae even if the CPR is successful.

(v) Cardiopulmonary resuscitation in terminal malignancy or in terminal hepatic, renal, or pulmonary diseases offers a cruel extension of life for a short span, and should be best avoided. The ethical issues involved are fairly clear, but should be decided in consultation with the patient's relatives, and one's own colleagues.

Management of the Individual Patient (Fig. 2.1.1)

The following steps are detailed for the management of the individual patient. In an in-hospital setting, and more so in an ICU setting, one step dovetails into the next, and more often than not,

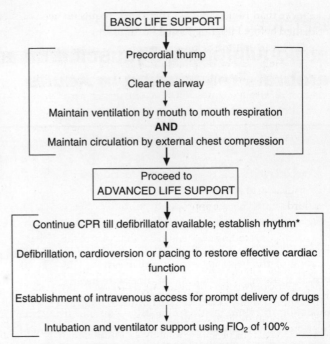

Note : In an ICU setting, each step dovetails into the next, and very often many steps are carried out simultaneously. Also Basic Life Support graduates almost *pari passu* to Advanced Life Support.
*If rhythm shows ventricular fibrillation (VF) or pulseless ventricular tachycardia (VT) proceed as in Fig. 2.1.3.
If rhythm shows asystole or electromechanical dissociation (EMD) proceed as in Fig. 2.1.4a.

Fig. 2.1.1. Steps in cardiopulmonary resuscitation.

many steps are in simultaneous operation. It is important that in an ICU setting each doctor, nurse or paramedical person knows exactly what is expected of him, and that there is one individual to supervise and direct operations.

I. Basic Life Support

(a) *An Ultra-quick Diagnostic Assessment.* It is vital to confirm that a collapsed, unconscious state is due to cardiac arrest. The patient is unresponsive to either a 'shout' or a 'shake'. Absence of pulsation in the carotid and femoral arteries is unquestionably the major diagnostic criterion. Auscultation in an emergency to confirm absence of heart sounds often wastes time, and in my opinion, is unimportant. Marked pallor of the skin followed by cyanosis is the rule, but may be difficult to ascertain in dark-skinned individuals. Absence of respiration or agonal respiratory efforts in conjunction with absent major pulses is diagnostic of cardiac arrest. On the other hand, stridor or apnoea in the presence of a palpable pulse points to a primary respiratory arrest, which if untreated would lead within a few minutes to a cardiac arrest. In such circumstances, an immediate exploration of the oropharynx with the finger to locate a foreign body, and a Heimlich manoeuvre should be carried out, particularly if the 'episode' has occurred against a background where aspiration of food is possible (e.g. Café Coronary).

Once a diagnosis of a cardiac arrest is made (and this should not take more than 10–12 seconds), three basic requisites need to be performed before initiating Basic Life Support.

The first is to call for help—e.g. a shout 'Cardiac arrest in Room 226—Help'. Every hospital should always have an alarm activity system that informs the emergency team, the ICU, the doctors on call within seconds. This not only brings experienced doctors to the site of emergency, but also the 'crash cart' containing the defibrillator. Early defibrillation in a patient with 'arrest' caused by VF or VT is the single most important factor in successful resuscitation.

The second requisite is to appropriately position the victim—on a hard surface, in a supine position.

The third requisite is the appropriate position of the rescuer—kneeling adjacent to the shoulder of the patient, if the patient is on the ground, or standing adjacent to the shoulder of the patient if on a hard bed.

(b) *Precordial Thump*. Once a diagnosis of cardiac arrest is established, one or two forceful blows are delivered from a height of 8–10 inches, roughly at the junction of the middle and lower third of the sternum. Such a thump delivers a low level electric depolarization current of approximately 25 Joules which is able to interrupt conduction along a re-entrant pathway if delivered at a correct time in the cardiac cycle (7, 8). Earlier, the American Heart Association recommended the use of a precordial thump only in monitored patients because of the fear of converting a ventricular tachycardia to a ventricular fibrillation (9). Caldwell and associates (7) in a prospective study on 5000 patients noted that this indeed does not occur, and there seems to be no contraindication to its use in unmonitored patients if there is no other option available. The present American Heart Association recommendations permit the use of a precordial thump if no defibrillator is available (10). One should of course not persist in 'thumps' or blows to the chest if the pulse and respiration do not return spontaneously after one or two attempts at 'thumpversion'.

(c) *Clearing of the Airway*. The next step is to clear the airway. This is achieved by tilting the head backwards, lifting the mandible forwards, and opening the mouth and removing any foreign body (including dentures) from the oropharynx (**Fig. 2.1.2**). Extension

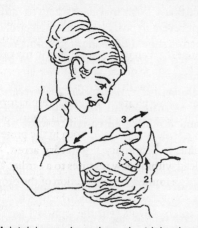

Fig. 2.1.2. Maintaining a clear airway by triple airway manoeuvre: (1) Tilt head backwards. (2) Lift mandible forwards. (3) Open the mouth and try to remove any foreign body.

of the neck in patients with traumatic fractures of the cervical spine is best avoided. If a foreign body is suspected of obstructing the larynx, the Heimlich manoeuvre is performed. This entails encircling one's arms around the patient from the back, and delivering an upward and backward thrust with a closed fist to the abdomen just below the costal angle (**11**). In a prostrate, unconscious individual, the Heimlich manoeuvre can be performed by delivering upward thrusts with the thumbs on the upper abdomen, in an attempt to mechanically dislodge the foreign body obstructing the airway. Undue force in performing the manoeuvre can lead to rupture of the upper abdominal viscera, including the liver (**12**).

(d) *Institution of Mouth to Mouth Respiration and External Cardiac Compression*. Time is of infinite importance, and there should be no delay between establishing the diagnosis and the earlier steps and the initiation of mouth to mouth respiration and external chest compression. The purpose of basic life support as provided by these measures is to maintain the viability of vital organs particularly the heart and brain, till such time as effective spontaneous circulation and respiration are restored, or till more definite 'advanced' intervention is achieved.

The heart and lungs work as a single unit and serve to transport oxygen to body tissues. It is pointless to quibble as to whether one should first initiate mouth to mouth respiration or cardiac compression; both should be carried out *pari passu*.

Maintaining Artificial Ventilation in an Out-of-Hospital Setting. Ventilation is maintained by mouth to mouth breathing. With a single resuscitator, mouth to mouth breathing is employed 2–5 times after every 15–20 cardiac compressions. If two resuscitators are available, two rescue ventilations are given over 4 seconds, adequate time being given (1 to 2 seconds per ventilation) to allow for exhalation. Ventilations with this slow inspiratory flow rate are recommended, so that the oesophageal opening pressure is not exceeded and the risk of gastric distension, regurgitation and aspiration are reduced. The correct technique of mouth to mouth respiration can be easily taught to paramedical staff as well as lay people. The resuscitator pinches the patient's nostrils with the index finger and thumb of the hand, which is firmly placed on the patient's forehead. After a deep inspiration, the resuscitator seals his opened mouth over the patient's mouth and blows in a fairly large volume of expired air sufficient to cause a moderate expansion of the patient's chest. He then separates his mouth from the patient's to allow a passive exhalation of air from the patient. The fear of acquiring the human immunodeficiency virus or the hepatitis B virus is a point of genuine concern for those engaged in resuscitative care, particularly during mouth to mouth respiration. The use of an 'S' shaped airway (Brooke's airway) or other protective barrier ventilation devices in mouth to mouth respiration afford a measure of safety to the resuscitator.

Maintaining Ventilation in an In-Hospital Setting, in an Intensive Care Unit or in a Mobile Intensive Care Unit (or a well-equipped ambulance). A fitting face mask connected to an AMBU bag which in turn is connected to an oxygen source enables 100 per cent oxygen to be administered to the patient till such time as endotracheal intubation is performed and the airway firmly secured. A bag-mask ventilation is most efficiently performed if one individual holds the face mask firmly covering the nose and mouth of the patient to ensure that there is no air-leak, and the other squeezes the AMBU bag. One should not wait idly till the AMBU bag and face mask or endotracheal tube are brought for the patient, but institute and carry on mouth to mouth respiration till more effective means of ventilation are available even in an in-hospital setting. *Each ward of every hospital should have an emergency tray which has a face mask with an AMBU bag, a laryngoscope with a light in working order and an endotracheal tube.*

External Chest Compression or External Cardiac Massage. This must be started as soon as possible after a cardiac arrest together with mouth to mouth breathing for artificial ventilation. The correct technique must be carefully adhered to.

With the patient lying on a hard surface the resuscitator places the heel of the proximal part of one hand over the lower part of the sternum. With arms held straight and locked at the elbow, the heel of the other hand is placed over the dorsum of the first. External cardiac compression is now started by forcibly depressing the sternum about 4–5 cm by a downward pressure followed by immediate relaxation and release of pressure. This cycle of depression and relaxation is performed 70–90 times per minute. It is important to check that external cardiac compression produces a palpable pulse in the carotids. If it does not, the technique is probably faulty, and the procedure will be of no avail.

Complications of External Cardiac Compression. These include fracture of ribs, sternum, flail chest, haemopericardium, cardiac lacerations, cardiac tamponade, pneumothorax, lacerations of the lung, injury to the liver and other abdominal organs, and fat embolism. The following guidelines help in minimizing or avoiding the traumatic complications listed above.

(i) Never exert pressure over the xiphoid cartilage as it can lacerate the liver.

(ii) The fingers of the hands should be lifted up and not be pressing on the ribs; pressure should only be exerted with the heel of the hand over the lower sternum.

(iii) Compression should be smooth, regular, and half the cycle should be used for compression and half for relaxation. Jerky irregular movements are more likely to result in fractures and other injuries.

(iv) Cardiac compression in a patient with a prosthetic valve often causes laceration of the valve area. If external cardiac compression over 3–4 minutes, together with the definitive procedures outlined later fail to resuscitate, it is better to open the chest for a direct cardiac massage.

II. Advanced Cardiac Life Support (ACLS)

ACLS should be considered a continuum of Basic Life Support or perhaps the other end of the spectrum of Basic Life Support. The objectives of ACLS are to revert the cardiac rhythm to one which is haemodynamically effective in maintaining and supporting the restored circulation, and to maintain adequate ventilation and gas exchange till effective spontaneous breathing is re-established. The earlier ACLS is initiated, the greater the chances of survival. In an intensive care unit, ACLS can be offered in a

matter of seconds or minutes. In an out-of-hospital arrest, ACLS can be offered only when trained resuscitators reach the patient or following transport to a hospital with ICU facilities.

Advanced Cardiac Life Support consists of the following:

(a) Defibrillation (cardioversion) or pacing to restore effective cardiac pumping action.

(b) Intubation with ventilator support on 100 per cent oxygen.

(c) Establishment of an intravenous line which allows prompt delivery of appropriate drugs.

Advanced Cardiac Life Support obviously necessitates the availability of proper equipment as well as trained staff, and the steps enunciated above are invariably carried out simultaneously by different members of the trained staff. Each member of the resuscitative team is assigned a specific task. The head of the team directs the resuscitative effort. The step which demands the utmost urgency and priority is the restoration of a haemodynamically effective cardiac rhythm by defibrillation and cardioversion in ventricular tachycardia or fibrillation (**Fig. 2.1.3**).

(a) *Restoring a haemodynamically effective cardiac rhythm (in VF/ VT)—defibrillation cardioversion. As soon as a defibrillator is available, it is attached to the patient, and if VT or VF is present, defibrillation is carried out with a shock of 200 Joules. A stable sinus rhythm is often restored.* If the first shock is unsuccessful, a 300—360 Joules shock is repeated, if still unsuccessful a third shock is administered. If three consecutive shocks fail to cardiovert the heart, CPR is continued and the patient promptly intubated and an intravenous access line is established (see below).

The importance of early defibrillation in the success of cardiopulmonary resuscitation in VT or VF cannot be overemphasized. Over 90 per cent of patients who survived cardiac arrest were resuscitated from ventricular fibrillation (**5, 13**). Also, the success of defibrillation is time-dependent. The probability of successful defibrillation declines by about 2 per cent to 10 per cent per minute, starting with an estimated probability of 70 to 80 per cent survival at time zero (**14**). Thus, if a patient with VF is not shocked (defibrillated) within ten minutes of the onset of collapse or 'arrest', the probability of survival approaches zero.

It is to be noted that VT/VF may be resistant to cardioversion in the presence of severe hypoxia, acidosis or electrolyte disturbances. These factors should be monitored during resuscitative efforts and corrected as far as possible (see use of intravenous sodium bicarbonate).

(b) *and* (c) *Intubation and ventilation with 100 per cent oxygen and establishment of an intravenous line.* One member of the resuscitative team should be entrusted to intubate and give ventilator support using 100 per cent oxygen to start with. Another member is entrusted to secure an intravenous line. Both these procedures are carried out more or less simultaneously. If peripheral venous access in the upper limbs is impossible because of collapsed veins, securing a central venous line is mandatory. Even if a peripheral venous line is promptly secured, we also prefer to insert a central line both for measuring central venous pressure and for injecting the required drugs during resuscitation. The insertion of a central line requires special expertise when

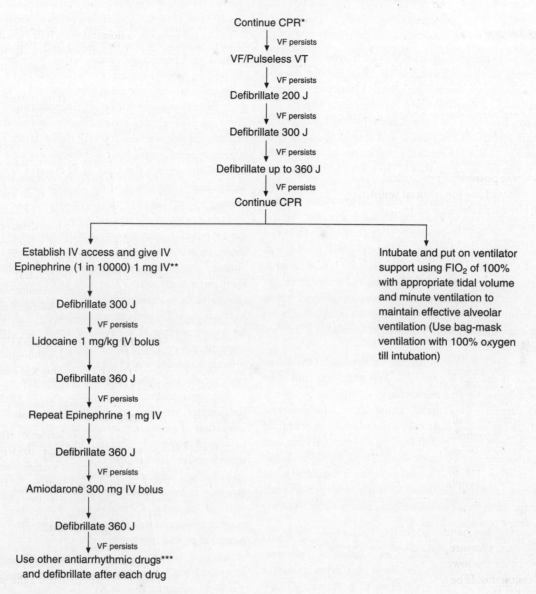

Continue CPR*

↓ VF persists

VF/Pulseless VT

↓ VF persists

Defibrillate 200 J

↓ VF persists

Defibrillate 300 J

↓ VF persists

Defibrillate up to 360 J

↓ VF persists

Continue CPR

Establish IV access and give IV
Epinephrine (1 in 10000) 1 mg IV**

↓

Defibrillate 300 J

↓ VF persists

Lidocaine 1 mg/kg IV bolus

↓

Defibrillate 360 J

↓ VF persists

Repeat Epinephrine 1 mg IV

↓

Defibrillate 360 J

↓ VF persists

Amiodarone 300 mg IV bolus

↓

Defibrillate 360 J

↓ VF persists

Use other antiarrhythmic drugs***
and defibrillate after each drug

Intubate and put on ventilator
support using FIO$_2$ of 100%
with appropriate tidal volume
and minute ventilation to
maintain effective alveolar
ventilation (Use bag-mask
ventilation with 100% oxygen
till intubation)

*Continue CPR till patient resuscitated or pronounced dead
**Epinephrine can be repeated 1 mg IV every 5 mins during CPR
***We use other anti-arrhythmic drugs in the following order: (i) Bretylium tosylate 5 mg/kg IV, repeated after 15 mins; (ii) Procainamide may be given IV as 100 mg boluses every 5 mins, to a total dose of 500–1000 mg. This is followed by a continuous infusion at the rate of 2–4 mg/min. However, we rarely use this drug in our set-up.

Fig. 2.1.3. Algorithm for treatment of ventricular fibrillation (VF), or pulseless ventricular tachycardia (VT).

performed during CPR; the latter should not be interrupted for more than 10–15 seconds while the line is being inserted. The use of intracardiac injections to administer drugs is best avoided, unless it has been impossible to secure a venous line quickly. Once venous access is available, and the patient is in VF in spite of receiving 2–3 shocks, 1 mg of epinephrine is administered intravenously as a bolus. Thirty to sixty seconds after the dose of epinephrine, the rhythm is reassessed and if VT/VF is still present, the patient is again shocked—a 'stack' of three shocks at 360 joules being delivered. The dose of epinephrine can be repeated every 3 to 5 minutes during subsequent resuscitative efforts. If this approach fails, the dose of epinephrine can be increased to 2 to 5 mg

every 5 minutes or an escalating dose of 1 mg–3 mg–5 mg 3 minutes apart can be tried (15). Each dose of intravenous epinephrine should be followed within 30 seconds by a DC shock if VF/VT persists. Cardiopulmonary resuscitation should continue unabated, except when DC shocks are being given. The resuscitation guidelines of the European Resuscitation Council (16) recommend four sets of three defibrillations with 1 mg epinephrine after each set. This approach results in 12 defibrillations and 3 mg of epinephrine before using pharmacotherapy described below. The AHA guidelines (17) however, continue to recommend a single shock after the first dose of epinephrine if intravenous medications are promptly available. Pharmacotherapy is used if the patient is still in VF/VT.

Pharmacotherapy

For the patient who continues to be in VT/VF in spite of attempts at DC cardioversion after epinephrine, electrical stability may be achieved by the intravenous administration of antiarrythmic agents during continued cardiopulmonary resuscitation. The modus operandi is to administer the chosen antiarrythmic medication which is likely to benefit the patient and then defibrillate with 360 Joules within 30 to 60 seconds after each dose of medication. The pattern should be drug-shock, drug-shock, drug-shock. Lidocaine is used first as an intravenous bolus of 1 mg/kg, with the dose repeated within 5 minutes if electrical instability persists. If lidocaine in a total dose of 2 to 3 mg/kg is unsuccessful, 300 mg of amiodarone is given intravenously over 10 minutes followed by an infusion of 10 mg/kg/day. Additional bolus dosing to a maximum of 500 mg can be tried if the initial bolus is unsuccessful.

Other drugs can also be tried if lidocaine and amiodarone are unsuccessful, but success with these drugs is uncommon. These drugs include bretylium tosylate which is given as an initial bolus of 5 mg/kg intravenously to be repeated in 5 minutes if the first bolus is unsuccessful.

We have never found procainamide of any use in the above circumstances. If used, it is given in a dose of 30 mg/min in an intravenous infusion up to a maximum of 17 mg/kg.

If hyperkalaemia is the cause of cardiac arrest, an intravenous infusion of 20 ml 10 per cent calcium gluconate is promptly administered over 5 minutes, followed by 100 ml of 7.5 per cent sodium bicarbonate given intravenously. Though calcium is not given in the routine protocol for cardiac arrest, it should be given as intravenous calcium gluconate to those who are severely hypocalcaemic or to those who have been poisoned by an excess of calcium entry blocking drugs.

Hypokalaemia can also lead to resistant VT/VF and should be corrected with 40 mEq of KCl as an infusion of 5 per cent glucose. A combination of hypokalaemia plus hypocapnia due to hyperventilation is an important cause of persistent VT/VF. Reducing minute ventilation and increasing serum K^+ may help restore electrical stability.

Some forms of VT, polymorphic VT or torsades de pointes, rapid monomorphic VT may respond to intravenous $MgSO_4$ (1 g given intravenously over 1 to 2 minutes). Metoprolol in a dose of 5 mg to 20 mg intravenously can also be tried under the above circumstances.

Use of Sodium bicarbonate. Till recently, frequent boluses of intravenous sodium bicarbonate were routinely administered early during resuscitation for cardiac arrest. This often resulted in an overuse of the drug with deleterious side-effects. If adequate CPR is initiated immediately in a witnessed cardiac arrest, and the patient ventilated with 100 per cent oxygen, a stable acid-base balance is generally maintained for over 30 minutes (18). Current studies show little benefit and possible harm associated with bicarbonate administration in lactic acid acidosis (19–21). Intravenous sodium bicarbonate is indicated in hyperkalaemia; prompt administration in this condition can restore electrical stability and is often life-saving. It is also indicated in bicarbonate-responsive acidosis and in arrest due to an overdose of tricyclic antidepressants. We also use intravenous sodium bicarbonate in patients with prolonged cardiac arrest who have a low arterial pH and in post-resuscitation acidosis. Intravenous sodium bicarbonate is administered in a dose of 1 mEq/kg; this is repeated every 10 to 15 minutes with careful monitoring of the arterial pH. The dangers of injudicious use of intravenous sodium bicarbonate include hyperosmolarity, alkalosis with hypokalaemia, hypernatraemia, paradoxical intracellular acidosis (because of faster diffusion into the cells of liberated CO_2 as compared to bicarbonate), and a shift of the O_2 dissociation curve to the left, causing a sharp fall in the $P\bar{v}O_2$ and the PaO_2.

Early intubation and ventilator support with 100 per cent oxygen to allow maximal O_2 saturation of blood is important and as far as possible should be accomplished simultaneously with the other measures outlined above. *It is however, more important to first defibrillate the heart (in patients with VF or VT) and to administer intravenous epinephrine in an attempt to quickly restore an effective cardiac rhythm and circulation.* Till such time as the patient is intubated and placed on ventilator support, a bag-valve-mask ventilation is continued using 100 per cent oxygen. It is preferable to have two persons to provide bag-valve-mask ventilation. One maintains the sealed open airway, the other ventilates the patient.

Improper technique in ventilating the patient can lead to progressive inflation of the stomach with increased risk of aspiration of stomach contents, or even rupture of the stomach or oesophagus from increased intragastric pressure. Bag-valve-mask ventilation is however greatly inferior to ventilation via an endotracheal tube which should be inserted at the earliest. No attempt at intubation should last for more than 20 seconds without restarting CPR and ventilation. After intubation, the position of the endotracheal tube should be checked by auscultating both lungs and observing the movements of the chest on ventilation. Minute ventilation should then be so adjusted as to keep the $PaCO_2$ between 35 to 40 mm Hg. Hypocapnia, when marked promotes instability of the heart, particularly in the presence of hypokalaemia. After correct placement, the endotracheal tube should be securely taped to prevent undue movement or dislodgement of the tube. It is important to bear in mind that if the endotracheal tube is in place and if the intravenous line has not been established, certain emergency drugs can be effectively administered via the tube (22). The drugs that can be administered via the tube are epinephrine, lidocaine and atropine. The dose of these drugs is 2.5 times that recommended for intravenous use and should first be diluted in N saline or distilled water (23). Drugs should not be injected directly into the endotracheal tube but through a long catheter (e.g. a central line catheter) whose tip extends beyond the tip of the endotracheal tube. External cardiac massage should be discontinued whilst the drug is being injected into the upper airways, and the injection is followed with a few manual inflations of the lungs. The drug, after this manoeuvre is effectively absorbed.

Approach to Pulseless Electrical Activity (PEA) (**Fig. 2.1.4a**). This form of 'arrest' is characterized by the absence of a detectable pulse and the presence of some type of electrical activity. The

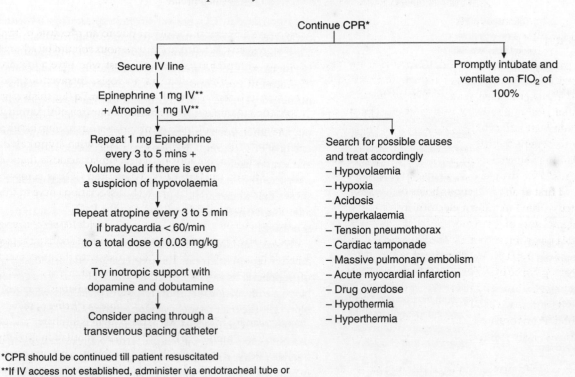

Fig. 2.1.4a. Algorithm for management of Pulseless Electrical Activity (PEA).

heterogenous group of rhythm disturbances includes electromechanical dissociation (EMD), pseudoEMD, idioventricular rhythm, ventricular escape rhythms and brady-asystolic rhythm. The term electromechanical dissociation is applied to a condition where the electrical acivity is characterized by narrow ventricular complexes with no mechanical contractions and no detectable pulse (24). Recent research with cardiac ultrasonography and indwelling pressure catheter has shown that in some of these patients electrical activity is associated with contractions too feeble to be detected by palpating the pulse or by using a sphygmomanometer (25–27). Paradis has termed this pseudoelectromechanical dissociation.

The most common cause of pulseless electrical activity is hypovolaemia. Other important causes are tension pneumothorax, cardiac tamponade, massive pulmonary embolism, severe acidosis, drug overdosage (digoxin, beta blockers, tricyclic antidepressants), hyperkalaemia, severe hypoxia, massive myocardial infarction, hypothermia, hyperthermia. Some of these can be promptly recognized and when corrected can salvage life. It is therefore imperative that clinicians search for reversible, treatable cause of PEA. Resuscitative measures include prompt intubation with ventilation using 100 per cent oxygen and the securing of an intravenous line if this has not already been done. CPR is vigorously continued till resuscitation succeeds or is abandoned. Adrenaline 1 mg intravenous is administered and if needs be, is repeated every 3 to 5 minutes.

If the veins are not obviously engorged, a volume load (N saline or a colloid) is given to prime the heart. Vasopressors like norepinephrine, inotropes like dopamine are started in separate intravenous infusions. In combination with a volume load, they may at times restore cardiac contractions. Intravenous sodium bicarbonate should be used to counter acidosis after prolonged resuscitation. Intravenous calcium chloride may also be considered. Pacing with an external pacemaker, followed by pacing through a pacing catheter may help in selected circumstances.

Approach to Asystole or Severe Bradycardia (**Fig. 2.1.4b**). There are two points to consider in the approach to an asystolic arrest. The first is to confirm asystole when faced with a straight line on the monitor. This can be done by changing to another lead on the lead select switch or by changing placement of the defibrillating panels by 90 degrees. A 'false' asystole, that is to say a VF masquerading as an asystole can thereby be quickly diagnosed. The second point is to quickly assess the possible treatable causes of asystole or severe bradyrhythm. These causes include pre-existing acidosis, hypoxia, hyperkalaemia, drug overdose, hypothermia, hyperthermia. Promptly treating the cause whenever possible can make the difference between life and death.

The treatment of asystole is rather similar to that of PEA. CPR is continued all through till resuscitation is successful or is abandoned. The patient is promptly intubated and ventilated with 100 per cent oxygen and an intravenous line secured if this has not already been done. If a transcutaneous external pacemaker is available, the patient is promptly paced, till such time as a pacing catheter is inserted and connected to a temporary pacemaker. Simultaneously 1 mg epinephrine is administered intravenously. Epinephrine can be repeated every 3 to 5 minutes to a total dose of 0.03 to 0.04 mg/kg. Intravenous calcium chloride 2 mg/kg may be tried in the hope that effective cardiac contractions may be restored.

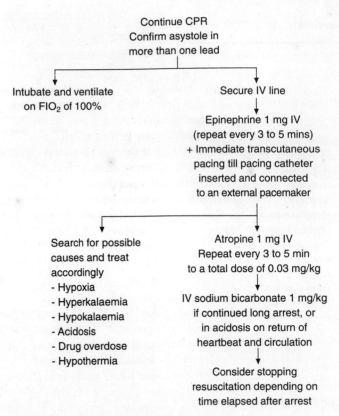

Fig. 2.1.4b. Algorithm for management of asystole.

Caution: It is important not to shock a patient in true asystole. On some occasions, high levels of parasympathetic tone may lead to cessation of supraventricular and ventricular pacemaker activity **(28, 29)**. Electrical shocks can produce a stunned myocardium with marked increase in parasympathetic tone. Such shocks to an asystolic heart could therefore render return of spontaneous cardiac contractions impossible.

It is generally accepted that the asystolic patient has the worst prognosis, despite all resuscitative measures including external cardiac pacing or pacing through the use of a quickly inserted pacing catheter **(30)**.

Maintaining and Supporting Circulation. Electrical stability in a patient is maintained with intravenous lidocaine 1 to 3 mg/min. in an infusion of N saline or intravenous amiodarone 1000 mg in an infusion over 24 hours. Catecholamines and inotropic drugs are very useful in maintaining and supporting circulation after effective cardiac action has been restored. Epinephrine, norepinephrine, dopamine, dobutamine or an appropriate combination of any two of these drugs given in separate intravenous infusions produce elevation of aortic diastolic blood pressure with increased cerebral and myocardial blood flow **(31)**. A satisfactory volume load must be given to prime the heart and to maintain an adequate filling pressure.

Clinical Monitoring of CPR. The purpose of CPR is to maintain an effective blood flow within the body. Monitoring electrical activity of the heart, the pulse, blood pressure (if recordable), urine output, arterial pH and blood gases is important. However, the presence of a palpable pulse and arterial blood pressure waves is not always an indication of blood flow. The end tidal pressure of carbon dioxide (CO_2 pressure in end-expiratory gas) is a useful parameter and bedside marker to help monitor cardiac output. This is because the excretion of carbon dioxide in expiratory gas is a function of the pulmonary blood flow i.e. of cardiac output. The level of concentration of CO_2 in expired gas is directly proportional to the cardiac output. A low cardiac output will be associated with a low end tidal PCO_2 and an increased cardiac output with an increasing end tidal PCO_2. Thus a steadily increasing end tidal PCO_2 during CPR denotes an increasing cardiac output and is more likely to be associated with a successful outcome than a persistently low end tidal PCO_2. Wayne and colleagues **(32)** have shown that when end tidal PCO_2 does not rise above 10 mm Hg after 15 to 20 minutes of resuscitation time, a successful outcome is unlikely.

Venous Blood Gases. Marino **(33)** believes that venous blood is a better representative of the oxygenation and acid-base status of peripheral tissues compared to arterial blood. Thus, arterial blood gas estimation may show respiratory alkalosis, while venous blood gas show a metabolic acidosis during CPR **(34, 35)**.

Results of Cardiopulmonary Resuscitation. In our unit at most 4 to 5 out of 10 patients with cardiac arrest are resuscitated—in that a stable cardiac rhythm with adequate circulation and perfusion is restored. However, only a third of these patients ultimately leave hospital and resume their normal lives. This poor outcome even after resuscitation is related to cardiac failure, or to brain damage with neurological sequelae. In some cases, brain damage leads to ultimate death or to a vegetative existence, and in others to neurological sequelae that prevent the patient from resuming his normal activities. *Preservation of the myocardium and of the brain during cardiopulmonary resuscitation is therefore of prime importance—* unfortunately, inherent changes in physiology during resuscitation render this task difficult, and at times even impossible.

Altered Physiology during CPR. Unfortunately, external cardiac massage (chest compression) does not generally result in an adequate blood flow to the vital organs. In fact, the blood flow in both systemic and regional circulations (e.g. coronary circulation), is less than one quarter of pre-arrest levels during closed chest compressions **(36–38)**. This explains the poor success results of CPR.

The brain and the heart are two organs that are most vulnerable to deprived blood supply. The brain accounts for just 2 per cent of body mass, and yet receives over 15 per cent of the cardiac output. Cerebral perfusion is maintained in preference to perfusion of the other organs in the face of decreasing flow and perfusion pressure. This is achieved through a process of 'autoregulation' and the chief autoregulator in the CNS is carbon dioxide. Accumulation of carbon dioxide within the CNS due to a falling perfusion pressure produces local cerebral vasodilatation with a resulting compensatory increase in cerebral blood flow. Autoregulation ceases to function effectively when the mean arterial blood pressure falls below 60 mm Hg **(39)**. Even so, cerebral function is sustained until blood flow to the brain falls below 25–30 per cent of normal levels **(40, 41)**. Open cardiac massage can achieve normal or even supranormal cerebral perfusion **(40)**. In practice, resuscitation by open cardiac massage is rare except in the theatre immediately following coronary artery bypass surgery, or when the chest is opened for an arrest during induction of anaesthesia, or during surgery. External chest compression achieves only around 5 per cent of normal cerebral flow rates (**40**) and this is clearly less than the flow needed to maintain cerebral metabolism. This inability to maintain adequate levels of cerebral blood flow during closed chest CPR is the reason for brain death, neurological sequelae and the overall poor survival rates, even when resuscitation is apparently thought to be successful. It was believed earlier that external chest compression maintained circulation as a result of a squeeze or pressure on the heart between the sternum and the thoracic spine. This 'squeeze' pushed blood out into the systemic and pulmonary circulations, followed by a filling of the heart when the pressure was released. The current concept is that external pressure on the chest leads to an increased intrathoracic and intrapleural pressure, and this positive pressure is responsible for propelling the blood forward. Release of external pressure leads to a fall in the intrathoracic and intrapleural pressures, allowing blood to fill the heart.

New techniques and protocols for CPR are under trial to further improve perfusion of the heart and brain during circulatory arrest (**42**). These chiefly include interposed abdominal compression (IAC-CPR) and phased thoracico-abdominal compression (PTAC-CPR). In IAC-CPR abdominal compressions (through pressure mid-way between the umbilicus and xiphisternum) are interposed with the usual chest compressions. Randomized trials have shown significant improvement in return of spontaneous circulation, survival to 24 hours, and to hospital discharge, when compared to standard CPR (**43**). The technique of PTAC-CPR improves circulation and vital organ perfusion. For this technique, an instrument (The Lifestick) has been devised to alternate thoracic and abdominal compression using a see-saw action between two suction pads (**44**). The above techniques require trained personnel and in our scenario are best avoided till results of further trials are conclusive.

Stopping Efforts to Resuscitate. Mere survival in a vegetative state can be an unfortunate sequel of CPR. The risk of organ dysfunction or failure is related directly to the duration of ischaemic insult. The ischaemic time following an 'arrest' includes the time from the onset of arrest to the start of CPR (arrest time) plus the duration of CPR efforts. In the study by the Brain Resuscitation Clinical Trial I Study group, Abramson et al. (**45**) found that if the arrest time is less than 6 minutes and the CPR time does not exceed 30 minutes, half of the survivors had a good neurological recovery. If however, the arrest time exceeds 6 minutes, a CPR lasting more than 15 minutes always resulted in a significant neurological impairment in the survivors. Though it is perhaps impossible to be dogmatic, this observation suggests that CPR should be continued for at least 30 minutes if the arrest time is less than 6 minutes. If the arrest time is longer than 6 minutes, the CPR should be terminated after 15 minutes (**42**).

III. Prolonged Life Support

Patients who do not recover within 24 hours may require prolonged life support. Overall critical care is vital under such circumstances. This involves support to all organ systems and also involves dealing with post-resuscitation problems, which may be trying to both the ICU staff and relatives of the patient.

Post-Resuscitation Problems. The two major concerns even after restoring spontaneous circulation are (a) the development of multiple organ dysfunction, and (b) possible neurological injury in patients who fail to recover consciousness after successful CPR.

Remarkably enough, inadequate perfusion with ischaemic damage to tissue cells can continue in the post-resuscitation period despite restoration of the blood pressure and circulation (**46**). This is due to a persistent state of vasoconstriction that follows the period of hypotension. This vasoconstriction with resulting hypoperfusion to organs is believed to be induced by the entry of calcium into the damaged vascular smooth muscle and is more marked in the cerebral and splanchnic circulation (**46**). Calcium channel blockers like verapamil and magnesium have been shown to abolish post-arrest vasoconstriction and hypoperfusion in animal models (**47**).

Another proposed mechanism for post-resuscitation injury is related to the accumulation of toxic products of oxygen metabolism (notably free oxygen radicals) during the ischaemic period. During reperfusion, these toxic products are disseminated into all organ systems producing widespread organ damage (**48**). Perhaps both the above mechanisms may play a significant role in post-resuscitation injury and have prompted the institution of clinical measures to enhance cerebral preservation.

Enhancement of Cerebral Preservation. The following measures have been proposed:

(a) *'New CPR'.* Modification of standard CPR techniques include techniques to increase intrathoracic pressure during CPR mentioned earlier. However the role of these measures in enhancing survival rates is as yet uncertain.

(b) *Avoidance of Intravenous Dextrose.* Recent evidence in animals shows that intravenous dextrose administered during CPR increases mortality (**49**). Glucose enters ischaemic areas in the CNS and is anaerobically metabolized to produce lactic acid which contributes to tissue damage. It has not been conclusively proven that the above theory holds true in human beings during CPR, but it is wise to avoid unnecessary dextrose infusions during resuscitation and in the immediate post-resuscitation period. Blood sugar levels should be kept within normal limits in the post-resuscitation period, and insulin should be used if necessary.

(c) *Avoidance of Calcium.* Calcium was invariably used in the past to initiate or augment cardiac contractions particularly in asystole or electromechanical dissociation. The possible role of calcium in promoting vasoconstriction and hypoperfusion in the immediate post-resuscitation period, has led to a re-evaluation of its use during CPR. Also ischaemia produces accumulation of intracellular calcium and this can lead to cell injury due to disruption of the cell membrane and uncoupling of oxidative phosphorylation (**50**). Intravenous calcium in any form should preferably not be routinely used during CPR, and should be administered only to counter (i) hyperkalaemia; (ii) a low ionised calcium after successful resuscitation; (iii) over-medication with calcium channel blockers.

(d) *Use of Calcium Channel Blockers.* In the post-resuscitation period, calcium blockade should be considered to counter vaso-constriction in vital organs. This is due to the prevailing concept that the entry of calcium into damaged vessel walls perpetuates vasoconstriction and hypoperfusion. We use intravenous nimodipine 30–60 mg four hourly in patients who do not require inotropic support after resuscitation, and are mentally obtunded or unconscious. Intravenous magnesium sulphate (2–4 ml of 50 per cent magnesiun sulphate solution given over 30 minutes) can also be used as a calcium channel blocker. Intravenous magnesium has been found to be effective in maintaining cerebral blood flow after CPR in animal experiments (51).

(e) *Measures against Cerebral Oedema:*

STEROIDS. We use steroids (dexamethasone 4 mg intravenously 6 hourly) routinely in post-resuscitation states particularly in obtunded patients as an anti-oedema measure. Though clinical trials have not shown a clear benefit following the use of steroids (40), we feel they may well be of use in patients with cerebral oedema.

MANNITOL. 150–300 ml intravenously can be given empirically in comatose patients following restoration of circulation after a cardiac arrest. Mannitol is also given if there is a sudden neurological deterioration after an initial improvement, in the level of consciousness.

Table 2.1.1. Guidelines for cerebral preservation in patients with coma following cardiac arrest

1. Maintain as normal a circulation as possible, with a systolic arterial blood pressure > 120 mm Hg, and a mean arterial pressure of 90 mm Hg. Use adequate inotropic support if necessary
2. Once the circulation has been restored and maintained, keep the head elevated between 10–30 degrees
3. Use controlled ventilation and maintain a PaO_2 close to 100 mm Hg, and $PaCO_2$ around 25–30 mm Hg. If necessary sedate patient with diazepam; in patients who are very restless and clashing with the machine, use pancuronium 2–4 mg IV as and when necessary.
4. Maintain a normal pH and normal electrolytes
5. Control blood sugar levels, if necessary with insulin—keep blood sugar < 150 mg/dl
6. Maintain normothermia; avoid hyperthermia
7. Avoid infusions of IV dextrose —use glucose saline or Ringer Lactate
8. Avoid IV calcium except to counter hyperkalaemia, hypocalcaemia, or overmedication with calcium antagonists
9. Consider the use of calcium-channel blockers (nimodipine 30–60 mg IV 4 hourly) in post-resuscitative coma, if circulation and blood pressure are stable
10. Implement measures against possible cerebral oedema:
    - IV dexamethasone 4–6 mg 6 hourly for 3–4 days
    - IV mannitol 150–300 ml as an empirical single dose
    - IV furosemide 40–60 mg
    - Maintain $PaCO_2$ around 25 mm Hg through controlled ventilation
11. Control coughing, straining, restlessness, myoclonic jerks and seizures, with appropriate medication
12. (a) Monitor the neurological state and depth of coma by the Glasgow Coma Score
    (b) Determine if brain-death is present. If so, confirm with EEG. Request for an independent assessment by a colleague. Explain the situation to the relatives. The law should permit the doctor to then remove ventilator and other support

FUROSEMIDE. 40–60 mg intravenously is also used as an anti-oedema measure.

INDUCED HYPOCAPNIA. We prefer to keep the $PaCO_2$ around 25 mm Hg with controlled ventilation, in the hope that this helps to reduce the cerebral oedema. The oxygen saturation of arterial blood is kept close to 100 per cent.

PREVENTING RISE OR FLUCTUATION IN INTRACRANIAL PRESSURE. Coughing and straining are prevented by the use of intravenous diazepam. Seizures are controlled by appropriate measures.

Guidelines for cerebral preservation in patients with coma following cardiac arrest are listed in **Table 2.1.1.**

Neurological Sequelae

In spite of expert management even in good centres, neurological sequelae are all too common:

(a) *Brain Death.* This is the most catastrophic and often unavoidable sequel. Till recently in our country the legal definition of death was restricted to cessation of the heart's activity and of respiration. The sequel of brain death with consequent inevitable prolongation of the end by hours, and even by days was agonising to doctors, nursing staff and relatives. Wisdom has at last dawned on the powers that be, and brain death has by a recent act of Parliament been accepted as the criterion for death, even in the presence of continuing heart action or beat.

Brain death is characterized by an unarousable state of coma, a flat EEG, and absent brain stem reflexes. These include absent doll's eye movements, no eye movements on stimulation of the labyrinth by cold water syringed into the auditory canal, and absent corneal, pupillary, gag and cough reflexes. There is also absence of spontaneous breathing. The apnoea test is considered positive if there is no evidence of spontaneous ventilatory efforts for at least 3 minutes, and the $PaCO_2$ is > 60 mm Hg at the end of the test.

The local spinal reflexes may be preserved in a brain-dead individual. Deep tendon reflexes may thus continue to be elicitable. The heart and circulation can function effectively for as long as two weeks or even longer if ventilatory support is continued. Pressure from concerned, and at times angry relatives, leaves one with no option other than to continue with life support, even though the futility and anguish of this has been explained to the relatives. The longest 'survival' we have recorded after brain death has been close to 3 weeks. Gradually, multiple organ failure sets in. An interesting feature is the occurrence of diabetes insipidus perhaps due to involvement or 'injury' to the hypothalamus and pituitary. Another noteworthy feature is the frequent occurrence of hyperglycaemia in these patients. Failure of gastrointestinal function is characterized by absent peristalsis, yet without any associated distension. Perhaps there is a decrease and virtual cessation of secretion of digestive and other fluids within the GI tract. Invariably there is a final and merciful fall in the blood pressure, or the development of a malignant arrhythmia which pulls the curtain on the tragic scene. Legislation to define brain death and to permit withdrawal of life support in such circumstances was long overdue. In our experience about 5–10 per cent of patients who survive cardiopulmonary resuscitation are left brain-dead.

(b) *Alteration in the state of consciousness* is a frequent sequel of cardiopulmonary resuscitation. This alteration may take the form of coma, a vegetative state, a 'locked in' state, or stupor. Coma is an unconscious state with absence of verbal communication, inability to respond to or to localise noxious stimuli, and an absence of spontaneous opening of the eyes. A vegetative state is similar to coma except that the patient opens his eyes spontaneously, and may appear to look around. A locked-in state is due to a brainstem lesion in which though there is no movement of the limbs, the patient is aware of his surroundings; he cannot speak but can communicate with his eyes. Stupor is a comparatively benign sequel in which the patient is arousable by a noxious stimulus; significant and at times complete recovery can ensue from this stage. Mental obtundation and amnesia for present as well as past events are often observed for 24–48 hours after successful resuscitation; here recovery is the rule.

(c) *Cortical blindness* is sometimes seen after recovery. This type of blindness is associated with an intact optic nerve and a normal retina. The condition usually improves over a period of time though full recovery may not occur. The longer it persists, the greater the likelihood of permanent impairment of vision.

(d) *Seizures* are an important sequel in the first 24 hours. In the worst form, they present as a status epilepticus, which may be impossible to control and which carry a grim prognosis of impending brain death. Epilepsy partialis continuosa is characterized by repetitive clonic movements of a limb. These often disappear as further recovery of the CNS ensues. Myoclonic jerks are irregular jerky movements which can be localized or generalized. Myoclonic jerks particularly when generalized, or involving the eyes and facial muscles, carry a grim prognosis and generally forecast impending brain death.

Anticonvulsant therapy as outlined in a later chapter should be given, but more often than not, is ineffective, particularly in status epilepticus or in generalized myoclonus. Seizures uncontrolled by the conventional use of dilantin, or by the use of diazepam in a continuous intravenous infusion, can at times be controlled by 500–1000 mg of thiopentone, given intravenously as a slow infusion over 24 hours.

Prognosis of Neurological Recovery Based on Clinical Examination

(a) Persistent coma in the first few hours after CPR does not necessarily denote prolonged or permanent neurological damage. However, coma persisting beyond 6 to 8 hours is associated with a poor prognosis. A study on 500 patients by Levy et al. (52) showed that if coma persisted for one day, only 10 per cent of patients showed good neurological recovery. The recovery rate was less than 5 per cent when coma persisted for a week; no patient recovered neurological function when coma persisted over two weeks. A Glasgow Coma Score of less than 5 on the third day of coma is also of ominous prognosis and almost always indicates a poor outcome or a permanent severe neurological deficit (53).

(b) Brain stem reflexes (doll's eye movements, response to cold water irrigation of the external auditory canal, pupillary and corneal reflexes) are often absent immediately after successful resuscitation. Their return within 1–2 hours is a good prognostic sign for possible recovery. The absence of pupillary or corneal reflexes at 6–24 hours after arrest carries a grim prognosis. Levy et al. (54) noted that not a single patient with absent pupillary or corneal reflexes 24 hours following CPR, was restored to a good quality of life.

The data given above is useful not only in predicting prognosis, but in identifying patients in whom critical care is likely to prove futile.

REFERENCES

1. Kuller LH, Lilienfeld A, Fisher R. (1967). An epidemiological study of sudden and unexpected deaths in adults. Medicine. 46,341.

2. Myerburg RJ, Castellanos A. (2001). Cardiac Arrest and Sudden Cardiac Death. In: Heart Disease—A Textbook of Cardiovascular Medicine (Eds Braunwald E, Zipes DP, Libby P). pp. 890–931. WB Saunders Company. Philadelphia, London, Toronto, Tokyo.

3. Eisenberg MS, Copass MK, Hallstrom AP et al. (1980). Treatment of out-of-hospital cardiac arrests with rapid defibrillation by emergency medical technicians. N Engl Med. 302,1379.

4. Cobb LA, Hallstrom AP. (1982). Community-based cardiopulmonary resuscitation: What have we learned? Ann N Y Acad Sci. 382,330.

5. Eisenberg MS, Bergner L, Hallstrom AP. (1979). Cardiac resuscitation in the community: Importance of rapid provision and implications of program planning. JAMA. 241,1905.

6. Ewy GA. (1984). Current status of cardiopulmonary resuscitation. Mod Concepts Cardiovasc Dis. 53,43.

7. Caldwell G, Miller G, Quinn E et al. (1985). Simple mechanical methods of cardioversion: A defense of the precordial thump and cough version. Brit Med J. 291,627.

8. Miller J, Trech D, Horwitz L et al. (1984). The precordial thump. Ann Emerg Med. 13,791.

9. Creed JD, Packard JM, Lambrew CT, Lewis AJ. (1983). Defibrillation and synchronized cardioversion. In: Textbook of Advanced Cardiac Life Support (Eds McIntyre KM, Lewis AJ). pp. 89–96. American Heart Association, Dallas.

10. American Heart Association, Advanced Cardiac Life Support (1997–1999). p. 1–15.

11. Heimlich HJ. (1975). A life-saving manoeuvre to prevent food-choking. JAMA. 234, 398.

12. Visintine RE, Baick CH. (1975). Ruptured stomach after Heimlich manoeuvre. JAMA. 234, 215.

13. American Heart Association, Advanced Cardiac Life Support (1997–1999) p. 1–12.

14. American Heart Association, Advanced Cardiac Life Support (1997–1999) p. 1–7.

15. American Heart Association, Advanced Cardiac Life Support (1997–1999) p. 16.

16. Advanced Life Support Working Party of the European Resuscitation Council (1992). Guidelines for advanced life support. Resuscitation 24:111–121.

17. American Heart Association, Advanced Cardiac Life Support (1997–1999) p. 1–18.

18. Bishop RL, Weisfeldt ML. (1976). Sodium bicarbonate administration during cardiac arrest: effect on arterial pH, PCO_2, and osmolality. JAMA. 235, 506.

19. Hindman BJ. (1990). Sodium bicarbonate in the treatment of subtypes of acute lactic acidosis: physiologic considerations. Anesthesiology 72:1064–1076.

20. Arieff AI. (1991) Indications for the use of bicarbonate in patients with metabolic acidosis. Br J Anesth. 67:165–177.

21. Ritter JM, Doktor HS, Benjamin N. (1990). Paradoxical effect of bicarbonate on cytoplasmic pH. Lancet 335:1243–1246.

22. Aitkenhead AR. (1991) Drug administration during CPR: what route? Resuscitation 22:191–195.

23. Emergency Cardiac Care Committee and Subcommittees, American Heart Association. (1992). Guidelines for cardio-pulmonary resuscitation and emergency cardiac care. JAMA. 268, 2171–2302.

24. Ewy GA. (1984). Defining electromechanical dissociation. Ann Emerg Med. 13:830–832.

25. Barryman CR. (1986). Electromechanical dissociation with a directly measurable arterial blood pressure. Ann Emerg Med. 15:625–626

26. Bocka JJ, Overton DT, Hauser A. (1988). Electromechanical dissociation in human beings: an echographic evaluation. Ann Emerg Med. 17:450–452.

27. Paradis NA, Mortin GB, Goetting MG, Rivers EP, Fungold M, Novak RM. (1992). Aortic pressure during human cardiac arrest: identification of pseudoelectromechanical dissociation. Chest 101:123–128.

28. Brown DC, Lewis AJ, Criley JM. (1979). Asystole and its treatment: the possible role of the parasympathetic nervous system in cardiac arrest. J Am Coll Emerg Phys. 8:448–452.

29. Vassale M. (1985). On the mechanisms underlying cardiac standstill and factors determining success or failure of escape pacemakers in the heart. J Am Coll Cardiology. 5:35B-42B.

30. Knowlton AA, Falk RH. (1986). External cardiac pacing during in-hospital cardiac arrest. Amer J Cardiol. 51,1295.

31. Holmes HR, Babbs CF, Voorhees WD et al. (1980). Influence of adrenergic drugs upon vital organ perfusion during CPR. Crit Care Med. 8, 137.

32. Wayne MA, Levine RL, Miller CC. (1995). Use of end-tidal to predict outcome in prehospital cardiac arrest. Ann Emerg Med. 25:762–767.

33. Marino PL. (1991). Cardiac Arrest. In: The ICU Book. p. 272. Lea and Febiger, Philadelphia, London.

34. Weil MH, Rackow EC, Trevino R. (1986). Difference in acid-base state between venous and arterial blood during cardiopulmonary resuscitation. N Engl J Med.315:153–156.

35. Steedman DJ, Robertson CE. (1992). Acid-base changes in arterial and central venous blood during cardiopulmonary resuscitation. Arch Emerg Med. 9:169–176.

36. Weil MH, Gazmuri RJ, Rackow EC. (1990). The clinical rationale of cardiac resuscitation. Dis Mon 36:423–468.

37. Barton CW, Manning JE. (1995). Cardiopulmonary resuscitation. Emerg Med Clin North Am. 13:811–830.

38. DeBehnke DJ, Swart GL. (1996). Cardiac arrest. Emerg Med Clin North Am 14:57–82.

39. Bruns FJ, Fraley DS, Haigh J et al. (1987). Control of organ blood flow. In: Oxygen transport in the critically ill (Eds Snyder JV, Pinsky MR). pp. 87–124. Year Book Medical Publishers, Chicago.

40. Koehler RC, Michael JR. (1985). Cardiopulmonary resuscitation, brain blood flow and neurologic recovery. Crit Care Clin. 1, 205–222.

41. Kirsch JR, Dean JM, Rogers MC. (1986). Current concepts in brain resuscitation. Arch Intern Med. 146, 1413–1419.

42. E Roland, H Binns.(2004). Resuscitation. In: Recent Advances In Anaesthesia And Intensive Care 1st Edition (Ed: AP Adams, JN Cashman, RM Grounds). pp. 279–283. Jaypee Ltd., N. Delhi.

43. Sack JB, Kesselbrenner MB, Jarrad A. (1992). Interposed abdominal compression cardiopulmonary resuscitation and resuscitation outcome during asystole and electromechanical dissociation. Circulation; 86: 1692–1700.

44. Wenzel V, Lindner KH, Prengel AW et al. (2000). Effect of phased chest and abdominal compression-decompression cardiopulmonary resuscitation on myocardial and cerebral flow in pigs. Crit Care Med; 28: 1107–1112.

45. Abramson NS, Safar P, Detre KM et al. (1985). Neurological recovery after cardiac arrest: effect of duration of ischaemia. Crit Care Med 13:930–931.

46. McNamara JJ, Suehiro GT, Suehiro A, Jewett B. (1983). Resuscitation from haemorrhagic shock. J Trauma. 23, 552–558.

47. White BC, Winegar CD, Wilson RF, Krause GS. (1983). Calcium blockers in cerebral resuscitation. J Trauma. 23, 788–794.

48. Babbs F. (1988). Reperfusion injury of postischemic tissues. Ann Emerg Med. 17, 1148–1157.

49. Yatsu FM, McKenzie JD, Lockwood AH. (1987). Cardiopulmonary arrest and intravenous glucose. (Editorial.) J Crit Care. 2, 1–3.

50. Rees AP, Valentino VA, Genton E. (1991). Pharmacological adjuncts to cardiopulmonary resuscitation. Intern Med 12:22–35.

51. White BC, Winegar CD, Wilson RF et al. (1983). Possible role of calcium blockers in cerebral resuscitation: A review of the literature and synthesis for future studies. Crit Care Med. 11, 202–207.

52. Levy DE, Bates D, Caronna JJ et al. (1981).Prognosis in nontraumatic coma. Ann Int Med. 94, 293–301.

53. Edgren E, Hedstrand U, Kelsey S et al. (1994). Assessment of neurological prognosis in comatose survivors of cardiac arrest. Lancet 343:1055–1059.

54. Levy DE, Caronna JJ, Singer BH et al. (1985). Predicting outcome from hypoxia-ischemic coma. JAMA. 253, 1420–1426.

SECTION 3

Basic Cardiorespiratory Physiology in the Intensive Care Unit

Basic Cardiorespiratory Physiology in the Intensive Care Unit

All important organs and organ systems in the human body are interrelated and interdependent. This interrelation and interdependence is most marked and evident between the heart and circulation on the one hand, and the lungs on the other. The heart (circulatory system) and the lungs (respiratory system) form a single inseparable unit whose purpose is to supply oxygen to the tissues, and to remove carbon dioxide produced during tissue metabolism.

In any and every critical illness, adequate oxygen delivery or oxygen transport to tissues is crucial for proper function of different organ systems, and for survival. Oxygen delivery is controlled by, and is dependent on the cardiorespiratory system as a whole. Poor function or failure of this system is a common theme in numerous critical illnesses in the ICU. Cardiorespiratory failure invariably heralds a decline in the clinical state of a critically ill individual. Cardiac failure has repercussions on pulmonary function and gas exchange. Respiratory failure sooner or later worsens cardiac function. A vicious spiral of deteriorating cardiorespiratory function spells death in any critical illness. It is therefore important for the intensivist to be aware of basic cardiopulmonary functions and the factors which affect these functions, particularly in relation to critical care medicine.

This chapter briefly describes factors regulating cardiac function. It then very briefly outlines basic concepts of gas exchange within the lungs, which relate to the assessment and care of critically ill patients. It then goes on to stress the importance of oxygen content of blood, oxygen transport, and the interrelationship, as illustrated by the Fick principle, between oxygen consumption, oxygen transport, and tissue needs for oxygen.

Factors Regulating Cardiac Output

The regulation of the cardiac output ($\dot{Q}_T$) is complex, particularly in critically ill individuals, and is dependent on tissue factors, neurohormonal factors, and on intrinsic cardiac mechanisms.

Tissue Factors

The cardiac output ($\dot{Q}_T$) is basically governed by the tissue needs for oxygen and nutrients. Each organ has a built-in autoregulation of blood flow through arteriolar dilatation and vasoconstriction.

The mechanism of this autoregulation is incompletely understood. It is related to local release of vasodilator substances and other locally operating vasoregulatory mechanisms.

Neurohormonal Influences

Neurohormonal factors also play a crucial role in regulating cardiac output. Increased sympathetic activity is very important for increased cardiac output in stressed states. Neural and hormonal influences mediate compensatory mechanisms in a patient in acute circulatory failure. These neurohormonal compensatory mechanisms are life-saving as they override local autoregulatory tissue mechanisms, reduce flow to the skin, muscles and the splanchnic circulation, and maintain an adequate flow to the brain, heart and other vital organs during shock.

Intrinsic Cardiac Mechanisms

The heart has a significant reserve which enables it to increase its cardiac output whenever necessary. This reserve may be impaired or totally absent in patients with cardiac disease. Increase in cardiac output can be brought about by an increase in the heart rate and in the stroke volume. The stroke volume is governed by the following factors:

(i) Preload or the end-diastolic fibre length, or the end-diastolic ventricular volume (Frank Starling's law).

(ii) Contractility or the force of myocardial contraction, as determined by inherent contractile properties of the myocardium, and by neurohormonal influences.

(iii) Afterload which is the degree of wall tension developed during ventricular ejection.

(i) Preload

This is the degree of stretch of myocardial fibres at end-diastole, just prior to myocardial contraction. The Frank Starling law states, 'the energy of contraction however measured, is a function of the length of the muscle fibres' (1, 2). The greater the stretch of muscle fibres within physiological limits, the stronger the force of contraction. The resting length of myocardial fibres is related to end-diastolic ventricular volume. Thus increased venous return increases the stretch of muscle fibres, increases the diastolic volume, and is translated into an increased cardiac output. The heart can therefore vary stroke volume and $\dot{Q}_T$ in response to changes in venous return and tissue needs. The Frank Starling mechanism is an intrinsic property of muscle, and is independent of neural and hormonal factors. The normal heart can handle an increase in venous return to 2–3 times normal, even if denervated (3). When a further increase in $\dot{Q}_T$ becomes necessary, neurohormonal factors must come into play.

Venous return by its influence on the preload, is one of the most important factors governing cardiac output. Venous return is governed by several factors. An important factor is the difference between the mean systemic pressure and the right atrial pressure. The mean systemic pressure is the volume weighted average pressure in the entire circulation—arteries, capillaries and veins, and is chiefly determined by the total blood volume and the tone of the vessels. It averages about 7 mm Hg. The greater the difference between the mean systemic pressure and the right atrial pressure, the greater the venous return. The relationship between the mean systemic pressure and the right atrial pressure is illustrated in graphic form by Guyton (4) (**Fig. 3.1.1**). An increase in right atrial pressure without a corresponding increase in the mean systemic pressure sharply reduces venous return. Venous return stops when right atrial pressure equals mean systemic pressure. This is exactly the circulatory disturbance underlying cardiac tamponade.

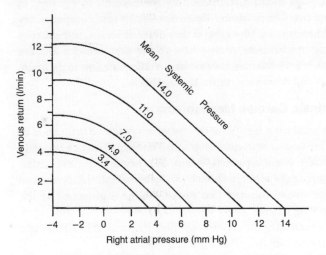

Fig. 3.1.1. Effects of mean systemic pressure and right atrial pressure on venous return to the right heart. The greater the difference between the mean systemic pressure and the right atrial pressure, the greater the venous return. Increase in right atrial pressure without a corresponding increase in the mean systemic pressure causes a sharp fall in venous return. (Adapted from Guyton AC, et al. 1973. Circulatory Physiology, Cardiac Output, and its Regulation. W B Saunders, PA, by Clemmer TP, 1988. Cardiopulmonary Critical Care Management, Elsevier, Inc.)

The veins are far more distensible than the arteries, so that a small increase in venous tone results in a large volume of blood being returned to the heart. Similarly a decrease in venous tone leads to pooling of blood in the peripheries, with a decrease in the volume of blood returned to the heart. Thus *venous pressure constitutes a very large portion of the mean systemic pressure, and is the most important factor in determining venous return. Venous pressure*

in turn is largely dependent on volume of blood within the veins, and on venous tone.

Measurement of Preload and its Significance in Critical Care Medicine. It is difficult to measure end-diastolic volume in critically ill patients in the ICU. The next best option is to measure end-diastolic pressure or the filling pressure of the ventricle, as an indirect measure of the preload. The higher the filling pressure within physiological limits, the greater the preload and the greater the force of ventricular contraction. The upper normal limit of the left ventricular end-diastolic pressure is 15–17 mm Hg. Cardiac output can be augmented in critically ill patients by increasing the left ventricular filling pressure to an optimum of 15–17 mm Hg, and in some instances to even 20 mm Hg. A further increase in the filling pressure will not increase cardiac output, but will lead to an increase in "backward pressure" and pulmonary oedema. In a critically ill patient, a high left ventricular filling pressure (measured clinically as the pulmonary capillary wedge pressure) is usually either related to myocardial dysfunction, or to fluid overload.

Can one equate left ventricular end-diastolic pressure (LVEDP) to left ventricular end-diastolic volume (LVEDV)? The relation between LVEDP and LVEDV is dependent on the following:

(a) The venous return and volume of blood distending the left ventricle at end-diastole;

(b) The compliance or degree of 'stiffness' or distensibility of the ventricle;

(c) The transmural pressure i.e. the pressure surrounding the ventricle;

(d) The volume of the right ventricle, which shares a common wall (the septum) with the left ventricle, and a common limiting pericardial sac.

Venous pressure and its relation to venous return has already been briefly discussed earlier. It is a major factor influencing both ventricular end-diastolic filling pressure and end-diastolic volume.

Compliance of the Ventricle. Altered compliance or distensibility is also important in determining fibre length. Compliance can be regarded as the change in end-diastolic volume (Δ EDV) in relation to change in end-diastolic pressure (Δ EDP).

$$\text{Compliance} = \Delta\, EDV\, /\, \Delta\, EDP$$

A fall in compliance (i.e. a decrease in diastolic distensibility), will lead to a rise in end-diastolic pressure for any given diastolic volume. If a ventricular function curve of stroke volume against end-diastolic filling pressure is plotted, the stroke volume will fall for the same filling pressure, if the compliance is reduced. When ventricular compliance is markedly reduced (stiff, very poor distensibility), two effects follow: (a) the stroke volume is sharply reduced because the ventricular end-diastolic volume is reduced; (b) the high left ventricular end-diastolic pressure needed to distend the stiff ventricle leads to pulmonary congestion and oedema. The decrease in stroke output that accompanies a decrease in ventricular compliance is termed diastolic dysfunction or diastolic heart failure, as it is independent of any change in the systolic function (i.e. contractility) of the ventricle. In clinical medicine it is important that a fall in stroke volume due to decreased compliance (poor distensibility) is not wrongly attributed to a reduction in contractility.

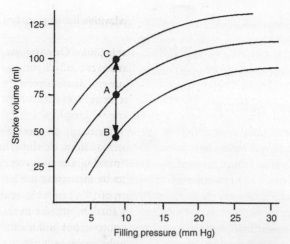

Fig. 3.1.2. Ventricular function curve showing effect of ventricular compliance on stroke volume and end-diastolic filling pressures. It should be noted that a reduction in ventricular compliance causes a fall in the stroke volume (A → B), without any change in the filling pressure. Similarly, an increase in ventricular compliance results in an increased stroke volume (A → C) for the same filling pressure.

In a similar fashion, a decrease in ventricular compliance would lead to an increase in end-diastolic volume, and to an increased stroke volume for the same filling pressure (**Fig. 3.1.2**).

Ventricular compliance does alter in critical illnesses. Compliance is reduced for example, in ischaemia to the ventricle, in haemorrhagic and septic shock, and following the use of inotropic drugs like dopamine, epinephrine, and isoproterenol (**5**). Compliance on the other hand is increased after relief of ischemia, in cardiac dilatation, and after drugs such as nitroglycerin and nitroprusside (**6–8**).

Transmural Pressure. Transmural pressure also influences the pressure-volume relationships in the ventricle. This is illustrated in **Fig. 3.1.3**. The intrapleural pressure has risen from –2 to +4 mm Hg; the intraventricular pressure (P) has increased to the same extent (from 10 to 16 mm Hg). The transmural pressure gradient remains the same, and therefore the intraventricular volume (v)

is unchanged. If however; the rise in intrapleural pressure (pressure surrounding the heart) is not associated with a corresponding rise in intraventricular pressure, the transmural pressure gradient is reduced, and the intraventricular pressure falls. The measured stroke volume is thus the same with a higher LVEDP. This could be wrongly interpreted as a fall in contractility, or to a decreased compliance, when in point of fact it is related to an increase in the intrapericardial or intrapleural pressure. The former can result from pericardial effusion, and the latter may occur in patients on ventilatory support, particularly when positive end-expiratory pressure (PEEP) is being used.

Volume of the Right Ventricle. Acute dilatation of the right ventricle can shift the interventricular septum towards the left ventricular cavity, reducing left ventricular end-diastolic volume without any apparent change in left ventricular end-diastolic pressure. This has been observed to occur following a sharp increase in pulmonary vascular resistance due to pulmonary embolism, in acute respiratory failure, and with use of high levels of PEEP. Acute right ventricular dilatation may thus reduce left ventricular filling and cardiac output.

In summary, the left ventricular filling pressure (the pulmonary capillary wedge pressure as measured through a Swan-Ganz catheter) is a good index of the preload. However when interpreting pressure readings, or when manipulating filling pressures through volume infusions, the influence of the compliance of the ventricle, as also of the intrapleural and intrapericardial pressures should be given due consideration. Septal shifts due to acute right ventricular dilatation may also compromise left ventricular end-diastolic volume, and interfere with left ventricular filling, for reasons stated above.

(ii) Contractility

Stroke volume can be increased not only by augmenting preload, but also by increasing contractility. This is accomplished by the use of inotropes which increase both isometric force, and the velocity of isotonic muscle shortening at all loads. Neurohormonal mechanisms within the body, by stimulating beta-1 agonist

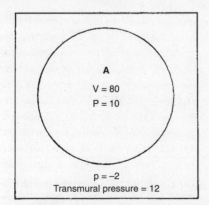

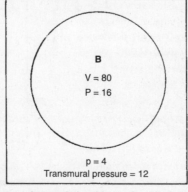

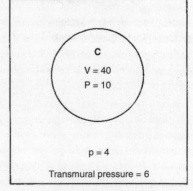

Fig. 3.1.3. Influence of transmural pressure on pressure-volume relationships in the ventricle. In **B**, as compared to **A**, the intrapleural pressure (p) has risen from – 2 to + 4 mm Hg, and the intraventricular pressure (P) has increased to the same extent (from 10 to 16 mm Hg). The transmural pressure gradient remains the same, and therefore the intraventricular volume (V) is unchanged. If however, as in **C**, the rise in intrapleural pressure (pressure surrounding the heart) is not associated with a corresponding rise in intraventricular pressure, the transmural pressure gradient is reduced, and the intraventricular volume falls (modified from Clemmer TP, 1988, as in Fig. 3.1.1.).

receptors in the ventricles, also increase contractility with improved emptying of the ventricles, for any given diastolic length.

(iii) Afterload

This is an important factor governing stroke volume. Afterload is the ventricular wall tension generated during systolic ejection of blood from the ventricles. The aortic pressure is an important determinant of left ventricular afterload. Increasing the afterload moderately in a normal heart, causes a slight fall in the ejection fraction. This results in a compensatory increase in fibre length and diastolic volume, with stronger contraction and an improved ejection fraction. On the other hand, an increased afterload in a diseased heart which has poor contractility, can be disastrous. It results in a profound fall in the ejection fraction, and in the forward flow from the heart.

The relationship of a changing afterload to a failing heart is more clearly illustrated by the application of Laplace's law,

$$T = \frac{Pr}{2h}$$

where T is the wall tension (afterload). T is not only directly related to the intracavitary pressure (P), but also directly related to the radius of the chamber (r), and inversely to (h), the thickness of the ventricular wall. Thus T (wall tension, or afterload) increases with the increased radius of a dilated heart. It is reduced with hypertrophy or increased thickness of the ventricular wall.

Influence of Pleural Pressure on Afterload

Negative intrapleural pressures increase transmural pressure and increase ventricular afterload. Negative pressure surrounding the heart acts by impeding the inward movement of the ventricular wall during systole (9). This is responsible for a reduced cardiac output and reduced systolic blood pressure during the inspiratory phase of spontaneous breathing. When the fall in inspiratory-related pressure during systole is > 15 mm Hg it is termed pulsus paradoxus. There is nothing paradoxical about this observation as it is merely an exaggeration of a normal response.

Positive intrapleural pressure can reduce the afterload, by promoting the inward movement of the ventricular wall during systole, thereby facilitating ventricular emptying. It is likely that the beneficial effects of closed chest massage performed during cardiac resuscitation are related to sharp swings in positive pleural pressure which exert a massage-like action and propel blood outwards from the heart into the systemic circulation.

It is to be however noted that the reduction in afterload effect produced by a positive intrapleural pressure during the inspiratory phase of positive pressure ventilation is negated by the obstruction to venous return caused by the inspiratory rise in intrapleural pressure. In fact the sum effect is a decreased inspiratory cardiac output because of decreased venous return (see Chapter on Mechanical Ventilator in the Critically Ill).

Cardiac Rate and Rhythm

The rate is also important in determining cardiac output. A rate > 100/min adversely affects cardiac output, and a marked

bradyrhythm acts likewise. Loss of atrial kick may sharply reduce cardiac output in patients with a poor cardiac reserve. Rhythm disturbances even in a normal heart can reduce output; they can be catastrophic in diseased hearts.

Heart Failure

This has been dealt with at length in subsequent chapters of the book. A few basic concepts need to be stressed at this juncture.

Cardiac failure, in brief, is a failure of the pumping action of the heart. Left ventricular failure leads to two recognizable features:

(a) Pulmonary oedema, with or without systemic venous congestion. Pulmonary oedema is associated with an increase in end-diastolic left ventricular pressure to > 15 mm Hg, and often as high as 30 mm Hg.

(b) Poor forward flow resulting in poor tissue perfusion.

Cardiac failure may produce pulmonary oedema, or poor forward flow, or both. It is important to consider these two aspects of cardiac failure as separate facets, even when both are present at the same time. Death from acute cardiac failure can be due to a severe fall in cardiac output, forward flow and tissue perfusion, without pulmonary oedema. This can only be appreciated if the inter-relation between left and right ventricular function curves is clearly understood (10), and if both ventricles are considered as an interlocked single functioning unit.

An explanation of the two above-stated facets of acute cardiac failure has been given in the chapter on Cardiogenic Shock.

A final thought provoking statement that needs to be made, is that the presence of increased filling pressures with pulmonary

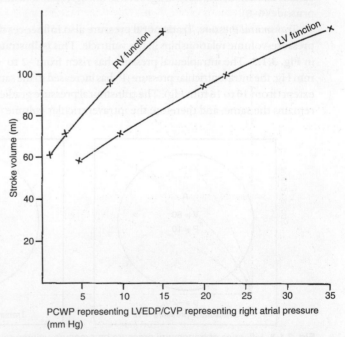

Fig. 3.1.4. Left and right ventricular function curves in an overinfused hypervolaemic patient. Note that very high left and right ventricular filling pressures that cause pulmonary oedema and systemic venous congestion, can occur in the presence of good pump function with high stroke volumes and cardiac output.

oedema and systemic venous congestion, does not necessarily mean failure of the heart as a pump. This situation (increased filling pressures with pulmonary oedema and systemic venous congestion), can also arise in an over-transfused or over-infused hypervolaemic patient. Measurements of cardiac output in such a patient show high stroke volume and cardiac output readings (in accordance with Frank Starling's principle), pointing to good pump function. This is illustrated in **Fig. 3.1.4**.

Left ventricular function curves in moderate and severe left ventricular failure are illustrated by plotting stroke volume against LVEDP, and stroke volume against increasing afterload (**Figs. 3.1.5 and 3.1.6**).

The description of the applied physiology of the circulatory system given above has been chiefly related to the heart and its function. There are other components to the circulatory system that need to be considered (**11**). These components include the following:

(i) Intravascular volume which regulates mean circulatory pressure and venous return.

(ii) The arteriolar bed, the tone of which chiefly determines afterload, arterial blood pressure and distribution of systemic blood flow. A marked fall in arteriolar tone causes severe hypotension. A marked rise impedes left ventricular ejection and tissue perfusion.

(iii) The capillary network where fluid and nutrient exchange between the intravascular and extravascular compartment occurs. Damage to capillary endothelium results in increased capillary permeability with loss of intravascular volume and tissue oedema.

(iv) The venules which are responsible for 10–15 per cent of the vascular resistance.

(v) Arteriovenous connections. Opening of these connections allows blood to bypass the capillaries and produces tissue hypoxia.

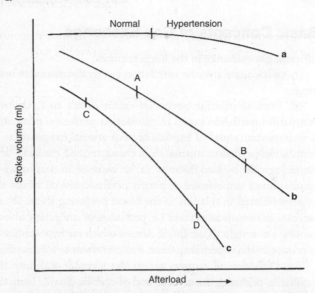

Fig. 3.1.6. Relationship of stroke volume to afterload in subjects with normal myocardial function (**a**), and in patients with moderate (**b**) and severe (**c**) myocardial dysfunction. In subjects with normal myocardial function, increase in afterload results in hypertension without much change in the stroke volume (SV) or cardiac output (CO). In contrast, in patients with moderate or severe myocardial dysfunction, an increase in afterload produces a sharp fall in the SV and CO, the SV being inversely proportional to the afterload or outflow resistance. It is important to note that the blood pressure may remain constant at points A and B on curve **b**, and points C and D on curve **c**, even though the SV is sharply reduced.

(vi) Venous capacitance which contains 80 per cent of the intravascular volume. Decrease in venous tone or increase in venous capacitance reduces mean circulating pressures, filling pressures within the heart, and effective circulating volume. Increase in venous tone or decrease in venous capacitance has exactly the contrary effects—an increase in the venous pressure and an increase in the filling pressures of the heart.

(vii) Viscosity of blood. Blood viscosity is chiefly due to circulating erythrocytes (haematocrit). Increase in the haematocrit means increased viscosity, entailing greater work for the heart to move blood through the circulatory system. This increase in work load may have significant clinical implications in patients with ischaemic heart disease or in patients with poor myocardial reserve.

Viscosity of blood increases following a loss of plasma or fluid from the vascular system. Blood viscosity also increases following repeated packed cell transfusions, a fall in body temperature, and a decrease in the flow rate of blood. This rise in viscosity can further reduce flow through the circulation and thereby promote ischaemic injury. Prevention of an undue rise in viscosity is therefore of particular importance in critically ill patients. The degree of viscosity is best gauged by monitoring haematocrit values which should not exceed 40–45 per cent as the upper limit.

Finally the right heart which pumps into the low resistance, low pressure pulmonary circuit, is intrinsically and inevitably locked to the left heart which pumps into the high resistance, high pressure systemic circuit. It is a closed system, and by sheer necessity the stroke volume pumped by the two sides of the heart must be equal.

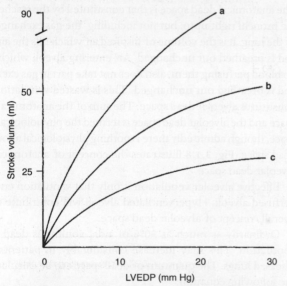

Fig. 3.1.5. Relationship of stroke volume to LVEDP in subjects with normal myocardial function (**a**), and in patients with moderate (**b**) and severe (**c**) left ventricular dysfunction. Note that in patients with myocardial dysfunction, a rising LVEDP produces a smaller degree of rise in the stroke volume, as compared to normal subjects.

Basic Concepts of Gas Exchange

Efficient gas exchange in the lungs requires:

(i) An adequate alveolar ventilation evenly distributed to both lungs.

(ii) Even ventilation-perfusion ratios of 0.8 to 1. Uneven ventilation-perfusion ratios or ventilation-perfusion mismatch is an important cause of hypoxia or poor arterial oxygenation. A ventilation-perfusion mismatch is characterized clinically and physiologically by two features: (a) an increase in dead space—ventilation of unperfused or poorly perfused alveoli which are hyperventilated in relation to the blood perfusing them; (b) an increase in venous admixture i.e. perfusion of atelectatic alveoli causing a true right to left shunt. Alveoli which are hypoventilated in relation to blood perfusing them, also contribute to a shunt effect.

(iii) Diffusion of oxygen across the alveolar wall into the capillaries perfusing the alveoli, and of carbon dioxide from the capillaries out into the alveolar space. A severe diffusion defect may contribute to a low PaO_2 but is hardly ever its sole cause. Most pathologies producing a diffusion defect also lead to an uneven compliance within the lungs and thereby to a ventilation-perfusion mismatch.

Alveolar Ventilation

The pressure of CO_2 in arterial blood ($PaCO_2$) is the best indicator of alveolar ventilation. This basic fact in respiratory physiology is explained below. Consider for purposes of illustration an alveolus of volume $\dot{V}_A$ (**Fig. 3.1.7**). It contains a volume of $CO_2 - \dot{V}CO_2$. The fractional concentration of CO_2 ($FACO_2$) in this alveolus is given by the volume of CO_2 divided by the volume of the alveolus.

$$FACO_2 = \frac{\dot{V}CO_2}{\dot{V}_A}$$

The CO_2 released into the alveolus from the blood perfusing it, will be cleared from the alveolus by ventilation; the greater the ventilation the lower the concentration of CO_2 in the alveolus. The alveolar concentration will be a balance between the alveolar ventilation and the rate at which the CO_2 is evolved ($\dot{V}CO_2$).

$$FACO_2 = \frac{\dot{V}CO_2}{\dot{V}_A}$$

The fractional concentration of CO_2, $FACO_2$ (0.05–0.06), exerts a pressure equal to the same fraction of the barometric pressure (PB).

$$\frac{PACO_2}{PB} = \frac{\dot{V}CO_2}{\dot{V}_A}$$

$$PACO_2 = \frac{\dot{V}CO_2}{\dot{V}_A} \times 0.863$$

0.863 is the correction factor that takes into account the barometric pressure and the different units in which $\dot{V}CO_2$ and $\dot{V}_A$ are expressed. This is the alveolar ventilation equation. It shows that the $PACO_2$ is directly proportional to the CO_2 produced, and

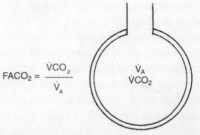

$$FACO_2 = \frac{\dot{V}CO_2}{\dot{V}_A} \qquad \dot{V}_A \quad \dot{V}CO_2$$

Fig. 3.1.7. Concept of alveolar ventilation.

inversely proportional to alveolar ventilation ($\dot{V}_A$). If $\dot{V}CO_2$ is constant, then $PACO_2$ is inversely proportional to $\dot{V}A$.

$$PACO_2 \; \alpha \; \frac{1}{\dot{V}_A}$$

There is good evidence to show that $PaCO_2$ is very close to the average alveolar PCO_2 i.e. $PACO_2$. Thus

$$PACO_2 = PaCO_2 = \frac{\dot{V}CO_2}{\dot{V}_A} \times 0.863$$

The $PaCO_2$ is thus inversely related to $\dot{V}_A$. A high $PaCO_2$ (> 48 mm Hg) denotes hypoventilation; a low $PaCO_2$ (< 35 mm Hg) denotes hyperventilation; a normal $PaCO_2$ (35–45 mm Hg) denotes normal alveolar ventilation. It should be evident from the above equation that if the normal $PaCO_2$ of 40 mm Hg is doubled to 80 mm Hg, it means that the alveolar ventilation is just half of what is normally necessary to deal with the CO_2 produced by the body. It is to be also noted that the $PaCO_2$ may rise if the $\dot{V}CO_2$ rises and if the patient for some reason cannot increase his alveolar ventilation to get rid of the extra CO_2.

Concept of Dead Space

The anatomical dead space is that constituted by the trachea and the bronchi right upto, but not including, the gas exchange unit of the lung. It is the volume of inspired air which fills the airways and is breathed out unchanged. Air entering alveoli which have no blood perfusing them, also does not take part in gas exchange and is breathed out unchanged. This is wasted ventilation and constitutes alveolar dead space. The sum of the anatomical dead space and the alveolar dead space is termed the physiological dead space, though admittedly there is nothing physiological about this dead space. **Fig. 3.1.8** illustrates the concept of anatomical and alveolar dead space.

Effective alveolar ventilation is only that ventilation entering perfused alveoli. Hyperventilated alveoli will contribute to the overall concept of alveolar dead space.

Ordinarily as much as 30% of tidal volume is dead space ventilation. This may increase considerably in patients with diseased lungs. The quantum of dead space can be calculated by the following equation:

$$\frac{V_D}{V_T} = \frac{PaCO_2 - P_{\bar{E}}CO_2}{PaCO_2}$$

where $P_{\bar{E}}CO_2$ is the pressure of CO_2 in expired gas.

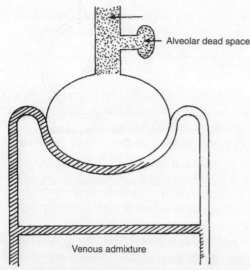

Fig. 3.1.8. Concept of anatomical and alveolar dead space and venous admixture (right to left shunt within the lungs). (From Udwadia FE. 1979. Diagnosis and Management of Acute Respiratory Failure. OUP, Mumbai.)

Alveolar Oxygen

Fresh oxygen from inspired gas enters alveoli during ventilation; the oxygen diffuses through the alveolar wall into the blood perfusing the alveoli. For any given concentration of oxygen in inspired gas (FIO_2), the alveolar concentration of oxygen (FAO_2) will be a balance between alveolar ventilation ($\dot{V}_A$) and the oxygen taken up ($\dot{V}O_2$) by the blood perfusing ventilated alveoli.

$$FIO_2 - FAO_2 = \frac{\dot{V}O_2}{\dot{V}_A}$$

In terms of partial pressure,

$$PIO_2 - PAO_2 = \frac{\dot{V}O_2}{\dot{V}_A} \times 0.863$$

We have already defined $\dot{V}_A$ (under Alveolar Ventilation) in terms of $PaCO_2$.

$$PAO_2 = PIO_2 - PaCO_2 \times \frac{\dot{V}O_2}{\dot{V}CO_2} \times 0.863$$

The ratio $\dot{V}O_2/\dot{V}CO_2$ is in fact the respiratory exchange ratio R, and R in a steady state equals the metabolic respiratory quotient. Thus

$$PAO_2 = PIO_2 - PaCO_2 \times \frac{1}{R}$$

If carbohydrates are preponderantly burnt as fuel, R = 1; if fats are burnt as fuel R = 0.7; if carbohydrates and fats are both burnt as fuel, as is usually the case, R = 0.8.

The above equation is a simplified form of the alveolar air equation. It is of great use because:

(a) It allows a quick determination of alveolar oxygen pressure (PAO_2) if the PIO_2 and the $PaCO_2$ are known.

(b) If the PAO_2 is known and the PaO_2 is available through an arterial blood gas measurement, the alveolar-arterial oxygen gradient can be calculated as the difference between PAO_2 and

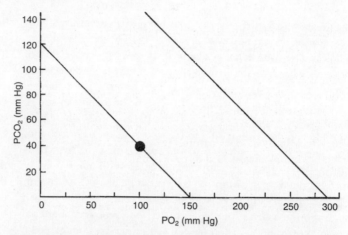

Fig. 3.1.9. O_2–CO_2 diagram. The slope of the line depends on the RQ (normally 0.8). For any given PCO_2 the alveolar PO_2 can be read, and for any given PO_2 the PCO_2 can be read. The line to the left illustrates the PO_2–PCO_2 relationship in alveoli when breathing air ($PIO_2 = 149$ mm Hg). The circle marked on this line shows the normal alveolar PO_2 and PCO_2 when breathing air (RQ = 0.8). The line to the right illustrates the PO_2–PCO_2 relationship with an RQ of 0.8 when breathing 40% oxygen ($PIO_2 = 285$ mm Hg). (From Udwadia FE. 1979. Diagnosis and Management of Acute Respiratory Failure. OUP, Mumbai.)

PaO_2. The upper normal of this gradient is 15 to at most 20 mm Hg. In most normal individuals it averages 10 mm Hg.

(c) The alveolar equation points to a linear relationship between PAO_2 and $PaCO_2$. The O_2–CO_2 diagram or line is further elaborated upon in the chapter on Acute Respiratory Failure in Adults (**Fig. 3.1.9**). From this diagram one can quickly plot the expected PAO_2 if the $PaCO_2$ is known for any given inspired oxygen concentration. If the alveolar arterial oxygen gradient is taken as 10–15 mm Hg, then for any given $PaCO_2$ one can read off the PaO_2. This is true provided the alveolar-arterial oxygen gradient is not abnormally increased.

(d) A consideration of the alveolar air equation shows that at a given inspired oxygen concentration and a given respiratory quotient, the alveolar PO_2 is dependent on alveolar ventilation. A lower alveolar ventilation would thus lead to a lowered alveolar PO_2, and hence a lowered arterial PO_2.

(e) The alveolar air equation helps the physician to check on blood gas measurements. If the value of the measured $PaCO_2$ is taken as correct, the alveolar equation allows one to compute the PAO_2. If the PaO_2 reported by the laboratory is higher than the PAO_2, it is obviously incorrect.

The Alveolar-Arterial Oxygen Gradient

The normal range of the alveolar-arterial oxygen gradient has already been mentioned. An increased alveolar-arterial oxygen gradient denotes an impairment of gas exchange across the alveolar capillary membrane. When however a low PaO_2 is due to hypoventilation, or is related to breathing at high altitudes, then there is no increase in the alveolar-arterial oxygen gradient since the PAO_2 is also proportionately low. A lowered PaO_2 from any other cause ($\dot{V}/\dot{Q}$ mismatch, increased shunt, impaired diffusion), is always associated with an increased alveolar-arterial oxygen gradient. Also the greater the alveolar-arterial oxygen gradient, the greater the disturbance in gas exchange within the lungs. This observation should however be viewed in its proper perspective. Thus an alveolar-arterial gradient of 20 mm Hg (upper limit of normal), when it occurs on the steep part of the oxygen dissociation curve will denote a gross disturbance in pulmonary gas exchange.

Let us consider a patient with chronic bronchitis in severe hypercapnic respiratory failure. If the PAO_2 of this patient is 50 mm Hg and the PaO_2 is 30 mm Hg, the gradient of just 20 mm Hg (upper limit of normal) would suggest that the hypoxia is chiefly due to alveolar hypoventilation. However at a PO_2 of 50 mm Hg the oxygen saturation is 85 per cent; at a PO_2 of 30 mm Hg the oxygen saturation is about 55 per cent. Thus the oxygen saturation has fallen 30 per cent between the alveoli and the arterial blood. Normally the fall in oxygen saturation does not exceed 2 per cent. It is evident that there is a serious disturbance in gas exchange in this patient, even though the alveolar-arterial oxygen gradient is not unduly increased.

Venous Admixture (Fig. 3.1.10)

If unoxygenated blood perfuses atelectatic alveoli and bypasses ventilated alveoli, the oxygen content of the blood leaving the lungs will be less than that leaving ventilated alveoli. This constitutes the concept of venous admixture. Venous admixture at the bedside has two components—a true right to left shunt due to perfusion of totally atelectatic alveoli, and a shunt effect observed in alveoli which are hypoventilated in relation to blood perfusing them i.e. alveoli with low ventilation-perfusion ratios. A true right to left shunt (also called a true venous admixture) is unchanged by increasing inspired concentration of oxygen. The shunt effect produced by alveoli with lowered ventilation-perfusion ratios will however be abolished by suitably increasing the inspired oxygen concentration. The simple bedside test of noting the degree of rise in PaO_2 with 100 per cent inspired oxygen, thus distinguishes between a true right to left shunt within the lungs, and a shunt effect produced by ventilation-perfusion inequalities. More often than not, a right to left shunt as also ventilation-perfusion inequalities are present in the same patient. This is further elaborated upon in the Chapter on Acute

Respiratory Failure. The mathematical calculation of the venous admixture or shunt is given by the following equation:

$$\frac{\dot{Q}_S}{\dot{Q}_T} = \frac{CcO_2 - CaO_2}{CcO_2 - C\bar{v}O_2}$$

Where $\dot{Q}_S$ is the shunt fraction, $\dot{Q}_T$ the cardiac output, CcO_2 the capillary oxygen content, CaO_2 the arterial oxygen content and $C\bar{v}O_2$ the mixed venous oxygen content.

In practice, end-capillary oxygen content is calculated from the alveolar PO_2 by assuming that PAO_2 is equal to end-capillary PO_2. Arterial oxygen content is either derived from the PaO_2, or estimated by an oximeter. Mixed venous oxygen content is obtained by sampling blood from the pulmonary artery through a Swan-Ganz catheter.

The normal $\dot{Q}_S / \dot{Q}_T$ is generally not more than 5 per cent. A shunt fraction exceeding 30 per cent is serious, and a shunt fraction approaching 50 per cent indicates a gross degree of venous admixture, and carries a grim prognosis.

Concept of Oxygen Content and Oxygen Transport

The heart lung combine working in unison ensures oxygenation of arterial blood. But this is not enough. Blood should have an adequate oxygen content, and what is more the oxygen within the blood should be efficiently delivered or transported to tissue cells all over the body. This principle should never be lost sight of in the management of critically ill patients in the ICU.

Oxygen Content

1 g of haemoglobin combines with 1.39 ml of oxygen at full saturation.

$$O_2 \text{ Content} = 1.39 \times Hb \times \frac{\% \text{ saturation}}{100} + 0.003 \times PO_2$$

where the solubility coefficient of oxygen at 37°C is 0.003 ml/100 ml blood/mm Hg.

The per cent saturation of Hb in arterial blood is related to the PaO_2. Oxygen content thus depends on Hb concentration and

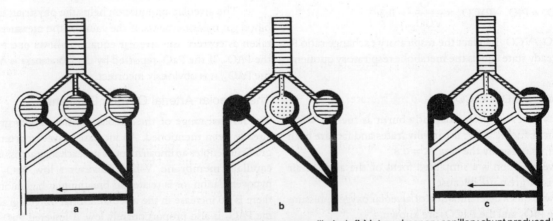

Fig. 3.1.10. (a) Anatomical shunt (portion of cardiac output bypassing pulmonary capillaries). **(b)** Intrapulmonary capillary shunt produced by perfusion of atelectatic alveoli (as in the alveolus to the left) or when $\dot{V}_A/\dot{Q}_C$ ratio is reduced (middle alveolus). **(c)** Overall physiological shunt which includes a true right to left shunt, as also a shunt effect produced by perfusion of poorly ventilated alveoli. (From Udwadia FE. 1979. Diagnosis and Management of Acute Respiratory Failure. OUP, Mumbai.)

the PaO_2. The amount of oxygen in solution in plasma is very low (0.3 ml) due to its relative insolubility. Anaemia will decrease O_2 content in a linear fashion so that a reduction in Hb from 15 g to 7.5 g/100 ml will reduce arterial oxygen content by one half— i.e. from 21 ml to 10.5 ml. However a fall in PaO_2 from 90 mm Hg to 45 mm Hg i.e. by 50 per cent results in just a 20 per cent reduction in the arterial oxygen content. It is evident that significant changes in haemoglobin concentration have a greater influence on CaO_2 than changes in PaO_2.

It is mentioned above that the PaO_2 has an important influence on arterial Hb saturation. There are two other situations (rare though they be) that can also influence Hb saturation. In methaemoglobinaemia, the iron in the Hb molecule is oxidized to its ferric state; reversible oxygen binding is not possible and Hb is unavailable for oxygen transport. Again in carbon monoxide poisoning, the Hb molecule avidly binds to carbon monoxide, and cannot bind to oxygen, nor offer effective transport. Both these situations are characterized by a normal Hb, a normal PaO_2, but a lowered per cent Hb saturation with oxygen, a poor oxygen content and transport.

Oxygen Transport

Transport of oxygen to tissues is a vital function of the cardiorespiratory system. A normal arterial oxygenation or oxygen content does not ensure adequate oxygen transport. The latter is crucially dependent on cardiac output.

Oxygen Transport = Cardiac Output × Arterial Oxygen Content
$$\dot{D}O_2 = \dot{Q}_T \times CaO_2 = \dot{Q}_T \times (1.39 \times Hb \times SaO_2) \times 10$$

It is to be noted that the dissolved oxygen component is removed and that the factor 10 converts the result to ml/minute. If the cardiac index (cardiac output / body surface area) is used instead of the cardiac output, the $\dot{D}O_2$ is expressed as ml/minute/m^2. The normal range for $\dot{D}O_2$ is 520–570 ml/minute/m^2.

Good critical care should therefore help provide both an adequate cardiac output and satisfactory CaO_2 to ensure the necessary oxygen transport for the needs of the tissues.

The Fick Principle

The interrelationship between oxygen transport and oxygen utilization ($\dot{V}O_2$) was described by Fick in 1872.

$$\dot{V}O_2 = \dot{Q}_T \times C\,(a\text{-}\bar{v})O_2$$

i.e. oxygen consumption = cardiac output × arteriovenous oxygen content difference.

The normal range for $\dot{V}O_2$ is 110–160 ml/minute/m^2.

An increase in oxygen consumption ($\dot{V}O_2$) by the tissues is brought about by an increase in the $\dot{Q}_T$, so that the arteriovenous oxygen content difference remains the same (normally about 4–5 ml). If for some reason the cardiac output does not increase appropriately, then the step-up in $\dot{V}O_2$ is met by an increase in oxygen extraction by the tissues i.e. by an increase in the arteriovenous oxygen content difference. The equation in Fick's principle thus remains unaltered, and well balanced. A widened arteriovenous oxygen content difference (i.e. a lowered $P\bar{v}O_2$ and $S\bar{v}O_2$) occurs in the following conditions in critical care medicine.

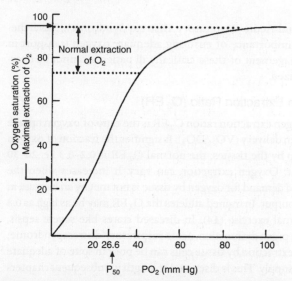

Fig. 3.1.11. The normal oxyhaemoglobin dissociation curve ($P_{50} = 26.6$ mm Hg). At a normal PaO_2, O_2 saturation is close to 100%. At a PaO_2 of 40 mm Hg (venous blood), O_2 saturation is about 75%. Maximum O_2 extraction allows a reserve down to about 25%, corresponding to a PaO_2 of 15–20 mm Hg.

(i) An inadequate cardiac output for tissue needs.

(ii) A very low arterial oxygen content, as with severe anaemia.

(iii) When tissue demands for oxygen are so great, that the normal circulatory system cannot keep pace with excessive tissue demands. This could happen for example in patients with uncontrolled seizures in fulminant tetanus.

As mentioned above, the increased extraction of oxygen by tissues from the blood, leads to a lowered $P\bar{v}O_2$ and $S\bar{v}O_2$. The normal $P\bar{v}O_2$ is 35–40 mm Hg, and the $S\bar{v}O_2$ is 75 per cent. There is a reserve which allows for a fall in $P\bar{v}O_2$ to 15–20 mm Hg, and the $S\bar{v}O_2$ to 25–30 per cent, in conditions characterized by a very low $\dot{Q}_T$, while still enabling diffusion of oxygen at a level that prevents cellular death (**Fig. 3.1.11**).

In critical care settings, the $P\bar{v}O_2$ and the $S\bar{v}O_2$ can thus act as indicators for adequacy or inadequacy of cardiac output and tissue perfusion (**Table 3.1.1**).

Table 3.1.1. $P\bar{v}O_2$ and $S\bar{v}O_2$ as indicators of cardiac output and tissue perfusion adequacy

$P\bar{v}O_2$ (mm Hg)	$S\bar{v}O_2$ (%)	Clinical State
36–42	71–79	Normal Range
> 45	> 80	Septic Shock
< 30	< 50	Lactic Acidosis
< 17	< 20	Neural Damage

Underlying Fick's principle is the concept that $\dot{V}O_2$ is governed by tissue needs and not by oxygen delivery ($\dot{D}O_2$). However as will be illustrated later, below a critical level of oxygen delivery, $\dot{V}O_2$ *does* depend on oxygen supply (**12, 13**). It was earlier believed that in certain pathological states like sepsis, septic shock, acute respiratory distress syndrome, $\dot{V}O_2$ was dependent on $\dot{D}O_2$ at all levels of oxygen delivery. The current though not universal consensus is that this is not really so (see Chapter on

Sepsis and Acute Respiratory Distress Syndrome). Nevertheless the importance of ensuring adequate oxygen transport in the management of these critically ill patients cannot be over-emphasized.

Oxygen Extraction Ratio (O_2 ER)

The oxygen extraction ration O_2 ER is the ratio of oxygen uptake to oxygen delivery ($\dot{V}O_2/\dot{D}O_2$). It signifies the fraction of oxygen taken up by the tissues; the normal O_2 ER is 0.2–0.3 i.e. 20–30 per cent. Oxygen extraction can vary. It increases when the increased demand for oxygen by tissue is not met by an increase in cardiac output. In trained athletes the O_2 ER may be as high as 0.8 at maximal exercise (14). In diseased states like severe sepsis, multiple organ dysfunction, acute respiratory distress syndrome, oxygen extraction by tissue cells can be poor in spite of adequate oxygen supply. This is discussed at length in subsequent chapters on these topics.

REFERENCES

1. Starling EH. (1918). The Linacre lecture on the law of the heart, given at Cambridge in 1915. Longmans, Green and Company, London.

2. Frank O. (1895). Zur Dynamik des Herzmuskels. Ztschr Biol. 32, 370.

3. Sibbald WJ, Calvin J, Driedges AA. (1982). Right and left ventricular preload and diastolic ventricular compliance: implications for therapy in critically ill patients. In: Critical Care, State of the Art, Vol. 3. (Eds Shoemaker WC, Thompson WL). pp. 1. Society of Critical Care Medicine. Fullerton, California.

4. Guyton AC, Jones CE, Coleman TG. (1973). In: Circulatory Physiology, Cardiac Output, and Its Regulation. WB Saunders, Philadelphia.

5. Alderman EL, Glantz SA. (1976). Acute hemodynamic interventions shift the diastolic pressure-volume curve in man. Circulation. 54, 662.

6. Braunwald E, Ross J Jr, Sonnenblick EH. (1967). Mechanism of contraction of the normal and failing heart. N Engl J Med. 277, 794.

7. Glantz SA, Parmley WW. (1978). Factors which affect the diastolic pressure-volume curve. Circ Res. 42, 171.

8. Brodie BR, Grossman W, Mann T, McLaurin LP. (1977). Effects of sodium nitroprusside on left ventricular diastolic pressure-volume relations. J Clin Invest. 59, 59.

9. Pinsky MR. (1991). Cardiopulmonary interactions: the effect of negative and positive changes in pleural pressures on cardiac output. In: Cardiopulmonary Critical Care (Ed. Dantzger DR). pp. 87–120. WB Saunders, Phildelphia.

10. Smith TW, Braunwald E, Kelly RA. (1992). The Management of Heart Failure. In: Heart Disease. A Textbook of Cardiovascular Medicine, 4th edition (Ed. Braunwald E). pp. 464–519. WB Saunders Company. Philadelphia, London, Tokyo.

11. Asitz ME, Rackow EC, Weil MH. (1993). Pathophysiology and Treatment of Circulatory Shock. Critical Care Clinics. 9(2), 183–189.

12. Cain SM. (1977). Oxygen delivery and uptake in dogs during anemia and hypoxic hypoxia. J Appl Physiol. 42, 228.

13. Danek SJ, Lynch JP, Weg JG, Dantzger DR. (1980). The dependence of oxygen uptake on oxygen delivery in the adult respiratory distress syndrome. Am Rev Respir Dis. 122, 387.

14. Leach RM, Treacher DF. (1994). The relationship between oxygen delivery and consumption. Dis Mon. 30, 301–308.

Procedures and Monitoring in the Intensive Care Unit

4.1 Procedures in the Intensive Care Unit
4.2 Cardiac Monitoring in Adults
4.3 Respiratory Monitoring in Adults

CHAPTER 4.1

Procedures in the Intensive Care Unit

Contributed by Dr J. D. Sunavala, MD, FCCP, Consultant Physician, Breach Candy Hospital, Jaslok Hospital and Parsee General Hospital, Mumbai.

Endotracheal Intubation

An endotracheal tube (ET) can be inserted orally or nasally through the larynx and into the trachea. The main indications of endotrachoal intubation are:

(i) Relief of airway obstruction e.g. facial burns, smoke inhalation, epiglottitis or vocal cord oedema.

(ii) Protection of airway e.g. prevention of aspiration, incoordination of swallowing muscles, obtunded and comatose patients.

(iii) Ventilatory support e.g. acute respiratory failure, during general anaesthesia, flail chest (also see Chapter on Airway Management).

Oral Endotracheal Intubation

Intubation by mouth is preferred over nasal intubation as it allows a larger ET with less airflow resistance. However, oral intubation is less comfortable to the patient producing excessive secretions. Conscious patients find it difficult to tolerate the ET and they may constantly gag or bite at the tube.

Instrument tray for oral endotracheal intubation should include the following:

(i) Laryngoscope with both straight (Miller) and curved (MacIntosh) blades, ranging from size 0 (neonates) to 4 (adults). It is vital to check that the blades attach to the handles well and that both batteries and the bulb are in place, so that it lights sharply (brightly) on snapping open the blade of the laryngoscope.

(ii) Endotracheal tubes, which come in sizes ranging from 2 to 10. The size refers to internal diameter (ID) of the tube in mm and it comes in 0.5 mm increments (see **Table 4.1.1**). Along the body of the tube, a radio-opaque line runs lengthwise for the proper verification of tube placement on X-ray. Markings in mm are also shown along the body for easy determination of the depth of insertion. Distal end of the tube has a cuff which is connected to a balloon at the proximal end which is used to regulate volume of air in the cuff via a 10 ml or larger syringe.

Portex tubes are the most commonly used tubes, but stiff rubber endotracheal tubes (Rush) should also be handy, as they may prove useful in difficult intubations.

(iii) Syringes, lubricants, securing tape, flexible guiding stylet, topical anaesthetic, Magill forceps, suction catheters and an AMBU bag with proper connections should also be provided.

Table 4.1.1. Estimation of size of ET

Patient	Size
Neonates < 1000 gm	2.5 mm
Neonates 1000–3000 gm	3–4 mm
Child 1–2 years	4–5 mm
Child 2–12 years	4.5 + (age/4) mm
Avg. adult female	7.5–8.5 mm
Avg. adult male	8–9 mm

Procedure for Oral Intubation

After assessing the patient, clearing the mouth of any foreign body such as dentures and checking the endotracheal tube and laryngoscope, place the patient in sniffing position by tilting the head back so that the oral, pharyngeal and laryngeal axes are aligned. This is usually achieved by raising the head by about 10 cm with pads under the occiput while shoulders remain on the table (**Fig. 4.1.1**). Always explain the procedure to the patient and reassure him if he is conscious. Next, lubricate the deflated cuff at the distal end of the ET. It is always best to ventilate and preoxygenate the patients with 100 per cent O_2 using an AMBU bag and a face mask. If endotracheal intubation is not successful in 30 sec, ventilate the patient once again using 100 per cent O_2. Now hold the laryngoscope handle with the left hand (**Fig. 4.1.1**) and insert the blade into the right side of the mouth; sliding the blade to the base of the tongue and simultaneously swapping the blade to the left. Manoeuvre the tip of the straight (Miller) blade underneath the epiglottis, or the tip of the curved MacIntosh blade at the vallecula. Lift the handle and blade up anteriorly to display the tongue and attached soft tissues. You should be able to now locate the larynx and vocal cords and under direct vision insert the ET. Check for airflow at the proximal end and auscultate for breath sounds and then inflate the cuff. It is always best to confirm proper tube placement on X-ray chest.

Nasal Intubation

The initial preparations and head positioning are the same as for oral intubation. This is a blind technique and intubation is done by inserting the ET (size smaller than one would use for oral intubation) through a nostril. This should be advanced slowly and

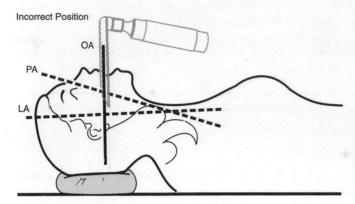

Incorrect Position

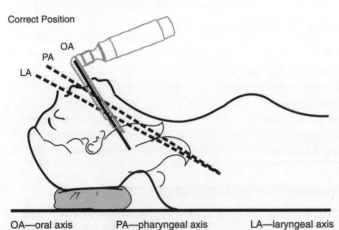

Correct Position

OA—oral axis   PA—pharyngeal axis   LA—laryngeal axis

Fig. 4.1.1. Position of head and neck for endotracheal intubation.

when the distal end can be seen through the mouth it is laryngoscopically guided by Magill forceps into the trachea. In a fully conscious and cooperative patient the tube may be advanced slowly during inspiratory efforts and when the distal end approaches the trachea air movement can be felt and heard through the tube. At this point the tube is gently pushed into the trachea releasing a gush of air almost audible through the tube. Tube placement should be immediately confirmed by ensuring bilateral breath sounds and later by X-ray chest.

Common Problems and Errors of ET Intubation

The commonest error is wrong placement of the tube. The tube could be wrongly pushed so that its tip lies in a bronchus (usually the right bronchus) instead of the trachea (above the carina). If undetected and uncorrected this could cause a disastrous collapse of the unventilated lung. The tube could also lie with its tip in the oropharynx, or pushed down into the oesophagus instead of the trachea. This is immediately detected by the absence of breath sounds on manually ventilating the patient. Instead one can see the stomach getting distended. It is mandatory to always confirm correct tube placement by auscultating both lungs for good air entry and confirming the location of the tip by an X-ray of the chest. Measurement of the end-tidal CO_2 (ETCO$_2$) is also useful in confirming the placement of the ET.

The ET should be *secured* firmly to avoid displacement. Usually an adhesive tape or a commercially made harness is used but too

often moisture and secretions gather between the tape and skin and loosen the tape creating a risk of self-extubation. It is hence important to check the fit frequently and to use adhesive tapes of good material.

Ischaemic injury and tissue necrosis may occur if the *cuff pressure* is too high and exceeds the capillary perfusion pressure in the trachea. The ET pressure should be less than 25 cm H_2O to allow adequate capillary pressure and for patients with hypotension, it should be kept even lower. To ensure and monitor proper cuff pressure, a Posey cufflator with an in-built manometer is available.

To avoid suction-induced hypoxia, the patient is pre-oxygenated and the suction time kept less than 15 seconds.

Certain specific problems can be encountered when using the laryngoscope, especially in oral intubation. A common mishap is aspiration of dentures if one has forgotten to check and remove them. Trauma to the teeth and soft tissue can also occur. This can be avoided by being more gentle and careful during the procedure. Also, with experience, one can guide and manoeuvre the tube over the laryngoscope's blade with greater skill, especially in difficult intubations. Complications of endotracheal intubation have been dealt with in the Chapter on Airway Management.

The general criteria for extubation are listed in **Table 4.1.2**. For care of ET tube and extubation see Chapter on Airway Management.

Table 4.1.2. General criteria for extubation

I Rapid breathing test
f / V$_T$ < 100 min/l
(V$_T$ is tidal volume in litres)
II ABG
Acceptable blood gases on FIO$_2$ less than 0.4 and spontaneous minute ventilation < 10 l/min.
PaO$_2$ / FIO$_2$ > 250 mm Hg
III Ventilatory pressure
Maximum inspiratory pressure > –20 cm H$_2$O
VC > 15 ml/kg
IV Cardiopulmonary assessment
Stable cardiac and pulmonary status

Cricothyroidotomy (1–3)

Cricothyroidotomy is a bedside surgical procedure which can be life-saving when performed for the correct indication.

Indications

Surgical cricothyroidotomy is indicated in all patients who require immediate intubation which cannot be performed because of the following problems: (i) severe maxillofacial problems; (ii) poor visualization of vocal cords due to local oedema, blood or abnormal anatomy; (iii) cervical spine lesions requiring immobilization and where the neck cannot be manipulated.

Equipment

(i) Kelly or Crile clamp;
(ii) Scalpel;

(iii) Antiseptic solution and surgical gloves;

(iv) Tracheostomy tube; No 6 size.

Procedure

The most important part of the procedure is the correct identification of the cricothyroid membrane. The cricoid cartilage is the first small notch on sliding the index finger upwards in the midline from the sternal notch. The firm membrane between it and the thyroid cartilage (Adam's apple) is the cricothyroid membrane.

The patient should be supine with the neck in neutral position and the thumb and index finger of the non-operating hand should stabilize the tracheo-laryngeal complex by firmly fixing the thyroid cartilage as shown in **Fig. 4.1.2**. A 3 to 4 cm vertical or transverse incision should be made through the skin, dermis and cricothyroid membrane. This should identify the cricothyroid space which should be dissected and opened transversely by means of a sharp knife. In spontaneously breathing patients, a successful incision of the membrane should immediately be followed by a gush of air. The index finger should be immediately inserted in the space and a clamp is next inserted to spread the membrane and enlarge the space. Now by pulling the clamp upwards the trachea is elevated and a no. 6 tracheostomy tube is inserted under the clamp and the clamp is removed.

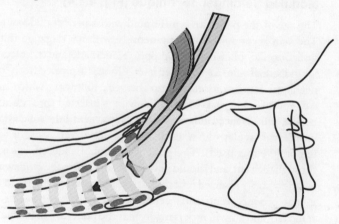

Fig. 4.1.2. Procedure for cricothyroidotomy. Tracheostomy tube advanced behind the clamp and trachea pulled up by clamp.

Complications

(i) Laceration of the anterior jugular veins is a potential complication because of their paramedian and superficial location which is in close proximity to the incision. With a vertical incision the likelihood of injury to the veins is less. However in the event it is injured the bleed can be stopped with manual pressure or may require suture ligation.

(ii) Oropharyngeal injury is a major complication and can occur if the scalpel penetrates the posterior wall of the trachea. This is avoided by dissecting the cricothyroid membrane with a finger or a blunt clamp but never by using a sharp and penetrating instrument like a knife. Observing proper fixation of the thyrolaryngeal complex and taking an adequate incision enabling good

visualization of the thyroid and cricoid cartilage is very important in avoiding this mishap.

(iii) Bleeding from adjacent structures is probably the most common problem but can be avoided or minimized by staying in the midline during the surgery.

Percutaneous Dilatational Tracheostomy (PDT)

Indications

(i) As an elective procedure when it is desirable to shift from endotracheal intubation to a tracheostomy. In this situation, the endotracheal tube is left in position and removed only at the appropriate time.

(ii) To secure an airway in an emergency, when endotracheal intubation fails or when endotracheal intubation is not considered feasible for technical or anatomical reasons.

It is to be noted that though PDT is perhaps more expedient than a formal tracheostomy in a dire emergency, it carries a greater risk of peri-operative cardiopulmonary complications and death. It requires not only expertise, but also experience and should not be performed if these are not available. PDT should also be avoided in children and in obese patients.

Procedure

The two most commonly available kits for this procedure are:

(i) Cook kit,

(ii) Portex kit.

In an elective PDT, the endotracheal tube is left in place throughout the procedure and removed only at the appropriate time. The procedure begins with a small 2 cm vertical incision made mid-distance between the cricoid cartilage and sternal notch. After separating the pretracheal muscles the trachea is palpated through the incision. Next a needle attached to a 10 ml syringe filled with saline is digitally guided and inserted in the midline through the second and third tracheal rings, with constant suction on the syringe while inserting. On entering the trachea bubbles of air are aspirated into the syringe and at this point it is vital to hold the needle still and disconnect the syringe (**Fig. 4.1.3**).

Once the needle is stabilized a guidewire is gently passed through its lumen and the needle then withdrawn. A dilator is next passed over the guidewire to dilate the existing tract. After removing the dilator a guiding catheter is passed over the guidewire and inserted into the trachea. Progressive dilatations are now done starting from 12 Fr dilator up to the largest 36 Fr and these are all done over the guidewire and the guiding catheter. Serial dilatations should be done at a correct angle and with minimal force to avoid injury to trachea or creating a false pretracheal passage. After the largest dilator is inserted and withdrawn a digit is inserted through the incision into the trachea for palpating the ET. An assistant is asked to withdraw the ET slowly and stop withdrawal when the tip of the tube is right over the palpating finger. A no. 8 Shiley tracheostomy

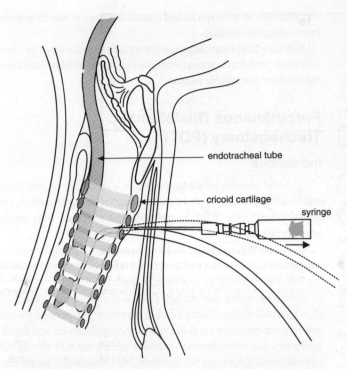

endotracheal tube

cricoid cartilage

syringe

Fig. 4.1.3. Procedure for percutaneous dilatational tracheostomy (PDT).

tube fitted snugly with a 28 Fr dilator is now introduced over the guidewire and guiding catheter complex into the trachea. Once the tracheostomy tube is in place the guidewire, the guiding catheter and the 28 Fr dilator are all withdrawn. The balloon of the tracheostomy tube is inflated and the tube placement is confirmed by auscultation and only then the ET is removed.

Complications

(i) Incorrect placement of needle. This may be avoided by introducing the needle under digital guidance.

(ii) Perforation of the posterior wall of the trachea by dilators. This can be avoided by not applying unnecessary force to the dilator whilst putting it into the trachea and placing the dilator at the correct angle.

(iii) Bleeding into the trachea. This can occur with a low placement of the tube causing injury to the thoracic inlet vessels; though rare the most lethal is an injury to the innominate artery. If such a complication should occur direct pressure should be applied until the patient is moved to the OT for surgical repair.

The sophistication, ease and safety of this technique has made it an increasingly popular procedure that can be performed by a trained intensivist at the bedside. There is however an ongoing debate whether this is truly as safe as it was predicted and whether it is cost effective. In any case, it is always an asset for an intensivist or the on-call surgeon to be familiar with the technique.

Percutaneous Techniques for Central Venous Catheterization (4)

Presterilized sets of special catheters with associated devices are now available as presterilized sets for percutaneous entry into larger veins e.g. the subclavian, internal jugular, femoral or brachial veins.

'Catheter-over-needle devices' are most commonly used, and are designed to eliminate the risk of the needle cutting through the catheter; the greatest danger of 'catheter-through-needle devices' is the shearing of the catheter if it is accidentally withdrawn through the needle. These devices consist of catheters of variable length which can be easily passed through the needle lumen, and can be advanced through the peripheral veins into the central veins.

Both these devices allow placement of a catheter in the central veins by direct puncturing of the vessel. However if a Swan-Ganz or a pacing catheter needs to be passed through the vein, one may have to use special 'Introducer Sets'. These are usually expensive units consisting of a needle, guidewire and a dilator over which a polythene sheath is tightly wrapped. These sets require use of the modified Seldinger technique for introduction of the wide-bore introducer sheath in the vein, through which the catheters can then be passed.

Modified Seldinger Technique (Fig. 4.1.4)

The site of the puncture is infiltrated with 1 per cent lidocaine. The vein is cannulated percutaneously with an 18-gauge thin-walled needle, following the appropriate landmarks and techniques for individual veins as described later. Blood is aspirated from the needle to confirm its entry into the vein, following which the soft end of a J-tip 0.035 inch guidewire is inserted through the needle, and advanced into the superior vena cava (if the subclavian or internal jugular vein is used), or the inferior vena cava (if the femoral vein is used). The guidewire should slide effortlessly through the vein, and should never be forced. After the guidewire is satisfactorily inserted (check that it is not inserted too far in as it may produce ventricular ectopics), the introducer needle is removed, and a small nick is made near the puncture to facilitate the passage of the dilator. The tapered vein dilator carrying an introducer sheath, is then advanced over the guidewire with a twisting motion through the skin and subcutaneous tissue, into the vessel. Finally the wire and dilator are removed, leaving the wide-bore introducer sheath in the vein, through which the Swan-Ganz or pacing catheter can be passed. The sheath should be secured well with sutures. Some of the introducer sheaths have a one-way valve at the proximal end to prevent backflow of blood, and a side port to allow continuous infusion of fluid to prevent clotting. Throughout this procedure, care should be taken to ensure that the proximal end of the guidewire always remains outside, and does not migrate into the vein. If for any reason during the procedure the guidewire needs to be removed and reinserted, the whole procedure should be repeated from the beginning; the needle should never be reintroduced over the guidewire as it can shear the wire.

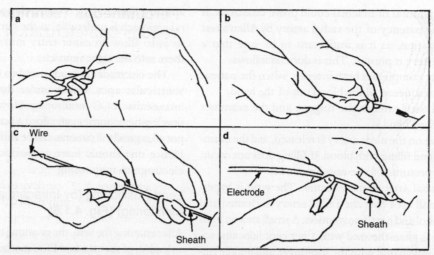

Fig. 4.1.4. Modified Seldinger technique of inserting a guidewire and introducer set via subclavian vein puncture. **(a)** Direction of needle and site of puncture. **(b)** Insertion of guidewire. **(c)** The introducer sheath (with dilator) is first advanced over the guidewire. Next, with the sheath well in, the guidewire and dilator are removed. **(d)** An electrode or catheter is inserted through the sheath. (From Vakil RJ and Udwadia FE. 1988. Diagnosis and management of Medical Emergencies, 3rd Edn. OUP, Mumbai.)

Techniques for Specific Veins

Subclavian Vein Catheterization

(Figs. 4.1.4 and 4.1.5)

The patient lies flat or in a slight head-low position. Correct positioning is important; both arms should be stretched straight by the sides, and the patient should be lying on a firm flat surface so that both the shoulders are in the same plane. The site of puncture is a point just below the junction of the middle and inner thirds of the clavicle.

The skin is now punctured at the selected site, with the point of the needle directed towards the suprasternal notch; the plane of the needle should be horizontal to the ground and parallel to the parietal pleura (**Fig. 4.1.5**). The needle is advanced with a gentle suction on the syringe until the subclavian vein is entered, often with a distinct give. It is sometimes necessary to slightly change the angle of the needle, in which case it is always essential that the needle is completely withdrawn before re-entering in a new

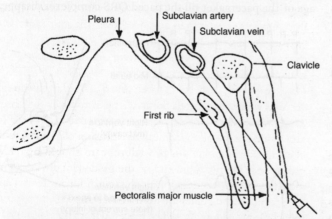

Fig. 4.1.5. Percutaneous subclavian vein puncture: anatomical relationship of the subclavian vein. (From Vakil RJ and Udwadia FE. 1988. Diagnosis and management of Medical Emergencies, 3rd Edn. OUP, Mumbai.)

direction. Once the needle is in the vein, depending on the catheter design, proceed either with the modified Seldinger technique, or directly introduce the catheter through the needle, or slide it from over the needle.

Complications. Pneumothorax is the commonest major complication of this procedure. The incidence of pneumothorax can be reduced by avoiding large-bore needles, multiple punctures, and by disconnecting the ventilator at the time of venepuncture. Other serious complications include air embolism, catheter-induced infection, perforation of the superior vena cava, and hemothorax (due to accidental puncture of the subclavian artery).

Internal Jugular Venepuncture (5)

The patient is placed in the Trendenlenburg position, and the skin cleaned and carefully draped. The site of puncture is located two finger breadths above the clavicle at the outer border of the sternomastoid, with the patient's head rotated to the opposite side. The needle with the syringe attached, is directed towards the suprasternal notch. Aspiration of blood indicates entry into the vein. Air embolism and thrombophlebitis are the main complications encountered in this procedure. Accidental puncture of the internal carotid artery can also occur. Pneumothorax is rarely observed following this procedure.

Femoral Venepuncture (6)

The femoral vein can also be entered percutaneously. The site of puncture is below the inguinal ligament, just medial to the point where the femoral artery pulse can be palpated. Wound infection is generally more common, and there is an increased risk of thrombophlebitis when the femoral vein is used.

Arterial Catheterization (7)

Except in unavoidable circumstances, it is wise to choose the radial artery for catheterization (8), as the risk of occlusion of a proximal artery such as the femoral or brachial could prove disastrous. It is vital to assess the patency of the radial artery by Allen's test prior to catheterization, as it is important to be sure that a competent ulnar artery is present. This is done as follows:

(i) The examiner compresses both arteries, when the patient makes a tight fist to squeeze all the blood out of the hand.

(ii) The patient then extends the fingers, and the examiner observes the blanched hand.

(iii) Compression on the ulnar artery is released, and the examiner observes the hand filling with blood. If filling does not occur, the ulnar artery is presumed to be non-functional.

Technique of Radial Artery Catheterization. The wrist is hyperextended and a small area over the radial artery is cleaned and prepared with alcohol and betadine solution. A small area on both sides of the artery is anaesthetized with 1 per cent lidocaine solution. The artery is palpated with the forefinger and middle finger of one hand, and the needle (we prefer a 'catheter-over-needle device'), is now inserted percutaneously towards the artery. As the needle touches the vessel wall the arterial pulsations are 'damped'; the needle is now advanced further through the wall into the lumen of the artery. As soon as the blood gushes out, the catheter is advanced slowly over the needle, and the needle is then removed. The catheter hub is attached to a continuous flush system ('intraflo') via a pressure tubing. The hub of the catheter should be fixed firmly to the skin, and an antibiotic ointment dressing applied over the point of arterial puncture.

Maintaining tight compression over the puncture site, and proper attention to asepsis will go far in avoiding the two commonest complications of arterial puncture viz. local hematoma formation and infection. Clotting of the catheter can be prevented by using a low dose continuous heparin infusion.

Temporary Bedside Pacing (9, 10)

The most commonly used external pulse generators are ventricular inhibited (demand) units; these generally permit programming of the rate between 50–150/min, and have a sensing facility which allows use in full demand or in the asynchronous mode. Temporary pacing leads (both unipolar and bipolar) are available in various sizes (5–7 French); however pacing with a bipolar lead is more common.

In extreme emergencies, transthoracic temporary pacing can be done by introducing a wire into the myocardium through a chest wall needle.

Technique

Lead Insertion

The pacing electrode may be introduced into the vein percutaneously or by venous cutdown. The commonly used veins are the basilic vein in the antecubital fossa, the subclavian, internal jugular or femoral veins. The choice of vein depends on the doctor's expertise. However it should be noted, that inserting a lead through a cutdown in the antecubital fossa usually involves considerable manipulation, whereas insertion through the internal jugular, subclavian or femoral veins provides a more direct route to the

atrium and requires less manipulation. A left subclavian or femoral approach is preferable, as the curvature of the lead is shaped so as to allow an easier entry into the right atrium, and from there into the right ventricle.

The electrode tip is advanced to its final position at the right ventricular apex, either under fluoroscopic guidance or by intracardiac ECG monitoring. However not many hospitals in developing countries can afford a portable image intensifier, and not all critically ill patients can be shifted to the X-ray department. Hence one should learn to position the lead by intracardiac electrogram monitoring.

Lead Positioning (by Intracardiac Electrogram Monitoring) (Fig. 4.1.6)

After entering the vein, the proximal tip of the electrode is attached to lead V_1 of the standard ECG machine with the aid of an alligator clip cable. Lead V_1 shows a prominent P wave as the pacing electrode advances towards the heart, being inverted in the high atrium and biphasic in the midatrium. Entry of the pacing electrode into the right ventricle is facilitated by forming a loop in the right atrium, and then rotating the catheter either clockwise or anticlockwise, so that the distal end of the lead flips across the tricuspid valve. As the electrode tip crosses the tricuspid valve and enters the right ventricular cavity, the intracardiac ECG changes markedly. A rS ventricular pattern with very deep S and deep T waves appears; this may necessitate decreasing the standardization by half. When the catheter tip abuts on the endocardial surface of the right ventricular wall, an elevated ST segment is observed due to a current of injury. Ventricular ectopic beats are commonly observed when the catheter tip traverses the tricuspid orifice; rarely ventricular fibrillation may occur, necessitating withdrawal of the pacing catheter tip and prompt defibrillation if necessary.

Once the electrode is correctly positioned at the apex of the right ventricle, the lead is connected to the battery-operated pacemaker box. It is now necessary to test the electrical threshold of stimulation, and if the pacemaker is set for demand mode, the ability of the electrode tip to sense the R waves.

The electrical threshold is tested by slowly reducing the amperage of the pacemaker till the paced QRS complexes disappear,

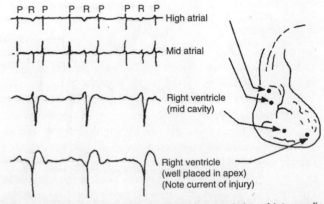

Fig. 4.1.6. Bedside intracardial pacing characteristics of intracardiac electrocardiograms. (From Vakil RJ and Udwadia FE. 1988. Diagnosis and management of Medical Emergencies, 3rd Edn. OUP, Mumbai.)

and only the pacemaker spikes and the patient's own spontaneous beats are present. The amperage is now slowly increased till pacing is re-established, this being the electrical threshold. If pacing does not occur at an electrical threshold of < 2 mA, it may be best to reposition the electrode. The pacemaker rate depends on the clinical needs of the patient, and is generally kept between 70–80 beats/minute.

To test the sensing function in the demand mode, the sensing dial is turned clockwise (in most pulse generators) to full demand mode, and then gradually turned towards the asynchronous mode till sensing is just lost. In this way we can measure the R wave amplitude to ensure adequate sensing of cardiac activity. Unfortunately, most temporary pulse generators do not write the exact values over the dial, but the full demand mode would usually indicate 1 mV, and the opposite asynchronous mode about 20 mV. Ideally a R wave < 6 mV should be 'sensed'. If this does not occur, indicating that the sensing threshold for the R wave exceeds 6 mV, the lead should be repositioned.

Indications for Temporary Pacing

Temporary pacing with an external pulse generator remains an important therapeutic option, and an experienced physician can readily initiate temporary pacing in emergency situations. The two main indications for this procedure are as follows:

1. Therapeutic

These can be broadly classified into 3 major groups:

(a) In patients with life-threatening bradyarrhythmias (e.g. severe sick sinus syndrome, second degree, third degree, or high degree AV blocks, slow junctional or idioventricular rhythms), where it is mandatory to maintain an adequate cardiac rate.

(b) In patients with symptomatic bradycardias or symptomatic conduction defects.

These patients commonly present with recurrent Stokes-Adams attacks, syncope or near syncope which may be due to second or third degree AV blocks or sinus dysfunction.

(c) In selected cases with intractable tachyarrhythmias, where overdrive temporary pacing is used to terminate or prevent the tachycardia. However this is only a temporary measure, and helps to buy time till the tachycardia can be controlled by medical therapy.

2. Prophylactic

Temporary pacing may help in preventing the occurrence of sudden death in the following subsets of patients with acute myocardial infarction:

(a) In patients with inferior myocardial infarction associated with Wenkebach's phenomenon or a second degree heart block, where the possibility of a complete heart block is anticipated.

(b) In patients with extensive anterior wall infarction with recently acquired bifascicular blocks (especially those with right bundle branch block associated with a block in the left posterior inferior division, or in patients with a new bundle branch block associated with transient complete heart block).

(c) Patients with underlying conduction defects such as chronic heart blocks, bifascicular blocks or bradyarrhythmias, who are otherwise asymptomatic, may require temporary pacing at the time of major surgery.

Complications of Pacing

Infection at the local site, phlebitis and thrombosis of peripheral veins are the commonest complications. Systemic infection, lead perforation through the ventricular wall, diaphragmatic pacing and pacemaker-induced arrhythmias, are other major complications that need to be promptly recognized and treated.

Pacing Failure

Malfunction of a temporary pacemaker may result in complete or intermittent failure to capture. Here the ECG will show regular pacing spikes without pacemaker captures; the commonest cause of this is a displaced lead which will require repositioning. A total lack of output on the other hand, manifests on the ECG as absence of both spikes and pacing captures, and is generally caused by either a loose connection, lead fracture, battery failure or a fault in the pacemaker itself.

Sudden cessation of pacing in a patient with marked bradyarrhythmia or absent intrinsic rhythm due to any of the above-mentioned causes, can result in cardiac arrest. In such an eventuality, the first priority should be the re-establishment of cardiac rate and rhythm. All ICU personnel should be familiar with the following emergency protocol in case of sudden pacemaker failure:

(i) Check if patient is asymptomatic.

(ii) Check whether all generator connections are tightly fitted.

(iii) Increase pulse generator output to highest setting.

(iv) Replace pulse generator battery.

(v) Turn patient on left side.

(vi) If cardiac arrest occurs, continue cardiopulmonary resuscitation till such time as the fault is corrected, or the lead is repositioned.

Other less common causes of pacemaker failure are failure to sense, and right ventricular (RV) perforation. Failure to sense occurs if the pacemaker continues to function at a fixed rate, even though it is set on demand mode. The commonest cause of sensing failure is a slight displacement (may be only a few mms) of the electrode tip; it is mandatory that the lead be repositioned immediately to avoid a potential though rare danger of ventricular tachycardia or fibrillation. Perforation of the RV by the electrode tip leads to a total loss of pacing, or frequent failure to 'capture' and to 'sense', and is seen on the ECG as a marked change (> 90 degrees) in the electrical axis of the pacemaker spike, or in the QRS axis of the paced ECG. Stimulation of the phrenic nerve may occur, producing contractions of the diaphragm or of the intercostal or abdominal muscles. A pericardial friction rub is heard at times; hemopericardium with cardiac tamponade is a rare complication.

Chest Tube Drainage (11)

Intercostal tubes are used to aspirate air or fluid from the intra-pleural space. At times, as in a tension pneumothorax, intercostal drainage needs to be performed as an emergency procedure. This is basically a bedside procedure which can be performed easily and safely in the ICU, and all senior resident doctors looking after ICU patients should familiarize themselves with the techniques of chest tube insertion.

Emergency Procedure

A tension pneumothorax can cause a very rapid haemodynamic deterioration, leading to cardiopulmonary collapse and death, if not relieved immediately. Inserting a chest tube may be time-consuming, and a needle should be immediately inserted to relieve the pressure. A 16 gauge angiocath (catheter-over-needle device) is inserted in the second intercostal space, anteriorly in the mid-clavicular line. Once the pleural space is penetrated, the air under tension is immediately released and the pneumothorax is decompressed. At this point the needle is removed, leaving the catheter in the pleural space. The catheter hub is connected to a long tubing, the other end of which is placed underwater—so that the air can bubble out in a more controlled manner. This is however a temporary procedure, and preparation for an immediate chest tube placement must be made for more efficient decompression of the pneumothorax.

Drainage System

A conventional 2 or 3 bottle system is commonly used for evacuation of intrapleural air and fluid as shown in **Fig. 4.1.7**. Each bottle is placed in a series. The first is the trap bottle which collects the fluid from the pleural space, and at the same time allows air to pass through to the next bottle i.e. the water seal bottle. This second bottle acts as a one-way valve, allowing air to escape from the pleural space, but preventing atmospheric air from entering the pleural space when negative pleural pressure is created during inspiration. The inlet tube in the second bottle is placed underwater, thereby creating a back pressure on the pleural space, which is equal to the submerged depth of the inlet tube. This back pressure, called the water seal pressure, is usually 1–2 cm of H_2O, and should ideally suffice to re-inflate the lung. Further negative pressure if required, can be provided by applying a central suction.

However for reasons of safety, a third bottle called the 'suction control bottle', is added in the series. This bottle has an underwater tube which is open to the atmosphere, as shown in **Fig. 4.1.7**. The depth of this tube column determines the safety, by setting a limit on the negative pressure that is imposed on the pleural space. For example, if this column is 15 cm under water, any negative pressure > -15 cm H_2O from a central suction, will result in a constant bubbling of air into the third bottle, and prevent the sub-atmospheric pressure from exceeding -15 cm H_2O.

Procedure for Chest Tube Insertion

A chest tube tray containing sterile drapes, local anaesthetic, medium and large Kelly clamps, and other material such as sutures, antiseptic solution, and dressing materials should be kept ready. Chest tubes of various sizes are available from 12 Fr to 42 Fr. Larger sized tubes are used for traumatic haemothorax or haemopneumothorax, whereas smaller tubes ranging from 12 to 22 Fr may be used for spontaneous pneumothorax. The tube itself is made of a transparent material, with multiple side holes over the distal third of its length; there is also a radio-opaque strip at the distal end of the tube to mark its placement in the pleural space. These tubes are available in a trocar for tunneling through the intercostal space. In case these special tubes are not available, a simple Malecot's catheter may be used.

The patient should lie flat with the involved side elevated by a pillow, and arms flexed over the head. After infiltrating the skin with lidocaine (1 per cent or 2 per cent solution), a skin incision is made at the appropriate site of tube insertion, which is usually in the fifth or sixth intercostal space in the anterior axillary line. Some operators prefer the second intercostal space in the mid-clavicular line, but the penetration of muscles and breast tissue is more difficult at this site. After incising the skin at the appropriate puncture site, the muscles and tissues are penetrated by either a blunt dissection using clamps and index finger to enter the pleural space, or the tube is directly inserted with the help of a trocar. Rotating movements are used whilst advancing the tube with the trocar.

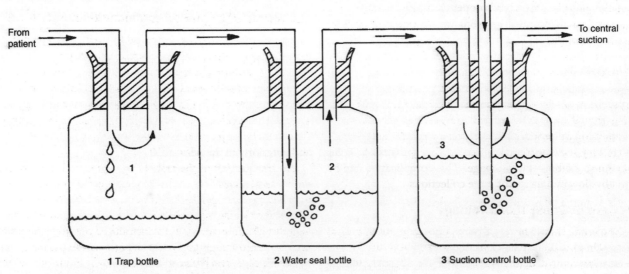

Fig. 4.1.7. Three-bottle pleural drainage system (see text for discussion). → = flow of air.

Once the pleural space is entered, the tube is advanced upward in the direction of the apex for treatment of a pneumothorax, and towards a post-basal position for drainage of fluid, with the last side hole inserted 2 or 3 mm into the chest to ensure dependent drainage. Prior to insertion, the approximate length of the tube that should lie within the thoracic cage is estimated, and the position where the tube should emerge from the chest wall is marked with a silk tie.

Once the tube is properly placed in the pleural space it is fastened to the skin with 1–0 or 2–0 silk sutures, using a mattress stitch. Before fixing the tube, ensure that the last side hole is in the pleural space. The ends of the suture are not cut, but are wrapped around the tube, and secured with a tape so that they can be used later to close the wound after the tube is removed.

Throughout the procedure the proximal end of the tube is kept clamped and is opened only when the tube is finally connected to the drainage system. The placement is confirmed by the drainage of fluid, or by the bubbling of air in the drainage bottle.

Precautions

There is no absolute contraindication for inserting a chest tube. Coagulation abnormalities however, should be corrected before insertion of the tube; in case of emergency, fresh frozen plasma or platelet transfusions may be given during the procedure.

A chest tube should never be inserted at the bedside for the purpose of draining a massive haemothorax. Accumulated blood in a massive haemothorax acts as a seal preventing further bleeding from the source, and insertion of a chest tube may precipitate catastrophic haemorrhage. Hence, a massive haemothorax should always be drained in the operation theatre where facilities for controlling such a bleed, if necessary with an open thoracotomy, are available.

Complications

Common complications of chest tube drainage include improper positioning of the chest tube, inadequate drainage, bleeding, nerve damage, injury to the diaphragm, infection, surgical emphysema, and problems in the drainage system. Use of the correct technique of insertion and placement, and proper chest tube management whilst the tube is in place, will go a long way in preventing most of these complications.

Incessant pain may occur after re-expansion of the lung and may evoke a vasovagal response manifesting as bradycardia or hypotension. Intercostal nerve blocks or intrapleural lidocaine may help; parenteral analgesics may be needed if pain persists. Strong sedatives should however be avoided. Another major complication is re-expansion pulmonary oedema following rapid evacuation of a large, long-standing pleural collection. Symptoms usually occur within 6 hours after rapid drainage. This complication can be avoided by slow evacuation of large collections.

After Care of Chest Tube Drainage

(i) The bottle should never be raised above the chest level, as fluid may drain back into the pleural space and lead to infection, or cause a drowning disaster in the presence of a bronchopleural fistula. However if the kind of drainage system demonstrated in Fig. 4.1.7 is used, this complication can be avoided, because the draining tube never comes in contact with the water in the bottle.

(ii) The fluid level in the tube should oscillate with each breath. Failure to oscillate may be due to blockage or a kink in the chest tube, or may be due to full expansion of the lung.

(iii) The intercostal tubes should always be clamped whilst changing the bottles.

(iv) The original level of water in the bottle should always be marked, so that hourly drainage can be measured.

(v) Very high negative suction via a suction pump should be avoided. Ideally a suction control bottle should be added to the drainage system as a safety measure, as described earlier.

Chest Tube Removal

Chest tubes should be removed when there is minimal drainage (less than 100 ml/24 hrs), and the chest X-ray shows complete re-expansion of the lung after clamping the outside tube for 24 hrs. Check X-rays of the chest should be repeated after removal of the tube. Appearance of a small pneumothorax or minimal surgical emphysema is common, and often resolves by itself.

Pericardiocentesis (12)

Pericardiocentesis carried a high risk of morbidity in the past, when done as a blind procedure. However in the last decade the incidence of complications has decreased dramatically, largely due to improved imaging and monitoring techniques. However bedside imaging facilities are not always available, and hence each and every resident doctor working in the ICU or emergency department of a hospital, should be familiar with the technique of blind pericardiocentesis, as this is the procedure of choice in the face of a life-threatening emergency like cardiac tamponade. Cardiac tamponade occurs when increasing accumulation of pericardial fluid produces cardiac chamber compression limiting ventricular filling, and significantly compromising the stroke volume. In such a situation, blind pericardiocentesis is justified as any delay in pericardial drainage may prove fatal.

Technique of Blind Pericardiocentesis (Fig. 4.1.8)

This procedure should always be performed in an intensive care setting with continuous ECG monitoring. The three approaches to the pericardium are subxiphoid, apical and parasternal.

The *subxiphoid approach* is probably the safest as it avoids the pleura, the coronary and internal mammary arteries. The patient should be premedicated with atropine, and placed in an upright or semi-reclining position, as this allows pooling of blood inferiorly and anteriorly in the pericardial sac.

An area just left of the xiphoid tip is prepared and infiltrated with a local anaesthetic. A 16–20 gauge spinal or cardiac needle attached to a syringe filled with local anaesthetic is used, and the hub of the needle is connected to the V lead of an ECG via an alligator clip. The needle tip is introduced between the xiphoid and the left costal margin, so that it passes under the inner aspect of the rib cage, and the needle is then slowly advanced, with the tip pointing towards the left shoulder.

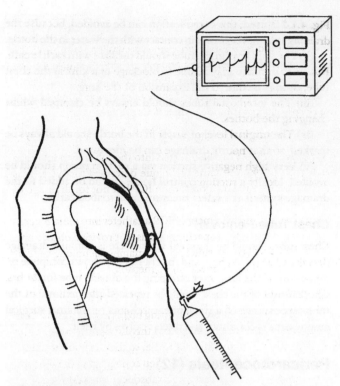

Fig. 4.1.8. Technique of blind pericardiocentesis.

Whilst advancing the needle, a gentle suction is continuously applied to the syringe, and periodically small amounts of local anaesthetic are injected. This helps to keep the needle patent, and also anaesthetises the deeper tissues. A resistance is felt on penetrating the diaphragm and pericardium. If a current of injury pattern, with ST-segment elevation, is recorded on the V lead tracing of the ECG (signifying the needle has touched the epicardium), the needle should be withdrawn slightly and readvanced in a more medial direction. Once fluid is aspirated, a soft catheter should be inserted with the help of a guidewire, and the needle withdrawn.

The apical approach is from the fourth or fifth inter-costal space, 2 cm medial to the outer edge of the cardiac dullness, perpendicular to the chest wall. The needle bore is aimed at the right sterno-clavicular joint. There is minimal risk of injuring the coronary arteries with this approach as there are no large vessels near the apex of the heart; however the risk of ventricular or pulmonary lacerations are greater with this method.

The parasternal route lies 2 cm lateral to the sternum in the fifth intercostal space. The greatest danger of this approach is injury to the internal mammary artery, and hence this method carries a significantly greater morbidity than the two other approaches described earlier.

Intra-aortic Balloon Pump (IABP) (13)

IABP is the only accepted method of mechanical circulatory assistance available at present. It is now being increasingly used for sustaining patients with potentially reversible cardiac problems affecting the pumping function of the LV, when pharmacological therapy has failed to restore adequate coronary artery and systemic perfusion. The goal of balloon assistance is to provide temporary support to the LV when corrective surgery is planned in the near future, or spontaneous ventricular recovery is anticipated.

IABP works on the principle that a balloon catheter inserted in the thoracic aorta inflates during diastole, and deflates during systole. The inflation improves diastolic-dependent coronary perfusion and myocardial oxygen consumption, whereas the sudden deflation occurring in systole decreases the aortic end-diastolic pressure and lessens the workload on the LV, thereby decreasing the myocardial oxygen demand. Common indications for the use of IABP are:

(i) Immediate post-operative support after CABG surgery or other open heart surgery.

(ii) In patients with unstable angina or impending infarction who are refractory to medical therapy, and are awaiting bypass surgery.

(iii) In acute myocardial infarction with cardiogenic shock.

(iv) In patients with mechanical complications of acute myocardial infarction which warrant surgical intervention e.g. acute ventricular septal rupture, papillary muscle dysfunction or rupture.

(v) In patients with high risk for PTCA.

(vi) In haemodynamically unstable patients who are awaiting surgery after a failed angioplasty.

Absolute contraindications for the use of IABP are dissecting aortic aneurysms, aortic regurgitation, irreversible brain damage, and end-stage heart disease.

Equipment and Procedure

The two basic equipments required for this procedure are (i) a drive unit and (ii) intra-aortic balloon catheters. The operation of a drive unit is based on recognition of the variability of the interval between the electrical and mechanical events of the cardiac cycle. Hence the precise timing of both inflation and deflation in relation to the events of the cardiac cycle, becomes the most important function of the drive unit. The large-bore catheter has a 30 cm long polyurethane balloon wrapped tightly around its intra-aortic end, and has two concentric lumens running through its length. The central lumen leads to the catheter tip allowing a J tip safety guidewire which helps to introduce the balloon. This central lumen also allows recording of critical arterial pressure in the proximity of the balloon tip, thus eliminating the need of a separate arterial pressure line to obtain waveforms required for balloon pump timing. Concentric to the central lumen is the helium channel, through which the balloon is inflated with helium to a capacity of 30 to 40 ml.

Before selecting the groin through which the balloon catheter is to be inserted, all the pulses in both lower extremities are compared and graded, and the leg with the greater pulse velocity is selected. A Swan-Ganz thermodilution catheter, and an intra-arterial line to record arterial waveforms, should also be inserted. However separate arterial lines may not be necessary in most catheters, which allow intra-aortic waveform recording through their central lumen. The entire balloon device is inserted into the femoral artery at the groin, either percutaneously or by performing an arteriotomy. The balloon is then advanced up the aorta until the tip lies 1 cm below the origin of the left subclavian artery. Fluoroscopic guidance should be used whenever available, as it assures more precise placement.

Complications

The most commonly encountered complications in order of frequency are vascular (limb ischaemia), infections, failure to place the balloon catheter, and bleeding.

Weaning

The balloon assistance should be withdrawn gradually by either decreasing the frequency of balloon inflations per cardiac cycle, or by stepwise reduction in the volume of the balloon. Weaning can usually be completed within 60 minutes provided the patient remains haemodynamically stable. If the patient's condition deteriorates, full volume IABP is resumed, and weaning may be reattempted after 6–24 hours.

Intracranial Pressure Monitoring (also see Chapter on Increased Intracranial Pressure)

Indications (14)

(i) Traumatic brain injury if Glasgow Coma Score < 8 (after resuscitation). In addition, there should be evidence of an abnormal CT scan or in case the CT scan is normal, two or more of the following should be present—(a) age > 40 years; (b) unilateral or bilateral posturing; (c) systolic blood pressure > 90 mm Hg.

(ii) In patients with metabolic and other causes known to cause elevated intracranial pressure, such as subarachnoid haemorrhage, stroke, intracranial mass, hydrocephalus, hepatic encephalopathy and coma, poisonings.

Methods

ICP monitoring can be done by 3 methods:

1. Ventriculostomy with intraventricular catheter (IVC);
2. Subarachnoid catheter;
3. Subdural bolt.

1. Ventriculostomy

In this technique, an IVC can be placed through a craniostomy in the operation theatre, or by a twist-drill ventriculostomy in the OT or in the ICU. The most preferred side is the posterior frontal lobe of the non-dominant hemisphere, and the catheter is passed through the brain to a depth of 6–8 cm. On finding CSF, the IVC is attached to a 3-way stopcock that leads to a pressure transducer through one port and an external drainage system through another. The pressure transducer is connected to a monitor which provides continuous digital and waveform display of the ICP.

The ICP baseline gently dips up and down with respiratory or ventilatory excursions. 'Zeroing' of the pressure transducer should be done at the level of the external auditory meatus.

The IVC is the most accurate method of measuring ICP (15). It can also be safely used to slowly drain CSF from the ventricles.

However, it is difficult to perform in cases of head trauma as the ventricles are shrunken in size and the catheter is then left in the brain parenchyma. The main disadvantage is that it is more invasive and there are increased chances of infection. Most units use prophylactic antibiotics when IVCs are used.

2. Subarachnoid catheters

A subdural catheter can be inserted into the subarachnoid space inside the skull by the same technique described for IVCs. This method can be used to monitor the ICP but not for drainage of CSF.

For one-time measurement of ICP, a catheter into the subarachnoid space in the L3–L4 space can be used, provided obstructive hydrocephalus has been ruled out by imaging techniques. However, CSF cannot be drained by this method.

3. Subdural bolt

In this technique, a hollow self-tapping bolt is inserted into a burr hole in the skull at the bedside, and the dura at the base of the bolt is perforated with a spinal needle, so that CSF fills the bolt. Pressure tubing filled with saline is then connected to the bolt and communication with an external transducer is established.

This technique is used when the first two techniques are difficult. Also, this method is associated with a lower infection rate as compared to ventriculostomy. However, this method cannot be used for drainage of CSF.

Fibreoptic ICP monitors which use miniature transducers incorporated into their ends can also be used to measure ICP.

Several parameters such as cerebral blood flow velocity (CBFV) in different parts of the brain circulation, measured through the use of transcranial Doppler have been suggested for estimating the ICP noninvasively (16). However, as yet, none of these methods are reliable enough to substitute for invasive ICP monitoring.

REFERENCES

1. Goumas P, Kokkinis K, Petrocheilos J et al. (1997). Cricothyroidotomy and the anatomy of the cricothyroid space. An autopsy study. J Laryngol Otol. 111:354–356.
2. Isaacs JH Jr, Pederson AD. (1999). Emergency cricothyroidotomy. Am Surg. 63:346–349.
3. Halsted Residents of the John Hopkins Hospital, Baltimore. (1996). In: Manual of Common Bedside Surgical Procedures. (Eds Chen H, Sola J, Lillemoe K). p. 20. Willaims & Wilkins, USA.
4. Rosen M, Latto IP, Ng WS. (1981). Handbook of Percutaneous Central Venous Catheterization. WB Saunders Company. London.
5. Denys BG, Uretsky BF. (1991). Anatomical variations of internal jugular vein location: Impact on central venous access. Crit Care Med. 19, 1516.
6. Swanson RS, Uhlig PN, Gross PL et al. (1984). Emergency intravenous access through the femoral vein. Ann Emerg Med. 13, 244.
7. Clark VL, Kruse JA. (1992). Arterial Catheterization. In: Critical Care Clinics, Procedures in the ICU (Guest Ed. Kruse JA). 8(4), 687–697.
8. Slogoff S, Keats AS, Arlund C. (1983). On the safety of radial artery cannulation. Anesthesiology. 59, 42.
9. Benotli JR. (1985). Temporary Cardiac Pacing. In: Intensive Care Medicine. (Eds Rippe JM et al.). Little Brown and Co. Boston.
10. Moses HW, Taylor GJ, Scheveiner JA, Dove JT. (1987). In: A Practical Guide to Cardiac Pacing, 2nd Edn, Little Brown and Co. Boston.

11. Miller KS, Sahn FA. (1987). Chest tubes: Indications, technique, management and complications. Chest. 91, 258.

12. Kirkland LL, Taylor RW. (1992). Pericardiocentesis. In: Critical Care Clinics, Procedures in the ICU (Guest Ed. Kruse JA). 8(4), 699–712.

13. Kantrowitz A, Cardona RR, Freed PS. (1992). Percutaneous Intra-aortic Balloon Counterpulsation. In: Critical Care Clinics, Procedures in the ICU. 8(4), 819–837.

14. Brain Trauma Foundation. (1996). Indications for intracranial pressure monitoring. J Neurotrauma. 13, 667.

15. Brain Trauma Foundation. (1996). Recommendations for intracranial pressure monitoring technology. J Neurotrauma. 13, 685.

16. Treib J, Becker SC, Grauer M, Haas A. (1998). Transcranial Doppler monitoring of intracranial pressure therapy with mannitol, sorbitol and glycerol in patients with acute stroke. Eur Neurol. 40, 212.

Cardiac Monitoring in Adults

Contributed by Dr J.D. Sunavala, MD, FCCP, Consultant Physician, Breach Candy Hospital, Jaslok Hospital and Parsee General Hospital, Mumbai.

General Considerations

The most important part of cardiac monitoring is frequent clinical assessment, which includes physical examination and intelligent observation. Proper evaluation of important symptoms such as chest pain, dyspnoea, cough, and of vital signs, is of prime diagnostic value in emergency situations. A correct technique of inspecting the jugular vein in the neck can give a good idea of the central venous pressure (CVP) in the absence of a central venous catheter. This clinical observation should also be used frequently to countercheck the reliability of any invasive CVP measurement. Repeated chest auscultation is essential, as it may reveal newly developed or increasing moist sounds indicative of early pulmonary oedema. Monitoring of urine output is essential for assessment of renal perfusion. Relevant blood tests and routine chest X-rays are also essential aspects of cardiac monitoring. However in this chapter, we have mainly discussed monitoring techniques which involve instrumentation.

ECG Monitoring (1)

Bedside detection of cardiac arrhythmias, and of ST segment changes to some extent, are the most important objectives of continuous ECG monitoring. There are certain technical points worth discussing to ensure the accuracy and the optimal benefit from the information obtained. These include:

Skin Preparation and Electrode Placement

Shaving and careful skin preparation to achieve proper electrode contact is essential. Further, electrodes should be so placed that they do not interfere with physical examination, the recording of a 12-lead ECG, or the use of a defibrillator. Electrode wires should always be checked for breaks or fractures, as this may result in artefacts.

Selection of the Monitoring Leads

The modified CL_1 (MCL_1) hook-up (**Fig. 4.2.1**) has been the most popular lead used for monitoring since many years, as it best represents V_1. The V_1 lead is excellent for studying atrial activity

and the QRS complex, but it is difficult to monitor, and hence MCL_1 is a simple, excellent alternative which gives similar information. Here the positive electrode is placed at the V_1 position, the negative electrode at the left shoulder, and the ground electrode may be placed at any site, but is usually placed at the right shoulder. As seen in **Fig. 4.2.1**, this leaves sufficient space over the precordium for physical examination and for emergency cardioversion. In addition since it closely resembles V_1, this lead offers several diagnostic advantages:

(i) It displays well-formed P waves.

(ii) It is easy to distinguish between left bundle branch block (LBBB) and right bundle branch block (RBBB).

(iii) It is the best lead for distinguishing between a ventricular ectopic originating from the left ventricle with a positive QRS deflection, and one originating from the right ventricle with a negative QRS deflection.

Most rhythm and conduction disturbances are easily recognizable, but there are a significant number of arrhythmias that defy

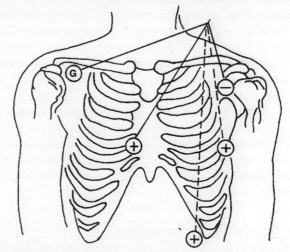

Fig. 4.2.1. MCL_1 hook-up shown by uninterrupted lines representing positive, negative and ground electrodes. MCL_6 and M_3 are obtained by simply changing the positive electrode from the V_1 position to the two positions as shown by broken lines, leaving the negative and ground electrodes undisturbed.

immediate recognition. Hence, if MCL$_1$ fails to provide enough information, a left chest lead MCL$_6$ (which reasonably simulates V$_6$), or M$_3$, a modified lead III, can be tried. This can be easily done without disconnecting the entire MCL$_1$ hook-up, by simply changing the positive wire from V$_1$ to V$_6$ for MCL$_6$, or from V$_1$ to the left lower chest, or down towards the left groin for M$_3$ (**Fig. 4.2.1**). Lead V$_6$ or MCL$_6$ is an important lead for differentiating between aberration and ectopy whenever V$_1$ fails to reveal this. A sinus beat in V$_6$ always begins with a small q wave; disappearance of this q wave with onset of tachycardia, is characteristic of left ventricular tachycardia rather than sinus tachycardia with aberrance. V$_6$ or MCL$_6$ is also very useful in monitoring ischaemic ST segment changes, especially in patients with unstable angina, as this lead represents the main left ventricular free wall.

In rare instances when one wants to demonstrate the polarity of the P wave, M$_3$ (which simulates Lead III), will have to be used. For instance a retrograde P wave will show up clearly in M$_3$ in case of a junctional rhythm, whereas both sinus and retrograde P waves are predominantly positive in MCL$_1$.

This easy method of changing leads comes handy in monitoring pacemaker patients, as one lead may not show a pacemaker artefact; however on changing the lead configuration, this will become clearly evident. This is commoner with bipolar pacing, where the pacemaker spikes or artefacts are not as prominent as in unipolar pacing.

Special Leads

As recognition of the P wave is the key to diagnosis of arrhythmias in bedside monitoring, all efforts should be made to magnify the P wave so as to render it easily recognizable. Certain invasive methods such as inserting intra-atrial electrode catheters or oesophageal electrodes can greatly enhance the P wave which may have been virtually indiscernible with surface leads. However, these forms of monitoring may not be feasible, particularly in very sick patients, and another non-invasive special lead, viz. S$_5$ should be tried. This was first introduced by French cardiologists, and is easily obtained by placing the positive electrode in the fifth intercostal space close to the sternum (just below V$_1$ position), and the negative electrode on the manubrium of the sternum. This lead may sometimes succeed in magnifying the P wave, and if so it is preferable to invasive means of monitoring.

There are some simple leads which are rarely used to diagnose an arrhythmia. One such lead is aVR, or any other lead which shows the smallest ventricular complex. Elusive P waves or small pacemaker spikes are often more prominently seen in leads having the smallest ventricular complexes, provided the lead has minimum baseline disturbance.

Haemodynamic Monitoring

Haemodynamic monitoring is in essence an invasive method of monitoring arterial, central venous and pulmonary artery pressures. Measurement of cardiac output (CO), and pressure of oxygen in mixed venous blood (P$\bar{v}$O$_2$) are other important aspects of haemodynamic monitoring. With the information gained from the above parameters, one can calculate the ventricular work load, vascular resistances, oxygen transport ($\dot{D}O_2$), and oxygen consumption ($\dot{V}O_2$); this data can be extremely useful in the management of critically ill patients. However, mere numerical values are of limited value, and a balanced clinical approach in the interpretation and application of these values cannot be overemphasized. Further, as doctors caring for seriously ill patients, we witness life at its most poignant, intimate and critical moments. It is thus obligatory, that we learn to use these invasive techniques with sensitivity and skill.

There are varied indications for haemodynamic monitoring which will be discussed under the appropriate procedures. However, the fundamental goal of monitoring remains constant—the early detection, and the prompt restoration to normal of inadequate perfusion.

Pressure Monitoring System

Equipment (Fig. 4.2.2)

The equipment required for direct pressure monitoring consists of 3 main components—the transducer, pressure lines and the pressure monitor.

A transducer is a device that converts the mechanical energy created by the arterial or venous pressure waves into electrical energy, which in turn gets displayed on the monitor as a waveform. Most transducers available are strain gauge devices or quartz transducers. Quartz transducers are more frequently used today as they are conveniently designed, more durable, and less affected by ambient conditions. The latest in transducer technology are the disposable or single-use units, and most of these are modifications of strain gauge devices (**2**).

Pressure lines include the tubings, connecting stop cocks, the pressure infusor bag and a continuous flush valve device also commonly known as 'intraflo' (**Fig. 4.2.2**).

The pressure infusor bag is a hollow pressure bag wrapped around a heparinized saline intravenous bag, which can be inflated to high pressures. 'Intraflo' is a flushing device which under constant pressure (around 300 mm Hg) assures a continuous flow of heparinized solution at a rate of 3 ml/hr through the system. This prevents clotting and backflow, and also provides for the manual flushing of the fluid column as and when necessary.

The pressure monitor is an amplifier system which can display wave forms and digital readouts on a screen, in addition to having recording facilities. With improving technology, the bedside pressure monitors available today are highly sophisticated, significantly smaller in size, and extremely reliable. Even so, monitors may not always be 100 per cent accurate; in fact, one recent study has shown that errors of 5–10 mm Hg are frequent, and gross errors of 30–40 mm Hg are not uncommon. In order to minimize such errors and obtain accurate pressure data, the ICU personnel must familiarize themselves with the equipment, and be able to set up the system with accuracy and speed; they should also be competent in detecting and solving problems encountered during monitoring.

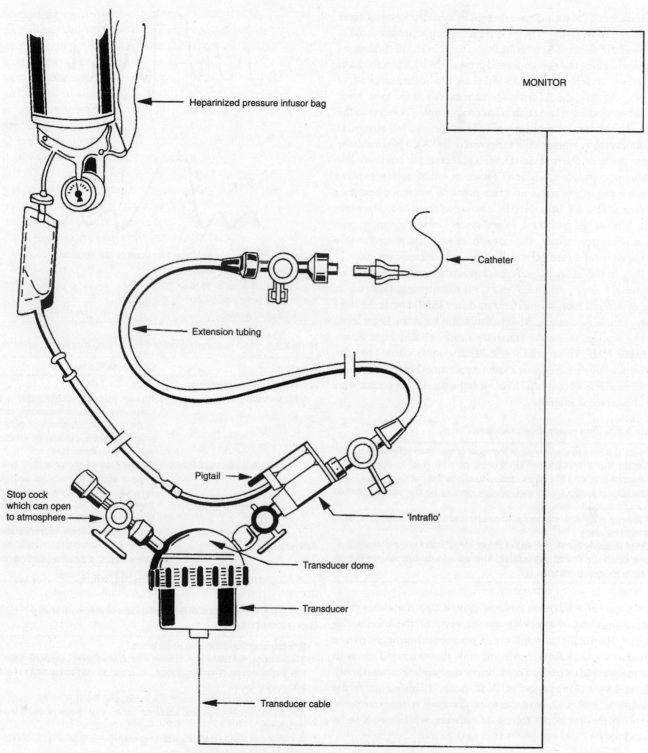

MONITOR

Heparinized pressure infusor bag

Catheter

Extension tubing

Pigtail

Stop cock
which can open
to atmosphere

'Intraflo'

Transducer dome

Transducer

Transducer cable

Fig. 4.2.2. Assembly of the pressure monitoring system.

Assembly and Calibration of the Monitoring System

The pressure monitoring system is assembled as shown in **Fig. 4.2.2**. Care should be taken to remove all air bubbles from the tubings and the dome of the diaphragm whilst setting up the pressure lines. The extension tube connecting the 'intraflo' to the catheter should be a stiff, non-distensible pressure tubing of approximately 100 cm length. Once the system is connected and ready for monitoring, it should be balanced, calibrated, and placed at the correct reference point.

Reference Point: There is always a hydrostatic pressure gradient in a fluid-filled system, consisting of blood in the vessels interfaced with a column of saline in the catheter, tubings and transducer.

For instance, if the transducer is manually raised or lowered, there are bound to be changes in pressure recordings, proportional to the weight of the fluid column applied to the transducer diaphragm. In order to eliminate this undesired pressure head, the transducer diaphragm and the catheter tip which are considered as 2 ends of the pressure line, should always remain exactly at the same level. By convention we relate central haemodynamic pressures to the level of the heart, or more specifically to the mid left atrium, at which level the catheter tip is supposed to lie. For a patient in the supine position, the mid-chest level is accepted as a reference line approximating the left atrial level. However, whilst nursing patients in semi-upright positions, an exact point of reference becomes necessary. This is represented by a point on the mid-axillary line at the level of the fourth intercostal space. Before beginning zero referencing procedures, the transducer must be placed at this appropriate reference point, called the zero reference point.

This is the accepted reference point for measurement of pulmonary artery pressures and CVP monitoring; however in case of arterial monitoring the transducer should be at the level of the cannulated artery, which should also be at the heart level.

The exact procedure for zero referencing or balancing is shown in **Table 4.2.1**. The transducer calibration procedure tests the transducer by exposing it to a known pressure (Hg manometer), unlike zero referencing, which balances the transducer output with the atmospheric pressure.

Table 4.2.1. Zero referencing procedure

* Place the transducer dome at the level of the zero reference point
* Adjust the 2 transducer stopcocks so that one is open to the atmosphere, and the other closed towards the patient
* The digital readout and oscilloscope display on the screen, should now both read 0 mm Hg
* If they do not, follow the particular machine instructions so as to achieve a zero balance
* Once properly zeroed, close the stopcock exposed to the atmosphere, and open the line to the patient. The waveform that follows is now ready for interpretation

'*Eliciting of a waveform response*' (**Fig. 4.2.3**) is another rapid bedside method of checking the integrity of the monitoring system. Normally on pulling and releasing the pigtail of the 'intraflo', the waveform on the monitor shows a rapid rise with an equally rapid return to a point below the baseline (undershoot), followed by a short period of oscillations. If this return to the baseline is slow with inadequate oscillations, it suggests some sort of occlusion in the tubing or catheter, which needs to be looked into.

Common Problems Related to Monitoring Systems

Distortion of the waveform, questionable pressure readouts, and artefacts are 3 common problems encountered whilst dealing with pressure monitoring systems, irrespective of venous or arterial catheterizations. **Table 4.2.2** enumerates the causes, and gives guidelines for solving most of these problems. Some general precautions which need to be taken for smooth and uncomplicated monitoring are listed in **Table 4.2.3**.

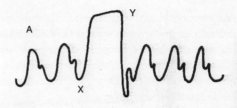

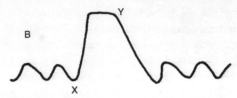

Fig. 4.2.3. Eliciting a waveform response at the bedside.
A = normal waveform response
B = dampened waveform response
X = 'intraflo' activated by pulling the pigtail
Y = release of pigtail

Table 4.2.2. Trouble-shooting guide for pressure monitoring systems

Problems	Check and Correct
Waveform Related Problems	
* No waveforms	Power supply, calibration and balancing, loose connections, clots in the tubings, stopcock direction, broken catheter, catheter tip abutting against the vessel wall
* Over-dampened waveforms	Air bubbles in the pressure lines, kinks or clots in the tubings, catheter tip abutting against the vessel wall
Questionable Pressure Readings	Balancing and calibration, reference level of transducer, loose connections in the pressure lines, faulty 'intraflo'
Artefacts	Patient movements, respiratory movements, electrical interference, catheter whip artefact

Table 4.2.3. General precautions and care of pressure lines during monitoring

* Employ aseptic technique at all times
* Select uncomplicated monitoring 'kits' (avoid long pressure lines or too many interconnecting tubes, in order to eliminate kinks, leaks and air bubbles)
* Once system is in use, avoid disconnecting the line for any reason
* Avoid blood collection and administration of IV drugs through these catheters
* Avoid use of sharp instruments when removing dressings around the catheter site
* Do zero referencing at the beginning of the procedure, and each time following interruption of continuous monitoring, whatever the reason. In any case, it is recommended that zero referencing be done 3–4 times a day

Arterial Pressure Monitoring (3)

The techniques and complications of arterial cannulation are described in the Chapter on Procedures in the Intensive Care Unit.

Arterial pressure monitoring is initiated in all patients with compromised haemodynamic status. In these cases, the cuff method of recording blood pressure is likely to be inaccurate as Korotkoff's sounds are less audible at low flow rates. It is also indicated in severely vasoconstricted patients, and in patients being treated with vasoactive or antihypertensive drugs, which require careful titration of dosage to avoid precipitous changes in arterial blood pressure.

The radial artery is usually the preferred site for placement of an arterial catheter, provided that the adequacy of collaterals to the ulnar artery has been assessed and determined to be sufficient by the Allen's test (see Chapter on Procedures in the Intensive Care Unit). In addition to the fact that the hand receives a generous collateral circulation, the radial artery is superficial, compressible and easily accessible. Cannulation of the artery involves little or no risk to neighbouring anatomical structures, and above all the surrounding skin area can be easily kept clean. The only drawback of the radial artery is its relatively small size which may limit the success of cannulation. For proper monitoring the placement catheter should be inserted right up to the hub to avoid kinking, and the wrist should be maintained in a neutral position.

The brachial, axillary and femoral arteries are other possible sites for cannulation, but they should never be the first choice for arterial catheterization as they have many disadvantages, and more serious complications may ensue.

During intra-arterial monitoring, the catheter should be properly secured to avoid accidental disconnection resulting in significant blood loss. Silent bleeds or oozing within the tissue spaces, which are most common following femoral punctures, may lead to huge haematomas. Aseptic measures should be strictly followed during catheterization, subsequent manipulation and blood sampling.

The extremity distal to the catheter site should be frequently assessed for adequacy of blood flow, and neurological integrity. The pressure infusor bag should always be pumped to a level higher than the systolic pressure so as to prevent reverse blood flow in the catheter, and prevent embolization at a peripheral site.

Waveform Interpretation and Clinical Applications

The normal arterial pressure produces a characteristic waveform, which has 2 main components. The initial upstroke (anacrotic limb) represents the rapid ejection of blood from the ventricle through the open aortic valve, the peak value representing the systolic pressure. This is followed by the downward trend (dicrotic limb) as the pressure begins to fall. This fall in pressure continues till it reaches a point where the pressure in the ventricle is less than the pressure in the aortic root; the aortic valve closes at this point, producing a characteristic dicrotic notch in the descending limb of the waveform. The closure of the aortic valve signals the onset of diastole, which progresses till it reaches its lowest resting level. The value at this level represents the diastolic pressure.

The configuration of the waveform and the actual pressure measurements vary depending on the catheterization site. Arteries more distal from the aorta show higher systolic and

lower diastolic pressures; hence, systolic and diastolic pressures in the peripheral arteries may not be an accurate reflection of the pressure in the aorta. However the mean pressure remains relatively constant irrespective of the anatomical site of catheterization, and it is this value which is most commonly used to derive various haemodynamic parameters. The mean pressure is measured electronically by dividing the area under the arterial waveform by the duration of the cardiac cycle. Mean pressure can also be estimated manually as the diastolic pressure + one-third the pulse pressure, but this estimate is often unreliable, and it is preferable to use the electronically derived measurement.

The size and configuration of the waveform can be altered due to abnormal physiological conditions such as severe hypertension, shock and aortic stenosis. Useful information can be obtained by careful observation of the waveform, the upstroke of the waveform being proportional to the contractility of the ventricle. The peak pressure may give a rough idea of the volume ejected, and the downstroke is proportional to both the compliance of the great vessels, and the systemic vascular resistance. However it must be noted that these observations are useful to the extent that they only roughly indicate changes in the haemodynamic status, depending on changes in an individual's waveforms over a period of time; mere interpretation of a waveform at a specific point in time cannot reflect on the patient's cardiovascular status, and may be most misleading.

An alternative approach was investigated by Parel and co-workers (4) based on the observation that significant systolic pressure variation (SPV) occurs during positive pressure ventilation. SPV is the difference between the maximum and minimum systolic blood pressures as measured from a graphic display of a waveform during one ventilatory cycle (**Fig. 4.2.4**). This experimental study (4), proposed that the raised SPV was a very sensitive marker for relative hypovolaemia, probably even more sensitive than changes in the PCWP or the CO, provided that the inspiratory airway pressure was not abnormally raised, and there were no arrhythmias during the measurements.

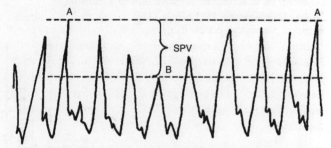

Fig. 4.2.4. Systolic pressure variation [SPV]. **A** is the maximum systolic pressure and **B** is the minimum systolic pressure during one ventilatory cycle (A-A').

Central Venous Pressure (CVP) Monitoring (5)

Central venous catheterization (see Chapter on Procedures in the ICU) provides venous access to one of the central veins, and can be used to monitor the CVP. Various anatomical sites may

Table 4.2.4. Advantages and disadvantages of various central venous sites

Site	Advantages	Disadvantages
Subclavian	* Accessible and secure * Affords unrestricted patient movements * Easy to keep the area sterile and maintain intact dressing * Allows very rapid flow	* Likely complications – Pneumothorax – Injury to subclavian artery – Haemothorax * Operator skill—advanced * Difficult to compress if bleeding occurs
Internal Jugular	* Low risk of pneumothorax * Short and direct pathway to the RA * Unrestricted arm movement * Allows very rapid flow.	* Likely complications—Injury to common carotid artery or trachea * Operator skill—advanced; more difficult in patients with short neck * Restriction of neck movements * Landmarks not very clear
Femoral	* Operator skill—easier techniques with high success rate * Most useful for emergency pacing as it is fastest pathway to the RV apex	* Likely complications – High infection rate – Ischaemia of lower limb * Difficult to maintain a sterile intact dressing.
Antecubital Site	* No major complications	* Difficult to advance the catheter * Restricted arm movements * Thrombophlebitis

be used to insert the catheter into the central vein. The advantages and disadvantages of the more commonly used sites are listed in **Table 4.2.4.** We find that the subclavian site is ideally suited for long-term monitoring, failing which the internal jugular vein is used.

Technique of CVP Measurement

The actual measurement can be done by using a simple water manometer or attaching the central line to a transducer.

Water Manometer Technique (Fig. 4.2.5) This is a simple bedside procedure which does not require any sophisticated equipment. The central venous catheter is connected to an extension tubing, the other end of which is connected to one port of a 3-way stop cock. The second port of the stop cock is connected to an intravenous fluid administration set, and the central third port is connected to a pliable tubing which is attached to a pre-calibrated manometer stand, as shown in **Fig. 4.2.5.** The zero marking on the manometer should begin at the level of the stop cock. Before proceeding with the actual measurement, the reference point should be established (see Subsection on Assembly and Calibration of the Monitoring System). In case the manometer is placed at a distance from the patient, a spirit level may be used to ensure the exact zero level. **Figs. 4.2.5 a, b** and **c** (in that order) show the 3 different positions of the stop cock in the stepwise measurement of the CVP. After turning the stop cock to the **c** position, the fluid column in the manometer which is in direct continuity with the blood in the central veins, starts falling. Observe the descent of the fluid column in the manometer tubing till it eventually stabilizes, and the reading at this level is the CVP measurement (in cm of water). Marked respiratory fluctuations in the fluid level are expected, and in fact the patient is at times encouraged to cough or breathe deeply to confirm the catheter placement in a central vein.

Transducer Monitoring Technique. The pulmonary artery catheter is used for continuous right atrial (RA) pressure and waveform monitoring. The proximal port of this multilumen catheter lies in the right atrium, and this can be directly connected to a separate transducer in a pressure monitoring system. However, an additional transducer and extra lines can be avoided by using an extra bridge tubing between the proximal (RA) port, and the distal (PA) port, as shown in **Fig. 4.2.6.** This method allows continuous pulmonary artery waveform recording, whilst the RA pressure and waveform can be easily obtained as and when required by simply turning the 2 stop cocks, situated at the 2 ends of the bridge tubing, as shown in **Fig. 4.2.6.**

Continuous RA pressure recording can also be done without the use of the pulmonary artery catheter, by directly connecting the ordinary CVP line to the pressure monitoring system.

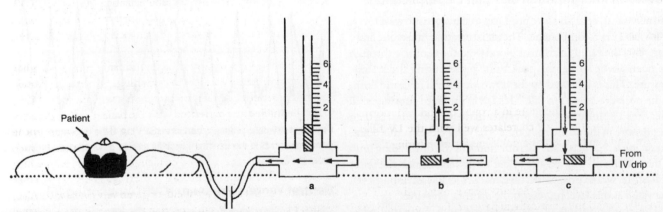

Fig. 4.2.5. CVP measurement using a water manometer with zero marking at the level of the patient's mid-axillary line. **(a)** Stop cock closed to manometer, IV to patient. **(b)** Stop cock closed to patient, IV to manometer. **(c)** Stop cock closed to IV, manometer to patient (this is the final position of the stop cock to measure CVP).

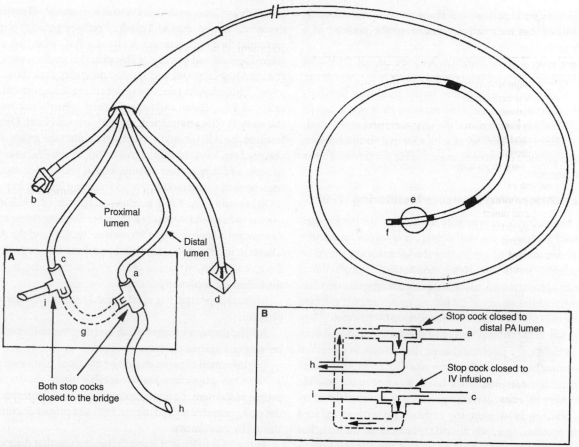

Fig. 4.2.6. Triple lumen pulmonary catheter. a = distal PA port, b = balloon inflation port, c = proximal RA port, d = thermistor hub, e = balloon, f = thermistor, g = bridge tubing connecting proximal and distal ports, h = line to 'intraflo' and transducer, i = IV infusion tubing connected to proximal lumen. **A** shows stop cock positions for continuous PA monitoring. **B** shows stop cock positions for CVP monitoring.

Clinical Application

The mean pressure in the right atrium is 0–6 mm Hg (using a transducer monitoring system), and 3–8 cm of H_2O (when using a simple water manometer), the conversion being 1 mm Hg = 1.36 cm of H_2O. The CVP catheter may be placed in the superior vena cava instead of the RA because it accurately reflects the right atrial pressure and waveforms. Placing the catheter tip in the right atrial cavity may inadvertently cause the tip to negotiate the tricuspid valve and momentarily record the higher RV pressure; this may also result in ventricular premature contractions (VPCs). However in the case of a pulmonary artery catheter, the proximal port would automatically lie in the RA.

The CVP or RA pressure reflects the right ventricular end-diastolic pressure (RVEDP). Ordinarily in healthy individuals the RVEDP and the left ventricular end-diastolic pressure (LVEDP) correlate rather well. Therefore in a young person with normal cardiac function, the CVP correlates well with the LV filling pressure, and can be used as a guideline for monitoring the LV preload during fluid therapy. *However in clinical practice, it is fallacious to assume that the CVP is a good guide to LV filling pressure in all cases;* in fact, there may be a disparity between the right and left ventricular function in critically ill patients, for more than one reason. Firstly this may occur due to right ventricular dysfunction

which may be caused by tricuspid or pulmonary valve defects, right ventricular infarcts or pulmonary hypertension. In all these conditions, the CVP will be high, and will not correctly reflect the LV preload. Secondly, it may occur due to LV dysfunction in which case the CVP will remain erroneously within normal limits instead of reflecting the high LVEDP. Because of this frequent disparity between right and left ventricular functions in critically ill patients, monitoring of the CVP alone is discouraged, and is largely being replaced by pulmonary artery catheterization (6). At best CVP monitoring may be used to urgently correct fluid depletion in hypovolaemic shock. If however the shock is prolonged, it is best to insert a pulmonary artery catheter.

CVP monitoring is of limited value, and can be most misleading if it is interpreted as an isolated reading. In order to obtain maximum benefits, serial measurements over a period of time should be studied and correlated with the patient's clinical status. This is most important when considering fluid replacement in elderly patients suspected of having cardiac dysfunction. In such patients small amounts of fluid challenge should be given whilst closely monitoring the rise in CVP. If there is a sharp rise, further fluid challenge should be withheld, or given very cautiously. Also, in such patients, a CVP value even in the lower limit of normal should be accepted as the endpoint, provided there is a significant clinical improvement in perfusion. If this is practised meticulously, CVP monitoring can be a safe alternative in the absence of a pulmonary artery catheter.

There are several other limitations to the use of CVP—for instance, if the venous tone is increased in severe hypovolaemia, the CVP may not fall in proportion to the fluid loss. Similarly patients on mechanical ventilator support may show falsely elevated CVP values due to raised intrathoracic pressure. Falsely raised CVP values may also occur with external compression of the vena cava because of a tumor mass, or due to increased intra-abdominal pressure.

Pulmonary Artery (PA) Pressure Monitoring (7–9)

As the left ventricle (LV) is primarily responsible for the forward flow of blood perfusing the vital organs, it is logical to assume that an accurate means of measuring the LV function would be the most essential part of critical care monitoring. Though clinical findings such as tachypnoea, moist lung sounds, or gallop rhythm are common manifestations of LV failure, unfortunately they are not sensitive indicators of rapidly deteriorating LV function. They may appear late in the natural history of the disease, and vital time may be lost before the haemodynamic disturbance is corrected (10). Measurement of the LV filling pressure (or LVEDP) without actually entering the left side of the heart, was first made possible by the discovery of a flow-directed pulmonary artery catheter by Swan and Ganz in 1970. Here the catheter tip with an inflated balloon just proximal to it, was floated far into one of the branches of the pulmonary artery and wedged, so that the catheter tip was in direct continuity with the left atrium (LA) via the pulmonary veins, and hence reflected the LA pressure which was the same as LVEDP, provided there was no LV inflow obstruction. In addition, the pulmonary artery catheter could measure the RA pressure through its proximal lumen, and the CO could also be measured by the thermo-dilution technique. Further, mixed venous blood could be collected from the distal lumen of the catheter for assessment of $P\bar{v}O_2$ and saturation of mixed venous oxygen ($S\bar{v}O_2$).

Indications (9, 10)

Though bedside monitoring with a balloon tip pulmonary artery catheter (PAC) has been in use since the last 30 years, controversy still persists regarding its value. However, in conditions such as septic shock or acute lung injury (ARDS), manipulation of certain haemodynamic parameters and of oxygen transport, have definitely changed the approach to therapy, with an improved outcome. There is also no dispute over the fact that constant monitoring of LV preload is mandatory whilst infusing large volumes of fluids or giving massive transfusions, especially in the elderly or in those with suspected cardiovascular dysfunction. Similarly, pulmonary wedge pressure measurements are of immense help in differentiating between cardiogenic pulmonary oedema and non-cardiogenic pulmonary oedema (11).

It is clear that PAC provides data that can be used to make therapeutic decisions as above. However, the critical question is whether these therapeutic decisions improve outcomes. Some studies have suggested that the use of PAC actually worsens outcome.

In a study by Connors et al. (12) involving critically ill patients from the intensive care units of 5 medical centres, patients with a PAC were matched with patients without a PAC who had a comparable diagnosis and severity of illness. In this analysis, patients with PAC had higher 30-day and 180-day mortality than those without a PAC. This rekindled the strong debate regarding the efficacy and safety of PAC. Dalen and Bone, in their editorial accompanying this study (13) recommended that the National Heart, Lung, Blood Institute (NHLBI) should immediately undertake an appropriately designed randomized clinical trial of use of the PAC in critically ill patients and they further recommended that if such randomized trials were not undertaken, the US Food and Drug Administration (FDA) should issue a moratorium on the use of the PAC. However, in response to the study by Connors, a joint statement by the American College of Chest Physicians (ACCP) and the American Thoracic Society (ATS) (14) stated that there was no indication for the moratorium on the use of the PAC at that time, but released the following recommendations:

(i) Further prospective randomized controlled trials of the PA catheter.

(ii) The decision to insert a PAC and its potential benefits should be weighed against the risks involved.

(iii) Informed consent should be obtained whenever possible.

(iv) Only physicians knowledgeable about the technique of proper placement, potential complications and interpretation of the data generated should use the PAC and proper documentation should be mandatory.

In the final analysis, it is worth mentioning that diagnostic tests

Table 4.2.5. Indications for pulmonary artery pressure monitoring

1. In critically ill, haemodynamically unstable patients:
   - Shock (of any aetiology)
   - Burns, sepsis, peritonitis, acute renal failure, acute lung injury, fulminant tetanus etc.
2. In cases where the diagnosis is uncertain:
   - Cardiogenic versus noncardiogenic pulmonary oedema
   - Acute respiratory failure with uncertain cardiac status
   - Acute myocardial infarction with a new loud murmur indicating acute rupture of the inter-ventricular septum, or of a papillary muscle
   - Suspected pulmonary embolism
   - In patients with acute myocardial infarction and shock, in whom hypovolaemia has to be differentiated from pump failure
3. As a therapeutic guideline under the following conditions:
   - Massive fluid replacement in patients with severe fluid loss, especially in elderly patients, or in those with a history of ischaemic heart disease
   - Fluid management in patients with non-cardiogenic pulmonary oedema (ARDS)
   - In acute haemorrhage necessitating massive transfusions, particularly in patients with associated cardiac or renal problems
   - Management of patients with shock, or other critically ill patients on inotropic and/or vasodilator drugs
   - In patients with pump failure who respond unsatisfactorily to initial therapy
4. Patients at risk of haemodynamic decompensation:
   - Pre-operative monitoring in all seriously ill patients (cardiac or non-cardiac surgery)
   - Patients with underlying cardiac disease on mechanical ventilator support with PEEP or continuous positive pressure

and monitoring devices do not alter clinical outcome, but treatment does. If PAC does not alter treatment decisions it can have no positive effect on the clinical outcome but may unnecessarily add to potential complications. Hence, to benefit patients, the PAC must provide information that is not otherwise available and that information should be useful in selecting a treatment plan that has proven clinical benefit (15). Secondly, time is of essence and there are studies which show significant improvement in outcomes, when therapy guided by PAC was given early, 8–12 hours post-operatively (16, 17).

The general indications for pulmonary artery pressure monitoring are listed in **Table 4.2.5**. These are only guidelines and there is no compulsion to adhere to them to the letter. Each individual patient should be carefully considered, and the anticipated benefits must clearly outweigh the possible risks (18). By and large this procedure should not be used too liberally in developing countries, and its use should be restricted to centres having the proper set-up, expertise and an assured aseptic environment.

Catheter Design

A wide range of catheters (from the adult to the pediatric size) are available for various clinical applications. They range from 60–110 cm in length, 4–7.5 Fr in calibre, with balloon inflation volumes ranging from 0.5–1.5 ml. The catheter material is polyvinyl chloride which is pliable at room temperature, and softens further at body temperature. The simplest type of catheter contains only 2 lumens, one to transmit pulmonary artery pressures, and the other for balloon inflation; however, the most commonly used one is the sophisticated triple-lumen thermodilution catheter. In fact, there are various types of catheters available and their use depends on the clinician's choice.

The triple lumen 7.5 Fr thermodilution PA catheter (**Fig. 4.2.6**) is 110 cm in length. The lumen of the distal PA port (a) runs through the length of the catheter to terminate at the tip, and is used to measure the pulmonary artery pressure (PAP), and the pulmonary capillary wedge pressure (PCWP); mixed venous blood can also be drawn from this lumen. Drugs and hyperosmotic solutions should never be administered from the distal lumen as they may induce a local vascular or tissue reaction in a small pulmonary artery segment. The balloon inflation port (b) opens to a lumen that terminates within the balloon (e), which is situated just proximal to the catheter tip. The proximal RA port (c) opens to a lumen that terminates 30 cm from the tip of the catheter and lies in the right atrium (RA), when the tip of the catheter is in the PA. The RA port is used for monitoring RA pressure and also for administration of fluids. The RA port is also used to inject ice-cold saline during CO measurement. (d) represents the thermistor hub which is connected by wires to a small thermistor (f) located 3.5–4 cm proximal to the catheter tip. The thermistor records changes in the temperature over change in time during CO measurement; this is then relayed to an outside computer via the thermistor hub.

Four-lumen thermodilution catheters are also available; these have an additional venous infusion lumen which provides separate access to the RA, and allows continuous infusion of fluids, even during CO measurement. The same four-lumen catheter has been recently modified by moving this venous infusion port distally so as to open 10 cm from the tip, and lie in the right ventricle (RV), when the catheter tip lies in the pulmonary artery. This lumen is not used now for infusing fluids, but for continuously monitoring the RV waveform. This modified catheter, referred to as a 'position monitoring catheter' is an excellent innovation as it prevents distal migration of the catheter into the small branches of the pulmonary arteries (19, 20). If the catheter should inadvertently migrate to a distal wedge position by even a few cm, there will be a change from RV waveform to PA waveform, signaling the need to withdraw the catheter back to a position that restores the RV waveform. Four-lumen thermodilution catheters are also available with a RV lumen that terminates 19 cm from the distal tip, to provide for passage of pacing wires whenever cardiac pacing is indicated during haemodynamic monitoring.

The newer 'S-tip' catheters are designed for femoral vein insertion; similarly stiffer catheters (Swan-Ganz Hi-Shore from Baxter) are available, and may be used when more torque control and manoeuvrability are needed, particularly during a femoral approach. Some new catheters available today are treated with antimicrobials and coated with heparin. A *fibreoptic thermodilution PA catheter* is also available for continuous monitoring of mixed venous oxygen (M$\bar{v}O_2$); this has an additional channel that contains 2 fiberoptic bundles for light transmission. The light transmitted from outside is reflected back from the haemoglobin in the blood to a photo-detector, which calculates the fraction of Hb saturated with oxygen, and displays it continuously on a bedside monitor.

Insertion Technique

Balloon catheters float easily from the vena cava to the pulmonary wedge pressure position, and knowledge of the various intracardiac waveforms is generally sufficient to be able to insert the catheter. Bedside fluoroscopy is not mandatory, and fluoroscopic equipment can be very cumbersome in an already small and cluttered ICU room. Besides, each patient's bed needs to be specially designed for imaging purposes, thereby adding to the overall cost. However in cases with abnormal intracardiac flow patterns due to raised right ventricular pressures, the flow direction of the catheter may become very difficult and fluoroscopic guidance becomes necessary.

Percutaneously, a Seldinger technique is usually employed, which leaves an introducer catheter in situ through which the PA catheter is easily passed. These procedures have been described in detail in the Chapter on Procedures in the Intensive Care Unit. There is no ideal site for pulmonary artery catheter insertion, and this choice depends entirely on the operator's preference and expertise. In our unit we prefer the subclavian site for reasons discussed earlier (**Table 4.2.4**). The jugular and femoral veins are the other two common accesses, particularly if subclavian puncture is contraindicated for any reason. Many operators prefer to use the left subclavian vein as this approach offers the easiest route from the site of insertion to the RV due to its unidirectional bend.

Before insertion of the pulmonary artery catheter, the pressure monitoring system should be set-up and kept ready as described earlier in this chapter. The catheter tip should be 'jiggled' before

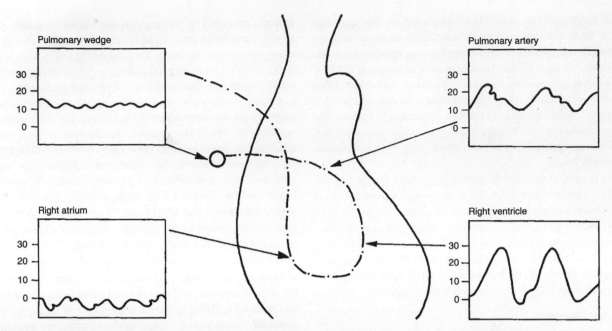

Fig. 4.2.7. Pressure waveform configuration as seen during the passage of the pulmonary artery catheter through the various chambers of the heart and in wedge position. The position of the catheter shown here is as seen on fluoroscopy.

insertion, and this produces sharp oscillations on the monitor. If no oscillations occur, there is probably an equipment malfunction which should be corrected. The balloon should be tested by inflating with air as per the manufacturer's recommendations. After ascertaining the integrity of the balloon, the catheter is flushed with a sterile solution to ensure its patency and to remove all air. The thermistor's electrical continuity should also be checked before insertion, by connecting the thermistor hub of the catheter to the CO monitor and checking for any faults. The external surface of the catheter is usually wiped with wet gauze soaked with sterile saline, as this helps to reduce vein irritation. However, one should avoid wiping heparin-coated catheters, as this may remove the heparin coating.

Now with the balloon deflated, introduce the catheter through the introducer sheath into a central vein. Before advancing the catheter further, it is advisable to follow the markings on the catheter, as this gives a fair idea of the distance the catheter has travelled from the insertion point. In a normal adult to reach the RA, the catheter has to be advanced 10–15 cm from the subclavian vein, 15–20 cm from the right jugular vein, and 30–40 cm from the femoral vein. Under continuous pressure monitoring, with or without fluoroscopy, gently advance the catheter into the RA. Entry of the catheter tip into the thorax is signaled by increased respiratory fluctuations of the waveform. Once in the RA, inflate the balloon with air or carbon dioxide to the recommended volume (printed on the catheter). Never use fluids to inflate the balloon. In the presence of intracardiac shunts, CO_2 should be used instead of air for inflation of the balloon, in order to avoid systemic air embolization in case of accidental balloon rupture. Further passage of the catheter from the RA to the pulmonary wedge position should normally not take longer than 30–40 seconds, provided there is no abnormal flow pattern in the heart or markedly elevated

RV pressures. The shape of the waveform and RV, PA and PCWP pressure readings are used as a guide in advancing the catheter (**Fig. 4.2.7**). On entering the RV, the waveform is characterized by a steep upstroke, which is normally 3–4 times higher than the RA pressure. The sharp downstroke without a dicrotic notch dips to near zero, and then rises to reach a baseline plateau which directly records the RVEDP, and is equal to the mean RA pressure. On advancing the catheter further into the pulmonary artery, another change in pressure waveform is noted, and this can be immediately differentiated from the RV waveform by the sudden elevation of the diastolic pressure and the appearance of the dicrotic notch. In the pulmonary vasculature the inflated balloon acts as a sail, and continues with the flowing stream into the more peripheral branch of the pulmonary circulation where it will wedge. The catheter tip will now record a pulmonary wedge pressure tracing which is very similar to the RA waveform (**Fig. 4.2.7**).

Correct Wedging Procedure

The balloon should not be allowed to remain inflated in the occluded position beyond 10–15 seconds. Inflation beyond this period can lead to pulmonary infarction. In addition, artefactually elevated pressures may result due to prolonged wedging. Upon deflating the balloon, the catheter recoils back towards the hilum into the main branch of the PA, and the PA waveform reappears. If the wedge tracings continue even after the balloon is deflated, the catheter should be carefully withdrawn to a point where PA waveforms reappear. The pulmonary wedge tracing should be obtained on reinflating the balloon to the recommended inflation volume; if the inflation volume is significantly lower than that recommended to produce a wedge trace, it implies that the catheter tip is still placed too far peripherally.

It is vital to remember that the mean pulmonary artery wedge pressure which is normally equal to pulmonary artery diastolic pressure (PADP), may be lower in certain conditions associated with increased pulmonary vascular resistance (PVR). However, the PCWP is never higher than the PADP, and if so, it represents an artefact.

Lastly the blood sample withdrawn from the catheter which is truly wedged, should represent and be equal to the oxygen saturation of arterial blood, whereas blood drawn from the pulmonary artery with the balloon deflated, gives the oxygen saturation of mixed venous blood, averaging 75 per cent.

Normally if there is a good correlation between PADP and PCWP, the PADP should be used to estimate the left atrial pressures instead of rewedging the catheter frequently. This reduces the risk of pulmonary vascular damage and pulmonary infarction, and also prolongs the balloon life.

Complications of Pulmonary Artery Catheterization (21)

All complications associated with a cutdown procedure or a percutaneous central venous catheterization can occur during PA catheterization. These complications have been discussed separately under the appropriate techniques in the Chapter on Procedures in the Intensive Care Unit. The following complications are directly attributable to pulmonary artery catheterization:

(i) Arrhythmias. The occurrence of arrhythmias, and of ventricular ectopics in particular, are common during insertion of the catheter. The incidence is higher in patients with ischaemic heart disease, ventricular failure, hypoxaemia, digitalis toxicity, metabolic and electrolyte imbalance, and in patients with shock. The risk of arrhythmias can be minimized by decreasing the insertion time; in the high-risk group it would be best to use fluoroscopy, so that less manoeuvring of the catheter is necessary. If arrhythmias persist even after ensuring that the catheter tip is well placed in the PA, and the catheter is not looped in any other cardiac chamber, it should be promptly removed.

(ii) Infection. A meticulous sterile technique during insertion, and strict attention to asepsis in the aftercare of the catheter, particularly during CO studies, is vital in order to reduce the incidence of infection. Among other factors that increase the potential risk of local and systemic infection, the most important ones are prolonged indwelling time, and repeated manipulation of the catheter with entry of the non-sterile portion of the catheter into the vascular system. Critically ill patients are commonly immunocompromised, and are frequently at a higher risk for catheter-induced infections.

(iii) Balloon Rupture. Inflation of the balloon is typically associated with a feeling of resistance, and absence of this resistance coupled with a failure to wedge, suggest balloon rupture. In case of balloon rupture, if there is a good correlation between PCWP and PADP the balloon does not need to be used; in such cases, the catheter need not be replaced, but a piece of tape labelled 'balloon rupture' should be stuck on to the balloon port. Nonetheless, a remote but potential risk of embolization of balloon fragments to the distal pulmonary circulation remains.

(iv) Knotting. Small calibre catheters are more likely to form knots within the cardiac chambers, around intracardiac structures, and around other intravascular catheters. Knots may be resolved by insertion of suitable guidewires and manipulation under fluoroscopy. If the knot does not include any intracardiac structure, gentle traction may be applied to tighten the knot, and then withdrawn slowly. In the worst cases, a thoracotomy and cardiotomy may be required for catheter removal.

(v) Thromboembolic Complications. Clots occluding the catheter lumen or the tip can result in inaccurate pulmonary artery pressure or CO measurements. This can be avoided by intermittent flushing of the catheter line with heparinized saline. Thrombotic occlusion can also occur in the systemic veins or in the RA due to long-standing catheter placements, and these patients are at high risk of pulmonary embolism. Heparin-coated catheters may reduce catheter thrombogenecity.

(vi) Pulmonary Infarction. Persistent or repeated wedging of the pulmonary artery catheter, inadvertent migration of the catheter tip into a small branch of the pulmonary artery, or prolonged inflation of the balloon in the wedged position, can lead to pulmonary infarction. Precautions mentioned below for preventing pulmonary artery rupture, if meticulously observed, will go a long way in preventing this complication as well.

(vii) Pulmonary Artery Rupture. PA rupture following PA catheterization though rare, is the most dreaded of all complications as it is associated with a very high mortality rate. Perforation of the artery can be caused by the catheter tip directly, if it is forcibly advanced into a peripheral branch, or by overinflation of the balloon. The risk of perforation is greater in older patients, in patients with pulmonary hypertension, or in those receiving anticoagulation.

PA rupture may clinically present as haemoptysis. In most cases there is mild haemoptysis to begin with, and if ignored this may progress to massive haemorrhage.

To avoid this catastrophic complication it is important to observe the following points: (a) Avoid overinflation or prolonged inflation of the balloon in the wedged position. (b) Avoid inserting the catheter too far peripherally into a branch of the pulmonary artery. If the catheter is more than 3 cm beyond the hilum, there is an increased chance of infarction or rupture, and the tip should be pulled back. Position-monitoring catheters as described earlier, are useful indicators of unsuspected distal catheter migration. (c) If PADP equals PCWP, it is best to continuously monitor the PADP instead of repeatedly wedging the catheter to measure the PCWP.

Pitfalls in Pulmonary Artery Pressure Measurement

Several practical factors may be crucial in obtaining meaningful information whilst performing haemodynamic studies. Problems related to pressure lines, transducers, and monitors which commonly manifest as overdamped or underdamped waveforms, are common to both arterial and venous catheterizations. Similarly improper 'zero levelling' and whip artefacts may be seen. All these problems have been discussed earlier in the Subsection on Pressure Monitoring System (**Table 4.2.2**). In addition to all these

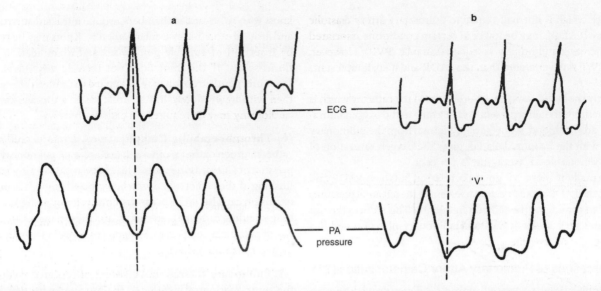

Fig. 4.2.8. Identification of 'v' wave by superimposing the ECG on the pressure tracings. (a) PA tracing with the balloon deflated; the upstroke of the PA systolic wave starts near to the end of the QRS. (b) Balloon-inflated wedge tracing with superimposed 'v' wave which is delayed by 200–300 msec after the QRS (see text).

problems PA waveforms in particular, are affected by cardiac dysfunction and by changes in intrathoracic pressures.

Cardiac Dysfunction. The PCWP waveforms consist of 2 distinct peaks—the 'a' and the 'v' waves. The first pressure peak, the 'a' wave, represents the increase in LA pressure during atrial contraction at the end of diastole. The 'a' wave correlates with the PR interval on the ECG, and may be elevated whenever there is increased resistance to LV filling as in LV failure, or in any condition with decreased LV compliance; the mean PCWP however may not rise proportionately to the LVEDP, thus making their interrelationship less reliable. In such a situation the 'a' wave peak pressure and not the mean PCWP, best reflects the LV filling pressure as it closely approximates the LVEDP.

More problematic during catheterization is the 'v' wave which occurs in the presence of mitral insufficiency or significant mitral valve prolapse. This is a large 'v' wave transmitted retrogradely from the LV, which is superimposed on the PCWP wave, thereby exaggerating its size; this may be wrongly interpreted as a pulmonary waveform even though the catheter is in the fully wedged position.

The 'v' wave should be suspected if no PCWP waveform is seen despite the catheter being properly positioned in the wedge position. This can be confirmed by superimposing an ECG strip on both the balloon-inflated and balloon-deflated pressure tracings (**Fig. 4.2.8**). The 'v' wave of the wedge waveform in the balloon-inflated tracing will be delayed by 200–300 msec after the QRS, whereas the upstroke of the PA systolic wave starts near the end of the QRS as shown in **Fig. 4.2.8**.

Clinically, identification of 'v' waves is important from 2 points of view. Firstly, once it is identified as a true PCWP waveform, and not a pulmonary artery waveform, the catheter need not be advanced any further into the peripheral pulmonary artery branch. Secondly, the correct pulmonary artery occlusion pressure should be read just prior to the upstroke of the 'v' wave.

Artefacts due to Ventilatory Effects

(i) Spontaneous Breathing. During normal quiet breathing, inspiration or chest expansion requires a slightly negative intrapleural pressure (subatmospheric), whilst expiration requires a slightly positive intrapleural pressure (near atmospheric). These cyclic changes in the intrathoracic pressure are transmitted to the intravascular pressure tracings, creating a minimally wandering baseline, with expiration producing positive deflections, and inspiration producing negative deflections. These pressure changes are insignificant, and minimally affect the mean PCWP. However, in case of marked laboured breathing, as in patients with acute lung injury or COPD, greater swings in pleural pressures are required to move air in and out of the lungs. As a result there is a wide fluctuation in the pressure waveform baseline. This leads to inconsistent and inaccurate recordings. In such a situation it is best to disregard the digital display and record a long tracing of the PAP or PCWP waveforms, and read that portion of the waveform that corresponds with end-expiration. It should however be noted that in patients on mechanical ventilation, the end-expiration is reflected by the negative deflection of the wandering pressure baseline.

(ii) Influence of Gravity (22). Pulmonary artery pressures increase progressively down the lung, as the blood flow increases in the lower parts of the lung due to the influence of gravity. However, the alveolar pressures remain equal throughout. West divided the lung model conceptually into 3 zones, called the West Zones (**Fig. 4.2.9**), which illustrated the interrelationship between the alveolar and vascular pressures and the effect of gravity.

Zone 1 is the uppermost portion of the lung or apex in an upright person. This is an area with potentially low vascular pressure, hence alveolar pressures here exceed both the PAP and the pulmonary venous pressure (PVP) (Alveolar pressure > PAP > PVP). If a wedged catheter tip is placed in this position, it will

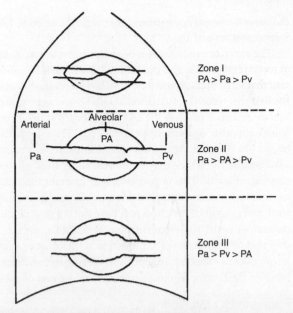

Fig. 4.2.9. Interrelationship between the alveolar and vascular pressures in the three West Zones. PA = alveolar pressure; Pa = pulmonary artery pressure; Pv = pulmonary venous pressure (see text for details).

not reflect the LA pressure as the continuous conduit between the catheter tip and the LA is occluded by the higher alveolar pressure, but will reflect only the alveolar pressure.

Zone 2 is represented by the middle portion of the lung and here too the alveolar pressure is > PVP, but < PAP. However, during end-expiration and inspiration the alveolar pressure is at its lowest, and does not occlude the pulmonary veins, thus allowing the wedged catheter tip to accurately reflect the LA pressure; however during end-inspiration and early expiration, the elevated alveolar pressure will pinch the pulmonary veins, and the wedged catheter once again shows an erroneously high PCWP.

Zone 3 is at the bottom of the lung, where there is increased blood flow due to gravity, and vascular pressures are greatest. Hence both the PAP and the PVP far exceed the pulmonary alveolar pressure, producing a constant open vascular conduit from the catheter tip to the LA which allows the PCWP to accurately reflect the LA pressure in all phases of respiration.

To confirm the Zone 3 catheter position one should constantly be able to identify the wedge waveform. A damp tracing in absence of other problems suggests a Zone 1 or Zone 2 position. A lateral chest X-ray can also ascertain the proper catheter position; a Zone 3 position can be confirmed if the catheter tip is seen to lie at, or below the left atrial level. Lastly in patients on positive end-expiratory pressure (PEEP), the PCWP should not be influenced by sudden increase or decrease in PEEP levels if the catheter is properly positioned in Zone 3 (**23**).

The three zones described above hold true for an individual in an erect position, and as measurements are so often made with the patient upright or semi-inclined, it is important to place the catheter tip at or below the left atrial level, confirming the Zone 3 condition. However, in the supine position, most of the alveolar capillary units fall in the gravity-dependent area of the lung having the characteristics of Zone 3 condition, and as most

of the blood flows in this area, the PA catheter invariably floats into Zone 3.

(iii) Effects of Mechanical Ventilation and PEEP. Positive changes in the airway pressures produced by mechanical ventilation reflect on the heart and vascular structures of the thorax. This can lead to inaccurate measurements and wrong interpretation of haemodynamic parameters for three reasons.

(a) Measured PAP and PCWP will increase during the delivery of each mechanical breath. However the pressure at end-expiration should be the same as with spontaneous breathing, and therefore it is important that the measurements are recorded at end-expiration.

(b) Mechanical ventilation has the potential to decrease cardiac output by increasing the intrathoracic pressure and thus reducing the venous return to the heart. In addition the positive pressure surrounding the heart may produce a tamponade effect, further interfering with the diastolic filling. Though the CO may fall, the CVP, PAP and PCWP may rise because of perivascular compression distorting the volume-pressure relationship. In other words, pressures that appear to be normal may be insufficient to ensure adequate preload and CO.

(c) Positive alveolar pressure may increase the Zone 1 and 2 conditions, so that a considerable anatomical area of Zone 3 now takes on the characteristics of Zones 1 and 2, especially if the PAP is low. This will lead to inaccurate measurements as PCWP will no longer reflect the LA pressure correctly, even though the catheter tip seems to lie in Zone 3 on X-ray.

All these above-mentioned effects of mechanical ventilation will be exaggerated in patients on either PEEP, or continuous positive airway pressure (CPAP). Generally PEEP levels < 10 cm of H_2O do not compromise the measurements of PCWP or CO very significantly. However, PEEP levels > 10–15 cm H_2O certainly increase the disparity between the PCWP and LA pressure relationship, and also compromise cardiovascular function.

In order to obtain more accurate LA pressure measurements by measuring PCWP in patients on high levels of PEEP, one has to assume that approximately 50 per cent of the PEEP is transmitted to the LA. As PEEP is measured in cm of water, and PCWP in mm Hg, a simple calculation would be to subtract 1.5 mm Hg pressure from PCWP for every 5 cm of H_2O of PEEP administered (as 1 mm Hg = 1.36 cm H_2O). For example if a PCWP of 28 mm Hg is recorded in a patient on PEEP of 20 cm H_2O, the patient's corrected LA pressure should read 6 mm Hg less i.e. 22 mm Hg.

Many clinicians prefer to disconnect the patient from the mechanical ventilator during PCWP measurements; this practice should however be discouraged. As long as the pressure tracings show the characteristic PCWP waveforms, and one-half of PEEP is approximately subtracted from the PCWP, it seems reasonable to measure the pressures that apply to the patient during therapy, rather than during a brief interval without it. On the other hand, on discontinuing mechanical ventilation or PEEP, a sudden change in haemodynamics occurs because of an increase in venous return, and the measured parameters may be different from those that exist when the patient is on ventilator support.

Cardiac Output Measurement by the Thermodilution Technique (24)

The Fick oxygen consumption method described by Adolph Fick in 1870, is usually considered to be the gold standard to which other methods are compared because of its extreme accuracy in measuring the CO. However this method is not practical for day-to-day use in the ICU as it is time consuming, and requires the patient to be in a steady metabolic state.

The indicator dye dilution technique is another method of measuring cardiac output, but this too is not a practical bedside procedure.

The thermodilution technique is currently the most widely used method in clinical practice. Though first introduced by Fegler in 1954, its first reported use in humans was published by Margaret Branthwaite and Ronald Bradley in 1968. The basic principle underlying this method is the detection of the change in temperature of blood over a period of time; this can be accomplished by injecting cold saline in the RA from a proximal port of the PA catheter, whilst the thermistor on the catheter tip detects the temperature change in the PA. This change is inversely proportional to the blood flow.

Procedure

The main equipment required for CO monitoring is the cardiac output computer, and a thermodilution pulmonary artery catheter. Also needed are five to six 10 ml sterile plastic syringes, an injectate solution (usually ice cold normal saline), an injectate temperature probe and catheter connecting cables. It goes without saying that aseptic precautions should be observed throughout the procedure. The patient should be preferably supine, but a semi-reclined position (< 20°) should not alter the CO. A more erect position, particularly in critically ill patients on potent vasodilators, can produce orthostatic hypotension; hence in such patients relative changes in position during serial measurements can affect the reliability of the cardiac output readings.

Prior to injection, the position of the thermodilution catheter should be ascertained. The catheter tip must lie in the pulmonary artery and should not be in the wedged position. The balloon must be deflated prior to injection and the thermistor hub should be connected to the CO monitor via the catheter connecting cable. The injectate probe should be connected to the CO computer, with the sterile probe dipped into the injectate solution.

10 ml of 0.9 per cent saline or 5 per cent dextrose (ice cold solution or solution at room temperature, depending on the method used), is injected within 4 seconds as a bolus through the proximal port of the PA catheter. Lesser volumes, or prolonged injection times can give unreliable measurements. The cold solution mixes with the blood in the right heart chamber lowering the blood temperature, the cooled blood flows into the PA, and the thermistor at the catheter tip records the temperature change and relays this information to the CO monitor. The CO computer calculates the temperature difference between the injectate solution and the blood, and displays the temperature-time curve. The area under the curve is inversely proportional to the flow rate in the PA, which is representative of the CO.

The injectate used need not be an ice cold solution, as solutions at room temperature also produce reliable results. It is also important that serial measurements should be obtained, after discarding the first trial which is often unreliable. The average value of three measurements is taken as the CO, provided that they do not differ from each other by more than 15 per cent. The injections should be always timed during end-expiration to avoid unacceptable variations in CO which may occur during different phases of the respiratory cycle. This is particularly important for patients on mechanical ventilator support. However it may be impossible to start and complete injection precisely during one phase of the respiratory cycle. To overcome this practical difficulty, it is reasonable to time the starting of the injection at the onset of inspiration; it may take 2–4 seconds to reach the thermistor, and this should produce the thermodilution curve close to the end of expiration.

Pitfalls in CO Monitoring

Erroneous CO readings may be produced by conditions such as tricuspid regurgitation, or by a clot partially blocking the catheter lumen, or due to intracardiac shunts. In case of right to left shunts, the CO is falsely high because part of the cold injectate crosses the shunt and the temperature difference sensed by the thermistor in the PA is less; in left to right shunts, falsely elevated readings are obtained as the blood volume in the right side of the heart is increased, and the injectate is diluted, once again decreasing the temperature difference in the PA, and producing a curve with a reduced height.

Besides other technical points, the temperature and volume of the injectate solution must be precisely determined to avoid errors in CO measurements. A larger volume will produce a greater temperature change in the pulmonary circulation, which is interpreted by the monitor as a low CO. Conversely, a lesser volume will produce a smaller temperature change, which will be interpreted as a high CO.

If the injectate solution is at room temperature, producing very minor temperature changes, the serial CO readings will be less reproducible. This is therefore the practical disadvantage of using a room temperature injectate instead of an ice cold solution. Similarly the reproducibility of the measurements may be affected despite using iced injectate, if there is a significant temperature change between the time the solution is drawn and the time it is injected. However several systems are available today that measure the injectate temperature at the time it enters the proximal port of the pulmonary artery catheter. This minimizes injectate temperature errors, and improves the reproducibility of the measurements.

Continuous CO Monitoring

Continuous CO measurements using thermodilution techniques are also available. Instead of cold water, a small heating filament at the end of the catheter warms pulmonary blood and a downstream sensor records changes in temperature. These measurements are found to lag behind by a few minutes, but they are reliable and able to provide near real-time cardiac outputs.

Minimally Invasive and Non-invasive Methods of Determining Cardiac Output (25)

Thoracic Electrical Bioimpedence (26, 27)

This is a non-invasive technique of measuring CO. The technique is based on correlating changes in aortic flow throughout the cardiac cycle with changes in electrical impedance of the thoracic cavity. This technique has shown good correlation with invasive methods in spontaneously breathing patients; however, this correlation may vary in patients on mechanical ventilation or on PEEP. Many other conditions resulting in electrical field distortions produced by pleural fluid, pulmonary oedema, haemothorax, pneumonia, etc. could result in appreciable differences in the CO readings as compared to thermodilution calculations. There is also a group of clinical conditions (e.g. end-stage cirrhosis, hyperdynamic states, tachyarrhythmias), where the percentage of aortic blood flow occurring in systole is appreciably less and in these conditions the estimation of CO by impedence method may be less than that calculated by thermodilution method.

Transoesophageal Doppler Monitoring (28, 29)

This involves inserting of a flexible probe into the mid-thoracic oesophagus. A pulse wave Doppler transducer in the probe tip calculates blood flow velocity from the Doppler frequency shift of RBCs in the descending aorta. By entering the age, gender, height and weight of the patient, the aortic diameter can be estimated. From this and the blood flow velocity, aortic blood flow is calculated, representing approximately 70 per cent of the total CO. Estimates of preload and afterload can be derived from the shape of the velocity waveforms. Modifications of this technique allow for the actual measurement of aortic diameter using M-mode ultrasound, eliminating the error associated with normogram-based estimates. The resulting values for aortic blood flow correlate well with those of thermodilution CO.

Lithium Dilution (30)

A relatively new technique, less invasive than PAC, but requires central venous and intra-arterial catheters. This method involves injection of a small dose of lithium chloride in a central venous catheter and the plasma concentration is then measured by a special sensor connected to an arterial line and the CO is calculated.

Lithium dilution compares well with thermodilution technique. However, the accumulation of lithium with repeated dosing is a potential concern which could probably limit its use.

CO_2 Based Techniques (31)

These provide a non-invasive measure of CO in patients receiving mechanical ventilation. This method, which is based on the Fick's principle, involves transient partial rebreathing of CO_2 and the measurement of changes in CO_2 elimination and end-tidal CO_2 (a measure of arterial CO_2). Based on these values, the CO component participating in gas exchange is calculated.

The main limitation of this technique is that it can only be done on intubated and mechanically ventilated patients.

In the future, it is possible that multiple non-invasive physiological methods may be used in the initial screening of acutely ill patients. These non-invasive monitoring systems seem to compare well with the invasive methods despite many limitations. However, the non-invasive display of early small changes can be assessed and treated before they progress to life-threatening proportions. Early deficits are usually easy to correct effectively, whereas late effects of shock and hypovolaemia may be irreversible.

Haemodynamic Variables and their Clinical Application

Determinants of Ventricular Performance

Pulmonary artery monitoring allows us to obtain various haemo-dynamic variables which are either directly measured, or derived by using specific calculations (**Table 4.2.6**). These help us to understand the determinants of cardiac performance, and factors influencing oxygen transport, thereby providing a better perception of cardiovascular haemodynamics at the bedside.

The *stroke volume* (SV) is the volume of blood ejected by the heart during each contraction, and is a very important indicator of ventricular performance. It is calculated by dividing the CO by the heart rate, and when indexed to the body surface area (BSA), the normal stroke volume index (SI) is arrived at (normal range is 35–45 ml/m^2). The three most important physiological determinants of SV are preload, afterload and myocardial contractility.

Table 4.2.6. Normal haemodynamic values

Variables	Abbreviations	Units	Normal range
Right atrial pressure	RAP	mm Hg	0–6
Mean pulmonary artery pressure	MPAP	mm Hg	11–15
Pulmonary capillary wedge pressure	PCWP	mm Hg	3–15
Cardiac index	CI	l/min-m^2	2.8–3.6
Left ventricular stroke work index	LVSWI	gm-m/m^2	44–68
Right ventricular stroke work index	RVSWI	gm-m/m^2	4–8
Systemic vascular resistance index	SVRI	dynes-sec/cm^5-m^2	1700–2600
Pulmonary vascular resistance index	PVRI	dynes-sec/cm^5-m^2	100–225
Oxygen delivery index	$\dot{D}O_2I$	ml/min-m^2	500–650
Oxygen consumption index	$\dot{V}O_2I$	ml/min-m^2	110–150

Preload refers to the length of the cardiac muscle fibres at the start of ventricular contraction; this is equal to the left ventricular end-diastolic volume (LVEDV), and is clinically measured as left ventricular end-diastolic pressure (LVEDP). The PCWP which is directly measured by a well-positioned pulmonary artery catheter, in the absence of left ventricular inflow obstruction, gives an indication of the relative changes in the preload. However this is true only if the ventricular compliance is static; in a diseased heart the LVEDP and the LVEDV may not correlate as the ventricular compliance is altered. For instance in dilated cardiomyopathy, the ventricular compliance increases, and a large increase in the ventricular filling volume is accompanied by only a small change in the filling pressure. On the other hand, in a stiff non-compliant ventricle seen in ischaemic or fibrotic heart disease, the ventricular filling pressure increases disproportionately to the ventricular filling volume. Hence the clinical importance of maintaining a slightly higher LVEDP in cases of acute myocardial infarction, in order to achieve an adequate CO, cannot be overstressed.

Afterload is defined as the impedance to blood flow from the ventricle. Whilst preload determines the force of the ventricular contraction, afterload denotes the tension developed by the cardiac muscle during systole as a result of systemic vascular resistance (SVR). Resistance is typically calculated as a pressure gradient divided by mean flow. Hence the resistances to the two ventricles (indexed to the BSA) are derived by the following equations:

$$SVRI = \frac{\text{Mean arterial blood pressure} - CVP}{\text{Cardiac Index}} \times 80$$

$$PVRI = \frac{\text{Mean pulmonary artery pressure} - PCWP}{\text{Cardiac Index}} \times 80$$

The normal range of values is given in **Table 4.2.6**.

The SVRI is usually raised in cardiogenic and hypovolaemic shock, in systemic hypertension, and with the use of vasoconstrictor drugs. It is characteristically low in septic shock, thyrotoxicosis, anaemia, cirrhosis and with vasodilator therapy. The PVRI is primarily raised in pulmonary oedema, following pulmonary embolism, and in some valvular or congenital heart diseases. It is also raised in hypoxaemia, due to pulmonary vasoconstriction.

Contractility is the inotropic state of the cardiac muscle, and may be expressed as the velocity of muscle fibre shortening during systole. It is important to realize that contractility is independent of preload or afterload, and at present we have no bedside method of monitoring cardiac contractility. However, if two of the three fundamental factors determining SV (viz. preload and afterload) can be kept constant, then obviously the changes in stroke work performed by the ventricle become the determinant of ventricular function, and give a good idea of the inotropic state of the heart. The stroke work for the two ventricles (indexed to the BSA), is calculated as follows:

$$LVSWI = SI \times (MAP - PCWP) \times 0.0136 \text{ gm.m/m}^2$$
$$RVSWI = SI \times (MPAP - CVP) \times 0.0136 \text{ gm.m/m}^2$$

The normal range of values is given in **Table 4.2.6**.

The basic relationship between preload, afterload and con-

tractility is best described by Starling's pressure curves, which are plotted by obtaining responses of LV filling pressure (PCWP) and SV to fluid challenge. LV performance can be judged by plotting such a curve; however, one cannot be sure if a good or poor response is due to increased or decreased contractility, or is secondary to an alteration in the afterload.

Determinants of Overall Circulatory Function and Tissue Perfusion

The overall measurement of peripheral circulation may be calculated using $\dot{D}O_2$, which is the product of CO and arterial O_2 content. This is the amount of O_2 delivered to the tissues per minute and can spontaneously increase in the face of trauma, sepsis and other forms of stress, representing a compensatory response to an inadequate tissue oxygenation. A limited circulatory reserve may be revealed by failure of the $\dot{D}O_2$ to increase even after adequate fluid challenge or inotropic support.

Indexed to BSA, $\dot{D}O_2$ is calculated as

$$\dot{D}O_2I = CI \times CaO_2 \times 10$$

where CaO_2 is the arterial O_2 content. The normal range of $\dot{D}O_2I = 500–650$ ml/min/m^2.

Tissue perfusion at present is difficult to measure directly but in routine practice it is conveniently inferred from the clinical signs of shock. However, quantitative measurement of tissue oxygenation, may be best evaluated by oxygen consumption ($\dot{V}O_2$) which is the product of CO and the arteriovenous O_2 content diffusion. Indexed to BSA, $\dot{V}O_2$ is calculated as

$$\dot{V}O_2I = CI \times C(a-\bar{v})O_2 \times 10$$

where $C(a-\bar{v})O_2$ is the arteriovenous O_2 content difference.

The normal range of $\dot{V}O_2I = 110–150$ ml/min/m^2. An increase in $\dot{V}O_2$ indicates an increase in metabolic demands as a result of sepsis, trauma, burns, etc. Because O_2 cannot be stored in the tissues, $\dot{V}O_2$ must match metabolic requirements of O_2 by the tissues. In conditions where $\dot{D}O_2$ can vary widely, adjustments in O_2 extraction by the tissues play an important role in maintaining O_2 uptake. This is accomplished by compensatory adjustments in O_2 extraction ratio (O_2ER) in response to changes in $\dot{D}O_2$. O_2ER is thus the balance between $\dot{V}O_2$ and $\dot{D}O_2$ i.e. $O_2ER = \dot{V}O_2/\dot{D}O_2$.

Haemodynamic parameters can be greatly influenced by drug therapy which may rapidly change the haemodynamic status of a critically ill patient. Hence it is important to know the pharmacological influence of the drugs commonly used in the ICU, on the haemodynamic variables (**Table 4.2.7**).

Table 4.2.7. Haemodynamic changes caused by some commonly used IV drugs

Drug	HR	MAP	PCWP	CO	SVR
Nitroprusside	↑	↓	NC or ↓	↑	↓
Nitroglycerin	↑	↓	↓	↑	↓
Norepinephrine	NC or ↑	↑	↑	↑ ↓, NC,↑	↑
Dopamine*	NC or ↑	NC or ↑	NC or ↑	↑	↑
Dobutamine	NC or ↑	NC or ↑	NC	↑	NC
Amrinone	NC	↓	↓	↑	↓

NC = No change; *Dose related; ↑ = increased; ↓ = decreased.

Mixed Venous Oxygen Saturation (SvO₂)

Saturation of mixed venous oxygen (SṽO₂) is the saturation of mixed venous blood returning from the systemic circulation to the pulmonary circulation to be reoxygenated. It is usually, though not always, a good indicator of the adequacy of tissue oxygenation and it reflects the balance between oxygen demand and supply in the tissues.

The saturation of oxygen in the pulmonary catheter, which represents the SṽO₂ can be monitored continuously by using special fibreoptic thermodilution catheters, or intermittently by obtaining serial samples of blood drawn from the distal lumen of the PAC. The technology for measuring SṽO₂ is based on reflection spectrometry. This involves sending light of selected wavelengths down one fibreoptic filament in the catheter body to blood flowing past the catheter tip. The reflected light is then transmitted back through the second fibreoptic filament to a photodetector located in the optical module. Haemoglobin and Oxyhaemoglobin absorb light at different wavelengths and the reflected light is analysed to obtain the SṽO₂.

In a normal individual, SṽO₂ ranges from 60–80 per cent. It is generally accepted that SṽO₂ should be considered clinically significant if the value is outside the normal range or if a change in SṽO₂ of 5–10 per cent from the baseline value persists for > 3–5 minutes, even if the value is in the normal range. A marked fall in SṽO₂ generally indicates inadequate tissue oxygenation, and the fall is attributed to a decrease in SaO₂, Hb concentration, or the CO or to a marked increase in V̇O₂. When thermodilution techniques are not available, serial measurements of this are frequently used to monitor changes in the CO, provided that the Hb concentration remains constant, and the PaO₂ does not fluctuate significantly.

Gastric Tonometry (32)

Gastric tonometry is a minimially invasive way to monitor splanchnic perfusion. It determines the perfusion status of the gastric mucosa by measuring the local PCO₂. Data suggest that tonometry is useful for outcome prognostication and for detection of early hypovolaemia in critically ill patients. Given the important role of the gut in the development of MOF, it appears that ability to recognize and correct ischaemia of the gut early and promptly should go a long way in treating critically ill patients and gastric tonometry is the only non-invasive technology that allows the clinician to do so.

Summary of Haemodynamic Monitoring

1. The main indication of haemodynamic monitoring, and more specifically of PA catheterization, will always depend on the risk-benefit ratio as judged by the clinician. However it is invaluable in monitoring fluid administration, and inotrope and vasodilator therapy in critically ill patients with shock, acute lung injury, or multiple organ dysfunction.

2. The accuracy and reliability of all invasive haemodynamic measurements depend mainly on the correct method of assembling and calibrating the pressure monitoring equipment.

3. In most centres in India CVP monitoring is common, and may be considered to be quite reliable, provided its limitations (as discussed earlier) are fully appreciated.

4. The following criteria should be fulfilled if PA pressure monitoring is to be used as a measure of preload: (a) A normal ventricular compliance, where the LV pressure-volume relationship can be predicted; (b) Absence of LV inflow obstruction; (c) Unobstructed vasculature in the pulmonary capillary bed.

5. It is not advisable to disconnect the mechanical ventilator or remove PEEP during PCWP measurements. On the contrary, the measurement of pressures during therapy (with appropriate correction for PEEP) is more relevant and meaningful.

6. Catheter-induced sepsis is the commonest of the long-term complications of pulmonary artery catheterization in our part of the world, and hence strict asepsis should be observed. Pulmonary artery rupture, though rare, is the most dreaded complication, and carries the highest mortality.

7. It is important to understand and differentiate the various determinants of cardiac and circulatory functions and measurements of tissue perfusion. It would be inappropriate to treat perfusion failure entirely with the concepts and therapy designed for cardiac failure. Hence, for overall management it is important to understand the failure of each circulatory component.

8. The goal of non-invasive monitoring is not just attaining comparable information vis-à-vis invasive monitoring, but the information attained should be continuous and in real time. Another important advantage of non-invasive monitoring would be to provide information early, possibly in pre-ICU locations such as in the casualty room. Once the hardware and software innovations of these monitoring devices attain acceptable accuracy, reliability and cost-effectiveness, it may change the standards of management of acutely ill patients with early haemodynamic impairment.

REFERENCES

1. Marriot HJL. (1984). Systemic Approach to Diagnosis of Arrhythmias. In: Practical Electrocardiography, 9th edn. pp. 216–221.

2. (1984). Disposable Pressure Transducers. Health Devices. 13, 268.

3. Maloy L, Gardner RMI. (1986). Monitoring Systemic Arterial BP: Cuff Recording versus Digital Display. Heart Lung. 15, 627.

4. Parel A, Pizov R, Cotev S. (1987). The systolic pressure variation is a sensitive indicator of hypovolemia in ventilated dogs subjected to graded hemorrhage. Anaesthesiology. 67, 498–502.

5. Bongard FS, Sue DY. (1994). Critical Care Monitoring. In: Current Critical Care Diagnosis and Treatment (Eds Bongard FS, Sue DY). pp. 170–190. Appleton and Lange. USA.

6. Samii K, Conseiller C, Viars P. (1976). Central venous pressure and pulmonary wedge pressure. Arch Surg. 111, 1122.

7. Ermakov S, Hoyt JW. (1992). Pulmonary Artery Catheterization. In: Critical Care Clinics, Procedures in the ICU (Guest Ed. Kruse JA). 8(4), 773–806.

8. Eisenberg PR, Jaffer AS, Schuster DP. (1984). Clinical evaluation compared to pulmonary artery catheterization in the haemodynamic assessment of critically ill patients. Crit Care Med. 12, 549.

9. Steingrub JS, Celoria G, Vickers-Lahti M. (1991). Therapeutic impact of pulmonary artery catheterization in a medical/surgical ICU. Chest. 99, 1451.

10. Sibbald WJ, Sprung CL. (1988). Pulmonary artery catheterization: The debate continues (editorial). Chest. 94, 899–901.

11. Gore J, Goldberg RJ, Spodick DH et al. (1987). A community-wide assessment of the use of pulmonary artery catheters in patients with acute myocardial infarction. Chest. 92, 721.

12. Connors AF, Speroff T, Dawson NV et al. (1996). The effectiveness of right heart catheterization in the initial care of critically ill patients. JAMA. 276, 889–897.

13. Dalen JE, Bone RC. (1996). Is it time to pull the pulmonary catheter? JAMA. 276, 916–918.

14. Pulmonary Artery Catheter Conference: Consensus Statement. (1997). Crit Care Med. 25, 910–925.

15. Dalen JE. (2001). The Pulmonary Artery Catheter: friend, foe or accomplice? JAMA. 286 (3), 348–350.

16. Shoemaker WC, Appel PL, Kram HB et al. (1988). Prospective trial of supranormal values of survivors as therapeutic goals in high risk surgical patients. Chest. 94, 1176–1186.

17. Boyd O, Grounds M, Bennett D. (1993). Pre-operative increase of oxygen delivery reduces mortality in high-risk surgical patients. JAMA. 270, 2699–2704.

18. Mathay MA, Chatterjee K. (1988). Bedside catheterization of the pulmonary artery: Risks compared with benefits. Ann Intern Med. 109, 826–834.

19. Robertie PG, Johnston WE, Williamson MK. (1991). Clinical utility of a position-monitoring catheter in the pulmonary artery. Anaesthesiology. 74, 440.

20. Santora T, Ganz W, Gold J et al. (1991). New method for monitoring pulmonary artery catheter location. Crit Care Med. 19, 422.

21. Smart FW, Husserl FE. (1990). Complications of flow-directed balloon-tipped catheters. Chest. 97, 227.

22. Culver BH. (1988). Hemodynamic monitoring: Physiologic problems in interpretation. In: Cardiopulmonary Critical Care Management (Eds Fallat RJ, Luce JM). pp. 165–177.

23. Teboul JL, Besbes M, Axler O et al. (1988). A bedside index for determination of zone 3 condition of pulmonary artery catheter tips during mechanical ventilation. Am Rev Respir Dis. 137(S), 139.

24. Gardner PE. (1989). Cardiac output: Theory, technique and troubleshooting. Crit Care Nurs Clin North Am. 1, 577.

25. Caruso LJ, Layon AJ, Gabriellei A. (2002). What is the best way to measure cardiac output? Who cares anyway? Chest. 122 (3), 771–774.

26. Raaijimakers E, Faes TJC, Scholfen RJ et al. (1999). A meta-analysis: three decades of validating thoracic impedance cardiography. Crit Care Med. 27, 1203–1213.

27. Shoemaker WC, Wo CJ, Bishop MH et al. (1994). Multicentre trial of a new thoracic electrical bioimpedence system for cardiac output estimation. Crit Care Med. 22, 1907–1912.

28. Cariou A, Monchi M, Joly LM et al. (1998). Noninvasive cardiac output monitoring by aortic blood flow determination: evaluation of the Sometec Dynemo-3000 system. Crit Care Med. 26, 2066–72.

29. Boulnois JLG, Pechoux T. (2000). Non-invasive cardiac output monitoring by aortic blood flow measurement with the Dynemo 3000. J Clin Monit Comput. 16, 127–140.

30. Kurita T, Morita K, Kato S et al. (1997). Comparison of the accuracy of the lithium dilution technique with the thermodilution technique for measurement of cardiac output. Br J Anaesth. 79, 770–775.

31. Guzzi L, Jaffe MB, Orr JA. (1998). Clinical evaluation of a new noninvasive method of cardiac output measurement: preliminary results in CABG patients. Anaesthesiology. 89, A543.

32. Heard SO. (2003). Conundrums in the management of critically ill patients. Gastric tonometry—the hemodynamic monitor of choice (Pro). Chest. 123(5 Suppl), 469S–74S.

Respiratory Monitoring in Adults

General Considerations

Respiratory monitoring is merely one facet in the overall monitoring of a critically ill patient (1–3). The degree of respiratory monitoring and the number of parameters monitored, depend on the nature of the critical illness. Close monitoring of the respiratory system is particularly essential in respiratory emergencies and in acute respiratory failure, problems so frequently encountered in busy intensive care units. Since the heart and lung function as a single interrelated unit, haemodynamic monitoring is often equally essential in these patients. Acute respiratory failure particularly when due to acute lung injury (ARDS) is often complicated by renal dysfunction. Monitoring renal function in these patients is essential for diagnosis and management.

Respiratory monitoring helps (a) in assessment of respiratory function; (b) in detecting complications involving the respiratory system in the course of any critical illness; (c) in detecting complications of mechanical ventilation. The information provided by this monitoring improves decision making ability, and hopefully should improve patient outcome. Monitoring techniques can also help to assess progression or regression of pulmonary disease, and the response to various therapeutic interventions. It is however important to bear in mind that decision making in the management of patients with acute respiratory problems should not rest solely on monitoring of the respiratory parameters. Decision making should also depend on overall patient assessment, particularly of the haemodynamic state and of renal function.

Monitoring Techniques

Monitoring techniques particularly in poor developing countries, should always invoke cost-benefit considerations. The potential risk and hazard of invasive monitoring procedures together with the added cost and added patient discomfort, should be balanced against the possible benefit of improved diagnosis and better management.

The simplest, most basic and perhaps the most valuable aspect of patient monitoring is the close observation of the patient by the medical and nursing staff. Physical examination and radiological examination from day to day, are of critical importance and provide a wealth of information. Sophisticated units unfortunately tend to neglect these basic, irreplaceable tenets of critical respiratory care. *All other monitoring techniques should supplement these basic tenets; they should never supplant them.*

An overall complete *physical examination* is of paramount importance. Special emphasis is placed on the heart rate, blood pressure, respiratory rate, examination of the chest and heart. A *radiological examination* of the chest is really a necessary appendage of the physical examination and merits equal importance. *Other basic monitoring techniques* include an arterial pH and blood gas analysis. ECG monitoring, monitoring of Hb and haematocrit, monitoring of urine output and of basic renal function parameters.

Other specific respiratory and haemodynamic parameters may need to be monitored at the bedside depending on the nature of the problem. These include tidal volume (V_T), minute ventilation ($\dot{V}_E$), maximum inspiratory force, the physiological dead space (V_D) and the V_D/V_T ratio. Patients on mechanical ventilation may need bedside measurements of lung mechanics—this includes measure-

Table 4.3.1. Bedside measurements in patients with acute respiratory failure

* Physical examination—heart rate, blood pressure, respiratory rate, clinical examination of the heart and chest
* Radiological examination and ultrasonography of the chest
* ECG monitoring
* Monitoring of arterial pH, arterial blood gas analysis, oxygenation indices
* Pulse oximetry
* Airway CO_2 monitoring
* Monitoring of renal function
* Monitoring of haemoglobin and haematocrit
* Monitoring of respiratory parameters—tidal volume, respiratory rate, minute ventilation, maximum inspiratory force, physiological dead space, V_D/V_T ratio
* Bedside measurement of lung mechanics—dynamic and static compliances, airways resistance
* Monitoring wave form and loop analysis in mechanically ventilated patients
* Measurement of physiologic shunt, oxygen delivery/transport, oxygen consumption
* Monitoring of mixed venous oxygen tension and mixed venous oxygen saturation
* Haemodynamic monitoring in selected cases

ments of dynamic compliance, static compliance and resistance to air flow. Physiological shunt ($\dot{Q}_S/\dot{Q}_T$) may also need to be measured together with measurements of oxygen delivery or transport ($\dot{D}O_2$), and oxygen consumption ($\dot{V}O_2$). Haemodynamic monitoring is essential in some patients; it provides a measure of the cardiac index, filling pressures of the right and left heart, the vascular resistances in the pulmonary and systemic circulation. It also enables measurements of the mixed venous oxygen tension and saturation, and enables the computing of the shunt equation and of $\dot{D}O_2$ and the $\dot{V}O_2$. Finally an analysis of expired gas, particularly with reference to carbon dioxide, may provide useful information in a few patients. **Table 4.3.1** lists bedside measurements which are useful in patients with acute respiratory failure.

Not all measurements are necessary in every patient. The clinician should selectively monitor those parameters which are of help either in diagnosis, in management, or in both, bearing in mind the cost-benefit ratio of each monitoring technique in a given patient.

Physical Examination (4, 5)

Tachycardia or bradycardia should be assessed in relation to the overall clinical situation. Both can occur in relation to increasing hypoxia.

Changes in arterial blood pressure may be due to several factors. These include hypoxia, hypercapnia, changes in effective circulating blood volume, and changes in cardiac contractility and in systemic vascular resistance due to various causes. Methods of measurement of arterial blood pressure have already been discussed in the earlier Chapter on Cardiac Monitoring in Adults.

Respiratory Rate

A careful count and monitoring of the respiratory rate is of crucial importance. The normal range is from 10–16/minute. A rate above 20/minute always demands a satisfactory explanation. Rates > 30/min signify respiratory distress and may cause significant hypocapnia.

An increase in the respiratory rate is an early feature of a fall in PaO_2 or a rise in $PaCO_2$. Pulmonary problems producing tachypnoea include atelectasis, pneumonia and pulmonary oedema. Pleural effusion and pneumothorax should also be carefully excluded. In a critical care setting, sudden tachypnoea may also be an early sign of sepsis, of increasing liver cell dysfunction, or of pulmonary embolism. Metabolic acidosis initially produces an increase in the depth of breathing followed by an increase in the rate. Increase in respiratory rate and minute ventilation are observed in patients on total parenteral nutrition who receive large carbohydrate loads. A large carbohydrate intake increases carbon dioxide production ($\dot{V}CO_2$), so that a higher minute ventilation ($\dot{V}_E$) is required to excrete the excess CO_2. In a critically ill patient this constitutes a significant stress demanding increased respiratory muscle work. Respiratory muscle fatigue can result, particularly in patients who already have chronic airways obstruction. Overfeeding with carbohydrates may make weaning (in a patient on mechanical ventilation) impossible, and this is manifested by tachypnoea and dyspnoea on a T-tube. Decreasing total caloric intake,

and increasing the ratio of fat : carbohydrate intake decreases the $\dot{V}CO_2$ and remedies the situation.

Clinical Examination of the Chest

The degree of chest movements during breathing often enables an astute observer to assess the adequacy of ventilation. Movements may however be deceptive in that adequate chest movement on clinical examination, may still be associated with alveolar hypoventilation, particularly when the physiological dead space is increased.

Asymmetrical movements with diminished breath sounds over the poorly moving side indicate pneumothorax, pleural effusion, pneumonia, atelectasis or uneven ventilation due to right main stem bronchial intubation.

Clinical examination should include a search for signs of respiratory muscle fatigue (see Chapter on Acute Respiratory Failure in Adults). A stony dull note over the base of the chest may confirm a doubtful radiological opacity to be related to fluid, rather than to a parenchymal lung lesion. Auscultation should determine the intensity of breath sounds, character of breath sounds and the presence of wheezes or crackles. Auscultation over the trachea may help in the detection of an inadequately inflated cuff of an endotracheal or tracheostomy tube.

Clinical Examination of the Cardiovascular System

This should be meticulous. Myocardial dysfunction may manifest with a diastolic gallop. A low cardiac output causing a low PaO_2 may be related to pump dysfunction or to mechanical problems like a valvular defect, or a ruptured septum or ruptured papillary muscle.

Radiological Examination

This as mentioned earlier, is an appendage or a continuation of a physical examination. A radiological examination helps (a) to check the position of various tubes, lines, catheters; (b) to detect early pulmonary oedema, atelectasis, pneumonia, pleural effusion; (c) to diagnose a pneumothorax which has been missed, or is undetectable on clinical examination; (d) to detect localized hyperinflation of a portion of the lung due to uneven lung compliance in patients on mechanical ventilation and positive end-expiratory pressure; (e) to detect other features of barotrauma; (f) to detect abnormalities in the cardiac silhouette.

Pneumothorax may be difficult to diagnose when only supine films are available for interpretation. Features which may help in diagnosis in such situations include (a) a sharp curvilinear change in density over the upper quadrant of the abdomen which becomes significantly radiolucent and (b) a deep lateral costophrenic angle on the affected side **(6, 7)**. A cross-table lateral or decubitus film in the above circumstance should be able to confirm the diagnosis of a pneumothorax.

A bedside ultrasound examination of the chest is extremely useful to confirm or detect fluid within the pleural space.

ECG Monitoring

Arrhythmias are frequent in patients with acute respiratory failure. Supraventricular tachycardia, chaotic atrial tachycardia, atrial flutter/fibrillation all occur. Ventricular rhythm disturbances including ventricular tachycardia, may be observed with increasing hypoxia particularly in patients with ischaemic heart disease (8). ECG monitoring techniques have been discussed in an earlier chapter.

Arterial pH and Arterial Blood Gas Analysis

A close monitoring of arterial pH and arterial blood gases is indispensable in the management of acute respiratory failure, as also in the management of any critically ill individual with multiple organ system dysfunction. The PaO_2 is an index of arterial oxygenation, and the $PaCO_2$ is an index of alveolar ventilation. The significance of a low PaO_2 and of changes in $PaCO_2$, have been discussed in the Chapter of Basic Cardiorespiratory Physiology in the Intensive Care Unit, as also in the Chapters on Acute Respiratory Failure in Adults and Mechanical Ventilation in the Critically Ill.

It is however extremely important to restress that a fall in PaO_2 in a critically ill patient could be due to either deteriorating pulmonary function, or to nonpulmonary causes—in particular to deteriorating cardiovascular function.

The PaO_2 / FIO_2 ratio is a good overall index of gas exchange (9). In a similar fashion the arterial oxygen tension divided by the alveolar oxygen tension (the a/A ratio) remains stable with a varying FIO_2 and is a reliable index of factors governing gas exchange (9). The normal a/A ratio is > 0.75. The ratio can predict the new PaO_2 that should result from a change in oxygen concentration (10). It is therefore a good pointer to a change in lung function when the FIO_2 administered to the patient is changed.

Pulse Oximetry

In critically ill patients the PaO_2 might fluctuate significantly, and a sharp fall in the PaO_2 may be missed during suctioning, during change in posture and following the administration of drugs. Continuous monitoring of PaO_2 by special electrodes in the radial, brachial, and femoral arteries, as also of mixed venous blood ($P\bar{v}O_2$) in the pulmonary artery can be done (11). These are invasive, expensive techniques and it is doubtful if they help to significantly decrease the morbidity and mortality of very ill patients. However, a universally accepted non-invasive method of measuring arterial oxygen saturation is by the use of the pulse oximeter (12, 13). A beam of light of appropriate wavelength is made to shine through a finger or ear lobe. The change in light absorption as blood traverses the vascular bed from beat-to-beat is dependent on the oxyhaemoglobin saturation, and this saturation is continuously displayed on the monitor. The sensor however needs to be in continuous contact with the finger or the ear lobe to which it is clipped. Monitoring oxygen saturation through pulse oximetry is today universally practised in all critical care units, emergency departments, and operation theatres. Pulse oximetry is also used during all minor procedures. A sharp fall in oxygen saturation should alert the physician or surgeon to potential disaster. There are however certain issues which need to be considered in this monitoring technique. Pulse oximetry is fairly accurate in the range of mild to moderate hypoxia. When hypoxaemia is severe, as with a fall in O_2 saturation below 75 per cent, its accuracy is suspect. In severe hypoxaemia the difference between measured oxygen saturation and the oxygen saturation obtained through pulse oximetry ranges from 5 to 12 per cent.

Pulse oximetry is also unreliable in patients with severe hypotension and in patients with poor perfusion of the peripheries, either from shock due to any aetiology, or from the use of vasopressors causing severe vasoconstriction. These factors impair blood flow to the site of the sensor of the oximeter and cause a variation in the contour and intensity of the pulse beats used to calculate oxygen saturation. Most oximeters are devised and programmed to stop recording O_2 saturation in states of low perfusion or when a poor pulse signal is being measured. However some oximeters continue to display O_2 saturation in spite of marked hypoperfusion and hypotension. These results are inaccurate, and the oxygen saturation readings under the above circumstances are misleadingly high.

Pulse oximetry though of great use in critical care medicine cannot and should not replace measurement of arterial blood gases. The measurement of PaO_2, pH remains of vital importance. The PaO_2 cannot always be accurately predicted from the O_2 saturation readings of the oximeter. When the O_2 saturation is between 95–100 per cent, the exact measure of the PaO_2 can only be made by an accurate blood gas (PaO_2) estimation.

Clinical Uses

(i) Monitoring oxygen saturation in all procedures—major and minor. Minor procedures would include bronchoscopy, endoscopies, haemodialysis, cardioversion, injection of dyes and contrasts for imaging purposes.

(ii) Keeping track on patients who are hypoxaemic.

(iii) Helping in ventilator support, as it enables, (a) adjustment of FIO_2 as per the O_2 saturation readings; (b) detection of effects on arterial oxygenation with different modes of ventilator support and with use of PEEP.

(iv) Aiding the weaning process, as it tracks the O_2 saturation when the patient is off ventilator support.

It is to be noted that the pulse oximeter cannot measure carboxyhaemoglobin nor measure oxyhaemoglobin in the presence of carboxyhaemoglobin. Unreliable readings are also observed in methaemoglobinaemia

Transcutaneous blood gas analysis is an important non-invasive method of monitoring infants with acute respiratory failure, and has been described in the Chapter on Respiratory and Cardiac Monitoring in the Critically Ill Child.

Airway CO2 Monitoring

Airway CO_2 monitoring is done non-invasively, either with a quickly responding infrared CO_2 analyser or a mass spectrometer, which measures CO_2 directly at the end of the endotracheal tube. Breath-by-breath analysis of the end tidal PCO_2 ($PETCO_2$) can thus be obtained from an endotracheal tube during mechanical ventilation. Non-intubated patients can have the $PETCO_2$ sampled by a catheter placed through the nares in the posterior nasopharynx. Continuous wave forms can be recorded by capnography and the expired CO_2 is thereby monitored. The end-tidal pressure of CO_2 is related to

$PACO_2$ (pressure of alveolar CO_2), which in turn is a measure of the $PaCO_2$. Thus when expired CO_2 waveforms are continuously monitored, an estimate of the end-tidal PCO_2 ($PETCO_2$) would amount to a non-invasive measurement of the $PaCO_2$. The $PETCO_2$ will be increased if there is alveolar hypoventilation, or an increase in the CO_2 production; it will be decreased if there is alveolar hyperventilation.

Analysis of the $PETCO_2$ thus helps in assessing the adequacy of alveolar ventilation, and guides ventilator adjustments to ensure that this is achieved. However the close correlation between $PETCO_2$ and $PaCO_2$ observed in normal subjects, does not always hold in patients with marked $\dot{V}/\dot{Q}$ abnormalities. In such patients there is a divergence between $PETCO_2$ and $PaCO_2$ values. The expired gas in the presence of a $\dot{V}/\dot{Q}$ abnormality is more influenced by lung units with high $\dot{V}/\dot{Q}$ ratios and increased dead space, whereas the arterial blood is more weighted by lung units with low $\dot{V}/\dot{Q}$ ratios and increased shunt. The $PETCO_2$ is thus an unreliable estimate of the $PaCO_2$ in these circumstances, though monitoring of changing trends may still be of use.

Capnography and end-tidal PCO_2 monitoring have been useful in the following other clinical situations:

(i) To provide a non-invasive method determining correct endotracheal tube placement. The capnograph should display an increased CO_2 concentration during expiration and the end-tidal PCO_2 reading should be plausible.

(ii) To assess the efficacy of cardiopulmonary resuscitation. A very low $PETCO_2$ during cardiopulmonary resuscitation points to a very poor return of venous blood to the right heart and central circulation.

Monitoring Renal Function

Renal function needs to be monitored in every critically ill individual. *Close monitoring is specially important in acute respiratory failure, as renal dysfunction is a frequent complication and this significantly adds to the mortality.* Sweet et al. (14) in a study of 400 critically ill patients noted a mortality of 32 per cent in respiratory failure alone, 44 per cent in renal failure alone, and 65 per cent in combined respiratory and renal failure. Hypoxaemia, acidosis, mechanical ventilation, use of PEEP may all disturb renal haemodynamics and tubular functions. Sepsis, hypovolaemia and the use of nephrotoxic drugs can also significantly add to renal dysfunction.

Urine output, blood creatinine, blood urea nitrogen and serum electrolytes require close monitoring. A urine sodium level $< 10–20$ mEq/l or a urine osmolality > 600 mOsm/l suggest hypovolaemia.

Renal function can also be monitored by measuring the urine osmolality, the plasma osmolality, and the osmolar clearance. The urine osmolality divided by the plasma osmolality is calculated; if > 1.7 the concentrating ability of the kidney is good.

The osmolar clearance (COsm) is calculated as follows:

$$COsm = \frac{Urine\ Osmolality}{Plasma\ Osmolality} \times Urine\ Output$$

The normal osmolar clearance is 120 ml/hour; it is decreased in renal dysfunction.

The normal calculated serum osmolality is between 275–295 mOsmoles/l (see Chapter on Fluid and Electrolyte Disturbances in the Critically Ill). The calculated osmolality is 5–8 mOsm less than the measured osmolality, the difference being related to anions like phosphate and lactate. The greater this difference between measured and calculated osmolality in a critically ill patient with acute respiratory failure, and the greater the increase in serum lactic acid, the poorer the prognosis.

Monitoring Haemoglobin and Haematocrit

Monitoring haemoglobin concentration is essential as oxygen content of the blood depends significantly on this parameter. It is best to keep the Hb concentration around 11 g/dl. The haematocrit is affected by a loss or gain in the red blood cells or in plasma volume. Sudden blood loss will not immediately change either Hb or the haematocrit. The haematocrit falls gradually as a result of shift of fluid from the interstitial compartment into the vascular compartment. This is a compensatory mechanism which helps to maintain an effective circulating volume. Blood loss of 500 ml is replaced by fluid from the interstitial compartment initially at a rate of 1 ml/min (15). The haematocrit needs to be monitored periodically; following haemorrhage it needs to be monitored every 4–6 hours.

Monitoring Specific Respiratory and Haemodynamic Parameters

Tidal Volume, Respiratory Rate, Minute Ventilation and Maximal Inspiratory Force

Bedside spirometers, as also dry gas meters are easily available to measure exhaled volumes. Tidal volume (V_T), respiratory frequency (f) and minute ventilation ($\dot{V}_E$) often need to be monitored, particularly in ventilatory failure and in patients who are to be weaned off ventilator support. As mentioned earlier, an increase in respiratory rate (f) may be the first sign of respiratory distress, and the degree of rise is proportional to the severity of underlying lung disease. Rapid shallow breathing is commonly observed in those who fail to be weaned from ventilator support. This can be quantitated by the ratio f/V_T; if the value is above 100 breaths per minute per litre weaning is generally unsuccessful (16).

A rapid respiratory rate with a low tidal volume may cause a fall in alveolar ventilation, particularly if the dead space is increased. A marked increase in $\dot{V}_E$ should lead to hypocapnia; if the $PaCO_2$ is within normal limits it points to a marked increase in dead space. A $V_T > 5$ ml/kg and a vital capacity (VC) > 10 ml/kg suggest a good chance of weaning the patient from ventilator support. A $\dot{V}_E \geq 10$ l makes weaning difficult and unlikely. A maximum inspiratory force < -20 cm H_2O generally necessitates the use of mechanical ventilatory support (see Chapter on Mechanical Ventilation in the Critically Ill).

Physiological Dead Space

As explained in the Chapter on Basic Cardiorespiratory Physiology in the Intensive Care Unit, an increase in physiological dead space points to wasted ventilation. Mechanical ventilation by itself leads to an increase in dead space (V_D). In respiratory failure and in many pulmonary pathologies, an increase in dead space is due to increased ventilation of alveoli which are poorly perfused or unperfused.

$$\frac{V_D}{V_T} = \frac{PaCO_2 - P_{\bar{E}}CO_2}{PaCO_2}$$

where $P_{\bar{E}}CO_2$ is the mixed expired CO_2 tension.

If the end-tidal PCO_2 ($PETCO_2$) is substituted for $PaCO_2$, anatomical dead space can be calculated by analysis of the expired gas. An increase in V_D or in the V_D/V_T ratio in acute respiratory failure due to severe lung injury (ARDS) correlates with an increase in mortality. The higher the V_D, the greater the mortality [17].

Bedside Measurement of Lung Mechanics

It is important to monitor lung mechanics in patients on ventilator support. The volume delivered by the ventilator divided by the peak airway pressure, constitutes the dynamic compliance. It includes the components of resistance to airflow, and resistance related to the elastic properties of the lung.

$$\text{Dynamic Compliance} = \frac{\text{Tidal Volume}}{\text{Peak Pressure}}$$

If PEEP is being used or if auto-PEEP is present, then

$$\text{Dynamic Compliance} = \frac{\text{Tidal Volume}}{\text{Peak Pressure} - \text{PEEP (if present)}}$$

Dynamic compliance correlates with changes in airway resistance.

If we occlude the outflow of the ventilator momentarily (by turning the knob to inspiratory hold or to pause), the pressure dial will show a momentary drop at which no air flow occurs. This pressure is the plateau pressure.

$$\text{Static Compliance} = \frac{\text{Tidal Volume}}{\text{Plateau Pressure} - \text{PEEP (if present)}}$$

Static compliance correlates with changes in elastic recoil.

The normal static compliance of the lung and the chest wall in mechanically ventilated patients is 70 ml/cm H_2O. When the static compliance of the lung and the chest wall is < 20 ml/cm H_2O, the lungs are very stiff, and the degree of respiratory failure is invariably severe. In very severe acute lung injury, the static compliance may be as low as 10 ml/cm H_2O.

Periodic monitoring of the peak inflation pressure and plateau pressure for a fixed tidal volume thus gives a good indication of lung mechanics. High plateau and peak pressures, and in particular progressively increasing plateau and peak pressures, are indicative of increasingly stiff lungs. This occurs in pulmonary oedema, atelectasis, pneumonia, acute lung injury and pneumothorax. It is also observed when for some reason the patient strongly clashes with the machine.

Normally the peak pressure exceeds the plateau pressure by < 5 cm H_2O. If the plateau pressure is significantly lower than the peak pressure, it indicates an increase in airways resistance. A normal plateau pressure with a markedly increased peak pressure points to a marked increase in airways resistance. This can be due to a blocked endotracheal or tracheostomy tube, to secretions within the bronchial tubes, or to bronchospasm (see Chapter on

Mechanical Ventilation in the Critically Ill). If air flow is measured, airways resistance (Raw) can be calculated as follows:

$$\text{Raw} = \frac{P_P - P_{ST}}{V}$$

where P_P is the peak pressure, P_{ST} is the static or plateau pressure, V is the volume of air flow measured at end-inspiration at the time of peak pressure. In normal subjects Raw is between 2–3 cm H_2O/l/sec. In severe airways obstruction, Raw may be more than 10 times the normal value.

It is sometimes important to chart on a graph the dynamic and static compliance of the lungs, by ventilating the lungs at different tidal volumes and recording the peak and plateau pressures for each volume. The dynamic compliance curve correlates with airways resistance and the static compliance curve with lung stiffness. The method of charting compliance is as follows:

(i) Select different tidal volumes—400, 600, 800, 1000, 1200 ml.

(ii) For each volume record spirometer volume, peak pressure, plateau pressure (ensure that the tracheostomy cuff is adequately inflated and that there is no air leak).

(iii) Calculate dynamic compliance and static compliance as explained earlier.

(iv) This procedure is repeated for each volume setting.

(v) If at any volume setting the peak pressure shows a marked increase, a further increase in tidal volume setting should not be done as barotrauma may result.

(vi) The data is charted on a graph so that dynamic and static compliance curves are obtained for varying tidal volumes (**Fig. 4.3.1**).

Peak and plateau pressures (with graphs of dynamic and static

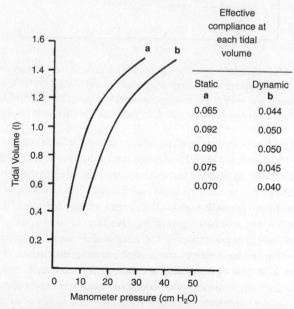

Fig. 4.3.1. Effective static and dynamic compliance curves calculated at varying tidal volumes. **(a)** Effective static compliance curve. **(b)** Effective dynamic compliance curve. Figures show effective static **(a)** and dynamic **(b)** compliance at each tidal volume. (Modified from Bone RC. 1981. In: Adult Respiratory Distress Medicine. Thieme Medical Publishers, New York.)

Procedures and Monitoring in the Intensive Care Unit

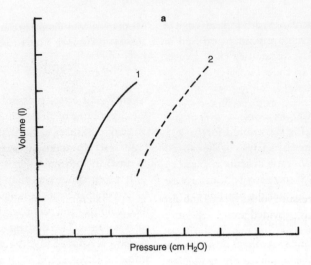

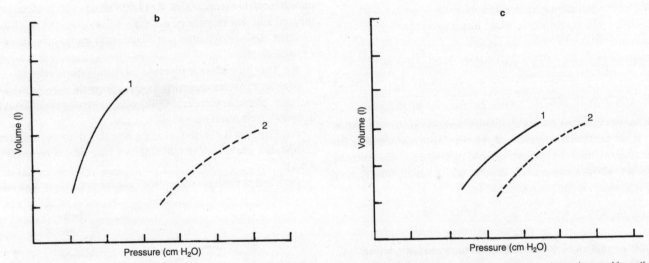

Fig. 4.3.2. (a) Static compliance curve (1) and dynamic compliance curve (2) in normal individuals. These curves remain unchanged in patients who are hypoxic due to pulmonary embolism. **(b)** Static (1) and dynamic (2) compliance curves in patients with increased airway resistance. Note flattening and shift of the dynamic compliance curve (2) to the right. **(c)** Static (1) and dynamic (2) compliance curves in patients with increased stiffness of the lungs. Note that both the static and dynamic compliance curves are flattened and shifted to the right.

compliance) can also be charted at a constant tidal volume with a gradual increase in PEEP. At high tidal volumes, or with higher PEEP levels, decreasing static compliance signals hyperinflation, and care must be taken to avoid barotrauma. The incidence of the latter increases with high tidal volumes or high levels of PEEP, which cause overdistension of the alveoli.

A careful examination of the static and dynamic compliance curves provides further information on lung mechanics (**Figs. 4.3.2 a, b** and **c**). Conditions causing an increase in airways resistance, shift the dynamic compliance curve to the right and flatten it. Conditions causing increasingly stiff lungs or causing chest wall stiffness, shift both the static and dynamic compliance curves to the right and flatten both (**18**). If the patient has a low PaO_2 and both compliance curves are unchanged, the possibility of pulmonary embolism should be entertained (**15**).

The charting of compliance graphs is subject to two possible errors (**15**). If the patient clashes with and resists the ventilator, the pressure required to inflate the lungs will be greater than when he is relaxed. Also, if the patient actively assists the ventilator in inspiration, the pressure shown on the ventilator dial will be less than the total pressure required.

Ordinarily compliance curve charts are rarely necessary, and mere monitoring of peak and plateau pressures in relation to tidal volume settings provide adequate information on lung mechanics in patients on ventilator support.

Intrinsic PEEP

Intrinsic PEEP (auto-PEEP) is dealt with at length in the Chapter on Mechanical Ventilation in the Critically Ill. Intrinsic PEEP is measured in relaxed patients on ventilator support by using the expiratory hold manoeuvre at the end of expiration. Intrinsic PEEP imposes an increase in the respiratory threshold load; this needs to be overcome by an increased inspiratory muscle effort, so that a sufficient negative pressure is created in the central airways to trigger the ventilator. The inspiratory effort needed to trigger the machine must overcome the set sensitivity plus the intrinsic PEEP. Monitoring intrinsic PEEP is important not only in ventilated patients who have airways obstruction, but also in patients with other lung pathologies, such as acute lung injury.

Wave Form and Loop Analysis in Mechanically Ventilated Patients

Modern ventilators are provided with gadgetry capable of displaying breath-by-breath wave forms, pressure volume loops and also flow volume loops. The wave forms provided are the pressure-time waveform, the volume-time wave form and the flow-time wave form. Analysis of wave forms and loops enables the clinician to determine changes in resistance and compliance of the patient's lungs while on ventilator support. A correct interpretation of wave forms and loops allows the intensivist to make a correct clinical decision on patient-ventilator relationship. It is our considered opinion that the display of wave forms and loops is of help; yet patient management can be as good and as effective with good clinical observation coupled with basic monitoring of respiratory mechanics discussed earlier (19).

Physiological Shunt

The true venous admixture is an index of the quantity of cardiac output perfusing unventilated alveoli. This has already been explained in the Chapter on Cardiorespiratory Physiology in the Intensive Care Unit.

$$\frac{\dot{Q}_S}{\dot{Q}_T} = \frac{CcO_2 - CaO_2}{CcO_2 - C\bar{v}O_2}$$

where $\dot{Q}_S$ is the shunt, $\dot{Q}_T$ the total blood flow to the lungs, and CcO_2, CaO_2 and $C\bar{v}O_2$ refer respectively to the oxygen content of pulmonary capillary, arterial and mixed venous blood.

Shunt is measured while breathing 100 per cent oxygen for 20 minutes. If inadequate time is given to wash out all nitrogen from poorly ventilating alveoli, the degree of shunt will be overestimated. On the other hand, prolonged breathing of 100 per cent oxygen promotes atelectasis and increases the $\dot{Q}_S/\dot{Q}_T$ value.

If the shunt is measured on a FIO_2 of < 1, ventilation-perfusion inequalities will contribute to the shunt. It needs to be stressed that a change in the degree of shunt may reflect either a change in pulmonary function influencing gas exchange, or may be related to a change in cardiac output. A decrease in the cardiac output in acute lung injury, can decrease the shunt within the lungs and thereby cause a rise in the PaO_2. A decrease in cardiac output on the other hand, could lower the $P\bar{v}O_2$ and thereby further decrease the PaO_2. The final effect on the PaO_2 depends on which of the above two haemodynamic changes predominates.

Oxygen Delivery

The importance of oxygen transport has been dealt with in a number of chapters.

Oxygen Delivery = Cardiac Output × CaO_2

where CaO_2 is the content of arterial oxygen (see Chapter on Cardiorespiratory Physiology in the Critical Care Unit).

Monitoring Mixed Venous Oxygen Tension ($P\bar{v}O_2$) and Mixed Venous Oxygen Saturation ($S\bar{v}O_2$)

The $P\bar{v}O_2$ and $S\bar{v}O_2$ are often used as indices of tissue oxygenation and of cardiac output. This can only be possible if a pulmonary artery catheter is in use. Fibreoptic catheters are available for continuous monitoring of $S\bar{v}O_2$. A $P\bar{v}O_2 < 30$ mm Hg invariably signifies severe hypoxia due to poor tissue perfusion. It is generally accepted that though the $P\bar{v}O_2$ accurately reflects tissue oxygenation in haemorrhagic and hypoxic shock, it often does not do so in septic shock and in patients with acute lung injury (ARDS). Misleadingly high $P\bar{v}O_2$ values may be obtained in these situations even when there is marked tissue hypoxia and lactic acid acidosis. This is probably related to a number of factors, chiefly perhaps to inability of the tissue cells to utilize oxygen (20–22).

Monitoring Serum Lactate Levels

The normal lactic acid levels in blood are ≤ 2 mM/l. Increase in serum lactic acid levels indicates tissue hypoxia. A normal or even an increased $\dot{D}O_2$ may however at times be associated with increase in lactic acid levels. This either indicates that the oxygen needs of the tissues are still relatively greater than the oxygen delivered to the tissues, or that the tissues are unable to effectively utilize oxygen (see Section on Clinical Shock Syndromes).

Haemodynamic Monitoring

This is indicated in select cases of acute respiratory failure. A stable cardiovascular function is essential for good respiratory function, the heart and lungs being inseparably linked in function. Haemodynamic monitoring is invasive, and should be done with circumspection after due consideration of potential risks versus the possible benefits. It is particularly helpful in acute lung injury as it enables the clinician to manipulate filling pressures, and adjust inotropic support so that oxygen transport to tissues is adequately maintained.

Computer Monitoring (23)

We have no experience with the mass spectrometer and of online simultaneous measurements of gas exchange and lung mechanics. The cost-effectiveness of this technology is doubtful, perhaps confusing, and at times unreliable. The data obtained does not substantially add to patient management and may well detract from it. More time may be spent in looking at computer data rather than in observing the patient. This is not to decry the use of computers; it is a plea to use them in a proper perspective particularly in poor countries.

REFERENCES

1. Tobin MJ. (1988). Respiratory monitoring in the intensive care unit. Am Rev Respir Dis. 138(6), 1625–1642.
2. Vaz Fragoso CA. (1993). Monitoring in adult critical care. In: Monitoring in Respiratory Care. (Eds Kacmarek RM, Hess D, Stoller JK). Mosby. St. Louis.

3. Scanlan CL. (1995). Patient Monitoring and Management. In: Egan's Fundamentals in Respiratory Care, 6th edn (Eds Scanlan CL, Spearman CB, Sheldon RL). pp. 920–967. Mosby. New York, London, Toronto.

4. Wilkins L, Sheldon RL, Krider SJ. (1990). Clinical Assessment in Respiratory Care, 2nd edn. Mosby. St. Louis.

5. MacIntyre NR. (1990). Respiratory monitoring without machinery. Respir Care. 35(6), 546–553.

6. Gordon R. (1980). The deep sulcus sign. Radiology. 136, 25.

7. Rhea JT, Sooenberg EV, McLoud TC. (1979). Basilar pneumothorax in the supine adult. Radiology. 133, 593.

8. Hall JB, Schmidt GA, Wood LDH. (1994). Principles of Critical Care for the Patient with Respiratory Failure. In: Textbook of Respiratory Medicine, 2nd edn (Eds Murray JF, Nadel JA). pp. 2545–2588. WB Saunders Company. Philadelphia, London, Toronto.

9. Nelson LD. (1993). Assessment of oxygenation: oxygenation indices. Respir Care. 38(6), 631–640.

10. Gilbert F, Keightley JF. (1974). The arterial/alveolar oxygen tension ratio: an index of gas exchange applicable to varying inspired concentrations. Am Rev Respir Dis. 109, 142.

11. Goecbenjan G. (1979). Continuous measurement of arterial PO_2—significance and indications in intensive care. Biotelem Patient Monit. 6, 51.

12. Welch JP, DeCesare R, Hess D. (1990). Pulse oximetry: instrumentation and clinical applications. Respir Care. 35(6), 584–596.

13. McCarthy K, Decker MJ et al. (1993). Pulse Oximetry. In: Monitoring in Respiratory Care (Eds Kacmarek RM, Hess D, Stoller JK). Mosby. St. Louis.

14. Sweet SJ, Glenney JP, Fitzibbons JP et al. (1981). Synergistic effect of acute renal failure and respiratory failure in the surgical intensive care unit. Am J Surg. 141, 492.

15. Bone RC. (1988). Respiratory Monitoring. In: Cardiopulmonary Critical Care Management (Eds Fallat RJ, Luce JM). pp. 89–111. Churchill Livingstone. New York, London.

16. Yang K, Tobin MJ. (1991). A prospective study of indexes predicting outcome of trials of weaning from mechanical ventilation. N Engl J Med. 324, 1445.

17. Shimada Y, Yoshiga I, Tamala K et al. (1979). Evaluation of the progress and prognosis of adult respiratory distress syndrome, simple physiologic measurement. Chest. 76, 180.

18. Bone RC. (1976). Diagnosis of causes for acute respiratory distress by pressure-volume curves. Chest. 70, 740.

19. Mancebo J, Benito S. (1993). Pulmonary mechanics in acute respiratory failure. Intensive Care World. 10: 64–67.

20. Phang PT, Russell JA. (1993). When does VO_2 depend on DO_2? Respir Care. 38(6), 618–626.

21. Pasquale MD, Cipolle MD, Cerra FB. (1993). Oxygen transport: does increasing supply improve outcome? Respir Care. 38(7), 800–825.

22. Robin ED. (1977). Dysoxia: abnormal tissue oxygen utilization. Arch Int Med. 137, 905.

23. Scanlan CL, Ruppel GL. (1995). Computer Applications in Respiratory Care. In: Egan's Fundamentals in Respiratory Care, 6th edn (Eds Scanlan CL, Spearman CB, Sheldon RL). pp. 150–175. Mosby. New York, London, Toronto.

Imaging in the Critical Care Unit

5.1 Introduction

5.2 Imaging Techniques in the Chest

5.3 Imaging Techniques in the Abdomen

5.4 Neuroimaging Techniques

CHAPTER 5.1

Introduction

Imaging procedures are extremely useful in the diagnosis and management of acute illnesses in the critical care unit. Therapeutic interventions using image guidance are being increasingly practised in selected problems, thereby considerably reducing both morbidity and mortality. Numerous imaging modalities are now available for diagnostic and therapeutic help. These include radiology, ultrasonography, echocardiography, computed tomography (CT scanning), magnetic resonance imaging (MRI), nuclear scintigraphy, Doppler study of blood flow through the arteries and veins, angiography and digital subtraction angiography (DSA). It is important for the critical care physician to be aware of the advantages, disadvantages, benefits, risks, and complications of each of these modalities. The mode or modes selected in a particular patient should thus increase the diagnostic and therapeutic yield at minimal cost. Cost is indeed an extremely important factor to be considered in our country. CT scans and MRI are expensive imaging procedures. To repeat them unnecessarily in a critically ill individual, is bad medicine.

Management of critically ill patients requires a close liaison and communication between the radiologist and the critical care physician. Good management would also entail early availability of results of imaging procedures. This entails rapid processing of images, immediate interpretation by the radiologist, and prompt availability of the films to the clinician. A daily discussion between the radiologist and the ICU physician of all X-rays and other imaging procedures is mandatory for the smooth, efficient functioning of a critical care unit.

Some imaging procedures like X-rays of the chest and abdomen, ultrasonography, echocardiography, and Doppler studies, can be performed at the bedside. Other investigations like CT scan, MRI, angiography, nuclear scintigraphy, unfortunately require the patient to be transported to the Imaging Department within the hospital. The risk of transfer of a critically ill individual to other departments, even if within the hospital, should be carefully assessed. All necessary safeguards and precautions must be ensured, and the risk-benefit ratio carefully considered before transfer.

The next chapter deals with imaging of the chest, followed by imaging of the abdomen and of the central nervous system. The imaging modalities considered are radiology, ultrasonography, CT and MRI. Echocardiography, Doppler studies, angiographic studies and nuclear scintigraphy are briefly discussed in relation to the relevant clinical problems in different chapters of this book. Nuclear scintigraphy is the one modality which has been infrequently used by our unit. This is because of logistic reasons— we do not have a nuclear medicine department, and the use of nuclear medicine would necessitate transfer of seriously ill patients to centres outside the hospital. Nuclear scintigraphy does however have important uses in the critically ill individual. These include ventilation-perfusion scanning in cases of suspected pulmonary embolism, myocardial perfusion scanning in cardiac disease, evaluation of an occult GI bleed, establishing the diagnosis of acute cholecystitis, and the localization of an occult infection.

It needs to be stressed that imaging procedures for diagnosis and management in a critically ill individual, should supplement and never supplant a good clinical examination. *A machine, particularly an expensive one, does not have to be used just because it is available. It should be used only when its use confers a clear benefit to the patient, and not merely to the institution which houses it.*

Note: All Figures in Section 5 appear as plates within this section.

Imaging Techniques in the Chest

Contributed by Dr Anirudh Kohli, MD, DNB, DMRD, Head of Department of Radiology, Breach Candy Hospital, Mumbai.

General Considerations

Radiology plays a key role in the successful management of critically ill patients. The chest radiograph, especially when performed at the bedside is an invaluable examination in identifying and evaluating pulmonary and cardiac problems.

It is often debated whether there is a need for daily chest radiographs or only 'stat' films. Many studies have shown that daily portable chest X-rays are very effective in diagnosing unexpected problems resulting in treatment alterations, which in turn affect the final outcome of the patient (1–3). The quality of portable chest X-rays however is a factor of major concern. The limited power output and longer exposure time required for portable chest X-rays result in poorer quality than departmental films. There are other factors which also contribute to non-consistent quality. In a large hospital with numerous radiographers, many different film screen combinations and multiple portable X-ray machines, the quality of portable films is bound to be inconsistent as each radiographer uses technical factors which he feels are appropriate. Similarly film screen combinations and portable machines require different settings. The ideal situation is for a single radiographer to use a single film screen combination and a single portable machine to take all the radiographs in the ICU, as this would eliminate the variations. Often in a large hospital this is not possible. For this reason it is advocated that the radiographer should note the radiographic factors used, the distance, the film screen combination and the portable machine used, on the film. As films are taken on a daily basis, the radiographer taking the next X-ray can view the previous day's films, note the factors and other technical details and repeat the same, so that there is no change in the consistency of the radiographs. In addition if the previous day's films were overexposed or underexposed, then the factors can be adjusted to achieve optimal quality.

The recent introduction of digital radiography has resulted in a dramatic improvement in image quality of radiographs in the critically ill patient especially at the bedside. Not only is there a marked improvement in image quality but also there is no need for retakes. The images being digital can be adjusted so as to correct any under or over exposure, thus helping to remove any variability. There are two means to go to digital. One is to have purely digital X-ray machines; these are very expensive and portable digital X-ray machines are not available. The best means available today is CR where routine X-ray machines are used and rather than recording the image on film, images are recorded on an imaging plate in pixels. Another advantage is that as soon as the imaging plate is processed in the X-ray department, the image can be visualized in the ICU as the images can be sent using the hospital computer networks or to the physician or radiologist at a remote location, even his home, via the internet.

Most of the X-rays taken in the ICU are an AP view with the patient upright. In this view, there is cardiac magnification and it is very difficult to comment on the cardiac size. It should also be kept in mind that in supine chest X-rays the lung volume appears smaller. Another point which is often overlooked is the difficulty encountered in getting a critically ill patient to sit upright. A pathology in the lung bases can easily be missed in an X-ray chest taken when a patient is not totally upright. Every effort should therefore be made to position the patient correctly.

CT scan has evolved over the last two decades and is now an integral part of the radiological work up. Its cross sectional display eliminates superimposition of structures, improves contrast, resolution and tissue characterization, thus allowing better diagnosis of diseases. The only disadvantage is the need to transport the patient to the CT scanner suite and back. This can be time-consuming and occasionally risky with the patient away from the intensive care unit. However the useful information offered by CT far outweighs the risks. In one study, evaluation of thoracic CT in critically ill patients provided useful additional information, which was not available on plain chest X-rays in 70 per cent of the cases (4, 5).

Pulmonary Oedema

This is one of the most important pathologies affecting the cardiovascular system and a very frequent cause of respiratory distress in the critically ill patient. There are three main causes for pulmonary oedema: (i) cardiogenic oedema; (ii) overhydration oedema due to overinfusion of fluids or renal failure; (iii) increased capillary permeability due to various insults to the capillary membrane. The initial treatment for pulmonary oedema is the same irrespective of the aetiology. Management however requires accurate assessment and correction of the underlying cause. The chest radiograph should therefore be evaluated not only for signs of pulmonary oedema, but also to identify the underlying aetiology.

The radiographic features of pulmonary oedema can be considered in three categories:

(a) Pulmonary venous hypertension

(b) Interstitial oedema

(c) Alveolar oedema

On an upright chest radiograph of a normal subject, the lower lobe vessels are more prominent than the upper lobe vessels. With elevation of pulmonary venous pressures the blood flow is redirected to the mid and upper zones. In addition non-perfused blood vessels in the upper zones are opened up and there is reflex vasoconstriction of the lower zone vessels, resulting in a vascular redistribution on the chest radiograph. The appearances can be classified into three types: (i) Normal or caudalization of blood flow i.e. normal flow patterns; (ii) balanced, essentially equal blood flow to apices and bases; (iii) inverted or cephalization of blood flow—when the upper lobe vessels are larger than the lower lobe vessels. These findings will only be observed on upright X-rays; recumbent or supine X-rays may show no evidence of vascular redistribution.

When the pulmonary capillary wedge pressure (PCWP) increases to 18–25 mm Hg there is transudation of fluid into the interstitium; when the PCWP is > 25 mm Hg, transudation of fluid occurs into the alveoli. Interstitial oedema is recognized by the presence of Kerley lines, perivascular cuffing, peribronchial cuffing and perihilar haze. The Kerley lines are of three types A,B,C. Kerley A lines are 2–6 cm in length and about 1 mm in thickness. These lines radiate from the hilum to the periphery of the lung and are best seen in the upper zones. Kerley B lines are 1–2 cm long and about 1 mm in diameter. These lines are seen in the subpleural regions of the lower zones adjacent to the costophrenic angles. Kerley B lines are more frequently seen than the Kerley A lines. Kerley C lines are considered as an overlap between A and B. These are not important as they are seldom detected on a chest radiograph. With transudation of the fluid into the interstitium around the vessels and bronchi, the sharp margin of these structures becomes indistinct and this is known as perivascular and peribronchial cuffing. Similarly exudation into the interstitium about the hilum results in a perihilar haze.

Alveolar oedema occurs with transudation of fluid into the alveoli and is characterized by fluffy ill-defined opacities in the lung, especially in the central zones giving rise to a bat's wing or butterfly appearance (**Fig. 5.2.1**). Often an air bronchogram pattern may be seen within these ill-defined fluffy shadows.

Unilateral pulmonary oedema is not an uncommon finding and poses a diagnostic dilemma, as the radiological appearances may be similar to those seen with an inflammatory pathology (**Fig. 5.2.2**). Pulmonary oedema may occur in one lung or lobe, either due to a disease process within that lung (e.g. patients lying on one side for prolonged periods, or unilateral veno-occlusive disease), or may be related to some pathology in the opposite lung which prevents pulmonary oedema from developing on the same side (e.g. cases with unilateral pulmonary emboli or the Sweyer-James syndrome). The distribution of unilateral pulmonary oedema may

be patchy, with some areas of the lung being more affected than others. This is usually due to underlying emphysema, scarring, or radiation injury. It is difficult to differentiate focal pulmonary oedema from focal inflammation radiologically, and a clinical correlation together with serial follow-up X-rays are often needed to confirm the diagnosis.

Differentiation between Cardiogenic Oedema, Overhydration Oedema and Capillary Oedema

Milne and co-workers (**6**) have reported that these could be differentiated on the basis of three principal features—distribution of pulmonary blood flow, distribution of pulmonary oedema, and width of the vascular pedicle. Systemic blood volume is accurately depicted by the vascular pedicle which is the portion of the superior mediastinum containing the great vessels. As these vessels are distensible they respond to changes in the circulating blood volume (**7**).

It has been found that the vascular pedicle was enlarged in 60 per cent of patients with cardiac oedema, and 85 per cent of patients with renal failure or overhydration; in contrast, 70 per cent of patients with capillary permeability oedema had a vascular pedicle of normal width (**6**). As regards the distribution of pulmonary flow, patients with overhydration oedema had balanced or cephalization of blood flow, while patients with capillary permeability oedema had normal or balanced flow. The distribution of oedema was symmetric, perihilar in patients with cardiac or overhydration oedema, whereas capillary permeability oedema appeared patchy and peripheral.

Acute Lung Injury (ARDS)

ARDS is a consequence of acute lung injury resulting in damage to the alveolar epithelium and pulmonary vasculature with resultant capillary permeability oedema. Three stages have been described in ARDS (**8**).

Stage I is the earliest and occurs within a few hours after the insult. Pathologically there is a pulmonary capillary congestion, endothelial cell swelling and extensive micro-atelectasis. As the fluid leakage into the interstitium is minimal the radiograph at this stage shows relatively clear lungs, though the lung volumes may appear small due to diminished compliance. If the acute lung injury is due to a primary lung pathology such as aspiration or pneumonia, then pulmonary opacities related to this condition will also be seen.

Stage II occurs about 2–5 days after the injury. The pathological features are of fibrin deposition, haemorrhagic fluid leakage and hyaline membrane formation. These are seen on the radiograph as diffuse ill-defined bilaterally symmetrical patchy areas of consolidation, which may have an air bronchogram pattern present in them. Asymmetrical shadowing can also occur. Rarely there may be associated pleural effusions, but these are usually small.

Stage III is characterized by collagen deposition, proliferation of fibroblasts and epithelial cells. Radiologically the appearance is of progressive lung destruction with a transition from alveolar to interstitial opacities. The treatment of ARDS includes positive pressure ventilation which may result in barotrauma, manifested by pneumothorax, pneumatocele, pneumomediastinum or pulmonary interstitial emphysema (**Figs. 5.2.3, 5.2.4**). With the use of PEEP, there may be areas of overinflation or barotrauma in the lung parenchyma which give rise to the appearance of disappearing opacities. However this is not accompanied by evidence of clinical or physiological improvement. After recovery there may be residual fibrosis and focal emphysema, but often the X-ray returns to normal.

Pneumothorax and pneumomediastinum are easily identified on radiographs. However CT helps in detecting the early features of barotrauma e.g. interstitial pulmonary emphysema and pneumatoceles. Interstitial pulmonary emphysema (IPE) is seen as thin streaks of air in the interstitium and should be differentiated from an air bronchogram. There is sharp delineation of the bronchovascular bundle in IPE. A CT examination can detect a large pneumatocele formed by the coalescing of small thin walled peripheral cysts.

In stage II ARDS the X-ray may resemble that of cardiogenic pulmonary oedema, and needs to be differentiated from it. In contrast to cardiogenic, uraemic and hypervolaemic pulmonary oedema, the alveolar oedema of ARDS is not associated with widening of the vascular pedicle, cardiomegaly or altered pulmonary blood flow distribution. The pulmonary vessels visualized are usually constricted because capillary leak occurs directly into the alveolar spaces and septal lines are absent.

Pneumonia

Aspiration Pneumonia

Aspiration pneumonia occurs as a result of endotracheal aspiration of oropharyngeal or gastric secretions. Tracheal and oesophageal intubation, depressed cough reflex, impaired mucociliary function, increased secretions, cardiopulmonary resuscitation events, and the supine posture, are factors which predispose the critically ill patient to aspirate. Radiologically the demonstration of suddenly appearing new focal pulmonary lesions, should raise the suspicion of aspiration. The areas of involvement are mainly in the dependent portion of the lung—superior segments of the lower lobes, or posterior segments of the upper and lower lobes when the patient is supine (**Fig. 5.2.5**). If the patient has been in the lateral decubitus position, aspiration causes collapse consolidation of multiple segments of one lung, while the other lung is spared. Patients who are prone in rotobeds show involvement of the anterior segments of the upper and lower lobes, the middle lobe and the lingula (**9**). Aspiration pneumonia may be complicated by a necrotizing lung abscess. Aspiration of gastric contents results in an acute pulmonary reaction with pulmonary oedema causing chemical pneumonitis. This type of pneumonitis may eventually progress to ARDS or secondary bacterial pneumonia.

Nosocomial Pneumonia

Nosocomial pneumonia is defined as a lower respiratory tract infection occurring after 72 hours of hospital admission, and is an important cause of death in hospitalized patients. A large study showed that 31 per cent of patients admitted to an ICU were at risk of developing pneumonia following intubation (**10**). Radiologically nosocomial pneumonia is seen as new or worsening multifocal parenchymal opacities. Nosocomial pneumonias are often complicated by a lung abscess or empyema. These complications help to differentiate nosocomial pneumonia from other conditions like atelectasis or pulmonary oedema which may present in critically ill individuals as new opacities on a chest radiograph.

Community-acquired Pneumonia

The appearances can be divided into three types—lobar pneumonia, bronchopneumonia and interstitial pneumonia. In lobar pneumonia there is usually alveolar inflammation resulting in a diffuse opacity with the presence of an air bronchogram pattern. The opacity usually involves a segment or a portion of a lobe; rarely it may involve the entire lobe. It is generally impossible on radiographic appearance to differentiate the various bacteriological organisms which cause pneumonia. However when there is evidence of increased lung volume in the affected portion of the lung, then the possibility of Klebsiella or Pneumococcal pneumonia should be considered. It is important to localize the consolidation to a specific lobe as this is helpful to the bronchoscopist. The 'silhouette sign' is used to determine the site of the consolidation. Whenever the consolidation is adjacent to a soft tissue structure it causes obliteration of the margin of that structure. When the consolidation is adjacent to the right border of the heart, it is localized to the right middle lobe; when the consolidation is in the left lingula it obliterates the left heart border. Lower lobe pneumonias may cause loss of the diaphragmatic contour.

Bronchopneumonia results from inflammation of the terminal end-respiratory bronchioles. Radiologically this is seen as patchy infiltrates involving multiple segments. There may be evidence of volume loss, but air bronchograms are usually not visualized.

Interstitial pneumonias are usually caused by viruses or Mycoplasma pneumoniae. Radiologically they appear as diffuse reticular opacities in both lung fields with peribronchial thickening. These changes may however progress to an alveolar inflammation thereby simulating a lobar pneumonia.

Parapneumonic fluid collections may accompany pneumonias. These are usually well seen on radiographs, though occasionally they may be difficult to separate from a consolidation. In such situations a sonography or CT examination accurately picks up fluid within the pleural space, and enables the interventional radiologist to perform a guided aspiration of the fluid. Examination of the fluid confirms the diagnosis of empyema. Mediastinal adenopathy is not usually present with bacterial pneumonias, but may be seen with tuberculosis, fungal and viral pneumonias. Pneumonia may be complicated by the formation of lung abscess or empyema. The diagnostic feature of a lung abscess is the presence of an air-fluid level. For this to be demonstrated the patient has to be in the erect position. Occasionally the abscess may have no significant fluid level and appears as a cavitatory lesion. This needs to be differentiated from a bulla, pneumatocele, or a cavitatory neoplasm. Bullae and pneumatoceles have thin walls whereas lung abscesses have relatively thick walls. A cavitatory neoplasm usually does not have any perilesional inflammation, as is usually seen with a lung abscess. It has been reported that lung abscesses may not be detected radiologically in 18 per cent of cases **(11)**. A CT in these patients becomes mandatory. CT clearly demonstrates the air-fluid level in an abscess **(Fig. 5.2.6)**. CT is also very useful in differentiating between pleural and parenchymal components which may be superimposed on a plain X-ray, and thus be difficult to differentiate.

Atelectasis

Atelectasis is one of the commonest findings on chest X-ray taken in the ICU. The left lower lobe is the most frequent location of atelectasis, especially in the post-bypass patient **(Fig. 5.2.7)**. The atelectatic portion of the lung has variable radiological appearances. It may be seen as plate-like or linear opacities known as plate atelectasis. Loss of volume is evidenced by shift of the fissures, hilum, diaphragm, trachea and heart. A bronchogram pattern may be seen within the opacity. This is an important finding because patients with an air bronchogram pattern within an atelectatic segment may not improve with bronchoscopy. If no air bronchogram is seen the patient is likely to improve with bronchoscopic aspiration **(12)**.

Pulmonary Embolism

The X-ray findings **(Fig. 5.2.8)** and spiral CT angiography scan abnormalities **(Fig. 5.2.9)** seen in critically ill patients with pulmonary embolism, have been discussed in the Chapter on Pulmonary Embolism.

Fig. 5.2.10 demonstrates a case with septic embolism which occurred in a patient with congenital heart disease.

Pleural Effusions

Free pleural effusions tend to gravitate to the most dependent portions of the pleural cavity. On erect chest X-rays these are seen as homogenous densities in the lower zone with a typical concave or upward-sloping contour, the lateral margin being higher than the medial margin. The posterior costophrenic (CP) sulcus is the deepest portion of the pleura. This is the site where the fluid tends to first accumulate. Radiologically this is seen as blunting of the costophrenic angle on the lateral view.

At least 200 ml of fluid is required to cause obliteration of the CP angle on a PA view of the chest, though in some cases there is no blunting of the angle even when 500 ml of fluid is present. The lateral decubitus view is the most sensitive X-ray to demonstrate free fluid. Fluid is seen layering in the dependent part of the chest wall as a thin uniform opacity. This view however may be technically difficult to obtain in a patient who is critically ill. In patients who are too critically ill to sit erect, a diagnosis of pleural effusion has to be made on a supine X-ray chest. The findings in moderate sized or large effusions are a homogenous opacity of the affected hemithorax with absence of the vascular markings. This is because the fluid is layering posteriorly along the chest wall.

Fluid also tends to accumulate along the apex, like an apical pleural cap, and in the base, as these are the most dependent areas on a supine film. Small pleural effusions can be easily missed on a supine radiograph. In fact only 67 per cent sensitivity and 70 per cent specificity have been reported for the detection of a pleural effusion on supine chest X-ray as opposed to a lateral decubitus view **(14)**.

In critically ill patients who cannot be positioned for a lateral decubitus view, or if a supine radiograph shows equivocal or negative findings, sonography is an excellent means for demonstrating pleural fluid. This imaging modality is portable and can be easily performed at the bedside. Pleural fluid is seen as an anechoic area separating the echogenic line of the diaphragm and the echogenic inferior margin of the lung. Sonography is also useful in differentiating a pleural effusion from atelectasis/consolidation which may simulate an effusion on the chest X-ray. Further it is an excellent guide for thoracocentesis markedly reducing the incidence of iatrogenic pneumothorax.

Occasionally free pleural fluid may accumulate in a subpulmonic location between the lung and diaphragm, with the lung floating on the fluid. The upper margin of the fluid may then take the appearance of the diaphragm. Left sided subpulmonic effusions may be detected by noting the wide distance between the stomach air bubble and diaphragm. On the right side differentiation from an enlarged liver pushing the diaphragm upwards may be difficult. In these cases either a lateral decubitus view or sonography is useful to clinch the diagnosis. A loculated effusion may occur when there are adhesions between the visceral and parietal pleura, as a result of which the fluid does not shift with change of the patient's position. Empyema and haemothorax may appear as loculated effusions.

CT is extremely sensitive in detecting even small pleural fluid collections. With the patient supine, free fluid accumulates posteriorly as a hypodense layer conforming to the contour of the chest wall. The presence of septae in the pleural fluid (denoting a likely exudate), is however brought out by a sonographic study rather than by a CT scan. Acute haemorrhage in the pleural space can be well identified by the hyperdensity of blood. CT is also useful in the assessment of the site, extent and wall thickening of the loculated effusions, and for loculated interlobar effusions. These may simulate a mass lesion on plain X-ray but can easily be differentiated on CT. CT with intravenous contrast medium is very useful in differentiating parenchymal from pleural lesions, especially when a plain radiograph has not helped. CT is also an effective guide for thoracocentesis except when the effusion is small and layering posteriorly in the dependent portion of the chest. In these conditions sonography is far superior to CT.

Empyema

On a chest radiograph an empyema is usually seen as a loculated fluid collection. It tends to be lenticular in shape as compared to a lung abscess which is rounded. Further, an empyema usually forms an obtuse angle with the chest wall while a lung abscess forms an acute angle. CT is very useful in the diagnosis and management of empyema. On CT an empyema appears as a well-defined fluid collection with enhancing parietal and visceral pleura (**Fig. 5.2.11**). This sign of separation of the pleura is known as the split pleura sign. CT is far superior to any other imaging modality in differentiating lung abscess from empyema, though occasionally the differentiation may be difficult. On CT a lung abscess is usually rounded whereas an empyema is lenticular in shape. Also, the lung margin is very sharp in relation to an empyema, whereas in a lung abscess there is usually peripheral consolidation around the abscess.

Traditionally empyemas have been treated with insertion of chest tubes. The success rate with chest tube drainage is 35 per cent to 71 per cent (**15**). However 35 per cent of all patients treated with conventional chest tubes are found to subsequently require either open chest tube drainage or decortication. Several studies estimated the success rate of fluoroscopy, sonography and CT in image-guided percutaneous insertion of chest tubes to be between 70–90 per cent. Under imaging the catheter can be placed accurately in the fluid collection. In fact image-guided percutaneous drainage of empyemas is advocated as the primary method of treating empyemas. Patients who show inadequate drainage or progressive persistent pleural thickening, may finally require decortication.

Pneumothorax

This is a relatively common complication seen in the ICU and should be very carefully looked for on every chest radiograph of a critically ill patient, especially following procedures such as thoracocentesis, central venous line insertions, endotracheal intubation, tracheostomy and in patients on positive pressure ventilation. Air in the pleural cavity is seen in the most non-dependent portion of the chest. On the erect chest X-ray it is therefore seen in the apical region. There are numerous radiographic signs to recognize a pneumothorax, the most important being demonstration of the visceral pleura as a thin opaque line. Other signs observed are hypertranslucency between the chest wall and the collapsed lung, this region being devoid of vascular markings (**Fig. 5.2.12**).

The degree of atelectasis of the underlying lung is variable and depends upon the size of the pneumothorax. The underlying lung shows a mild increase in density but appears opaque only when total collapse has occurred. The size of the pneumothorax may be measured, but is usually depicted as small (< 25 per cent), moderate (25–50 per cent) and large (> 50 per cent). Routine X-rays obtained in the ICU are usually inspiratory films and in these films a small pneumothorax may be missed. If there is a high index of suspicion, then an expiratory film should be taken to demonstrate a small pneumothorax. Another important point to bear in mind is that a pneumothorax following a procedure may take up to four hours to develop; thus the ideal X-ray to determine a post-procedure pneumothorax is a delayed (4 hrs) expiratory film.

Often patients are critically ill and cannot be radiographed in the upright position. The appearance of a pneumothorax on a supine film is different. As air collects in the most non-dependent portion (this being the anteroinferior portion on a supine film) this is seen as a hypertranslucency over the upper quadrant with a deep costophrenic sulcus. If these signs are doubtful a cross-table

lateral view is obtained, which clearly shows the collection of air.

Occasionally tubes and skin folds may mimic a pneumothorax; these can however be differentiated by visualizing lung markings beyond these structures. Also skin folds are usually in pairs, bilateral, do not have a sharp margin like the visceral pleura and often extend outside the thorax.

Two unusual types of pneumothorax need to be considered. The more important one is a tension pneumothorax which is an absolute emergency and if untreated will result in death. A tension pneumothorax occurs when air enters during inspiration but cannot exit during expiration due to a check valve mechanism. On a chest X-ray, the entire hemithorax is hypertranslucent, the mediastinum is shifted to the opposite side and the ipsilateral lung is compressed. In addition the diaphragm on the affected side may be deeply inverted. The second unusual type of pneumothorax is when there is collapse or lobar atelectasis. There is diffusion of gas into the pleural space due to volume loss. In this scenario the pneumothorax is essentially an exvaco occurrence, and resolves spontaneously as the affected portion of lung is better aerated by suctioning or bronchoscopy (**16**).

Pneumomediastinum

This may occur following oesophageal rupture, tracheobronchial injuries or alveolar rupture with air tracking into the hilum via the interstitium. Air in the mediastinum is seen as a lucency about the mediastinal structures, bounded laterally by an echogenic line—the mediastinal pleura, which is now visualized as it has air on both sides. Air tracking inferiorly in a pneumomediastinum permits visualization of the infracardiac surface giving rise to the continuous diaphragm sign. In children the mediastinal air elevates the thymus and outlines it, producing a triangular opacity along the lateral mediastinal border, known as the 'spinnaker sail' sign.

Pulmonary Interstitial Emphysema

Pulmonary interstitial emphysema occurs due to elevated intra-alveolar pressure causing rupture of the alveoli, with consequent leak of air into the interstitium. This air then dissects along the bronchovascular bundle which is the path of least resistance. This may extend to the mediastinum or peripherally to the visceral pleura, resulting in pneumomediastinum or pneumothorax. It may also track superiorly into the neck as subcutaneous emphysema, or rarely decompress into the retroperitoneum as a pneumoperitoneum.

On X-ray, pulmonary interstitial emphysema is difficult to detect and can be seen only when it is superimposed on an area of air space consolidation. It is then seen as thin streaky and bubbly radiolucencies. In fact when visualized and compared with previous X-rays, it may falsely suggest an improvement in an air space consolidation, as the density of the consolidation becomes less due to the superimposed radiolucencies. This is one paradoxical situation where the patient clinically deteriorates and yet the radiograph shows an apparent improvement. When there is no air space consolidation and the lung is normally aerated these radiolucencies are not visualized, as they are contrasted against a dark lung. In these cases a CT is very helpful as it demonstrates the linear and cystic areas of air trapping.

Tubes and Supporting Devices

There are numerous tubes and devices used in the ICU for monitoring and support of the critically ill patient. It is important to monitor the position, possible malpositions, and complications of these tubes and devices. Portable chest bedside X-rays usually provide adequate information on these devices/tubes.

Airway Tubes

Endotracheal and tracheostomy tube position should be checked immediately after placement and periodically thereafter to ensure proper positioning, as airway tubes if malpositioned may cause serious complications. These tubes usually have a radiopaque line running along their entire length or may be totally opaque. The correct site for the tip of an endotracheal tube is 5–7 cm above the carina with the head in the neutral position (17). If the carina is not easily delineated, then it is assumed that the carina is between T_5 and T_7 and the endotracheal tube should end 5–6 cm above the T_4/T_5 disc space i.e. between T_2 and T_4. Changes in head position can alter the site of the tip of the endotracheal tube seen on the radiograph as the tube is usually fixed to the nose or mouth. The tube shifts approximately by 2 cm in flexion or extension. It is therefore important to determine the position of the head on the radiograph first. If the tube is too inferior in position it may be seen to extend into the main bronchus especially the right main bronchus resulting in a bronchial intubation (**Fig. 5.2.13 a**). This results in overinflation of the intubated lung which is therefore at increased risk of barotrauma and pneumothorax. The opposite lung may show changes of atelectasis and collapse. Conversely an endotracheal tube not inserted inferior enough may extubate or cause vocal cord damage. To prevent vocal cord damage the tip should be at least 3 cm below the vocal cords. Oesophageal intubation may rarely occur. This is detected by visualizing the tube outside the tracheal lumen and the presence of gross overdistension of the stomach (**Fig. 5.2.13 b, c**). Occasionally it is difficult to determine if the tube is outside the trachea on the frontal radiograph as the oesophagus lies behind the trachea. In these cases a right posterior oblique view, with the patient's head turned to the right allows separation of the oesophagus and trachea.

A tracheostomy tube tip is ideally situated between half and two-thirds the distance from the stoma to the carina, and the width of the tube should be approximately 2/3rd the tracheal width. Tracheal intubation may result in injury to the trachea and consequent tracheal stenosis. Endotracheal intubation may result in subglottic stenosis or stenosis at the cuff site. AP and lateral radiographs of the neck and trachea may demonstrate the site and level of stenosis. CT scan is very useful in the demonstration of subglottic and tracheal stenosis, depicting the level, extent and degree of narrowing. MRI demonstrates the larynx and trachea well and may also be used to demonstrate the site, extent and degree of narrowing.

Nasogastric Tubes

These tubes usually have small rounded radiopaque balls at their lower end denoting the inferior extent of the tube. The ideal location of the tube is in the duodenum as this prevents gastro-oesophageal reflux; it should also be kept in mind that the last 10 cm of the tube has side holes; therefore at least 10 cm should be below the oesophageal hiatus. After introduction of a nasogastric tube a radiograph should be taken to determine its location. Occasionally tubes may be coiled in the pharynx or oesophagus, or worse still, they may be in the tracheobronchial tree, which may result in pneumonia, lung abscess, pneumothorax or a hydropneumothorax. Inadvertent tracheobronchial insertion of a nasogastric tube may occur in patients with endotracheal intubation especially in those with low pressure, high volume balloons, as these do not prevent passage of a feeding tube into the tracheobronchial tree. If inadvertent placement of the tube has occurred into the tracheobronchial tree as seen on X-ray, then the tube is withdrawn and repositioned. A rare malposition has been a perforation of the nasopharynx and base of the skull with an intracranial placement of the nasogastric tube. Rarely oesophageal perforation may result in pneumomediastinum, mediastinal haematoma or pleural effusion. This may occur with a Sengstaken-Blakemore tube when the gastric balloon is inadvertently inflated in the oesophagus.

Thoracotomy Tubes

These tubes are frequently used to evacuate air/fluid from the pleural cavity. This is a clear plastic tube with a radiopaque line along its length which is interrupted by the proximal-most side hole. When used to drain air it is ideally placed in the second intercostal space anteriosuperiorly and directed to the apex. To drain fluid it is ideally located in the 6th, 7th or 8th intercostal space in the midaxillary line and directed posteriorly. Ideally the tubes take a gentle curve within the thorax at the site of penetration of the pleura. The tube may be malpositioned in the lung parenchyma or fissures. Malposition in the lung parenchyma usually leads to the formation of a haematoma, bronchopulmonary fistula or parenchymal laceration. Placement of the tube in a fissure results in poor drainage. The malposition may not be appreciated on a frontal radiograph, but is usually well seen on a lateral radiograph, as the tube is seen to turn sharply medially when in a minor fissure, and obliquely when in a major fissure. Occasionally the tube may be malpositioned within the extrapleural soft tissue resulting in inadequate drainage and subcutaneous emphysema. Rapid decompression of the pleural space by the tube may result in a unilateral re-expansion pulmonary oedema. A pulmonary infarct may occur if lung tissue is sucked into the tube. Fibrous adhesions may occur around an indwelling tube, so that when the tube is removed a track persists and may be confused with a pneumothorax. Fluid may accumulate in this tract and appear as an abscess on a chest X-ray. These tracks usually decrease in size over a few days and then finally disappear.

Central Venous Pressure (CVP) Catheters

Central venous catheters are commonly used in ICU patients to monitor central venous pressure and provide a venous access. These catheters are seen as thin radiopaque tubes extending peripherally from the subclavian, internal jugular or femoral vein into the superior vena cava (SVC). The ideal location of the tip of a CVP tube is in the SVC. This is because the tip should be outside the right atrium and beyond the most proximal venous valves which are usually situated in the subclavian and internal jugular veins.

The CVP catheter may be malpositioned in the internal jugular, opposite subclavian, azygous, brachiocephalic, axillary, hepatic veins or in the right atrium / ventricle. Rarely there may be a possibility of intra-arterial introduction of a CVP catheter. This may be seen in a hypoxic / hypotensive patient in whom the arterial blood is non-pulsatile and dark, simulating venous blood. As the SVC is a right-sided structure, visualization of the catheter on the left side or in the midline should raise the possibility of an intra-arterial placement.

The main complication of CVP catheter insertion is a pneumothorax (**Fig. 5.2.13 d**). This may occur immediately, or may be delayed for a few hours or even days after insertion due to the slow accumulation of pleural air (**18, 19**). Therefore radiographs immediately after placement of CVP catheters may not totally exclude a pneumothorax, and delayed films are required. Haemothorax, perforation of the vessel, mediastinal haemorrhage (**Fig. 5.2.13 e**) and ectopic infusion of intravenous fluids may occur resulting in radiographic appearances of fluid accumulation at these sites. Venous air embolism is another uncommon complication which may be visualized on a chest X-ray as air in the main pulmonary artery, with associated signs of pulmonary embolism. Other complications which may occur, and which are diagnosed on an X-ray are catheter knotting, catheter fragmentation and the 'catheter pinch-off' syndrome. Catheter knotting and fragmentation are serious complications. To visualize the catheter fragments, both frontal and lateral views are required as some fragments may be overlapped on the frontal view. The 'catheter pinch-off' syndrome occurs due to kinking of the catheter between the clavicle and the first rib resulting in poor catheter function and increased incidence of catheter fracture. This is seen on the radiograph as a focal narrowing of the catheter at the site of kinking.

Pulmonary Artery Catheter

The pulmonary artery catheter is a thin radiopaque tube with a balloon at its terminal end. When in situ it is seen to pass from either the internal jugular vein or subclavian vein into the superior vena cava, right atrium, right ventricle and into the pulmonary outflow tract. The tip of this catheter should lie beyond the pulmonic valve in the right or left pulmonary artery. The catheter tip however should not be more than 2 cm lateral to the pulmonary hilum on the frontal chest radiograph (**Fig. 5.2.13f, g**). When the balloon is inflated to measure pulmonary wedge pressure, it is seen as a rounded radiolucency at the tip of the catheter.

Complications which may occur due to the catheter are pulmonary infarction if the catheter is placed too distally and the balloon inflated, thereby occluding a pulmonary vessel. Intracardiac placement of the catheter can result in arrhythmias or perforation. A rare complication is the formation of a pulmonary artery pseudo-aneurysm which is seen on a chest X-ray as a rounded well defined opacity in relation to the pulmonary artery. This can be easily confirmed with a CT pulmonary angio.

Intra-aortic Counterpulsation Balloon

The distal tip of this catheter is visualized as a small radiopaque rectangle. The ideal location for this balloon is at the proximal portion of the descending aorta just distal to the left subclavian artery. If the catheter is advanced too far, it may obstruct the left subclavian artery or carotid artery leading to ischaemic changes. An abdominal location of the catheter may occur in extensively atherosclerotic or tortuous aorta, resulting in occlusion of the intra-abdominal vessels and consequent renal / mesenteric ischaemia. Rarely this catheter may cause aortic dissection.

Cardiac Pacemakers

These are used in the treatment of bradyarrhythmias and various degrees of heart block. They are usually implanted by either epicardial placement or transvenous placement, the latter technique being more commonly used. On frontal radiographs the right ventricular electrode of a pacing catheter should point just to the left of the midline, and on the lateral view the catheter projects anteriorly and inferiorly with the electrode seen behind the sternum.

The electrode may be malpositioned in the right atrium, pulmonary outflow tract, inferior vena cava or coronary sinus. This may occur in 3–14 per cent of cases (**20**). Most of the above sites of malposition are well identified on frontal radiographs. A pacing catheter malpositioned in the coronary sinus is difficult to appreciate on a frontal radiograph. A lateral radiograph however shows the catheter directed to the posterior aspect of the heart rather than the anterior.

Thoracic Aortic Aneurysm

Spiral CT angio is the modality of choice in the evaluation of thoracic aortic aneurysms. Spiral CTA demonstrates the exact extent of the aneurysm in multiple planes. Further the mural thrombus and true lumen are well visualized. Through angiography has been considered the gold standard in evaluation of thoracic aortic aneurysms, it only demonstrates the true lumen of the aneurysm. The mural thrombus and aortic wall are not demonstrated on angiography. Spiral CTA also visualizes the arch vessels and defines the relationship of the arch vessels with the aneurysm, the effect of the aneurysm on adjacent structures, and in case of aortic rupture demonstrates a periaortic haematoma. Spiral CTA provides information regarding lumen / wall / structures outside the wall, rules out other clinical conditions which may simulate dissection.

Aortic Dissection

Spiral CTA is the ideal technique to evaluate aortic dissection. The definitive diagnosis of aortic dissection requires the identification of the intimal flap, which is seen as a linear density within the lumen of the aorta separating the true and false lumens (**Fig. 5.2.14**). In chronic dissection CTA can also demonstrate thrombosis within the false lumen. MRI also demonstrates whether the aortic branches arise from the true or false lumen, and also identifies the most serious complication of dissection, viz. aortic rupture.

A diagnostic problem which affects CT, MRI and angiography, is the differentiation between a completely thrombus-filled false channel, and a thoracic aortic aneurysm with a mural thrombus. If the patent lumen is eccentric and appears to be compressed, if the thrombus extends for > 7 cm, and if the thrombus changes position within the aorta at different levels, then it is more likely to be related to dissection.

REFERENCES

1. Henschke CI, Pasternack GS, Schroeder S et al. (1983). Bedside chest radiography: Diagnostic efficacy. Radiology. 149, 23–26.
2. Janower ML, Jennas-Nocera Z, Mukai J. (1984). Utility and efficacy of portable chest radiographs. Am J Roentgenol. 142, 265–267.
3. Bekemeyer WB, Crapo RO, Calhoon S et al. (1985). Efficacy of chest radiography in a respiratory intensive care unit. A prospective study. Chest. 88(5), 691–696.
4. Mirvis SE et al. (1987). Thoracic CT in detecting occult disease in critically ill patients. Am J Roentgenol. 148, 685–689.
5. Snow M, Bergin KT, Horrigan TP. (1990). Thoracic CT scanning in critically ill patients. Information obtained frequently alters management. Chest. 97, 1467–1470.
6. Milne ENC et al. (1985). The radiologic distinction of cardiogenic and non-cardiogenic pulmonary oedema. Am J Roentgenol. 144, 879–894.
7. Milne ENC, Pistolesi M, Miniati M et al. (1984). The vascular pedicle of the heart and the vena azygous. Part I—The normal subject. Radiology. 152, 1–8.
8. Bachogen M, Weibel ER. (1977). Alterations of the gas exchange apparatus in adult respiratory insufficiency associated with septicaemia. Am Rev Respir Dis. 116, 589–615.
9. Carlson RW, Geheb MA. (1994). Imaging in the intensive care unit. Critical Care Clinics. 10(2), 260.
10. Ruiz-Santana S et al. (1987). ICU pneumonias: A multi-institutional study. Crit Care Med. 15, 930–932.
11. Brown K, Raman SS, Kallman C. (2002). Imaging Procedures. In: Current Critical Care Diagnosis and Treatment (Eds Bongard FS, Sue DY). pp. 146–203. McGraw-Hill, USA.
12. Harns RS. (1985). The importance of proximal and distal air bronchograms in the management of atelectasis. Can Assoc Radiol J. 36, 103–109.
13. Habscheid W, Hohmann M, Wilhelm T et al. (1990). Real time ultrasound in acute deep vein thrombosis of the lower extremity. Angiology. 41(8), 599–608.
14. Ruskin JA, Gurney JW, Thorsen MK et al. (1987). Detection of pleural effusions on supine chest radiographs. Am J Roentgenol. 148, 681–683.
15. Muller NL. (1993). Imaging of the pleura. Radiology. 186, 297–309.
16. Patz EF Jr. (1993). Radiographic evaluation of extra-alveolar air. In: Imaging and Invasive Radiology in the Intensive Care Unit (Ed. Ravin CE). pp. 39. Churchill Livingstone.
17. Zarshenas Z, Sparaschu RA. (1994). Imaging in the intensive care unit. Catheter placement and misplacement. Critical Care Clinics. 10(2), 418.
18. Sivak SC. (1986). Late appearance of pneumothorax after subclavian venepuncture. Am J Med. 80, 323–324.
19. Plaus WJ. (1990). Delayed pneumothorax after subclavian catheterization. J Parent Entr Nutrition. 14, 414–415.
20. Steiner RM, Legtmeyer CJ, Morse D. (1986). The radiology of cardiac pacemakers. Radiographics. 6, 373–399.

Imaging Techniques in the Abdomen

Contributed by Dr Anirudh Kohli, MD, DNB, DMRD, Head of Department of Radiology, Breach Candy Hospital, Mumbai.

General Considerations

The radiologist is now well armed with a full complement of diagnostic modalities to evaluate the abdomen in a critical care setting. These modalities are also an excellent guide for therapeutic procedures. A plain X-ray of the abdomen (erect and supine) is usually the first investigation ordered. These films are very useful in diagnosing perforation, bowel obstruction, bowel ischaemia and other bowel pathologies. Calcification, calculi, foreign bodies and information regarding position and placement of tubes, are easily detected on plain X-rays.

A chest X-ray is also mandatory as this is the best view to demonstrate a pneumoperitoneum with gas under the diaphragm. A number of chest pathologies may present clinically as an acute abdomen e.g. pneumonia, congestive heart failure, myocardial infarction, dissecting aortic aneurysm, pulmonary infarction and pericarditis. Acute abdominal conditions can also cause respiratory complications, chiefly pleural effusion, atelectasis, and aspiration pneumonia. Finally, an X-ray of the chest on admission, provides a good baseline study. Post-operative complications like a subphrenic abscess may cause subtle changes on an X-ray, which may be evident only on comparison with a baseline X-ray.

Sonography is indispensable in the evaluation of the abdomen and pelvis in critically ill patients with acute abdominal problems, as it can be performed at the bedside. In fact it is the modality of choice for evaluation of the gallbladder, free fluid, genitourinary system, and compares well with CT in evaluation of the liver. Unfortunately bowel gas, obesity, wound dressings, and abdominal scars interfere with sonographic evaluation.

A CT scan is the modality of choice as it can image the entire abdomen and pelvis, and factors which interfere with sonographic evaluation do not hamper a CT scan. The only disadvantage is the need to transport the patient to the CT scanner suite. However the information that is gained far outweighs the risk of transportation of the patient.

Spiral CT angiography is an excellent non-invasive modality to visualize the abdominal vasculature especially aortic aneurysms.

MRI of the abdomen and pelvis has not shown the promise it has demonstrated in the evaluation of the brain and the spine. It is a lengthy procedure with poor visualization of most abdominal

pathologies; however it is useful in vascular pathologies where spiral CT angiography is contraindicated such as when serum creatinine is elevated or there is known allergy to contrast media. Angiography is now mainly used as a combined diagnostic and therapeutic procedure for the treatment of GI haemorrhage.

Acute Cholecystitis

Sonography is the modality of choice in evaluating acute cholecystitis. The hallmark of acute cholecystitis is the presence of gallstones with a positive sonographic Murphy's sign. These features are present in 92 per cent of cases of acute cholecystitis [1]. The sonographic Murphy's sign is similar to the clinical Murphy's sign, the only difference being that pressure is applied by the sonography transducer instead of the clinician's hand. This sign is more sensitive than the clinical sign as the transducer is applied exactly over the site of the gallbladder. Gallstones are seen as echogenic (bright) dependent shadows which are accompanied by acoustic shadowing below the calculi due to reflection of the sound waves by the calculi. The calculi are usually mobile and move with change in the patient's position; occasionally they may be impacted at the neck of the gallbladder and in these situations do not move with change of position. Other sonographic findings are gall bladder wall thickening, presence of sludge and pericholecystic fluid. These signs are not specific as they are seen in a variety of other conditions. The gallbladder wall is considered to be thickened when it exceeds 3 mm in diameter. Sludge in the gallbladder may be seen as echogenic material layering the dependent portion of the gallbladder with no shadowing. Pericholecystic fluid is seen as a thin halo around the gallbladder.

Complications of acute cholecystitis are gangrenous cholecystitis, emphysematous cholecystitis and perforation. Gangrenous changes are reported to occur in 2–38 per cent of cases of acute cholecystitis [2]. On sonography this appears as marked asymmetry of the gallbladder wall evidenced by focal wall thickening and irregularity of the wall. These changes are due to mucosal oedema, necrosis, ulcers, intramural haemorrhage and microabscesses in the gallbladder wall. There may also be intraluminal echoes due to sloughing of the gall bladder mucosa and fibrous/mucosal debris. An important sonographic sign in gangrenous cholecystitis is the conversion of a positive sonographic Murphy's sign to a negative sonographic Murphy's sign due to denervation of the gallbladder. This is usually accompanied by diffuse abdominal pain. Emphysematous cholecystitis is a severe variant of acute cholecystitis which occurs due to gas-forming bacteria invading and devitalizing the gallbladder wall. More than one-third of patients with emphysematous cholecystitis are diabetics; gangrene and perforation of the gallbladder are important complications. The sonographic findings depend upon the demonstration of gas which is released by the bacteria into the lumen or wall of the gallbladder. Air in the lumen is seen as an echogenic (bright) non-dependent area, whereas air in the gallbladder wall is seen as a curvilinear or arc-like echogenic area (**Fig. 5.3.1**).

Perforations occur in 5–10 per cent of cases with acute cholecystitis (**3**). It can present in three forms: (i) an acute form which results in generalized peritonitis; (ii) a subacute form which results in the formation of a pericholecystic abscess; (iii) a chronic form which results in an internal biliary fistula. Most cases are of the subacute variety resulting in abscess formation at the fundus of the gallbladder. It is important to differentiate an intraperitoneal abscess from a gallbladder bed/intramural abscess, as the former requires surgery and the latter can be managed conservatively. Abscesses are seen as ill-defined hypoechoic to echogenic collections in relation to the gallbladder. CT is considered superior to sonography in the evaluation of pericholecystic abscesses. Contrast enhanced CT reveals a thick walled irregular enhancing lesion with a necrotic core, adjacent to the gall bladder.

Acalculous Cholecystitis

In 5–10 per cent of cases of acute cholecystitis no calculi can be demonstrated in the gallbladder (**4**). This form of cholecystitis has a higher mortality and morbidity rate, and is seen particularly in patients following trauma, surgery, sepsis, and burns; it is also observed in critically ill patients with shock and poor perfusion, in patients with diabetes mellitus, and in hyperalimentation. Gangrene and perforation are common complications. The sonographic signs are limited by the absence of calculi and diagnosis rests on demonstration of the sonographic Murphy's sign, gallbladder wall thickening, presence of sludge and pericholecystic fluid. When there is a high index of suspicion on clinical grounds but imaging findings are negative, an imaging-guided aspiration of the gallbladder contents may be performed and the fluid sent for bacteriology and leucocyte count. In patients who are too ill to undergo surgery, a percutaneous cholecystostomy may be performed by introduction of a catheter into the gall bladder under imaging guidance. Using sonography a 97.5 per cent success rate has been reported for cannulating the gallbladder (**5**). Complications that may occur with this procedure are biliary peritonitis, bilioma, haemobilia, and vagal reaction. However the reported complication rate in elderly patients is 10 per cent which is far better than the surgical complication rate for cholecystectomy which is 24 per cent (**5**). Therefore in a critically ill patient percutaneous cholecystostomy can be used as a temporizing procedure till such time as the patient is ready for cholecystectomy.

Pancreatitis

CT is the imaging modality of choice for evaluation of acute pancreatitis. It is not limited by gaseous shadows in the intestinal loops, by abdominal bandages, or by an obese abdominal wall; it also evaluates the retroperitoneum extremely well.

Sonography has limited use in the evaluation of acute pancreatitis. It is useful for detecting biliary calculi as a cause of pancreatitis and helps in the follow-up of pancreatic fluid collections. It is also useful as a guide for aspiration of fluid collections. The inflamed pancreas may be visualized on sonography as an enlarged gland with a decrease in its echogenicity due to oedema of the gland. However as necrotic areas are not evaluated well by sonography, CT becomes mandatory.

MRCP—Magnetic Resonance Cholangio-Pancreatography—is particularly useful in evaluation of the aetiological cause of acute pancreatitis. It has a sensitivity of close to 100 per cent in detecting calculi as small as 2 mm. It is also useful to detect pancreas divisum.

There are two distinct forms of pancreatitis—acute oedematous pancreatitis and acute necrotizing pancreatitis. In acute oedematous pancreatitis there is only mild swelling of the pancreas with loss of normal lobulations and a diffuse decrease in attenuation of the pancreas. This form of pancreatitis runs a mild course and rarely progresses to acute necrotizing pancreatitis with its associated complications.

Acute necrotizing pancreatitis is a fulminant form of pancreatitis in which there is necrosis of the pancreas. These areas of necrosis may be diffuse or focal, consisting of non-viable pancreatic parenchyma which vary in size, location and extent. A dynamic contrast enhanced CT accurately defines the extent of pancreatic necrosis (**Fig. 5.3.2**); this has been found to correlate very well with the extent of necrosis found at surgery. Necrosis is seen on CT as areas within the pancreas which exhibit no enhancement. These necrotic areas have a very important bearing on the course of pancreatitis, as they are liable to undergo secondary infection and form pancreatic abscesses. The more extensive the pancreatic necrosis the greater is the morbidity and mortality. Patients with no pancreatic necrosis have been found to have a 0 per cent mortality and a 6 per cent complication rate, whereas patients with pancreatic necrosis have a 23 per cent mortality rate and a 82 per cent complication rate (**6**).

Patients with acute necrotizing pancreatitis usually have accompanying peripancreatic changes in the form of oedema, effusions and phlegmon. Oedematous changes in the peripancreatic region are manifested by a subtle increase in the density of the peripancreatic fat which on CT has a non-homogenous appearance with strands and thickened fascial planes. The anterior pararenal fascia is often thickened; this is more evident on the left than on the right side. Effusions or acute fluid collections are enzyme rich pancreatic juice collections seen in about 40 per cent of patients with acute pancreatitis (**7**). The fluid collections usually develop around the inflamed gland; they are localized only by the anatomic space in which they collect (**Fig. 5.3.3**). Peripancreatic fluid collections are very well demonstrated by CT scans, and are most commonly seen in the anterior pancreatic region, the lesser sac, the anterior pararenal, perirenal, posterior pararenal regions, and rarely in the mesocolon and root of the mesentry. These fluid collections are usually limited by the thickened pararenal or Gerota's fascia. The quantity of fluid in these effusions is variable and can range from a small amount to large quantities. Of these collections, 50 per cent resolve spontaneously; the remainder may evolve into pseudocysts (8).

Sepsis

Sepsis is a major complication of pancreatitis and is accompanied by a high incidence of mortality and a prolonged hospital stay. Pancreatic abscesses occur following secondary infection of parenchymal pancreatic necrosis, phlegmon, effusions and pseudocysts. Detection of the development of sepsis in these areas is very difficult even with a CT, the only sure sign being the presence of gas due to secondary infection by coliform bacteria. Gas is seen in the fluid collection as very dark well-defined bubbles (**Fig. 5.3.4**). Occasionally gas may be present due to a gastrointestinal fistula or previous surgery. It is important to note that a small amount of fat may be seen interspersed with a pancreatic phlegmon as a result of fat necrosis; this should not be confused with air bubbles which are indicative of abscess formation. The differentiation is easy by CT, the values of fat ranging between –20 Hu to –80 Hu, and of air being $\geq$ –300 Hu. Also air bubbles have well-defined margins and are homogenously jet black, whereas fat is non-homogenously grey with ill-defined margins.

Since the presence of air is seen only in a small per cent of patients with pancreatic abscesses, the diagnosis of pancreatic sepsis has to be made by CT-guided aspiration. All sites of fluid collection, parenchymal necrosis and peripancreatic phlegmon are subjected to CT-guided aspiration. This is a tedious process and requires a dedicated interventional radiologist as there are often more than 5–6 sites from which it may be necessary to obtain samples. The sites of aspiration are marked and guided by CT, a fresh needle and syringe being used for each site. Care is taken not to go through the large bowel as the colon has a large number of bacteria, and transgressing it could result in colonic bacteria contaminating the CT-guided aspiration sample, with false positive results. Further, colonic bacteria may be inoculated into the effusion or phlegmon thereby converting a sterile collection into an infected one. Technical expertise is therefore of utmost importance. Complications of the procedure include pnuemothorax/ empyema if the pleura is transgressed, haemorrhage due to trauma to a vessel, and secondary infection.

It is crucial from the management point of view, to differentiate an abscess from infected necrosis. An abscess may be treated by percutaneous drainage, whereas infected necrosis developing in relatively solid tissue, can be treated by surgical debridement alone. On CT an abscess is seen as a peripancreatic fluid collection which is composed of liquid pus, as determined by needle aspiration. Infected necrosis is seen on CT as a non-enhancing solid or partly liquefied soft tissue which reveals infected material on needle aspiration. As the CT appearances of an abscess and infected necrosis may be similar, needle aspiration is crucial in differentiating between the two conditions.

Pancreatic sepsis is treated by surgical debridement, necrosectomy and drainage through thick tubes. CT is invaluable in surgical planning and in the follow-up of post-operative patients to evaluate any fresh collection, and to determine whether the drains are well sited or not. Patients who are too critically ill to undergo surgery for pancreatic sepsis, may benefit from CT guided introduction of pigtail and sump catheters. These CT guided procedures are extremely successful elsewhere in the abdomen; however in pancreatitis they have met with only limited success. This is due to the fact that the sepsis of pancreatic necrosis and phlegmon, usually causes infection in solid tissues which requires manual debridement, and attempts to drain this prove futile. Interventional radiology is mainly a temporizing procedure which helps to tide the patient over a period of time, till the patient is deemed fit for surgery.

Pseudocysts

Pseudocysts are round or oval encapsulated fluid collections containing necrotic material, proteinaceous debris and enzymatic material. On CT, a pseudocyst appears as a well-defined fluid collection with a thin capsule. The most common location for pseudocysts is the lesser sac, though they may be found anywhere in the mediastinum, abdomen or pelvis as they may dissect along fascial planes, along vessels and through capsules of solid organs. Complicated, enlarging or symptomatic pseudocysts require percutaneous catheter or surgical drainage.

Infected pseudocysts are treated by percutaneous drainage. The management of a noninfected psudocyst is controversial. Surgical treatment is only undertaken when the wall is mature after several weeks. Large pseudocysts greater than 5 cm in size can easily be drained percutaneously. The cure rates are reported to be 85 per cent with percutaneous drainage, the drainage period averaging about 20 days (9).

Retroperitoneal Haemorrhage

Retroperitoneal haemorrhage may occur as a late complication due to vascular injuries produced by the extravasated pancreatic enzymes. These injuries result in the formation of a pseudoaneurysm which may rupture resulting in massive haemorrhage. This is seen on CT as high density fluid in the retroperitoneum, or as a pseudocyst. The commonly involved vessels are the splenic or pancreatoduodenal arcade. The diagnosis is usually confirmed by angiography and subsequently treated by embolization of the bleeding vessel.

Grading

CT may be used as a prognostic indicator of the severity of acute pancreatitis. The patients are classified into 5 grades:

Grade A—Normal CT of pancreas.

Grade B—Diffuse pancreatic enlargement with or without parenchymal necrosis.

Grade C—Pancreatic enlargement with necrosis and peripancreatic oedema.

Grade D—Pancreatic involvement with a single ill-defined peripancreatic fluid collection or phlegmon.

Grade E—Two or more fluid collections and/or the presence of gas.

Most complications of acute pancreatitis occur in Grade D and E patients. A more accurate grading system is the CT Severity Index (CTSI), in which patients are assigned 0–4 points depending upon their grade (from A to E). To this 2, 4 or 6 points are added depending upon the extent of pancreatic necrosis—30 per cent necrosis or less is given 2 points; 30 per cent to 50 per cent necrosis is given 4 points, and > 50 per cent necrosis is given 6 points. Thus the patients are graded on a scale of 0 to 10. Those with a score of 0 to 1 showed no mortality or morbidity. Patients with a score of 2 had no mortality and only a 4 per cent morbidity. Patients with a score between 7 and 10 had a 17 per cent mortality and a 92 per cent complication rate (8).

It is often confusing to the clinician when to order a CT scan in acute pancreatitis. It has been suggested that an initial CT study should be done (i) in patients in whom the diagnosis is in doubt; (ii) in patients with severe pancreatitis accompanied by fever, tenderness and leucocytosis; (iii) in patients who do not improve within 72 hours of conservative treatment; (iv) in patients with a Ranson score > 3 or a APACHE II score > 8; (v) in patients who show initial good improvement, but then rapidly deteriorate. A follow-up CT study is done (i) in patients with CT scan Grade A to C, or CTSI of 0–2, only if there is a clinical suspicion of a complication; (ii) in patients with CT scan Grade D or E, and CTSI of 3–10 after 7–10 days. Further CT scans of patients with Grade D/E, and CTSI 3–10, are performed only if the clinical status deteriorates or does not improve. A final CT is done in this group of patients at the time of discharge as important complications may develop without clinical symptoms. It must be remembered that the resolution of the CT features of pancreatic / peripancreatic inflammation lag behind clinical improvement.

Appendicitis

This is the most common surgical emergency with a lifetime risk of 6.7 per cent in women and 8.6 per cent in men (10). A careful history and thorough physical examination are adequate in most cases to make a diagnosis, imaging having no role to play in these cases. However, approximately 20 per cent of cases have an atypical presentation especially in elderly patients where there may be minimal pain, in children where an accurate history is not available, and in ovulating women who have a misdiagnosis rate of about 40 per cent, due to a pathology in the ovaries, fallopian tubes, uterus or bladder (11). In these cases imaging is useful to clinch the diagnosis, or exclude other conditions which may be mistaken for appendicitis.

The plain film seldom provides much help in the diagnosis; the presence of a distended caecum with an air/fluid level, or terminal ileal ileus are non-specific and unreliable signs. Appendicoliths are specific findings on a plain film that generally confirm a diagnosis of appendicitis. These are seen as round/oval opacities, 0.5–2 cm in diameter, with a calcified laminated rim. In 10 per cent of cases of acute appendicitis an appendicolith may be seen; however 50 per cent of these cases are usually associated with perforation

(11). Over the past 5 years improvements in US/CT technology, techniques and interpretations have substantially improved the sensitivity, specificity and accuracy of US/CT in diagnosing acute appendicitis. Graded compression sonography has shown a sensitivity of 77–89 per cent and a specificity and accuracy in 90 per cent of cases of acute appendicitis (11–14).

A high resolution (5–7.5 Hz) transducer is placed over the area of maximal tenderness and pressure is applied slowly and gently to minimize pain and discomfort. This procedure of graded compression sonography displaces bowel loops and gas, reducing the distance between the transducer and the appendix and thereby providing better resolution, as well as information regarding compressibility of the appendix. On sonography an inflamed appendix is seen as a tubular fluid-filled structure > 6 mm in diameter, devoid of peristalsis and non-compressible (**Fig. 5.3.5**).

CT is superior to sonography with a 98 per cent sensitivity, 83 per cent specificity and 93 per cent accuracy as it directly visualizes the appendix, the pericaecal region and other intra-abdominal structures (15). Sonography is not able to image well in the obese patient and in those with significant tenderness preventing adequate compression. On CT the inflamed appendix is seen as a tubular fluid-filled structure approximately 0.5–2 cm in diameter with a thickened enhancing wall which is usually 3 mm or more in diameter. Pericaecal inflammatory changes may be seen in the form of pericaecal fascial thickening, altered density of pericaecal fat, ill-defined phlegmonous soft tissue, and occasionally a fluid containing area representing an abscess (**Fig. 5.3.6**). The presence of pericaecal inflammatory changes alone, without visualization of the inflamed appendix is not diagnostic but makes the diagnosis highly probable. Adnexal cysts, masses, salpingitis, tubo-ovarian abscess, ureteric calculi, lymphadenitis and ileitis may clinically mimic appendicitis, but ultrasonography/CT help to differentiate between these conditions.

In women of child bearing age an ectopic pregnancy or a ruptured ectopic pregnancy must be kept in mind as a differential diagnosis. Sonography is the modality of choice in evaluating an ectopic pregnancy, and is preferably done by both the transabdominal and transvaginal routes. The surest sign of an ectopic is the presence of an extra-uterine gestational sac; this is seen in only 20 per cent of cases. The other important sign is the extra-uterine sac sign seen in 70 per cent of cases (16). A ruptured ectopic is seen as an adnexal haematoma; on ultrasound this appears as a complex hyperechoic adnexal lesion often accompanied by echogenic free fluid.

Pneumoperitoneum

Demonstration of a pneumoperitoneum is one of the most important signs in medicine, as it generally warrants emergency surgery. The best view to demonstrate a pneumoperitoneum is the erect frontal chest X-ray, which demonstrates gas under the domes of the diaphragm better than an erect abdominal X-ray (**Fig. 5.3.7**). This is because the exposure factors used are higher in abdominal X-rays and the X-ray beam is tangential to the diaphragm, resulting in a darker appearance of the diaphragmatic region with consequent difficulty in demonstrating gas under the diaphragm. In nearly 75–80 per cent of perforations of a hollow viscus, free air is demonstrated on a radiograph and 75 per cent of these cases are visible on a frontal chest X-ray. In a small percentage of patients (10 per cent), when the frontal chest radiograph fails to demonstrate free air, a left lateral decubitus view may be used. This view is very useful to demonstrate small quantities of free air. The patient is positioned on his side with the left side down and the right side up. At least 10 minutes must elapse to permit the free air to migrate to a nondependent position i.e. between the right margin of the liver and the lateral abdominal wall, and a horizontal radiograph is taken with the X-ray cassette behind the patient. Free air is seen as a crescent between the liver and right abdominal wall. This position is difficult as it may be cumbersome for the patient to lie in this position for 10 minutes, and at least 2–3 attendants are needed to position the patient for this view. Therefore in patients who are critically ill, traumatized, or comatose, erect and left lateral decubitus views may be technically difficult. In such patients only a supine radiograph of the abdomen is possible. However this view is not very useful and a pneumoperitoneum can be easily missed.

Post-operative pneumoperitoneum may be seen for a few days (generally about 3 days), after which time the free air is resorbed. Occasionally, free air may be seen for up to 24 days. The resorption rate is said to be much greater in obese individuals than in thin individuals. It is important to detect a fresh post-operative leak of air which is diagnosed by an increase in the amount of air, or with help of contrast studies/CT scan.

Intestinal Obstruction

Mechanical obstruction of the bowel is produced by occlusion or constriction of the lumen; this may progress to strangulation, interruption of blood supply with subsequent mucosal ulceration, bowel necrosis and perforation. Obstruction may occur in the small or large bowel.

Small Bowel Obstruction

The most common cause of small bowel obstruction is adhesions (occurring in 75 per cent of cases). In fact 5–20 per cent of patients who have undergone abdominal surgery will develop small bowel obstruction. On an erect abdominal X-ray dilated small bowel loops with multiple air fluid levels are visualized. Usually the dilated loops are in the form of an inverted U with fluid levels in both limbs. Occasionally in a non-obstructed patient a few air-fluid levels may be seen, but if more than 3 levels are seen, or if they are present in the left hypochondrium, there is strong possibility of obstruction. When there is a high jejunal obstruction dilated loops may show a typical appearance known as the 'string of pearls' sign. In this sign the obstructed bowel loops are fluid-filled and small bubbles of air collect on the surface giving rise to the 'string of pearls' sign.

The site of obstruction in the small bowel, whether jejunal or ileal can be differentiated by noting the pattern of the dilated bowel loops. Jejunal loops have a typical appearance in the form of concentric bands extending across the lumen, known as valvulae conniventes. Ileal loops have a featureless appearance, appearing like a tube (**Fig. 5.3.8**). A barium enema may used to differentiate a colonic from a distal small bowel obstruction.

CT is very useful in the evaluation of a small bowel obstruction and has a sensitivity of 94 per cent and specificity of 96 per cent (**17–19**). A small bowel diameter of more than 3 cm indicates that the bowel is dilated. CT also demonstrates a transition zone between the dilated proximal loops and the decompressed distal bowel, this sign being diagnostic of small bowel obstruction. As CT is also able to demonstrate the peritoneal surface of the bowel, tumor or inflammatory mass lesions can thereby be detected or excluded. Absence of tumor or inflammatory processes suggests that the cause of obstruction is an adhesion.

A rare form of small bowel obstruction is gallstone ileus. This occurs due to erosion of a gallstone into the duodenum, the gallstone lodging in the ileum and causing ileal obstruction. The radiological features are the presence of a gallstone in the lower abdomen, dilated small bowel loops and air in the biliary tree.

A diagnosis of intussusception can also be made on CT which shows a typical appearance. As the intussusceptum enters the intussuscipiens, there is trapping of the fatty mesentery and a complex composed of the intussusceptum and the intussuscipiens is seen on CT as concentric cylinders with fat density interposed between them.

Large Bowel Obstruction

The commonest cause of large bowel obstruction is carcinoma, about 60 per cent of growths being situated in the sigmoid colon. Other causes are diverticular disease and volvulus of the colon. The radiographic signs of large bowel obstruction depend upon the state of the iliocaecal valve. If the iliocaecal valve is competent (Type I), there is gross distension of the caecum and the large bowel. If the ileocaecal valve is incompetent (Type II), there is no distension of the large bowel, and the appearance is that of a small bowel obstruction. The caecum may perforate in a Type I obstruction. A distended colon is evidenced by the presence of its haustral markings which are seen as asymmetric folds. This is an important distinguishing feature from small bowel obstruction.

Paralytic Ileus

Paralytic ileus occurs commonly following surgery especially where excessive bowel manipulation has been performed, and in peritonitis. Fluid and gas accumulate in the dilated small and large bowel loops as a result of cessation of intestinal peristalsis. On plain radiographs these features are seen as dilated small and large bowel loops with multiple air-fluid levels. In view of the dilated large bowel loops, it is difficult to differentiate a distal large bowel obstruction from a paralytic ileus. The differentiation is possible if air is demonstrated in the rectum or distal large bowel. If this is not demonstrated on a plain film then a right lateral decubitus and/or prone film may be taken. In the right lateral decubitus view air rises into the distal colon and in a prone film air migrates into the rectum. If these are not conclusive then a contrast enema may be required to exclude distal obstruction. Alternatively, a CT

Imaging in the Chest

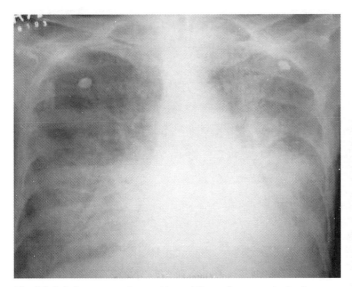

Fig. 5.2.1. Pulmonary oedema—Frontal X-ray shows marked pulmonary oedema with diffuse opacities in hilar/parahilar regions.

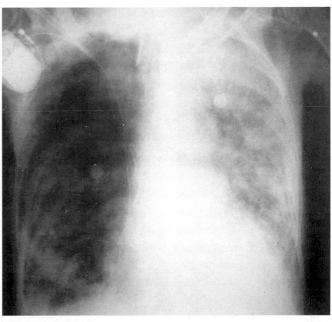

Fig. 5.2.2. Unilateral pulmonary oedema—Frontal X-ray shows diffuse opacity of left lung due to unilateral pulmonary oedema as a result of COPD changes in right lung.

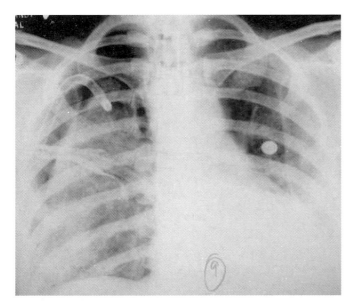

Fig. 5.2.3. Barotrauma in ARDS: Frontal X-ray reveals a right pneumothorax with intercostal tube in situ.

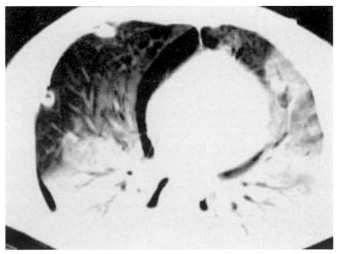

Fig. 5.2.4. ARDS with barotrauma—CT scan demonstrates pneumomediastinum, pneumothorax, subcutaneous emphysema and pulmonary interstitial emphysema seen as linear air streaks along vessels.

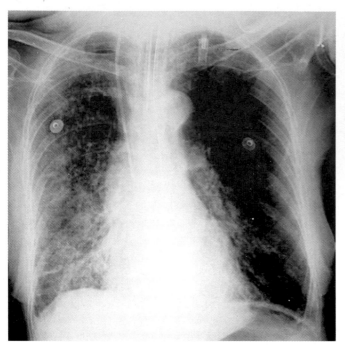

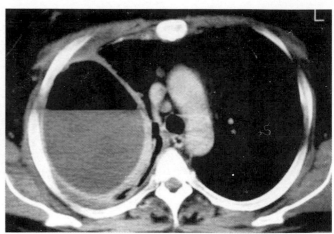

Fig. 5.2.6. Lung Abscess seen on CT as a large cavity with an air-fluid level.

Fig. 5.2.5. Aspiration pneumonia—Areas of consolidation are seen in the lower portions of the right upper and lower lobes due to aspiration.

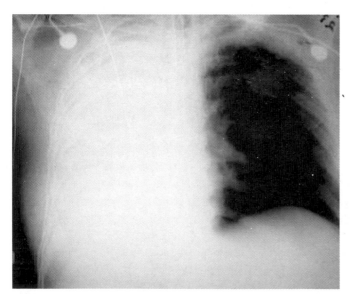

Fig. 5.2.7. Mucus plug in Right Bronchus causing collapse of right lung. The entire right hemithorax is opaque with a shift of the mediastinum to the right. Following Bronchoscopic aspiration the right lung reexpanded totally.

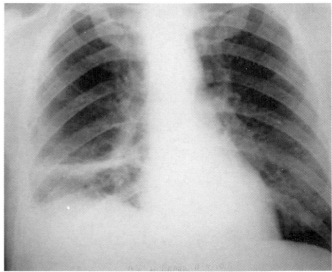

Fig. 5.2.8. Pulmonary infarct seen as plate like atelectasis in right lower lobe. Right lobe of diaphragm is elevated.

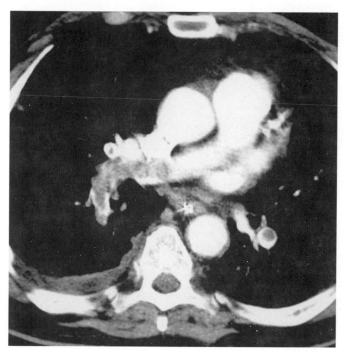

Fig. 5.2.9. Spiral CT angio showing bilateral pulmonary thromboemboli (arrows).

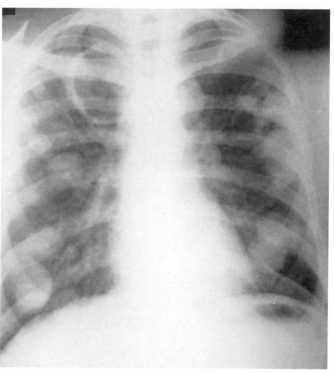

Fig. 5.2.10. Septic emboli—Chest X-ray reveals numerous rounded nodular lesions with air-fluid levels in a case of congenital heart disease.

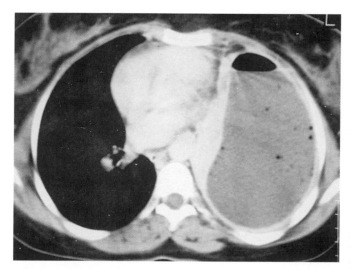

Fig. 5.2.11. Empyema—CT scan shows large loculated fluid collection with a thickened enhancing wall, which on aspiration revealed thick pus.

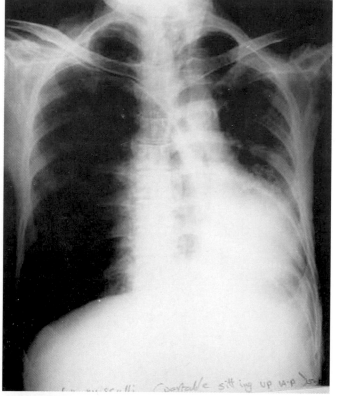

Fig. 5.2.12. Tension Pneumothorax—Chest X-ray shows a large right pneumothorax with shift of mediastinum to left and herniation of right lung into left hemithorax.

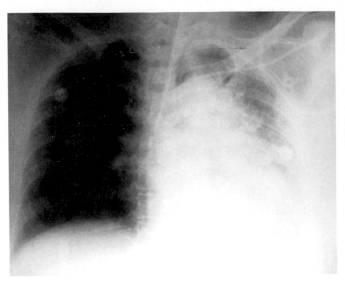

Fig. 5.2.13a. Portable chest X-ray demonstrates an ET tube in the right main bronchus, too low in position. There is gross over inflation of the right lung. There are diffuse opacities in the left lung due to hypoventilation of the left lung.

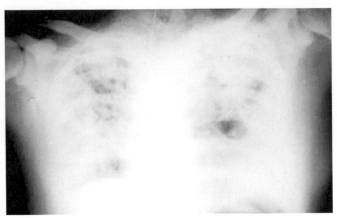

Fig. 5.2.13b. Chest X-ray showing bilateral small poorly ventilated lungs due to oesophageal intubation.

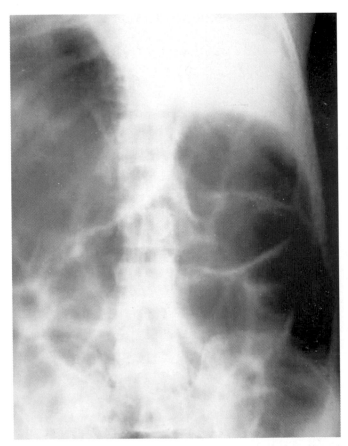

Fig. 5.2.13c. X-ray abdomen showing gross gaseous distension of bowel loops due to oesophageal intubation.

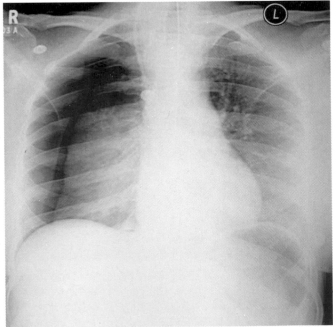

Fig. 5.2.13d. Portable chest X-ray showing a right pneumothorax following right jugular central line placement.

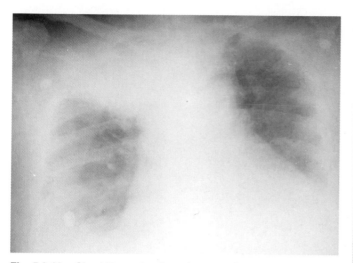

Fig. 5.2.13e. Chest X-ray showing a large mediastinal opacity which was a mediastinal haematoma following malposition of CVP line.

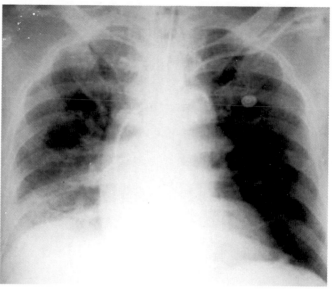

Fig. 5.2.13f. Chest X-ray showing Swan-Ganz catheter in perfect position.

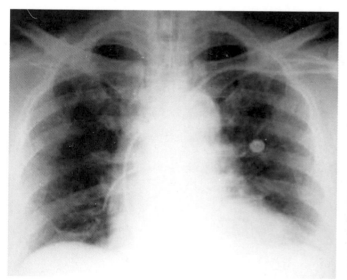

Fig. 5.2.13g. Chest X-ray showing Swan-Ganz catheter inserted too far in the right pulmonary artery.

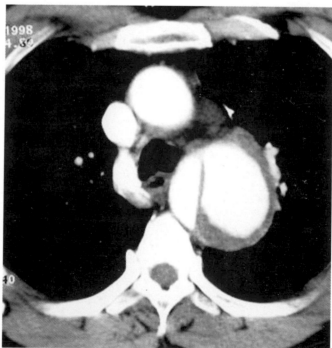

Fig. 5.2.14. Spiral CT angiogram showing intimal flap (arrow) in descending aorta indicating a dissection.

Imaging in the Abdomen

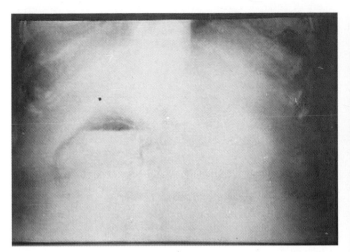

Fig. 5.3.1. Emphysematous Cholecystitis—Plain abdominal X-ray reveals a curvilinear air in region of gall bladder due to emphysematous cholecystitis.

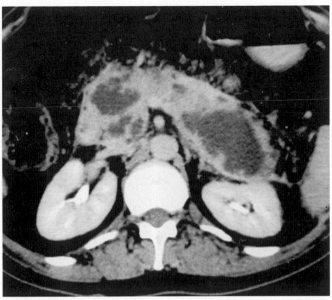

Fig. 5.3.2. Pancreatic necrosis—CT demonstrates large area of necrosis in the body and head of the inflamed pancreas.

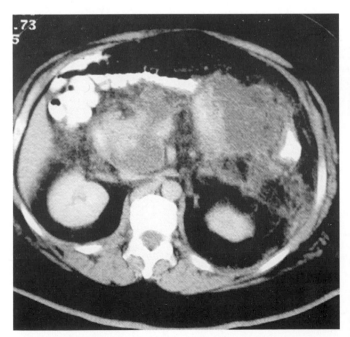

Fig. 5.3.3. Acute pancreatitis with fluid collections in peripancreatic and paracolic regions.

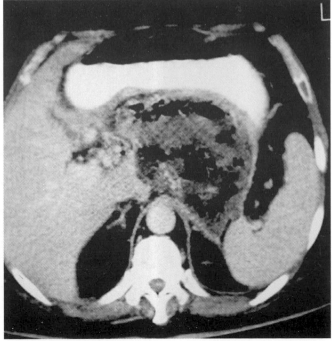

Fig. 5.3.4. Sepsis in acute pancreatitis—CT scan shows a large fluid collection in the lesser sac with multiple air bubbles within the collection. CT guided aspiration revealed pus.

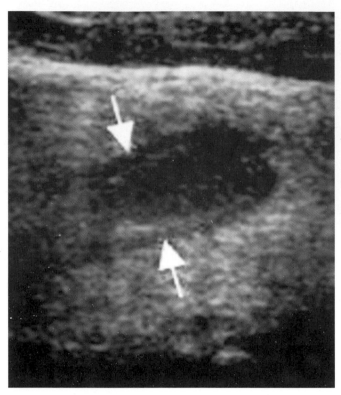

Fig. 5.3.5. Acute appendicitis—Sonography shows dilated appendix as tubular structure with thickened oedematous wall.

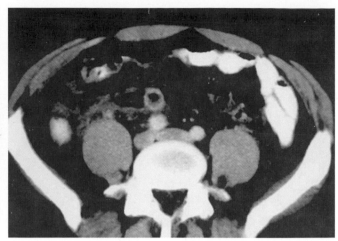

Fig. 5.3.6. Acute appendicitis—CT scan shows dilated inflamed appendix (arrow) with periappendicular inflammation.

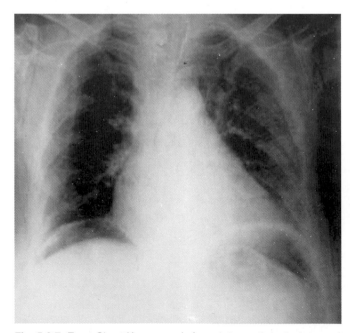

Fig. 5.3.7. Erect Chest X-ray reveals free air beneath both domes of the diaphragm due to perforation.

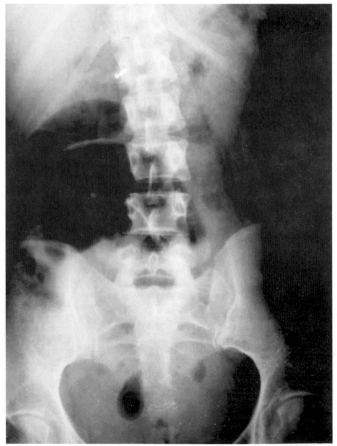

Fig. 5.3.8. Dilated small bowel loops on supine abdominal X-ray. These are ileal loops as the have a featureless appearance.

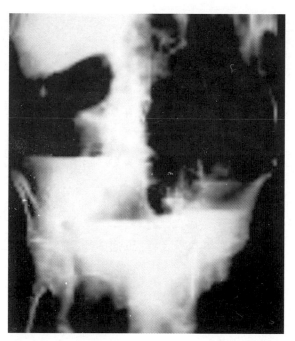

Fig. 5.3.9. Toxic megacolon—Erect abdominal X-ray shows gross distension of colon with a small fluid level in the colon.

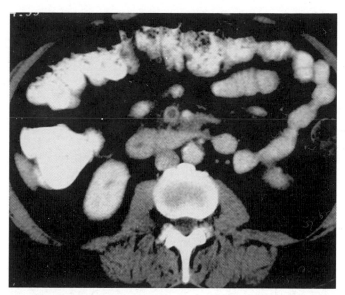

Fig. 5.3.10. Mesenteric ischaemia—CT scan with contrast shows thrombosis of superior mesenteric vein.

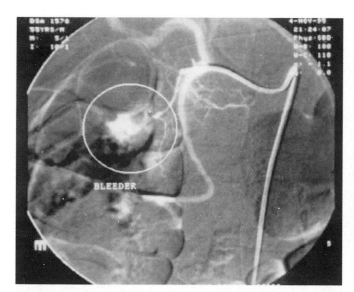

Fig. 5.3.11. Digital subtraction angiography demonstrating extravasation of contrast due to acute gastrointestinal haemorrhage.

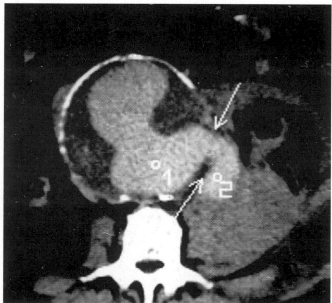

Fig. 5.3.12. Aortic aneurysm rupture—CT scan shows a large aortic aneurysm with calcification of its wall. Note there is leak of contrast into the retroperitoneum on the left side due to rupture of aneurysm.

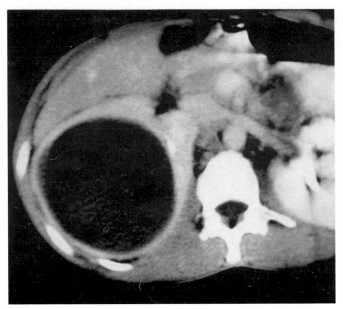

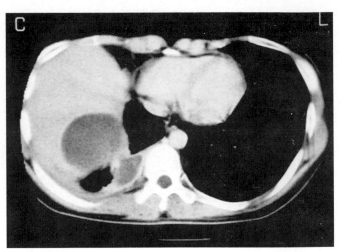

Fig. 5.3.14. Amoebic abscess rupture—CT scan shows rupture of right lobe amoebic abscess into right pleura (arrow).

Fig. 5.3.13. Large well defined fluid collection in right kidney on CT scan representing a large renal abscess.

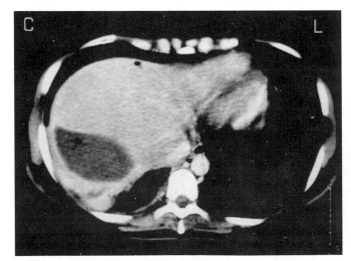

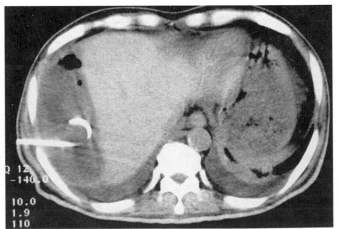

Fig. 5.3.16. Pigtail catheter inserted in situ liver abscess as seen on CT scan.

Fig. 5.3.15. Subphrenic abscess seen on CT as well defined fluid collection posterior and superior to right lobe of liver with specks of air within it due to anaerobic infection.

Neuroimaging

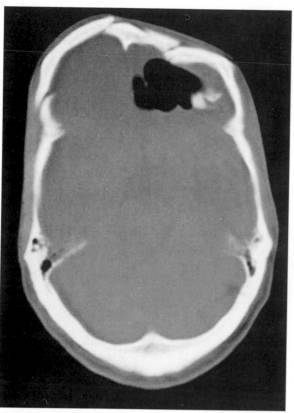

Fig. 5.4.1. Depressed fracture seen as displaced fragment compressing brain parenchyma.

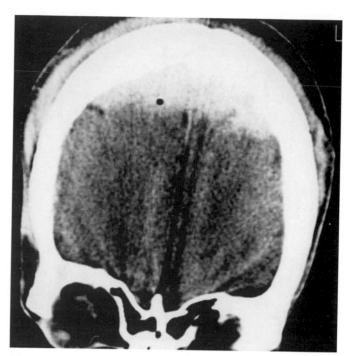

Fig. 5.4.2. Extradural haematoma seen as large biconvex hyperdense extra-axial lesion causing mass effect and crossing the midline on a coronal CT.

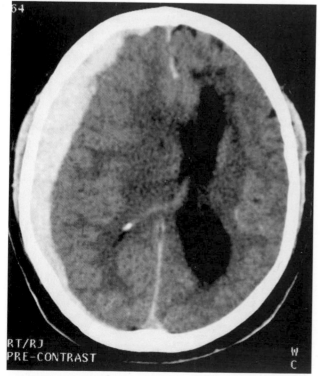

Fig. 5.4.3. Subdural Haematoma seen as a concavo convex hyper density causing mass effect on the right lateral ventricle and shift of midline structures to the left.

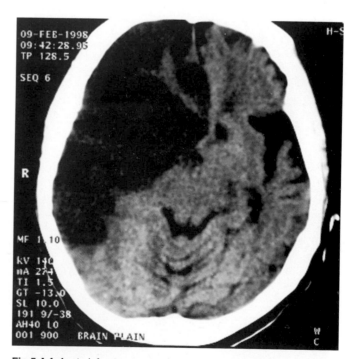

Fig 5.4.4. Acute infarct seen as a large hypodensity in right frontal and middle cerebral arterial territories with associated mass effect.

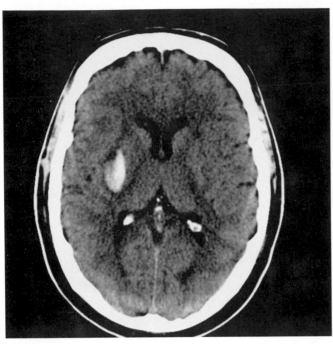

Fig. 5.4.5. Right lentiform nucleus hemorrhage seen as Hyperdense area in right lentiform nucleus.

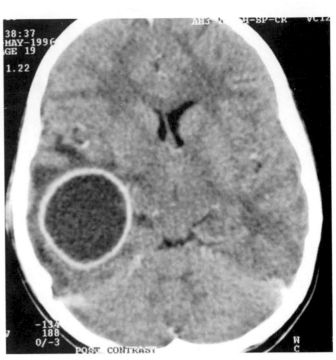

Fig. 5.4.6. Large abscess seen as rounded hypodensity with peripheral ring enhancement and perifocal oedema in right temporal lobe.

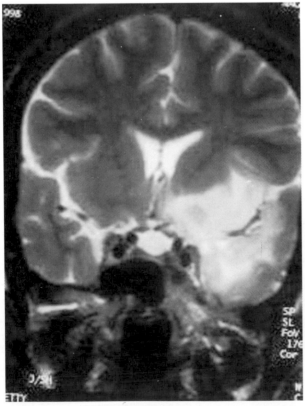

Fig. 5.4.7. Herpes encephalitis seen as hyper intensities in left temporal lobe on coronal T2 Weighted MRI.

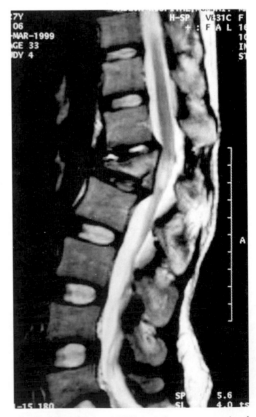

Fig. 5.4.8. Sagittal T2 Weighted MRI reveals a compression fracture of D12 with compression of thecal sac and altered attenuation in conus due to an intramedullary contusion.

can be performed to demonstrate air in the rectum/sigmoid; this excludes an obstruction. If there is suspicion of a perforation or if the colonic diameter exceeds 5.5 cm, a water-soluble contrast should be used instead of barium.

Localized ileus is seen adjacent to the site of inflammation e.g. cholecystitis, pancreatitis, appendicitis, and is visualized as isolated dilated small bowel loops with a few fluid levels. Ogilvie's syndrome is a condition seen in elderly debilitated patients who have a major underlying systemic abnormality such as severe infection, recent surgery or cardiac disease. There is marked dilatation of the colon and occasionally there is associated small bowel ileus. This condition is also known as pseudo-obstruction. In view of the markedly distended large bowel, these patients are prone to caecal perforation especially when the caecum is dilated to more than 9 cm for two to three days. Colonic and caecal distension can be treated by colonoscopic decompression.

Toxic Megacolon

Toxic megacolon is a fulminant form of colitis in which there is marked dilatation of the colon (diameter > 5.5 cm). The radiographic features are most commonly seen in the transverse colon as this is the region where gas accumulates in the supine posture (**Fig. 5.3.9**). In addition to marked distension of the colon, there is thickening of the wall/mucosa with numerous nodular areas projecting into the bowel lumen representing mucosal islands (spared mucosa), adjacent to the areas of ulceration. The haustrae are effaced and a thumb-printing pattern may be seen. A contrast enema is contraindicated due to the high risk of perforation, but a CT may be useful in demonstrating the wall thickening.

Ischaemic Colitis

Ischaemic colitis may be caused by primary ischaemia due to mesenteric arterial stenosis, thrombosis or venous occlusion. Occasionally strangulation or obstruction of the bowel may lead to ischaemic changes. Any part of the small bowel may be involved, but in the colon it is usually localized to the distal colon supplied by the inferior mesenteric artery. Segmental ischaemia may result in strictures and occasionally transmural infarction may progress to perforation. On radiographs the characteristic signs are oedematous thickened loops with a thumb-printing pattern due to submucosal haemorrhages. There may be air in the bowel loop wall (pneumatosis intestinalis), and air in the portal venous system. Other non-specific findings are small bowel ileus, or an X-ray plate which remains 'dark' through lack of gas within the small gut.

CT is very useful in the evaluation of ischaemic bowel (**Fig. 5.3.10**); it may demonstrate the direct signs of mesenteric arterial/venous thrombosis and secondary signs of thickened bowel loop walls, pneumatosis intestinalis and portal venous air. Ascites and bowel distension may also be seen. A non-diagnostic CT/plain film does not exclude ischaemic colitis and if there is a strong clinical suspicion, angiography should be performed. Angiography may be both diagnostic and therapeutic; vasodilators and thrombolytic therapy may be used as therapeutic interventions.

Gastrointestinal Haemorrhage

Angiography has a useful role to play in detecting the cause, and the subsequent management of upper and lower gastrointestinal bleeds. The cause of upper GI bleeds is usually evident on an upper GI endoscopy; if this fails, then angiography is used to determine the site of bleeding (**Fig. 5.3.11**). The limitation of angiography is that the rate of blood loss should be at least 5 ml per minute, or if superselective catheters are used at least 1 ml per minute, to be able to detect the site of bleeding. The site of bleeding is identified on angiography as a diffuse blush of extravasating contrast. Once the site is localized vasopressin may be injected through the catheter at the rate of 0.2 units per minute, to help control the bleeding. The duration of the therapy is 20 to 40 minutes. Occasionally it may be longer in elderly atherosclerotic individuals.

Epinephrine may also be used in a dosage of 8 to 30 µg/min. Infusions into the left gastric artery usually control bleeding from Mallory-Weiss tears, gastritis, and stress ulcers of the upper part of the stomach. An infusion into the common hepatic artery is useful for antral lesions, and gastroduodenal arterial infusions usually control duodenal bleeding.

An infusion of vasopressin into the superior mesenteric artery may be used to control bleeding due to portal hypertension by lowering the venous pressure. Complications of vasopressin therapy are water retention, abdominal cramps, diarrhoea, and occasionally cardiotoxicity. Vasopressin effectively controls bleeding from small vessels and capillaries as seen in mucosal tears and stress ulcers. However bleeding from large arteries, as in duodenal ulcer, may not be controlled and may require embolization of the vessel.

Different materials have been used for embolization—coils, glue, gelatin or fibre, each having its own advantages and disadvantages. Coils and glues are most commonly used. These are injected through the catheter at the site of bleeding in an attempt to occlude the bleeding vessel. As bleeding from large arteries is not effectively controlled by vasopressin, embolization is advocated as the primary procedure. Lower GI bleeds usually occur as a result of bleeding from colonic diverticuli. These usually respond well to vasopressin therapy.

Abdominal Aortic Aneurysms

Abdominal aortic aneurysms are usually infrarenal in location and may be fusiform or saccular. Sonography usually detects nearly all abdominal aortic aneurysms; however CT is required for further evaluation to determine the extent of the aneurysm. On CT, abdominal aortic aneurysms are usually more than 3 cm in diameter with calcification of their walls. There is usually an associated mural thrombus which is seen as a circumferential thrombus along the wall of the aorta. Occasionally it may be eccentric along the anterolateral wall, and may be difficult to differentiate from a chronic dissection.

CT is very useful in determining the extent of the aneurysm—whether it is infrarenal, or involves the renal or superior mesenteric arteries, or if there is any inferior extension into the iliac vessels. These points are very important in planning surgical intervention.

MRI is a useful modality for evaluating the aorta, its main advantage being its ability to image in multiple planes; also there is no need to inject intravenous contrast medium as flowing blood is seen as a signal void. Angiography has been the age-old modality for evaluating abdominal aortic aneurysms, but with the current imaging modalities available, it is no longer necessary. In fact angiography is limited to defining only the patent lumen of an aneurysm, as the extraluminal thrombosed component, which is well visualized on ultrasound/CT/MRI, is not demonstrated on angiography.

Abdominal Aortic Dissection

Aortic dissection is fortunately a rare complication of aortic aneurysms, and usually occurs as an inferior extension of a dissecting thoracic aneurysm. The CT, MRI, and angiographic imaging characteristics are similar to those of dissecting aneurysms of the thoracic aorta, and have been discussed earlier.

Abdominal Aortic Rupture

This is a catastrophic event requiring emergency surgery. The crux of the diagnosis lies in the demonstration of a retroperitoneal haematoma adjacent to an abdominal aortic aneurysm. In this emergency situation in a critically ill patient with rapidly dropping blood pressure, sonography is invaluable as it is portable and can be performed at the bedside. A retroperitoneal haematoma is seen as an ill-defined mixed echoic lesion adjacent to the aorta. However sonographic examination is often hampered by bowel gas especially if the patient is obese. CT is an ideal investigative modality and will demonstrate a mildly hyperdense collection in the pararenal regions adjacent to the aorta. Occasionally a discontinuity of the aortic wall may be seen on CT (**Fig. 5.3.12**). MRI similarly is useful in detection of a retroperitoneal haematoma which is seen as a mixed intensity retroperitoneal lesion. T_1 weighted images are only required to detect the haematoma, a breach in the aortic wall may also be seen on MRI. MRI has a disadvantage of being a much longer procedure with difficulty in monitoring the patient, and therefore CT is the modality of choice.

Renal Inflammatory Processes

Acute pyelonephritis usually follows infection in the bladder which ascends to involve the renal pelvis and renal parenchyma secondarily. Sonography is usually negative though occasionally may demonstrate an enlarged hypoechoic kidney. CT is more sensitive and specific. The affected kidney is seen to be enlarged; following administration of intravenous contrast medium the nephrogram has a striated and blotchy appearance due to areas of decreased enhancement or non-enhancement, which subsequently on delayed scans show filling in of contrast. In acute bacterial nephritis the changes are similar but are more marked. Occasionally the changes seen on CT may be more lobar extending to the hilum.

Acute lobar nephroma (pre-abscess) usually occurs due to a partially treated infection and appears as a focal area of inflammation with small necrotic areas. On sonography these changes may appear as a mass like hypoechoic lesion mimicking a neoplasm. On CT they appear as a hypodense lesion with small necrotic areas within it, of near water density. These may resemble renal infarct/ischaemic areas.

Sonography is usually effective in the detection and evaluation of renal abscesses which are greater than 2 cm in size. They appear as relatively well-defined hypoechoic or mixed echoic lesions which may be uni- or multi-loculated. The presence of debris is very suggestive of an abscess. CT has a much better sensitivity and specificity for renal abscesses as it also depicts the perinephric and retroperitoneal inflammatory changes. On CT these appear as well-defined hypodense collections which may have debris in the form of a fluid level (**Fig. 5.3.13**). Perinephric changes may be present in the form of fascial thickening or perinephric/psoas extension of the abscess.

Pyonephrosis occurs when there is infection of an obstructed collecting system. Sonography is an excellent modality for evaluating pyonephrosis and shows evidence of debris layering in the dilated pelvicalyceal system. Sonography can also be used as a guide for aspiration as well as percutaneous nephrostomy.

Emphysematous Pyelonephritis

This is the most severe necrotizing renal infection and mainly occurs in diabetics, immuno-compromised patients, or patients with urinary tract obstruction. The hallmark of this condition is the presence of air in the renal parenchyma or renal pelvis. On sonography air is seen as echogenic areas but may be missed at times. Occasionally differentiation of echogenic foci from calculi may be difficult. CT is far more sensitive than sonography or plain X-ray in detecting air which are seen as jet black specks. Gas may also be seen in the perinephric regions.

Acute Renal Failure

The question to be answered by imaging is whether the urinary system is obstructed or not. Sonography adequately answers this question where dilatation of the pelvicalyceal system is seen as separation of the renal sinus echo. Occasionally in acute obstruction there may be no evidence of dilatation of the pelvicalyceal system. This may be due to the fact that the obstruction is too early to manifest, or the obstruction may have led to forniceal rupture with leakage of fluid into the perirenal region. Therefore the presence of perirenal fluid in acute renal failure indicates obstruction. Occasionally there may be pre-existing dilatation of the pelvicalyceal system due to an old obstruction, and the clinician has to determine whether this dilatation is due to a new obstruction, or is due to an old lesion. In this condition, a duplex Doppler of the intrarenal vessels is very useful. An estimate of the renal vascular resistance known as the resistive index (RI), is obtained by the formula:

$$RI = \frac{(\text{Peak Systolic FS} - \text{Minimum Diastolic FS})}{(\text{Peak Systolic FS})}$$

(FS stands for frequency shift).

An elevated RI is seen in fresh obstruction (**20**).

In acute renal failure due to non-obstructive causes the

sonogram is usually negative or may show alteration in renal size and echogenicity. These changes however are non-specific and not helpful as regards the aetiology. A duplex Doppler sonography is however helpful in differentiating acute tubular necrosis from acute prerenal failure (21). The resistive index (RI) is elevated in most patients with acute tubular necrosis, but is also raised in a fifth of patients with prerenal failure.

Liver

Hepatic Abscess

Both CT and sonography are very useful in the evaluation of hepatic abscesses. CT is slightly superior in the detection of small abscesses. Abscesses may be solitary/multiple, small or large. Amoebic abscesses have a predilection for the posterosuperior portion of the right lobe of the liver and are seen on sonography as ill-defined hypoechoic areas with a wall of varying thickness. In the early stages of an abscess the abnormal area may be seen as an isoechoic or mildly echogenic area. Later the abscess becomes better defined and more hypoechoic. Often there is debris present in the abscess seen as layering of echogenic material. On CT abscesses are seen as ill-defined hypodense / non-enhancing areas with a wall of varying thickness (**Fig. 5.3.14**).

Large abscesses should be subjected to sonographic or CT guided aspirations. Of particular importance is the approach used in the aspiration of these abscesses. A liver abscess should not be approached posteriorly as the inferior margin of the posterior recess of the pleura is not known, and inadvertently the pleura may be transgressed; seepage of purulent material from the liver abscess could result in an empyema. Abscesses in the posteriosuperior quadrant of the right lobe of the liver are very difficult to tackle, and are best aspirated under CT guidance. Very large abscesses are best treated with catheter drainage as they would otherwise necessitate a long hospital stay and multiple aspirations.

Immunosuppressed patients with AIDS or those on chemotherapy may have multiple disseminated fungal abscesses—the most common incriminating organism being Candida albicans. These abscesses have a relatively classical appearance on CT—a hyperdense core with peripheral hypodensity (bull's eye lesion). On sonography the appearances vary: (i) 'wheel in wheel' appearance with a hypoechoic centre, a hyperechoic wall and a hypoechoic periphery; (ii) 'bull's eye' lesion with hyperechoic centre and hypoechoic outer margin. Occasionally these abscesses may be uniformly hypoechoic or hyperechoic.

Imaging modalities may help in the diagnosis of a number of other intra-abdominal or gastrointestinal problems in immunosuppressed patients, particularly in AIDS. Thus cytomegalovirus infections, infections with Mycobacterium avium intracellulare, or Cryptosporidium infections in patients with AIDS, can cause an ascending cholangitis recognizable on CT by the presence of dilated intrahepatic biliary radicles. Kaposi's sarcoma, non-Hodgkin's lymphoma may involve the gut. Splenomegaly may be related to a lymphoma. AIDS enteritis may involve the jejunum with effacement of the jejunal folds. CT is the ideal imaging modality as it evaluates visceral organs, adenopathies, and bowel loops. A CT guided biopsy in visceral disease or in lymphadenopathy also helps in arriving at an exact diagnosis.

Liver Trauma

After the spleen and the kidney, the liver is the third most common organ likely to be injured in abdominal trauma. Most cases result from blunt trauma. The lesions can range from a small tear to a large laceration with an intrahepatic haematoma. CT is the imaging modality of choice in abdominal trauma. An acute haematoma is seen as a bright area (brighter than the liver parenchyma) on the unenhanced scan. After administration of intravenous contrast medium, the lesion does not enhance, the lesion thereby appearing darker than the liver.

Peritonitis

Diagnosis of peritonitis is nearly always clinical, the role of imaging being merely to demonstrate (i) free fluid in the peritoneal cavity; (ii) intraperitoneal abscess; (iii) the aetiology of peritonitis. Sonography is usually adequate to detect free fluid. Small amounts of fluid may be seen in the hepatorenal pouch and/or in the pelvic cul de sac. When there is a large amount of fluid, the liver, spleen and bowel loops are pushed to the centre of the abdomen, with the fluid being peripheral. The fluid if not grossly infected may be sonolucent. Severely infected fluid is echogenic with loculations or debris.

Intraperitoneal abscesses occur due to a variety of causes. Most occur between the transverse colon and the diaphragm. Nearly 60 per cent of these are on the right side, 15 per cent bilateral and 25 per cent on the left. Abscesses can occur anywhere in the abdomen or pelvis, and are often distant from the site of perforation or primary pathology (**Fig. 5.3.15**). Therefore the whole abdomen and pelvis need to be imaged in detail when looking for intraperitoneal abscesses. Sonography has been found to be superior to CT in evaluating subphrenic abscesses as these tend to be more plaque-like, spreading along the surface of the liver or spleen. Therefore a coronal form of imaging is useful to demonstrate these plaque-like abscesses, and determine their relation to solid visceral organs. MRI scanning (which gives good coronal images) is also a useful modality in localizing these abscesses. However the ability of MRI to image the rest of the abdomen is poor. CT is far superior to sonography for detection of abscesses in other portions of the abdomen/pelvis, as well as interloop abscesses which may be missed on sonography. When a search for an intra-abdominal abscess is undertaken with CT scan, it is very important that a large quantity of oral contrast (1.5 to 2 l) is given to the patient and this is supplemented with intravenous contrast. This is because dilated fluid-filled bowel loops can mimic abscesses and vice versa. False-negative or false-positive results may at times occur when there is inadequate opacification of the bowel loops.

On sonography abscesses appear as relatively well-defined hypoechoic lesions with or without a layering of debris in the collection. On CT, abscesses appear as well defined phlegmonous mass lesions which undergo central liquefaction and have thick peripheral enhancing walls. Occasionally there may be gas within the collection indicating infection by a gas forming organism. This is the surest sign of an abscess. The differential diagnosis of abscesses are pseudocysts, cysts, urinomas, biliomas, loculated ascites, old haematomas and necrotic tumors. The clinical setting as well as radiographic appearances help to differentiate the varying pathologies. Differentiation can sometimes only be achieved by percutaneous aspiration.

Imaging-Guided Procedures

Over the years, technological improvements in imaging modalities and catheter design have considerably helped to improve the safety, simplicity and effectiveness of imaging-guided procedures. This has therefore led to a greater acceptance of these procedures.

Drainage of Localized Intra-Abdominal Suppuration

Drainage of an intra-abdominal abscess is commonly performed in critically ill patients under either ultrasound or CT guidance.

Sonography is also useful for percutaneous transhepatic drainage, cholecystostomy and percutaneous nephrostomy. These procedures may be performed under sonographic guidance or with the help of fluoroscopy.

Contraindications

Contraindications for drainage of a collection are: (i) lack of a safe access route i.e. through bowel or vascular structures; (ii) associated coagulopathy; (iii) sub-diaphragmatic abscesses which cannot be approached without traversing the pleura; (iv) poorly formed abscesses—such as pancreatic phlegmons; (v) multiloculated and multicompartment abscesses.

Methods of Drainage

There are two main methods employed in the insertion of drainage tubes—one being the Seldinger technique and the other the Trocar technique. In the Seldinger technique a 22 gauge needle is introduced first and fluid is aspirated to confirm that the needle is in the collection. Once this is confirmed by imaging, the needle is removed and dilators passed over the guidewire to dilate the tract. Dilators (from size 6 French upwards) are used progressively in increments of 2 French and constantly watched under fluoroscopy. Depending on the size of the pigtail catheter, the track is dilated to a 2 French size above the size of the catheter required. Generally for thin fluid collections/bile an 8 French size catheter is adequate, while for thicker collections like pus 10 to 13 French size is necessary. For even thicker material a catheter up to about 24 French size can be inserted. The catheter is advanced over the guidewire into the collection. Once in the collection the guidewire is removed and fluid/pus aspirated and drained via the catheter. Following complete aspiration, contrast is injected and a cavitogram is performed to ensure that the cavity is totally drained, as well as to see if there are any other pockets of collection or fistulas opening into the GI tract. The catheter is then secured to the skin. An important point to note is that at all times the guidewire should be held at the skin site so that it is not dislodged from the collection.

The Trochar technique is a very convenient technique as it does not involve a guidewire, and hence the chances of the guidewire slipping are absent. Also it is a rapid technique and can be performed under sonography/CT guidance. The main limitation is that only catheters up to 8/10 or 12 French can be used. However this thickness has been found to be more than adequate for drainage of thick pus. In this technique the pigtail catheter is loaded on the needle. The needle is introduced into the collection, the stylet removed, pus aspirated and the pigtail advanced over the needle into the collection. The pigtail coils in the collection and the needle is then removed (**Fig. 5.3.16**). The pigtail is then fastened to the skin and a drainage bag is attached.

When selecting the guidance system for drainage, it is important to keep the following points in mind: (i) note if the patient can be transported; (ii) check regarding availability of the equipment; (iii) check whether adjacent structures are adequately visualized; (iv) localize the anatomical area to be aspirated or drained. The most important factor is safety and accuracy of the guidance system. CT is the best modality for guidance as it can visualize the extent of the abscess, visualize the bowel, lung and free air, display the entire abdomen, visualize through post-operative drains and dressings, and can confirm accurate and adequate drainage. The main disadvantage of CT is the need to transport the patient to the CT scanner suite.

REFERENCES

1. Sherman M, Ralls PW, Quin M et al. (1985). Real time sonography in suspected acute cholecystitis. Radiology. 155, 767–771.

2. Jeffrey RB, Laing FC, Wong W et al. (1983). Gangrenous cholecystitis: diagnosis by ultrasound. Radiology. 148, 219–221.

3. Strohl EL, Dyfenbaugh WG, Baker JH et al. (1962). Collective reviews: gangrene and perforation of the gall bladder. Gynec Obstet Surg. 114, 1–7.

4. Laing FC. (1992). Ultrasonography of the acute abdomen. Radiol Clin North Am. 30(2), 389–404.

5. Brown K, Raman SS, Kallman C. (2002). Imaging Procedures. In: Current Critical Care Diagnosis and Treatment (Eds Bongard FS, Sue DY). pp. 146–203. McGraw-Hill, USA.

6. Balthazar E, Robinson D, Megibow A et al. (1990). Acute pancreatitis. Value of CT in establishing prognosis. Radiology. 174, 331–336.

7. Kourtesis G, Wilson S, Williams R. (1990). The clinical significance of fluid collections in acute pancreatitis. Am Surg. 56, 769–799.

8. Balthazar E, Pratick F, van Sonnenberg E. (1994). Imaging and intervention in acute pancreatitis. Radiology. 193, 297–306.

9. van Sonnenberg E, Wittich G, Carola G et al. (1989). Percutaneous drainage of infected and non-infected pancreatic pseudocysts. Experience in 101 cases. Radiology. 170, 757–761.

10. Goldman CD. (1992). Acute appendicitis. In: Gastrointestinal Emergencies (Ed. Taylor MB). pp. 426–436. Williams and Wilkins. Baltimore.

11. Gore R, White M, Port R et al. (1994). Acute appendicitis: A practical approach. The Radiologist. 1(1), 1–10.

12. Rioux M. (1992). Sonographic detection of the normal and abnormal appendix. Am J Roentgenol. 158, 773–778.

13. Sivit CJ. (1993). Diagnosis of acute appendicitis in children. Spectrum of sonographic findings. Am J Roentgenol. 161, 147–152.

14. Carlson JM, Pierce JC, Ellinger DM et al. (1989). The validity and utility of sonography in the diagnosis of acute appendicitis in the community setting. Am J Roentgenol. 153, 687–691.

15. Balthazar EJ, Megibow AJ, Siegel SE et al. (1991). Appendicitis: Prospective evaluation with high resolution CT. Radiology. 180, 21–24.

16. Hertzberg B. (1994). Ultrasound evaluation for ectopic pregnancy. The Radiologist. 1, 11–18.

17. Megibow AJ et al. (1991). Bowel obstruction evaluation with CT. 180, 313–318.

18. Frazer D, Medwid S, Baer JW et al. (1994). CT of small bowel obstruction. Value of establishing the diagnosis and determining the degree and cause. Am J Roentgenol. 162, 37–41.

19. Giazelle S, Goldberg M, Wittenberg J et al. (1994). Efficacy of CT in distinguishing small bowel obstruction from other causes of small bowel dilatation. 162, 43–47.

20. Platt JF, Rubin JM, Ellis JH. (1989). Distinction between obstructive and non-obstructive pyelocalyctasis with Duplex Doppler Sonography. Am J Roentgenol. 153, 997–1000.

21. Platt JF, Rubin JM, Ellis JH. (1991). Acute renal failure:Possible role of duplex doppler ultrasound in distinction between acute prerenal failure and acute tubular necrosis. Radiology. 179, 419–423.

CHAPTER 5.4

Neuroimaging Techniques

Contributed by Dr Anirudh Kohli, MD, DNB, DMRD, Head of Department of Radiology, Breach Candy Hospital, Mumbai.

General Considerations

CT scanning was introduced in the mid-seventies and enabled a direct visualization of the brain parenchyma, ventricles and cisterns. CT imaging thus replaced invasive diagnostic radiology techniques such as air encephalography, ventriculography and cisternography; it also decreased the use of carotid/vertebral angiography. Magnetic Resonance Imaging (MRI) was introduced in the mid-eighties, and this became another important modality in the evaluation of the CNS. MRI has a better intrinsic contrast of images and a higher sensitivity for pathologic changes on T_2 weighted images (T_2WI). One of the important advantages of MRI over CT is its ability to image soft tissues in the absence of artefacts from overlying bone. This makes MRI the modality of choice in evaluating the brain stem, posterior fossa, extra-axial regions and the spinal cord.

The advantages of CT over MRI are that bony abnormalities, calcification and hyperacute haemorrhage are well detected. Another important advantage is that critically ill patients can be more easily monitored during CT than during MRI. Though MRI compatible ventilators, pulse oximeters and respiratory monitors have now been introduced, they are not widely available, and further in the event of a cardiorespiratory arrest, the patient needs to be removed from the MRI room because defibrillation and ECG monitoring cannot be performed close to the magnet. MRI is contraindicated in patients with cardiac pacemakers, implanted auto defibrillators, thermodilution Swan-Ganz (S-G) catheters, and cochlear implants (1). Implanted drug infusion pumps may also stop during imaging (2). Ferromagnetic objects in a patient may move or become dislodged producing damage to the patient, or artefacts in the images. The majority of intracranial aneurysmal clips are ferromagnetic; movement of these clips in the MRI can have disastrous consequences. Non-ferromagnetic clips are now available. However most haemostatic vascular clips, staples, carotid artery clamps (except Poppen-Blalock carotid artery clamp) (1), wire sutures, vascular access ports, plastic endotracheal tubes, chest tubes, catheters (except S-G catheters), orthopaedic devices, prosthesis, prosthetic heart valves (except Starr-Edwards 6000 valve), intravascular coils, stents and filters are safe in the MRI. Most bullets are non-ferromagnetic (3) (in doubtful cases, a similar bullet is taken to the MRI suite and checked). Another disadvantage

of MRI is the longer examination time as compared to CT, though newer MRI machines with echoplanar MRI are as fast or even faster than CT.

With the advent of carotid Doppler, MRI angiography, and spiral CT angiography, the use of angiography has reduced considerably. However none of these techniques can totally replace angiography, as angiography is required prior to surgery in carotid stenosis, intracranial aneurysms and angiomatous malformations. Cerebral angiography is also being now used for interventional purposes—carotid angioplasty, embolization of aneurysms and angiomatous malformations.

Head Injury

CT is far superior to MRI in the evaluation of patients with acute head injury as it is more sensitive than MRI in the detection of acute haemorrhage and fractures. Further, patients who have polytrauma require CT for imaging the thorax and abdomen; CT head can be done at the same time. MRI is useful in the evaluation of subacute/chronic subdural haematomas, and is far superior in the evaluation of diffuse axonal injury. A plain X-ray of the skull can only demonstrate the presence of a fracture, and help determine if the fracture is depressed. If there is a fracture, a CT must be performed. A basal fracture may not be seen on a skull X-ray. However air in the subarachnoid space points to a fracture of the base of the skull. Other areas that can be evaluated for fractures on a plain X-ray are the orbit/paranasal sinuses and upper cervical spine.

On CT, fractures appear as linear breaks in the calvarium. A depressed fracture is seen as a bony fragment compressing the underlying brain (**Fig. 5.4.1**). It is important to see if there is any underlying haematoma or haemorrhagic contusion, because elevation of the fragment can cause an increase in the size of an underlying haematoma.

Extradural Haematoma

An extradural haematoma occurs due to a tear of an artery traversing between the dura and the calvarium, resulting in a haematoma which strips the dura from the inner table of the skull. There is usually an associated overlying fracture, the common sites being the frontal and temporal regions near the branches of the middle meningeal artery. On CT, extradural haematomas are seen as very hyperdense, well-defined collections which have a biconvex or lenticular appearance (**Fig. 5.4.2**). They may cross the midline as they are limited only by sutural margins. Internally they may contain areas of lower attenuation due to presence of unclotted blood. These haematomas tend to be brighter than other haemorrhages as there is no mixing with CSF. Of particular importance are posterior fossa epidural haematomas, as they have a mortality rate of 37–69 per cent (4). Fortunately they are relatively uncommon.

Subdural Haematoma

Subdural haematomas are the most common of post-traumatic intracranial haematomas. They occur due to a tear of a bridging vein in the subdural space resulting in a haematoma between the dura and arachnoid. Rarely they may occur in the posterior fossa due to a tear of a venous sinus. The most common cause of a subdural haematoma is head injury. However rarely they may occur following shunt placement, coagulopathy, arteriovenous malformations or aneurysmal bleeding. Subdural haematomas are concavoconvex in shape conforming to the contour of the brain (**Fig. 5.4.3**); they are limited by the falx cerebri and therefore do not cross the midline but may extend into the interhemispheric fissure. It is important to note that subdural haematomas lying over the convexity below the frontal/occipital lobes, or above/below tentorium are much better imaged by coronal scans. Subdural haematomas are classified according to their age into three types—acute (1–3 days old), subacute (3–22 days old), and chronic (more than 22 days old).

Acute subdural haematomas are best imaged by CT as MRI is relatively insensitive to acute haemorrhage. These appear as crescentic high attenuation lesions causing mass effect on the ipsilateral cortex with effacement of the sulci and a shift of the midline structures to the opposite side. Rarely in severe anaemia with haemoglobin < 5 g/dl, acute subdural haematomas may appear to be of low attenuation, resembling chronic haematomas. As subdural haematomas age, they decrease in attenuation appearing in a spectrum between mildly hyperdense to mildly hypodense, with a certain proportion being isodense with brain parenchyma. Due to the minimal density differences between these haematomas and brain parenchyma they may be difficult to detect.

There are indirect signs which may help to detect a subacute or isodense subdural haematoma. These are: (i) effacement of the cortical sulci; (ii) a subtle inbuckling of the grey/white matter interface on the ipsilateral side, as the brain parenchyma is displaced away from the calvarium; (iii) compression of the ipsilateral ventricle. Rarely but not uncommonly bilateral isodense subdurals may be present; as the ventricular system is compressed from both sides it appears very small and pinched. In doubtful cases intravenous contrast may be used as this enhances the membrane of the subdural haematoma along with the cortex of the brain, thereby helping to define the subacute subdural easily. If doubt still exists an MRI is warranted. Due to the presence of methaemoglobin in subacute subdural haematomas, these

haematomas appear very bright on MRI resulting in very easy depiction.

Chronic subdural haematomas are often not accompanied by a clinical history of head injury as the patients are usually elderly, alcoholic or have psychiatric problems. On CT they are seen as crescentic hypodense fluid collections causing effacement of the sulci, shift of the midline structures and compression of the ipsilateral ventricle. On MRI these appear as hypointense on T_1 weighted images (T_1WI) and hyperintense on T_2 weighted images. These may be difficult to differentiate from subdural hygromas which appear similar on CT and MRI. The only differentiating factor is the presence of a membrane which is present in haematomas. Occasionally a chronic subdural may mimic an acute subdural due to rebleeding into the subdural.

Contusions

Contusions occur due to a shearing injury and are most commonly seen in the anterior portions of the frontal and temporal lobes. They may be haemorrhagic or non-haemorrhagic. They may be small or very large causing significant mass effect, and are often multiple and bilateral. On CT they appear as ill-defined hyperdense areas with peripheral hypodensity, or multiple ill-defined hyperdense areas which tend to get confluent with peripheral hypodensity. The non-haemorrhagic contusions appear hypodense and are better detected on MRI than CT.

MRI is far superior in the evaluation of diffuse axonal injury especially in patients with severe post-cognitive disorders in whom the CT is often negative. These axonal injuries are seen as multiple ovoid/round areas of altered signal intensity in the corpus callosum, centrum semiovale and at the grey/white matter interfaces. 80 per cent of these lesions are non-haemorrhagic. The cortex is usually spared but larger lesions may involve the cortex. Occasionally these lesions are seen on the dorsolateral aspect of the brainstem and the cerebellum.

A rare form of subcortical haemorrhage is seen with focal areas of haemorrhage in the upper brainstem, basal ganglia, thalamus and around the third ventricle. Patients with these findings are usually comatose, have a low Glasgow Coma Score, and often die early.

Stroke

The primary purpose of imaging in acute stroke is to differentiate a non-haemorrhagic infarct from acute haemorrhage. The modality which best meets this purpose is CT, as MRI is relatively insensitive to the detection of acute haemorrhage. Infarcts are detected earlier on MRI—as early as 6 hours after the cerebrovascular accident. Also, small lacunar infarcts in the basal ganglia, internal capsule and posterior fossa may never be seen by CT, and may be visualized only by MRI. On CT the infarcted area is seen as an ill-defined hypodense area with associated mass effect which becomes more hypodense as it ages (**Fig. 5.4.4**). In the subacute phase the infarct may become isodense and may be missed on a plain CT. This is due to revascularization of the infarct and is known as the fogging phase. In this situation intravenous contrast may be useful as it will demonstrate dense peripheral gyral enhancement. This is also known as luxury perfusion, which starts at 6 days and persists till 6 weeks. Flooding of an infarct with ionic contrast has been known to increase the incidence of necrosis of the infarct. Non-ionic contrast however has not shown any of these adverse effects; therefore in cases of stroke if contrast is to be administered, non-ionic contrast should be used (**5**). If the infarct is deep in the brain (as for example in the basal ganglia), then instead of peripheral gyral enhancements, ring enhancement may be seen. Chronic infarcts appear as very hypodense (CSF attenuation) areas with associated gliosis.

Infarcts typically conform to a vascular territory, unless they lie between vascular territories and are known as watershed infarcts e.g. in the frontoparietal region between the anterior cerebral artery and the middle cerebral artery, and in the parieto-occipital region between the middle cerebral artery and the posterior cerebral artery. These infarcts are commonly seen in hypoxia or due to hypoperfusion distal to a high grade carotid stenosis. Occasionally large infarcts may be seen involving the anterior cerebral artery, middle cerebral artery territory, with or without the ipsilateral posterior cerebral artery territory or the opposite anterior cerebral artery territory. These are usually due to internal carotid artery occlusion. On MRI an echogenic area may be seen in the internal carotid artery representing a thrombus.

On MRI infarcts appear iso- to hypointense on T_1 weighted images, and bright on T_2 weighted images. As the infarct ages, it becomes more hypointense on the T_1 weighted images. A chronic infarct is of CSF intensity on the T_1 weighted images with associated gliotic changes. When larger areas of haemorrhage are seen within an infarct i.e. haemorrhagic infarct, the possibility of a venous infarct or embolic infarct should be considered. The possibility of an embolic infarct should be also considered when there are infarcts in multiple vascular territories. Venous infarcts are often haemorrhagic and do not conform to any vascular territory. They are often cortical or deep such as bilateral thalamic infarcts. MRI is useful in demonstrating an associated venous sinus thrombosis, as venous sinuses are seen as flow void areas. Thrombosis of a venous sinus replaces this flow void with isointense or hyperintense signals.

Intracerebral haemorrhage occurs most commonly in hypertensive patients due to rupture of a small deep vessel. There are five typical sites—basal ganglia, thalamus, grey/white matter junction, cerebellum and pons. On CT, haemorrhage is seen as a confluent high density area with mass effect and oedema (**Fig. 5.4.5**). Progressive expansion of the haematoma may cause hydrocephalus or cerebral herniation. There may be associated intraventricular or subarachnoid extension of the haemorrhage. As the haemorrhage resolves the clot becomes smaller, and the oedema, mass effect and density of the haematoma become less. In this subacute stage if intravenous contrast is administered there may be ring enhancement of the capsule or haematoma. In the chronic stage only a gliotic area is seen with no enhancement. The appearances of haemorrhage on MRI are very complex as they depend upon the paramagnetic effects of the blood degradation products. The blood degradation products are oxyhaemoglobin, deoxyhae-

moglobin, intracellular and extra-cellular methaemoglobin, haemosiderin and ferritin. These are serially formed as the haematoma evolves. Hyperacute haemorrhage (first 24 hrs) mainly consists of the first breakdown product oxyhaemoglobin, which has no paramagnetic properties; it may not be detected by MRI at all, or may be hypointense on T_1WI and hyperintense on T_2WI, thus resembling an infarct. Therefore in the acute stage of a stroke, a CT and not an MRI should be performed, as only a CT will detect a haemorrhage.

Deoxyhaemoglobin, intracellular and extracellular methaemoglobin, haemosiderin and ferritin have relatively typical appearances. Deoxyhaemoglobin appears hypointense on T_1WI and more hypointense on T_2WI. Methaemoglobin appears hyperintense on T_1WI, the appearance on T_2WI depending on whether the methaemoglobin is intra- or extracellular. Intracellular methaemoglobin is dark or hypointense, whereas extracellular methaemoglobin is bright or hyperintense on T_2WI. Haemosiderin and ferritin are similar to deoxyhaemoglobin; hypointense on T_1 and becoming more hypointense on T_2 weighted images, with some associated blooming due to paramagnetic effects.

A significant number of strokes occur as a result of a shower of emboli from atherosclerotic disease at the carotid bifurcation. Carotid endarterectomy is currently recommended in cases of symptomatic high grade carotid stenosis to prevent a stroke. The gold standard for evaluating carotid stenosis is angiography. Duplex color Doppler, MRI angiography and spiral CT angiography are non-invasive imaging techniques which are proving very useful in the evaluation of carotid stenosis. These are essentially used as screening techniques. Doppler ultrasound is the most widely used screening modality. Its limitations are that it is operator-dependent resulting in a wide variability of interpretation. Tortuous carotid arteries may in addition cause diagnostic problems, and difficulties may arise in differentiating subtotal from total occlusion. Colour Doppler sonography is used to determine the sites of flow abnormality and grade the severity of stenotic lesions (**6**).

MR angiography has been recently demonstrated to be a sensitive non-invasive tool in the diagnosis of internal carotid artery stenosis. The major advantage of MR angiography is that it displays the carotid bifurcation anatomy in a format similar to carotid angiography. The degree of stenosis may however be overestimated by both MR angiography, as well as carotid Doppler in a non-proportional manner (**7**). Therefore a conversion factor cannot be calculated to correct this overestimation. Arteriography is a road mapping procedure; in addition it can detect tandem lesions such as intracranial stenosis and stenosis of the origin of the carotid artery. Recently it has been proposed that a combination of colour Doppler and MR angiography can almost totally replace the need for angiography. In addition to lowering the pre-operative diagnostic costs, the use of colour Doppler and MR angiography reduces the complication rate to nearly nil. This has been countered by the recent development in angiography of Digital Subtraction Angiography (DSA), which involves the use of thinner catheters, and the use of nonionic contrast medium. The use of DSA has helped to reduce the complication rate from 1–4 per cent with traditional angiography, to 0.09–0.3 per cent (**8**).

Subarachnoid Haemorrhage

Subarachnoid haemorrhage (SAH) occurs following rupture of an aneurysm, arteriovenous malformation, or due to trauma. A CT scan is very sensitive in detecting SAH, which is seen as hyperdensity in the sylvian fissures, the interhemispheric fissures, and along the cortex or basal cisterns. Some amount of blood may also be seen layering in the ventricles. It must be remembered that 10 per cent of SAH may have a negative CT and if the clinical suspicion for SAH is high, a lumbar puncture is mandatory for diagnosis.

Following the demonstration of SAH, a DSA is required to detect an aneurysm. The common sites for aneurysms are at the junction of the anterior cerebral artery/anterior communicating artery, bifurcation of middle cerebral artery and junction of internal carotid artery and posterior cerebral artery. If an aneurysm is detected, it is important to demonstrate the neck of the aneurysm for surgical purposes. MRI can detect aneurysms as small as 3 mm in diameter. As flowing blood is seen as a flow void on MRI, an aneurysm appears as a circular flow void area. A partially thrombosed aneurysm is seen as a signal void area with a peripheral thrombus. This is important as on angiography only the signal void portion i.e. the patent lumen is demonstrated. Following surgery or in the follow-up of SAH patients, a CT is necessary to monitor ventricular size, strokes (due to vasospasm) or rebleeding. The presence of a clot helps to localize the site of an aneurysm.

Angiomatous malformations are best evaluated by MRI where they are seen as serpiginous/curvilinear signal void areas. There may be associated areas of haemorrhage or brain atrophy due to the 'steal' phenomenon. CT scan with contrast can demonstrate enhancing curvilinear/serpiginous areas with large draining veins and feeding arteries. Angiography is useful to provide a vascular map of the arteriovenous malformation with special reference to feeding/draining vessels. This information is necessary prior to embolization/radiotherapy or surgery.

CNS Infections

Both CT and MRI are extremely useful in the evaluation of CNS infections; however MRI is more sensitive than CT in the evaluation of both meningeal and parenchymal inflammation. Intravenous contrast enhancement is mandatory with CT and provides valuable information in an MRI scan as well.

Meningitis

Imaging in bacterial and viral meningitis is usually negative. Occasionally leptomeningeal enhancement with intravenous contrast may be seen along the convexity of the brain. In granulomatous diseases like tuberculous meningitis, sarcoid and fungal meningitis, intravenous contrast enhanced CT or MRI may demonstrate dense enhancement in the region of the basal cisterns. The main role of imaging in meningitis is to detect complications such as communicating hydrocephalus, cerebritis, abscess, subdural effusion/empyema, ventriculitis and cortical or subcortical infarcts. Infarcts may be seen in the basal ganglia due to involvement of perforating basal vessels by associated vasculitis. Venous infarcts may occur due to venous sinus thrombosis.

Cerebritis and Abscess

There are four stages in the formation of an abscess—early cerebritis stage, late cerebritis stage, early capsule stage, late capsule stage. Most cases are detected in the late cerebritis stage or early capsule stage. MRI is considered superior to CT in the evaluation of these lesions as it is much more sensitive to subtle parenchymal changes, especially to white matter changes. On CT, cerebritis appears as an ill-defined hypodense lesion with associated mild to moderate mass effect with usually no enhancement. Occasionally in this stage there may be ring enhancement which fills in later on delayed scans. On MRI, cerebritis appears as an ill-defined area which is hypointense on T_1WI and hyperintense on T_2WI. Abscesses appear on CT as necrotic hypodense rounded areas with perifocal oedema (**Fig. 5.4.6**). After administration of intravenous contrast the capsule/wall of the abscess enhances; the capsule is well formed on the cortical side but the ventricular side is usually thinner. This helps to differentiate abscesses from metastases, which usually have thicker, shaggier, more nodular enhancing walls. Occasionally abscesses may be multilocular or may be associated with multiple peripheral daughter abscesses. On MRI abscesses appear as rounded hypointense areas on T_1WI and turn hyperintense with a thin well-defined dark capsule on T_2WI. There is a fair amount of perifocal oedema about the abscess. As on CT, the capsule enhances with intravenous contrast on MRI.

Encephalitis

Parenchymal infections are usually most often due to a viral aetiology. MRI detects changes earlier than a CT; it also provides a better estimate of the extent of the lesion, particularly when lesions involve the white matter.

Herpes simplex type I infection is an important treatable infection of the neuraxis. Herpes simplex encephalitis occurs due to latent herpes simplex virus in the Gasserian ganglion which spreads along the trigeminal nerve retrogradely to involve the temporal and inferior frontal lobes. Rarely there may be brain stem involvement due to retrograde spread of the virus along IX, X, XI cranial nerves. MRI is far superior to CT in the detection of the subtle changes associated with herpes simplex virus (HSV) encephalitis. The changes seen on imaging are classically in the temporal and inferior frontal lobes and are seen on T_2 weighted images as ill-defined hyperintense areas (**Fig. 5.4.7**). Often there is bilateral involvement of both cortex and white matter. As the lesion progresses medially it is limited by the basal ganglia which are spared giving rise to a characteristic sharp medial margin. The disease may extend superiorly across the Sylvian fissure to involve the island of Reil. Small petechial haemorrhages are often present and are seen as hyperintensities on T_1WI or hypointensities on T_2WI. CT scan usually demonstrates the changes much later than MRI. The lesions are seen as hypodense areas in the temporal and inferior frontal regions. The subtle bilateral involvement seen on MRI is usually not picked up on CT. On contrast studies there is no significant enhancement. When HSV affects immunocompromised patients, especially HIV positive patients, there may be multiple sites of involvement and it does not conform to the typical appearance as described above. Following resolution of the HSV encephalitis, necrotic and gliotic areas are seen.

Varicella zoster virus encephalitis is usually seen as a brainstem encephalitis due to spread along the V and VII cranial nerves to the brainstem. On MRI similar changes are seen on T_2WI in the form of hyperintense areas in the brainstem with more involvement of white matter than grey matter. This form of encephalitis may be accompanied by vasculitis.

Cytomegalovirus encephalitis which is usually seen in immunocompromised patients is seen to affect both white and grey matter, with areas of altered signal intensity on T_2WI. This form of encephalitis is usually accompanied by ependymitis. Post-contrast MRI reveals considerable enhancement along the ependyma. This form of enhancement may make it difficult to differentiate this pathology from primary CNS lymphomas which also show diffuse ependymal enhancement. Usually CNS lymphomas are accompanied by diffuse nodular enhancing lesions in the centrum semiovale and the periventricular region.

Progressive Multifocal Leukoencephalopathy (PML)

PML is an encephalitis due to infection by JC virus (papovirus) in the immunocompromised patient. The early lesions of PML are small, round, begin in the subcortical white matter and spread to deeper white matter, becoming larger and confluent. There is sparing of the cortical grey matter giving rise to a typical scalloped appearance of the grey white matter junction. PML is usually bilateral but asymmetrical, with a predilection for involvement of the posterior centrum semiovale. Periventricular and grey matter (basal ganglia, thalamic) involvement is rare. 10 per cent of cases may have lesions which are purely infratentorial. These lesions rarely show enhancement with contrast.

HIV Encephalitis

The clinical diagnosis of HIV encephalitis usually antedates convincing radiologic evidence of the disease. On MRI there may be diffuse areas of altered signal intensity seen in the supratentorial white matter which may be solitary or confluent. With progression of the disease there is involvement of the cortex, basal ganglia, brainstem and cerebellum. MRI mainly displays the secondary changes of HIV encephalitis—atrophy and demyelination.

Acute Disseminated Encephalomyelitis (ADEM)

MRI demonstrates diffuse, ill-defined, patchy hyperintensity in the deep/subcortical white matter of the cerebrum. Occasionally changes are seen in the midbrain, pontine and cerebellar regions, and spinal cord white matter. The lesions are few, asymmetrically distributed, without evidence of mass effect and haemorrhage. Embolic infarction, vasculitis, acute haemorrhagic leukoencephalopathy and acute multiple sclerosis need to be differentiated from ADEM. Embolic infarction usually conforms to a vascular distribution. Vasculitis is not necessarily limited to white matter. There are haemorrhagic changes in acute haemorrhagic leukoenceph-

alopathy; no haemorrhagic changes occur in ADEM. Acute multiple sclerosis and ADEM are not easily differentiated on plain MRI, but on contrast MRI all the lesions in ADEM enhance, whereas in multiple sclerosis only active plaques enhance.

Toxoplasmosis

This is one of the most common opportunistic infections seen in patients with AIDS. Parenchymal lesions in toxoplasmosis are seen on CT as mildly hyperdense nodular lesions with perifocal oedema. On a contrast study there is ring or nodule enhancement. These lesions are typically seen in the basal ganglia, periventricular region and the brainstem. On MRI the lesions appear iso- to hypo-intense on T_1WI, and turn hypo- or hyperintense on T_2WI with perifocal oedema. With gadolinium DTPA there is ring or nodular enhancement of the lesions. Occasionally evidence of haemorrhage may be detected within the lesions on MRI. The presence of enhancement on CT/MRI helps to differentiate active from inactive lesions. As these lesions resemble and may coexist with other parenchymal granulomas and lymphomas, the best confirmation of the diagnosis lies in the response of the lesions to antitoxoplasmal therapy. Following resolutions of the lesions the scans may return to normal, or there may be residual gliosis. Rarely toxoplasmosis can present as a fulminant, necrotizing meningoencephalitis in which CT/MRI can be negative.

Cryptococcosis

Intraparenchymal cryptococcal granulomas are seen typically in the basal ganglia as hypodense non-enhancing areas appearing similar to lacunar infarcts on CT, or bright areas on T_2W MRI. These are in fact gelatinous masses of cryptococcal organisms inciting minimal or no inflammatory response. These may be associated with cryptococcal meningitis.

Neurocysticercosis

Disseminated neurocysticercosis is an important cause of status epilepticus in our part of the world. The cysts may be in the live, dying, dead stages, or in a combination of all three stages. Both CT and MR are very useful in demonstrating these lesions. However MR is considered superior to CT as it is able to demonstrate the scolex better, as well as detect small live cysts thereby giving a more accurate depiction of the cyst burden. Live cysts appear as rounded CSF attenuation/intensity lesions with an eccentric scolex; no perifocal oedema or cyst wall enhancement is seen with administration of intravenous contrast. Dying cysts have a similar appearance as live cysts (CSF attenuation/intensity lesions), but perifocal oedema and cyst wall enhancement are present. As the scolex is often not visualized in dying cysts, they may resemble other granulomatous lesions. Dead cysts are seen as calcified foci, which are better detected on CT than MR. In disseminated neurocysticercosis, cysts are also often present in striated muscles as in the thigh, calf, tongue, myocardium, and the orbital muscles. The thigh is the commonest extracranial site; clinically there is enlargement of the thigh muscles resulting in a pseudotumour appearance. The cysts can be demonstrated easily in these locations on imaging (CT/MR).

Spinal Cord Infarction

Infarction of the cord is most often the result of inadvertent occlusion of the anterior spinal artery during the repair of thoracic aortic aneurysms. Other causes are embolic disease, vasculitis, cardiac arrest and dissecting aortic aneurysm. MRI is the only imaging modality which will demonstrate a spinal cord infarction which is seen on T_1 weighted images as a generalized swelling of the cord; on T_2WI there is increased signal intensity in the involved region of the cord.

Transverse Myelitis (TM)

The role of imaging in TM is to exclude spinal cord compression. Occasionally in cases of TM intrinsic abnormalities may be seen in the cord on MRI. T_1 weighted images may show no change, but on T_2WI ill-defined hyperintensities will be seen at the level of the affected segment. With gadolinium there may be subtle enhancement in these regions.

Spinal Trauma

Plain X-rays of the spine are extremely useful in evaluating vertebral body fractures and dislocations. However CT provides far more information regarding the extent of the fracture, intraspinal fragments, posterior element fractures, thecal sac compression and presence of intraspinal or paraspinal haematomas. MRI is useful as it demonstrates the cord. Intrinsic cord abnormalities are not uncommon in spinal trauma and MRI is the only modality which can demonstrate them. Intrinsic cord abnormalities may be in the form of oedema of the cord due to compression by vertebral fracture; this is seen as a hyperintensity in the cord on T_2WI. Other abnormalities may be the presence of haemorrhagic or non-haemorrhagic cord contusions. Haemorrhagic contusions are seen as bright areas within the cord on T_1WI, and non-haemorrhagic contusions as hypointense (dark) areas on T_1WI which turn bright on T_2WI. Rarely there may be transection of the cord which is best appreciated on sagittal images as a discontinuity of the cord (**Fig. 5.4.8**). The presence of intrinsic abnormalities in the cord is of importance as it provides prognostic information. Extradural haematomas may occasionally cause cord compression and are best appreciated on axial MRI images as well defined hyperintense areas compressing the cord. A traumatic disc protrusion is not uncommon, and this is also well evaluated on a sagittal or axial MR image. As bony abnormalities are well visualized on CT, this modality has an advantage over MRI in the evaluation of posterior arch fractures, as well as in the visualization of intraspinal fragments.

REFERENCES

1. Shellock FG, Curtis JS. (1991). MR imaging and biomedical implants, materials and devices: an updated review. Radiology. 180, 541.

2. von Roemeling R, Canning RM, Cames FA. (1991). MR imaging of patients with implanted drug infusion pumps. J Magn Reson Imaging. 1, 77.

3. Teitelbaum GP, Yee CA, van Horn DD et al. (1990). Metallic ballistic fragments: MR imaging safety and artefacts. Radiology. 175, 855.

4. Tobias JA. (1989). MRI of intracranial vascular diseases with emphasis at low intermediate field strengths. In: Craniospinal Magnetic Resonance Imaging (Ed. Pomeranz SJ). pp. 315. WB Saunders Co. Philadelphia.

5. Alberts M, Gray L. (1993). Neuroimaging, Imaging and Invasive Radiology in the Intensive Care Unit (Ed. Ravin CE). pp. 13. Churchill Livingstone.

6. Polak JF, Kalina P, Donaldson MC et al. (1993). Carotid endarterectomy: Pre-operative evaluation of candidates with combined Doppler sonography and MR angiography. Radiology. 186, 333–338.

7. Huston J III, Lewis B, Wiebers DO et al. (1993). Carotid artery prospective blinded comparison of two dimensional time of flight MR angiography with conventional angiography and duplex ultrasound. Radiology. 186, 339–344.

8. Polak JF. (1993). Noninvasive carotid evaluation: Carpe Diem. Radiology. 186, 329–331.

SECTION 6

Clinical Shock Syndromes

6.1 Overview of Shock Syndromes
6.2 Hypovolaemic and Haemorrhagic Shock
6.3 Cardiogenic Shock
6.4 Septic Shock
6.5 Cardiac Compressive Shock
6.6 Anaphylactic Shock

CHAPTER 6.1

Overview of Shock Syndromes

General Considerations

Shock is a state of acute circulatory failure that leads to tissue hypoxaemia. It is a syndrome, a symptom-complex recognized by clinical features many of which are subjective and therefore imprecise. Shock on a close analysis is not a single physiological entity, but a group of life-threatening circulatory syndromes with varying physiological profiles. Though hypotension is a feature of severe shock, the shock syndromes cannot just be equated to hypotension or to a fall in cardiac output or to accompanying changes in circulatory haemodynamics. It is a major misconception that correction of hypotension and restoration of a normal haemodynamic profile is the be-all and end-all in the management of shock. Shoemaker (1) evaluated the significance of restored haemodynamic parameters in a series of critically ill survivors and nonsurvivors with shock. With therapy, mean arterial blood pressure (ABP mean), heart rate (HR), central venous pressure (CVP), pulmonary capillary wedge pressure (PCWP) and cardiac output (CO) were restored to normal in 76 per cent of non-survivors who still went on to die. Obviously, though restoring the haemodynamic profile in shock to as near normal as possible is important, it is simply not enough. Thus a restored haemodynamic profile in shock may for various reasons be associated with an impaired microcirculation to various organs leading to persistent hypoperfusion and hypoxia to tissue cells. There is more to the management of shock than the mere restoration of circulatory haemodynamics.

What needs to be stressed is the concept that every form of severe shock is characterized by inadequate tissue oxygenation. Marino (2) expresses this succinctly when he points out that shock is buried in the tissues and that an approach that helps assess tissue oxygenation should be central to its management. What complicates matters is that in shock different tissues may have different or varying needs for oxygen. To accurately evaluate the effects of restoration of the circulation on tissue oxygenation particularly in critically ill individuals, may therefore seem an impossibly difficult task. How does one ensure that the oxygen uptake by tissues ($\dot{V}O_2$) is matched to metabolic needs? The balance between $\dot{V}O_2$ on the one hand, and the metabolic rate or needs on the other, can be indirectly determined by measuring the lactate levels in arterial blood (2). A blood lactate level well above normal points to anaerobic tissue metabolism, which again suggests that tissue requirements for oxygen are not being met.

Another important manifestation of shock (besides hypoperfusion, hypoxia detected by increased lactate levels in blood), is the inducement of the systemic inflammatory response syndrome (SIRS) (3). Hypoperfusion and resuscitation (ischaemia—reperfusion) can initiate SIRS which then literally feeds upon itself through various mechanisms briefly touched upon in a later chapter. The inflammatory component may be less marked (as in quickly resuscitated hypovolaemic or cardiogenic shock), large (as in septic shock), or intermediate (as in many patients with traumatic shock). This inflammatory component of shock often determines the final outcome as it sets into motion a vicious downward spiral that can lead to progressive multiple organ dysfunction, failure and death.

In clinical practice the two chief factors that determine the outcome of any form of shock are oxygen transport or supply to tissues ($\dot{D}O_2$), and oxygen uptake or consumption by tissues ($\dot{V}O_2$). $\dot{V}O_2$ may be inadequate or limited because of hypovolaemia, a reduced $\dot{D}O_2$, hypermetabolism and/or maldistribution of blood flow observed in sepsis, trauma, surgery, post-operative states, endocrine and metabolic catastrophes. The relation of $\dot{D}O_2$ to $\dot{V}O_2$ may vary in different shock states, and also from time to time in the same patient with shock.

Survival in shock is determined by the ability of the circulation to match oxygen supply to tissue needs for oxygen. It is important that this is achieved before permanent tissue damage has occurred. Therapy which is adequate but delayed, may be ineffective for *there comes in the natural history of shock a point beyond which there is no return.*

Shock can be due to a number of aetiological factors. Basic forms of shock include Hypovolaemic Shock, Cardiogenic Shock and Vasogenic or Distributive Shock. Shock due to cardiac compression (Cardiac Compressive Shock), is also discussed later in this section. The different types of shock have been classified in **Table 6.1.1**. The basic haemodynamic profiles of each of these shock syndromes are briefly described below.

Table 6.1.1. Classification of shock

1. Hypovolaemic and Haemorrhagic
2. Cardiogenic
   * Acute myocardial infarction
   * Cardiomyopathy
   * Cardiac arrhythmias
   * Mechanical causes e.g. valvular disease, outflow tract obstruction, ruptured ventricular septum
3. Distributive or Vasogenic
   * Septic shock; toxic shock syndrome
   * Anaphylactic
   * Neurogenic
4. Cardiac Compressive

Hypovolaemic Shock

Shock due to hypovolaemia is characterized by a loss in circulatory volume which results in a decreased venous return, a decreased filling of the cardiac chambers, and hence a decreased cardiac output which leads to an increase in the systemic vascular resistance (SVR). *The haemodynamic profile on monitoring of flow pressure variables, shows a low central venous pressure (CVP), a low pulmonary capillary wedge pressure (PCWP), a low cardiac output (CO) and cardiac index (CI), and a high SVR. The arterial blood pressure may be normal or low.*

Cardiogenic Shock

This is primarily dependent on poor pump function. *Cardiogenic shock due to acute catastrophic failure of left ventricular pump function is characterized by a high PCWP, a low CO and CI, and generally a high SVR.* When overall pump function of both right and left ventricles fails, the haemodynamic profile is more complex (see Chapter on Cardiogenic Shock).

Vasogenic or Distributive Shock

This shock syndrome occurs with a number of aetiological factors and is characterized by a poor vascular tone in the peripheral circulation (low SVR). There is also a maldistribution of blood flow to organs within the body. The CO varies but is usually raised. *A common haemodynamic profile is a low or normal PCWP, a high CO, a low arterial blood pressure, and a low SVR.* Vasogenic shock is typified by septic shock and the toxic shock syndrome. It is also observed in traumatic shock, neurogenic shock following spinal cord trauma, in post-operative shock, shock in pancreatitis, and in anaphylactic shock. Septic shock, toxic shock syndrome and anaphylactic shock have been described in subsequent chapters.

Though the above profiles are easily understood and generally accepted for teaching purposes, in actual practice, problems in assessment and management of shock syndromes are often complex and difficult. For one thing, the features of hypovolaemia, myocardial dysfunction and sepsis may all be present in the same individual. Similarly, hypovolaemic shock is not uncommonly associated with cardiogenic shock. For another, acute circulatory failure triggers a chain of compensatory responses, chiefly mediated by neurohormonal mechanisms. These compensatory responses alter the haemodynamic profile induced by the initial insult to the circulation. Compensatory features in shock, particularly changes in SVR vary from patient to patient. Old age, neu-ropathies and diabetes mellitus are some important background factors that can blunt the systemic vascular response and other compensatory responses. Then again, various therapeutic modalities instituted in the management of shock can alter the haemodynamics of shock and its haemodynamic profile, and this alteration may last for only a short period of time. Finally, not only compensatory mechanisms but also decompensation within the circulatory system can further produce varying haemodynamic profiles in different shock syndromes.

Hence the assumption that each cause of shock necessarily has a characteristic profile, and that therapeutic principles in management are dependent on analysing one single profile at any one point in time, is simplistic and beset with difficulties. Various permutations and combinations of the above basic haemodynamic profiles can lead to a number of possible patterns. However, familiarity with the basic profiles described above helps the intensivist analyse the haemodynamic changes that can occur in shock syndromes, and aids in management.

An Overview of Management Strategies in the Shock Syndromes (Table 6.1.2)

The principles of management are as follows:

(i) *Treat the Cause Whenever Possible.* In haemorrhagic shock it is important to arrest the source of bleeding in so far as this is possible. Sepsis should be managed by draining local pockets of infection surgically, ensuring that the source of sepsis (e.g. a perforated viscus) is eradicated, and by using appropriate antibiotics. Traumatic shock, shock in an adrenal crisis and in anaphylaxis need appropriate specific therapy outlined in other chapters of this book.

(ii) *Interpretation of the Haemodynamic Pattern.* At the outset it should be mentioned that not every patient with shock requires invasive haemodynamic monitoring. For example, moderately severe hypovolaemic shock due to vomiting and diarrhoea, can well be managed without resorting to invasive procedures. When appropriate treatment however does not result in a quick reversal of the shock state, or in cases of shock of obscure aetiology, further management is unquestionably helped by monitoring

Table 6.1.2. Overview of management strategies in the shock syndromes

1. Treat cause whenever possible
2. Interpret and manage haemodynamic abnormality
   a. Low PCWP & CVP—Volume load to raise PCWP to 15–18 mm Hg
   b. Low CO, hypotension and normal SVR—
      * If PCWP in upper limit of normal or slightly raised—use inotropic support
      * If PCWP normal, push it to upper limit of normal with volume load, before starting inotropic support
   c. Low CO, hypotension and increased SVR—
      * Inotropic support
      * Lower SVR by IV nitroglycerin/IV nitroprusside
   d. Low CO, hypotension, normal filling pressures and reduced SVR—
      * Raise filling pressures to upper limit of normal
      * Inotropic support
3. Ensure adequate tissue oxygenation
   * Increase $\dot{D}O_2$ to maximal levels if possible—thereby ensure adequate $\dot{V}O_2$

circulatory haemodynamics—arterial blood pressure (ABP), the filling pressures (CVP and PCWP), the CO, CI, pulmonary artery pressures (PAP), the systemic and pulmonary vascular resistance (SVR and PVR), stroke volume, and if necessary the right and left ventricular stroke work indices. These values should enable one to determine the nature of the haemodynamic abnormalities or problems present in a given patient. Thus a pattern of a low CVP, low PCWP, low CO, hypotension, and a low SVR points to hypovolaemia plus poor vascular tone. Therapy would therefore comprise a volume load together with drugs that increase the sympathetic tone. A pattern of a normal PCWP, a low CO, a low arterial pressure and a normal SVR, can only be sorted out by noting the response of the cardiac output to a volume load which pushes the PCWP to a little above normal. An inadequate rise in CO would point to myocardial dysfunction. A normal SVR would indicate an inadequate compensatory response of the peripheral circulation, or a blunting and partial reversal of the compensatory response by other factors, such as sepsis.

Should one hazard a diagnosis of the aetiology of the shock syndrome on the basis of the haemodynamic profile? It is wise not to necessarily expect any particular or fixed profile in the different aetiological forms of shock mentioned earlier. Though in difficult cases the cause of shock may well be suggested by the profile observed, this need not be so. The aetiology and the nature of circulatory disturbances causing shock in a patient, should be arrived at by an overall perspective of background factors, clinical features, laboratory investigations and the haemodynamic profile observed over a period of time. The sum total of evidence is far more important than the mere consideration of the haemodynamic pattern observed at a given point in time.

(iii) *Haemodynamic Management.* This is based on correct interpretation of the haemodynamic findings. As mentioned earlier, a number of permutations and combinations of these variables are seen in clinical practice.

A management protocol, dependent on some of the important parameters observed, is summarized below merely as a guide to patient care.

(a) Low filling pressures (low PCWP and CVP). Therapy should always include a volume load to raise the filling pressures to normal or just above normal i.e. PCWP is raised to 15–18 mm Hg.

(b) Low CO, hypotension, and a normal SVR. If the PCWP is in the upper limit of normal, or even moderately raised, a low CO deserves to be treated with inotropic support. Dopamine would be the drug of choice, as besides providing inotropic support it can increase the SVR. If the PCWP is normal, it should be pushed to the upper limit of normal or even above normal by a suitable volume load, before starting inotropic support.

(c) Low CO, hypotension, and a raised SVR. In the presence of high normal or raised filling pressures, inotropic support is provided by dobutamine or a combination of dopamine and dobutamine, or a combination of dobutamine and amrinone. The raised SVR is lowered by appropriate drugs—by intravenous nitroglycerin if the filling pressures are raised, or by intravenous nitroprusside provided the systolic blood pressure is not below 90 mm Hg, and can be maintained at this level by the above therapy.

(d) A low CO, hypotension, normal filling pressures, with a low SVR. Filling pressures should be raised by a volume load to the upper limit of normal or even to a little above normal. If the CO still remains low, the use of inotropic agents is indicated—dopamine besides being an inotropic agent, also increases the SVR.

As a general rule, vasoconstrictors must be used with caution, as they can elevate a low blood pressure, but can reduce blood flow to vital organs. Dopamine is the drug of choice in most instances because of its triple action—a dopaminergic effect on the kidneys in low doses which stimulates urinary excretion, an inotropic effect, and a vasoconstrictor action on the peripheral circulation. Norepinephrine or vasopressin is preferred as first choice by some units. We use norepinephrine or vasopressin only when dopamine fails to produce the desired effect. Adrenaline infusions may also be administered particularly during resuscitation following cardiac arrest. Details of drugs used in the shock syndromes are described in subsequent chapters.

It has already been mentioned earlier that the mere restoration of the haemodynamic profile to normalcy does not predict recovery in shock. The period following restoration of blood pressure and even cardiac output to within the normal range can often be associated with continued ischaemia and progressive organ damage. The pathogenesis of progressive ischaemia, injury to tissue cells and to multiple organs within the body under these circumstances, continues to be the subject of intense research. 'Post-resuscitation injury' is perhaps related to the following factors:

(a) No Reflow (2). There is persistent hypoperfusion following an ischaemic insult (4, 5). The mechanism is believed to be due to a calcium influx into the vascular smooth muscle during the period of ischaemia, leading to intense, persistent vasoconstriction of the small vessels within various organs. This persists for hours after the blood pressure and cardiac output are restored to normal, and results in progressive multi-organ dysfunction and multi-organ failure which carry a high mortality.

(b) Reperfusion Injury. Reperfusion of organs after the ischaemic insult leads to the distribution of toxic substances (which accumulate during the ischaemic period) to various organs of the body. These toxic substances are oxygen metabolites and free oxygen radicals which readily produce widespread cellular injury (6).

(c) Oxygen Debt. During the shock state when hypotension or poor tissue perfusion is the key feature, oxygen uptake and oxygen consumption may be inadequate for tissue needs. This represents an ongoing ischaemia and it is during this ischaemic period that the tissues accumulate an oxygen debt. This debt must be repaid by a compensatory period during which oxygen delivery and oxygen consumption are well above normal. Patients in whom this compensatory mechanism does not occur are at greater risk of increasing cellular injury, multiple organ failure and death (2). In addition to the development of oxygen debt, circulatory shock results in an increase in tissue carbon dioxide, and hence an increase in the tissue PCO_2 (7). The significance of hypercarbonic acidosis in tissues (resulting from poor perfusion) in relation to cell and organ function, is not yet elucidated.

The above considerations lead to an extremely crucial feature in the management of shock states.

(iv) *Ensuring Tissue Oxygenation.* Patients having a lower than normal $\dot{V}O_2$ have a higher mortality than those with a normal or supranormal $\dot{V}O_2$ (**8, 9**). Also the $\dot{V}O_2$ may be within the normal range, yet be insufficient for tissues having an increased metabolic rate as in sepsis. An inadequate $\dot{V}O_2$ in relation to tissue needs can be determined, as mentioned earlier, by estimating blood lactate levels.

The normal lactate levels in arterial blood in healthy individuals is $\leq 2\,mM/l$ and in 'stressed' individuals $> 4\,mM/l$ (**10**). It has been shown that mortality in shock increases as lactate levels increase above $2\,mM/l$ (**11**). If after the blood pressure and cardiac output are restored the $\dot{V}O_2$ is still low ($< 110\,ml/min\text{-}m^2$), then the CO should be further increased by either volume infusion (if PCWP $< 18\,mm\,Hg$), or by inotropic support (if PCWP $> 18\,mm\,Hg$). A combination of volume load and inotropic support may be used. It has been further suggested, that if the $\dot{V}O_2$ is normal or even above normal, but the lactate level is $> 4\,mM/l$, the CO and with it $\dot{V}O_2$ should be even further increased to supramaximal or supranormal levels, using a further volume load and/or by inotropic support of dopamine and dobutamine. Shoemaker (**1**) is the champion advocate of supranormal increase in cardiac output and oxygen consumption in shock. In his opinion, if this is achieved survival is more likely. Yet there are others who feel that attempting to achieve supramaximal cardiac outputs and oxygen consumption in shock does not improve survival and may even have an adverse effect (**12**). It is possible that pushing cardiac output and $\dot{V}O_2$ to supranormal levels may help in the small subset of intra-operative and post-operative patients who develop the haemodynamic features of shock (**1**). Perhaps the above policy is successful if it is used very early in the natural history of shock and is unsuccessful if used later in the natural history when organ failure has already set in.

From the practical point of view, at least in the medical ICU, we have often found it impossible to raise both CO and $\dot{V}O_2$ to supranormal levels. When we have managed to do so, we have not observed any improvement in morbidity and mortality.

Criteria for Tissue Oxygenation

The measurements of oxygen transport $(\dot{D}O_2)$, *oxygen consumption* $(\dot{V}O_2)$ *and blood lactate give an overall global estimate of tissue oxygenation. The adequacy or inadequacy of tissue oxygenation in individual organ systems remains undetermined.* All forms of shock, including septic shock are associated with splanchnic hypoperfusion. The latter is therefore a very important feature of many critical illnesses and may constitute an early warning of impending multiple organ failure. Gastric tonometry is a method of evaluating oxygenation in the gastrointestinal tract which is supplied by the splanchnic circulation (**13**).

Gastric Tonometry. The method is inherently simple. A saline filled silicone balloon permeable to CO_2 is affixed to the end of a nasogastric tube and is allowed to remain in contact with gastric mucosa for 20 minutes so that the CO_2 of the mucosa equilibrates with the saline in the balloon. The PCO_2 of the saline is taken as a measure of the PCO_2 in the mucosa. The higher the PCO_2 the poorer the perfusion of the mucosa. The intramucosal pH can be calculated by the Henderson-Hasselbach equation

$$pH = 6.1 + \log_{10} \frac{\text{Arterial } HCO_3}{\text{Saline } PCO_2 \times 0.03}$$

The bicarbonate concentration of arterial blood is used as a measure of the bicarbonate in the gastric mucosa. The normal gastric intramucosal pH has a mean of 7.38 with a range of 7.35 to 7.41. A pH < 7.32 is abnormal and indicates acidosis due to poor mucosal perfusion. It is believed that estimating gastric mucosal pH is a better method of predicting outcome in critically ill individuals than estimating $\dot{V}O_2$ and blood lactate levels (**14**).

We are not familiar with gastric tonometry. It has a few drawbacks. Intramucosal pH is influenced by gastric acidity, as also by systemic acid-base disorders. Also the use of arterial bicarbonate as a measure of mucosal bicarbonate may be inaccurate, particularly in situations associated with poor splanchnic blood flow.

Management decisions on gastric mucosal pH or PCO_2 in critically ill patients are ill-defined. Splanchnic blood flow can be improved by volume infusions and in some patients by dobutamine. In any case it is bad medicine to rely on a single parameter for the diagnosis, prognosis and management of a complex problem.

In conclusion, stress on adequate oxygenation of tissues in relation to their needs is probably the key factor that determines survival in severe shock states. The sooner this is achieved in the natural history of shock, the more likely are we to succeed. The difficulty lies in devising easily ascertainable methods to determine oxygen consumption and tissue oxygen requirements in critically ill patients. The practical approach of meeting the oxygen demands of the tissues in severe shock is difficult, debatable and needs further study.

REFERENCES

1. Shoemaker WC. (1998). Diagnosis and Treatment of Shock and Circulatory Dysfunction. In: Textbook of Critical Care, 4th Edn (Eds Shoemaker WC, Ayres S, Grenvik A, Holbrook PR). pp. 92–114. WB Saunders Company, Philadelphia, London, Toronto, Montreal, Sydney, Tokyo.

2. Marino PL. (1998). Haemodynamic Monitoring: Tissue Oxygenation. In: The ICU Book. pp. 187–203. Williams and Wilkins, USA.

3. Bone RC. (1996). Toward a theory regarding the pathogenesis in the systemic inflammatory response syndrome: What we do and do not know about cytokine regulation. Crit Care Med. 24, 163.

4. McNamara JJ, Suehiro GT, Suehiro A et al. (1983). Resuscitation from haemorrhagic shock. J Trauma. 23, 552–558.

5. White BC, Winegar CD, Wilson RF et al. (1983). Possible role of calcium blockers in cerebral resuscitation: A review of the literature and synthesis for future studies. Crit Care Med. 11, 202–207.

6. Waxman K, Nolan LS, Shoemaker WC. (1982). Sequential perioperative lactate determination. Physiological and clinical implications. Crit Care Med. 10, 96–99.

7. Johnson B, Weil MH. (1991). Redefining ischemia due to circulatory failure as dual defects of oxygen deficit and carbon dioxide excess. Crit Care Med. 19, 1432–1438.

8. Shoemaker WC. (1987). Relationship of oxygen transport patterns to the pathophysiology and therapy of shock states. Intensive Care Med. 13, 230–243.

9. Weber K, Janicki JS, Hunter WC et al. (1982). The contractile behaviour of the heart and its functional coupling to the circulation. Prog Cardiovasc Dis. 24, 375–400.

10. Haljmade H. (1987). Lactate metabolism. Intensive Care World. 4, 118–120.

11. Weil MH, Affizi DA. (1970). Experimental and clinical studies on lactate and pyruvate as indicators of the severity of acute circulatory failure (shock). Circulation. 41, 989–1001.

12. Alia I, Esteban A, Federico G et al. (1999). A Randomized and Controlled Trial of the Effect of Treatment Aimed at Maximizing Oxygen Delivery in Patients with Severe Sepsis or Septic Shock. Chest. 115, 453–61.

13. Gutierrez G, Brown SD (1995). Gastric tonometry: a new monitoring modality in the intensive care unit. J Intensive Care Med. 10, 34–44

14. Maymard N, Bihari D, Beale R et al. (1993) Assessment of splanchnic circulation by gastric tonometry in patients with acute circulatory failure. JAMA. 270, 1203–1210.

Hypovolaemic and Haemorrhagic Shock

Hypovolaemic shock results from a decrease in circulating volume which results in poor tissue perfusion. The commonest cause of hypovolaemic shock is trauma resulting in external or concealed haemorrhage from blunt or penetrating injuries. Blood loss into surrounding tissues following fractures of long bones or the pelvis is an important cause of haemorrhagic shock. Non-traumatic causes of bleeding constitute an important cause of haemorrhagic shock. Important non-traumatic causes include bleeding from a peptic ulcer, acute mucosal erosions, oesophageal varices or from other pathologies into the GI tract, dissection of the aorta, rupture of an aneurysm of a large vessel (e.g. a ruptured aortic aneurysm), and rarely bleeding into a viscus in blood dyscrasias.

Hypovolaemic shock is also frequently due to loss of water and electrolytes, with a fall in effective circulating volume. This is seen in burns, in vomiting and/or diarrhoea from any cause, in severe water loss as in diabetes insipidus, in diabetes mellitus, adrenocortical insufficiency, exfoliative dermatitis, and following excessive sweating in hot, humid climates. Sequestration of fluid with loss of effective circulating volume and hypovolaemic shock can occur in intestinal obstruction, pancreatitis and peritonitis. Quick reaccumulation of a large volume of ascitic fluid after paracentesis can also occasionally lead to a fall in effective circulating volume with features of hypovolaemic shock. **Table 6.2.1** lists the important causes of haemorrhagic and hypovolaemic shock.

Physiopathology

Hypovolaemia from any cause if severe and untreated, causes increasingly poor perfusion of tissues, ischaemia and injury to tissue cells, and ultimately death.

A fall in circulating volume leads to decreased venous return, decreased filling pressures on the right and left sides of the heart, and a decreased cardiac output, which leads to tissue hypoxaemia. The loss of intravascular volume initiates several compensatory mechanisms, the ultimate purpose of which is directed towards maintaining perfusion of vital organs such as the heart and the brain. The effectiveness of these mechanisms is dependent on the rate of fluid loss, and the degree of volume depletion present.

Table 6.2.1. Causes of haemorrhagic and hypovolaemic shock

Haemorrhagic shock

Traumatic	Non-Traumatic
* Blunt or penetrating injury * Fractures specially of long bones and pelvic fractures	* GI bleeds (e.g. peptic ulcer, gastric mucosal erosions, oesophageal varices, typhoid bleeds, bleeds in sepsis, DIC) * Aortic dissection * Rupture of aneurysm of a large vessel e.g. aorta * Erosion of a large vessel e.g. in pancreatitis or due to tumour infiltration * Diffuse inflammation of mucosal surfaces e.g. ulcerative colitis

Hypovolaemic Shock

Traumatic	Non-Traumatic
* Burns * Crush injuries	* Fluid loss from vomiting and/or diarrhoea e.g. in cholera, other GI infections * Fluid loss in diabetes mellitus, adrenal insufficiency, excessive sweating, exfoliative dermatitis, diabetes insipidus, reaccumulation of ascites after tapping * Sequestration of fluid e.g. in intestinal obstruction, pancreatitis

Neurohormonal Compensatory Mechanisms

Volume depletion stimulates baroreceptors within the intrathoracic vessels and the carotids, as also organ-specific baroreceptors within the kidneys resulting in an increased sympathetic discharge, increased release of stress hormones like catecholamines and cortisol, increased secretion of antidiuretic hormone, and activation of the renin-angiotensin system. The increased sympathetic discharge leads to tachycardia, increased SVR, maintenance of systemic blood pressure, and maintenance of perfusion to the brain and the heart at the expense of perfusion to other organs (skin, muscles, kidneys, gut).

Shift of Fluid from the Extravascular to the Vascular Compartment

Total body water comprises 60 per cent of the lean body weight (or 600 ml/kg) in man and 50 per cent of the lean body weight (or 500 ml/kg) in woman. 55 per cent of the total body water is intracellular, and 45 per cent extracellular. The interstitial fluid content is 20 per cent of the total body water, while plasma constitutes just 7.5 per cent of total body water, and in a 70 kg male amounts to 3–3.2 litres (1). With a haematocrit of 45 per cent, the blood volume in a 70 kg male would be about 5.5 to 5.7 litres (or 66 ml/kg) and in a female would be about 60 ml/kg. The blood volume thus constitutes just 13 per cent of the total body fluids. Ordinarily, an acute loss of 35–40 per cent of the blood volume can be fatal, which means that human survival is determined by about 4 per cent of the fluid in the body (1). Therefore to reduce mortality, it is imperative to prevent a bleeding patient from losing this 4 per cent fluid volume.

Besides the neurohormonal compensatory mechanisms, shift of fluid from the interstitial compartment into the vascular compartment helps in some measure to restore blood volume in haemorrhagic shock. This occurs in 3 phases (**Fig. 6.2.1**).

Phase 1. Within an hour of blood loss, there is a shift of fluid from the interstitial compartment into the capillaries. This continues for 40 hours and the volume shift can be as high as one litre. The interstitial compartment however stands depleted due to this shift.

Phase 2. A depleted blood volume activates the renin system, leading to sodium retention. Sodium diffuses into the extravascular compartment, and the retained sodium leads to water retention, thus helping to replenish the interstitial fluid.

Phase 3. Blood loss stimulates erythropoiesis within a few

hours. 15–50 ml of cell volume is produced daily, and complete replenishment of depleted cells takes as long as 2–3 months (2).

The neurohormonal changes described above and the shift of interstitial fluid into the vascular compartment, work hand in hand to preserve tissue perfusion particularly to vital organs. Compensatory mechanisms however can only work up to a point. Severe volume loss if not adequately and quickly replaced, inevitably leads to tissue ischaemia and metabolic acidosis. Tissue damage results and this induces cellular and humoral inflammatory responses which further exacerbate circulatory abnormalities that ultimately lead to irreversible widespread cell injury, and death. The importance of early restoration of a depleted blood volume by vigorous infusions of intravenous fluids cannot be overstressed, if haemorrhagic and hypovolaemic shock are to be reversed.

Clinical Features

Clinical features of haemorrhagic and hypovolaemic shock are similar, and depend on the age of the patient, pre-existing background medical problems, the degree of volume loss, the time period over which the volume loss has occurred, and the ability of a patient to bring the compensatory mechanisms outlined above into play.

The earliest features are tachycardia, pallor (when there is blood loss), and a slight anxiety with restlessness. The skin may be cold and clammy. Sudden, inexplicable, profuse sweating may be the first symptom or sign of an occult or fairly severe blood loss as in an upper GI bleed. Unless blood or volume loss is very severe and acute, the blood pressure is often initially maintained. Even so, orthostatic hypotension may be demonstrated by a drop in systolic blood pressure > 10 mm Hg on changing from the supine to the sitting posture. The neck veins are collapsed, unlike patients in cardiogenic shock where the neck veins are full. Oliguria is present (urine output < 0.5 ml/kg/hour), and may progress to well-nigh complete anuria.

Compensatory mechanisms in severe shock ultimately fail. The systolic blood pressure then drops and the patient's mental state may get progressively obtunded. In an otherwise uncomplicated case of haemorrhagic shock, a significant drop in pressure (> 30 mm Hg) in the supine position, together with marked oliguria, suggests a loss of 30–40 per cent of blood volume, or an effective loss of about 2 l in a 70 kg patient. Increasing metabolic acidosis is the classic sign of increasingly poor tissue perfusion. Towards the end, the patient is pulseless, pressureless and almost anuric. If cerebral perfusion is preserved to some extent, the patient may remain alert; more often than not, he is obtunded and confused.

The expected clinical findings will depend on the degree of blood or volume loss, and the degree of compensatory mechanisms in the patient. Three categories of haemorrhagic shock have been described based on the degrees of volume lost, and the expected clinical findings. These three categories or classes have been briefly tabulated in **Table 6.2.2** (3). Compensatory responses chiefly in the form of tachycardia and vasoconstriction (increased SVR), may be blunted in elderly patients, diabetics, alcoholics, in patients with chronic renal and liver cell dysfunction, and in patients

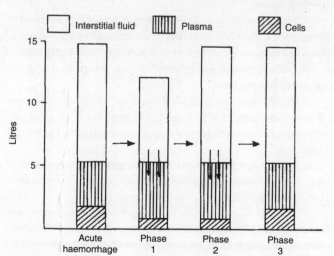

Fig. 6.2.1. Response to mild haemorrhage (from Marino PL. 1991. The ICU Book, Lippincott Williams & Wilkins, MD.)
Phase 1: Shift of fluid from interstitial fluid compartment into capillaries with decrease in volume of the interstitial fluid compartment.
Phase 2: Depletion of blood volume activates the renin system, resulting in sodium retention, water retention and replenishment of interstitial fluid compartment.
Phase 3: Erythropoiesis stimulation due to blood loss.

Table 6.2.2. Haemorrhagic Shock: clinical features and their relation to estimated blood loss and to fluid replacement therapy*

	Mild	Moderate	Severe
Heart rate	100/min	100–140/min	> 140/min (as high as 160–200/min)
Blood pressure	Normal or slightly reduced; postural drop present	Decreased; marked postural drop present	Markedly decreased; may be unrecordable
Respiratory rate	< 20/min	20–35/min	> 35/min
Skin	Mild pallor	Increasing pallor, cold, clammy	Severe pallor, sweating, hypothermic
Urine output	< 30 ml/hr	< 20 ml/hr	<10 ml/hr; may be anuric
Mental state	Anxious	Increasingly anxious; confused	Obtunded, may be comatose
Arterial pH	Normal	Slightly reduced	≤ 7.2
Blood loss (approx.)	≤ 700 ml	700–1750 ml	> 1750 ml
Fluid replacement**	Crystalloids	Crystalloids + blood	Crystalloids + blood

*It is to be noted that every clinical feature listed above need not necessarily be present at the same time in the different grades of haemorrhagic shock. Clinical features are dependent on the compensatory haemodynamic responses to blood loss.

**The empiric fluid replacement for most patients in haemorrhagic shock is 300 ml of electrolyte solution for 100 ml blood loss. This is a general guideline which should never be followed blindly as it could result in either hypervolaemia or inadequate volume replacement. Fluid therapy should be guided by clinical response and by careful monitoring of haemodynamic changes. Colloid infusions could be used to urgently increase blood volume till blood is available for patients with severe haemorrhagic shock.

enfeebled by debilitating illnesses. Tachycardia may be less marked or even absent in these situations, and hypotension may occur early with little blood loss.

Monitoring Hypovolaemic Shock

Clinical monitoring of vital parameters like the pulse, blood pressure, respiratory rate, skin and core temperature, capillary refill, urine output, oxygen saturation, jugular venous pressure, arterial pH and blood gases is essential. An arterial line is indicated if the blood pressure is low, as otherwise false very low readings are obtained with the non-invasive blood pressure measurement technique.

Monitoring the haematocrit, the haemodynamic pattern, oxygen extraction, and the end-tidal CO_2 are briefly described below. It needs to be mentioned, particularly for our part of the world, that it is not necessary to measure oxygen extraction and end tidal CO_2 for the proper management of hypovolaemic shock. Even the pulmonary artery catheter to monitor the haemodynamic profile is being used with increasing infrequency in our unit. Yet there are occasions when these measurements are of help to understand the nature of a difficult problem confronting the intensivist.

The Haematocrit

It is important to remember that acute blood loss produces no immediate change in the haemoglobin (Hb), RBC count, or the haematocrit. This is because if whole blood is lost, the concentration of RBCs, Hb and the proportion of RBCs to plasma remains unchanged. It may take 24 hours for sufficient interstitial fluid to enter the vascular compartment and significantly reduce the Hb and the haematocrit. On the other hand, if the patient has bled slowly, if recognition of blood loss is delayed, or if fluid resuscitation has been prompt, the haematocrit will be low. When hypovolaemia results from loss of fluids as in vomiting, diarrhoea, fistulae involving the GI system, or in sequestration of fluids as in intestinal obstruction, the haematocrit is high.

Haemodynamic Pattern

The classic haemodynamic pattern as has already been stated, is a low CVP, a low PCWP, a low CO and a high SVR. Tachycardia is generally present, and the blood pressure may be maintained within normal limits because of compensatory increase in systemic vascular resistance. It is important to interpret haemodynamic findings with circumspection, and not necessarily let them take precedence over clinical findings. The filling pressures, and in particular the central venous pressure, are not always very reliable in assessing the degree of volume loss in critically ill patients. The following features may interfere with the correct interpretation of the clinical state:

(i) The CVP is influenced by the compliance of the veins and of the ventricles, and both these may be decreased by hypovolaemia. The excessive venoconstriction resulting from sympathetic activation may produce a higher CVP than is expected with the degree of volume loss.

(ii) Higher than expected CVP readings are observed if vasopressors have been used to counter hypotension. This is not uncommon when the aetiology of hypotension has been incorrectly diagnosed.

(iii) Higher than anticipated CVP readings may also be observed when the hypovolaemia is associated with cardiac tamponade or a tension pneumothorax (as in severe trauma).

(iv) A CVP below +2 cm H_2O signifies volume depletion. However, the CVP is ordinarily low (between 2–10 cm H_2O), and there is little margin for change with hypovolaemia. Single pressure readings at a given point in time can be misleading. It is important to interpret changes in trends in pressure readings over a period of time, particularly after fluid resuscitation has commenced, and to correlate these changes with improvement in clinical findings.

Oxygen Extraction

According to Fick's principle (see Chapter on Cardiopulmonary Physiology), the usual response to a lowered cardiac output is an increase in oxygen extraction from the blood perfusing the tissues. This can continue only to a point, after which an oxygen debt occurs and tissue metabolism switches from aerobic to anaerobic. Ideally, mixed venous oxygen saturation and pressure are estimated from blood samples withdrawn from the pulmonary artery via the pulmonary artery catheter. However, there is now a tendency to use blood samples drawn from a central venous line, on the assumption that the results of $S\bar{v}O_2$ thus obtained are close to those obtained by the more accurate estimation of $S\bar{v}O_2$ of blood drawn through a pulmonary artery catheter. There is however considerable dispute over this assumption.

The expected changes in oxygen extraction and mixed venous oxygen saturation in hypovolaemia progressing to hypovolaemic shock are given below.

	SaO_2	$S\bar{v}O_2$	O_2 extraction $(SaO_2 - S\bar{v}O_2)$
Normal	> 95%	65 to 70%	about 30%
Hypovolaemia	> 95%	50 to 65%	30 to 50%
Shock	> 95%	< 50%	> 50%

An increasing difference between SaO_2 and $S\bar{v}O_2$ is ominous and a difference over 50 per cent generally denotes shock with tissue hypoxia.

End-tidal CO_2

A decrease in cardiac output results in a decrease in PCO_2 of the expired gas (4). This is a simple method of monitoring a falling cardiac output in hypovolaemic shock. The end-tidal CO_2 is normally 3 to 4 mm Hg less than the arterial $PaCO_2$. It may drop to below 10 mm Hg in severe shock and shows a progressive rise with successful volume resuscitation. End-tidal PCO_2 can be measured and monitored using standard nasal cannula used to provide oxygen to the patient.

Differential Diagnosis

Hypovolaemic shock may be mistaken for shock due to other causes if bleeding or fluid loss is not externally evident. Cardiogenic shock has similar features except that it is usually associated with distended neck veins. Spinal injury following trauma may produce vasodilatation which is relatively refractory to fluid administration. Shock following trauma is however invariably due to hypovolaemia, and other causes should only be entertained after adequate fluid replacement therapy has first been instituted. A state of shock can occur following hypoglycaemia due to excessive insulin administration. The patient is cold, clammy, has tachycardia, and may be hypotensive. Brain stem signs and decerebrate states when present, are seen more frequently in hypoglycaemia than in hypovolaemic shock. A history of insulin administration should always arouse suspicion. After blood has been sent for glucose estimation, administration of 50 ml of 50 per cent dextrose should promptly produce marked improvement in the patient's condition.

Management

The principles of management are as follows:

I. Fluid resuscitation. Rapid fluid resuscitation is the keystone of therapy in hypovolaemic (including haemorrhagic) shock. Restoring the volume within the vascular compartment increases venous return, increases and supports cardiac output, raises blood pressure and improves tissue perfusion. It reverses the effects of hypovolaemic shock.

II. Replacement of haemoglobin with blood transfusions when shock is due to significant blood loss.

III. Monitoring fluid and blood resuscitation clinically, and re-evaluating the overall condition after initial fluid resuscitation. CVP monitoring is essential; in difficult cases (see below), haemodynamic monitoring through a Swan-Ganz catheter may further help management.

IV. Determining the aetiology of hypovolaemic shock and treatment of the cause in so far as this is possible. In haemorrhagic shock without external bleeding, it is important to determine the site of blood loss, and arrest a continuing bleed. External haemorrhage should be controlled by prompt pressure over the site, and surgical control of the bleed. One should never wait for laboratory tests, but should start fluid resuscitation promptly. In a well equipped ICU, investigations to determine the cause of severe hypovolaemic shock are carried out after, or *pari passu* with emergency resuscitation.

I. Fluid Resuscitation

A. Principles

The ultimate objective in fluid resuscitation is to restore and maintain O_2 uptake in vital organs of the body so as to preserve organ function.

$$\dot{V}O_2 = \text{Cardiac Output } (\dot{Q}_T) \times Hb \times 13 \times (SaO_2 - S\bar{v}O_2)$$

In acute severe fluid loss it is the cardiac output alone which needs to be urgently restored and sustained. In severe acute blood loss, $\dot{V}O_2$ is compromised both by a low cardiac output and a low Hb. Unquestionably a low cardiac output has far more dangerous consequences than anaemia. The prime objective therefore in shock due to acute blood loss is to first restore cardiac output and improve blood flow; correcting Hb deficit is the next objective.

Therefore in severe hypovolaemic or haemorrhagic shock, fluids should be infused rapidly to quickly correct the volume deficit and thereby increase cardiac output and blood flow.

In young, previously healthy patients, the infusion in severe hypovolaemic shock is given at the maximal rate permissible by the catheter, and the size of vein cannulated for infusion. In older patients, or in those with cardiac disease, the infusion should be given less rapidly with a close watch for hypervolaemia and complicating pulmonary oedema.

B. Cannulation Site

In severe shock, it is mandatory to have access to two veins through two large bore (16 gauge) intravenous catheters. Central venous catheters do not permit rapid fluid replacement in severe hypovolaemic shock, simply because of their long length, and because the lumen of the usual central lines is too small to allow rapid fluid flow (see below). It is best therefore, to insert a short 16 gauge catheter into a peripheral vein. If this is impossible because of totally collapsed peripheral veins, a large bore catheter can be placed in the femoral vein, or a central line necessarily has to be secured.

C. Catheter Dimensions and Relation to Flow Rate

Severe hypovolaemic shock requires rapid infusion of intravenous fluids. It is important to remember that the maximum infusion rate is dependent on the size (i.e. lumen) of the catheter, and not on the size of the vein that is cannulated. To be more precise, the infusion rate is directly related to the pressure gradient along the catheter, and the fourth power of the radius of the catheter. It is inversely related to the length of the catheter and the viscosity of the fluid infused (5). The relationship stated above is illustrated in **Table 6.2.3**. It is to be noted that the infusion rate is almost four times greater in the 2" short peripheral 16 gauge catheter, than in the usual 12" long central venous catheter. This table illustrates the importance of the short 2" peripheral catheters for rapid infusions and quick fluid replacement, as compared to the long central venous catheters.

Table 6.2.3. Influence of catheter size on infusion rate

Infusion device	Length (inches)	Flow rate* (ml/min)
9-French Introducer	5 1/2	247
IV Extension Tubing	12	220
Peripheral		
14-Gauge Catheter	2	195
16-Gauge Catheter	2	150
Central		
16-Gauge Catheter	5 1/2	91
16-Gauge Catheter	12	54

*Gravity flow of tap water.
From Mateer JR et al. Rapid fluid resuscitation with central venous catheters. Ann Emerg Med 1983, 12:149–152, with permission from American College of Emergency Physicians.

Use of Introducer Catheters in Central Veins. Marino (1) has correctly stressed that the adverse effect of catheter length on infusion rate in central venous cannulation, can be overcome by the use of large bore introducer 'sheath' catheters. These introducer sheaths in sizes of 8.5 French (2.7 mm internal diameter), and 9 French (3 mm internal diameter), are normally used as conduits for multilumen catheters or the Swan-Ganz catheters, but can be used by themselves for rapid volume replacement.

D. Relation of Fluid Viscosity to Flow Rate

Dula and co-workers (6) have studied the influence of viscosity on flow rates (**Table 6.2.4**). It was shown that the infusion rates

Table 6.2.4. Influence of fluid type on infusion rate

Fluid	Flow rate (ml/min)*
Tap Water	100
5% Albumin	100
Whole Blood	65
Packed Cells	20

*Gravity flow through a 16-gauge, 2-inch catheter.
From Dula DJ, et al. Flow rate variance of commonly used IV infusion techniques. J Trauma 1981, 21:480–482, Lippincott Williams & Wilkins, MD.

of water and 5 per cent albumin were similar. The infusion rate of whole blood was slower, and that of packed red blood cells was the slowest. The importance of using crystalloids and/or colloids for emergency fluid replacement is therefore evident.

E. Estimating Volume Requirements in Hypovolaemic Shock

There is always a tendency to underestimate volume or blood loss in hypovolaemic shock. The following approach has been proposed by Marino (1) for a rough estimation of fluid loss:

(i) *Estimate Normal Volume.* In adults the normal blood volume is estimated at 66 ml/kg for males, and 60 ml/kg for females. Lean body weight is used for this estimate. For obese patients, the blood volume is first estimated on the actual body weight, and 10 per cent is then subtracted from the value obtained initially.

(ii) *Estimate the Percentage of Volume that is Depleted.* This is calculated according to the classification system tabled earlier (**Table 6.2.2**).

(iii) *Calculate the Volume Deficit.* This done by multiplying the estimated normal blood volume and the per cent lost. This quantifies the volume that requires to be replaced.

(iv) *Resuscitation with reference to the Fluids Used.* The volumes are estimated roughly as follows:
– If whole blood is used for resuscitation, then the volume to be replaced is 1 × volume deficit.
– If colloids are used for fluid resuscitation, then the volume necessary is 1 × volume deficit.
– If crystalloids (normal saline, Ringer Lactate) are used for fluid resuscitation, the volume that needs to be infused is 3 × volume deficit.

F. Fluids used in Volume Replacement

Shoemaker (7) studied the ability of different resuscitation fluids to promote cardiac output. Each of the fluids was administered over an hour and the change in cardiac index was noted at the end of infusion. The resuscitation fluids studied were whole blood (500 ml), packed cells (500 ml), dextran-40 (500 ml), Ringer Lactate (1 l). The maximum increase in cardiac index was observed with the colloid dextran-40, the next with whole blood, then with Ringer Lactate and the least (little or no increase) with packed RBCs. The obvious inference was that colloids were superior to blood products and crystalloids for increasing cardiac output and blood flow. Also, erythrocyte concentrates should not be used to increase blood flow. As has already been stated, the volume of crystalloid fluid should be three times greater than the volume of colloid infusion. Even so, there is still debate as to whether crystalloids or colloids should be used for emergency fluid resuscitation.

We generally use rapid infusions of crystalloids, either normal saline or Ringer Lactate. In our country, these fluids are cheap, readily available, and provide quick though transient intravascular expansion. When signs and symptoms of shock are apparent, 2 l of crystalloid solution is administered to the adult, and 20 ml/kg to a child. As quick equilibration occurs with the extravascular fluid compartment in about 30 minutes, only 25 per cent of the infused fluid can be presumed to remain in the vascular compartment after an infusion of crystalloids. Hence the rough rule that the volume to be replaced is at least three times the volume deficit as calculated in the manner described earlier.

Colloid solutions (Haemaccel or 5 per cent or 25 per cent albumin) are probably equally good or even better for effective volume replacement, and have been shown to improve and increase cardiac output more quickly than crystalloid solutions (7). Colloid solutions in our country, are however extremely expensive and not easily available. When hypovolaemic shock is associated with hypotension, we prefer to infuse crystalloid solutions through one vein and colloid solutions through another. The colloid solution helps to augment cardiac output and blood pressure quickly, whilst the crystalloids further help replenish the depleted volume, and also correct the sodium loss in the extracellular compartment which is an invariable feature of moderate to severe hypovolaemic shock.

The major complication associated with the use of crystalloid solutions is either underhydration due to inadequate volume replacement, or overhydration resulting in a hypervolaemic state. Excessive administration of crystalloids can result in generalized oedema. Pulmonary oedema is however rare in previously healthy individuals unless overinfusion results in a sharp increase in the PCWP to > 25–30 mm Hg. A careful monitoring of pulmonary hydrostatic pressure (PCWP) is important, and should prevent this complication. Since the chloride concentration of normal saline is significantly higher than the chloride concentration of plasma, patients resuscitated with large infusions of normal saline develop a hyperchloraemic metabolic acidosis which requires renal excretion of chloride for correction. After infusing the first 1.5–2 l as normal saline in severe hypovolaemic shock, we then prefer to alternate normal saline with either Ringer Lactate solution or 5 per cent dextrose saline for further correction of the volume deficit. Ringer's solution is preferred to normal saline infusions in some units for replacing volume deficits. Ringer's solution has a more physiological electrolyte content; the lactate within it is converted to bicarbonate by the liver, except in very ill patients or in those with marked hepatic dysfunction.

It is important not only to replace volume, but to ensure that the concentration of electrolytes in plasma is kept normal. Hypokalaemia is very frequent in hypovolaemia produced by vomiting, diarrhoea, by fluid loss from fistulae involving the GI tract, or by sequestration of fluids within the gut. 40–60 mEq of potassium (K^+) in a dextrose or dextrose-saline infusion are given over 4 hours through a separate vein, and repeated if necessary after monitoring serum K^+ levels. It is a mistake to give large volumes of 5 per cent dextrose for fluid resuscitation as severe hyponatraemia results, and this may be difficult to correct against a background of shock.

Occasionally hypovolaemic shock due to vomiting and diarrhoea is associated not only with a severe hypokalaemia, but also by excessive loss of bicarbonates in the stools with a resulting metabolic acidosis. Cholera (due to the gram-negative Vibrio cholerae), is a classic example where severe hypovolaemic shock due to fluid loss from vomiting and diarrhoea, is associated both with hypokalaemia and metabolic acidosis, with low plasma bicarbonate levels. Intravenous fluid replacement is best undertaken by using a special solution containing 5 g sodium chloride, 4 g sodium bicarbonate, and 1 g potassium chloride in one litre of distilled water. If the above solution is not available, infusion of 1 l of isotonic saline is alternated with 500 ml of either isotonic sodium bicarbonate (1.4 per cent in 500 ml), or 1/6th molar sodium lactate. This is continued till volume replacement is judged adequate. In fulminant cases with uncontrolled vomiting, and the continuous passing of large volume 'rice water' stools, 10–12 l of fluid may need to be replaced in the first 12 hours. Potassium losses may need to be separately replaced in a dextrose-saline drip. The patient needs critical care, but it is advisable to provide this in an isolation ward rather than in an all-purpose critical care unit. Fluid and electrolyte replacement as outlined above, and tetracycline 500 mg four times a day for 10 days, form the cornerstones of therapy. Oral rehydration therapy is both cheap and extremely effective in moderately severe cases. The solution used orally, if necessary through a nasogastric tube, should contain glucose 30 g, sodium chloride 3.5 g, and potassium bicarbonate 2.5 g in 1 l of water. The rate of administration is 750 ml/hr for patients weighing > 25 kg, and 500 ml/hr for patients weighing < 25 kg.

The Colloid Crystalloid Controversy. The controversy on the choice of colloids or crystalloids for volume replacement in hypovolaemic, and in particular haemorrhagic shock, continues.

Colloids because of their increased oncotic pressure and because of their very low permeability through capillary walls, produce as mentioned earlier, quick volume expansion, as well as a quicker and greater increase in cardiac output. This is an advantage as improved circulatory effects are produced by a smaller volume of colloid infusions as compared to larger volumes of crystalloid infusions. However, the recent SAFE study (8) concluded that the use of either 4 per cent albumin or normal saline for fluid resuscitation in ICU patients resulted in similar outcomes at 28 days.

The disadvantages of colloids are that when shock is associated with increased capillary permeability, they may initiate or worsen the acute respiratory distress syndrome (ARDS). There is some evidence that albumin given intravenously may accumulate in the lung interstitium.

Infusions of Hetastarch (an effective volume expander) may result in a decreased platelet count, and a prolongation of the partial thromboplastin time due to its anti-factor VIII effect. Allergic reactions, including anaphylaxis, have been reported with all colloid solutions, though they are comparatively rare with human albumin. Dextrans (Dextran 40 with a molecular weight of 10,000–80,000, and Dextran 70 with a molecular weight of 25,000–125,000) are powerful plasma expanders. We rarely use them for volume expansion because they may produce numerous problems—chiefly anaphylaxis, renal failure and bleeding. Dextrans inhibit platelet adhesion and aggregation, and the clinical effect produced is similar to Von Willebrand's disease.

The colloid used for volume expansion in our unit is generally a starch solution (Haemaccel) or intravenous albumin. We do not use colloids routinely but restrict their use for the following special conditions:

(i) As stated earlier, in severe hypovolaemic shock with well-marked hypotension, colloids are used in conjunction with crystalloid solutions (given through a separate vein). A quicker restoration of blood volume, a more rapid rise in cardiac output and blood pressure, and a quicker improvement in tissue perfusion is observed.

(ii) In fluid restoration for burns patients, intravenous albumin infusions are used after 24 hours to minimize the formation of oedema which would result from further continued administration of large volumes of crystalloids.

(iii) After volume restoration with crystalloids, colloids may be used in patients who are waterlogged or who have well-marked pitting oedema. The increased plasma oncotic pressure mobilizes accumulated extravascular fluid into the vascular compartment, the extra fluid being then excreted via the kidneys.

G. Monitoring Fluid Replacement and Endpoints in Therapy

Volume replacement by fluids should reverse shock. Clinical parameters such as a fall in heart rate, increase in blood pressure, restoration of urine output, increased warmth of the skin with evidence of improving or good capillary refill should be taken into account to determine the adequacy of volume replacement. Restoration of the mental state to normal, and correction of metabolic acidosis are good indicators of improving circulatory function.

The quantum of volume replacement should be guided by, but not solely determined by the estimated volume loss (**Table 6.2.2**). This is particularly important in haemorrhagic shock in older patients. Severe blood loss causing shock in these patients is associated with a marked compensatory increase in venous tone. Blood transfusions to replace lost blood ordinarily reverse shock, and simultaneously cause a reduction in venous tone. However, in some patients the venous tone remains persistently high. An increasing volume in the vascular compartment in association with a raised venous tone, can cause a rise in the filling or right atrial pressures to above normal, even when volume replacement is incomplete. In young individuals with normal hearts, this does not matter. In older individuals with poor depressed left ventricular function curves, a rise of right atrial pressure by even 3–4 mm Hg above normal, can induce a three-fold increase in the left ventricular filling pressure. The latter may rise from 8 mm Hg to 24 mm Hg, and cause acute pulmonary oedema.

Overinfusions resulting in pulmonary oedema can be clinically detected by noting an increased respiratory rate, by careful auscultation for crackles at the lung bases, and by pulmonary congestion which is evident on a chest X-ray. Detailed haemodynamic monitoring of PCWP, CO, SVR by a Swan-Ganz (S-G) catheter is not indicated in every case. We use invasive haemodynamic monitoring in the following circumstances:

(i) When hypovolaemia complicates other forms of shock e.g. septic or cardiogenic shock.

(ii) When the cause of shock is not clearly evident.

(iii) Hypovolaemic shock occurring in patients with known poor cardiac function, or in patients with suspected myocardial dysfunction.

(iv) When during fluid replacement, pulmonary congestion is evident, even though the replaced volume seems to be inadequate.

(v) In cases where the CVP is persistently higher than expected in the face of shock.

(vi) In cases where inotropic support is required even after adequate volume replacement.

The end-point of volume replacement with haemodynamic monitoring is to maintain a PCWP around 12–15 mm Hg and a CVP within the normal range.

H. The $\dot{V}O_2$ and Serum Lactate

In individuals with severe hypovolaemic shock, volume repletion may still (see Chapter 6.1) be associated with persistent tissue ischaemia, either due to the severity of the shock to start with, delay in resuscitation, or perhaps to 'reperfusion injury'. In patients where clear evidence of one or more organ dysfunction persists after volume replacement, $\dot{V}O_2$ and serum lactate measurements should be monitored. If the $\dot{V}O_2$ is found low and the serum lactate measurements are > 4 mM/l, further volume infusion with or without inotropic support is advocated. Shoemaker (see Chapter 6.1) is a strong advocate of increasing both cardiac output and $\dot{V}O_2$ to even supranormal levels to help recovery. There is however dispute and debate over this issue, and we have ceased attempting to do so.

Vasopressors are not indicated in pure hypovolaemic shock. If however, hypovolaemic shock is complicated by myocardial infarction, or poor myocardial function, inotropic agents may be used after volume repletion is complete. A fall in filling pressures after fluid replacement with a relapse into a 'shocked state', should suggest continuing fluid or blood loss. A persistent need for vasopressors or inotropic agents after fluid resuscitation should also alert the physician to continuing volume loss or myocardial infarction, and in patients with traumatic shock, to pump failure from myocardial contusion, cardiac tamponade or aortic dissection. The clinical features, relevant investigations and response to therapy should help to detect these problems.

II. Replacement of Hb in Shock due to Blood Loss

Once depleted volume has been replaced, and cardiac output and blood pressure supported by fluid resuscitation, the lost haemoglobin (Hb) should be replaced. Whole blood is rarely available promptly for the immediate resuscitation of the patient with haemorrhagic shock. A complete cross-matching of the blood takes about one hour. If the patient is stable after fluid resuscitation, fully cross-matched blood can be given. Blood compatible for ABO and Rh antigens is however available within minutes and is given to patients who have lost > 20 per cent blood volume, or those who still continue to bleed. If type specific blood is unavailable, and the situation is an extreme emergency produced by exsanguinating blood loss, Type O Rh negative blood may be obtained from the blood bank. In acute emergencies blood and fluid can be infused by pressure infusion devices, or in the set-up prevailing in poor countries, by hand—infusion with large syringes through large sized catheters inserted in peripheral or central veins.

Blood transfusions or transfusions of packed RBCs are ordinarily given to maintain a Hb of 10–11 g/dl. This should improve the oxygen-carrying capacity of blood significantly and should help tissue oxygenation. This is probably true in many patients, but not necessarily in all. McCormick and associates studied the influence of an increase in cardiac output and an increase in haematocrit by blood transfusions on oxygen uptake by tissues ($\dot{V}O_2$) during resuscitation from haemorrhagic shock (9). They noted that the $\dot{V}O_2$ increased after the cardiac output was raised, but did not increase when the haematocrit was raised by blood transfusions. This may well be possible if the $\dot{V}O_2$ is on the flat portion of the curve relating oxygen delivery to oxygen consumption. Marino (1) is of the opinion that indications for transfusions in normovolaemic patients are: (i) $\dot{V}O_2$ below the normal range; (ii) Blood lactate levels > 4 mmol/l; (iii) Oxygen extraction ratio > 0.5. To physicians practising in poor countries, these conditions for infusing packed cells in haemorrhagic shock (after restoring fluid volume and cardiac output) are absurd. We strongly feel that the traditional dictum of maintaining the Hb at around 10 to 11 g/dl holds true.

III. Monitoring Fluid and Blood Resuscitation

This has already been discussed.

IV. Determining and Treating the Aetiology of Hypovolaemic or Haemorrhagic Shock.

In the tropics and in the poor developing countries, cholera is an important cause of acute vomiting and diarrhoea. Salmonella infections or violent gastrointestinal infections with gram-negative organisms (in particular Klebsiella or E. coli), can also cause severe hypovolaemic shock. Relevant investigations and specific treatment are available for such infections (see Section on Fever and Acute Infections in a Critical Care Setting).

Profuse haemorrhage from the GI tract may produce profound collapse, and if the patient does not have haemetemesis, the source of bleeding may not be evident for as long as 24 hours. A rectal examination in these patients often reveals the presence of malaena by the jet black stools staining the examining finger. Haemorrhage from a leaking aneurysm may be missed if a careful clinical examination has not been performed.

Definitive therapy might first require diagnostic studies after the patient has been resuscitated and stabilized. Important diagnostic techniques to detect the site of the GI bleed are endoscopy and imaging techniques like arteriography. Definitive therapy might include surgical intervention, endoscopic therapeutic procedures like laser photocoagulation and injection of gastro-oesophageal varices by sclerosing agents, selective embolization of bleeding vessels, or mechanical balloon tamponade of bleeding varices.

Intravenous hydrocortisone is mandatory and lifesaving in hypovolaemic shock of adrenocortical insufficiency. Hypovolaemic shock in diabetic ketoacidosis cannot be fully reversed without the use of insulin.

REFERENCES

1. Marino PL. (1998). Clinical Shock Syndromes: Haemorrhage and Hypovolaemia. In: The ICU Book. pp. 207–227. Williams and Wilkins, USA.
2. Moore FD. (1965). The effects of haemorrhage on body composition. N Engl J Med. 273, 567–577.
3. Committee on Trauma. (1989). Advanced trauma life support student manual. Chicago: American College of Surgeons. 57.
4. Weil MH, Bisera J, Trevino RP, Rackow EC. (1985). Cardiac output and end-tidal carbon dioxide. Crit Care Med. 13, 907–909.
5. Chien S, Usami S, Skalak R. (1984). Blood flow in small tubes. In: Handbook of Physiology. Section 2: The Cardiovascular System. Volume IV. The microcirculation (Eds Renkin EM, Michel CC). American Physiological Society, Bethesda.
6. Dula DJ, Muller A, Donovan JW. (1981). Flow rate of commonly used IV techniques. J Trauma. 21, 480–482.
7. Shoemaker WC. (1987). Relationship of oxygen transport patterns to the pathophysiology and therapy of shock states. Intensive Care Med. 13, 230–243.
8. SAFE Study Investigators. (2004). A Comparison of albumin and saline resuscitation in the Intensive Care Unit. N Engl J Med. 350, 2247–2256.
9. McCormick M, Feustel PJ, Newell JC et al. (1988). Effect of cardiac index and haematocrit changes on oxygen consumption in resuscitated patients. J Surg Res. 44, 499–505.

CHAPTER 6.3

Cardiogenic Shock

Cardiogenic shock is due to a failure of the pumping action of the heart (pump failure), resulting in a lowered cardiac output and an inadequate tissue perfusion. Progressive tissue hypoxia ultimately leads to irreversible shock and death.

Unquestionably, the commonest cause of pump failure leading to cardiogenic shock is acute myocardial infarction (1). Other cardiac pathologies including acute myocarditis, congestive cardiomyopathy and hypertrophic cardiomyopathy may also progress to a low-output state, finally ending in shock. Mechanical problems that interfere seriously with myocardial function and contractility, and which therefore can lead to cardiogenic shock, include critical aortic stenosis, severe mitral and aortic valvular incompetence, ruptured ventricular septum, ruptured free wall of the ventricle and a ruptured papillary muscle. The picture of cardiogenic shock may also be observed in severe tachyarrhythmias or severe bradyarrhythmias, and in patients with poor myocardial preservation and myocardial dysfunction following open heart surgery. Massive pulmonary embolism and cardiac compression due to tamponade may also lead to a low-output state with shock. These are considered separately though the clinical picture may be indistinguishable from cardiogenic shock. The important causes of cardiogenic shock are listed in **Table 6.3.1**.

Table 6.3.1. Important causes of cardiogenic shock

* Acute myocardial infarction (commonest cause)
* Acute myocarditis
* Congestive cardiomyopathy
* Hypertrophic cardiomyopathy
* Mechanical causes impairing myocardial function and contractility
  - Critical aortic stenosis
  - Severe mitral and aortic valvular incompetence
  - Ruptured interventricular septum/ruptured free wall of ventricle / ruptured papillary muscle
* Severe tachyarrhythmias or bradyarrhythmias
* Patients with myocardial dysfunction following open heart surgery

Physiopathology

A low cardiac output due to the various causes listed above is the primary reason for shock. The present brief discussion is limited to cardiogenic shock in myocardial infarction. The onset and severity of shock are closely related to the quantitative damage

and loss of functional myocardium (2). An infarction involving > 40 per cent of the wall of the left ventricle invariably spells fatal cardiogenic shock. Shock primarily results from death of the muscle leading to poor ventricular contractility and a low cardiac output. Contributory cardiac factors which potentiate the low-output state include an early increase in the compliance of the infarcted area which bulges during systole, and a dyssynergy of contraction in the peri-infarcted area.

Proximal obstruction of just the left anterior descending artery can well infarct > 40 per cent of the left ventricular wall. The majority of patients with cardiogenic shock due to myocardial infarction, present however with critical three vessel disease and with an acute massive left ventricular infarction (3). Inferior wall infarction, when it involves the right ventricle, can also cause cardiogenic shock (4). A patient may evolve into cardiogenic shock from one single massive infarct. Alternately, he could have suffered more than one or two infarcts. The most recent one (even if small), adds to the sum total of non-functioning myocardium, and if this exceeds a critical level (35 per cent), shock results. Global myocardial ischaemia in a patient with ischaemic heart disease can also result in severe pump failure with shock (**Fig. 6.3.1**).

Cardiogenic shock in myocardial infarction still carries a mortality of over 80 per cent (5). It generally does not occur

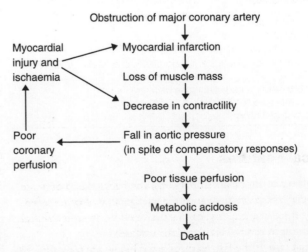

Fig. 6.3.1. Pathogenesis of cardiogenic shock in acute myocardial infarction.

immediately following infarction, but evolves within the first 24–48 hours and at times during the first week of infarction. This is because ischaemic injury, necrosis and death of myocardial tissue continue to increase over a period of time; haemodynamic deterioration may therefore be slow but progressive and ultimately culminates in shock.

There are specific haemodynamic complications other than the loss of viable myocardium that can precipitate or worsen shock in myocardial infarction. These include a ruptured interventricular septum, ruptured free wall of the ventricle with cardiac tamponade, or a ruptured papillary muscle. It is also important to bear in mind other factors that may trigger or potentiate shock in acute myocardial infarction simply because they are treatable to a varying extent. These include:

(i) Hypovolaemia, either due to the use of diuretics, sweating, restricted salt and water intake, vomiting or sometimes for no apparent reason.

(ii) Tachyarrhythmias or bradyarrhythmias.

(iii) Depressant action of drugs. The use of propranolol in the setting of an early or insidious pump failure can be particularly disastrous. It must be remembered that depressant drugs may far outlast the biological half-life of the agent, since positive feedback mechanisms during the use of the drug may become self-perpetuating even when the drug is withdrawn. Oversedation with narcotics and tranquillizers can also induce hypotension and worsen shock.

(iv) Metabolic acidosis (lactic acid acidosis) and electrolyte disturbances potentiate myocardial dysfunction.

(v) Severe prolonged unrelieved pain may worsen the shock state.

(vi) Unrelieved hypoxia worsens shock.

(vii) Pulmonary embolism can aggravate the shock state in myocardial infarction.

Factors aggravating cardiogenic shock in acute myocardial infarction are given in **Table 6.3.2**.

Table 6.3.2. Factors aggravating cardiogenic shock in acute myocardial infarction

* Severe unrelieved pain
* Hypovolaemia
* Tachyarrhythmias or bradyarrhythmias
* Depressant action of drugs e.g. propranolol, overuse of narcotics and sedatives
* Metabolic acidosis and electrolyte disturbances
* Unrelieved hypoxia
* Pulmonary embolism

Clinical Features

The features of shock develop against the background of acute myocardial infarction, or against the background of other severe low output states due to myocardial dysfunction, or to mechanical problems (as in severe valvular heart disease).

At least two of the five features listed below are present:

(i) Hypotension with a systolic pressure below 90 mm Hg or a mean arterial pressure < 55 mm Hg. There are a few points wor-

thy of note in relation to hypotension. Blood pressure readings taken by the cuff method are unreliable in the presence of severe vasoconstriction. They are often much lower and often unobtainable by the cuff method under the above circumstances, even though pressure measurements via an intra-arterial cannula show satisfactory readings. It is equally important to remember that shock can exist with a systolic pressure > 90 mm Hg, particularly in the presence of compensatory vasoconstriction which raises the peripheral vascular resistance. Also, a patient may at times remain well perfused with a systolic blood pressure between 70–90 mm Hg. Tachycardia is frequently associated with hypotension but shock can exist with a bradyrhythm, or even with a normal heart rate.

(ii) Cold, pale, clammy or sweaty skin. The skin over the peripheries, forehead, nose, lips, face, first turns cold and clammy; the coldness then extends to the trunk.

(iii) A fall in urine output to < 25 ml/hour with a sodium content < 30 mEq/l.

(iv) Impaired cerebration—anxiety, restlessness, agitation, confusion and later, obtundation.

(v) Metabolic acidosis due to lactic acid accumulation.

When life support systems keep a patient in severe cardiogenic shock alive for a few days, signs of increasing multiple organ dysfunction are observed.

Diagnosis

The diagnosis of cardiogenic shock is evident when it evolves against the clinical features, ECG and serial enzyme changes of a myocardial infarction. When shock follows very soon after a myocardial infarction, or if for any reason the history is unavailable, or the ECG changes are atypical, the diagnosis is more difficult. A patient in severe shock may never complain of chest pain pointing to an underlying myocardial infarction, and yet a patient with hypovolaemic shock due to a massive GI bleed may complain of ischaemic cardiac pain and thus mislead the clinician into arriving at a wrong diagnosis.

The diagnosis of cardiogenic shock due to low-output states related to cardiomyopathy and severe valvular heart disease, should be evident on a clinical examination and relevant investigations. An aetiology which is often missed is the low-output state due to a very tight aortic stenosis. The typical murmur may be absent in these patients because of the sharp reduction in the forward flow. An echocardiography is mandatory in all patients, and should aid in making a convincing diagnosis of aortic stenosis under the above circumstances. Acute aortic incompetence as a cause of a low-output state, may also be missed as the aortic diastolic murmur is short (due to high left ventricular end-diastolic pressures), and the left ventricle is not enlarged. The diagnosis is confirmed by echocardiography, and by catheter studies on the heart.

Cardiogenic shock can be mistaken for:

(i) *Shock due to a severe internal bleed.* A common site for an internal bleed is the GI tract. The bleed may not be evident for some hours, and blood loss for the first 6 to 12 hours is not manifested by an appreciable fall in the Hb or the haematocrit. The diagnosis becomes obvious when there is malaena or there is massive bleeding from the rectum or when the gastric aspirate through the nasogastric tube contains blood. A ruptured aortic aneurysm can also produce a rapidly evolving hypovolaemic shock that may be mistaken for cardiogenic shock. A clinical examination however, will always reveal collapsed neck veins in the former. Quick investigations should localize the source of bleeding. In difficult cases, a haemodynamic profile (low CVP and low PCWP) obtained through a Swan-Ganz catheter can confirm hypovolaemia as the cause of shock.

(ii) *Massive pulmonary embolism.* This produces the picture of cardiogenic shock. The ECG may simulate a myocardial infarct because of evidence of subendocardial injury. An S_1Q_3 pattern, right bundle branch block, a right ventricular strain pattern with a P pulmonale and clockwise rotation should point to a correct diagnosis. Pressure readings show a raised CVP, a high pulmonary artery end-diastolic pressure and a low to normal PCWP.

(iii) *Dissecting aneurysm of the aorta.* A dissection of the thoracic aorta can result in pain indistinguishable from an acute myocardial infarction and a picture of rapidly evolving shock. A suspicion of this diagnosis is aroused when the patient complains of excruciating pain chiefly in the back, and the ECG does not reveal the typical changes of infarction. An echocardiogram would help in the diagnosis; a CT of the chest and aortic angiography are confirmatory tests.

(iv) *Cardiac tamponade.* This is characterized by an increasing heart rate, a rising CVP and a falling blood pressure. A pulmonary artery catheter reveals an equilibration in the mean right atrial, pulmonary artery diastolic and pulmonary capillary wedge pressures.

(v) *Other conditions* which mimic cardiogenic shock are hypotension following drugs, and septic shock, where the source of sepsis is not evident, and where there is an associated severe myocardial dysfunction. Shock following acute fulminant pancreatitis can also mimic cardiogenic shock, specially when the former is associated with grossly abnormal ST segment changes in the ECG. A full clinical examination and an evaluation of basic investigations point to the correct diagnosis.

The emphasis in the diagnosis of cardiogenic shock should be on the early recognition of signs of reduced tissue perfusion. Thus a patient with myocardial infarction who has an unexplained change in the pulse rate, pulse volume, blood pressure, urine output, or skin temperature, is suspect as being in 'preshock', even though the clinical features do not fulfill the criteria listed earlier.

Haemodynamic Changes and Haemodynamic Profile

A failure of pump function is followed by a failure of forward flow, resulting in poor perfusion and poor tissue oxygenation. This is the essence of cardiogenic shock. A failure of pump function of the left ventricle is also associated with increased left ventricular end-diastolic pressure, increased left atrial pressure and increased pulmonary capillary wedge pressure. When the latter clearly exceeds the oncotic pressure exerted by the plasma proteins, pulmonary oedema results. The picture of cardiogenic shock as will be explained below, is associated with the following haemodynamic effects and profiles.

(a) Hypoperfusion and Pulmonary Oedema (Fig. 6.3.2)

Varying degrees of hypoperfusion ranging from moderate to very severe, with varying degrees of pulmonary oedema ranging from moderate to fulminant are observed. The severest form of this situation is exemplified by a patient who is pulseless, pressureless, anuric, hypothermic with lactic acid acidosis and with evidence of failure of other vital organs due to very poor forward flow and perfusion; fulminant pulmonary oedema is simultaneously present. Death in such instances is inevitable. However as explained, varying gradations in both tissue hypoperfusion and in the degree of pulmonary oedema are encountered. The haemodynamic profile shows the following:

(i) Normal or elevated CVP.

(ii) Increase in PCWP > 18 mm Hg—the greater the rise in

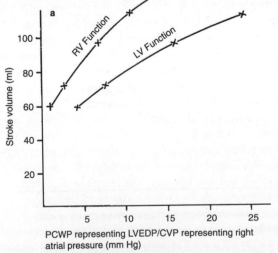 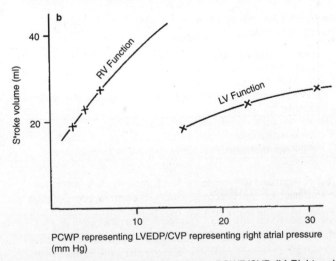

Fig. 6.3.2. (a) Normal right and left ventricular function curves in a healthy volunteer as plotted by stroke volume against PCWP/CVP. **(b)** Right and left ventricular function curves in a patient with cardiogenic shock due to massive anterior wall infarction. Note (i) the wide separation of the RV and LV function curves resulting in a susceptibility to pulmonary oedema; (ii) the marked flattening in the LV function curve resulting in poor forward flow with poor tissue perfusion and shock.

PCWP, the greater the degree of pulmonary oedema. Fulminant oedema is generally associated with a PCWP approaching or exceeding 30 mm Hg.

(iii) A lowered CI < 2.5 l/min/m² — the lower the CI, the poorer the tissue perfusion. In very severe cases, the CI is < 1.8 l/min/m² and terminally may even approach 1 l/min/m². In patients with early cardiogenic shock, the CI may only be slightly less than normal because of compensatory mechanisms.

(iv) A systolic blood pressure often < 90 mm Hg. In early shock, the blood pressure may be maintained at or above 100 mm Hg because of a raised SVR. In severe shock with failure of forward flow, the systolic blood pressure is < 70 mm Hg.

(v) A raised SVR. This is a compensatory mechanism to keep the blood pressure close to normal.

(b) Isolated Hypoperfusion

It is very important to realize that pump failure should not necessarily be equated solely to increasing PCWP and pulmonary oedema. In fact, pump failure may be solely characterized by poor flow of blood in the forward direction from the left ventricle causing severe shock, without a rise in the PCWP to an extent that leads to pulmonary oedema. This was beautifully illustrated and first brought to our notice by Bradley in his excellent small book on Studies in Acute Heart Failure (6). Bradley showed through his haemodynamic studies, that when right ventricular function curves (representing stroke volume equations) were severely depressed and shifted to the right so that they overlapped the left ventricular function curves, the lungs were protected from pulmonary oedema, even though the patient was in shock. We were subsequently able to demonstrate this on our patients as well. The stroke

volume equations of the right and left ventricles in these patients are illustrated in **Fig. 6.3.3**.

The haemodynamic profile in patients with shock due to isolated hypoperfusion is as follows:

(i) Increase in mean atrial pressure or CVP

(ii) PCWP ≤ 15 mm Hg.

(iii) Low CI < 2.2 l/min/m² and often below 1.8 l/min/m²

(iv) Hypotension with systolic BP < 70–90 mm Hg

(v) Increase in SVR

The above haemodynamic effects and profiles can be brought about in the following conditions:

(i) A global infarct when the left ventricular wall as well as the right ventricle are both infarcted and the right ventricular function curve is even below the left ventricular function curve.

(ii) An infarct of the left ventricular wall where the overall pump function of not only the left ventricle but also of the right ventricle is grossly disturbed. This occurrence stresses the importance of not always considering the heart to be consisting of two separate pumps (the right and the left), but as an overall, single, interdependent functioning unit so that gross disturbance in the left side can also affect the function of the right heart. Perhaps this is because of the septal wall which is common to the left and right ventricles; poor function consequent to a massive septal infarct would affect both ventricles. A further contributory factor is that even though the left ventricle may be infarcted, right ventricular function may be seriously prejudiced because of overall global ischaemia. This is generally related to critical narrowing of the right coronary artery with poor collateral flow from the branches of a blocked left anterior descending artery to the right coronary vessels, and also to a falling aortic pressure leading to a poor circulation through the right coronary artery.

(iii) In pure severe right ventricular infarction, the haemodynamic profile shows a marked increase in the CVP or in the mean right atrial pressure, a normal or low PCWP, a marked fall in the CI to less than 2 l/min/m², and severe hypotension with a rise in the SVR (**Fig. 6.3.4**).

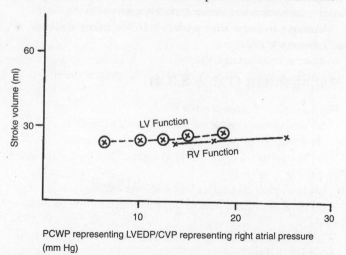

Fig. 6.3.3. Right and left ventricular function curves in a patient with myocardial infarction and cardiogenic shock with extremely poor perfusion and shock but no pulmonary oedema. Note (i) The flattening of both right and left ventricular function curves resulting in poor perfusion and shock. (ii) The right ventricular function curve overlaps, and is below and to the right of the left ventricular function curve, in contrast to the normal curves. The relation between right and left atrial pressure is such that the patient is protected from pulmonary oedema. This is observed in a global infarct (right and left ventricular wall involved), and in a massive anterior wall (LV) infarct with severely depressed right ventricular function (see text).

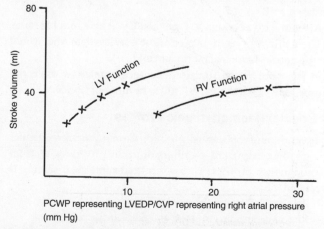

Fig. 6.3.4. Right and left ventricular function curves in a patient with inferior wall infarction and cardiogenic shock, but no pulmonary oedema. Note right ventricular function curve is flattened and transposed below and to the right of the left ventricular function curve. Relation between right and left atrial pressures is such that the patient is protected from pulmonary oedema.

Clinical Shock Syndromes

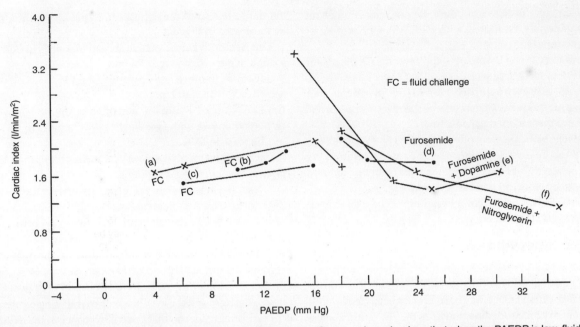

Fig. 6.3.5. LV performance curves in patients with acute myocardial infarction. Curves a, b, and c show that when the PAEDP is low, fluid challenge raises both the PAEDP and the CI; however, the degree of rise is far less than what would be expected with normal pump function. Also, it is worth noting that the use of furosemide alone (d), or in combination with dopamine (e), or with nitroglycerin (f), can reduce a raised PAEDP with an increase in the CI.

(c) Hypovolaemia and Pump Failure

The association of hypovolaemia with pump failure also adds a new dimension to the haemodynamic profile of pump failure. Typically hypovolaemia in these patients as stated earlier, results from a combination of vomiting, very poor fluid intake or the use of diuretics.

The haemodynamic profile shows:

(i) A lowered CVP.

(ii) A PCWP ≤ 15 mm Hg.

(iii) A lowered CI of < 2.5 or even < 2.2 l/min/m².

(iv) Hypotension—systolic pressure ≤ 90 mm Hg with an increased SVR.

A volume load enough to raise the PCWP ≥ 18 mm Hg raises the CI significantly, yet the degree of rise is far less than what would be expected with normal pump function.

In fact poor pump function becomes unmasked when the volume load raises the PCWP to 15–18 mm Hg (**Fig. 6.3.5**).

(d) Special Haemodynamic Profiles

Complications of myocardial infarction like a ruptured ventricular septum or a ruptured papillary muscle produces distinct haemodynamic profiles. Thus a ruptured ventricular septum is associated with:

(i) Rise in CVP and right atrial pressure.

(ii) Rise in pulmonary systolic and diastolic pressures.

(iii) Rise in PCWP > 18 mm Hg to often as high as 30 mm Hg.

(iv) Fall in CI < 2.2 l/min/m².

(v) Arterialization of blood sampled from the right ventricle and pulmonary artery (i.e. a marked step-up of SaO₂ of blood from the right ventricle and pulmonary artery compared to blood in the superior vena cava or right atrium).

Papillary muscle dysfunction will show a high PCWP, a low CI, hypotension and prominent 'v' waves with characteristic morphology in pressure tracings obtained from the pulmonary artery and pulmonary artery occlusive sites.

Various haemodynamic profiles described above are detailed in **Table 6.3.3**.

Management (Table 6.3.4)

The principles of management are:

(a) To improve cardiac output and tissue perfusion.

(b) To reduce or relieve severe pulmonary oedema.

(c) To maintain a clear airway and maintain a PaO₂ of at least 70 mm Hg.

(d) To correct electrolyte and acid-base balance.

(e) To recognize and treat factors which aggravate or potentiate shock.

(f) To improve the patient's haemodynamic profile, as elaborated below.

A patient with cardiogenic shock due to a recent myocardial infarction characterized by ST elevation on the ECG should be promptly thrombolysed provided there is no absolute contraindication for doing so. If thrombolysis is successful, coronary artery perfusion is restored. Pump function should then improve further, aided by the medical management outlined below. Thrombolysis may however be unsuccessful and the state of shock then persists or even worsens.

Table 6.3.3. Haemodynamic (HD) profiles in cardiogenic shock

HD Profiles	CVP mm Hg	Systolic BP mm Hg	CI l/min/m²	PCWP mm Hg	SVR dynes-sec/cm⁵
(a) Hypoperfusion with pulmonary oedema	Normal or ↑	< 90; often < 70	< 2.2	20–30 or more	↑ to ↑ ↑ ↑
(b) Isolated hypoperfusion (global infarct)	↑ or ↑ ↑	< 70–90	< 2.2	≤ 15	↑ to ↑ ↑ ↑
Hypoperfusion with severe right ventricular infarction	↑ ↑	< 70–90	< 2.2	< 15	↑ to ↑ ↑ ↑
(c) Hypovolaemia with pump failure	Normal or low	< 90	< 2.2	≤ 15	↑ to ↑ ↑ ↑
(d) Ruptured ventricular septum or papillary muscle	↑ ↑	< 90	< 2.2	> 15; may be 20–30	↑ to ↑ ↑ ↑

Under these circumstances, *the current trend in the management of cardiogenic shock in acute myocardial infarction is to improve the patient's haemodynamic profile to an acceptable state, so that diagnostic testing and intervention whenever possible, either through angioplasty or in selected cases through surgery, become feasible. Improvement in the haemodynamic profile and the general circulatory state is brought about by the prompt use of medical measures outlined below, and by using the support of the aortic balloon pump. The latter assist device should be used early and not late in the management of severe cardiogenic shock.* In an ideal set-up, this policy should be judiciously followed. However, most set-ups in third world countries do not have an infrastructure where diagnostic and therapeutic intervention in such patients can contribute to overall improvement in the mortality. Where optimum facilities are available, and where after angiography an appropriate angioplastic repair or opening up of

the 'culprit' lesion is carried out, the prognosis improves and the mortality rate falls (7–9). Our personal experience is too small to determine whether open heart bypass surgery is of any benefit in these patients. We feel that surgery following a fresh infarction more often results in death, and only rarely is rewarded by recovery.

Good treatment is only possible in a well-equipped ICU. The patient is nursed flat, or if pulmonary oedema is marked, in a propped-up position. *Oxygen* is administered through a tight fitting mask or through nasal prongs at 6–8 l/minute. An obtunded or hypoxic patient in shock should be intubated and given ventilator support. Pain if present, is relieved by morphine 2–4 mg intravenously, or buprenorphine 0.3 mg intramuscularly or intravenously, or pethidine 25 mg intravenously. A central venous line is promptly secured both for administration of fluids and drugs, as also for monitoring the central venous pressure.

Table 6.3.4. Principles of management in cardiogenic shock

Objective: Improve haemodynamic profile to an acceptable state, so that diagnostic testing and intervention, whenever possible through angioplasty, or rarely through surgery, become feasible.
(a) Maximizing preload: volume challenge if PCWP is < 15 mm Hg. Increase PCWP to 15–20 mm Hg provided there is no pulmonary oedema
(b) Use of vasodilators: Principle—reduce abnormally high preload to optimal levels (15–18 mm Hg); reduce increased afterload.
  – IV nitroglycerin in patients with high PCWP and well marked pulmonary oedema
  – IV nitroprusside if marked increase in SVR, PCWP > 20 mm Hg, poor tissue perfusion, systolic blood pressure > 90–100 mm Hg.
(c) Increasing cardiac contractility:
  – Dobutamine or dopamine by IV infusion or both
  – Digoxin; other inotropes in rare instances
(d) Judiciously combine a, b and c.
(e) IV furosemide combined with b and c if there is pulmonary oedema.
(f) Maintain oxygenation: administer oxygen at flow rate of 6–8 l/min. If PaO₂ still < 60 mm Hg, or if respiratory distress (rate > 35/min.), intubate and put on ventilator support.
(g) Correction of electrolyte and acid-base abnormalities
(h) Correction of factors aggravating cardiogenic shock

Monitoring the Patient in Cardiogenic Shock (Table 6.3.5)

Half hourly pulse, and one hourly skin and rectal temperature, as well as hourly urine output through an indwelling Foley's catheter should be charted. The blood pressure may need to be checked very frequently and in patients with clinical evidence of peripheral vasoconstriction, it is important to cannulate the radial artery and connect the cannula or catheter to a pressure monitor so that correct pressure readings are obtained and recorded. The ECG is continuously monitored. The blood count, PCV, serum electrolytes, blood urea, NPN, creatinine, other blood chemistry, arterial pH and arterial blood gases are done on admission and repeated as and when necessary. A chest X-ray is mandatory, and follow-up X-rays are done to check in particular for radiological evidence of pulmonary oedema.

Clinical monitoring is extremely important with particular reference to all signs of shock (see Clinical Features). These should include respiration, pulse volume and rate, central venous pressure, mental state, respiratory rate and the degree of pulmonary congestion as judged by crackles on auscultation and by assessment of serial chest X-rays.

Table 6.3.5. Monitoring patients in cardiogenic shock

* Half-hourly heart rate, blood pressure and respiratory rate
* Hourly skin and rectal temperature; clinical monitoring
* Hourly urine output through indwelling catheter
* Continuous ECG monitoring
* Blood count, serum biochemistry, arterial pH and arterial blood gases done on admission and repeated as and when necessary
* Chest X-ray
* Haemodynamic monitoring
  – Central venous pressure
  – Pulmonary artery pressures—pulmonary artery end-diastolic pressure, pulmonary capillary wedge pressure
  – Cardiac output, cardiac index, stroke volume index, systemic vascular resistance, left and right ventricular stroke work indices

Central Venous Pressure (CVP)

It is important to learn to gauge CVP on clinical examination. In fact, one should easily recognize a raised or normal jugular venous pressure (JVP); with a little practice one should also detect a low JVP. But for an accurate measurement of the CVP, a central venous line connected to a pressure monitor is necessary. If a pressure monitor is unavailable, the central line is connected through a bivalve to a water manometer. The zero level measurement is in the plane of the mid-axillary line, midway between the sternum and the back. Most units in the country cannot afford the use of pulmonary catheters with the gadgetry to measure right-sided pressures, PCWP and CO; but a central venous line can be easily arranged with a bare minimum of facilities.

Left Ventricular Filling Pressure

The preload is ideally determined by measuring the end-diastolic volume. This is difficult in an ICU setting in a patient with myocardial infarction. A practical method of gauging the preload is by measuring the pulmonary artery end-diastolic pressure, which in myocardial infarction approximates the pulmonary occlusive or the pulmonary capillary wedge pressure. The latter in turn, corresponds reasonably with the left ventricular filling pressure. The compliance of the ventricular wall in myocardial infarction may be decreased so that the relation between the filling pressure and the end-diastolic volume is altered. Even so, measurement of the pulmonary artery diastolic pressure or the PCWP remains the most readily available method of gauging preload in these patients. Serial measurements are of greater value than isolated readings. It is important to stress that the CVP cannot be relied upon to give an idea of the left ventricular filling pressure in cardiogenic shock. The CVP may in fact be perfectly normal in some patients even though the left ventricular filling pressures are markedly raised.

Cardiac Output (CO)

Ideally all patients with cardiogenic shock should have their CO measured and monitored. Serial measurements of CO are made through the S-G catheter using the thermodilution technique. Samples of mixed venous blood from the pulmonary artery are also serially obtained through the S-G catheter. A lowered pressure of mixed venous oxygen ($P\bar{v}O_2$), or a lowered mixed venous oxygen saturation ($S\bar{v}O_2$) points to a lowered CO. Serial values of $P\bar{v}O_2$ or $S\bar{v}O_2$ help to indicate the trend in changing cardiac output. There are comparatively few centres in developing countries including India, that can afford the luxury of measuring cardiac outputs. When facilities are lacking, changes in the CO should be clinically gauged by observing changes in tissue perfusion, blood pressure, urine output, and changes in the function of other vital organs.

Monitoring the patient in cardiogenic shock should be done early by trained personnel. Except in an immediate crisis, it helps to monitor the above-mentioned parameters before starting inotropic agents.

(a) Increasing Cardiac Output and Improving Tissue Perfusion

This is the basic principle and forms the essence of therapy. Factors which determine cardiac output are: (i) end-diastolic fibre length i.e. end-diastolic volume or preload. Roughly in clinical practice (with the exceptions stated above), this is equated to the filling pressure of the ventricles, which in turn is equated to the measured pulmonary artery end-diastolic pressure or the measured PCWP; (ii) contractility of the ventricular muscles; (iii) heart rate and rhythm; (iv) afterload—in shock due to myocardial infarction this is clinically related (again roughly) to the outflow resistance offered by the constricted peripheral vessels.

Management should be directed to the skillful manipulation of the factors stated above so that cardiac output and perfusion improve.

Maximizing Preload. It has been shown that the optimal filling pressures of the left ventricle in shock following myocardial infarction, range between 15–24 mm Hg (4). If therefore in a hypotensive 'shocked' patient the PCWP is normal to low (< 15 mm Hg), and the CVP is also low or on the lower side of normal, the patient is hypovolaemic and needs a volume load. Boluses of 100–150 ml of dextrose or dextravan or Haemaccel are rapidly infused over 5–10 minute intervals till such time as the low blood pressure and other signs of shock improve. One should aim to maintain a PAEDP or PCWP between 15–20 mm Hg. The degree to which CO, blood pressure and signs of shock improve will depend on the underlying myocardial dysfunction. If hypovolaemia is a major contibutory factor in shock, then increasing the preload (PCWP or PAEDP) will produce a significant improvement in the CO, blood pressure and the clinical features of shock. If on the other hand hypovolaemia is a minor or incidental finding, then raising the PCWP to 18–20 mm Hg may produce only a slight improvement in the CO and blood pressure, thus unmasking the severity of underlying myocardial dysfunction (**Fig. 6.3.5**).

If to start with the PAEDP or the PCWP is < 20 mm Hg, one may still maximize the preload by judiciously pushing intravenous fluids so that the PAEDP increases to around 18–20 mm Hg. The patient should however be under constant clinical and frequent radiological monitoring, to determine increasing crackles within the lungs and increasing radiological evidence of pulmonary oedema. Some degree of pulmonary oedema may be acceptable if improvement in CO and tissue perfusion is obviously manifest. In our experience in Mumbai, in most patients with cardiogenic shock the optimum PAEDP is between 15–18 mm Hg, these values being a little lower than those reported from the West. If during the process of maximizing the preload frank pulmonary oedema ensues, the volume challenge is stopped and 40–100 mg intravenous furosemide administered intravenously.

If an increase in the PAEDP to above 18 mm Hg brings no improvement in either the CO or tissue perfusion (ideally gauged both clinically and by sequential CO measurements), then further management consists of the manipulation of the afterload and cardiac contractility. Also, if to start with the PAEDP is very high (> 20 mm Hg), volume infusion is pointless and will only add to the existing pulmonary oedema, without increasing the CO or tissue perfusion. In such cases, measures to reduce a very high preload to optimal levels, and measures to improve cardiac contractility, should immediately be resorted to. Intravenous furosemide should also be given to decrease preload and reduce pulmonary oedema.

Use of Vasodilators. If the haemodynamic profile shows a raised PAEDP (> 18 mm Hg), a systolic blood pressure ≥ 90 mm Hg, a lowered cardiac index and systemic hypoperfusion, vasodilator therapy is indicated.

Vasodilators reduce the abnormally high preloads and afterloads, thereby improving pump function. Nitroglycerine in a slow monitored intravenous infusion and/or sublingual nitrites, or a slow, closely monitored intravenous infusion of nitroprusside can be used for urgent intervention. The fall in peripheral resistance improves CO (as the outflow impedance is significantly reduced), and therefore in many patients there is no significant fall in blood pressure. Even when there is a slight fall in arterial blood pressure, the tissue perfusion may well improve, as judged clinically.

Sodium nitroprusside is the vasodilator of choice as it reduces both venous tone (thus decreasing preload) and arteriolar tone (thus decreasing afterload). It is the drug of choice when the SVR is markedly increased, and tissue perfusion is severely jeopardized. It should however not be used if the systolic blood pressure is < 90 mm Hg. When administered, it is best to start with an infusion rate of 2 μg/minute, and then gradually increase the concentration of the infusion. The end-point aimed at is a reduction of PAEDP to 15–18 mm Hg. The infusion should be stopped if the systolic BP falls to < 80 mm Hg or the patient becomes symptomatic from hypotension. The effect of nitroprusside disappears within 5–10 minutes of stopping the infusion. If the vasodilator infusion clearly improves peripheral flow as judged by the volume of the pulse, urine output, skin temperature and overall improvement in tissue perfusion, it is continued at a stable infusion rate for 12–24 hours. The patient is then gradually weaned off the infusion.

Excessively prolonged use of nitroprusside in cardiogenic shock can cause cyanide poisoning. It is recommended not to exceed a dose of 1–3 mg/kg. Metabolic acidosis is an early indication of overdosage resulting in cyanide toxicity. Nitroprusside infusions should never be used if the filling pressures (PAEDP or PCWP) are not distinctly raised, else severe hypotension and fall in CO may result. Use of vasodilator therapy is best not attempted without adequate monitoring facilities—an arterial cannula in the radial artery, an S-G catheter to monitor PAEDP or PCWP, and if possible the CO. It is also imperative to control and monitor the infusion rate if disaster is to be avoided. Once the patient has improved

haemodynamically and remains stable, captopril starting with 6.25 mg orally twice or thrice daily, is substituted for intravenous nitroprusside.

Nitrites chiefly reduce the preload and have a much smaller effect on the afterload. With a marked increase in PAEDP and frank pulmonary oedema, intravenous nitroglycerin (0.3–4 μg/kg/minute) is the drug of choice. The initial dose of nitroglycerin should be 10 μg/minute given through a microdrip. This is gradually increased till the optimal effects are achieved. The end-point here is a PAEDP of about 15 mm Hg. The infusion may have to be stopped or sharply reduced if there is a significant reduction in the systolic blood pressure. Tachycardia and severe headache are important side effects of nitroglycerin. Once the patient's haemodynamic profile has improved, we prefer to use oral or sublingual nitrites.

In our experience, it is rare in cardiogenic shock to register and maintain a significant improvement solely through the use of a volume load and the use of vasodilators. In our opinion, *inotropic drugs also need to be used to further improve the clinical picture and the haemodynamic profile of the patient.*

Increasing Cardiac Contractility. When the haemodynamic profile of a patient in cardiogenic shock shows hypotension (systolic BP between 70–90 mm Hg or even lower), a reduced CI (generally < 2 l/min/m²), a raised PCWP (well above 15 mm Hg), with increased SVR and poor tissue perfusion, inotropic drugs must be used to improve cardiac contractility (**10**). As far as possible, it is unwise to use inotropic drugs before first determining the CVP and the PAEDP—which means that it is wrong to use inotropic drugs without first determining whether volume loading by intravenous infusions would be helpful or not. Inotropic drugs often produce both central venous constriction (by increasing venous tone) thereby raising the CVP, and also at times pulmonary venous constriction, thereby raising the PAEDP. A wrong picture of iatrogenically induced high filling pressures may then be obtained after the use of inotropic drugs, and the major therapeutic intervention of increasing effective circulatory volume in cardiogenic shock may not be availed of.

The inotropic drugs most frequently used to augment contractility are dobutamine and dopamine.

(**i**) When the haemodynamic profile described above is associated with *moderate hypotension* (systolic blood pressure between 70–100 mm Hg), *we prefer to use dobutamine* as it is the most selective inotropic agent available with comparatively few side effects. In the presence of a low CI due to poor LV function, a raised PCWP, moderate hypotension and reduced peripheral perfusion, dobutamine (given in an infusion at a rate of 2–15 μg/kg/minute), improves stroke volume, CO and ventricular performance. The overall improvement in ventricular performance and function leads to decreased ventricular filling pressures. Dobutamine also increases the systolic blood pressure through an increase in stroke volume and pulse pressure, and improves peripheral tissue perfusion. These favourable haemodynamic effects are often achieved without undue tachycardia, ventricular ectopy, and with little increase in myocardial oxygen consumption. Dobutamine directly reduces ventricular afterload and wall stress by a direct reduction in systemic and pulmonary vascular resistances, ventricular systolic volume and ventricular filling pressures (11). Thus dobutamine has a favourable effect on the myocardial oxygen consumption to myocardial oxygen supply ratio. Dobutamine increases diastolic time (through a reduced systolic time), and increases perfusion pressure through the coronaries (through reduction in ventricular filling pressures and normal or increased diastolic blood pressure), thereby leading to increased myocardial oxygen supply, when this is vitally necessary (11). These effects have been proven in animal experiments and in humans with ischaemic heart disease (11). Dobutamine should be started at an infusion rate of 2–3 µg/kg/minute and the rate progressively increased till the patient improves haemodynamically and remains stable. It is best not to exceed the upper limit of 15–20 µg/kg/minute. If dobutamine fails to increase the systolic blood pressure beyond 80 mm Hg, dopamine may be added to the therapeutic regime, the infusion rate being titrated to maintain systolic BP > 90 mm Hg, and preferably at or above 100 mm Hg. Many prefer to add a low dose dopamine infusion to dobutamine even when the latter has achieved a satisfactory increase in systolic blood pressure. The purpose is to avail of the dopaminergic renal effect of dopamine and further augment urine output.

(ii) When a low CI (< 2 l/min/m²), a high PCWP or PAEDP, a high SVR and poor tissue perfusion is associated with *well-marked hypotension* (systolic BP ≤ 70 mm Hg), *we would rather use dopamine*. At such low perfusion pressures, blood supply to vital organs like the brain, gut, kidneys and myocardium is markedly prejudiced. Dopamine combines powerful inotropic properties with vasopressor properties (due to stimulation of alpha receptors), and effectively raises the perfusion pressure. It is started in a dose of 5 µg/kg/minute and the dose is progressively increased every 10–15 minutes (to a maximum of 20–30 µg/kg/minute) till the systemic arterial pressure rises to acceptable levels for reasonable perfusion to the brain and the myocardium. Cerebral and renal perfusion necessitate a systolic perfusion pressure > 75–80 mm Hg; adequate coronary perfusion necessitates a systemic diastolic pressure of 65 mm Hg with a left ventricular filling pressure of 15 mm Hg (11). Once the systolic pressure rises to 80 mm Hg, a combination of dopamine and dobutamine may be tried to further improve the haemodynamic state of the patient.

If dopamine and dobutamine fail to improve hypotension, a trial is given to noradrenaline or adrenaline. We generally use noradrenaline at 1 to 5 µg/minute, slowly increasing the dose to obtain satisfactory systolic pressure. However, these drugs being strong vasoconstrictors, may in fact worsen tissue perfusion and aggravate the state of shock. An absent or poor response to inotropes and vasopressors is associated with a mortality well beyond 90 per cent.

Isoprenaline is rarely used because though it is an inotrope with a vasodilatory effect on the systemic circulation, it produces tachycardia and a marked increase in the myocardial oxygen consumption. Though it increases coronary blood flow, it may actually shunt blood away from the ischaemic area and increase the infarct size. Isoprenaline may be used temporarily when hypotension and cardiogenic shock are associated with a severe bradyrhythm or when a shock-like state is due to severe aortic valvular insufficiency and a bradycardia (12). It is not likely to prove effective in cardiogenic shock if dopamine and dobutamine have failed. Intravenous administration is started in a dose of 0.01 mg/kg/minute and increased till the desired effect is achieved.

(iii) *Digoxin* is probably of little value in the management of cardiogenic shock except for the control of a rapid ventricular rate resulting from atrial fibrillation. It may also be used when left ventricular failure is chiefly characterized by pulmonary oedema rather than by poor tissue perfusion. A dose of 0.25 mg is given intravenously and repeated 4–6 hourly till a digitalizing dose of 0.75 mg to a maximum of 1 mg is reached.

(iv) *Other Inotropes. Amrinone* is a far weaker inotrope as compared to dopamine or dobutamine. It increases cardiac contractility independently of catechol pathways. It is believed to act by increasing cAMP and calcium concentrations. The increased cAMP in smooth muscle, decreases peripheral and pulmonary vascular resistances as also resistance in the coronary circulation. It increases stroke volume without producing a tachycardia. The initial dose is 0.75 mg/kg given over 5 minutes, followed by an infusion of the drug at 5–10 µg/kg/minute. The total daily dose should not exceed 10 mg/kg. A combination of dobutamine plus amrinone is often employed immediately after bypass surgery to counter myocardial depression in patients who to start with have a poor ejection fraction.

Glucagon is an inotrope which increases cardiac contractility and decreases peripheral resistance. The dose is 4–6 mg intravenously in a bolus followed by an infusion of the drug at a rate of 4–12 mg/hour. It could be used when dopamine or dobutamine fail to change the haemodynamic effects of severe cardiogenic shock or when dysrhythmias develop. Glucagon may be particularly useful when depressed left ventricular function is related to the previous use of beta-blockers. Glucagon could induce well-marked hyperglycaemia as a side effect.

A list of commonly used inotropic drugs with their doses and site of action, is given in **Table 6.3.6**.

Combination of Inotropic Drugs and Vasodilator Therapy. We generally combine vasodilator therapy comprising intravenous nitroglycerin or intravenous nitroprusside with dopamine or dobutamine in a dose sufficient to allow of the benefits of vasodilatation and yet maintain an adequate systolic perfusion pressure of 90–100 mm Hg. Close monitoring of the PAEDP, arterial blood pressure, CO, tissue perfusion and the infusion rates of drugs is mandatory.

Mechanical Cardiac Assistance (13). Mechanical cardiac assistance in the form of an aortic balloon counterpulsation is today being used with increasing frequency, early in the natural history of cardiogenic shock. It is inadvisable to persevere with conservative measures alone in severe cardiogenic shock. Arrangements for insertion of an aortic balloon pump are promptly made if facilities are available. In the meanwhile, monitoring procedures including the insertion of a pulmonary artery catheter are urgently carried out and treatment with respect to optimizing preload and cardiac contractility (as outlined earlier) promptly started. Improvement in blood pressure, coronary artery perfusion and in the general

Table 6.3.6. Commonly used inotropic drugs with their doses and main actions

Drug	Dose (μg/kg/min)	Alpha – 1 (Peripheral Vasoconstriction)	Beta – 1		Beta – 2 (Peripheral Vasodilatation)	Dopaminergic (Arterial Vasodilatation)
			Heart Rate	Cardiac Contractility		
Dopamine	1–10	0	++	++	++	++++
	> 10	+++	++	++	+	0
Dobutamine	1–10	+	+	++++	+	0
Amrinone	5–10	0	0	+++	+	0
Norepinephrine	2–8	++++	+++	+++	0	0
Epinephrine	1–8	++++	++++	++++	++	0
Isoproteronol	1–4	0	++++	++++	++++	0

circulatory state following the use of an aortic balloon pump renders the patient more fit for interventional procedures. The effects of an aortic balloon pump are almost always short-lived, unless a successful interventional procedure has improved or restored perfusion to the damaged myocardium.

Emergency Interventional Procedures. All interventional procedures should be preferably performed with an aortic balloon in place. Ideally a patient in cardiogenic shock should first be brought to a reasonably stable haemodynamic state to allow a diagnostic angiography. If there is a culprit lesion which is responsible for increasing ischaemia to the myocardium, and if the expertise to 'open' this lesion is available, an angioplasty should be done (**7–9, 14, 15**). This is provided the culprit lesion is a major artery, and is anatomically capable of being opened up by an invasive procedure.

We generally advise open heart surgery in patients with a ruptured intraventricular septum. If possible, they should first be improved haemodynamically with medical treatment, or failing this, with the use of intra-aortic balloon counterpulsation. The sooner these patients are taken up, the better the results. Waiting for 2–3 weeks often results in a deteriorating haemodynamic state with multiple organ failure and a hopeless prognosis (**16**).

Barring exceptional circumstances, we do not advocate open heart bypass surgery in patients with recent myocardial infarction and cardiogenic shock.

Ventricular Assist Device. In patients with acute myocarditis or cardiomyopathy who are in cardiogenic shock and who fail to improve with vigorous conservative measures, the use of a ventricular assist device might buy time, while they await a possible cardiac transplant. In Mumbai, there is no centre which has a ventricular assist device and we have no experience with its use.

(b) Management of Fulminant Pulmonary Oedema in Cardiogenic Shock (Table 6.3.7)

The prognosis in these patients is hopeless. The PAEDP is invariably raised above 30 mm Hg and the CO ≤ 1.5 l/min/m^2. Management consists of:

(i) Increasing cardiac contractility with a dopamine infusion and other inotropes.

(ii) Reducing preload with intravenous nitroglycerin or sub-lingual nitrites.

(iii) Intravenous furosemide given as 200 mg bolus, followed by an infusion at the rate of 20–40 mg/hour.

(iv) Reducing the preload and afterload with nitroprusside in-fusion provided the systolic blood pressure is not < 90 mm Hg. If

nitroprusside infusion is preferred, nitroglycerin should not be used.

(v) Intubating the patient and using positive pressure breathing with a FIO$_2$ of 100 per cent to maintain oxygenation, and to attempt to perhaps force back oedema fluid into the capillaries and veins, or at least reduce the rate of oedema formation within the alveoli.

Table 6.3.7. Management of fulminant pulmonary oedema in cardiogenic shock

* Morphine 2–5 mg IV
* Reduce preload with IV nitroglycerin
* Increase cardiac contractility with inotropic support (dopamine, dobutamine)
* IV furosemide 100–250 mg, repeated if necessary
* In suitable cases, reduce preload and afterload with IV nitroprusside infusion
* Intubate and put on ventilator support with a high FIO$_2$

(c) Maintaining Oxygenation

It is important to ensure proper oxygenation by administering oxygen at a flow rate of 6–8 l/minute. A PaO$_2$ of less than 60 mm Hg, or respiratory distress of > 35/minute are clear indications for intubation and ventilator support. In fact, severe shock in itself is an indication for respirator support. Mechanical ventilation rests respiratory muscles and reduces the oxygen cost of breathing, thus enabling oxygen to be used by the vital organs of the body. It also ensures adequate oxygenation and helps combat severe pulmonary oedema. The FIO$_2$ should be set to allow an oxygen saturation over 95 per cent. PEEP should, if possible, be gradually increased, watching its effect on the blood pressure.

(d) Correction of Electrolytes and Acid-Base Balance

Metabolic acidosis (lactic acidosis) is frequently observed and is due to poor tissue perfusion. Acidosis improves when tissue perfusion improves. If the pH is < 7.15, it may need correction with an appropriate dose of intravenous sodium bicarbonate. A PaO$_2$ > 70 mm Hg should be maintained through the use of ventilator support using a high FIO$_2$ and PEEP. Increasing metabolic acidosis leads to cellular injury and further impairs myocardial function. Hypokalaemia predisposes to ventricular dysrhythmias including ventricular tachycardia and fibrillation.

(e) Correction of Factors that Aggravate Shock

Hypotension in myocardial infarction may be potentiated by severe unrelieved pain, or it could also be partly related to the overuse of intravenous morphine or pethidine, sedatives and tranquilizers. Excessive use of diuretics can cause hypovolaemia and hypokalaemia leading to hypotension and weakness. Both, supraventricular and in particular ventricular arrhythmias with fast ventricular rates need to be recognized and treated with drugs or if the need arises, by electroversion. Arrhythmias can cause a serious deterioration in the haemodynamic profile of such individuals. Bradyrhythms due to inferior wall infarction when marked, cause a sharp fall in CO and need to be corrected by intravenous atropine or by pacing. Persistent mild hypoxia can aggravate the dangers of hypotension as it is associated with decreased oxygen transport to tissues. The oxygen saturation must be maintained well over 90 per cent. The danger of nosocomial infection is always present in a shock state particularly in patients with pulmonary oedema who are on ventilator support. Such infections can tilt the balance against a patient who could have otherwise recovered. Finally, the deleterious haemodynamic changes produced by dysfunction and death of the myocardial wall can worsen into an irreversible state following a complicating pulmonary embolism. This may be difficult to diagnose against the background of cardiogenic shock. Pulmonary embolism if sufficiently severe, is characterized by a high CVP, a high PAEDP and a PCWP which is significantly lower than the PAEDP. These are some of the contributory factors which singly or in combination can worsen the severity of shock in myocardial infarction.

A great deal of attention continues to be paid over the last many years to attempts at myocardial preservation—i.e. providing better blood supply to ischaemic muscle surrounding an area of infarction and thereby preventing ischaemic muscle from undergoing further damage or death. Improvement of blood supply to ischaemic muscle should improve pump function and help in relieving the state of shock. This, in principle is theoretically sound, but is difficult to translate into practice. There are a number of unknown factors in relation to anatomy, collateral circulation, local blood flow within the coronaries, and metabolic requirements of ischaemic or damaged myocardium, that operate in a given individual with myocardial infarction. The best known method of helping to increase coronary blood flow is by administering an intravenous nitroglycerin drip which can reduce the workload of the heart and which directly dilates the coronary vessels. We use a slow titrated infusion of nitroglycerine routinely, unless of course, the marked hypotension prevents its use, as is often the case. Some units continue to use intravenous glucose-potassium-insulin infusions (500 ml of 20 per cent dextrose, 20 units insulin, 40 mEq KCl) in the hope that this may improve myocardial function. Short of interventional procedures like angioplasty which opens a 'culprit lesion' within a coronary artery and directly improves blood supply, other methods of myocardial preservation are of dubious value.

Management of Cardiogenic Shock in the Absence of Invasive Monitoring Procedures (Fig. 6.3.6 and Table 6.3.8)

Most ICUs or coronary care units in the country lack the facilities to monitor intra-arterial pressure through an intra-arterial cannula, or the PAEDP via the S-G catheter. Facilities for cardiac output

measurements are even more scarce. Fortunately, both gadgetry and technical expertise have improved significantly over the last decade, particularly in the large metropolitan cities. Even so, they are still in short supply.

Almost all units can measure the CVP through a central line connected to a water manometer. The JVP, can also be gauged clinically from the upper limit of pulsations of the internal jugular vein (with the head and neck elevated to an angle of about 45 degrees from the horizontal). It is good clinical practice to tally the clinical measurement of the JVP with the actual measurement of the CVP through a central line connected to a pressure gauge or to a manometer. Unfortunately, the CVP does not predict the PAEDP, a normal CVP being often associated with a high PAEDP in cases of cardiogenic shock.

A high PAEDP or PCWP is indirectly confirmed thus:

(i) *Clinically*, by noting the presence or absence of crepitations over the bases. If present, the degree and extent of crackles are noted. A left ventricular diastolic gallop is always related to a raised left ventricular filling pressure. An audible third heart sound generally indicates a PAEDP > 18 mm Hg.

(ii) *Radiologically* by a chest X-ray which can diagnose both interstitial and alveolar pulmonary oedema. The chest X-ray is vital because on occasions (in our experience in about 30 per cent of cases), the radiograph shows clear pulmonary congestion and even pulmonary oedema which is not evident on auscultation. Gross pulmonary oedema generally signifies a PAEDP > 30 mm Hg; varying but gradually increasing degrees of pulmonary oedema are observed as the PAEDP rises above 20 mm Hg.

The arterial blood pressure by the cuff method is quite unreliable in the presence of severe vasoconstriction. Pressures may be unobtainable by the cuff method, but on monitoring via an intra-arterial catheter may be shown to be > 90 mm Hg. Impalpable radials or even brachials do not therefore signify irreversible shock in these individuals, but if the femorals are impalpable, or are barely felt, it always points to severe hypotensive shock. The CO and tissue perfusion can be judged clinically as best as possible by noting the skin temperature, the degree of sweating, the urine output, volume of peripheral pulses, general sensorium, the presence or absence of lactic acid acidosis and the overall clinical picture.

(a) When the CVP judged clinically or on actual measurement

Table 6.3.8. Monitoring of patients with cardiogenic shock in absence of invasive monitoring facilities

---

* Measure CVP via central line
* High PAEDP or PCWP evidenced by
  – CXR showing pulmonary oedema
  – Clinically—crepitations over lung bases, left ventricular diastolic gallop (audible third heart sound)
* Estimate CO and tissue perfusion clinically by noting
  – blood pressure
  – skin temperature
  – degree of sweating
  – volume of peripheral pulse
  – hourly urine output
  – general sensorium, and absence or presence of lactic acidosis

---

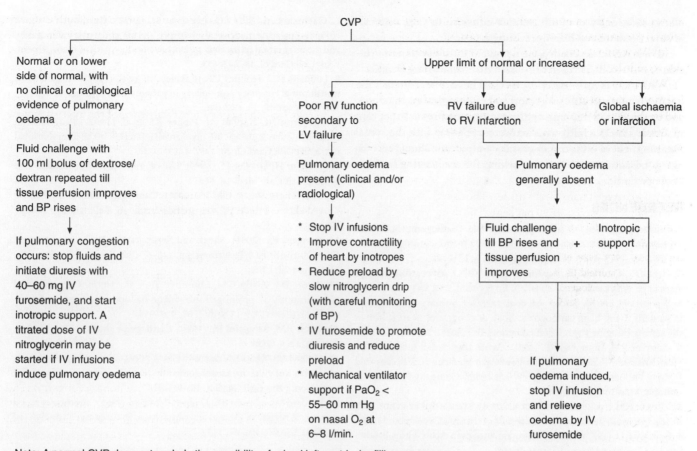

Note: A normal CVP does not exclude the possibility of raised left ventricular filling pressures.
Use mechanical ventilation in patients with severe shock, respiratory distress or when O₂ saturation < 90 per cent on O₂ at 6 l/min.

Fig. 6.3.6. Algorithm for management of cardiogenic shock in the absence of invasive monitoring facilities.
(CVP = central venous pressure; RV = right ventricle; LV = left ventricle)

is normal or on the lower side of normal, volume replacement is imperative and should be given a good try, unless the patient is in pulmonary oedema as judged on auscultation or on chest X-ray. Volume replacement in the form of bolus doses of 100 ml of dextrose or dextravan are given over 10 minutes and are repeated till the blood pressure rises and tissue perfusion improves. Tachypnoea and crackles on auscultation over the bases and mid-zones warn of pulmonary congestion and impending pulmonary oedema. This can be correlated with a chest X-ray. If pulmonary congestion increases, the infusion is stopped and intravenous furosemide 40–60 mg is given.

(b) A CVP which is on the upper limit of normal or clearly raised in a patient with cardiogenic shock, can be due to three possibilities: (i) Poor right ventricular function secondary to left ventricular failure; (ii) Right ventricular failure due to right ventricular infarction; (iii) Severe overall depressed myocardial function due to global ischaemia or global infarct.

The first instance is generally associated with clinical and radiological evidence of pulmonary oedema and fluid infusions are dangerous as they can increase the pulmonary oedema. The second and third situations are associated with a raised CVP but little or no pulmonary congestion. It should however be noted that a raised CVP might be iatrogenically produced by inotropic

agents which increase venous tone. A raised CVP may also be seen in pulmonary embolism, or when the CVP catheter is partially blocked, or when it is lodged in a tributary of the superior vena cava like the jugular vein, or in a patient who has pulmonary hypertension due to an associated chronic lung disease.

Clinically even if the CVP is raised, a fluid challenge is a must, provided that there is no evidence of pulmonary congestion or oedema clinically or on radiological examination. Volume load is continued till the BP rises and tissue perfusion improves.

(c) If pulmonary oedema is already present or if it develops during intravenous volume loading, intravenous infusions are stopped and the contractility of the heart is increased by using dopamine and dobutamine singly or in combination. These drugs are carefully titrated to increase perfusion pressure and to improve urine output and tissue hypoxia. An attempt is also made to reduce the preload by a slow titrated drip of nitroglycerin with a careful watch on the arterial blood pressure. Sublingual or oral nitrites or a liberal application of nitrobid ointment on the skin, may be used instead of intravenous nitroglycerin. Intravenous furosemide can also reduce preload and may also promote a much desired diuresis. Endotracheal intubation with mechanical ventilator support may be life-saving in severe pulmonary oedema as it increases PaO₂, perhaps mechanically limits alveolar oedema, and allows judiciously used intravenous infusions to raise systemic arterial pressure and improve tissue perfusion.

(d) We would never advocate the use of intravenous nitroprusside to reduce afterload in the absence of monitoring facilities.

With increasing experience, we have been able to predict the haemodynamic profile on clinical and radiological examination, and by the clinical response to therapeutic measures in 70 per cent of cases. This is a fairly satisfactory correlation with the actual measurement of pressures and cardiac output, and should encourage good patient care in units lacking the monitoring facilities outlined earlier.

REFERENCES

1. Goldberg RJ, Gore JM, Alpert JS et al. (1991). Cardiogenic shock after myocardial infarction: Incidence and mortality from a community-wide perspective, 1975–1988. N Engl J Med. 325, 1117–1122.

2. Page DL, Caulfield JB, Kastor JA et al. (1971). Myocardial changes associated with cardiogenic shock. N Engl J Med. 285, 133.

3. Wackers FJ, Lie KI, Becker AE et al. (1976). Coronary artery disease in patients dying from cardiogenic shock or congestive heart failure in the setting of acute myocardial infarction. Br Heart J. 38, 906.

4. Antman EM, Braunwald E. (2001). Acute Myocardial Infarction. In: Heart Disease—A Textbook of Cardiovascular Medicine (Eds Braumwald E, Zipes DP, Liby P). pp. 1114–1231. WB Saunders Company, Philadelphia, London, Montreal, Tokyo.

5. Gunnar RM, Cruz A, Boswell J et al. (1966). Myocardial infarction with shock. Haemodynamic studies and results of therapy. Circulation. 33, 753.

6. Bradley RD. (1977). Heart Failure. In: Studies in Acute Heart Failure. pp. 35–57. Edward Arnold, Great Britain.

7. Gacioch GM, Ellis SG, Lee L et al. (1992). Cardiogenic shock complicating acute myocardial infarction: The use of coronary angioplasty and the integration of the new support devices into patient management. J Am Coll Cardiol. 19, 647–653.

8. Hibbard MD, Holmes DR Jr, Bailey KR et al. (1992). Percutaneous transluminal coronary angioplasty in patients with cardiogenic shock. J Am Coll Cardiol. 19, 639–646.

9. Bengston JR, Kaplan AJ, Pieper KS et al. (1992). Prognosis in cardiogenic shock after acute myocardial infarction in the interventional era. J Am Coll Cardiol. 20, 1482–1489.

10. Lollgen H, Drexler H. (1990). Use of inotropes in the critical care setting. Crit Care Med. 18, 556.

11. Hollenberg SM, Parillo JE. (2001). Cardiogenic Shock. In: Critical Care Medicine, 2nd edn. pp. 421–36 (Eds Parrillo JE, Dellinger RP). Mosby, USA.

12. Bongard FS. (2001). Shock and Resuscitation. In: Current Critical Care Diagnosis and Treatment. pp. 242–67 (Eds Bongard FS, Sue DY). McGraw-Hill, USA.

13. Lazar JM, Ziady GM, Dummer SJ et al. (1992). Outcome and complications of prolonged intraaortic balloon counterpulsation in cardiac patients. Am J Cardiol. 69, 955–958.

14. Califf RM, Bengston JR. (1994). Cardiogenic shock. N Engl J Med. 330(24), 1724–1730.

15. Moosvi AR, Khaja F, Villanueva L et al. (1992). Early revascularization improves survival in cardiogenic shock complicating myocardial infarction. J Am Coll Cardiol. 19, 907–914.

16. Radford MJ, Johnson RA, Daggett WM et al. (1981). Ventricular septal rupture: A review of clinical and physiologic features and an analysis of survival. Circulation. 64, 545.

Sepsis and Septic Shock

General Considerations

Septic shock is the result of overwhelming sepsis or infection. It can evolve with frightening suddenness and severity and is frequently lethal. Severe sepsis is one of the most important causes of death in our unit. However sepsis and septic shock occurring from community-acquired infections outnumber sepsis and septic shock due to nosocomial infections. The epidemiological data from our country is lacking, but there are more than 750,000 cases of sepsis per year in the USA and more than 200,000 deaths per year from this entity. The mortality in septic shock ranges from 40 to 60 per cent despite the advances in antimicrobial treatment, and despite the intensive care provided to these patients (1).

The incidence of sepsis and septic shock appears to be increasing all over the world. Inadequate immune responses to infection due to underlying background diseases such as malignancy, lymphomas, leukaemias, HIV infection, chronic hepatic or renal failure, diabetes, predispose to sepsis and septic shock. Infections in the aged and in the malnourished are also frequently followed by severe sepsis, septic shock and death. Iatrogenic infections induced by procedures or their complications in critical care units can also cause septic shock (2, 3).

Septic shock chiefly follows gram-negative bacterial infections. There is however, an increasing incidence of gram-positive infections producing septic shock (4). The use of broad-spectrum antibiotics over prolonged periods of time, and organ transplantation, have brought in their wake fungal and viral infections which can also produce the picture of severe sepsis and septic shock (5).

Table 6.4.1. Important predisposing factors and causes of septic shock

* Infections in the aged, or malnourished
* Inadequate immune responses to infection due to underlying background disease e.g. hepatic or renal failure, diabetes mellitus, malignancy, antimitotic drugs, HIV infection, lymphoma
* Iatrogenic infections induced by procedures in critical care units
* Virulent gram-negative and gram-positive infections
* Opportunistic infections (including fungal, viral) after prolonged antibiotic therapy, or following organ transplants, or in other immunocompromized patients, such as those with HIV infection and lymphoma.
* Fulminant tetanus
* Disseminated haematogenous tuberculosis
* Severe Pl. falciparum infections
* Fulminant B. typhosus, salmonella and amoebic infections

Important causes of severe sepsis associated with mutiple organ failure in the tropics, in our experience, include fulminant tetanus, severe infections produced by Pl. falciparum, acute disseminated haematogenous tuberculosis, fulminant typhoid, salmonella and other gram-negative infections. Rarely, fulminant amoebic infections produce a similar picture. These have been discussed at length in other sections of the book.

The important factors predisposing to the development of septic shock are listed in **Table 6.4.1**.

Definitions

Definitions are a matter of semantics but it is important that clarity is introduced into the terminology used to describe various clinical profiles associated with sepsis. This would certainly help evaluate the results of management protocols in septic states. It has been increasingly realized over the last several years that the clinical features of gram-negative sepsis with complications of shock and multiple organ failure can occur in other widely different conditions, which are unrelated to infection. An ACCP-SCCM consensus conference held in 1991, proposed semantic terms that attempt to clearly define sepsis, and sepsis-related clinical states. This conference also proposed the use of the term 'systemic inflammatory response syndrome' (SIRS) to include patients in whom the clinical features resembled sepsis, even though the aetiology was due to non-infective causes. The proposed semantic definitions at this consensus conference are briefly described below (6).

The *systemic inflammatory response syndrome (SIRS)* is characterized by 2 or more of the following features: body temperature > 38°C or < 36°C; heart rate > 90 / minute; hyperventilation > 20/ minute or a $PaCO_2$ < 32 mm Hg; or a white blood cell count > 12000/mm^3 or < 4000/mm^3 or > 10 per cent band forms. A SIRS can occur following non-infectious causes e.g. trauma, crush injuries, pancreatitis and burns. Also, SIRS even when primarily unrelated to infection, can lead to hypotension, shock and to multiple organ failure. The consensus conference suggested that *the term sepsis be used exclusively when a SIRS is due to infection*. The interrelationship between SIRS, sepsis and infection is illustrated in **Fig. 6.4.1**.

Severe sepsis is defined as sepsis associated with organ dysfunction, hypoperfusion or hypotension. *Septic shock* is defined as

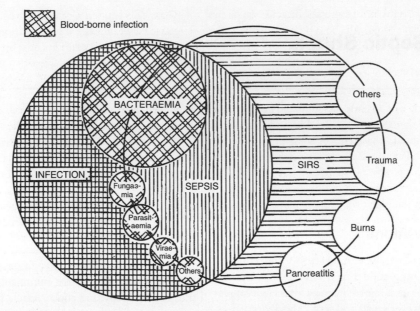

Fig. 6.4.1. The interrelationship between systemic inflammatory response syndrome (SIRS), sepsis and infection (from Bone RC et al. Chest, June 1992; 101:1644).

severe sepsis with hypotension that does not respond to adequate fluid replacement. It is associated with evidence of hypoperfusion and/or organ dysfunction.

These groupings, though arbitrary, are useful, and have been globally adopted both by clinicians and investigators. Their chief value lies in the evaluation and comparison of studies in patients with sepsis. The pathophysiological significance of these groupings remains to be established. Though the concept of the systemic inflammatory response syndrome (SIRS) is excellent in that it can arise as an innate immune response to noninfectious causes and to infections, the criteria used to define SIRS are both nonspecific and mild in degree. Judging by the present criteria, most patients in a large teaching hospital in our country would not only have SIRS but would be dubbed as 'septic'. The concept of SIRS, in our opinion, should be retained but its criteria either changed or abandoned.

Several North American and European Intensive Care Societies agreed in 2001 to take a re-look at the definitions of sepsis and sepsis related conditions (7). This consensus conference came to the following conclusions: (i) current concepts of sepsis, severe sepsis and septic shock should remain unchanged; (ii) current definitions do not allow for precise staging of the host response to infections; (iii) signs and symptoms of sepsis are more varied than the initial criteria stated in 1991; the consensus included in the clinical features of sepsis, subtle changes involving one or more organ systems either detected clinically, or on relevant laboratory tests (7); (iv) the future, according to this consensus conference lies in developing a staging system that will characterize progression of sepsis. They suggest the PIRO concept of staging sepsis. This concept stratifies patients on the basis of their Predisposing conditions, the nature and extent of the Insult (Infection), the nature and magnitude of the host Response, and the degree of concomitant Organ dysfunction. This consensus conference emphasized that the PIRO concept is

rudimentary; extensive testing and refinement would be necessary before its clinical application to patients with sepsis.

The recent consensus noted the relative nonspecificity of the clinical features decided under SIRS. SIRS is often associated with increased levels of inflammatory markers in the blood—notably, the circulating concentrations of IL-6, procalcitonin, and C reactive protein are increased. Thus it may be possible in the future to use purely biochemical and/or immunological markers rather than clinical criteria to identify the inflammatory response. However, as yet, no large prospective studies lend support to such a hypothesis.

Clinical Features

The clinical features of severe sepsis and septic shock include the following:

(i) Features of a SIRS due to an infection. These features include fever (or rarely hypothermia), tachycardia, tachypnoea, and leucocytosis (or leucopaenia < 4000/ mm^3).

(ii) Systolic arterial BP < 90 mm Hg, or a mean arterial BP (MAP) < 60 mm Hg. In hypertensive individuals, a fall of systolic arterial BP > 40 mm Hg below baseline is significant.

(iii) Evidence of poor tissue perfusion as judged by a lactic metabolic acidosis or a sharp fall in urine output, and/or evidence of dysfunction of one or more organs or organ systems, either detected clinically or through laboratory tests.

The circulatory state is generally hyperdynamic, so that in addition to tachycardia, the pulse is bounding and of good volume, and the peripheries are warm.

There are certain important clinical pointers to impending shock that need to be considered in a patient with infection or sepsis. These include the onset of unexplained tachypnoea, the presence of a mild icterus, a change in the mental state generally due to cerebral hypoperfusion and to metabolic changes, a sharp fall in the urine output (< 25–30 ml/hour), metabolic acidosis, or the presence of purpura or bleeding. All these point to early organ dysfunction and may precede hypotension.

Laboratory Features

Besides showing leucocytosis or leucopaenia, a coagulation profile may show evidence of an early disseminated intravascular coagulopathy (DIC). This includes an elevated prothrombin time, a decreased platelet count, decreased fibrinogen, increased fibrin degradation products, and increased thrombin index. Thrombocytopaenia may often occur without evidence of DIC.

Hyperglycaemia is common. Sudden marked elevations of serum glucose levels in patients on hyperalimentation may be the first indication of severe impending sepsis. Hypoglycaemia is observed in the pre-terminal or terminal state of septic shock and signifies severe hepatic dysfunction. A slight rise in serum bilirubin, serum aminotransferases, and in the alkaline phosphatase, occurs very frequently and points to hepatic dysfunction.

The hypermetabolic state is evinced by a marked increase in the urinary urea or urinary nitrogen over 24 hours, and a negative nitrogen balance.

The arterial pH may be low in the presence of metabolic acidosis and early involvement of the lung is manifested by a mild to moderate hypoxia with hypocapnia.

Recently, cytokines (specially IL-6 and IL-8), C reactive protein, and procalcitonin levels have been noted to rise significantly in sepsis. Procalcitonin (PCT) levels hold promise as they correlated better with the severity of inflammation. PCT is reported to be superior to the other markers in the diagnosis of a bacterial focus complicated by symptoms of severe sepsis and septic shock (8).

Physiopathology (9, 10) (Fig. 6.4.2)

A description of current research on this subject would fill a volume. This section merely gives a brief description of the physiopathology of septic shock to enable a better comprehension of sepsis and its complications; difficulties in management would then be more easily appreciated.

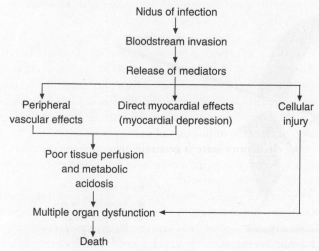

Fig. 6.4.2. Pathogenesis of septic shock.

Classically septic shock is due to endotoxins released by gram-negative bacteria. Recent investigations have implicated cell wall components of both gram-negative and gram-positive organisms. Septic shock can also occur with fungal infections as well as protozoal infections notably Pl.falciparum infections. Studies on septic shock have however been chiefly in relation to endotoxin produced by gram-negative bacteria. Endotoxin is a lipopolysaccharide component of the outer membrane of the bacterial cell. It consists of oligosaccharide side chains, a core polysaccharide and Lipid A, the latter being highly antigenic and believed to be responsible for the features of clinical sepsis. Endotoxin is directly toxic to endothelium and tissue cells, contributing to diffuse endothelial and tissue injury that characterizes the sepsis syndrome (11). Endotoxin interacts with normal host defences and triggers the release of numerous mediators—IL-1, granulocyte monocyte-colony stimulating factor, tumour necrosis factor (TNF) and procoagulant activity factor (12). Recent work suggests that endotoxin initiates the release of cytokines from mononuclear cells, in particular of TNF which is responsible for a number of features of the sepsis syndrome (13–15). Endotoxin also activates neutrophils with the subsequent release of proteases and oxidants which promote endothelial and tissue cell damage, degrade matrix and generate other pro-inflammatory mediators. A degradation of arachidonic acid is observed in cell walls through phospholipase. The mobilized arachidonic acid from the leucocyte cell can follow 2 pathways—the cyclo-oxygenase pathway leading to the formation of thromboxanes and prostaglandins, and the lipo-oxygenase pathway leading to the formation of leukotrienes. These mediators have various actions, some of them deleterious to tissue integrity and function. Phospholipase A_2 also releases membrane bound phospholipids which are converted to the platelet activating factor (PAF). The latter is known to increase vascular permeability, increase production of toxic oxygen free radicals, and activate platelets and phagocytes.

Endotoxin also activates factors within the serum. It thus activates and stimulates the coagulation pathway. This can occur at multiple sites (16). Recent work has focused increasing attention on the roles of endothelial injury and coagulation in sepsis. Sepsis can be conceptualized as a loss of homeostasis, caused by an imbalance of opposing mechanisms that normally maintain this homeostasis. On one side are coagulation and inflammation, actively promoted by endothelial injury, thrombin production, tissue factor expression and proinflammatory mediators. On the opposite side is fibrinolysis. Fibrinolysis normally counters the procoagulant factors, but is suppressed in sepsis. The suppression of fibrinolysis is perhaps related to several factors, notably increased levels of plasminogen activator inhibitor-1 (PAI–1), thrombin activatable fibrinolysis inhibitor (TAF.Ia) and decreased levels of Protein C. The homeostatic imbalance prevailing in sepsis is believed to lead to microvascular thrombi in various organ systems. This could well be the driving force that culminates in increasing multiple organ dysfunction and death.

In summary, invasive infection of the body by micro-organisms and their products or toxins elicits a strong response from the host defences. The response is characterized by activation of cellular elements and of the plasma protein systems. The cells activated include the mononuclear cells, lymphocytes, macrophages, neutrophils and endothelial cells. The activated cells produce numerous cytokines and mediators, some of which are proinflammatory and some anti-inflammatory. The host defence system also activates complement, the coagulation cascades and the kallikrein-kinin systems. Current thinking conceptualizes sepsis as a loss of homeostasis in which procoagulant forces predominate over fibrinolysis.

If the host defence response is disorganized, unorchestrated, unbalanced and unchecked it fails to defend the host and paradoxically enough inflicts injury on the host. This injury is widespread because of the toxic effect of numerous mediators, and also because of endothelial damage and the dominance of procoagulant factors leading to microvascular thrombi in various organ systems. The clinical features of severe sepsis, septic shock, and the evolution of multiple organ dysfunction and failure are a consequence of the changes described above. Figure **6.4.3a** illustrates the role of mediators in severe sepsis and septic shock. Figure **6.4.3b** illustrates the loss of homeostasis in severe sepsis.

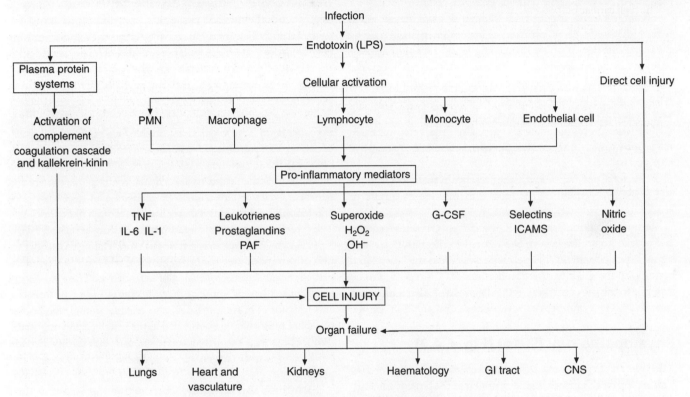

Fig. 6.4.3a. The role of mediators in severe sepsis and septic shock.

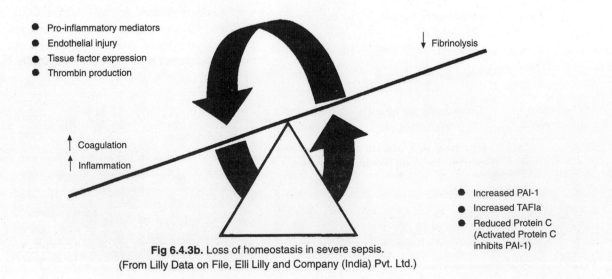

Fig 6.4.3b. Loss of homeostasis in severe sepsis.
(From Lilly Data on File, Elli Lilly and Company (India) Pvt. Ltd.)

Haemodynamic Effects

The haemodynamic effects of severe sepsis typically result in a high output hyperdynamic circulatory state with tachycardia and hypotension. Septic shock in addition to the above is characterized by systolic blood pressure ≤ 90 mm Hg not responding to fluid replenishment. It is associated with evidence of hypoperfusion and/or organ dysfunction. The haemodynamic state outlined holds not only for bacterial infections but also for fulminant infections peculiar to the tropical and developing countries of the world.

The high cardiac output and the hyperdynamic circulatory state in severe sepsis and septic shock could well be a compensatory response to increased tissue metabolism (17). This is certainly true for the haemodynamic profile of severe tetanus where a hyperdynamic circulatory state is observed even in paralysed patients on ventilator support (18, 19).

The haemodynamic effects of severe sepsis and septic shock can be considered under the following heads:

(a) The Peripheral Vascular System

(i) There is a marked decrease in the arterial and venous tone resulting in venous and arteriolar dilatation with a fall in peripheral vascular resistance, and therefore a fall in the systemic arterial blood pressure. The smaller arterioles are chiefly affected whereas venous tone is most reduced in the larger capacitance vessels (20, 21). These changes are greatest in the areas of active infection and inflammation (22). Hypotension in septic shock is associated with complement activation and with increased TNF, IL-1 levels (23, 24). Other vasodilating substances include nitric oxide, endothelial relaxing factor and platelet activating factor (25). Bernard et al. (26) have provided further insight into the mechanism of sepsis induced vasodilatation and hyporesponsiveness to vasoconstrictor drugs. Their study implicates macrophage derived mediators that affect smooth muscle contractility via nitric acid synthesis. Catecholamine alpha-receptor down-regulation has been experimentally reported, and if applicable to humans, may account for the poor vasoconstrictor response to vasopressors (27).

The microvascular circulation has been shown to be adversely affected, contributing thereby to tissue hypoxaemia and the frequent evolution of multiple organ failure. De Becker and colleagues (28) noted that the density of the microvasculature was markedly reduced in severe sepsis, with a sharp reduction in the proportion of perfused small vessels. A new technique, termed orthogonal polarization spectral imaging was used to measure sublingual microcirculation, as representative of the vascular bed. This new technique may help to elucidate the mechanisms involved in reduced microvascular blood flow in severe sepsis and septic shock.

(ii) A generalized increase in vascular permeability is also noticed in septic shock with increase in interstitial fluid and tissue oedema. A peripheral pooling, hepatosplanchnic pooling, and at times fluid loss from the gastrointestinal tract is responsible for a fall in effective circulatory volume.

(iii) The combined effect of the above two factors leads to hypovolaemia which may not be overt; this can at times mask the underlying hyperdynamic state, which becomes evident on fluid repletion.

(iv) There is a change in the pattern of blood flow distribution in septic shock. Some organs receive a supranormal supply of oxygen, whereas others are rendered ischaemic. This is of particular importance in the splanchnic circulation. Hepatovenous desaturation has been reported in septic patients (29).

(v) Changes in oxygen delivery, oxygen uptake and oxygen use or consumption by tissues are dealt with later.

(b) The Heart

Myocardial depression is present in almost all patients with septic shock (30, 31). Decreased compliance with decreased left ventricular diastolic function is observed. Left ventricular systolic function is also reduced as evinced by a dilated cardiomyopathy with a low ejection fraction and a reduced ventricular stroke work index. Cardiac output is usually increased because of marked tachycardia. Myocardial depressant factors include TNF, low molecular weight soluble molecules and lipid soluble substances (32, 33). There is no evidence of myocardial ischaemia, the coronary blood flow being well maintained. There is evidence of beta-receptor downgrading and this may be responsible for the poor response to inotropic drugs which is often observed in these patients (34, 35). In the absence of severe hypovolaemia, the net result is a hyperdynamic circulation with increased cardiac output due to increased heart rate.

(c) Pulmonary Hypertension

Pulmonary hypertension due to increased pulmonary vascular resistance is frequently present particularly when septic shock produces ARDS (36, 37). When significant pulmonary hypertension develops, right ventricular function may be markedly affected due to an increased afterload.

(d) Tissue Oxygenation

Tissue oxygenation eventually always suffers in septic shock. There is an increase in lactic acid production with metabolic acidosis.

Haemodynamic Profiles in Septic Shock (38)

The haemodynamic profile is dependent on the stage of shock—early or late, on the compensatory mechanisms present, on the presence and degree of myocardial dysfunction in the septic state, on the presence and degree of associated hypovolaemia, and the therapy the patient may have received prior to admission to the ICU.

(i) The most characteristic pattern in the early stage is a hyperdynamic circulation characterized by a high CI (at times as high as 7 l/m²) with tachycardia, a low systemic vascular resistance (SVR), a low pulmonary capillary wedge pressure (PCWP) and hypotension. The early stage of severe sepsis and septic shock is characterized by peripheral vasodilatation so that the pulse is bounding and the peripheries warm (**39**). The high CI is due to tachycardia and not to increased contractility. In fact, as has been discussed already under Haemodynamic Effects, both systolic and diastolic function of the heart are depressed in spite of the high cardiac output (**40**). The left ventricular ejection fraction (LVEF) typically falls to as low as 20–30 per cent in the first 24–48 hours. During this period the left ventricle dilates and abnormalities in both systolic and diastolic function are observed. Recent studies have shown that the left ventricle responds abnormally to a volume load, in that the reduced left ventricular stroke work increases marginally or to a very small extent. In survivors, a reversal of this abnormal function is observed over 7–10 days.

(ii) In the late stage of severe sepsis and septic shock, particularly in patients who are likely to succumb, the cardiac function remains poor or continues to deteriorate. The profile likely to be observed is a normal or a slightly low CI, an increasing PCWP, a normal SVR or a SVR showing a trend towards a slow increase. Persistent or increasing hypotension poorly responsive or unresponsive to therapy is observed.

(iii) The pre-terminal stage of septic shock is often associated with a low CI, a high PCWP and an increased systemic vascular resistance. Marked tachycardia, with hypotension unresponsive to all therapy is observed.

We feel that though the last profile is pre-terminal or in the late stages of septic shock, some patients with fulminant septic shock may have a very low CI with a high SVR to start with. At times, hypovolaemia may strongly contribute to this profile and this is recognized by low filling pressures. However, in a few individuals the PCWP is high, so that the haemodynamic profile is similar to that seen in severe cardiogenic shock.

The various haemodynamic profiles in septic shock are shown in **Table 6.4.2**.

Table 6.4.2. Various haemodynamic profiles in septic shock

1. Early stage—tachycardia, hypotension, low PCWP, high CI, and low SVR
2. With progression of the syndrome and deteriorating cardiac function—hypotension, high PCWP, normal or slightly low CI, normal to rising SVR
3. Late (preterminal) stage—hypotension, high PCWP, low and progressively decreasing CI, and increased SVR
4. Rarely, very low CI, high PCWP and high SVR is seen at the start in fulminant septic shock (profile resembles cardiogenic shock)

Table 6.4.3. Frequently observed right heart pressures and CO in septic shock, cardiogenic shock, cardiac compressive shock, hypovolaemic shock and anaphylactic shock

Types of Shock	PCWP mm Hg	CO ml/min
Septic Shock	↓ or Normal	↑ ↑ or Normal
Cardiogenic Shock (following acute MI)	↑ ↑	↓ ↓
Cardiac Compressive Shock (Cardiac Tamponade)	↑ ↑	↓ or ↓ ↓
Hypovolaemic Shock	↓ ↓	↓ ↓
Anaphylactic Shock	↓ or Normal	↑ or Normal

Frequently observed right heart pressures and cardiac output in septic shock vis-à-vis the values in cardiogenic, cardiac compressive, hypovolaemic shock and anaphylactic shock are detailed in **Table 6.4.3**.

Oxygen Delivery ($\dot{D}O_2$) and Oxygen Uptake ($\dot{V}O_2$) in Severe Sepsis and Septic Shock (41)

In the early and evolving phase of severe sepsis and septic shock, there is an increase both in $\dot{D}O_2$ and in $\dot{V}O_2$ (**42**). Even though there is an increase in oxygen consumption it may not be enough for the increased tissue need for oxygen, so that tissue hypoxia can still occur. Oxygen extraction ratios may be increased at this stage. Shoemaker (**43**) in a large prospective study of patients in septic shock, reported that survivors had a higher cardiac index, a higher $\dot{D}O_2$ and a higher $\dot{V}O_2$ than non-survivors. In the late phase of septic shock, oxygen consumption may fall sharply even though $\dot{D}O_2$ is satisfactory, resulting in a low oxygen extraction ratio. The reason for decreased oxygen extraction is debatable. It could well be due to damaged endothelial cells in capillaries, with oedema, resulting in increased distance necessary for diffusion of oxygen into tissue cells. More importantly, it could be due to damaged tissue cells which find it difficult to use the oxygen for their metabolic needs.

The Relation between Oxygen Uptake ($\dot{V}O_2$) and Oxygen Delivery ($\dot{D}O_2$) in Septic Shock

In normal subjects oxygen uptake is governed by tissue needs for oxygen (i.e. by tissue metabolism). In fact, oxygen uptake ($\dot{V}O_2$) is maintained constant over wide ranges of oxygen delivery (**44, 45**) (**Fig. 6.4.4**). This is accomplished by means of local compensatory mechanisms, chiefly by increased extraction of oxygen and increase in the cross-sectional area of capillaries perfusing an organ. When these compensatory mechanisms are exhausted, the $\dot{V}O_2$ falls in a manner directly related to oxygen delivery. The level of oxygen delivery below which the $\dot{V}O_2$ begins to fall, is aptly termed the critical threshold for oxygen delivery ($\dot{D}O_2$ crit.). It signifies the point of oxygen delivery below which supply and demand are no longer balanced.

It is claimed by several investigators that in patients with severe sepsis and septic shock, the relationship between oxygen delivery ($\dot{D}O_2$) and oxygen consumption ($\dot{V}O_2$) described above does not apply (**46–49**). In fact, in septic shock $\dot{V}O_2$ is believed to be dependent on $\dot{D}O_2$ at nearly all levels of $\dot{D}O_2$, including levels that are normally more than sufficient to meet tissue demands. If a rise in $\dot{V}O_2$ were dependent solely on a rise in $\dot{D}O_2$, it could denote the presence of an oxygen debt in the tissues in patients with severe sepsis and septic shock. This dependence of $\dot{V}O_2$ on $\dot{D}O_2$ at all levels in septic shock has however been disputed by several workers, and this has been elaborated upon in the chapter on ARDS.

As the severity of sepsis and septic shock increase, oxygen extraction (the slope of the $\dot{V}O_2/O_2$ delivery relationship) may decrease. This is not related to increased cardiac output and oxygen transport causing a luxuriant perfusion; it reflects the inability of the tissues to utilize oxygen (**Fig. 6.4.5**).

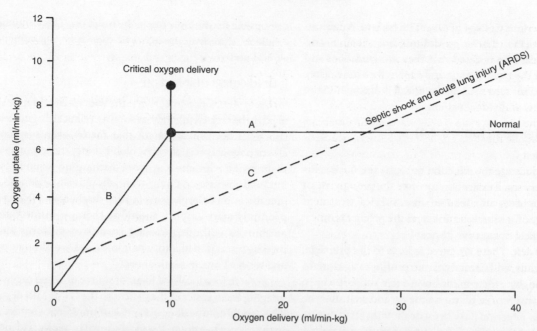

Fig. 6.4.4. Oxygen uptake-oxygen delivery relationships in normal subjects and in patients with ARDS (from Dorinsky PM, Gadek JE, Chest, 1989; 96: 885). Note: A similar relationship is also observed in patients with septic shock. In septic shock and ARDS, oxygen uptake is dependent on oxygen delivery at almost all levels of oxygen delivery (C). In normal subjects oxygen uptake is dependent upon tissue needs, and remains constant over a wide range of oxygen delivery (A). However once oxygen delivery falls below a critical level (critical oxygen delivery), there is a reduction in the oxygen uptake (B).

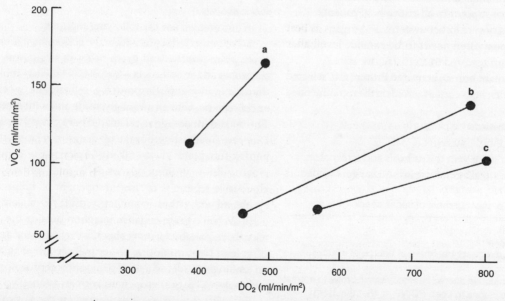

Fig. 6.4.5. Oxygen consumption ($\dot{V}O_2$) plotted against oxygen availability ($\dot{D}O_2$) in normals (**a**), and in patients with septic shock (**b** and **c**). Note that as the severity of septic shock increases (**b** and **c**), the slope of the $\dot{V}O_2$-Oxygen availability relationship decreases, pointing to an inability of the tissues to utilize oxygen in spite of adequate oxygen availability.

Management (50, 51)

Septic shock requires to be urgently treated and reversed, else it leads to worsening multi-organ failure and death. Though the patient should be urgently transferred to the ICU, treatment should commence wherever the patient is at the time of diagnosis (in the ambulance, emergency department or ward). This is particularly with reference to the prompt use of appropriate antibiotics and the start of cardiovascular resuscitation.

Guidelines for management of severe sepsis and septic shock have been published recently as a joint effort by eleven societies, which include Critical Care Societies of America, Europe, Australia,

New Zealand, American College of Chest Physicians, American Thoracic Society (51). These guidelines are sensible and instructive; yet it must be realized that they are guidelines and not 'diktats'. Guidelines will change and evolve with time. They should supplement but never supplant clinical judgement in the management of each individual patient.

Principles of Therapy (Table 6.4.4)

These are as follows:

I. To find and eradicate the infection or sepsis responsible for the state of septic shock. Eradication involves the prompt use of appropriate antibiotics in an adequate dose, surgical treatment of a proven localized focus of infection, and the prompt removal of an infected surgical or invasive device.

II. To reverse shock. There are three aspects to this principle: (a) To restore the altered haemodynamic profile to as close to normal as possible, by efficient cardiovascular support; (b) to maintain this restored profile till such time as, and well after the ravages of sepsis or infection have been dealt with; (c) to ensure as far as possible that the increased tissue demand for oxygen is more than adequately met; this is indeed the goal towards which cardiovascular support is directed.

Both I and II are set into motion together. In severe shock resuscitation takes pride of place; yet resuscitation would come to naught if prompt use and continuation of antibiotics is delayed, or if a pocket of pus remains undetected and undrained.

III. To use ventilator support in all critically ill patients.

IV. To support function of other systems and organs as best as possible. This support often needs to be extended well after the circulation has been restored to a satisfactory state.

V. To use recombinant human activated Protein C in selected patients, and to use intravenous corticosteroids in the recommended dose.

VI. To support nutrition.

VII. To provide metabolic support.

VIII. Prophylaxis for deep vein thrombosis and stress ulcer.

IX. To attempt to neutralize endotoxins and harmful mediators

Table 6.4.4. Principles of management of septic shock

I. Eradicate infection
  (a) Use of antibiotics
  (b) Identification and direct treatment of source of infection
II. Reverse Shock
  (a) Restore and maintain altered haemodynamic profile to normal
    (i) Volume infusions to keep PCWP at 15–18 mm Hg
    (ii) Inotropic support and vasopressors to ensure adequate DO_2 and VO_2 (dopamine and dobutamine or both; if these are ineffective, norepinephrine, vasopressin or epinephrine used)
  (b) Objectives: MAP $\geq$ 65 mm Hg, $S\bar{v}O_2$ 70 per cent, urine output $\geq$ 1 ml/kg, no base deficit
III. Ventilator support to all critically ill patients
IV. Use recombinant human activated protein C in selected patients with severe sepsis
V. Provide support to other organ systems
VI. Provide nutritional support
VII. Provide metabolic support
VIII. Prophylaxis for deep vein thrombosis and stress ulcers

---

responsible for multiple organ dysfunction. This continues to be a field of extensive research and cannot be recommended for clinical use.

I. Eradication of Infection

(a) Use of Antibiotics. Infection is the root cause of septic shock. It needs to be tackled urgently, as soon as a clinical diagnosis of septic shock has been made, or for that matter even suspected. The clinician should promptly send blood, urine, and any other cultures that may be relevant—e.g. from discharging wounds, loculated fluid and abscesses. A Gram's stain should also be done for a quick identification of organisms in such discharges. He should then promptly start empiric antibiotic therapy. Immediate use of antibiotics without awaiting results of cultures and other investigations is mandatory, as it improves the ultimate outcome and survival rate in septic shock.

A search for a localized focus or source of sepsis might warrant imaging and transfer of the patient to the CT or MRI department. This should only be done if the risk of transfer at a particular point in time is not too great. If a focal source of sepsis is identified (be it an abscess, or an infected invasive device, or necrotic tissue or a perforated viscus), it should be surgically tackled. The opportune time for doing this is a matter of experience and judgement. The sooner this is done the greater the chance of survival.

The antibiotics chosen in severe sepsis or septic shock will depend on the clinical picture and on the background against which shock evolves.

In our unit we use the following regimes :

(i) For suspected sepsis within the abdomen, it is important to cover gram-positive and gram-negative organisms, as well as anaerobes and streptococcus faecalis. We use a combination of a third generation cephalosporin e.g. ceftazidime or cefoperazone or ceftriaxone, with an aminoglycoside and with metronidazole. The maximum dosage as calculated per kg body weight, is used. Due care in adjusting dosage of drugs in relation to renal and hepatic function is always taken. An alternative regime is to use piperacillin + an aminoglycoside + metronidazole. Another alternative regime is to use meropenem or imipenem cilastin combined with either an aminoglycoside or vancomycin.

(ii) When a gram-negative infection outside the abdomen is felt to be responsible for septic shock, we recommend a combination of at least two antibiotics, either piperacillin or ticarcillin with an aminoglycoside, or a third generation cephalosporin with an aminoglycoside, or meropenem with an aminoglycoside.

(iii) In life-threatening situations where the source of infection is unknown, it is always wise to use a combination of two or more antibiotics. We use a third generation cephalosporin + an aminoglycoside, or ciprafloxacin + vancomycin + metronidazole or clindamycin. If the possibility of a streptococcal or pneumococcal infection cannot be excluded, we add ampicillin 2 g intravenously 4 hourly, till such time as the aetiology is known. A frequently used combination in the above situation is meropenem + vancomycin.

(iv) In nosocomial infections, the antibiotics used depend on the organisms prevailing and producing such infections in a particular ICU. In our unit, it is invariably a gram-negative infection which responds to a combination of a third generation cephalosporin + an aminoglycoside or ciprofloxacin. Methicillin resistant staphylococcal infections are uncommon, yet do occur in our unit with increasing frequency. In some other ICUs, methicillin resistant staphylococcal infections constitute an important and frequent nosocomial infection, so that vancomycin needs to be added to the above combination right from the beginning. Antifungal agents must always be used under appropriate conditions, particularly when the patient fails to improve with a powerful combination of antibiotics.

(v) In neutropaenic or immunocompromized patients, we use the same combination as for life-threatening infections. In suspected gram-negative infections we use ticarcillin with clavulanic acid or piperacillin tazobactum + an aminoglycoside. If fever does not settle within 36 hours, we add vancomycin to cover a possible staphylococcal infection. If the patient still remains febrile, we generally use amphotericin B with or without fluconazole to cover a possible fungal infection. The possibility of fulminant disseminated haematogenous tuberculosis causing the picture of sepsis and severe septic shock in immunocompromized patients, should always be kept in mind in our country, and in other poor countries where tuberculosis is rampant. This subject is discussed in the Section on Fever and Acute Infections in a Critical Care Setting.

(b) Identification of the Source of Infection and its Direct Treatment. After sending the requisite cultures and then starting an empirical antibiotic regime, an intensive search for possible sources of infection should be made. This should include an extremely thorough clinical examination, laboratory tests, and should utilize current imaging techniques. Any localized collection of pus within the body should be promptly drained. Intra-abdominal abscess, an empyema of the gall bladder, paracolic abscess, pelvic abscess, an appendicular abscess, an empyema tucked away in the paravertebral space are some localized collections of pus that should be avidly searched for. No amount of antibiotics can salvage a situation if a localized abscess is left undrained—the sooner it is drained the better. The possibility of iatrogenic haematogenous sepsis arising from contaminated central lines should always be kept in mind. Suspect central lines should be removed and the tips sent for culture.

In our experience, in close to 50 per cent of patients, no source of infection could be definitely identified. The frequency of positive blood cultures varies with different clinical situations, and with different microbiological laboratories. In our set-up, the incidence of positive blood cultures is less than 25 per cent. Again patients who have already received, or are receiving antibiotics, are less likely to have positive cultures. It is to be remembered that death from septic shock can result from a focus of sepsis which for many reasons need not yield positive blood cultures—this is particularly true in patients with abdominal sepsis.

Difficulties in the diagnosis and location of a source of sepsis may be immense in critically ill individuals, particularly if modern diagnostic and imaging facilities are unavailable, as is to be expected in many third world countries. These difficulties need special emphasis in the following situations :

(i) In Pregnancy and Parturition. During pregnancy and soon after delivery the source of sepsis can be easily missed. An acute appendicular abscess in a patient with advanced pregnancy often produces discomfort in the right hypochondrium, and in the tropics can be mistaken for an amoebic hepatitis or cholecystitis. A pelvic abscess can also be easily missed during pregnancy if not specifically looked for. Diagnosis is doubly difficult because of constraints on imaging procedures.

Perforation of the gut due to any aetiology soon after a caesarean delivery, is a disaster which is often missed. The subject has been discussed under Intra-Abdominal Sepsis in the Section on Surgical Infections.

(ii) In the Aged and the Infirm. Problems of identifying the source of sepsis in the aged are invariably extremely difficult. The body responses to sepsis are blunted, and this is one reason why the diagnosis is delayed. Localizing signs are few and sometimes ill-defined and indeterminate. For example, perforation of the large bowel may produce very few signs, and may therefore be missed till too late. A pneumonia, or an empyema tucked away in the paravertebral space may also remain undiagnosed for a period of time in the old and the infirm.

(iii) In Neutropaenic and Immunocompromized Patients. The problems in these patients are often impossibly difficult. In fact, neutropaenic patients with sepsis, in our experience, often have no identifiable source of infection. In these patients, the source of infection is believed to be a small or even microscopic focus in the bowel or perhaps in some other organ system.

II. Reversal of Shock: Support to the Cardiovascular System (50–52)

Resuscitation should commence promptly as soon as the diagnosis is made and not await transfer to the ICU. However the optimal management of septic shock requires transfer to a critical care unit. The description of the management of septic shock that follows is chiefly in relation to a critical care setting.

(a) Haemodynamic Monitoring. When facilities are available, haemodynamic monitoring is of immense value in management. The central venous pressure (CVP) is measured through a central venous line. In critical states, arterial pressure is monitored through a catheter inserted preferably in the radial artery—intra-arterial pressures are thus displayed from beat to beat. Septic shock is a prime indication for the use of a pulmonary artery (Swan-Ganz [S-G]) catheter. Mixed venous blood is sampled through the S-G catheter, and the $P\bar{v}O_2$ and $S\bar{v}O_2$ estimated and monitored. The haemodynamic parameters monitored are the heart rate, the arterial systolic, diastolic and mean pressures (MAP), CVP, PCWP, CO, CI, pulmonary artery pressure, systemic vascular resistance (SVR) and the pulmonary vascular resistance (PVR). The right and left ventricular stroke work indices (RVSWI and LVSWI) are also often monitored.

(b) Monitoring of Cardiac Rhythm. Though rhythm disturbances are not a special feature of septic shock, arrhythmias can occur in septic hypotensive patients who are on inotropic support and who have indwelling intracardiac catheters. Electrolyte disturbances contribute to or often cause dangerous ventricular arrhythmias.

These need to be recognized and corrected according to standard practice.

(c) *X-ray of the chest* on a daily or more frequent basis is imperative in critically ill patients.

(d) *Laboratory Monitoring*. Blood counts, routine biochemical tests, coagulation profile, serum lactate levels, arterial pH and blood gases are done and repeated as and when necessary.

(e) *Optimal Cardiovascular Support*. Optimal circulatory support should be planned and executed as follows:

(i) Volume Resuscitation. The initial goal is to maintain a PCWP of 15–18 mm Hg and a MAP ≥ 65 mm Hg. Volume infusions to prime or fill the pump (i.e. the left ventricle) to an optimal level are almost always necessary. The MAP as far as possible should not be < 65 mm Hg as coronary, renal and cerebral circulations then become slowly but surely jeopardized. The objectives of 'volume resuscitation' are a urine output ≥ 1 ml/kg, a MAP of ≥ 65 mm Hg, a SⅴO$_2$ of 70 per cent, no base deficit, normal or reduced serum lactate level, a significant reduction in tachycardia and a normal sensorium. The first four objectives are of crucial importance and they should if possible be achieved quickly within the first 6 to 8 hours.

In our experience, we have found it wise not to exceed a PCWP of 15 mm Hg in patients over 50–55 years of age, as otherwise the chance of pulmonary oedema and subsequent ARDS increases. In younger individuals, we generally keep to an upper limit of 18 to 20 mm Hg to provide an optimal filling pressure to the left ventricle. The optimal filling pressure varies—in a given patient it is that pressure which ensures adequate oxygen transport (DO$_2$) and increases arterial pressure, without causing pulmonary oedema. However when ARDS complicates septic shock, we prefer not to exceed a PCWP of 10–12 mm Hg, for fear of increasing the severity of ARDS. As explained later in this section, if facilities for a PA catheter are not available (as when resuscitation commences outside the ICU), volume infusions are so titrated as to keep the CVP at 8–12 mm Hg, oxygen saturation of venous blood drawn from the superior vena cava at 70 per cent, the MAP ≥ 65 mm Hg and a urine output ≥ 1 ml/kg. 4 to 8 litres of fluid or more may be required for initial emergency resuscitation.

There remains a controversy as to whether crystalloids or colloids need to be used for volume infusion in these patients. Crystalloids as explained earlier, are safe and inexpensive. Colloids (including albumin) are better volume expanders but are more expensive and can cause hypersensitivity reactions. Earlier work suggested that colloids were more effective than crystalloids in improving both cardiac output and oxygen delivery (53). Colloids were shown to improve VO$_2$ only in patients with elevated serum lactate levels (54, 55). They do not appear to influence the VO$_2$ when serum lactate levels were normal. However, the recent SAFE study (56) concluded that in patients in the ICU, use of either 4 per cent albumin or normal saline for fluid resuscitation resulted in similar outcomes at 28 days. Even so, for quick resuscitation we initially use 500–1000 ml of a colloid solution, and then switch over to crystalloids. Whole blood may need to be infused for replacing blood loss; packed RBCs are transfused only if necessary, to keep the haematocrit around 35 per cent.

(ii) Use of Inotropes and Vasopressors. If after volume infusions have raised the PCWP to 15–18 mm Hg, the MAP still remains < 65 mm Hg, inotropes and vasopressors need to be used. *We offer inotropic and vasopressor support in varying degrees to every patient, to increase and maintain an adequate cardiac index, an adequate blood pressure, oxygen transport and VO$_2$, but only after the heart has been sufficiently primed with a volume load. However, when the patient's condition is very critical, rapid volume infusions and inotropes and vasopressors need to be given simultaneously to sustain life and maintain tissue perfusion in the presence of life-threatening hypotension.*

The vasopressor in general use is norepinephrine and the inotropes used are dopamine and dobutamine. We prefer to use a combination of dopamine and dobutamine in our patients, starting at 5 µg/kg/min and titrating upwards if necessary to not more than 20 µg/kg/min. The emphasis should be on dopamine if the blood pressure is low and on dobutamine if the cardiac output is low. Vincent and colleagues (57) are of the opinion that when combined with volume infusion, dobutamine is superior to dopamine for increasing VO$_2$. Dopamine when increased to beyond 10 µg/kg/min, has an increasingly strong peripheral vasoconstrictor action in addition to its inotropic effect. Both dopamine and dobutamine are titrated upwards (not exceeding 20 µg/kg/min) to achieve an adequate oxygen transport (DO$_2$), oxygen consumption (VO$_2$), a systolic blood pressure ≥ 110 mm Hg, a mean arterial pressure > 65 mm Hg, SⅴO$_2$ 70 per cent, urine output > 1ml/kg, with normal lactate levels and no base deficit.

If dopamine > 10 µg/kg/min and dobutamine are ineffective, norepinephrine is used. Many critical care units use norepinephrine as the first line drug, and then if necessary use inotropic support with dopamine and/or dobutamine. This is indeed the recommendation in the recently formulated Surviving Sepsis Guidelines (51). *Almost always in critically ill individuals both inotropic and vasopressor support are necessary, and more often than not both these supports are used simultaneously.*

Norepinephrine can unquestionably increase the blood pressure, but its powerful vasoconstrictor properties due to its α adrenergic effects, could produce increasing organ ischaemia, and adversely affect cardiac output by increasing the afterload. However, several recent studies have shown that norepinephrine can reverse hypotension resistant to volume load and the use of dopamine and dobutamine. The usual dose ranges from 2–4 µg/min with a maximum of 10–12 µg/min (58).

Another vasopressor recently used in patients with septic shock resistant to inotropes and catecholamines is vasopressin (59). When given in a dose of 0.01 to 0.04 units/minute, it raises blood pressure and decreases the requirement of other vasopressors. Vasopressin increases urine output; pulmonary vascular resistance may decrease (60, 61). Vasopressin is best tried only if noradrenaline is ineffective. We have very little experience with this drug in patients with septic shock.

Epinephrine in a dose of 0.01 to 0.1 µg/kg/min has also been tried as a vasopressor but has the disadvantage of contributing to tachycardia and to splanchnic vasoconstriction.

Vasopressors and inotropes (given in a dose that produces a vasopressor effect) should always be administered through a central venous line. Sinus tachycardia and tachyarrhythmias are important complications of these drugs. A feared complication, particularly with dopamine administration, is ischaemic limb necrosis. Phentolamine in an intravenous bolus dose of 5 mg followed by an infusion at 1 mg/min should be given at the earliest sign of limb ischaemia.

It is not enough to restore the haemodynamic profile; it is important to *maintain* this improved circulatory state through the judicious use of volume load, inotropes, vasopressors as the circulatory state may remain in peril for some days after sepsis appears to be under control.

(iii) Ensuring an adequate oxygen supply to meet the tissue needs. The basic objective of cardiovascular support in patients with septic shock is to ensure, as far as possible that there is an adequate oxygen supply to meet the tissue needs of oxygen. In septic shock, because of the hypermetabolic state, tissue hypoxia can exist in spite of an increased $\dot{V}O_2$. The parameters that generally signify adequate $\dot{D}O_2$ and adequate tissue oxygenation are a systolic blood pressure > 110 mm Hg, mean arterial pressure > 65 mm Hg, a normal pH and no base deficit, a serum lactic acid level not > 4 mM/l and a mixed venous oxygen saturation close to 70 per cent. Inability to achieve these objectives is invariably observed in non-survivors of septic shock.

There are some investigators, notably Shoemaker and his colleagues (62) who believe that supranormal delivery of oxygen ($\dot{D}O_2$) to ensure supranormal consumption of oxygen ($\dot{V}O_2$) significantly improves survival in septic shock. This is achieved by pushing both volume load and inotropic support to very high levels. The specific goals for cardiac output, $\dot{D}O_2$, $\dot{V}O_2$ suggested by Shoemaker are tabled below (**Table 6.4.5**).

We attempted this strategy earlier and found no improvement in mortality. What is more, it was a strategy that was, at times, impossible to achieve. Perhaps the above strategy may hold for a select group of patients who develop shock after trauma or soon after surgery.

Recent studies suggest that aggressive management to raise $\dot{D}O_2$ to supramaximal levels does not help. Gattinoni and his colleagues (63) found no difference in survival in patients receiving supramaximal $\dot{D}O_2$ as compared to those who received standard care. Hayes and colleagues (64) in fact reported a reduced survival rate in patients receiving supranormal oxygen deliveries. Our present policy is to manipulate cardiovascular support so as to achieve, as far as possible, a $\dot{D}O_2$ at the upper limit of normal. Packed RBC infusions to keep a PCV of 35 per cent and/or intravenous

Table 6.4.5. Management goals in septic shock

Parameters	Normal	Optimal
Cardiac Index (l/min-m²)	2.8–3.6	> 4.5
Oxygen Delivery (ml/min-m²)	500–600	> 600
Oxygen Uptake (ml/min-m²)	110–160	> 170

(From : Shoemaker WC, Intensive Care Medicine, 1987, 13: 230–43, Spring-Verlad, NY)

infusion of dobutamine are of help in achieving this objective.

Successful management of cardiovascular support in the absence of a PA catheter is well illustrated by the work of Rivers and his colleagues (65). These workers achieved a significant increase in survival rate if treatment for severe sepsis and septic shock was early, as soon as the patient reached the emergency department, and was specifically *goal oriented*.

The specific goals that these workers achieved through volume load, the use of inotropes (in particular dobutamine) and vasopressors were as follows : a CVP of 8 to 12 mm Hg, a mean arterial blood pressure ≥ 65 mm Hg, a normal pH with no base deficit, a central venous oxygen saturation (measured and continuously displayed through a specially devised central venous catheter) of 70 per cent, and a PCV of at least 30 per cent. The goal of a CVP of 8–12 mm Hg was achieved by boluses of intravenous volume infusions; vasopressors were given to achieve a mean arterial pressure > 65 mm Hg. Dobutamine was titrated to a maximum of 20 µg/kg/min if the central venous oxygen saturation was < 70 per cent. Packed cell infusions were given to achieve a PCV of at least 30 per cent. The successful use of measurements of venous oxygen saturation in the superior vena cava (central venous oxygen), through a central venous line, in place of mixed venous oxygen saturation estimated through a PA catheter, though debatable, is of great interest to units that do not use a PA catheter.

III. Ventilator Support

Patients critically ill with septic shock need more than just supplemental oxygen. They need ventilator support. These patients often have a PaO_2 < 60 mm Hg, because of a low $P\bar{v}O_2$ and because of ventilation-perfusion inequalities within the lung (Type IV respiratory failure). Even otherwise, these patients are generally tachypnoeic with a respiratory rate > 30–35/minute. Ventilator support rests the muscles of respiration, sharply lowers the oxygen cost of breathing, enabling more oxygen to be diverted to the vital organs of the body. ARDS is an important complication of severe sepsis necessitating ventilator support. (see Chapter on Mechanical Ventilation in Critically Ill Patients).

IV. Support of Other Organ Systems

Septic shock often leads to multiple organ failure. Each organ system requires adequate support. Renal replacement therapy to counter acute renal failure is often necessary and should not be unduly delayed. The mortality in patients with ≥ 3 organ failure lasting for more than 5 to 7 days is horrendous in severe bacterial sepsis, but is not so forbidding in severe tropical infection or in multi-organ failure due to non-infective causes (see Chapter on Multiple Organ Dysfunction)

V. The Use of Human Recombinant Activated Protein C in Severe Sepsis

In experimental models of sepsis, activated Protein C has been shown to prevent organ damage by limiting microvascular coagulation, leucocyte activation and cytokine elaboration (66). This experimental work has been successfully translated to clinical use. Using properly evaluated inclusion and exclusion criteria, the

Protein C Worldwide Evaluation in Severe Sepsis (PROWESS) demonstrated that the use of drotrecogin alfa (activated), the recombinant form of human activated Protein C (APC) resulted in a 6.1 per cent absolute reduction and 19.4 per cent relative risk reduction in 28–day all cause mortality (67). Until recently, numerous interventions to help reduce 28–day all cause mortality in severe sepsis proved of no avail except perhaps in very small subsets of patients. The use of APC is the first intervention to have been proven useful in severe sepsis. The PROWESS study showed that 16 patients with severe sepsis would require to be treated to save one life.

APC is indicated in patients with severe sepsis or septic shock who have one or more organ dysfunction. It is given as a continuous intravenous infusion in a dose of 24 µg/kg/hour for 4 days. The major side-effect is bleeding, which can be particularly dangerous if the drug is used in patients with sepsis who have a deranged coagulation profile. The major contraindication to its use is a well-marked bleeding tendency. Unquestionably, the major disadvantage in poor developing countries is the cost (Rs. 3.5 lakhs for a 60 kg individual).

Corticosteroids in Severe Sepsis and Septic Shock (68)

High dose corticosteroids are contraindicated in severe sepsis and septic shock, except for special entities such as severe B. typhosus infection, pneumocystis carini pneumonia in HIV infection or in bacterial meningitis in children. However, recently, hydrocortisone acetate (administered as a 100 mg intravenous bolus three times a day for 5 days and tapered off over the next 6 days) was associated with a 31 per cent absolute reduction in 28–day mortality (69). The rationale for its use is as follows : (a) The existence of a relative adrenocortical deficiency in some patients with severe sepsis as judged by lowered cortisol levels after stimulation with ACTH (70). Such patients benefit with the use of hydrocortisone given in a dose of 50 to 100 mg every 6 to 8 hours. (b) It is conceivable that some patients with severe sepsis may be resistant to the use of glucocorticoids at the tissue level.

The present consensus is to use hydrocortisone in a dose of 50 mg intravenously 8 hourly, preferably in the early stage of severe sepsis and septic shock, for 5 to 10 days.

VI. Nutritional Support

This is vital for survival in the hypercatabolic state that characterizes sepsis and septic shock. Hyperalimentation is frequently necessary to supply adequate calories, proteins, carbohydrates, minerals and vitamins (see Chapter on Nutrition in The Critically Ill Adult).

VII. Metabolic Support

Glucose Control. Following initial stabilization in severe sepsis, insulin therapy is advocated to keep the blood sugar < 140 mg/dl. This has been reported to reduced morbidity and mortality among critically ill patients in the surgical intensive care unit (71).

Use of Bicarbonate. There is no evidence to support the use of bicarbonate therapy in the treatment of hypoperfusion-induced acidaemia associated with sepsis. Even so we use bicarbonate in severe acidosis with pH < 7.10. At times use of bicarbonate in patients with a very low pH has a salutary effect on myocardial function and arterial pressure.

VIII. Prophylaxis for Deep Vein Thrombosis and Stress Ulcers

Patient with severe sepsis need prophylaxis against deep vein thrombosis either with low molecular weight heparin, or if this is inappropriate, with the use of a mechanical protective device (intermittent compression device or compression stockings). Prophylaxis for stress ulcers in severe sepsis is provided by the use of H_2 receptor—anatgonists and anatcids, in preference to sucralfate.

IX. Immunotherapy—Neutralization of Toxic Mediators, Cytokines in Sepsis

Septic shock is mediated by numerous interacting endogenously produced mediators and cytokines, triggered by the action of bacterial toxins, chiefly endotoxins derived from gram-negative bacteria. A search is on for pharmaceutical agents which can directly counter these harmful endogenous mediators, or their noxious effects on tissues. Agents tried include nonsteroidal anti-inflammatory drugs, nalaxone, pentoxiphylline, anti-tumour necrosis factor, surfactant (to replace depleted surfactant in ARDS). The use of antibodies against pro-inflammatory interleukins or of monoclonal antibodies to the core antigen of the J-5 strain of E. coli has yielded unsatisfactory results. High dose corticosteroids and the use of a number of agents to inhibit activity of nitric oxide synthetase have proved futile. It is unlikely that a single inhibitor or antagonist to the numerous interacting mediators in severe sepsis is ever likely to succeed. Perhaps a multipronged attack on the important proinflammatory cytokines and mediators that inflict damage on the host seems a more rational approach.

Toxic Shock Syndrome

This is a form of septic shock produced by the exotoxin of Staphylococcus aureus. These pathogens remain localized usually in the skin or vagina, but the toxin is absorbed into the circulation and produces the features of septic shock. The toxic shock syndrome classically occurs against the background of tampon use in menstruating females. It can also occur at or after childbirth, and following pelvic infections. Any staphylococcal infection occurring at any site can produce this syndrome if the strain concerned produces the toxin causing toxic shock (72).

Clinical Features

Fever, headache and other non-specific symptoms are followed within 24–48 hours by a rapid clinical deterioration, characterized by hypotension and multiple organ failure (73). An erythematous rash, blanching on pressure is often observed in the early phase of the syndrome; this should suggest the correct diagnosis in the presence of clinical features described above. A desquamative rash involving the palms and soles appears after 1–2 weeks.

In critically ill patients, haemodynamic monitoring is a useful aid to management. The haemodynamic profile is the same as in septic shock—a low or normal PCWP, a high CO, and a low SVR.

Therapy

This remains the same as in septic shock. When shock is related to the use of tampons, immediate tampon removal is mandatory. Volume infusions to restore filling pressures to optimal levels should be given. If hypotension persists, inotropic support with dopamine or dobutamine is given. Antibiotic therapy with antistaphylococcal agents e.g. cloxacillin, first generation cephalosporins, or vancomycin should be promptly started. Mortality from the toxic shock syndrome is about 5 per cent (73).

REFERENCES

1. Rackow EC, Astiz ME. (1993). Mechanisms and Management of Septic Shock. Critical Care Clinics. 9(2), 219–237.

2. Bryan C, Reynolds K, Brenner E. (1983). Analysis of 1186 episodes of gram-negative bacteremia in non-university hospitals: the effects of antimicrobial therapy. Rev Infect Dis. 5, 629–630.

3. Kreger BE, Craven DE, McCabe WR. (1980). Gram-negative bacteremia III: reassessment of etiology epidemiology in 612 patients. Am J Med. 68, 332–343.

4. Tuchschmidt J, Fried J, Swinney R et al. (1989). Early haemodynamic correlates of survival in patients with septic shock. Crit Care Med. 17, 719–723.

5. O'Krent D, Abraham E, Winston D. (1987). Cardiorespiratory patterns in viral septicemia. Am J Med. 83, 683–686.

6. Bone RC. (1992). Definitions for sepsis and organ failure and guidelines for the use of innovative therapies in sepsis. The ACCP/SCCM Consensus Conference Committee. American College of Chest Physicians/Society of Critical Care Medicine. Chest. 101, 1644–1655.

7. Levy MM, Fink MP, Marshall JC et al. (2003). 2001 SCCM/ESICM/ACCP/ATS/SIS International Sepsis Definition Conference. Crit Care Med. 31 (4), 1250–1256.

8. Reinhart K, Mesner M, Hartag K. (2001). Diagnosis of sepsis : Novel and conventional parameters. Advances in Sepsis. 1(2), 42–51.

9. Shapiro L, Gelfand JA. (2000). Cytokines in Disease. In: Textbook of Critical Care (Eds Shoemaker WC, Grenvik A, Stephen MA, Holbrook P et al.). pp 578–586. W B Saunders and Company, Philadelphia.

10. Parrillo JE.(1993). Pathogenetic mechanisms of septic shock. N Engl J Med. 328(20), 1471–1477.

11. Danner RL, Elin RJ, Hosseini JM et al. (1991). Endotoxemia in human septic shock. Chest. 99, 169–175.

12. Niemetz J, Morrison DG. (1977). Lipid A as the biologically active moiety in bacterial endotoxin (LPS) initiated generation of procoagulant activity by peripheral blood leukocytes. Blood. 49, 947–956.

13. Hesse DG, Tracey KJ, Fong Y et al. (1988). Cytokine appearance in human endotoxemia and non-human primate bacteremia. Surg Gynecol Obstet. 166, 147–153.

14. Tracey KJ, Lowry SF, Fahey TJ III et al. (1987). Cachectin/tumor necrosis factor induces lethal shock and stress hormone response in the dog. Surg Gynecol Obstet. 164, 415–422.

15. Heard SO, Perkins MW, Fink MP. (1992). Tumor necrosis factor-alpha causes myocardial depression in guinea pigs. Crit Care Med. 20, 523–527.

16. Fein A, Wiener-Kronish JP, Niederman M et al. (1986). Pathophysiology of ARDS: What have we learned from in human studies? Crit Care Clin. 2, 429–453.

17. Shoemaker WC. (2000). Invasive and noninvasive hemodynamic monitoring of acutely ill sepsis and septic shock patients in the emergency department. Eur J Emerg Med. 7 (3), 169–175.

18. Udwadia FE. (1994). Haemodynamics in Severe Tetanus. In: Tetanus. pp. 88–100. Oxford University Press, Mumbai.

19. Udwadia FE, Sunavala JD, Jain MC et al. (1992). Haemodynamic studies during the management of severe tetanus. Q J Med. 83, 449–60.

20. Cryer H, Garrison W, Kaebnick H et al. (1987). Skeletal microcirculatory responses to hyperdynamic Escherichia coli sepsis in anesthetized rats. Arch Surg. 122, 86–92.

21. Dorio V, Whalen C, Naldi M et al. (1989). Contribution of peripheral blood pooling to central haemodynamic disturbances during endotoxin insult in intact dogs. Crit Care Med. 17, 1314.

22. Hermeck A, Thal A. (1969). Mechanisms for high circulatory requirements in sepsis and septic shock. Ann Surg. 170, 677–695.

23. Dammas P, Reuter A, Gysen P et al. (1989). Tumor necrosis factor and interleukin-1 serum levels during severe sepsis in humans. Crit Care Med. 17, 975–978.

24. Vadas P, Pruzanski W, Stefanski E et al. (1988). Pathogenesis of hypotension in septic shock: Correlation of circulatory phospholipase A2 levels with circulatory collapse. Crit Care Med. 16, 1–7.

25. Ochoa J, Udekwa A, Billiar T et al. (1991). Nitrogen oxide levels in patients after trauma and during sepsis. Ann Surg. 214, 621–626.

26. Bernard C, Szekely B, Philip I et al. (1992). Activated macrophages depress the contractility of rabbit carotids via an L-arginine/nitric oxide-dependent effector mechanism: Connection with amplified cytokine release. J Clin Invest. 89, 851–860.

27. McMillan M, Chernow B, Roth B. (1983). Hepatic alpha-adrenergic receptor alteration in a rat model of chronic sepsis. Circ Shock. 19, 185–193.

28. De Becker D, Creteur J, Preuseur JC et al. (2002). Microvascular blood flow is altered in patients with sepsis. Am J Resp Crit Care Med. 166, 98–104.

29. Bongard FS. (2002). Shock and Resuscitation. In: Current Critical Care Diagnosis and Treatment (Eds Bongard FS, Sue DY). pp 242–267. McGraw-Hill, USA.

30. Ellrodt A, Riedinger M, Kimichi A et al. (1985). Left ventricular performance in septic shock: reversible segmental and global abnormalities. Am Heart J. 110, 402–409.

31. Romano FD, Jones SB. (1986). Characteristics of myocardial beta-adrenergic receptors during endotoxicosis in the rat. Am J Physiol. 251, R359–R364.

32. Baumgartner J, McCutchan J, Melle G et al. (1985). Prevention of gram-negative shock and death in surgical patients by antibody of endotoxin core glycolipid. Lancet. 2, 54–63.

33. Parrillo JE, Burch C, Shelhamer JH et al. (1985). A circulating myocardial depressant substance in humans with septic shock. J Clin Invest. 76, 1539–1553.

34. Archer L, Black M, Hinshaw L. (1975). Myocardial failure with altered response to adrenaline in endotoxin shock. Br J Pharmacol. 154, 145–155.

35. Nasraway SA, Rackow EC, Astiz ME et al. (1989). Inotrope response to digoxin and dopamine in patients with severe sepsis. Cardiac failure and systemic hypoperfusion. Chest. 95, 612–615.

36. Brigham KL, Meyrick B. (1986). Endotoxin and lung injury. Am Rev Respir Dis. 133, 913–927.

37. Zapol W, Snider M. (1977). Pulmonary hypertension in severe acute respiratory failure. N Engl J Med. 296, 476–480.

38. MacKinzie IM. (2001). The hemodynamics of human septic shock. Anaesthesiology. 56 (2), 130–144.

39. Hess ML, Nastillo A, Greenfield LJ. (1981). Spectrum of cardiovascular function during gram-negative sepsis. Prog Cardiovasc Dis. 4, 279–298.

40. Parker MM, Shelhammer JH, Bacharach SL et al. (1984). Profound but reversible myocardial depression in patients with septic shock. Ann Intern Med. 100, 403–490.

41. Marino PL (1998). Infection, Inflammation and Multiorgan Injury. In: The ICU Book. pp 502–515.Williams and Wilkins, USA.

42. Rackow EC, Astiz ME, Weil MH. (1988). Cellular oxygen metabolism during sepsis and shock. JAMA. 259, 1989–1993.

43. Shoemaker WC, Appel PL,Kram HB. (1992). Sequence of physiological patterns in surgical septic shock. Chest. 102, 208–15.

44. Cone JB. (1987). Oxygen transport from capillary to cell. In : Oxygen Transport in the Critically Ill (Ed. Snyder JV). p 153. Year Book Medical, Chicago.

45. Dorinsky PM, Gadek JE. (1989). Mechanisms of multiple nonpulmonary organ failure in ARDS. Chest. 96, 885.

46. Cain SM. (1986). Assessment of tissue oxygenation. Critical Care Clinics. 2, 537.

47. Dorinsky PM, Costello JL, Gadek JE. (1988). Oxygen uptake-oxygen delivery relationships in non-ARDS respiratory failure. Chest. 93, 103.

48. Schumacher PT, Samsel RW. (1989). Oxygen delivery and uptake by peripheral tissues: Physiology and pathophysiology. Critical Care Clinics. 5, 255.

49. Kariman K, Burns SR. (1985). Regulation of tissue oxygen extraction is disturbed in adult respiratory distress syndrome. Am Rev Respir Dis. 132, 109.

50. Parrillo JE. (1991). Management of septic shock: present and future. Ann Intern Med. 115, 491–493.

51. Dellinger RP, Carlet JM, Masur H et al. (2004). Surviving sepsis campaign guidelines for management of severe sepsis and septic shock. Crit Care Med. 32,858–871.

52. Natanson C, Hoffman WD, Parrillo JE. (1989). Septic shock: the cardiovascular abnormality and therapy. J Cardiothorac Anaesthesia. 3, 215–227.

53. Waxman K, Nolan LS, Shoemaker WC. (1992). Sequential perioperative lactate determination. Crit Care Med. 10, 96–99.

54. Haupt MT, Gilbert EM, Carlson RW. (1985). Fluid loading increases oxygen consumption in septic patients with lactic acidosis. Am Rev Respir Dis. 131, 912–916.

55. Gilbert AM, Haupt MT, Mandanas RY et al. (1986). The effect of fluid loading, blood transfusion and catecholamine infusion on oxygen delivery and consumption in patients with sepsis. Am Rev Respir Dis. 134, 873–878.

56. SAFE Study Investigators. (2004). A comparison of albumin and saline for fluid resuscitation in the Intensive care unit. N Engl J Med. 350. 2247–2256.

57. Vincent JL, Van der Linden P, Domb M et al. (1987). Dopamine compared with dobutamine in experimental septic shock: Relevance to fluid administration. Anesth Analg. 66, 565–571.

58. Hoffman BB (2001). Catecholamine, sympathomimetic drugs, and adrenergic receptor antagonists. In: Goodman & Gilman's The Pharmacologic Basis of Therapeutics (Eds Hardman JG, Limbird LE). pp 215–268. McGraw-Hill, New York.

59. Patel BM, Chittcock DR et al. (2002). Beneficial effect of short-term vasopressin infusion during severe septic shock. Anaesthesiology. 96, 576–82.

60. Malay MB, Ashton RC, Landry DW et al. (2000). Low-dose vasopressin in the treatment of vasodilatory septic shock. J Trauma. 47, 699.

61. Romand JA, Treggiari-Venzi M. (2000). Is vasopressin an ideal vasopressor to treat hypotension in septic shock? Intens Care Med. 25, 763.

62. Shoemaker WC. (1987). Relation of oxygen transport patterns to the pathophysiology and therapy of shock states. Intensive Care Med. 13, 230–243.

63. Gattinoni L, Brazzi L, Pelosi P, et al. (1995). A trial of goal-oriented hemodynamic therapy in critically ill patients. N Engl J Med. 333, 1025.

64. Hayes MA, Timmons AC, Yau EHS, et al. (1994). Elevation of systemic oxygen delivery in the treatment of critically ill patients. N Engl J Med. 330, 1717.

65. Rivers E, Nguyen B, Havstad S et al. (2001). Early Goal-directed Therapy in the Treatment of Severe Sepsis and Septic Shock. N Engl J Med. 345 (19), 1368–77.

66. Esmon CT. (2001). Protein C anticoagulant pathway and its role in controlling microvascular thrombosis and inflammation. Crit Care Med. 29 (7)S, 48–51.

67. Bernard GR, Vincent JL, Laterre PF et al. (2001). Efficacy and safety of recombinant human activated protein C for severe sepsis. N Engl J Med. 344 (10), 699–709.

68. Annare D. (2001).Corticosteroids for septic shock. Crit Care Med. 29 (7)S, 117–20.

69. Bollaert PE, Charpentier C, Levy B et al. (1998). Reversal of late septic shock with supraphysiologic doses of hydrocortisone. 26, 645–50.

70. Schroeder S. (2001). The hypothalamic-pituary-adrenal axis of patients with severe sepsis: altered response to corticotropin-releasing hormone. Crit Care Med. 29(2), 310–6.

71. Berghe GV, Wouters P, Weekers F et al. (2001). Intensive insulin therapy in critically ill patients. N Engl J Med. 345.1359–1367.

72. Sperber SJ, Francis JB. (1987). Toxic shock syndrome during an influenza outbreak. JAMA. 257, 1086–1088.

73. Ciesielski CA, Broome CV. (1986). Toxic shock syndrome: Still in the differential. J Crit Illness. 1, 26–40.

Cardiac Compressive Shock

Compression of the heart and the great veins opening into the right heart can restrict and sharply reduce diastolic filling of the ventricles. This results in a low output state with inadequate tissue perfusion akin to the picture of cardiogenic shock. The classical cause of acute cardiac compression resulting in shock is cardiac tamponade due to accumulation of fluid within the pericardial sac. This chapter is devoted to the description of cardiac tamponade. Before we give the description, it should be noted that acute severe cardiac compression resulting in a shock-like low output state can also result from a tension pneumothorax. The problems here are further compounded by disturbances in pulmonary function and respiratory exchange due to acute compression collapse of one lung, with a marked shift of the mediastinum to the opposite side and by mediastinal flutter during inspiration and expiration. Acute cardiac compression can also occur in mechanical ventilation with PEEP. In the presence of very high intrathoracic pressures, the large veins opening into the right heart and the heart chambers are sufficiently compressed to sharply restrict diastolic filling and produce a low output state. A major contributory factor in this situation is the strain imposed on the right ventricle by increased vascular resistance within the pulmonary capillaries, and perhaps a further impairment of filling of the left ventricle by a septal shift that encroaches on the left ventricular volume.

Cardiac Tamponade

General Considerations

The pericardium has very little elasticity when acutely stretched. Therefore a very rapid accumulation of as little as 300–500 ml of fluid within the pericardial sac can result in a sharp rise in the intrapericardial pressure, and cause compression or 'tamponade' of the chambers of the heart. Fluid with a higher specific gravity, like blood or thick pus, will cause greater compression and greater tamponade. As little as 300 ml of thick pus formed acutely within the pericardial sac can lead to death from tamponade in children. On the other hand, a slow accumulation of fluid within the pericardial sac allows the pericardium to stretch maximally so that intrapericardial pressures may not be sufficiently raised to produce a serious tamponade even with an effusion of one litre or more.

Cardiac tamponade can result from pericardial effusions due to any cause. The important medical causes include acute viral (idiopathic) pericarditis, pericarditis secondary to metastatic neoplastic disease, uraemic pericarditis, purulent pericarditis, tuberculous pericarditis, pericarditis occurring in patients with myocardial infarction who have been anticoagulated, and occasionally in systemic lupus erythematosis. In tropical countries, a left lobe amoebic liver abscess rupturing into the pericardium, is a rare but important cause of tamponade.

In an emergency setting, unquestionably the most important cause is haemopericardium resulting from trauma and accidents. A dissection of the aorta which ruptures into the pericardial sac can also result in immediate tamponade and quick death.

In the ICU, post-operative bleeding following open heart or cardiothoracic surgery, and haemopericardium in sepsis and septic shock are important causes.

Diagnostic and therapeutic procedures performed in a critical care unit can sometimes be complicated by acute cardiac tamponade. Perforation of the right atrium by a central venous line, particularly when the line is used to administer fluids or is used for parenteral alimentation, is an important cause of acute cardiac tamponade. Perforation of the heart by a pacing catheter, or tear of the coronary artery during balloon angioplasty, or of the heart by catheters used for balloon valvuloplasty, can all cause haemopericardium, resulting in cardiac tamponade and death (**Table 6.5.1**).

Table 6.5.1. Iatrogenic causes of cardiac tamponade

* Post-operative haemorrhage following cardiac surgery
* Use of anticoagulants
* Barotrauma during mechanical ventilation
* Upper GI scopy or sclerotherapy resulting in oesophageal perforation
* Internal jugular or subclavian vein puncture
* Perforation of the heart by indwelling catheter (used for haemodynamic monitoring, pacing) or during angiography
* Perforation of the heart or coronary artery during balloon angioplasty

Physiopathology

A rapid accumulation of fluid within the pericardial sac leads to an acute increase in intrapericardial pressure. When this intrapericardial pressure rises to equal the atrial and the right ventricular diastolic pressures, the transmural pressure distending these chambers declines to about zero. A further accumulation of pericardial fluid leads to a further increase in the intrapericardial pressure and the right ventricular diastolic pressure, so that they now equal the left ventricular diastolic pressure. Cardiac tamponade thus occurs on equalization of the intrapericardial and ventricular filling pressures. This results in a marked fall in the distending pressure and therefore in the diastolic volumes of both ventricles, resulting in a fall in the stroke volume (1, 2). This reduction in stroke volume is initially compensated for by an increased adrenergic drive that causes tachycardia and an increase in the ejection fraction. To a lesser extent, it is also compensated for by an increase in circulatory volume due to salt and water retention induced by a decreased urinary excretion of sodium. A fall in sodium excretion is related to the reflex inhibition of the release of the atrial natriuretic factor (3) produced by a rise in intrapericardial pressure. With severe cardiac tamponade, the compensatory mechanisms do not suffice to prevent a sharp fall in cardiac output and in the systemic blood pressure, so that perfusion of vital organs is impaired. Reduced coronary perfusion results in subendocardial ischaemia (4). Sinus tachycardia is usually present, but sinus bradycardia may also occur through a reflex mediated by the cardiac depressor branches of the vagus nerve or through non-vagal mechanisms (5). Severe bradyrhythms foreshadow electromechanical dissociation and death in patients who are almost 'pressureless' because of severe tamponade.

Haemodynamic Profile

The haemodynamic profile in cardiac tamponade is characterized by a marked rise in the central venous and right atrial pressure, and by equalization of the right atrial, right ventricular diastolic and the pulmonary capillary wedge pressures. The PCWP is an index of the left ventricular diastolic pressure. If the intrapericardial pressure were to be measured, it would be found to be equivalent to the right atrial pressure, the right ventricular diastolic pressure and the PCWP. Tachycardia, hypotension and a raised systemic vascular resistance with poor tissue perfusion characterize the clinical haemodynamic profile.

A point worthy of note is that the rise in the right atrial (and intrapericardial) pressure is less marked in the presence of hypovolaemia, so that cardiac tamponade unless very severe, may be masked in hypovolaemic states.

Another point of note is that if the left ventricular diastolic pressure is elevated to start with because of left ventricular disease, then cardiac tamponade occurs when the intrapericardial, right atrial and right ventricular diastolic pressures become equal, but these pressures will be lower than the left ventricular diastolic pressure as gauged by the PCWP (6).

Clinical Features

The clinical features of acute cardiac tamponade are:

(i) A progressive rise in the central venous pressure as gauged by a clinical estimation of the jugular venous pressure, to +15 to +20 mm Hg. When hypovolaemia is associated with cardiac tamponade (as after trauma or accidental injuries), the central venous

pressure may not show the degree of rise normally expected. Such a 'low pressure tamponade' may pose difficulties in diagnosis. The liver is not usually enlarged in acute cardiac tamponade.

(ii) A falling arterial pressure. There is a progressive fall (initially in the systolic pressure), with an increasing inadequacy in tissue perfusion. This is characterized by oliguria, cold, sweating peripheries, restlessness, together with all the features of a rapidly evolving shock state.

(iii) A small quiet heart; the apex is not felt and the heart sounds are faint or inaudible. Clearly audible sounds do not however negate the diagnosis of cardiac tamponade.

(iv) A pulsus paradoxus. The volume of the pulse falls perceptibly during inspiration and increases during expiration and this can be best elicited by a sphygmomanometer. The cuff pressure is raised well above the systolic pressure, and is then very slowly lowered till Korotkoff's sounds are first heard only in expiration. The cuff is slowly further deflated so that the sounds are equally well heard both during inspiration and expiration. The difference between these pressures gives the magnitude of pulsus paradoxus—it exceeds 10 mm Hg in cardiac tamponade.

Complete disappearance of the pulse on inspiration can occur in severe tamponade. A pulsus paradoxus on palpation is often better appreciated in the carotids or femorals rather than in the radials, particularly when the volume of the pulse is low. At times a pulsus paradoxus not appreciated clinically or with a sphygmomanometer, can be demonstrated on recording the arterial pressure via an intra-arterial cannula. The degree of paradoxus in the arterial pulse is often significantly greater in direct arterial pressure recordings as compared with a clinical estimation using the sphygmomanometer.

A pulsus paradoxus in cardiac tamponade is merely an exaggeration of the normal physiology during inspiration which is characterized by a slight decrease in the left ventricular stroke volume and in the systolic arterial pressure. In cardiac tamponade, inspiration causes a decrease in the intrapericardial and right atrial pressures, with increased blood flow to the right ventricle. This increase in venous flow to the right ventricle during inspiration results in an increase in the dimensions and size of the right ventricle, the septum being straightened and pushed to the left. There is a resulting decrease in the left ventricular volume and size, with decrease in left atrial and left ventricular diastolic pressures. This leads to a fall in aortic flow and in systolic arterial pressure. Pulsus paradoxus in cardiac tamponade is thus chiefly related to increased inspiratory venous return and increasing flow into the right ventricle. Inspiratory pooling of blood within the lungs may result in a reduced gradient between the pulmonary venous circulation and the left heart, and this may be a minor contributory factor towards the observed inspiratory fall in left ventricular stroke volume and systolic arterial pressure.

(v) Tachycardia with a feeble pulse volume is invariably present. Bradycardia is often a pre-terminal event and precedes electromechanical dissociation and death.

(vi) Inspiratory swelling of the neck veins may be noted. Cardiac dullness may be increased on percussion, if there is a sufficiently large collection of fluid in the pericardial sac.

(vii) Patients with acute cardiac tamponade are tachypnoeic, restless, in 'shock', and may complain of precordial discomfort. A pericardial or a pleuropericardial rub may be heard. If hypotension is marked, the patient is generally obtunded.

Diagnosis (Table 6.5.2)

A well-marked rise in the CVP is a requisite for the diagnosis of cardiac tamponade, except in rare instances where hypovolaemia is associated with tamponade. In the latter situation, diagnosis is difficult and can only be arrived at if the background factors (trauma, injury) are kept in mind, and further relevant investigations done. It is important to recognize cardiac tamponade at a point in time when the chief physical finding is a rising CVP. A rise in CVP to + 15 mm Hg in the presence of a moderate sized pericardial effusion suffices for a diagnosis of cardiac tamponade. The diagnosis can be made with a lesser degree of rise in CVP if pulsus paradoxus > 10 mm Hg is present, or if the atrial and the right and left sided diastolic filling pressures are equalized. It is obviously unwise to wait for a falling blood pressure before making a correct diagnosis. Unfortunately, a rise in the CVP in a critical care setting can be due to several factors—notably overinfusion of intravenous fluids and myocardial dysfunction.

Acute right heart failure, due to right ventricular infarction, or massive pulmonary embolism may on clinical examination mimic acute cardiac tamponade as it produces a rise in the central venous pressure. Acute increase in the heart size with clear lung fields may further confuse the issue. However, the other clinical features of acute myocardial infarction and the presence of background features against which pulmonary embolism occurs, should help in the diagnosis. Pulsus paradoxus in the presence of a rising CVP always points to cardiac tamponade. Pulsus paradoxus is not observed in acute congestive heart failure, but may rarely be observed with massive pulmonary embolism.

The diagnosis of acute cardiac tamponade is frequently missed in acute bacterial pericarditis complicating acute pneumonias or sepsis. This is because a rapid accumulation of 250 ml of pus will demonstrate no clinical signs of fluid within the pericardial sac. A sudden clinical deterioration in a patient with lobar pneumonia or sepsis in the presence of a raised jugular venous pressure, should always suggest the correct diagnosis.

Chest X-Ray. A normal heart size does not rule out cardiac tamponade. A rapidly increasing cardiac silhouette with clear lung fields is however a feature of cardiac tamponade. Following open heart surgery, the presence of hypotension, raised CVP, and enlarged mediastinal shadow on an X-ray of the chest, strongly suggest cardiac tamponade.

ECG. The ECG may show features of electrical alternans of P, QRS and T waves but this is not commonly observed. A sudden fall in voltage in the ECG tracing should also suggest the development of pericardial effusion. A myocardial rupture following infarction is often associated with a slow junctional rhythm, promptly followed by electromechanical dissociation.

Echocardiography. Echocardiography is an accurate non-invasive test for demonstrating fluid within the pericardial sac. Certain echocardiographic signs are useful in the diagnosis of cardiac tamponade. These include reduced size of the right ventricular cavity, persistent distension of the inferior vena cava both during inspiration and expiration, inward movement of the free wall of the right ventricle in early diastole, and exaggerated variation of flow through the tricuspid orifice during respiration (7). Collapse of the right atrium and right ventricle in diastole is a fairly sensitive sign of pericardial effusion causing haemodynamic compromise.

Haemodynamic Profile. In an intensive care setting, provided that time is available, a haemodynamic study would show a raised atrial pressure and equalization of the atrial, right ventricular diastolic and left ventricular diastolic pressures. Equalization should always be measured at the end-expiratory phase, and it should be noted that the equalization need not be exact or perfect, particularly if the pulmonary capillary wedge or pulmonary artery end-diastolic pressure is used (as it invariably is) as a measure of the left ventricular diastolic pressure.

Management

(i) *Pericardiocentesis.* Acute cardiac tamponade particularly when due to haemopericardium as a result of trauma or injury, should be dealt with on an emergency basis. An immediate pericardiocentesis is mandatory. The technique of this procedure is described in a separate chapter.

Cardiac tamponade after open heart surgery necessitates resurgery to remove blood clots and fluid causing tamponade. Most surgeons prefer to relieve tamponade from other causes by a surgical procedure, wherein a 'pericardial window' is fashioned surgically and a drain left within the pericardial sac. The drain is removed when it stops draining. An antibiotic cover is generally necessary for a few days.

(ii) *Supportive Treatment.* Intravenous infusions and the use of catecholamines to raise the blood pressure play a very limited role, and may be used in the interim period between the recognition of tamponade and the relief of the condition by pericardiocentesis. This supportive therapy may help preserve perfusion to vital organs for a short period of time, but is never a substitute for relief of the tamponade by removal of the fluid compressing the chambers of the heart.

It is important to keep a close clinical watch after pericardiocentesis has been done to determine if tamponade recurs. A rising CVP is again an ominous sign. If a Swan-Ganz catheter is in situ, demonstration of an equalization of the atrial, right ventricular diastolic and pulmonary capillary wedge pressures should point to a recurrence of the tamponade.

Table 6.5.2. Diagnosis of cardiac tamponade

* Marked rise in CVP, tachycardia, hypotension
* Pulsus paradoxus > 10 mm Hg
* Chest X-ray—rapidly increasing cardiac silhouette with clear lung fields; increasing size of mediastinum after open heart surgery
* ECG—electrical alternans of P, QRS and T waves; sudden fall in voltage of tracing
* Echocardiography—collapse of the right atrium and the right ventricle in diastole is a very sensitive sign of pericardial effusion causing haemodynamic compromise
* Haemodynamic profile—raised atrial pressure; equalization of atrial, right and left ventricular diastolic pressures.

REFERENCES

1. Spodick DH. (1983). The normal and diseased pericardium: Current concepts of pericardial physiology, diagnosis and treatment. J Am Coll Cardiol. 1, 240.

2. Manyari DE, Kostuk WJ, Purves P. (1983). Effect of pericardiocentesis on right and left ventricular function and volumes in pericardial effusion. Am J Cardiol. 52, 159.

3. Mancini GBJ, McGillem MJ, Bates ER et al. (1987). Hormonal responses to cardiac tamponade: Inhibition of release of atrial natriuretic factor despite elevation of atrial pressures. Circulation. 76, 884.

4. Wechsler AS, Auerbach BJ, Graham TC, Sabiston DC. (1974). Distribution of intramyocardial blood flow during pericardial tamponade: Correlation with microscopic anatomy and intrinsic myocardial contractility. J Thorac Cardiovasc Surg. 68, 847.

5. Kostreva DR, Castaner A, Pedersen DH, Kampine JP. (1981). Nonvagally mediated bradycardia during cardiac tamponade or severe haemorrhage. Cardiology. 68, 65.

6. Reddy PS, Curtiss EI, O'Toole JD, Shaver JA. (1978). Cardiac tamponade: Hemodynamic observations in man. Circulation. 58, 265.

7. Hancock EW. (2001). Pericardial Tamponade. In: Critical Care Medicine, 2nd edn pp. 435–464 (Eds Parrillo JE, Dellinger RP). Mosby, USA.

Anaphylactic Shock

General Considerations (1)

The incidence of anaphylactic shock in hospitalized patients is around 1 in 10,000, and the fatality rate is as high as 10–20 per cent. Anaphylactic shock is an anamnestic response in which a sensitized individual comes in contact with an antigen. The antigen combines with specific IgE antibodies on mast cells and basophils, and induces the release of mediators such as histamine, platelet activating factor, and other mediators that mediate the anaphylactic response. The latter is characterized by severe vasodilatation, bronchoconstriction, pruritus and increased vascular permeability. The common precipitating agents for anaphylaxis include drugs, particularly penicillin. Other antibiotics can also give rise to anaphylaxis. Contrast material and blood products are important causes of anaphylaxis. In fact, almost any and every drug including steroids have been shown to cause an acute anaphylactic reaction at one time or another (2).

Anaphylactoid reactions are different from anaphylactic shock. The former are related to the direct release of mediators by the offending agent from mast cells and basophils without IgE antibodies coming into play. This direct release of mediators may be brought about by complement-mediated reactions, or by non-immunological activation of mast cells. Products of arachidonic acid breakdown include leukotrienes which increase vascular permeability and induce bronchoconstriction, as also thromboxanes and prostaglandins. Prostaglandin D_2 can further cause bronchoconstriction. Common etiological agents that result in anaphylactic shock and anaphylactoid reactions are listed in **Table 6.6.1**.

Clinical Features

Symptoms may occur instantaneously or within a few minutes after an intravenous injection of the offending agent. At times the reaction may develop after $1/_2$–1 hour of the exposure. Anaphylaxis to oral drugs may take 1–2 hours, but in many patients can be instantaneous.

The major features of anaphylactic shock include hypotension and circulatory collapse due to widespread peripheral vascular dilatation. Severe laryngeal oedema and obstruction, angio-oedema, overwhelming bronchoconstriction and fulminant

Table 6.6.1. Commonly used agents implicated in anaphylactic and anaphylactoid reactions

1. Antibiotics
   * Penicillin and analogs
   * Sulfonamides
   * Tetracyclines
   * Streptomycin
2. Local anaesthetics
   * Lidocaine
3. General anaesthetics and muscle relaxants
   * Thiopental
   * Tubocurarine
4. Nonsteroidal anti-inflammatory agents
5. Blood products and vaccines
   * Red blood cell, white blood cell and platelet transfusions
   * Gamma-globulin
   * Rabies
   * Tetanus
   * Diphtheria antitoxin
   * Snake and spider antivenoms
6. Diagnostic agents
   * Iodinated radiocontrast agents
7. Venoms
   * Bees, wasps, spiders, jelly fish
8. Hormones
   * Insulin
   * Hydrocortisone
   * Pituitary extracts
   * Vasopressin
9. Extracts of allergens used for desensitization
10. Foods
    * Eggs
    * Milk and milk products
    * Legumes (peanuts, soyabeans, kidney beans, chick peas)
    * Nuts
    * Shellfish
    * Citrus fruits
11. Other drugs
    * Protamine
    * Parenteral iron
    * Dextrans

pulmonary oedema may also occur either singly or in combination. Tachycardia, arrhythmias, syncope and seizures at times constitute the predominant clinical features. Diaphoresis, abdominal pain with cramps and diarrhoea may occur if death does not ensue following the sinister picture described above. Urticaria is often observed but may be totally absent in patients with fatal anaphylactic shock.

An increased haematocrit is often found due to haemoconcentration resulting from increased vascular permeability.

Differential Diagnosis (Table 6.6.2)

In a critical care setting, anaphylactic shock in a seriously ill patient may be mistaken for myocardial infarction, hypovolaemic or septic shock, or pulmonary embolism. Bronchoconstriction due to anaphylaxis may be wrongly imputed to aspiration of gastric contents. A sudden seizure with hypotension may be mistaken for a cerebrovascular accident. A temporal relationship to the administration of intravenous fluids, drugs or blood products should always arouse suspicion of the correct diagnosis.

Table 6.6.2. Conditions in the ICU to be distinguished from severe anaphylaxis

1. Cardiac problems in the ICU—acute myocardial infarction
2. Shock from any other cause—septic shock, hypovolaemic shock
3. Bronchoconstriction due to aspiration, asthmatic attack, pulmonary oedema from other causes
4. Pulmonary embolism
5. Cerebrovascular accident—causing seizures, hypotension
6. Vasovagal syncope

Treatment (3, 4) (Table 6.6.3)

The two immediate emergency measures to be instituted in anaphylactic shock are:

(i) Intubation to secure the airway before it is blocked by laryngeal oedema. Oxygen at high flow rates should be administered. Intubation may be extremely difficult even for an expert. If expert help is unavailable, or intubation fails and there is danger of asphyxia, an emergency airway must be secured (however inadequate this be), by puncturing the cricothyroid membrane by a large bore needle. A tracheostomy should be performed if intubation is impossible, as soon as surgical help is available.

(ii) Epinephrine which is the first drug to be administered, should be promptly given to every patient with anaphylaxis. We prefer to give it subcutaneously 0.5–1 ml of a 1 in 1000 solution. This may be repeated every 5–10 minutes if necessary. If the patient does not respond to the initial dose, or if laryngospasm or frank cardiovascular collapse is present, 5–10 ml of 1 in 10,000 solution of epinephrine is given intravenously. If intravenous access is not possible, 0.5–1 ml of a 1 in 1000 solution is given intramuscularly, or 10 ml of a 1 in 10,000 solution of epinephrine may be instilled through the endotracheal tube. A maintenance intravenous infusion of epinephrine may be necessary after the initial bolus dose.

Volume Load. This is the next most important aspect of therapy. In a critical care setting, a venous line is generally already present. We prefer to use crystalloids, though colloids produce quicker volume expansion, for fear of inducing further allergic reactions to colloidal solutions. Short, wide peripheral catheters permit quicker fluid infusions than long, thin central venous lines. Again, collapse of large veins due to circulatory shock increases the risk of iatrogenic complications associated with the insertion of central lines. An iatrogenic pneumothorax for example, in such a patient, would compound difficulties in management.

Table 6.6.3. Management of anaphylactic shock

1. Intubate and administer oxygen at high flow rates. If intubation not possible, emergency tracheostomy, or puncture of cricothyroid membrane.
2. Epinephrine 0.5–1 ml of 1:1000 solution subcutaneously; this can be repeated every 10 minutes, and is followed by a maintenance infusion of epinephrine.
3. If no response to subcutaneous epinephrine, or if laryngospasm or cardiovascular collapse present, 5–10 ml of 1:10,000 solution of epinephrine given IV.
4. If intravenous access unavailable, 0.5–1 ml of 1:1000 solution of epinephrine given IM, or 10 ml of 1:10,000 solution instilled through endotracheal tube.
5. Administer volume load.
6. Use antihistaminic e.g. diphenhydramine 1 mg/kg IV, and repeat 6 hourly.
7. Relief of bronchospasm by IV aminophylline 250 mg in 20 ml dextrose.
8. Hydrocortisone 300 mg IV stat, followed by 100 mg IV 6 hourly.
9. If hypotension persists despite epinephrine, volume load and antihistaminics, start dopamine infusion. If this also does not raise the BP, start epinephrine infusion.
10. Ventilatory support with high FIO_2 may be required in critically ill patients.

After the above management protocol has been instituted, one can use an antihistaminic like diphenhydramine 1 mg/kg intravenously, and repeat the dose 6 hourly if necessary. Aminophylline 250 mg intravenously in 20 ml dextrose helps reduce the bronchospasm. Hydrocortisone 300 mg intravenously, followed by 100 mg 6 hourly may prevent the late manifestations of anaphylaxis. Steroids have little or no role in the immediate alleviation of anaphylactic shock.

If hypotension persists after the use of epinephrine, volume load and antihistaminics, a dopamine infusion starting with 5 µg/kg/minute and titrated if so required to 10–20 µg/kg/minute, is infused to increase the blood pressure. If dopamine proves ineffective, then an infusion of epinephrine in a concentration of 3–4 µg/min is started and slowly increased till a rise in blood pressure is observed. Patients receiving beta-blockers at the time of acute anaphylaxis may fail to respond adequately to epinephrine. Intravenous atropine and glucagon are useful aids to reverse circulatory shock in such patients. Critically ill patients may need both cardiovascular support and ventilatory support with a high FIO_2 till such time as recovery slowly ensues.

REFERENCES

1. Haupt MT, Fujii TK, Carlson RW. (1998). Anaphylactic Reactions. In: Textbook of Critical Care, 4th edn (Eds Shoemaker WC, Grenvik A, Ayres SM, Holbrook PR). pp. 246–258. WB Saunders Company, Philadelphia.

2. Fisher M. (1987). Anaphylaxis. Volume 8. Disease-a-Month. Year Book Medical Publishers, Chicago.

3. Perkin RM, Anas NG. (1985). Mechanisms and management of anaphylactic shock not responding to traditional therapy. Ann Allergy. 54, 202–208.

4. Haupt MT. (2001). Anaphylaxis and Anaphylactic Shock. In: Critical Care Medicine, 2nd edn (Eds Parrillo JE, Dellinger RP). pp. 513–526. Mosby, USA.

Cardiovascular Problems Requiring Critical Care

7.1 Acute Coronary Syndromes

7.2 Unstable Angina

7.3 Acute Myocardial Infarction

7.4 Acute Left Ventricular Failure with Pulmonary Oedema

7.5 Tachyarrhythmias in the ICU

7.6 Bradyrhythms and Heart Blocks in the ICU

7.7 Antiarrhythmic Drugs Used in the ICU

7.8 Hypertensive Crisis and Aortic Dissection in the ICU

7.9 Pulmonary Embolism

Acute Coronary Syndromes

General considerations

Acute coronary syndromes are due to an acute disturbance in coronary artery circulation resulting in myocardial ischaemia which if severe or prolonged could progress to myocardial infarction. The syndromes include the classical triad of unstable angina, non Q-wave myocardial infarction and Q-wave myocardial infarction. These are not separate entities but form a related continuum of the same disease process. Even so, each of these three acute coronary syndromes has a differing prognosis and specific strategies in management. (**Fig. 7.1.1**).

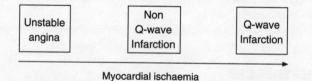

Fig. 7.1.1. Acute coronary syndromes—spectrum of clinical manifestations of myocardial ischaemia.

Critical care therefore demands that patients presenting with ischaemic cardiac pain be placed into one of these three syndromes. This can be achieved by integrating the history and clinical findings with the evolution in time of the 12 lead electrocardiogram and the quantification over time of the biological markers of myocardial cell necrosis. Since acute coronary syndromes form a dynamic continuum, patients diagnosed to start with as unstable angina, may during observation and investigation over time, ultimately develop into a non Q-wave or Q-wave myocardial infarct. Similarly, patients categorized as non Q-wave myocardial infarcts may also occasionally develop Q-wave infarcts. The dividing line between unstable angina and non Q-wave myocardial infarct may at times be tenuous. Microinfarction detected by a slight rise in the newer sensitive biological cardiac markers may well be an additional event between unstable angina and non Q-wave infarction. (**1**).

Acute myocardial ischaemia, besides producing unstable angina, non Q-wave myocardial infarction and Q-wave myocardial infarction (the classic triad of acute coronary syndromes), can also result in other clinical presentations. These include sudden death, cardiac arrhythmias causing palpitation, presyncope or syncope,

acute pulmonary oedema due to severe left ventricular failure. These presentations of myocardial ischaemia should logically also be included under acute coronary syndromes. They may present without anginal pain and without ECG or biochemical evidence of myocardial infarction.

Physiopathology

Most patients with acute coronary syndromes have significant obstructive atherosclerotic lesions in the coronary arteries. Acute myocardial ischaemia can be precipitated either by a sharp reduction in supply of oxygen (e.g. a thrombus obstructing the coronary lumen or vasospasm), or a significant increase in oxygen demand (e.g. an acute rise in the blood pressure or tachycardia). Both a reduction in oxygen supply and an increase in oxygen demand may operate in the same patient.

The major precipitants of the acute coronary syndrome are briefly described below (**2**):

(i) Rupture or erosion of an atherosclerotic plaque with a resulting thrombus obstructing the lumen of a coronary artery. This is the most frequent and important pathogenic mechanism. Remarkably enough, the vulnerable plaques (i.e. plaques prone to rupture) are not the tightly stenotic lesions but lesions with usually less than 50 per cent stenosis (**3**). These lesions may not be visualized by a coronary angiography.

Plaque rupture or erosion is precipitated by biochemical causes. These include liquid lipid content within the plaque, inflammation with erosion of a thin fibrous cap overlying the plaque and local shear stress forces. A ruptured atherosclerotic plaque exposes the underlying subendocardial matrix to the circulating blood. Initially, this leads to platelet adhesion followed by platelet activation. The latter results in the release of Thromboxane A_2, serotonin and other chemotactic agents which are strong vasoconstrictors. Platelet activation also results in expression and activation of glycoprotein II B/III A receptors on the platelet surface so that it can bind fibrinogen. The final step is platelet aggregation with the formation of a platelet plug over the plaque rupture site. Together with the formation of a platelet plug, there is activation of the coagulation system within the plasma initiated through the release of tissue factor. Activation of factor X to factor Xa leads to the generation of thrombin which converts fibrinogen to fibrin. Thrombin once formed acts as a powerful stimulus for platelet aggregation; thrombin also activates factor XIII which leads to stabilization of the fibrin clot. The pivotal role of a thrombus partially or completely occluding a coronary artery in the pathogenesis of acute coronary syndromes is supported by substantial evidence (4).

(ii) Inflamation and infection. Inflammation may well play an important role in the formation of atherosclerotic lesions and in the erosion or rupture of vulnerable plaques. (5). The role of infectious agents, in particular chlamydia pneumoniae in causing such inflammation is the subject of current research (6).

(iii) Coronary vasoconstriction. Coronary vasoconstriction reduces coronary blood flow and occurs in the following situations:

(a) in the presence of coronary atherosclerotic lesions, particularly with plaques;

(b) in 'microcirculatory angina', caused by spasm of intramural vessels;

(c) in Prinzmetal angina. The latter is associated with severe focal spasm either at the site of a mild to moderate obstructive lesion, or at the site of a non-obstructive plaque, or in patients without coronary atherosclerosis. These patients typically present with severe rest angina with transient ST elevation occuring during episodes of anginal pain.

(iv) Progressive mechanical obstruction. Progressive luminal narrowing is most frequently observed when restenosis occurs after a coronary angioplasty. However, it can also occur in patients who have no intracoronary procedures performed on them. It is due to rapid proliferation of cells within the stenotic lesion leading to a critical obstruction of the lumen.

(v) Increased myocardial oxygen demand. In patients with stable coronary artery disease, a sharp increase in myocardial oxygen demand due to extrinsic factors may precipitate the acute coronary syndrome, particularly unstable angina. Increased myocardial oxygen demand occurs in:

(a) sudden increase in blood pressure, in increasing aortic stenosis;

(b) tachycardia due to fever, anaemia, thyrotoxicosis, supraventricular tachycardia, atrial fibrillation with a fast ventricular rate, other hyperdynamic circulatory states.

The acute coronary syndrome could also be precipitated or worsened by:

(a) impaired oxygen delivery as in patients with a low output syndrome, anaemia, hypoxia from any cause, hyperviscosity states;

(b) metabolic derangements—in particular hypoglycaemia.

The clinical determinants of the acute coronary syndromes are related to the severity and duration of myocardial ischaemia.

Unstable angina is generally induced by a temporary, nonoccluding thrombus within the coronary artery lumen (7). Thrombus formation is a dynamic process—a thrombus after being

formed may in time be fibrinolysed. Temporary and repeated accretions of fresh thrombi over the site of plaque rupture may critically narrow the lumen to produce rest angina. Partial spontaneous resolution of the thrombus within 10 to 20 minutes would provide relief and this generally occurs in unstable angina.

In a non Q-wave myocardial infact, the thrombus is larger and generally does not completely occlude the lumen. It may cause significant obstruction for 20 to 30 minutes before being partially, or at times completely resolved. The degree of myocardial ischaemia is significantly great to cause myocardial necrosis with liberation of cardiac enzymes. However, the degree of necrosis and the infarct size is small compared to the Q-wave myocardial infarct.

In a Q-wave myocardial infarct, there is a thrombus that completely occludes a coronary vessel in over 95 per cent of patients. This can lead to fairly extensive necrosis (a Q-wave infarct), surrounded by an area of injury, which is in turn, surrounded by an area of ischaemia.

Whether a partially or a completely obstructing thrombus in a coronary artery results in unstable angina, a non-Q wave infarct or a Q-wave infarct, will to an extent be also influenced by the presence or absence of coronary collaterals, by the degree of coronary vasoconstriction and by associated increase in myocardial oxygen demand.

It is to be noted that the earlier classification of myocardial infarction into subendocardial and transmural has been given up, as these descriptions are clinically inaccurate when correlated with autopsy findings.

The subsequent sections now deal with the diagnosis and management of unstable angina and myocardial infarction.

REFERENCES

1. American Heart Association, Advanced Cardiac Life Support. (1997–99). p. 91.

2. Cannon CP, Braunwald E. (2001). Unstable Angina In: Heart Disease—A Textbook of Cardiovascular Medicine, 6th edn (Ed. Eugene Braunwald). pp. 1232–1236. W B Saunders Company, Philadelphia.

3. The TIMI IIIA Investigators. (1993). Early effects of tissue-type plasminogen activator added to conventional therapy on the culprit lesion in patients presenting with ischemic cardiac pain at rest: Results of the Thrombolysis in Myocardial Infarction (TIMI) III Trials. Circulation. 87, 38–52.

4. Falk E. (1985). Unstable angina with fatal outcome: Dynamic coronary thrombus leading to infarction and/or sudden death. Circulation. 71, 699–708.

5. Berk BC, Weintraub WS, Alexander RW. (1990). Elevation of C Reactive protein in "active" coronary artery disease. Am J Cardiol. 65, 168–172.

6. Danesh J, Collins R, Peto R. (1997). Chronic Infection and coronary heart disease: Is there a link? Lancet. 350, 430–436.

7. Foster V. (1994). Mechanisms leading to myocardial infarction: Insights from studies of vascular biology. Circulation. 90, 2126–2146.

CHAPTER 7.2

Unstable Angina

Unstable angina can be defined as new onset or worsening angina within the past 60 days, or post-infarction angina occurring 24 hours after the onset of myocardial infarction. Unstable angina signifies a seriously prejudiced circulation in the coronary arteries and carries with it a risk of myocardial infarction, serious cardiac arrhythmias, cardiac failure and sudden death. The problem is therefore of immense concern and of great importance to the critical care physician.

The diagnosis of unstable angina depends on the presence of one or more of the following:

(i) New-onset angina—i.e. angina occurring for the first time within a one month period, and brought on by minimal exertion.

(ii) Increasing severity of a previously stable angina. This may take the form of more protracted anginal pain, or pain with more extensive radiation, or more frequent angina (more than 3 times a day), or angina brought on by less effort or by other precipitating factors which previously had not produced any discomfort. Angina which is incompletely relieved or unrelieved by nitroglycerin, also denotes a worsening pattern and constitutes unstable angina. The increase in frequency and severity of angina is superimposed on a pattern of a relatively stable exertion-related angina.

(iii) Rest angina denotes anginal episodes at rest. In the acute or emergent form, many such anginal episodes may occur over 24 hours. At times angina at rest may occur more frequently at night. In the less emergent (yet dangerous) situations, rest angina may occur at infrequent intervals after lapses of 2 or more days.

Braunwald (1) has proposed a clinical classification taking into consideration three degrees of clinical severity, three clinical circumstances, the response to medical therapy and the presence or absence of ECG changes. The increasing degree of clinical severity is classed as follows (1):

Class I—severe or frequent new onset angina (< 2 months).

Class II—rest angina in the past month, but not during previous 48 hours.

Class III—anginal attacks at rest within prior 48 hours.

The three 'clinical circumstances' considered by Braunwald are as follows (1):

(i) Patients with secondary angina (Class A); there is a secondary cause that exacerbates angina (e.g. anaemia, fever, hypoxaemia, tachyarrhythmia, thyrotoxicosis, hypoglycaemia).

(ii) Patients in whom no precipitating cause can be found (Class B).

(iii) Patients with post-infarction angina (within 2 weeks of a myocardial infarct).

Braunwald (1) also considered symptom severity and clinical circumstances of a given patient in relation to treatment—whether the patient was not on treatment prior to unstable angina, on treatment for previous stable angina, and finally whether unstable angina persisted in spite of maximal treatment. Braunwald's classification has been shown to correlate with clinical outcomes. Patients with severe angina (class III), poor response to full medical treatment, ST-T changes on the ECG, and those with post-infarction angina have poorer outcomes (2). A higher clinical grading was predictive of plaques with thrombus at angiography (2).

The diagnosis of unstable angina rests chiefly on a good clinical history. The basic characteristics of the pain are similar to those observed in stable angina. The pain is substernal and often precordial, and is described as heaviness, constriction, and at times as just severe pain. It is often interpreted as a feeling of choking in the chest or throat. In unstable angina the duration of pain may be as long as 15 minutes and may extend to even 30 minutes. The typical sites of radiation include the left shoulder, arm, forearm, hand, right shoulder and upper arm, both shoulders and arms, the jaw, the neck, the back and the upper abdomen. On occasion, the pain may not be felt in the chest at all, but may only be experienced at one or more sites of radiation mentioned above.

The diagnosis of unstable angina in a patient with a past history of myocardial infarction, or a typical history of angina on effort, generally presents no difficulty. New onset angina characterized by frequent chest pain at rest may require careful evaluation of the history and a close follow-up, to help distinguish it from non-anginal or noncardiac pain. There are some important negative points which help in the diagnosis of ischaemic heart pain: (i) pain localized to the apex is almost always non-anginal; (ii) jabbing or pricking pain is also generally non-anginal in aetiology; (iii) pain which worsens on local pressure, or pain which is clearly aggravated by movement is also definitely non-anginal.

Physical findings in unstable angina are more often than not negative. During an attack of pain, one may hear a third heart sound at the apex, a reversed split of the second sound at the base, and a mid to late mitral systolic murmur of papillary muscle dysfunction. Rarely, frequent extrasystoles or even supraventricular or ventricular arrhythmias occur after the onset of pain, and may disappear after the pain subsides.

ECG. Transient ST elevation or depression, or T wave inversion may occur during the pain. However, absence of ECG changes even during periods of severe cardiac pain in no way rules out a diagnosis of unstable angina. Continuous ECG monitoring may at times reveal ST depression characteristic of myocardial ischaemia or may detect transient arrythmias. In patients with a past history of ischaemic heart disease or when previous investigations clearly denote ischaemic heart disease, the diagnosis of unstable angina can be confidently made on a history alone, even in the absence of ECG changes during episodes of pain. It is only in the group of patients without a history of previous stable angina or previous ischaemic heart disease, that the diagnosis of unstable angina without any ECG changes becomes difficult or inaccurate.

Serum Enzyme Levels. The enzyme levels of CK-MB, Troponin I and T and LDH are generally normal. By definition, if the CK-MB and Troponin levels are significantly elevated, the patient has suffered a myocardial infarction even though the clinical manifestation is that of unstable angina and the ECG shows no or little evidence of infarction. Some patients of severe unstable angina may however show a small rise in cardiac enzymes. We still categorize them as unstable angina even though these patients may in fact well have experienced small discrete areas of microvascular infarction (see Pathogenesis of Acute Coronary Syndromes). It is to be noted that even a slight rise in the CK-MB and Troponin levels in these patients is predictive of subsequent cardiac complications.

Specific Unstable Angina Syndromes

(i) Unstable angina after angioplasty. Unstable angina after angioplasty is related to restenosis and occurs in over 30 per cent of patients. It may present as angina at rest.

(ii) Unstable angina after bypass surgery. If this occurs within 6 months after surgery it may signify a single active lesion. Later it often signifies obstruction to venous grafts.

(iii) Prinzmetal angina is a vasospastic variant of unstable angina (see Acute Coronary Syndromes). The pain in this variant typically occurs at night or in the early hours of the morning. It is characterized by transient ST elevation during pain and is relieved by nitroglycerine and by calcium channel blockers.

Principles of Management (Table 7.2.1) (3)

These are as follows:

(i) Treat active myocardial ischaemia.

(ii) Prevent further or recurrent episodes of myocardial ischaemia.

(iii) Attempt to dissolve and/or prevent platelet aggregation or a thrombus which may block a coronary vessel.

(iv) Explore the possibility of invasive procedures e.g. angioplasty or bypass surgery in patients not responding to medical treatment.

General Principles

Unstable angina spells danger and the patient must be admitted for critical care in an intensive care unit. The ECG should be continuously monitored, an intravenous line secured and serial enzyme estimations of CK-MB and Troponin I and T should be done to exclude a myocardial infarction. Thallium scans, or 2D echocardiograms are not helpful in the immediate management, and are best deferred as they may exhaust the patient and worsen his angina.

Table 7.2.1. Management of unstable angina

* General Measures
  - Critical care monitoring
  - Serial estimations of Troponin T, Troponin I, CK-MB to exclude acute myocardial infarction
  - Sublingual nitroglycerin to relieve myocardial ischaemia
  - Diazepam for relief of anxiety
  - Morphine 2–4 mg IV if pain severe
* Nitrates
  - Nitroglycerin drip at 10 µg/min, and gradually increased till angina controlled. Systolic BP should not fall < 100 mm Hg
  - Later oral isosorbide dinitrate 10 mg 6 hrly, or sublingual isosorbide dinitrate or nitroglycerin
* Beta-blockers
  - For ongoing severe pain—metoprolol 5 mg IV repeated at 5 min intervals—watch heart rate, BP; then oral metoprolol or propranolol titrated to maintain heart rate between 55–60/min
* Calcium Antagonists
  - use only if ischaemia persists in spite of nitrates and β-blockers, diltiazem 30–60 mg 8 hourly or verapamil 40 mg 8 hourly
* Anticoagulants, Antiplatelet drugs, Gp IIb-IIIa receptor inhibitors
  - Either unfractionated heparin (IV 5000 units bolus, followed by 500–1000 units/hour) for 3–7 days or low molecular weight heparin (enoxaparin 1 mg/kg 12 hourly) for 3–7 days + aspirin 300 mg + clopidogrel 75 mg daily. Eptifibatide (180 µg/kg IV, followed by infusion of 2 µg/kg/min for 96 hours) or tirofiban (loading dose 0.4 mg/kg/min for 30 min, followed by 0.1 mg/kg/min for 96 hours, together with unfractionated heparin could be used in refractory or high-risk unstable angina. Risk of bleeding with this therapy
* Treat factors precipitating/aggravating unstable angina
* Coronary Angiography—Indicated if pain is unrelieved or marginally relieved with the above treatment, or if anginal episodes worsen

Emergency Management

The patient is given 300 mg aspirin to be chewed and swallowed. Oxygen is given through nasal prongs or a mask at 4 l/min. Sorbitrate 5 mg is given sublingually for relief of angina; this can be repeated after 5 minutes while closely monitoring the blood pressure and clinical effects. If pain is unrelieved, or even otherwise with a history of protracted cardiac pain, intravenous nitroglycerine is started. Severe pain may require the initial use of intravenous morphine (2–4 mg) or intravenous buprenorphine (0.3 mg). It is crucial to relieve pain; pain induces an increased catecholamine state which increases anxiety, heart rate, blood pressure and cardiac contractility, thereby increasing myocardial oxygen demand and myocardial ischaemia.

A quick but careful search for possible factors aggravating or precipitating unstable angina should be made and if possible these should be corrected. Increased myocardial oxygen demands with resulting angina can occur with fever, tachycardia, thyrotoxicosis, tachyrhythms, bradyrhythms or hypoglycaemia. Hypovolaemia due to fluid loss in vomiting and diarrhoea can also precipitate unstable angina. In patients with asthma or chronic lung problems, exacerbation of their pulmonary disease can produce hypoxaemia, which in turn worsens the angina. Recent blood loss (as after a GI bleed) or anaemia from any cause, can also precipitate unstable angina. A careful assessment of the associated problems outlined above may help in overall management and results in a quick stabilization of the angina. Acute mental stress from whatever cause should be promptly recognized, and benzodiazepines given to relieve anxiety. **Table 7.2.2** lists the important aggravating or precipitating factors of unstable angina.

Table 7.2.2. Important aggravating/precipitating factors of unstable angina

* Conditions increasing myocardial oxygen demand eg. fever, thyrotoxicosis, hypoglycaemia, tachyrhythmias including sinus tachycardia, severe bradyrhythmias
* Hypovolaemia due to fluid loss as in diarrhoea/vomiting
* Exacerbation of chronic lung problems eg. in patients with asthma or COPD
* Recent blood loss (e.g. GI bleed), or anaemia from any cause
* Acute mental stress

Nitrates

Nitrates act as coronary vasodilators and also act by reducing the preload, and therefore the work performed by the heart. They can be given sublingually (nitroglycerin or isosorbide dinitrate), orally (isosorbide dinitrate 10 mg 6 hourly), or intravenously. Intravenous nitroglycerin is preferred in patients with recurrent or protracted pain, as the onset of action is immediate, the duration of action short, and the drug can be titrated with a fair degree of precision. Recent studies in humans suggest that intravenous nitroglycerin in therapeutic doses has an inhibitory effect on platelet aggregation (4). The drip should be started at 10 μg/minute, and increased gradually till the angina is controlled. We never exceed a dose of > 100 μg/minute. Systolic arterial blood pressure is often reduced following a nitroglycerin infusion, but should not be allowed to drop to < 100 mm Hg. Nitrate induced hypotension is countered by reducing the dose or temporarily stopping the infusion. If needs be a small volume load of 150–250 ml may be necessary to restore a sudden sharp reduction in blood pressure.

Tachyphylaxis is often observed with nitroglycerin in that its anti-anginal effect is reduced despite a constant drug infusion. The infusion rate should be increased slightly by about 10 per cent every 24 hours to maintain efficacy. We generally wean the patient off nitroglycerin 3–7 days after the last episode of angina. Oral isosorbide dinitrate can then be started in a dose of 10 mg 6 hourly, or a topical nitrate paste can be applied on the skin as a 1 to 2 inch patch, every 8 hours.

Beta-blockers

Beta-blockers are useful in the management of unstable angina. The combination of nitrates and beta-blockers has been shown to reduce symptoms of myocardial ischaemia (5–7) and the occurrence of myocardial infarction (5, 6) in patients with unstable angina. Beta-blockers reduce myocardial oxygen demand by decreasing the heart rate and arterial blood pressure. They are particularly useful in those who have a well-marked tachycardia, provided the latter is not due to left ventricular failure or to volume depletion. Beta-blockers are recommended for patients with unstable angina (and non ST elevation myocardial infarction) provided there are no contraindications. Contraindications to beta-blockers include bradycardia, pulmonary oedema, hypotension, advanced atrio-ventricular block and a history of bronchial asthma or well marked chronic airways obstruction. A mild to moderate reduction of the ejection fraction is no longer a contraindication to the use of beta-blockers. In the presence of ongoing ischaemic pain, metaprolol is given in a dose of 5 mg intravenously at 5 minute intervals, while closely monitoring heart rate and blood pressure. Subsequently 50 mg metaprolol is given orally twice daily. The dose should be titrated to provide adequate beta-blockade. The pulse rate should not fall below 60/minute and the systolic blood pressure not less than 100 mm Hg. A careful watch should also be kept over the lung bases for evolving pulmonary oedema, particularly in those with lowered ejection fraction. Esmolol is a beta-blocker with a very short duration of action and can be given in titrated doses intravenously when contraindications to the use of beta-blockers (e.g. history of possible bronchospasm) are suspected. Untoward effects of beta-blockade are reversed soon after Esmolol is stopped.

Calcium Antagonists

Calcium antagonists are currently recommended only in patients who have persistent ischaemia in spite of the use of nitrates and beta-blockers or in patients in whom beta-blockade is contraindicated.

Diltiazem or verapamil are calcium channel blockers which slow the heart rate. They are given in a dose of 30 to 90 mg four times a day, both in unstable angina and in non Q-wave myocardial infarct (8). Amlodipine or felodipine can also be used safely but nifedepine has been shown to increase adverse events when not co-administered with a beta-blocker (9). Diltiazem is best avoided in patients with left ventricular dysfunction or congestive cardiac failure because of its negative inotropic effect.

Anticoagulant Therapy

Unfractionated intravenous heparin reduces the risk of death, myocardial ischaemia, myocardial infarction in acute coronary syndromes. A bolus dose of 5000 U is followed by an intravenous infusion of 450 to 1000 U/hour titrated to prolong the activated partial thromboplastin time to $1\frac{1}{2}$ to 2 times the control. Treatment is generally continued for 2 to 5 days till the patient is stable or until after an interventional procedure is carried out in patients with persistent or recurring angina. Several studies have shown lower death rates and lower incidence of myocardial infarction with the use of unfractionated heparin in addition to aspirin, than with aspirin alone (10).

Low molecular weight heparins (heparin chains with a molecular weight of less than 5400 daltons) are produced by different methods of depolymerization. Low molecular weight heparins inhibit factor Xa reducing both thrombin (IIa) and thrombin generation (Xa). They have a longer half life and are given subcutaneously twice daily. They do not require monitoring or dose adjustments. Heparin induced thrombocytopenia is less common with low molecular weight heparins than with unfractionated heparin.

The efficacy and safety of subcutaneous Enoxaparin (a low molecular weight heparin) in non Q-wave coronary events (ESSENCE) trial (11) demonstrated a benefit of Enoxaparin over unfractionated heparin in non ST segment elevation acute coronary syndromes. The Thrombolysis in Myocardial Infarction (TIMI) IIB study (12) also showed Enoxaparin to be superior to unfractionated heparin. A meta-analysis of the ESSENCE and TIMI IIB trials (13) showed that Enoxaparin therapy resulted in a 20 per cent reduction in rates of death and major ischaemic events that was sustained till 30 days.

Thus low molecular weight heparin (e.g. Enoxaparin in a dose of 1 mg/kg 12 hourly subcutaneously for 3–7 days) can safely and effectively replace fractionated heparin. It must however be remembered that there is no easily available assay to measure the effect of low molecular weight heparin on factor Xa levels. Interventional cardiologists prefer the use of unfractionated heparin to low molecular weight heparin in patients going immediately to the catheterization laboratory.

The major danger of both low molecular weight heparin and unfractionated heparin is bleeding and in our experience occurs with equal frequency with either therapy.

Antiplatelet Therapy

Antiplatelet therapy is important and effective in unstable angina.

Aspirin

Aspirin is useful during the acute phase and also in secondary prevention. An immediate dose of 300 mg is followed by a dose of 150 mg daily. The use of aspirin prevents the formation of thromboxane A_2 by platelets. Thromboxane A_2 is a powerful vasoconstrictor and activator of platelet aggregation.

Ticlopidine and Clopidogrel

Both these drugs inhibit adenosine diphosphate mediated platelet activation. Their action is independent of the arachidonic acid pathway and their antiplatelet activity is synergistic to that of aspirin.

Ticlopidine. Ticlopidine has a slow action reaching a plateau effect after 2 weeks. It produces neutropaenia in 1–3 per cent patients, can cause dermatologic side effects and in rare instances results in severe cholestatic hepatitis. Its use has been largely replaced by clopidogrel.

Clopidogrel. Originally clopidogrel was recommended only in patients who were intolerant to aspirin or in those in whom aspirin was contraindicated. It is now recommended as an addition to aspirin therapy (14). There is however an increased risk of bleeding when aspirin and clopidogrel are used together (14). The dose of clopidogrel is 300 mg for the first day, followed by 75 mg daily. Its antiplatelet activity is manifest in 2 hours and reaches its peak

between 4 to 7 days. The optimal duration of clopidogrel treatment has not been determined. We have used it in high risk patients for well over a year without running into serious problems.

Gp IIb-IIIa receptor antagonists

Platelet activation plays a crucial role in thrombus formation over a ruptured atheromatous plaque. Regardless of the reasons for platelet activation, Gp IIb-IIIa receptors on the platelet surface constitute the final common pathway for interaction between platelets and thrombus. The Gp IIb-IIIa receptor antagonists inhibit platelet activation and prevent thrombus formation.

The Gp IIb-IIIa receptor antagonists commercially available are: abciximab (ReoPro), eptifibatide (Integrelin) and tirofiban hydrochloride (Aggrastat). They have been approved for the treatment of refractory or high-risk unstable angina. However, abciximab is currently approved only for use during planned percutaneous coronary intervention or cardiac catheterization. Both eptifibatide or tirofiban are administered with unfractionated heparin in a dose titrated to increase the partial thromboplastin time to $1^1/_2$ to 2 times normal. Eptifibatide is administered as an intravenous bolus dose of 180 µg/kg followed by an infusion of 2 µg/kg/min for 72 to 96 hours. Tirofiban is given as an intravenous loading dose of 0.4 mg/kg/min for 30 minutes, followed by an infusion of 0.1 µg/kg/min for 48 to 96 hours.

Bleeding due to thrombocytopaenia is the major complication and occurs in up to 0.7 per cent of cases. Eptifibatide and tirofiban must be dose-adjusted in patients with raised creatinine levels; they are best avoided if the serum creatinine level is > 2 mg/dl.

Contraindications to Gp IIb-IIIa receptor antagonists include surgery or GI haemorrhage within less than 6 weeks, cerebrovascular accidents or neurosurgical interventions within less than 6 months and platelet count < 100,000/mm³.

The use of intravenous abciximab has significantly decreased major cardiac events in patients undergoing coronary angioplasties (15–17).

Both eptifibatide and tirofiban are reported to reduce mortality, myocardial infarction and the need for urgent revascularization (18). They are indicated only for a certain subset of severe unstable angina as also in non-elevated ST-segment myocardial infarction. In the present state of our knowledge and experience, the use of these drugs should be considered only in high risk cases presenting with refractory chest pain, dynamic ST segment changes, with slight elevation of the cardiac enzymes.

Thrombolytic Therapy

Thrombolytic therapy is not indicated in unstable angina or in non Q-wave myocardial infarct. In fact, there is evidence to suggest that thrombolytic therapy in the above subset of acute coronary syndromes may be associated with an increase in the incidence of adverse cardiac events (19).

Intra-aortic Balloon Counter Pulsation

This modality of treatment is indicated in:

(i) Patients with severe unstable angina refractory to maximal medical therapy—particularly when these patients are haemodynamically unstable. The above-mentioned therapy improves myocardial blood flow and reduces the myocardial oxygen demand by simply reducing resistance to left ventricular ejection in early systole. It is required in less than 1 per cent of patients with severe unstable angina.

(ii) It is also used in high-risk patients at the time of coronary angiography and angioplasty to provide support and a margin of safety during these procedures.

Intra-aortic balloon counter pulsation can cause lower limb ischaemia in about 10 per cent of cases. This generally resolves after removal of the device.

Indications for Coronary Angiography and Invasive Interventional Strategies in Unstable Angina

In our unit, over 50 per cent of patients settle down and are relieved of the symptoms of unstable angina by conservative medical management. Conservative management may however, prove ineffective. In conservatively managed patients, the indications for coronary angiography are:

(a) unrelieved or worsening angina;

(b) persistent angina at rest;

(c) haemodynamic instability;

(d) pump failure;

(e) ventricular arrhythmias.

The risks of coronary angiography are greater in patients with unstable angina particularly in the presence of some degree of haemodynamic instability (20). It is important

(i) to have an experienced cardiologist perform the angiography;

(ii) to correct as far as possible haemodynamic instability prior to the procedure;

(iii) if this is not possible, an angiography can however still be done after first placing the patient on intra-aortic balloon support.

Coronary angiography in unstable angina not responding to conventional medical therapy helps to identify several sub-groups (21) (**Table 7.2.3**).

(i) Patients with a left main stenosis who require emergency bypass surgery.

(ii) Patients with severe triple or multi-vessel disease who are advised bypass surgery within 7–10 days on a semi-urgent basis.

(iii) Patients having multi-vessel disease with left ventricular dysfunction, or diabetes with multivessel disease, who also will require bypass surgery to help prolong their life-span.

(iv) Patients with single or two vessel disease with an identifiable 'culprit' lesion. These patients are suitable for angioplasty. Current angioplasty success rates are over 95 per cent (**22**). Yet, there is an increased rate of acute complications in the form of abrupt closure of the vessel or myocardial infarction, following angioplasty in patients with unstable angina, or in those with a visible occluding thrombus, when compared to patients with stable angina or in those in whom a thrombus is not visible. The use of coronary stents has, however, reduced the incidence of emergency bypass surgery, and the increasing use of glycoprotein IIb-IIIa inhibitors has reduced the incidence of death and myocardial infarction (**23**).

(v) Patients with diffuse distal coronary artery disease for whom only medical therapy is advocated, as surgery shows poor results.

Table 7.2.3. Subgroups (with management) identified by coronary angiography in patients with unstable angina

* Patients with left main coronary artery disease—urgent bypass surgery indicated
* Patients with severe triple or multivessel disease (including proximal LAD)—bypass surgery advised on semi-urgent basis (7–10 days)
* Patients with multivessel disease and LV dysfunction; Patients with multivessel disease and diabetes—bypass surgery required to improve long-term survival
* Patients with single or double vessel disease with identifiable 'culprit' lesion in form of proximal discrete stenosis—angioplasty with stenting is procedure of choice
* Patients with diffuse distal coronary artery disease—medical therapy indicated as surgery gives poor results
* Small minority of patients (5 %) with no demonstrable organic coronary artery disease—medical management indicated

(vi) A small minority of patients (in our experience 5 per cent) with no significant organic coronary artery disease, who should continue with medical treatment.

After a successful angioplasty, the patient is monitored in the ICU. Sudden occlusion of the vessel on which angioplasty is done results in cardiac pain, and ECG changes of impending infarction. This constitutes an emergency which is tackled by either attempting to reopen the vessel by performing a fresh angioplasty, or by doing an emergency coronary artery bypass surgery. A standby surgical team should always be present when an angioplasty is done.

Patients with unstable angina who respond to medical treatment will subsequently require a work-up to determine the nature and extent of their coronary artery disease so that elective treatment can be planned. This is done in our opinion preferably 3 weeks after the angina has been well controlled. Many prefer to investigate these patients much earlier.

REFERENCES

1. Braunwald E. (1989). Unstable angina: A classification. Circulation. 80, 410–414.

2. van Miltenburg, van Sijli AJM, Simmons ML et al. (1995). Incidence and follow-up of Braunwald subgroups in unstable angina pectoris. J Am Coll Cardiol. 25, 1286–1292.

3. Braunwald E, Antman EM, Beasley JW et al. (2000). ACC/AHA guidelines for the management of patients with unstable angina and non-ST-segment elevation myocardial infarction: a report of the American College of Cardiology/ American Heart Association Task Force on Practice Guidelines (Committee on the Management of Patients with Unstable Angina). J Am Coll Cardiol. 36, 970–1062.

4. Diodati J, Theroux P, Latour JG et al. (1990). Effects of nitroglycerin at therapeutic doses on platelet aggregation in unstable angina pectoris and acute myocardial infarction. Am J Cardiol. 66, 683–687.

5. Hint Research Group. (1986). Early treatment of unstable angina in the coronary care unit: A randomized, double blind, placebo controlled comparison of recurrent ischaemia in patients treated with nifedipine or metoprolol or both. Br Heart J. 56, 400.

6. Tijssen JG, Lubsen J. (1988). Early treatment of unstable angina with nifedipine and metoprolol—the HINT trial. J Cardiovasc Pharmacol. 12(suppl. 71).

7. Muller JE, Turi ZG, Pearle DL et al. (1984). Nifedipine and conventional therapy for unstable angina pectoris: a randomized, double-blind comparison. Circulation. 69, 728.

8. Ryan TJ, Anderson JL, Antman EM et al. (1996). ACC/AHA guidelines for the management of patients with acute myocardial infarction: a report of the American College of Cardiology/American Heart association Task Force on Practice Guidelines (Committeee on Management of Acute Myocardial Infarction). J Am Coll Cardiol. 28, 1328–1428.

9. Wilcox RG, Hampton JR, Banks DC et al. (1986). Trial of Early Nifedepine in Myocardial Infarction: The TRENT study. BMJ. 293, 1204–1208.

10. The RISC Group. (1990). Risk of myocardial infarction and death during treatment with low dose aspirin and intravenous heparin in men with unstable coronary artery disease. Lancet. 336, 827–830.

11. Cohen M, Demers C, Gurfinkel EP et al. (1997). A comparison of low-molecular weight heparin for unstable coronary artery disease. Efficacy and safety of subcutaneous enoxaparin in non Q-wave coronary events (ESSENCE) study group. N Engl J Med. 337, 447–452.

12. Antman EM, McCabe CH, Gurfinkel EP et al. (1999). Enoxaparin prevents death and cardiac ischemic events in unstable angina/ non Q-wave myocardial infarction; results of the thrombolysis in myocardial infarction (TIMI) IIB trial. Circulation. 100, 1593–1601.

13. Antman EM, Cohen M, Radley D, et al. (1999). Assessment of the treatment effect of enoxaparin for unstable angina/non-Q-wave myocardial infarction. TIMI IIB ESSENCE meta-analysis. Circulation. 100, 1602–1608.

14. Yusuf S, Zhao F, Mehta SR. (2001). Effects of clopidogrel in addition to aspirin in patients with acute coronary syndromes without ST segment elevation. N Engl J Med. 345, 494–502.

15. Cannon CP, Weintraub WS, Demopoulos LA et al. (2001). Comparison of early invasive and conservative strategies in patients with unstable coronary syndromes treated with glycoprotein IIb/IIIa inhibitor tirofiban. N Engl J Med. 344, 1897–1987.

16. Anderson KM, Califf RM, Stone GW et al. (2001). Long-term mortality benefit with abciximab in patients undergoing percutaneous coronary intervention. J Am Coll Cardiol. 37, 2059–2065.

17. Boersma E, Akkerhuis KM, Theroux P et al. (1999). Platelet glycoprotein IIb/IIIa receptor inhibition in non-ST-elevation acute coronary syndromes: early benefit during medical treatment only, with additional percutaneous coronary intervention. Circulation. 100, 2045–2048.

18. Januzzi JL, Cannon CP, Theroux P et al. (2003). Optimizing glycoprotein IIb/IIIa receptor antagonist use for the non ST-segment elevation acute coronary syndromes: risk stratification and therapeutic intervention. Am Heart J. 146(5), 764–774.

19. Effects of tissue plasminogen activator and a comparison of early invasive and conservative strategies in unstable angina and non-Q-wave myocardial infarction; results of the TIMI IIIB Trial. Thrombolysis in Myocardial Ischemia (1994). Circulation. 89 (4), 1545–1556.

20. Myler RK, Shaw RE, Stertzer SH et al. (1990). Unstable angina and coronary angioplasty. Circulation. 82 (Suppl II), II-88–II-95.

21. Cannon CP, Braunwald E. (2001). Unstable Angina. In: Heart Disease— A Textbook of Cardiovascular Medicine (Eds Braunwald E, Zipes DP, Libby P). pp. 1232–1263. W B Saunders Company, Philadelphia, London, Toronto, Montreal, Sydney, Tokyo.

22. de Feyter PJ, Suryapranta H, Serruys PW et al. (1987). Effects of successful percutaneous transluminal coronary angioplasty on global and regional left ventricular function in unstable angina pectoris. Am J Cardiol. 60, 993–997.

23. Buller CE, Dzavik V, Carere RG et al. (1999). Primary stenting versus balloon angioplasty in occluded coronary arteries: the Total Occlusion Study of Canada (TOSCA). Circulation. 100, 236–242.

CHAPTER 7.3

Acute Myocardial Infarction

General Considerations

Acute myocardial infarction (AMI) signifies ischaemic necrosis or death of a portion of the myocardium. Atherosclerotic narrowing of the coronary vessels is the basic underlying pathology in most patients, and an occluding thrombus is usually present in a major coronary artery or its branch. Myocardial infarction still carries an overall mortality between 30–40 per cent. Prompt diagnosis and early transfer to a critical care unit whenever possible, are essential if mortality is to be reduced. The importance of quick diagnosis and early transfer to a well-equipped intensive care unit is related to two factors:

(i) 50 per cent of deaths in acute myocardial infarction occur within the first 2 hours, and 80 per cent within the first 24 hours. Early deaths occurring during this period are invariably due to primary ventricular fibrillation which can be promptly treated with good results in an ICU setting.

(ii) The present day management of acute myocardial infarction involves not only the relief of pain and other supportive treatment, but an active interventional approach directed towards restoring blood flow to the ischaemic myocardium. This interventional approach is chiefly through the use of thrombolytic agents with a view to dissolving a thrombus occluding a coronary artery, and/or in selected instances the use of angioplasty to physically open an occluded vessel. The earlier this is done after the onset of myocardial infarction, the better the results.

A patient with an acute myocardial infarction may be admitted to the ICU from the community. On the other hand, a patient who is already being treated in the ICU for some other serious ailment, may develop acute myocardial infarction as an added complication. It is not the purpose of this chapter to extensively detail the physiopathology, clinical features and diagnosis of acute myocardial infarction. Only the basic features of diagnosis are touched upon so that mistakes are perhaps less frequent and management is not unnecessarily delayed.

Diagnosis

The diagnosis of acute myocardial infarction is based on a positive history of cardiac pain, ECG changes, and elevated cardiac enzymes. A diagnosis should be made if any two of these three factors are present. In those patients who show no early serial ECG changes, a 4 hourly serial estimation of the cardiac enzymes (in particular the Troponin T, Troponin I, CK and the CK-MB fraction), should be monitored. A rise in the enzymes, even if a little delayed, confirms the diagnosis. If however, quick interventional therapy is to be instituted to salvage myocardium, a diagnosis has to be made on the history (and clinical findings), and on the ECG changes, as the rise in cardiac enzymes may take time to detect.

Cardiac pain is the most important clinical feature of acute myocardial infarction. In some, the pain is agonizingly severe, while in others it may be so mild as to be totally ignored by the patient and overlooked by the doctor. It is not necessarily the severity of pain, but the site and radiation of pain, as well as its character, which are diagnostic. The pain is similar to the one described in unstable angina, only it is more protracted and is often accompanied by associated features like sweating, pallor, breathlessness due to left ventricular failure, fall in the blood pressure, and disturbances in the rate and rhythm of the heart. Clinical examination may be essentially normal, or may reveal a diastolic gallop and basal crepitations denoting left ventricular failure, or early evidence of shock in the form of pallor, sweating, hypotension, or evidence of arrhythmias. Any one or more of these features may be present.

There are a few points to be kept in mind in relation to the clinical diagnosis of acute myocardial infarction:

(i) In diabetics, elderly patients, and at times for no apparent cause, there may be little or no pain.

(ii) A number of other non-cardiac conditions can cause severe, protracted chest pain. To give just a few examples, chest pain may be due to musculoskeletal problems, oesophageal spasm, a lower oesophageal tear, acute abdominal problems, pulmonary embolism, pneumothorax, pleurisy, acute pericarditis and dissecting aneurysm of the aorta. It is particularly important to exclude acute pericarditis and dissecting aneurysm of the aorta, as the use of thrombolytic therapy by mistake in either of these conditions can have disastrous consequences.

(iii) Acute myocardial infarction may occasionally present with the following clinical variants: (a) acute left ventricular failure; (b) acute shock of unexplained aetiology; (c) cardiac arrhythmias; (d) embolic complications which draw attention to an underlying infarction.

(iv) Clinical examination may be perfectly normal with no

change in the pulse or blood pressure even in the presence of an extensive infarction.

ECG Changes

ECG changes are very useful in the diagnosis of an acute myocardial infarction. It should however, be made clear that an acute myocardial infarct cannot be excluded even if the initial ECG is normal. The ECG should be repeated as changes may take hours or at times even a couple of days to manifest. The earliest change in the ECG is an ST elevation in the leads overlying the infarcted area (anterior, posterior, inferior, lateral). A pathological Q develops later, and its presence is associated with absent or low voltage R waves, denoting the occurrence of a transmural infarct. A non-Q infarct is characterized either by elevated or depressed ST segments and/or T wave changes. Differentiating between a Q-wave and a non Q-wave infarct is not just a matter of academic interest. Patients with Q-wave infarction have a worse immediate prognosis compared to those with non Q-wave infarction. What is even more important is that Q-wave infarcts with ST elevation benefit from coronary reperfusion therapy, whereas non Q-wave infarcts without ST segment elevation do not. The recognition of ST segment elevation of ≥ 1 mm in at least two contiguous leads is therefore crucial in management and outcome. In fact, from the point of view of the applicability or not of measures for coronary reperfusion, myocardial infarcts are best looked upon as ST segment elevation myocardial infarction (STEMI) or non ST segment elevation myocardial infarction (NSTEMI).

The importance of serial changes on the ECG, even if minor, cannot be overemphasized, as these changes may constitute the only ECG evidence of myocardial infarction. Again, since the characteristic ECG changes of acute myocardial infarction occasionally evolve much later in the course of the attack, and on rare occasions may be even totally absent, the possibility of such a diagnosis must be entertained even in the absence of ECG changes, provided a clear-cut clinical picture is present, and corroborative evidence of myocardial necrosis exists in the form of raised cardiac enzymes, particularly in the Troponin T, Troponin I and in the CK and the CK-MB fraction. Posterior and high lateral infarction may also take time to evolve and are then recognized late.

Electrocardiography may also not be always helpful in the diagnosis of patients with multiple previous infarcts, in LBBB block, or the WPW syndrome, and in patients on digitalis therapy. The occurrence of a new or fresh bundle branch block, and in particular a new LBBB in a patient with cardiac pain should be taken as a sign of a fresh infarct. Unfortunately, lack of a rapid ECG corroboration in some patients necessitates a delay in diagnosis, and this delay may well deprive a patient of thrombolytic or other interventional therapy to help salvage ischaemic myocardium.

Cardiac Enzymes

Myocardial necrosis results in the release of creatinine kinase and of Troponin T and Troponin I into the blood. A rise in the MB fraction of creatinine kinase (CK-MB) is more specific for myocardial necrosis than a rise in total CK. It should be measured immediately on admission and then serially every 4 to 6 hours for the next 36 hours. Plasma CK exceeds normal levels within 4 to 6 hours after onset of infarction, peaks at 10 to 20 times normal within 24 to 36 hours and then gradually declines to normal within 4–5 days. If the CK-MB fraction is 15 per cent or more of the total CK value, it points to a myocardial infarct. Recent research has identified isoforms of CK-MB. These are CK-MB$_1$ and CK-MB$_2$. An absolute value of CK-MB$_2$ greater than 1.0 U/l or a ratio of CK-MB$_2$/CK-MB$_1$ greater than 2.5 has a sensitivity for diagnosing AMI of 46 per cent at 4 hours and 96 per cent at 6 hours [1].

The rise of cardiac-specific troponins (Troponin T and I) in the blood is now considered the preferred biomarker for the diagnosis of acute myocardial infarct. The Troponins begin to rise within 3 hours of the onset of AMI. The rise in Troponin I may persist for 7–10 days and Troponin T for 10–14 days. The prolonged period of elevation of these enzymes is of advantage in the late diagnosis of AMI. It is of interest that Troponin assays are capable of detecting small areas of myocardial necrosis beyond the detection limit of the CK-MB assays. The term microinfarction has been used to describe a situation where the Troponin levels are raised and CK-MB levels are normal [2].

Principles of Management (Table 7.3.1)

An acute myocardial infarction does not necessarily evolve instantaneously, nor for that matter in minutes. In fact, it may evolve slowly, generally over hours, and at times over a period of a few

Table 7.3.1. Management of acute myocardial infarction

A. Medical Supportive Therapy
* Complete bed rest
* Relief of pain, anxiety and restlessness initially with 2 mg intravenous morphine or 0.3 mg buprenorphine
* Secure IV line and start 5% dextrose patency drip
* Administer oxygen at 2–4 l/min
* Monitor vital parameters (heart rate, blood pressure, urine output)
* ECG monitoring
* Use of nitrates:
  (i) For persistent pain or recurrent pain intravenous nitroglycerin infusion starting with 5–10 μg/min—can cause hypotension, tachycardia, headache
  (ii) Isosorbide dinitrate 10 mg 8 hrly or application of nitroglycerin paste used for mild pain, or after severe pain has been controlled
* Use of beta-blockers (see **Table 7.3.2**)

B. Interventional Therapy
* Thrombolytic therapy—streptokinase 1.5 million units intravenously over 1 hour, given within 6 hours of the infarct. May be given well after 6 hours, if pain and ST changes point to ongoing ischaemic injury
* Adjunctive medical therapy with thrombolytic therapy
  – Aspirin—165–325 mg/day orally
  – Heparin—5000 units IV bolus, followed by intravenous infusion at rate of 1000 units/hr; PTT should be kept at 1.5–2 times the control
* Coronary angiography with SOS angioplasty in patients who continue to have chest pain with persistent ST elevation in spite of thrombolytic therapy
* Primary angiography and SOS angioplasty in patients in whom thrombolytic therapy is contraindicated, in patients with typical ischaemic chest pain but no ECG changes, and in patients in whom acute pericarditis or aortic dissection cannot be ruled out

---

days. The objectives in management are two-fold—to limit infarct size as best as possible, and to support the heart as a pump and ensure adequate perfusion to tissues. In the first few hours after an acute myocardial infarction, myocardial preservation merits prime importance.

In practical terms the principles of management are as follows:

A. Medical Supportive Therapy. This includes relief of pain, the use of drugs, in particular aspirin, nitrates and beta-blockers, the management of life-threatening arrhythmias and conduction defects and the treatment of other complications of myocardial infarction.

B. Interventional Therapy. This is advocated with a view to directly promote reperfusion through a blocked coronary vessel, and thereby salvage ischaemic and injured myocardium. Interventional therapy chiefly takes the form of thrombolytic therapy but in selected cases may also include angioplasty to open up a blocked vessel. Rarely, coronary artery bypass surgery is performed as an emergency procedure to revascularize the jeopardized myocardium.

A. Medical Supportive Therapy

Following admission to the ICU, the priority procedures are complete bed rest, the prompt use of 300 mg aspirin, relief of pain, securing an intravenous line (and simultaneously sending blood for the relevant investigations), administering oxygen, and connecting the patient to an ECG monitor. These can all be done within a matter of a few minutes. The initial history taking should be brief and relevant. A quick clinical examination is then performed with special reference to the cardiovascular and respiratory systems, and an ECG is recorded. Points in diagnosis touched upon earlier are considered, to determine whether the referral diagnosis of a suspected myocardial infarction is probable or certain. Acute dissection, acute pericarditis and acute pleural and pulmonary problems need special consideration in the differential diagnosis. Complications of acute myocardial infarction are then carefully looked for—in particular left ventricular failure, arrhythmias, and features of early shock; if present these are promptly treated.

It is of vital importance to determine during this early assessment whether a patient with myocardial infarction qualifies for the use of thrombolytic therapy. If so, the latter should be initiated as a matter of urgent priority. The earlier thrombolysis is achieved the better, as it offers the best chance for reduction of infarct size and of myocardial preservation. Thrombolytic therapy is instituted side by side with other medical supportive treatment. The details of thrombolytic therapy are discussed later in this chapter.

Aspirin

The prompt use of 300 mg of aspirin is an essential feature in the management of AMI and the earlier it is administered the greater the benefit. Subsequently 300 mg aspirin is given once daily on an indefinite basis.

The use of thrombolytic agents does not contraindicate the use of aspirin and the drug is administered regardless of changes in the ST segments. The only contraindication to its use is an allergy to the drug or an active peptic ulcer. Aspirin therapy alone showed

a 23 per cent reduction of vascular mortality; the combined use of aspirin and streptokinase resulted in an astonishing 42 per cent reduction in overall vascular mortality (3). Aspirin with successful thrombolysis also reduces the risk of reocclusion and in-hospital reinfarction by 50 per cent (3).

Bed Rest

Complete bed rest is essential to start with. Most patients are nursed flat in bed; those with left ventricular failure need to be slightly propped up. The patient is encouraged to turn and move in bed from the very first day to minimize the risk of phlebothrombosis of the leg veins and hypostatic pulmonary congestion. In the absence of cardiac failure, arrhythmias, or shock, we encourage the patient to use a bedside commode to move his bowels. Most Indians find the bedpan an uncomfortable contraption; in fact, straining over a bedpan can prove disastrous and we tend to avoid its use as far as possible. If the patient is too ill to get out of bed, and is unfamiliar with the bedpan, he is encouraged to move his bowels in bed into a large pad of cotton.

Relief of Pain

Severe unrelieved pain can lead to increasing anxiety, shock and may even trigger dangerous arrhythmias. The best drug to relieve both pain and anxiety in acute myocardial infarction is morphine. In patients with severe pain, we always administer morphine intravenously—2–4 mg being diluted and given slowly. Morphine is unfortunately not always easily available. The next best drug is buprenorphine, 0.3 mg intravenously. A careful watch is kept on respiration and blood pressure. 2 mg morphine (or 0.3 mg buprenorphine) may need to be repeated every 15–30 minutes till the pain is relieved, or there is evidence of toxicity. Severe vomiting, respiratory depression, or hypotension preclude its further use. In patients with mild or moderately severe pain, 15 mg morphine given subcutaneously suffices for pain relief. This can be repeated as necessary, though we generally do not use more than 60 mg morphine over 24 hours.

Morphine by relieving pain, anxiety and restlessness associated with acute myocardial infarction, results in a decrease in the myocardial oxygen demand. It also has a beneficial action in patients with pulmonary congestion due to left ventricular failure. This is because it produces vasodilatation and reduces the preload (particularly in those with excessive sympathetic activity), reduces the heart rate through increased parasympathetic activity and reduced sympathetic tone, and decreases the work of breathing by slowing respiration.

Hypotension following morphine can be countered by nursing the patient flat in bed or in the head-low position. A bolus or volume load of 150–200 ml dextrose saline generally suffices to raise the systolic pressure to above 100 mm Hg. The use of atropine 0.5–1 mg intravenously together with morphine counters the parasympathomimetic effect of the drug, particularly if bradycardia and a lowered systolic blood pressure are present to start with. Vomiting is countered by the use of 25 mg intramuscular promethazine. Respiratory depression is surprisingly uncommon even with repeated doses of morphine in the presence of severe pain or tachypnoea due to pulmonary congestion. It should however be always watched for, specially in the aged and the feeble, and when present can be reversed by naloxone 0.1–0.2 mg intravenously. This dose can be repeated every 15 minutes till the respiration is no longer depressed.

Initially morphine suffices to relieve anxiety. When pain is no longer present, anxiety should be relieved by benzodiazepine (diazepam 5 mg twice or thrice daily orally).

Establishing an Intravenous Line

An intravenous line is essential and is secured as soon as the patient is admitted, through an indwelling catheter in a peripheral vein. A 5 per cent dextrose infusion is started at a very low flow rate through the intravenous line. This is a patency drip to be used for administering drugs. It is important to ensure that large quantities of fluids are not given intravenously (except for a specific purpose), for fear of inducing or aggravating pulmonary oedema. If peripheral veins are unobtainable due to shock, a central line (either subclavian or internal jugular) is secured percutaneously. Blood samples for blood count, glucose, creatinine, CK, CK-MB, Troponin I and T, SGOT and other relevant biochemical tests are collected when the intravenous line has been secured. It is best to avoid injections prior to sending blood CK levels to the laboratory, as intramuscular injections can by themselves cause a rise in the CK, and this can be misleading in diagnosis.

Oxygen

We routinely administer oxygen at 2–4 l/minute in a patient with a fresh myocardial infarction for the first 24 hours. Oxygen is imperative in the presence of severe or persistent pain, or in the presence of breathlessness or shock, and in these situations it is given at a higher flow rate of 6 l/minute.

ECG Monitoring

This is an extremely important aspect of critical care, as prompt detection of arrhythmias and their response to treatment can only be determined by continuous ECG monitoring. A high rate audiovisual alarm should be set at 110/min, and a low rate signal at 50/min. Monitoring of blood pressure, temperature, urine output are other important features of critical care in myocardial infarction.

Use of Nitrates

Nitrates are useful in the management of acute myocardial infarction provided there is no hypotension (systolic < 100 mm Hg or a fall of > 40 mm Hg from the baseline). In patients with severe or protracted pain, or when pain waxes and wanes, a slow infusion of nitroglycerin should be started at a rate of 5–10 µg/min, the infusion rate being gradually increased every 10–15 minutes. There is no fixed optimal dose, but the infusion is titrated so that there is substantial pain relief or a drop in the systolic arterial pressure by 10–20 per cent. The blood pressure should not be allowed to fall below 100 mm Hg, and should be carefully monitored. Titration to total pain relief may be impossible in acute myocardial infarction. Intravenous nitroglycerin infusions can be continued

for 4–7 days if so required. Generally after 2–3 days the infusion is substituted by the application of nitroglycerin paste (1.5–2 inches) every 8 hours or by oral nitrates e.g. isosorbide dinitrate 10 mg 8 hourly. It is best to avoid long-acting nitrates following acute myocardial infarction as titration of the dose is difficult. Patients who are stable from the start and whose pain has been virtually relieved by morphine, are treated in many units initially with oral nitrates or local application of nitroglycerin paste, without prior use of intravenous nitroglycerin infusions. Flaherty and colleagues (4) have shown in a prospective randomized trial that the use of intravenous nitroglycerin for 48 hours followed by the use of nitroglycerin paste for 72 hours, enhanced post-infarction improvement of myocardial function in a scintigraphic study.

Nitrates are vasodilators. They reduce the venous return, the preload and therefore the workload on the heart. Myocardial oxygen demands are reduced, and this in turn leads to a reduction in myocardial ischaemia. Nitrates also have a direct coronary vasodilator action and enhance blood supply to the ischaemic myocardium. Both these modes of action contribute therefore to the relief of pain, and to preservation of ischaemic myocardium. A reduction in preload also leads to reduced filling pressures in the left ventricle, and may be of great benefit in patients with pulmonary congestion and oedema due to left ventricular failure.

Unfortunately, the prior presence of hypotension or a sharp hypotensive response soon after starting nitrates, at times limits the use of these drugs. They should be used with great caution in patients with inferior wall infarction as even a small dose may cause a precipitous fall in blood pressure and heart rate—a reaction which can be promptly treated by intravenous atropine if recognized early. Nitrates, and in particular intravenous nitroglycerin are best avoided in patients with suspected right ventricular infarction. These patients often develop severe hypotension following their use because of inadequate right ventricular filling produced by vasodilatation. Hypotension induced by nitrates is dangerous; it reduces coronary perfusion, aggravates ischaemia, and potentiates myocardial injury and death.

Headache is common with nitrates but only rarely is it severe enough to warrant discontinuation of the drug. Prolonged use of large doses has been known to cause methaemoglobinaemia. Elevated methaemoglobin levels impair the oxygen-carrying capacity of the blood, and may increase myocardial ischaemia. If ethanol is used as a diluent in nitroglycerin solutions, ethanol intoxication may occur with prolonged intravenous use.

Beta-blockers

Beta blockers are of proven benefit when given in the early hours of AMI (5, 6), provided there are no contraindications to their use. Beta-blockers act by causing a reduction in the heart rate, blood pressure, myocardial contractility and hence in myocardial oxygen demand, thereby relieving chest pain and limiting infarct size. They may also help to reduce the incidence of post-infarction angina, ventricular arrhythmias, myocardial rupture and ventricular remodeling, thus reducing the overall mortality in AMI (5, 6).

It is however to be remembered that in third world countries, it is rare for patients to be admitted to the ICU within a few hours of an infarct. Patients are often admitted late, after several hours of chest pain. Beta-blockers could easily precipitate left ventricular failure if administered late in the natural history of the disease, after a massive infarct has evolved in its entirety.

Contraindications

Beta-blockers are contraindicated in patients with left ventricular failure, hypotension (systolic BP < 100 mm Hg), bradycardia (heart rate < 60–65/min) or heart block. They are also contraindicated in a patient with a history of asthma, or of significant chronic airways obstruction. Except under special circumstances, they are unlikely to be of use when used more than 6 hours after the onset of AMI.

Indications for use (Table 7.3.2)

1. In patients admitted within 6 hours of an AMI. We prefer to initiate therapy intravenously provided no contraindications exist.

2. Later in the natural history of AMI we use beta-blockers in the following circumstances.

(a) In patients with marked sinus tachycardia particularly when associated with anxiety and hypertension. It is important to first ascertain that the tachycardia is not due to left ventricular failure.

(b) In patients whose infarction is complicated by persistent or recurrent ischaemic pain, particularly when associated with tachycardia.

(c) In patients with tachyrhythms refractory to the usual antiarrhythmic drugs.

(d) In patients who have been beta-blocked prior to infarction, a sudden withdrawal of the drug may produce severe tachycardia. In such cases beta-blockers should be continued in smaller doses.

Table 7.3.2. Indications for using beta-blockers in acute myocardial infarction

* Within the first 4–6 hours after AMI (early use), provided no contraindications exist
* Later in the natural history of AMI
   - In patients with marked sinus tachycardia
   - In patients with marked sinus tachycardia (not due to left ventricular failure), particularly when associated with anxiety and hypertension
   - In patients in whom infarction is complicated by persistent/recurrent ischaemic pain, specially if associated with tachycardia and/or hypertension
   - In patients with tachyarrhythmias refractory to conventional antiarrhythmic drugs
   - In patients who have been beta-blocked prior to acute myocardial infarction

Mode of use

When patients are admitted within a few hours of AMI, metaprolol is given intravenously in three 5 mg bolus doses to a total of 15 mg. The patient is observed for 5 minutes after each bolus dose. No further dose is given if the heart rate falls below 60 beats/min or systolic BP falls to less than 100 mm Hg or the PR interval is prolonged beyond 0.24 sec, or basal crackles or a diastolic gallop appear. If the patient remains haemodynamically stable for 30 minutes after the last bolus dose, metaprolol is continued orally,

50 mg 12 hourly. The dose needs to be titrated to ensure that hypotension, bradycardia, heart block or LVF do not occur. The drug is also promptly stopped if there is bronchospasm.

If beta-blockers are used later in the natural history of AMI, we always prefer to use propranolol orally, starting with 5 to 10 mg thrice daily and then titrating the dose for optimal effect. The drug is stopped if breathlessness, a diastolic gallop or any of the untoward effects listed above are observed.

Calcium Antagonists

Both verapamil and diltiazem are best avoided immediately after Q-wave and non Q-wave AMI. They may be tried in post-myocardial infarction angina or in slowing the ventricular rate in atrial fibrillation when beta-blockers are ineffective or contraindicated. Calcium channel blockers have a negative inotropic effect on the heart.

Intravenous Magnesium

It has now been shown that intravenous magnesium is an inexpensive and relatively safe means of reducing serious arrhythmias and deaths from acute myocardial infarction (7, 8). 8 mmol of magnesium sulfate is given intravenously over 5 minutes, followed by 65 mmol over 24 hours. It probably acts by preserving myocardial tissue as well as by suppressing arrhythmias.

ACE Inhibitors

They are avoided during the immediate phase of AMI but may be of benefit after a few days. ACE inhibitors are of particular use in patients with clinical evidence of heart failure, in those with an ejection fraction < 40 per cent, and in those with a history of previous myocardial infarction. We prefer to use captopril 6.25 mg orally twice daily titrating the dose slowly to 25 mg thrice daily, provided there is no significant hypotension, nor a rise in the serum creatinine. Lisinopril, enalapril or ramipril could also be used in appropriate titrated doses. ACE inhibitors reduce the afterload and thereby the work of the heart. One should aim to reduce the systolic blood pressure by approximately 10 per cent in normotensive individuals and by 30 per cent in hypertensive individuals. ACE inhibitors should not be used when the systolic pressure is ≤ 100 mm Hg.

B. Interventional Therapy

Thrombolytic Therapy

Numerous clinical trials provide overwhelming evidence that thrombolytic agents administered early in the course of acute myocardial infarction reduce infarct size, preserve left ventricular function and substantially reduce mortality (9, 10, 11).

The benefit accrues from the ability of thrombolytic agents to lyse clots within a coronary artery and thereby re-establish perfusion of blood to the affected area of the myocardium. The Fibrinolytic Therapy Trialists Collaboration Group (FTTCG) (12) showed that mortality in Q-wave infarction is reduced by 25 to 30 per cent, if fibrinolytic therapy is instituted in patients with either ST segment elevation or new bundle branch block up to 12 hours, and possibly as much as 18 to 24 hours after the onset of symptoms.

The maximum benefits were observed in patients with anterior ST segment elevation but patients with inferior ST segment elevations also benefit. Patients with Q-wave infarction who are at the greatest risk, have the greatest benefit. The sooner treatment is instituted, the better the results.

This is beautifully illustrated by a study of pooled findings from 22 randomized controlled trials of thrombolytic therapy published between 1983 to 1993 (13).

This study noted the following:

Time when thrombolysis started	Additional lives saved per 1000 people treated with thrombolytics compared with 1000 people treated with standard therapy
In the first hour	65
In the second hour	37
In the third hour	26
Between 3 to 6 hours	26
Between 6 to < 12 hours	18
Between 12 to < 24 hours	9

The imperative need to use thrombolytic agents as early as possible in patients with AMI where thrombolytic therapy is indicated, and where no contraindications to this therapy exist, is clearly evident.

Indications

When a patient with AMI (suspected or proven) is referred to the ICU, the immediate question is to determine whether the patient is a candidate for thrombolytic therapy. The following criteria for the use of thrombolytic agents in AMI must be considered.

1. Chest pain for more than 30 minutes, consistent with AMI.

2. ECG changes showing

(a) ST segment elevation > 1–2 mm in at least 2 contiguous frontal leads (leads I, aVL, II, III, aVF) or 2 precordial leads (the V leads) or in ST segment elevation infarction (STEMI) with or without Q waves. It is to be noted that a right ventricular infarct may manifest with an elevated ST in V_4R, and a tall R in V_4R. It is often associated with elevated ST in leads II, III, aVF. The ST deviation in all patients should be measured 0.4 second after the J point, using the PQR segment as the isoelectric line.

(b) New or presumed new left bundle branch block, because this invariably denotes an acute anterior myocardial infarct.

3. Age < 75 years. It is to be however noted that the FTTCG overview suggests that age is not an absolute bar to fibrinolysis and that the benefit is greater than the risk even in patients over 75 years.

4. The therapy to be effective should be given early in the course of AMI. It is most beneficial if given within 6 hours of the onset of pain (or pain equivalent). It is less beneficial but is still used between 6 to 12 hours of pain. It may be used between 12 to 24 hours after onset of pain particularly if pain persists, but with decreasing benefits.

Thrombolytic therapy is not indicated in patients with unstable angina, in non Q-wave myocardial infarcts with ST depression or non-specific ST changes i.e. in non-STEMI.

5. There is however, a subset of patients eligible for thrombolysis even though they do not present either with ST elevation or LBBB. These are patients with:

(a) True posterior wall infarction who may have a tall R in V_1 and V_4R or present with marked ST segment depression in V_1 to V_4 which represents a posterior current of injury. The infarction is generally due to an occlusion of the circumflex artery, or occlusion of the posterior descending branch of the right coronary artery.

(b) Anterior myocardial infarction which in the very early phase may show hyperacute giant T waves without ST segment elevation.

Contraindications

The major danger in the use of thrombolytic therapy is bleeding. Contraindications to its use are outlined in **Table 7.3.3**.

These include a bleeding diathesis, an active peptic ulcer, active recent internal bleeding, history of a cerebrovascular accident in the recent past (3 to 4 weeks), recent major surgery, recent intracranial or spinal surgery, recent trauma, recent head injury, severe uncontrolled hypertension (diastolic > 110 mm Hg), known presence of an aneurysm or an arteriovenous malformation, aortic dissection and proliferative diabetic retinopathy. Relative contraindications include a recent arteriotomy or puncture of a major vessel, poorly controlled hypertension, recent organ biopsy (2 to 3 weeks), recent obstetric delivery, recent protracted cardiopulmonary resuscitation.

Table 7.3.3. Contraindications to thrombolytic therapy

Absolute
* Bleeding diathesis or chronic liver disease with portal hypertension
* Active recent internal bleeding
* Cerebrovascular accident in the recent past (3 weeks)
* Recent trauma, head injury or major surgery
* Aortic dissection
* Proliferative haemorrhagic diabetic retinopathy
* Uncontrolled severe hypertension
* Known presence of aneurysm/arteriovenous malformations

Relative
* Serious organic disease associated with increased risk of bleeding/embolization
* Poorly controlled hypertension
* Prolonged cardiopulmonary resuscitation
* Pregnancy/post-partum/menstruating women
* Diabetic proliferative retinopathy

Risks of thrombolytic therapy

1. Bleeding

Bleeding generally occurs from puncture wounds (arteries and veins). However, the general fibrinolysis caused by thrombolytic agents can occasionally cause catastrophic bleeding leading to death. The most dreaded of all complications is an intracranial bleed.

2. Reperfusion arrhythmias

Reperfusion arrhythmias are occasionally observed in patients during or immediately after thrombolytic therapy. These take the form of accelerated idioventricular rhythm and frequent ventricular ectopics. Rarely ventricular fibrillation may occur abruptly. Marked sinus bradycardia and hypotension may be observed following reperfusion in inferior wall infarction. There is considerable interest in the physiopathology of reperfusion arrhythmias. Metabolites accumulate in the ischaemic and injured myocardium following occlusion of a coronary vessel. A washout of these metabolites following reperfusion results in electrical and chemical gradients across cell membranes, resulting in arrhythmias (14).

Assessing the Efficacy of Thrombolytic Therapy

Thrombolytic therapy can be gauged to have succeeded, if there is relief of pain, a reduction in ST elevation by about 50 per cent, and by an improved haemodynamic state. The occurrence of an accelerated idioventricular rhythm after thrombolysis generally denotes successful reperfusion. Persistent pain, an unimproved haemodynamic state, with no change in the elevated ST segments, and even perhaps an extension of the infarct size, point to a failure of thrombolytic therapy.

Thrombolytic Drugs

The two thrombolytic drugs in wide use today are streptokinase (SK) and tissue plasminogen activator (TPA). There is little to choose between the two from the point of view of efficacy in re-establishing perfusion of a thrombosed coronary artery (15, 16).

The GUSTO trial (16) showed a small but significant survival benefit (1.1 per cent absolute) in the TPA regime as compared to the SK regime. But this is controversial and there was a slight increase in the incidence of cerebral haemorrhage (2 per cent increase) in the TPA regime. Also, the TPA regime is prohibitively expensive for third world countries.

It appears that for cost-effectiveness the SK regime is to be preferred in India and the poorer countries of the world.

Other drugs less commonly used are urokinase and anisoylated plasminogen streptokinase activator complex (APSAC). These have no special advantage over streptokinase or TPA except that they can be administered as a bolus intravenous injection. Both are far costlier than streptokinase.

Dosage Protocol
Streptokinase

SK is administered in a continuous intravenous infusion of 1.5 million units over one hour.

The administration of SK occasionally causes anaphylactic reactions which range from itching and urticaria to bronchospasm and severe hypotension. If severe, the drug is stopped and the anaphylactic reaction countered by intravenous hydrocortisone.

Tissue Plasminogen Activator

A 10 mg intravenous bolus is followed by 50 mg given by continuous infusion over the next hour. This is followed by an infusion of 20 mg over the second and third hour, to a total of 100 mg over three hours. TPA does not cause hypersensitivity reaction because it is synthesized by recombinant techniques. However, both SK and TPA can cause serious bleeding. If this occurs the drug is promptly stopped.

Urokinase

0.5–0.75 million units are administered intravenously as a bolus.

APSAC

It is given intravenously as a 35–50 units bolus over 2–5 minutes.

Table 7.3.4. Comparison between intravenously administered streptokinase, and recombinant tissue-type plasminogen activator (rt-PA)

	Streptokinase	rt-PA
Dose	1.5 million units in in 30–60 minutes	60 mg during 1st hr, 40 mg during 2nd & 3rd hours.
Patency of infarct-related artery	50–60%	75–85%
Reocclusion rate	5–20%	10–20%
Improvement of LV function	+	+
Improvement of survival	Yes	Yes
Hypotension	Severe in < 5%	Absent
Half-life	Long	Short
Allergic reactions	+	–
Fibrinogenolysis	Severe	Moderate
Intracranial bleeds	< 0.5%	< 0.5%
Periaccess bleeding	Common	Common
Repeated dosing	Not possible, because of antibodies	Possible
Approximate cost	Cheapest (Rs 3000)	Most expensive (Rs 35,000)

Adjunctive Therapy

The use of aspirin has already been commented upon. Unfractionated heparin should also be administered after the thrombolytic infusion is over. A bolus of 5000 IU is followed by a continuous infusion of 1000 U/hr. The dose of heparin is titrated so as to keep the aPTT to 1.5 to 2 times the control. Heparin is generally continued for 3–7 days. Recent data suggest that low molecular weight heparin in the form of enoxaparin 1 mg/kg subcutaneously twice daily may be as effective as unfractionated heparin (17).

The results of published randomized trials indicate that the combination of thrombolytic agents (SK or TPA), aspirin and heparin significantly reduces morbidity in acute myocardial infarction (18, 19). *In patients with non Q-wave and NSTE myocardial infarct, heparin is used alone (without thrombolytic therapy) exactly as outlined in the management of unstable angina. Heparin can also be used along with Gp IIb-IIIa inhibitors in severe cases of NSTE (see Chapter on Unstable Angina).*

Reuse of thrombolytic therapy

If thrombolytic therapy fails to afford relief, a rescue angioplasty is generally indicated. If however, facilities for a rescue angioplasty are lacking, thrombolysis may be attempted again. The following points need to be stressed:

1. If streptokinase is used for initial thrombolysis, it should not be used again as it can cause severe anaphylaxis.

2. Reuse thrombolytic therapy should therefore always be with TPA. If prior thrombolytic therapy was given 12 hours back for TPA or 24 hours back for SK, 25 to 50 per cent of the usual dose of TPA is administered. If more time has elapsed after initial therapy, the full dose of TPA can be given.

Coronary Angioplasty as an Interventional Post-thrombolysis Procedure

Patients who in spite of thrombolytic therapy continue to experience intermittent or continuous discomfort in the chest with persistent or increasing ST segment elevation, should be considered for coronary angiography. An angiographic study often shows a complete occlusion of the infarct-related vessel. A rescue coronary angioplasty aimed at opening up and if possible stenting the infarct-related vessel should then be considered (20). This requires good equipment and expertise, as the risk of doing more harm than good is always present. We would therefore strongly discourage the rescue interventional procedure except in those few centres in the country which have the necessary equipment, expertise and experience to use it optimally.

Primary Coronary Angioplasty (not preceded by Thrombolytic Therapy)

Primary coronary angioplasty is performed by many well-equipped centres, to restore myocardial perfusion immediately after an acute myocardial infarct (21–26). Points in favour of this procedure are:

(a) it ensures a reperfusion rate of 90 to 95 per cent compared to the reperfusion rate of 70 to 80 per cent with thrombolytic therapy;

(b) bleeding complications of thrombolytic therapy are avoided;

(c) the reocclusion rate in patients undergoing thrombolytic therapy is higher than those undergoing PTCA;

(d) PTCA is feasible in all patients with AMI including those who are not eligible for thrombolytic therapy;

(e) an 'open artery' with a TIMI flow grade 3 is an excellent predictor of a reduced 30 day mortality and this is more often achieved with a primary angioplasty than with thrombolysis.

Points against this strategy are:

(a) the logistic difficulty of performing a PTCA preferably within 4 hours, or at most within 12 hours of the onset of AMI—a time period when its efficacy is proven;

(b) the unavailability of the necessary equipment, expertise, experience and logistic support in many centres in developing countries.

Thrombolysis and primary angioplasty have an equal status as reperfusion strategies. The equivalence, however, only holds if primary angioplasty can commence within 30 minutes of a patient's entry into the emergency department, and is completed within 90 minutes of his entry into the emergency department. Very few hospitals in our country can claim to possess 24 hour facilities that satisfy the above criteria.

The present indications for primary angioplasty are:

(i) in patients in whom there are specific contraindications to thrombolytic therapy;

(ii) in patients with severe ischaemic cardiac pain, with a marked rise in the cardiac enzymes, or those with a possible 'stuttering infarction', and yet with no typical ECG features of a myocardial infarct;

(iii) in patients in whom acute pericarditis or a dissecting aneurysm of the aorta cannot be ruled out. A coronary angiography followed by an angioplasty (if there is occlusion to a major coronary artery) can be done;

(iv) in patients who are haemodynamically unstable or in cardiogenic shock;

(v) in patients who have had coronary artery bypass surgery in the past and in whom a recent occlusion of a vein graft may have occurred.

In experienced and expert centres a primary angioplasty is preferred to thrombolytic therapy in patients with ECG and echocardiographic evidence of an extensive infarct involving the anterior wall of the left ventricle. Underlying provisos are the availability of a well equipped centre, staffed with experienced, skilled, motivated interventional cardiologists and the logistics to enable this procedure to be performed preferably within 4 hours, and not later than 12 hours after the onset of myocardial infarction and within 60 minutes of admission to the hospital.

If primary angioplasty is decided upon, the angiographer generally commences the glycoprotein IIB-IIIA receptor inhibitor abciximab. It is administered as a bolus dose of 0.25 µg/kg, followed by 10 µg/min continuous infusion. This regime helps to prevent ischaemic events during and after the angioplasty procedure. Major bleeding can occur after the use of abciximab, particularly in combination with heparin.

An algorithm for the management of STEMI is given in **Fig. 7.3.1**.

Pharmacological Reperfusion with Combined Thrombolytic and GP IIb/IIIa Inhibitor Therapy

Clinical studies have evaluated combination therapy using both thrombolytics and GP IIb/IIIa inhibitors as a reperfusion strategy. It was noted that full doses of the thrombolytic agent and GP IIb/IIIa inhibitor improved flow (TIMI grade 2 or 3) as judged by a study of the infarct-related artery on follow-up angiography. There was however the unacceptable major risk of increased bleeding.

The TIMI 14 trial (27) demonstrated that abciximab combined with half the usual dose of TPA (50 mg) facilitated the rate and extent of thrombolysis (with TIMI 3 flow to infarct-related artery) without the risk of major bleeding. However if half the dose of streptokinase was used in place of TPA the risk of bleeding was again significantly increased. Eptifibatide has been used (in place of abciximab) in combination with half dose of TPA with improved quality and speed of reperfusion in an obstructed coronary artery, and is associated with a satisfactory safety profile (28). If thought necessary this combination therapy can be followed by a coronary angiography and an angioplasty. This constitutes a 'facilitated primary angioplasty' and is used in some units in patients with ST elevated AMI. The advantages of this double-pronged therapy are

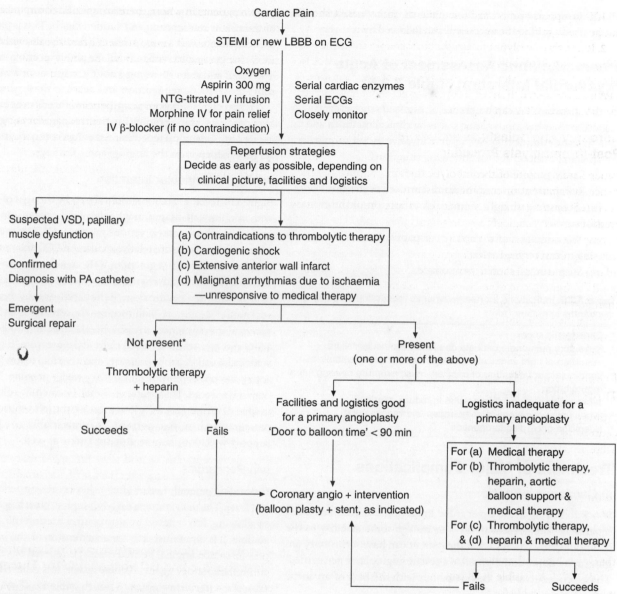

Fig. 7.3.1. Algorithm for management of STEMI.
*Some well equipped units may prefer primary angioplasty to thrombolytic therapy (if door to balloon time < 90 minutes).

available only for patients admitted to a hospital with angioplasty facilities. In patients admitted late into hospital after the cardiac event, or if facilities for coronary angioplasty are not available an approach that combines the use of a fibrinolytic agent plus a IIb/IIIa platelet inhibitor may prove to be more advantageous than the use of a thrombolytic agent alone. We need additional data not only on efficacy but also on safety and cost-effectiveness before this multi-pronged approach can be recommended. The cost of therapy plus the logistics involved in our country are major handicaps for this therapy.

Surgical Reperfusion (Coronary Artery Bypass Surgery)

Coronary artery bypass surgery has indeed a very small place in the management of acute myocardial infarction. It is indicated under the following conditions:

(i) When coronary dissection with occlusion develops during cardiac catheterization, coronary angiography or during percutaneous transluminal coronary angioplasty (PTCA).

(ii) Surgical reperfusion is to be considered in a small subgroup of patients who are undergoing or have completed thrombolytic therapy, but who continue to have ischaemic pain and are haemodynamically unstable. Rescue angioplasty is to be preferred but if this fails or is not feasible, or if the angiography shows left main disease or multivessel disease, emergency surgical revascularization is of benefit. Good centres report a low mortality and morbidity (**29, 30**).

(iii) Surgical reperfusion after an infarct has fully evolved is invariably unsafe, unwise and contraindicated. However in some patients, infarction appears to occur in a 'stuttering' manner over a period of days producing increasing haemodynamic instability and shock. Revascularization in these patients, though fraught with danger, may at times be successful and followed by recovery.

Haemodynamic Assessment of Acute Myocardial Infarction (Table 7.3.5)

With experience, most patients can be assessed satisfactorily with regard to their haemodynamic status by clinical methods and by non-invasive monitoring. We reserve invasive monitoring with a Swan-Ganz catheter for the following situations:

(i) Cardiogenic shock.

(ii) Refractory pulmonary oedema due to left ventricular failure.

(iii) Suspicion of right ventricular infarction or pulmonary embolism.

(iv) Ventricular septal rupture, or papillary muscle rupture causing mitral regurgitation.

(v) Suspicion of cardiac tamponade.

Table 7.3.5. Indications for haemodynamic monitoring in acute myocardial infarction (AMI)

* Cardiogenic shock
* Refractory pulmonary oedema due to left ventricular failure
* Suspicion of right ventricular infarction or pulmonary embolism
* Ventricular septal rupture or papillary muscle rupture causing mitral regurgitation
* When using sodium nitroprusside to reduce afterload
* When using combination of inotropes and vasodilators
* Suspicion of cardiac tamponade

Treatment of Major Complications

(i) Cardiogenic Shock

Shock following acute myocardial infarction has been discussed separately. The present trend is to restore some stability to the haemodynamic state so that the patient can have a coronary angiography done, and if possible a rescue angioplasty performed. These procedures may be carried out with the help of an aortic balloon assist device.

(ii) Left Ventricular Failure

This has been discussed separately.

(iii) Congestive Cardiac Failure

The principles of management have been dealt with in a separate chapter.

(iv) Arrhythmias

Arrhythmias need to be promptly detected and controlled. Ventricular arrhythmias are particularly common during the first 24 hours. Some units prefer to start prophylactic intravenous lidocaine in all patients with fresh infarcts. We prefer to treat arrhythmias as and when they arise (see Chapter on Arrhythmias).

(v) Post-Infarction Angina

Post-infarction angina requires prompt return to the ICU and the administration of intravenous nitroglycerin and restarting of intravenous heparin. An aggressive approach is important because of the risk of reinfarction and sudden death. This is particularly true in patients with a non-Q infarct where the absence of marked ECG changes to start with may lull the physician into complacency. The use of diltiazem 30–60 mg 8 hourly, may reduce the immediate short-term risk of reinfarction and death in these patients (**31**).

Persistent post-infarction angina always needs to be investigated by a coronary angiography. Further management (whether an angioplasty or surgical reperfusion through coronary artery bypass surgery) depends on the angiographic findings.

(vi) Right Ventricular Infarction

Right ventricular infarction should always be thought of in patients with inferior wall infarction who develop hypotension with poor perfusion, whose central venous pressure (CVP) is raised, and in whom the lung fields are relatively clear. An ECG shows an elevated R and an elevated ST segment in V4R; this change may disappear within 24 hours. Bradyrhythms may occur, necessitating the use of a temporary pacemaker. Echocardiography reveals right ventricular dilatation, wall motion abnormalities and often left ventricular dysfunction. Invasive haemodynamic studies through a S-G catheter reveal a raised right atrial pressure, a raised right ventricular end-diastolic pressure, and a normal to low pulmonary artery diastolic or pulmonary capillary wedge pressure. The cardiac output is reduced. These patients should be carefully volume loaded in spite of an increased CVP, to increase the left ventricular filling pressures and cardiac output. They invariably need inotropic support with dobutamine and dopamine as well.

(vii) Pericarditis

Pericarditis generally occurs after 48 hours causing pericardial pain, and fever. The pain is worse on lying supine, breathing deeply, and swallowing. It is relieved by sitting up; a friction rub is generally audible. It is often mistaken for an extension of the infarct or for post-infarction angina. In mild cases it is relieved by non-steroidal anti-inflammatory agents. When severe, it is relieved by dexamethasone 4 mg intravenously 8 hourly, tapered off within a week. Rarely, pericardial effusion is large enough to cause a cardiac tamponade; this necessates a pericardial paracentesis. Heparin should be withheld in the presence of pericardial effusion.

(viii) Rupture of the Interventricular Septum

Septal rupture is characterized by the sudden appearance of a pansystolic murmur generally best heard in the fourth left intercostal space, close to the left sternal border or midway between the left sternal border and the apex. Biventricular failure always follows. The diagnosis can be confirmed by 2D Doppler echocardiography. A S-G catheter will help demonstrate a step-up of oxygen saturation from the right atrium to the right ventricle (due to a left to right shunt at the ventricular level). Immediate management is concerned with restoring haemodynamic stability. Afterload and preload are reduced by a slow infusion of intravenous nitroprusside, and inotropic support is provided by dopamine or dobutamine to maintain the systolic blood pressure > 90–100 mm Hg. An intra-aortic balloon pump is often used to help stabilize the circulation.

Ventilatory support is often required. It is important to opt for quick surgical repair, and it is wrong to wait for days or weeks before undertaking surgery (32, 33). Invariably, delay results in a progressive worsening of the haemodynamic state, and the evolution of multiple organ failure. Once the latter complication ensues, surgery, even if attempted, is almost always unsuccessful.

(ix) Rupture of a Papillary Muscle

Papillary muscle rupture produces a pansystolic murmur at the apex due to severe mitral incompetence. It needs to be distinguished from a ruptured interventricular septum. There is no step up in the oxygen saturation from the right atrium to the right ventricle in this condition, and large 'regurgitant' V waves are observed in the pulmonary wedge tracing. A papillary muscle rupture leads to left ventricular failure with pulmonary oedema together with failure of forward flow and impaired tissue perfusion. Management is on the same lines as for intraventricular septal rupture. A combination of afterload and preload reduction by using sodium nitroprusside, together with inotropic support with dopamine, is necessary. Preload may need to be further reduced by furosemide. An aortic balloon pump may need to be used to help restore a semblance of haemodynamic stability. Urgent surgical repair should be considered in these patients.

(x) Myocardial Rupture

Rupture of the free wall of the ventricle typically occurs 3–5 days after an infarction. It usually presents with rapid hypotension and pericardial tamponade progressing quickly to electromechanical dissociation and death. Patients are almost never salvageable. If there is a comparatively slow leak of blood into the pericardium, time for possible rescue measures may be available. The diagnosis of tamponade should be made on clinical grounds. Echocardiography, if available, can be extremely useful. Treatment consists of emergency pericardiocentesis, infusion of fluids, inotropic and vasopressor support, ventilatory support and rapid transfer to the theatre for surgical repair. We have never had the good fortune of salvaging a patient with rupture of the ventricular wall following a myocardial infarction.

(xi) Embolic Complications

Embolic complications can arise from mural thrombi that may form within the ventricle over the infarcted area. Clinical features depend on the site of embolization. Neurological deficits due to

Table 7.3.6. Major complications of acute myocardial infarction

* Cardiogenic shock
* Left ventricular failure
* Congestive cardiac failure
* Arrhythmias
* Post-infarction angina
* Right ventricular infarction
* Pericarditis
* Rupture of interventricular septum
* Rupture of a papillary muscle
* Myocardial rupture
* Embolic complications

emboli in the cerebrovascular circulation may at times be the presenting feature of an underlying myocardial infarction. Anticoagulation is recommended in such patients. Rarely a saddle block due to an embolus straddling the aortic bifurcation, produces a loss of blood supply to both lower limbs. Removal of the obstructing clot through a Fogarty's catheter introduced through the femoral artery should be promptly done; this is followed by anticoagulation.

Myocardial Stunning or Hibernation

These entities have attracted considerable attention. In myocardial stunning, systolic dysfunction persists for a time after an ischaemic episode even though reperfusion has been established. It can occur after thrombolysis in AMI and after cardiopulmonary bypass. A hibernating myocardium is poorly contractile but still viable area of myocardium due to poor coronary blood flow. The myocardial dysfunction improves when coronary blood flow to the area is reestablished.

Duration of Intensive Care

An uncomplicated anterior myocardial infarct can be transferred out of the ICU after 2 days. An acute myocardial infarction with complications should stay till such time as intensive care is necessary. The need for haemodynamic monitoring, use of inotropes or of drugs to reduce afterload or preload, and close nursing supervision necessitate a stay in the ICU.

REFERENCES

1. Panteghini M, Apple FS, Christenson RH et al. (1999). Use of biochemical markers in acute coronary syndromes. IFCC Scientific Division, Committee on Standardization of Markers of Cardiac Damage, International Federation of Clinical Chemistry. Vclin Chem Lab Med. 37, 687–693.

2. Zimmerman J, Fromm R, Meyer D et al. (1999). Diagnostic marker cooperative study for the diagnosis of myocardial infarction. Circulation. 99, 1671–1677.

3. ISIS-2 (Second International Study of Infarct Survival) Collaborative Group. (1988). Randomized trial of intravenous streptokinase, oral aspirin, both or neither among 17,187 cases of suspected acute myocardial infarction. Lancet. 2, 349.

4. Flaherty JT, Becker LC, Bulkley BH et al. (1983). A randomized prospective trial of intravenous nitroglycerin in patients with acute myocardial infarction. Circulation. 68, 576.

5. The Miami Trial Research Group. (1985). Metoprolol in acute myocardial infarction (MIAMI). A randomized placebo-controlled international trial. Eur Heart J. 6, 199.

6. ISIS-1 (First International Study of Infarct Survival) Collaborative Group. (1986). Randomized trial of intravenous atenolol among 16,027 cases of suspected acute myocardial infarction. ISIS-I. Lancet. 2, 57.

7. Horner SM. (1992). Efficacy of intravenous magnesium in acute myocardial infarction in reducing arrhythmias and mortality: Meta-analysis of magnesium in acute myocardial infarction. Circulation. 86, 774–779.

8. Teo KK, Yusuf S, Collins R et al. (1991). Effects of intravenous magnesium in suspected acute myocardial infarction: Overview of randomized trials. Br Med J. 303, 1499–1503.

9. The ASSET Study Group. (1988). Trial of tissue plasminogen activator for mortality reduction in acute myocardial infarction. Lancet. 2, 525.

10. Gruppo Italiano per lo Studio della streptokinasi nell'Infarto Miocardico (GISSI). (1986). Effectiveness of intravenous thrombolytic treatment in acute myocardial infarction. Lancet. 2, 397.

11. The TIMI Study Group. (1985). The thrombolysis in myocardial infarction (TIMI) trial. N Engl J Med. 312, 932.

12. Fibrinolytic Therapy Trialists' (FTT) Collaborative Group. (1994). Indications for fibrinolytic therapy in suspected acute myocardial infarction: Collaborative overview of early mortality and major morbidity results from all randomized trials of more than 1,000 patients. Lancet. 343, 311–322.

13. Maggioni AP, Franzosi MG, Santoro E et al. (1992). The risk of stroke in patients with acute myocardial infarction after thrombolytic and antithrombotic treatment: Gruppo Italiano per lo Studio della streptokinasi nell'Infarto Miocardico II (GISSI-2) and the International Study Group. N Engl J Med. 327, 1–6.

14. Sobel BE, Corr PB, Robinson AK et al. (1978). Accumulation of lysophosphoglycerides with arrhythmogenic properties in ischaemic myocardium. J Clin Invest. 61, 109.

15. The GUSTO Investigators. (1993). An international randomized trial comparing four thrombolytic strategies for acute myocardial infarction. N Engl J Med. 329, 673–682.

16. GUSTO Angiographis Investigators. (1993). The effects of tissue plasminogen activator, streptokinase, or both on coronary artery patency, ventricular function, and survival after acute myocardial infarction. N Engl J Med. 329, 1615.

17. Théroux P. (2003). Meta-analysis of randomized trials comparing enoxaparin versus unfractionated heparin as adjunctive therapy to fibrinolysis in ST-elevation acute myocardial infarction. Am J Cardiol. 91(7), 860–864.

18. Gruppo Italiano per lo Studio della Sopravvivenza nell'Infarto Miocardico. (1990). GISSI-2: a factorial randomised trial of alteplase versus streptokinase and heparin versus no heparin among 12490 patients with acute myocardial infarction. Lancet. 336, 65–71.

19. ISIS-3 (Third International Study of Infarct Survival) Collaborative Group. (1992). ISIS-3: a randomised comparison of streptokinase vs tissue plasminogen activator vs anistreplase and of aspirin plus heparin vs aspirin alone among 41299 cases of suspected acute myocardial infarction. Lancet. 339, 753–770.

20. Califf RM, Topol EJ, Stack RS et al. (1991). Evaluation of combination thrombolytic therapy and timing of cardiac catheterization in acute myocardial infarction: results of thrombolysis and angioplasty in myocardial infarction—phase 5 randomised trial. Circulation. 83, 1543–1556.

21. Grines CL, Browne KF, Marco J et al. (1993). A comparison of immediate angioplasty with thrombolytic therapy for acute myocardial infarction. N Engl J Med. 328(10), 673–679.

22. Zijlstra F, Jan de Boer M, Hoorntje JCA et al. (1993). A comparison of immediate coronary angioplasty with intravenous streptokinase in acute myocardial infarction. N Engl Med. 328(10), 680–684.

23. Gibbons RJ, Holmes DR, Reeder GS et al. (1993). Immediate angioplasty compared with the administration of a thrombolytic agent followed by conservative treatment for myocardial infarction. N Engl J Med. 328(10), 685–691.

24. Eckman MH, Wong JB, Salem DN, Pauker SG. (1992). Direct angioplasty for acute myocardial infarction: A review of outcomes in clinical subsets. Ann Intern Med. 117, 667.

25. O'Neil WW, Broche BR, Ivanhoe R et al. (1994). Primary coronary angioplasty for acute myocardial infarction (The primary angioplasty registry). Am J Cardiol. 73, 627.

26. Grives CL, Browne KF, Marco J et al. (1993). A comparison of immediate angioplasty with thrombolytic therapy for acute myocardial infarction. N Engl J Med. 328, 673.

27. Antman EM, Giugliano RP, Gibson CM et al. (1999). Abciximab facilitates the rate and extent of thrombolysis: results of the thrombolysis in myocardial infarction (TIMI) 14 trial. Circulation. 99, 2720–2732.

28. Brenner SJ, Zeymer U, Adgey AAJ et al. (2002). Eptifibatide and low-dose plasminogen activator in acute myocardial infarction: The integrilin and low-dose thrombolysis in acute myocardial infarction (INTRO AMI) trial. J Am Soc Cardiol. 39(3), 377–386.

29. Meyer J, Merx W, Dorr R et al. (1985). Sequential intervention procedures after intracoronary thrombolysis: balloon dilatation, bypass surgery and medical treatment. Int J Cardiol. 7, 281.

30. Kereiakes DG, Topol EG, George BS et al. (1989). Favourable early and long-term prognosis following coronary bypass surgery therapy for myocardial infarction: results of a multicentre trial. Am Heart J. 118, 199.

31. The Multicenter Diltiazem Postinfarction Trial Research Group. (1988). The effect of diltiazem on mortality and re-infarction after myocardial infarction. N Engl J Med. 319, 385–392.

32. Held AC, Cole PL, Lipton B et al. (1988). Rupture of the interventricular septum complicating acute myocardial infarction: A multicenter analysis of clinical findings and outcome. Am Heart J. 116, 1330–1336.

33. Gaudini VA, Miller DG, Stinson EB et al. (1981). Post-infarction ventricular septal defect: An argument for early operation. Surgery. 89, 48–54.

Acute Left Ventricular Failure with Pulmonary Oedema

Acute left ventricular failure with pulmonary oedema is always associated with a marked increase in the left ventricular end-diastolic pressure and the pulmonary capillary wedge pressure. The increased pressure in the pulmonary capillaries and veins leads to a transudation of fluid into the interstitial tissues of the lung (interstitial oedema), and later into the alveoli producing alveolar flooding. Acute left ventricular failure may vary in severity. When mild, it is characterized by paroxysmal attacks of breathlessness which abate spontaneously; these attacks are related to sharp but transient rise in the left ventricular end-diastolic and the capillary wedge pressures. When severe, it is associated with frank pulmonary oedema, the patient literally drowning in his own secretions. Fulminant pulmonary oedema is associated with an increase in the left ventricular filling pressure (left ventricular end-diastolic pressure) close to or > 30 mm Hg **(1, 2)**.

Acute left ventricular failure with pulmonary oedema constitutes an important cause for emergency admission to an intensive care unit. Also, patients admitted to an ICU for other critical illnesses may suddenly develop acute pulmonary oedema due to left ventricular dysfunction. The latter may be pre-existing but may have gone undetected, and could well be unmasked by the stress of a critical illness (e.g. fever, tachycardia, seizures), or by therapy used to treat a critical illness e.g. fluid infusions which cannot be easily handled by a diseased or poorly functioning left ventricle. Left ventricular dysfunction and failure can also be induced in a previously healthy heart by an acute illness e.g. overwhelming sepsis, or a fulminant viral infection for which the patient has been admitted to the ICU.

Haemodynamic Profiles in Left Ventricular Failure

Failure of the pumping action of the left ventricle leads to two basic disturbances in the haemodynamics of the circulation:

(i) An increase in 'backward pressure' from the failing left ventricle which results in pulmonary oedema.

(ii) A failure of forward flow which leads in time to a decreasing cardiac output, decreasing arterial blood pressure, and above all to a fall in tissue perfusion.

Both the above features may be present in varying degrees in the same individual. Also each one of these disturbances may occur independently of the other (see Chapter on Cardiogenic Shock). The following haemodynamic patterns may be observed:

(i) An increased left ventricular end-diastolic pressure and pulmonary capillary wedge pressure with resulting pulmonary oedema; an adequate forward flow with a cardiac index not less than 2.5 l/min/m^2 and adequate tissue perfusion. To start with, the cardiac output in acute left ventricular failure may be normal in spite of pulmonary oedema, because the ventricle still responds to the increase in preload, as per Starling's law—a basic compensatory mechanism in cardiac failure. The arterial pressure is unchanged and for various reasons may even show a temporary rise.

The mechanics of this haemodynamic change is illustrated by **Fig. 7.4.1** which shows the right and left ventricular function curves in a patient with acute pulmonary oedema due to poor left ventricular function. Two features worthy of note in this figure are: (a) a normal right ventricular function curve; (b) a left ventricular function curve which is shifted to the right, and whose slope is moderately reduced.

(ii) Increased pulmonary capillary wedge pressure causing pulmonary oedema; a failure of forward flow with a drop in the cardiac index to less than or equal to 2.2 l/min/m^2, and a fall in tissue perfusion. As failure of forward flow increases, the arterial blood pressure drops in spite of compensatory mechanisms.

The mechanics of this haemodynamic change is the same as in (i) except that the slope of the left ventricular function curve is markedly reduced, pointing to a more severe dysfunction than in the first case (see Chapter on Cardiogenic Shock).

(iii) No pulmonary oedema as the PCWP is not raised; however there is marked failure of forward flow with a low cardiac index (often < 1.8 l/min/m^2), a low arterial blood pressure and poor tissue perfusion often causing a lactic acid acidosis. The picture is akin to that of cardiogenic shock without pulmonary oedema. This haemodynamic profile has been dealt with in the Chapter on Cardiogenic Shock.

(iv) Increased right sided heart pressures together with the increased left sided heart pressures noted above. Thus, in addition to an increased left ventricular end diastolic pressure and pulmonary capillary wedge pressure, there is also an increased pulmonary

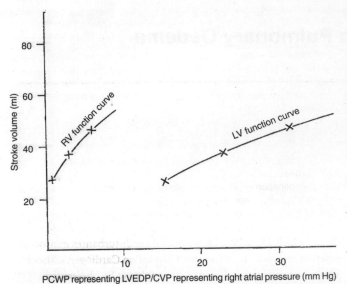

Fig. 7.4.1. Right and left ventricular function curves in a patient with acute left ventricular failure causing fulminant pulmonary oedema. Note that the left ventricular function curve is shifted to the right, and has a lesser slope compared to the right ventricular function curve. Fulminant pulmonary oedema occurs when PCWP exceeds 30 mm Hg, at which time the right atrial pressure is about 7 mm Hg. Note that a rise in right atrial pressure from 2 to 7 mm Hg is associated with a rise in the left ventricular filling pressure from 15 to 32 mm Hg.

artery pressure, increased right ventricular end diastolic and right atrial pressure and a rise in the central venous pressure. This is due to a progressive increase in pressure 'backwards' from the failing left ventricle, ultimately resulting in right heart failure. The clinical picture is not only that of pulmonary oedema, but also includes raised jugular venous pressure, enlarged tender liver and pitting oedema of the feet. This picture of congestive cardiac failure (left and right sided heart failure) can evolve rapidly as after a massive anterior myocardial infarct or evolves subacutely if a patient with left ventricular failure is inadequately treated or brought late to the intensive care unit.

Systolic and Diastolic Left Ventricular Dysfunction and Failure

Systolic dysfunction and heart failure is due to impaired contractility of the myocardium. Diastolic dysfunction and failure is characterized by a decrease in ventricular distensibility (reduced compliance of the ventricle). Inadequate ventricular filling results, and is then responsible for a fall in cardiac output, though cardiac contractility is normal. Diastolic ventricular dysfunction and failure are seen in left ventricular hypertrophy (due to hypertension or aortic stenosis), myocardial ischaemia, restrictive cardiomyopathy, positive pressure mechanical ventilation or pericardial effusion (3–5). However, in many patients, systolic and diastolic dysfunction co-exist. This is classically seen in patients with coronary artery disease. Systolic dysfunction and systolic failure in these patients can be caused by new or old myocardial infarction (loss of contractile muscle tissue), and by active or acute myocardial

ischaemia. Diastolic dysfunction and failure can result from replacement of muscle by fibrous tissue following infarction and by the acute reduction in myocardial distensibility during ischaemia. Measurement of the pulmonary capillary wedge pressure does not distinguish between systolic dysfunction from diastolic dysfunction as the wedge pressure is increased in both. However, the left ventricular end diastolic volume for a given end diastolic pressure is significantly greater in systolic dysfunction when compared to diastolic dysfunction.

Diagnosis (1)

The diagnosis of pulmonary oedema due to acute left ventricular failure is generally easy. The patient is breathless and often orthopnoeic (6). Pulmonary oedema is clinically manifest by crackles which may be restricted to only the lung bases. In severe oedema, loud crackles or bubbling moist sounds are heard all over both lungs; in fulminant oedema, pinkish frothy oedema fluid may well out of the mouth and nose, the patient literally drowning in his own secretions. Occasionally, there are more of polyphonic wheezes than crackles. In rare instances, wheezing with prolonged expiration is indistinguishable from that heard in severe bronchial asthma. If the chest is not too noisy, a diastolic gallop may be generally heard; a diastolic third heart sound signifies a left ventricular end-diastolic pressure ≥ 18 mm Hg. There is often, though not always, clinical evidence of underlying left heart disease. Hypertension, acute myocardial ischaemia, myocardial infarction, aortic valve disease, mitral incompetence, acute myocarditis, supraventricular and ventricular arrhythmias, complete heart block and cardiomyopathy are important causes of acute left ventricular failure. Acute pulmonary oedema can also occur when there is a sudden, sharp rise in left atrial pressure in patients with mitral stenosis. Positive pressure ventilation, particularly when associated with high PEEP may cause left ventricular diastolic dysfunction and failure. High output failures are characterized by arteriovenous shunting or increased demand for oxygen by tissues. They are observed chiefly in arteriovenous fistulas, severe anaemia, thyrotoxicosis, and beriberi. In our experience, they more often act as aggravating or precipitating factors of heart failure in patients with underlying cardiac disease. Diagnosis of the underlying aetiopathology during an attack of acute pulmonary oedema may be difficult, as in severe cases heart sounds and murmurs are inaudible due to the loud bubbling moist sounds which are heard even at some distance from the patient.

A *chest X-ray* shows clear evidence of pulmonary oedema. Interstitial oedema is observed in mild cases; alveolar oedema leads to homogenous alveolar shadows generally spreading from the hilum to the periphery. Occasionally one lung is considerably more involved than the other. It is important to note that there can be a short time lag between the sudden rise in left ventricular end-diastolic pressure (and with it in the pulmonary capillary wedge pressure), and the clinical and radiological appearances of pulmonary oedema (7).

An *ECG* may show evidence of ischaemic heart disease or of left ventricular hypertrophy.

An *arterial blood gas analysis* in well-marked pulmonary oedema shows a low PaO_2 (as low as 30–40 mm Hg), with hypocapnia. In the moribund patient or when the use of morphine has suppressed the respiratory drive, the $PaCO_2$ rises, and some degree of respiratory acidosis results. In patients with a failing forward flow and impaired tissue perfusion, there is a superadded metabolic (lactic acid) acidosis. A combination of metabolic and respiratory acidosis is of sinister prognosis.

Echocardiography. A transthoracic echocardiogram provides information of ventricular size and systolic function, wall motion, valvular structure and function, presence of intracardiac clots or masses, intracardiac flow, pericardium and ascending and transverse aorta. A normal or near normal left ventricular ejection fraction should never preclude the diagnosis of acute pulmonary oedema, as diastolic dysfunction may occur with normal or near normal ventricular systolic function in 40 per cent of patients with heart failure (**3–5**).

Differential Diagnosis

When acute left ventricular failure is associated with wheezing and prolonged expiration, it closely resembles a late-onset bronchial asthma. The diagnosis becomes doubly difficult when a patient with a past history of long-standing bronchial asthma develops left ventricular disease. In fact, these are just the patients who when they develop acute left ventricular failure, will manifest with wheezing rather than auscultatory crackles. We have been convinced over the years, that individuals with increased bronchial reactivity 'wheeze' rather than 'crackle' during left ventricular failure.

Rarely it is difficult to distinguish between pulmonary oedema resulting from left ventricular failure, and non-cardiogenic pulmonary oedema. A careful clinical history, the evolution of the disease and relevant investigations generally clarify the diagnosis. A pulmonary capillary wedge pressure > 18 mm Hg as measured by a Swan-Ganz catheter points to left ventricular failure. It must be remembered that a patient with left ventricular dysfunction may well suffer from an unrelated illness that can cause non-cardiogenic pulmonary oedema; in such individuals more than one cause may be responsible for the pulmonary oedema.

Management (Table 7.4.1) (8)

The patient with acute pulmonary oedema due to left ventricular failure is nursed propped up in bed. If possible, he should be made to sit up with his legs dangling over the side of the bed. If pulmonary oedema is associated with marked failure of forward flow and features of shock, he may need to be nursed flat in bed with the head slightly raised.

Morphine Sulphate (9)

This is an invaluable drug for use as the first immediate emergency measure. 15 mg can be given subcutaneously in moderately severe left ventricular failure. Alternatively, 2–4 mg of the drug is administered intravenously and the dose repeated after half to one hour if necessary, so that the desired effect of morphine is obtained.

Table 7.4.1. Management of acute pulmonary oedema due to left ventricular failure

* Morphine 2–4 mg IV, or buprenorphine 0.2–0.4 mg IV, repeated after half to one hour if necessary. If morphine is not available, pethidine 75–100 mg IM can be used. Patients with fulminant pulmonary oedema and alveolar hypoventilation, should first be put on mechanical ventilator support and then administered morphine
* Oxygen at 6–8 l/min through nasal prongs
* Measures to reduce preload
  – Furosemide 40–100 mg IV
  – Aminophylline 250 mg diluted with dextrose and given IV over 10–15 min
  – Application of rotating tourniquets or BP cuffs to extremities may be used during transport to hospital
* Digitalis—improves cardiac contractility and pump function 0.25 mg given IV slowly and repeated 4–6 hourly till digitalising dose of 0.75–1 mg given in 24 hrs
* Vasodilators
  – IV Nitroglycerin in a slow titrated drip starting at 15 µg/min—reduces preload
  – IV Sodium Nitroprusside in a slow titrated drip starting at 5 µg/min—reduces both preload and afterload
* Inotropic Agents (Dopamine/Dobutamine) Used
  – when pulmonary oedema associated with hypotension and/or reduced tissue perfusion
  – in patients with pulmonary oedema refractory to the above-mentioned treatment
* Ventilator support
  – in fulminant pulmonary oedema
  – when respiratory drive fails and patient breathes poorly
  – respiratory muscle fatigue

Morphine helps in several ways: (a) it allays anxiety, restlessness, and slows the respiratory rate, thereby reducing the work of breathing, and also the overall oxygen demand by the peripheral tissues (through sedation and quietening of the patient); (b) it dilates both arterioles and venules thereby increasing venous capacitance and reducing the preload. A reduced preload causes a drop in the pulmonary capillary wedge pressure and in the filling pressure of the left ventricle. This results in a reduction of pulmonary oedema.

Morphine is often impossible to obtain in hospitals and intensive care units in India. A useful substitute (but not an equally effective one), is buprenorphine given slowly intravenously in a 0.2–0.4 mg dose. This may need to be repeated till the desired effect is achieved.

Pethidine 75–100 mg intramuscularly can also be used, but lacks the overall efficacy of morphine. The only situation where we prefer to use pethidine is in patients in acute left ventricular failure who present with severe wheeze and prolonged expiration. In a few of these patients, morphine instead of relieving the wheeze, actually worsens it. The major side effects of morphine include hypotension, vomiting, and increased parasympathomimetic activity evinced by bradycardia and bronchospasm. Some patients with acute left ventricular failure may show a strong hypertensive response during the period of failure, even though they are not basically hypertensive. Morphine acts beautifully in such patients and lowers the blood pressure effectively. Vomiting can be controlled by the use of phenargan 25 mg intramuscularly. Most patients with acute left ventricular failure and pulmonary oedema have tachycardia, so that a lowering of the heart rate by morphine is a decided advantage. If parasympathomimetic effects are observed, the administration of atropine 0.5 mg intravenously easily reverses these effects.

There is just one strong contraindication to the use of intravenous morphine in patients with acute left ventricular failure. It should not be used as an immediate measure in a patient with fulminant pulmonary oedema who is literally frothing with oedema fluid. Such patients have ineffective breathing and in fact, their blood gases always show a raised $PaCO_2$ pointing to alveolar hypoventilation. A few of these patients are also so severely hypoxic, that they are obtunded. The use of morphine as the first measure in these patients invariably produces a respiratory arrest. As will be discussed below, these patients should be promptly intubated and ventilated; morphine should be given only subsequent to this emergency procedure.

Oxygen

This is promptly started to combat hypoxia, either through a nasal catheter or nasal prongs at 6–8 l/min, or through a well-fitting oronasal mask at 5–6 l/min. In patients with well-marked pulmonary oedema, oxygen can be given under continuous positive pressure using a well-fitting oronasal mask. This may provide satisfactory oxygenation, and may at times prevent the need for emergency intubation and ventilatory support.

Measures to Reduce Preload

A. Use of Diuretics—Furosemide (10–12)

Intravenous furosemide is useful in the management of acute pulmonary oedema. 40–100 mg or even more of the drug is given intravenously, depending on the severity of pulmonary oedema. Furosemide reduces preload in 2 ways:

(i) It produces almost within minutes a sharp increase in venous capacitance through a venodilating effect, which results in a significant lowering of the preload (as measured by the pulmonary artery end-diastolic and pulmonary capillary wedge pressures). Pulmonary congestion thereby decreases even before the onset of the diuretic action of the drug. We have observed a fall of 5–8 mm Hg in the left ventricular filling pressures after intravenous furosemide.

(ii) It has an excellent diuretic action. Diuresis starts within 15 minutes and is maximal for 4–6 hours. Some patients are exquisitely sensitive to even small doses (40 mg) of furosemide, and respond with profuse diuresis. Therefore unless the pulmonary oedema is gross, it is wiser to give only 40 mg furosemide initially and then repeat a larger dose if diuresis is inadequate in the first 2 hours. At times, patients require massive doses of furosemide (1 g over 24 hours) to promote an effective diuresis. When more than 100 to 120 mg of intravenous furosemide are required to produce an effective diuretic effect, we prefer to administer the drug by a continuous infusion at a rate of 10 mg–40 mg/ hour.

The diuresis induced by furosemide reduces the water content of the lungs and thus reduces pulmonary oedema. It is important to note that diuretics do not significantly increase cardiac output. In fact, over-diuresis with an over-reduction in the preload is a disadvantage, as this may initially cause a fall in the cardiac output. It is currently believed that a fall in the cardiac output may be further contributed to by an increase in systemic vascular resistance. The latter effect is due to a lasix-induced stimulation of release of rennin and raised circulating angiotensin levels (13). **Fig. 7.4.2a** illustrates the effect of furosemide on the left ventricular function curve in left heart failure. In contrast, the administration of dopamine to these patients improves the cardiac contractility to almost normal levels (**Fig. 7.4.2b**).

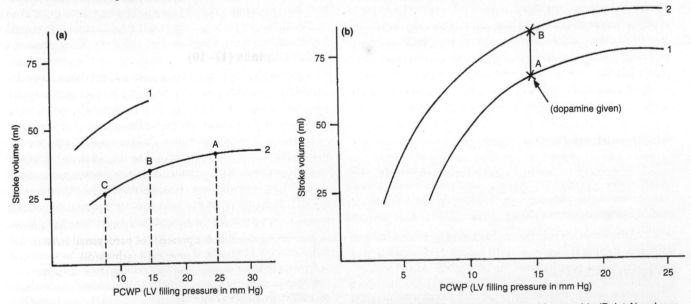

Fig. 7.4.2. (a) 1—Normal LV function curve; 2—LV function curve in patient with LV dysfunction. Administration of furosemide (Point A) reduces preload, causes a fall in PCWP (Point B), and relieves pulmonary oedema, but does not influence stroke volume or cardiac output. Overuse of furosemide will further reduce PCWP (to Point C) and though pulmonary oedema is further relieved, there is now a fall in the already low cardiac output. **(b)** LV function curves—(1) before administration of dopamine; (2) after dopamine administration. In contrast to **(a)**, the use of dopamine improves the cardiac contractility to almost normal levels (point A to point B).

The danger of overuse of furosemide is two-fold—it renders the patient hypovolaemic and can reduce the cardiac output, the sum total of these effects being an impairment of tissue perfusion. The above problems may prove dangerous if the kidneys continue to be 'whipped' by increasing doses of furosemide, in an attempt to increase a falling urine output in a hypovolaemic patient. Features of hypovolaemic shock (which may include oliguria and even renal shutdown), may thus be wrongly attributed to cardiogenic shock produced by poor pump function.

B. Use of Vasodilators

Vasodilators are important in the management of cardiogenic pulmonary oedema. Nitrates chiefly act by reducing the preload, whilst sodium nitroprusside when used in selected cases, acts by reducing both the preload and the afterload.

Nitrates (14, 15)

A slow drip of intravenous nitroglycerin is always used in patients with well-marked cardiogenic pulmonary oedema, starting with 15 µg/minute and progressively increasing the concentration till the desired relief is obtained. The blood pressure is carefully monitored, and as described under the management of cardiogenic shock, should not be allowed to fall below 100 mm Hg systolic. In previously hypertensive patients the systolic blood pressure should not be allowed to fall below 130–140 mm Hg. The other side effects of intravenous nitroglycerin have been discussed at length under cardiogenic shock. It is not always necessary to use a Swan-Ganz catheter for monitoring the right sided pressures and the pulmonary capillary wedge pressure when using intravenous nitroglycerin; non-invasive monitoring with careful clinical assessment generally suffices. However invasive haemodynamic monitoring is resorted to, when pulmonary oedema is associated with poor forward flow and impaired tissue perfusion.

In less severe cases of cardiogenic pulmonary oedema, the use of isosorbide dinitrate 10 mg four hourly suffices. One can use the drug either sublingually or orally with a careful watch on the arterial blood pressure.

The liberal use of a trinitrate ointment (2–2.5" patch) applied on the skin is also helpful in reducing preload. This method can be used after the patient has been weaned off the intravenous nitroglycerin infusion, which may take from 1–4 days. The trinitrate ointment can be applied on the skin concurrently with oral isosorbide therapy. The ointment can be promptly rubbed off if the arterial blood pressure starts to drop.

Sodium Nitroprusside (16)

Sodium nitroprusside may be used as a slowly titrated intravenous drip (starting at 5 µg/minute). It reduces both arteriolar and venous resistance thereby reducing both afterload and preload. Reduction of preload relieves pulmonary congestion and oedema; reduction of afterload improves the pumping action of the heart.

Sodium nitroprusside is particularly useful in patients who have well-marked hypertension, or in those who have poor pump function with inadequate tissue perfusion, provided the systolic blood pressure is > 100 mm Hg. Under the above circumstances, use of the drug is indicated if:

(i) there is gross pulmonary oedema—which means that there is markedly increased preload;

(ii) the use of morphine, intravenous furosemide, intravenous nitroglycerin infusions and intravenous digoxin have not promptly controlled the situation;

(iii) there are facilities to monitor the pulmonary artery pressures through a Swan-Ganz catheter, and the systemic arterial pressure through an intra-arterial catheter. The use of intravenous nitroprusside in the absence of these monitoring facilities can be tricky and dangerous, particularly in the hands of the inexperienced.

The side effects of nitroprusside, particularly a precipitous fall in blood pressure, should be carefully monitored. These side effects have already been elaborated upon in the Management of Cardiogenic Shock.

C. Aminophylline (1)

We use aminophylline (0.5 g in a slow intravenous infusion) only in the presence of severe bronchospasm. Aminophylline however, also has a venodilating effect, thereby reducing venous return and preload.

D. Use of Rotating Tourniquets or Blood Pressure Cuffs to the Extremities

Wide soft rubber tubings or blood pressure cuffs are used as tourniquets, and these are applied 6" below the groin and 4" below the shoulders. Three extremities are compressed by the tourniquets or blood pressure cuffs at one time, and every 15–20 minutes one tourniquet or blood pressure cuff is released and placed over the free extremity. The blood pressure cuffs are inflated to a pressure which is less than the systolic blood pressure (the pulse must be palpable distally). This is an emergency measure that may help to reduce venous return and preload during transport to the ICU of a hospital.

Use of Digitalis (17–19)

Digitalis improves cardiac contractility and therefore improves pump function in left ventricular failure. For prompt effect, digoxin is given in a dose of 0.25 mg very slowly, intravenously. This is repeated every 4–6 hourly till a total digitalising dose of 0.75–1 mg is given over 24 hours. If the patient has already been taking adequate doses of oral digitalis prior to the onset of acute left ventricular failure with pulmonary oedema, it is best to avoid intravenous use of the drug. However if it is given, no more than 0.125 mg is administered. Determination of serum digoxin levels helps in titrating the dose of digitalis. In a patient who has already been receiving digitalis, the presence of paroxysmal atrial tachycardia with a 2:1 block, A-V junctional tachycardia, or recurrent ventricular bigeminy are all suggestive of digitalis toxicity.

Inotropic Agents (20, 21)

An intravenous infusion of dopamine or dobutamine is used under the following conditions in patients with cardiogenic pulmonary oedema (see **Fig. 7.4.2b**). Their dosage and manner of use have been described under Cardiogenic Shock.

(i) When acute pulmonary oedema is associated with hypotension and/or evidence of impaired tissue perfusion.

(ii) When pulmonary oedema does not relent quickly in spite of the measures outlined above.

Dobutamine is preferred unless the systolic blood pressure is well below 90 mm Hg, in which case dopamine is used. In patients who do not diurese easily with furosemide, a low-dose dopamine infusion (2–3 μg/kg/min) in dextrose exerts a dopaminergic effect and helps urinary excretion.

Recognition of Factors Frequently Precipitating LV Failure and Pulmonary Oedema in the ICU (Table 7.4.2)

Important precipitating factors causing cardiogenic pulmonary oedema in patients being treated for some other critical illness in the ICU include:

(i) Increased salt intake.

(ii) Overloading patients with fluids through intravenous infusions. Pulmonary oedema may be triggered in patients with underlying poor LV function by the rapid infusion of fluids, even if the fluid intake is by no means excessive. This is particularly common when intravenous infusions of whole blood, plasma or colloid are given rapidly to patients with poor left ventricular function.

(iii) The occurrence of tachyrhythms. Sinus tachycardia produced by fever, marked restlessness, involuntary movements, or seizures, increases the workload on the heart in critically ill patients, and triggers cardiogenic pulmonary oedema, thereby unmasking left ventricular failure in these patients. Supraventricular tachycardias, atrial fibrillation with a fast ventricular rate, or ventricular tachycardias can have an even more disastrous effect in critically ill patients.

(iv) A marked bradyrhythm can also result in increased filling pressures and cardiogenic pulmonary oedema. Pacing may be required to increase the heart rate and reverse the pulmonary oedema, particularly if intravenous atropine proves ineffective.

(v) Severe anaemia, thyrotoxicosis and vitamin B1 deficiency may act as precipitating or contributory factors in acute heart failure.

Table 7.4.2. Important factors precipitating left ventricular failure and pulmonary oedema in critically ill patients in the ICU

* Increased salt intake
* Overloading patients with fluids through IV infusions. In patients with LV dysfunction, rapid infusion of fluids (particularly whole blood, plasma, colloids, even if not excessive), may trigger pulmonary oedema
* Occurrence of tachyrhythms eg. supraventricular tachycardia, atrial fibrillation with fast ventricular rate, or ventricular tachycardia. In critically ill patients, even sinus tachycardia due to fever, seizures, can increase the workload of the heart, and precipitate pulmonary oedema
* Occurrence of marked bradyrhythm can increase the filling pressure, and precipitate pulmonary oedema

Acute Left Ventricular Failure Presenting with Severe Bronchospasm (True Cardiac Asthma)

Patients with a background of asthma or hyperreactive bronchi often present with severe bronchospasm when they develop acute left ventricular failure due to underlying left ventricular disease. In addition to the treatment outlined above, we also administer methyl prednisolone 20 to 40 mg 8 hourly intravenously, and judiciously nebulize with salbutamol. Aminophylline 0.5 g administered in an intravenous infusion over 24 hours is of use.

Use of Ventilator Support in Cardiogenic Pulmonary Oedema

This is indicated in the following conditions:

(i) Fulminant pulmonary oedema in which secretions bubble within the trachea and the larger bronchi. The patient is grossly hypoxic, often cyanosed, with a $PaO_2 < 45$ mm Hg, and often as low as 30 mm Hg. These patients almost always hypoventilate because of ineffective respiration, and this is evinced by a $PaCO_2 > 50$ mm Hg. Prompt endotracheal intubation and the use of a volume cycled ventilator with an FIO_2 of 100 per cent is life-saving. Oxygenation improves, ventilation is satisfactory and the positive pressure forces the oedema fluid back against the alveolar walls, and at least prevents further transudation of fluid. A positive end-expiratory pressure (PEEP) of +5 to +10 cm of water is of help. The therapy described above is often life-saving in a patient with fulminant pulmonary oedema who has a palpable pulse and a satisfactory arterial blood pressure (> 90 mm Hg). It buys valuable time and gives other therapeutic measures, particularly the use of morphine, digoxin, furosemide, intravenous nitroglycerin infusion and intravenous dopamine support, a chance to take effect. If however ventilator support is delayed to a point in time when the pulse is barely perceptible and the arterial blood pressure unrecordable, the prognosis is poor. In less fulminant cases, non-invasive ventilator support through an orofacial mask is equally effective.

(ii) When the respiratory drive fails, and the patient is observed to breathe poorly. This occurs terminally in severe pulmonary oedema, or is the result of respiratory muscle weakness in critically ill patients. It also occurs when the respiratory drive has been excessively depressed by the use of morphine or pethidine. A poor respiratory drive is noted clinically and confirmed by blood gas analysis which shows increasing hypoxia and a rise in $PaCO_2$. The average patient with cardiogenic pulmonary oedema is hypocapnic; hence a $PaCO_2$ of 45–50 mm Hg can portend disaster.

Mechanical Support

In patients with pulmonary oedema and severe shock unresponsive to conventional methods, mechanical support with an intra-aotic balloon pump or rarely with a ventricular assist device may help to temporarily tide over a crisis.

Invasive Monitoring in Cardiogenic Pulmonary Oedema

Clinical judgement with routine non-invasive tests (which should include chest X-ray and arterial blood gas analysis) generally suffice to guide management. A Swan-Ganz catheter with monitoring of pulmonary artery and pulmonary capillary wedge pressures (and indirectly of left ventricular filling pressures), and measurement of cardiac output is indicated under the following circumstances:

(i) When the diagnosis of cardiogenic versus noncardiogenic pulmonary oedema is uncertain on clinical grounds.

(ii) When the knowledge of a patient's volume status is of vital importance, but cannot be determined from the history and clinical examination.

(iii) In severe cases of pulmonary oedema which do not respond to conventional therapy.

(iv) On the rare occasions when intravenous sodium nitroprusside is used to reduce both afterload and preload.

(v) When acute pulmonary oedema is associated with a sharp fall in arterial blood pressure, reduced tissue perfusion or with obvious shock.

(vi) When in a patient presenting as acute heart failure it is important to exclude cardiac tamponade or an acute left to right shunt.

Improvement in cardiogenic pulmonary oedema is gauged clinically and by chest X-rays. In patients with a Swan-Ganz catheter one can titrate therapy to maintain the pulmonary capillary wedge pressure close to 15 mm Hg to 18 mm Hg, ensuring that a fall in preload does not cause a sharp fall in the cardiac index. It is important to remember that there is a significant time lag between reduction of preload with a fall in the pulmonary capillary wedge pressure to safe levels, and the radiological clearing of oedema fluid. It is therefore important not to overdiurese these patients merely because of persistent alveolar shadows in the lung fields, as this could lead to unwanted hypovolaemia.

REFERENCES

1. Givertz MM, Colucci WS, Braunwald E. (2001). Clinical Aspects of Heart Failure: High-Output Failure; Pulmonary Oedema. In: Heart Disease. A Textbook of Cardiovascular Medicine (Ed. Braunwald E). pp. 553–561. WB Saunders Company, Philadelphia, London, Tokyo.

2. Schuster DP. (1998). Pulmonary Oedema. In: Pulmonary Diseases and Disorders (Ed. Fishman AP). pp. 1331–1356. McGraw-Hill Book Company, New York.

3. Bonow RO, Udelson JE. (1992). Left ventricular diastolic dysfunction as a cause of congestive heart failure. Ann Intern Med. 117, 502–510.

4. Goldsmith S, Dick C. (1993). Differentiating systolic from diastolic heart failure: pathophysiologic and therapeutic considerations. Am J Med. 95, 645–655.

5. Gaasch WH. (19994). Diagnosis and treatment of heart failure based on left ventricular systolic or diastolic dysfunction. JAMA. 271, 1276–1280.

6. Geltman EM. (1989). Mild heart failure: Diagnosis and treatment. Am Heart J. 118, 1277.

7. Steiner RM. (2001). Radiology of the Heart and Great Vessels. In: Heart Disease—a Textbook of Cardiovascular Medicine (Eds Braunwald E, Zipes DP, Libby P). pp. 237–272. WB Saundes Company, Philadelphia, London, Tokyo.

8. Bristow MR, Port JD, Kelly RA. (2001). Treatment of Heart Failure. In: Heart Disease. A Textbook of Cardiovascular Medicine (Eds Braunwald E, Zipes DP, Libby P). pp. 562–599. WB Saunders Company, Philadelphia, London, Tokyo.

9. Vismara LA, Leaman DA, Zelis R. (1976). The effects of morphine on venous tone in patients with acute pulmonary oedema. Circulation. 54, 335.

10. Wilson JR, Reichek N, Dunkman WB et al. (1981). Effect of diuresis on the performance of the failing left ventricle in man. Am J Med. 70, 234.

11. Anand I, Veall N, Kalra GS et al. (1989). Treatment of heart failure with diuretics: Body compartments, renal function and plasma hormones. Eur Heart J. 10, 445.

12. Wilcox CS. (1991). Diuretics. In: The Kidney (Eds Brenner BM, Rector FC). pp. 2123–2147. WB Saunders Company, Philadelphia.

13. Francis GS, Siegel RM, Goldsmith SR et al. (1986). Acute vasoconstrictor response to intravenous furosemide in patients with chronic congestive heart failure. Ann Intern Med. 103, 1–6.

14. Packer M. (1985). Mechanisms of nitrate action in patients with severe left ventricular failure: Conceptual problems with the theory of venosequestration. Am Heart J. 110, 259.

15. Cohn JN. (1990). Nitrates are effective in the treatment of chronic congestive heart failure: The protagonist's view. Am J Cardiol. 66, 444.

16. Franciosa JA, Guiha NH, Limas CJ et al. (1972). Improved left ventricular function during nitroprusside infusion in acute myocardial infarction. Lancet. 1, 650.

17. Arnold SB, Byrd RC, Meister W et al. (1980). Long-term digitalis therapy improves left ventricular function in heart failure. N Engl J Med. 303, 699.

18. Gheorghiade M, St Clair J, St Clair C et al. (1987). Hemodynamic effects of intravenous digoxin in patients with severe heart failure initially treated with diuretics and vasodilators. J Am Coll Cardiol. 9, 849.

19. Murray RG, Tweddel AC, Martin W et al. (1982). Evaluation of digitalis in cardiac failure. Br Med J. 284, 1526.

20. Rajfer SI, Borow KM, Lang RM et al. (1988). Effects of dopamine on left ventricular afterload and contractile state in heart failure: Relation to the activation of beta 1-adrenoceptors and dopamine receptors. J Am Coll Cardiol. 12, 498.

21. Robie NW, Goldberg LI. (1975). Comparative systemic and regional hemodynamic effects of dopamine and dobutamine. Am Heart J. 90, 340.

Tachyarrhythmias in the Intensive Care Unit

Tachyrhythms occur very frequently in patients under intensive care. They are not restricted to patients with underlying heart disease; in fact, they occur against a wide spectrum of background diseases—in shock from any cause, acute infections, acute respiratory problems, during ventilator support, following hypoxia and fluid and electrolyte disturbances. The sudden appearance of a tachyrhythm in a critically ill patient or in a patient on his way to recovery from a critical illness invariably makes even an experienced critical care physician's heart skip a beat! What is it due to? Should one react to it and if so how? Some tachyrhythms come and go all in a flash and produce no problems; others portend disaster. The answer to the two questions listed above, in spite of experience and wisdom gathered over the years, can sometimes be unfortunately given only by hindsight rather than by foresight.

Tachyrhythms can result from enhanced automaticity, triggered activity as in ectopic impulses or from a process called 're-entry'. In the 're-entry phenomenon', a triggered impulse encounters a 'block' when being propagated forwards through a conducting pathway. The impulse however is permitted to pass in the return or retrograde direction. Retrograde transmission can allow such a triggered impulse to result in a continuous self-sustained tachycardia. The re-entry phenomenon is an important underlying mechanism in many paroxysmal tachycardias (1, 2).

This chapter will not deal in detail with the electrophysiology and detailed mechanisms underlying tachyrhythms. It briefly deals with the quick recognition of the nature of different tachyrhythms, and describes the urgent management strategies in an identified tachyrhythm occurring in an ICU setting. This is followed by a brief section on digitalis-induced arrhythmias. The next chapter details relevant aspects of important and commonly used drugs in the management of tachyarrhythmias.

Quick Recognition of Tachyrhythms

A quick study of the rhythm strip is of great help in identifying the nature of the tachyarrhythmia. The features that should be quickly noted are the rate, the regularity or irregularity of the RR intervals, and the width of the QRS complex—whether < 0.12 seconds, equal to, or > 0.12 seconds (**Fig. 7.5.1**).

Narrow complex (QRS < 0.12 seconds) regular tachycardias are sinus

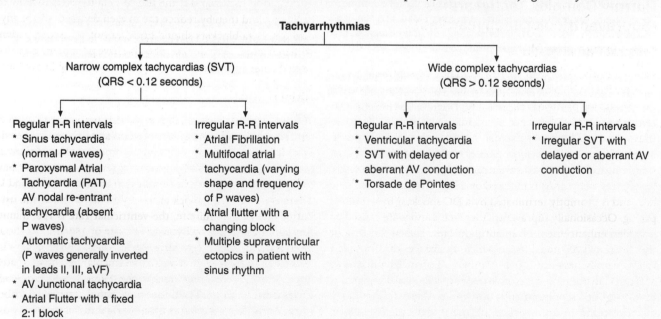

Fig. 7.5.1. Algorithm for quick recognition of tachyrhythms commonly encountered in the ICU.

tachycardia, atrial flutter with a fixed block, paroxysmal atrial tachycardia, junctional (nodal) tachycardia or AV nodal re-entrant tachycardia. A look at the P waves in a rhythm strip can help in further identification. Uniform P waves suggest a sinus tachycardia, saw-tooth P waves an atrial flutter, inverted P waves a junctional (nodal) tachycardia, absent P wave activity a paroxysmal atrial tachycardia, multiple varying P waves a multifocal atrial tachycardia. It is preferable to monitor V_1 so that the rhythm strip will depict a V_1 tracing where the P wave configuration, particularly in atrial flutter, is quickly discernible. A 12-lead tracing to study P waves and their configuration is however, often necessary.

Marked irregularity of a narrow complex tachycardia is observed in atrial fibrillation, multifocal atrial tachycardia, atrial flutter with varying block and when there are many supraventricular ectopic beats in patients with sinus rhythm.

The rate as computed from a rhythm strip is of comparatively less value. It of course distinguishes a tachyrhythm (> 100/min) from a bradyrhythm (< 60/min). Sinus tachycardia is uncommon with rates > 200/min. Again, the higher the rate in a tachyrhythm, the greater the chance of a compromised circulatory system.

Wide complex (QRS > 0.12 seconds) tachycardias can be ventricular tachycardias, supraventricular tachycardia with delayed or aberrant conduction, or torsade de pointes which is a particularly dangerous form of ventricular tachycardia. To distinguish between ventricular tachycardia and supraventricular tachycardia with delayed or aberrant conduction can be extremely difficult. Relevant distinguishing features are discussed later. As a matter of principle, a wide QRS tachyarrhythmia should be considered to be a ventricular tachycardia unless clearly proved otherwise.

A short description of narrow QRS complex tachycardias and management strategies to counter them is now given. This is followed by a similar description of wide QRS tachyrhythms.

Narrow Complex Tachycardias (Supraventricular Tachycardias)

General Considerations

Patients in the ICU with narrow complex or supraventricular tachycardias (SVT) often have underlying cardiac disease involving the conduction pathways. However, supraventricular arrhythmias can also occur in the absence of organic heart disease. They can thus be caused by hypokalaemia, hypomagnesaemia, hypoxia, increased adrenergic activity or tone, or by drugs. Most paroxysmal supraventricular tachyrhythms are caused by re-entry mechanisms. Re-entrant tachycardia is initiated by a supra-ventricular ectopic beat and is promptly terminated by a DC shock or by overdrive pacing. Occasionally supraventricular tachycardias are caused by a sudden enhancement of an autonomous focus in the atria or the junctional AV nodal tissue which 'discharges' or 'fires' at a rate generally between 150–220/minute. Enhanced autonomic activity of an ectopic focus is often due to metabolic derangements or to drugs, and supraventricular tachycardias due to this aetiology often respond to a correction of the underlying metabolic derangement. Though all SVT are sudden in onset and offset, SVT

due to enhanced autonomic activity are not as sudden as those due to re-entry mechanisms.

As mentioned briefly earlier, identification of the atrial activity (P waves) and its form is of crucial importance. It helps, as will be discussed later, to distinguish between SVT with delayed conduction and ventricular tachycardia, and also helps to arrive at the nature of a SVT with narrow QRS complexes. A full 12 lead ECG aided by carotid sinus massage (a vagal manoeuver that slows the heart and thereby brings out the P wave) may be necessary. If no emergency exists, the use of an oesphageal lead will invariably identify atrial activity.

Sinus Tachycardia

This is the commonest supraventricular tachycardia seen in the ICU. Though the rate is generally below 200/minute, in young patients with acute infections (and in severe tetanus in particular), the rate may exceed 200/minute. The P wave has a normal configuration. Sinus node re-entry tachycardias and atrial tachycardias due to autonomic activity from an ectopic focus close to the SA node may be indistinguishable from sinus tachycardia. Tachycardias decrease diastolic filling time; in a normal heart, the heart rate must exceed 180/minute before the cardiac output falls (3). In poorly compliant ventricles, diastolic filling and cardiac output are reduced with comparatively smaller increases in the heart rate. The management of sinus tachycardia is to first identify and then treat its cause. An unexplained rise in an otherwise stable pulse rate in a critically ill individual is a matter of common concern. Important causes of sinus tachycardia are severe anxiety, unrelieved pain, hypovolaemia, hypoxaemia, sepsis, infection, early shock from any cause, blood loss, pneumothorax, pulmonary embolism, the use of adrenergic drugs, myocardial ischaemia or infarction and thyrotoxicosis. Once the cause is treated, the sinus tachycardia disappears. Sinus tachycardia in patients with myocardial ischaemia or infarction may warrant the use of beta-blockers to slow the heart rate and thereby reduce the oxygen demands of the myocardium. Beta-blockers should however not be used in patients with ischaemic heart disease who also have poor pump function. (see Chapters on Unstable Angina and Myocardial Infarction).

Atrial Flutter

This is a common tachyrhythm in the ICU particularly in patients with severe chronic airways obstruction and ischaemic heart disease. It is also an important and common problem following major surgery, particularly coronary artery bypass surgery. Saw-tooth flutter waves are best identified in Leads II, III, aVF and V_1. There is usually a 2:1 block at the AV node so that at the usual flutter rate of 300/minute, the ventricular rate is 150/minute. Any supraventricular tachycardia at a rate of 150/minute should be considered to be due to atrial flutter unless proved otherwise. Occasionally there is an irregular ventricular response to atrial flutter due to a changing block in the AV node which typically varies from 2:1 to 4:1. The flutter may then resemble atrial fibrillation. Atrial flutter is often an unstable rhythm that spontaneously converts to atrial fibrillation or to sinus rhythm.

Management Strategies

The acute or emergency management of atrial flutter is determined by the haemodynamic state of the patient. In patients who are haemodynamically unstable, as judged by a low blood pressure, restlessness, tachypnoea, acidosis and evidence of decreasing perfusion to the major organ systems, emergency treatment consists of cardioversion. DC cardioversion with low energy levels of 25–50 joules generally converts atrial flutter to sinus rhythm. Atrial flutter can also be converted to sinus rhythm by pacing the atria at a frequency higher than the flutter rate. It is important not to wait for all the features of a failing circulation described above, before using cardioversion therapy. One should anticipate the likelihood of an increasingly unstable haemodynamic state from the early signs, and use DC cardioversion well before a very poor haemodynamic state evolves.

In the haemodynamically stable patient with adequate ventricular function, the goal is to reduce the ventricular rate if possible to below 100/minute. Intravenous therapy is necessary if the ventricular rate is > 140/minute; oral therapy suffices when the ventricular rate is between 100–140/minute. When the ventricular rate is already < 100/minute, there is no need to further reduce the rate.

When the heart rate is > 140/minute and there is no evidence of left ventricular dysfunction, we prefer to first use intravenous verapamil. The dose used is 0.075–0.15 mg/kg over 2–3 minutes—thus in a 60 kg patient, 5 mg to 10 mg is given intravenously initially. A second bolus of the same dose may be repeated if necessary after 15 to 30 minutes. The action of verapamil is short lived; hence the bolus dose should preferably be followed by a continuous infusion at the rate of 5 to 20 mg/hour. The advantages of verapamil are that (i) it acts very promptly within 2 minutes (4); and (ii) it may convert the flutter to sinus rhythm—if it does not do so, it effectively reduces the ventricular rate to a significant extent. The disadvantage is that it occasionally produces marked hypotension and precipitates heart failure because of its peripheral vasodilatory effect and its negative inotropic action on the heart, particularly in patients with underlying left ventricular dysfunction. The hypotensive effect of verapamil can be controlled with intravenous calcium (5, 6). Verapamil is particularly useful when atrial flutter complicates chronic airways obstruction, as it also acts as a mild bronchodilator. The drug is metabolized by the liver and its dose should therefore be reduced by 50 per cent in patients with liver cell disease.

If a patient with atrial flutter and a fast ventricular rate has evidence of left ventricular systolic dysfunction, diltiazem is preferred to verapamil to slow the ventricular rate. Diltiazem has a lesser negative inotropic effect than verapamil. It is given intravenously in a dose of 0.25 mg/kg over 2 minutes. If there is little or no response, a second dose of 0.35 mg/kg is administered. If necessary, a slow intravenous infusion of 10–15 mg/hour is continued to control the heart rate.

Beta-blockers have been used to slow the ventricular rate or in place of verapamil or diltiazem, particularly in hyperadrenergic states observed in some patients with myocardial infarction or in post-operative atrial flutter. The drugs of choice are esmolol and metoprolol. Esmolol is a very short acting beta-blocker with a half-life of just 9 minutes; any adverse effect caused by this drug is therefore transient. Esmolol is given in a loading dose of 0.5 mg/kg and then as a slow intravenous infusion of 50–300 µg/kg/minute with careful monitoring of the blood pressure. Metoprolol, if used, is given in a dose of 5 mg over 3 minutes. If necessary, it is repeated in the same dose every 5 minutes to a maximum of 15 mg. Hypotension and the precipitation of acute left ventricular failure are the two most important dangers encountered in the use of beta-blockers. These should not be given in patients with obvious ventricular systolic dysfunction or in asthmatics.

One should never combine verapamil or diltiazem with beta-blocker therapy in an attempt to reduce ventricular rate. In the presence of even mild left ventricular dysfunction, such a combination could result in a disastrous fall in arterial pressure and a cardiovascular collapse because of a strongly negative inotropic effect.

If atrial flutter with a fast ventricular rate cannot be electrically cardioverted or if the above mentioned drugs fail to slow the ventricular rate, digoxin should be tried alone, or with a calcium channel blocker or with a beta-blocker. Digoxin is of particular advantage in the presence of left ventricular systolic dysfunction and failure as besides slowing the ventricular rate, it can enhance ventricular contractility. Its slowing action may however take 60 to 120 minutes or even more to develop (4). An initial dose of 0.25 mg–0.5 mg is given intravenously; 0.25 mg is repeated every 4–6 hours to a maximum total digitalizing dose of 1–1.5 mg in 24 hours. Frequently atrial flutter converts to atrial fibrillation after digitalization, and the atrial fibrillation reverts to sinus rhythm upon withdrawal of digitalis. Occasionally digoxin induces a reversal of atrial flutter to sinus rhythm without intervening atrial fibrillation.

In a number of patients, controlling the ventricular rate results in reversion to sinus rhythm. One should not be unduly perturbed if atrial flutter with a controlled ventricular rate (<100/min) persists, despite the aforementioned measures being instituted. If however, reversion to sinus rhythm is desired, quinidine in a dose of 0.4 g is given every 2 hours for 4 to 5 doses on the first day and the same repeated, if necessary, on the next day. This generally produces a reversion to sinus rhythm. A maintenance dose of quinidine 0.2 g 6 hourly or 0.4 g 8 hourly may be necessary to prevent atrial flutter from recurring. Procainamide can be used instead of quinidine—500 mg 4 hourly on the first day, reduced to 500 mg 6 hourly subsequently. Reversion to sinus rhythm often occurs.

Quinidine or procainamide should never be used in atrial flutter till the ventricular rate has first been controlled and slowed by either verapamil or diltiazem or by digoxin, as these drugs by potentiating AV conduction could further increase an already rapid ventricular rate.

If in spite of the use of calcium blockers or digoxin, the ventricular rate in atrial flutter quickly returns to > 140/min, an elective DC cardioversion with a low level electrical energy (< 50 joules) can be performed. Overdrive pacing with an electrode in the right atrium (as has already been mentioned) can also convert flutter into sinus rhythm.

An algorithm for the management of atrial flutter is given in **Fig. 7.5.2a**.

Atrial Fibrillation

With the exception of sinus tachycardia, atrial fibrillation is the most commonly observed tachyrhythm in ICU patients. This supraventricular arrhythmia is easily recognized by an irregularly irregular rhythm (and the irregularly irregular spacing of the RR intervals). High frequency variable amplitude atrial fibrillatory waves are generally observed on the ECG. Atrial fibrillation generally signifies underlying cardiac disease. Paroxysmal atrial fibrillation lasting for brief periods may however occur in acute infections and post-operatively in patients with otherwise normal hearts. In the absence of AV nodal disease, the ventricular response to atrial fibrillation varies from 100–200 beats/minute. Increased adrenergic tone is associated with a faster ventricular rate. However even at very rapid rates, the ventricular response is irregularly irregular.

Adverse Effects of Atrial Fibrillation

The loss of effective atrial contraction in atrial fibrillation together with the decrease in diastolic filling time of the ventricles due to a fast and irregularly irregular ventricular rate impairs cardiac filling. The normal atrial 'kick' (contraction) is responsible for 25 per cent of the end-diastolic ventricular volume (preload). When this is lost as in atrial fibrillation, cardiac performance is hampered, particularly in patients with a non-compliant left ventricle as also in patients with left ventricular systolic dysfunction. Left atrial pressures rise followed by a rise of pressure in the pulmonary circuit causing pulmonary oedema. Right sided pressures also rise causing engorged neck veins or enlarged tender liver and with pitting oedema of the feet.

The other important adverse consequence of atrial fibrillation (and to a lesser extent in atrial flutter) is the strong possibility of the formation of mural thrombi in the atria. This could lead to either systemic embolism (if a mural clot is present in the left atrium) or pulmonary embolism (if a mural clot is present in the right atrium).

Management Objectives

1. The immediate objective of management in recent or acute atrial fibrillation with a fast ventricular rate is to reduce and control the ventricular rate to < 100/min and to abolish the pulse deficit (the difference between the ventricular rate and the pulse rate in a peripheral artery). A reduction of the heart rate to < 100/min invariably abolishes the apex pulse deficit.

2. The next objective is to revert the atrial fibrillation to sinus rhythm when possible.

3. The third objective is to prevent mural thrombi and consequent embolic episodes.

4. Finally, in critically ill patients, causes outside the heart may precipitate atrial fibrillation. These include hypoxia, pH, fluid and electrolyte abnormalities, pulmonary embolism and thyrotoxicosis.

Unsuspected cardiac causes include mitral valve disease, a recent silent myocardial infarct or myocardial ischaemia and pericardial disease. A quick but careful evaluation should unearth and help treat these underlying precipitating or causative factors.

Management Strategies (Fig. 7.5.2b)

Brief paroxysms of atrial fibrillation do not merit treatment. Verapamil or a beta-blocker may be used orally as a preventive measure.

A persistent paroxysm in a critically ill patient may lead to sudden haemodynamic instability if the ventricular rate is high. Management strategies are very similar to those outlined for atrial flutter, and are summarized below for the sake of convenience (**Fig. 7.5.2b**).

(i) In atrial fibrillation with a heart rate between 170–200/minute, *and in the presence of a rapidly deteriorating haemodynamic state*, DC cardioversion is necessary. Higher energy levels are needed as compared to atrial flutter. One should start with 50–100 joules, and if necessary increase the energy level to 200 joules. More than 50 per cent of cases will convert to sinus rhythm at energy levels of 200 joules or less (7).

(ii) When the ventricular rate is 110 to 150/min but the situation is not so emergent or critical, slowing the ventricular rate markedly improves cardiac performance. Patients in intensive care units who develop acute atrial fibrillation often do so against a background of left ventricular dysfunction. The drug of choice to rapidly and effectively slow the ventricular rate is diltiazem as it has a less negative inotropic effect than verapamil. Diltiazem is given intravenously in the same dosage as in atrial flutter. Verapamil may however be used intravenously if left ventricular function is normal.

Digoxin should be given intravenously in addition to diltiazem in patients with a rapid heart rate who develop clinical or other evidence of left ventricular failure. Digoxin must also be used promptly in emergency situations with fast ventricular rates and unstable or poor haemodynamic states (hypotension, shock, pulmonary oedema) when attempts at DC cardioversion have failed. The initial or loading dose required to control the very fast ventricular rate in atrial fibrillation is often larger than that recommended in patients with congestive cardiac failure who are in sinus rhythm. The drug is given in a dose of 0.25 to 0.5 mg intravenously and is repeated 6 hourly till the required effect on ventricular rate is achieved or a total dose of 1.5 mg to a maximum of 1.75 mg is given over 24 hours. Digoxin acts by depressing AV conduction, thereby reducing the ventricular rate and allowing proper filling of the ventricles. This effect, together with its direct positive inotropic action on the heart muscle, results in increased contractility and produces a dramatic improvement in the haemodynamic state. The slowing effect of digoxin on the heart is however not as rapid as with calcium channel blockers such as diltiazem, hence the need to use both diltiazem and digoxin in acute atrial fibrillation with rapid ventricular rates, particularly when there is impaired left ventricular function.

Digitalis may not be effective in the control of a fast ventricular rate in the presence of high fever, acute infection and thyrotoxicosis.

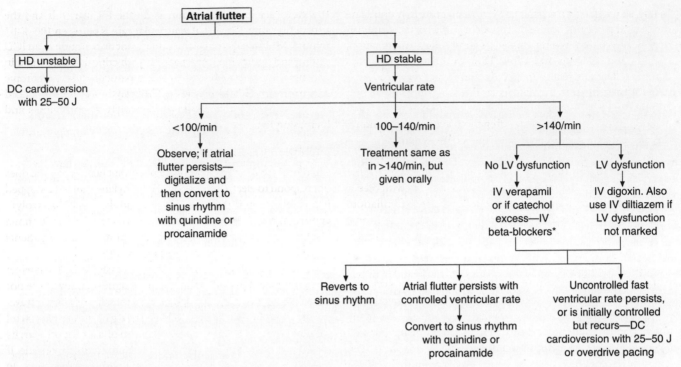

HD = haemodynamically
*Avoid combining verapamil with beta blockers.

Fig. 7.5.2a. Algorithm for the management of atrial flutter.

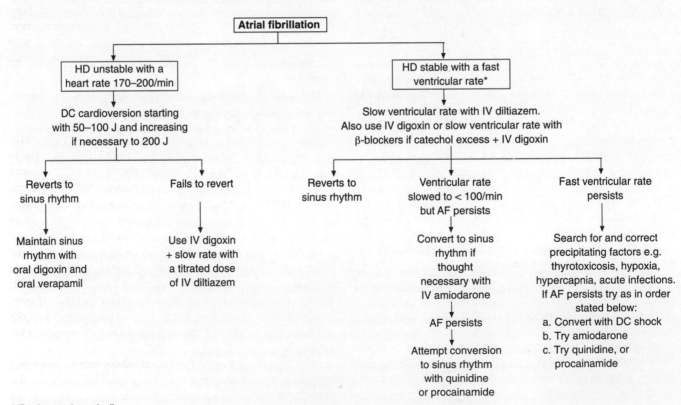

HD = haemodynamically
Note: For contraindications for conversion of atrial fibrillation to sinus rhythm, see text.
*Many units use IV amiodarone in a bolus dose of 300 mg followed by an infusion of 750 mg as the first choice in preference to IV diltiazem + digoxin.

Fig. 7.5.2b. Algorithm for the management of atrial fibrillation.

In fact, an irregularly irregular fast ventricular rate may dominate the clinical picture of severe thyrotoxicosis; the correct diagnosis of hyperthyroidism is often missed. A good clinical examination, high T_3 and T_4 levels and a low TSH level should clarify the diagnosis. Digitalis is also ineffective and in fact may produce a paradoxical increase in the ventricular rate when atrial fibrillation complicates a WPW syndrome. Failure of digitalis to act or an increase in the ventricular rate after the use of digitalis should therefore always suggest an underlying WPW syndrome.

Beta-blockers like esmolol and metoprolol can be used in place of diltiazem to slow rapid ventricular rates in patients with atrial fibrillation. They are particularly useful in patients with recent myocardial infarction and in post-operative atrial fibrillation. Their dosage is the same as in atrial flutter. Asthma, chronic airways obstruction and obvious left ventricular dysfunction are contraindications to their use.

Once the ventricular rate in atrial fibrillation is slowed to < 100/minute, there is no urgent need to convert to sinus rhythm. Conversion can be attempted (if thought necessary) by amiodarone or quinidine or procainamide. Amiodarone is preferred in many units; an intravenous bolus dose of 150 to 300 mg being followed by a slow intravenous infusion of 750 mg to 1 g over 24 hours. The drug is given orally, 200–400 mg thrice daily from the next day and the intravenous infusion tapered and stopped by 4 to 7 days. A maintenance oral dose of 200 mg twice or thrice daily may be necessary to prevent a recurrence of atrial fibrillation. Quinidine or procainamide are also used to convert atrial fibrillation into sinus rhythm. The dosage of these drugs is given under atrial flutter.

Elective electrical cardioversion to sinus rhythm is an alternative to pharmacotherapy once the emergent situation has come under control. Electrical cardioversion is however avoided or delayed if a large dose of intravenous digoxin has already been given. Cardioversion in atrial fibrillation is known to be associated with a 1–2 per cent risk of systemic embolism. Embolism is more frequent in high-risk patients (as in those with mitral valve disease, or cardiomyopathy), but can occur in any patient with atrial fibrillation lasting for more than a couple of days. It is therefore always safer to anticoagulate a patient before elective cardioversion—first with heparin and then with oral anticoagulants. Current recommendation is to avoid elective cardioversion till 2 weeks of anticoagulation therapy has been given. We have never encountered embolic episodes even if cardioversion has been carried out within 2–4 days of anticoagulation provided (i) the partial thromboplastin time or the prothrombin time are adequately raised; (ii) cardioversion is not attempted in patients with chronic atrial fibrillation, cardiomyopathy and LV dysfunction, in patients with significant enlargement of the left ventricle, or in those with echocardiographically proven thrombi in the atria or ventricles. In the last condition, the risk of embolism is significantly high, and in the remaining conditions, sinus rhythm is not restored and if restored, is ill-sustained.

Multifocal Atrial Tachycardias

This tachycardia as the name suggests is due to multiple foci of ectopic atrial activity. It is also called chaotic atrial tachycardia. The P waves vary in configuration as do the PR intervals and the ventricular rate. The usual ventricular rate is between 100–140/minute. Multifocal atrial tachycardia is not uncommon in an ICU setting and occurs in elderly patients with critical illnesses, and in patients with severe pulmonary disease, particularly severe chronic airways obstruction with hypoxia. The arrhythmia can be produced or aggravated by theophylline, electrolyte abnormalities and increasing hypoxia.

Management Strategies

Multifocal atrial tachycardia is not a re-entrant tachycardia and does not respond to electroconversion. Theophylline should be stopped if possible, even if the levels are not unduly raised. Electrolyte abnormalities, if present, should be corrected. The arrhythmia resolves with conversion to sinus rhythm in 50 per cent of patients with the discontinuation of theophylline (8).

Intravenous magnesium has been successfully used to correct this arrhythmia provided that serum magnesium levels are not raised (9). 2 g magnesium sulphate in 50 ml saline is given intravenously over 15 to 30 minutes, followed by 6 g of the drug in 500 ml N saline over 6 to 8 hours. The mechanism of action is unclear; its antiarrhythmic action may be due to calcium channel blockade. If multifocal atrial tachycardia is associated with hypokalaemia, 40 mEq of potassium chloride is given in an intravenous infusion over 4 hours. Magnesium may need to be given prior to potassium in order to correct hypokalaemia. Metoprolol has also been shown to be effective (10) but one should always avoid beta-blockers (however selective in action) in the presence of airways obstruction. Verapamil has also proved effective, particularly in patients with bronchospasm (11). This arrhythmia does not respond to digitalis or to Class I antiarrhythmic agents.

Paroxysmal Atrial Tachycardia (PAT)— AV Nodal Re-Entrant Tachycardia

Typical or classical PAT comprises two separate re-entry mechanisms that involve conducting tissues below the atria. In most cases, PAT is due to AV nodal re-entry; in a small minority PAT is related to a concealed 'accessory' pathway between the atria and the ventricles, which conducts only in a retrograde fashion.

AV nodal re-entrant tachycardia involves dual pathways in the AV node—generally a slow pathway conducting antegradely, and a rapid pathway conducting retrogradely. A premature atrial ectopic sets off a re-entry loop, and since the atria are depolarized retrogradely, the P waves are inverted in Leads II, III and aVF, and are usually buried and indiscernible within the QRS complex. In a few instances, the P wave may be seen just beyond the QRS complex. The usual atrial and ventricular rates are between 150–200/minute.

This arrhythmia is seen in young individuals with no underlying organic heart disease. Vagal manoeuvres usually terminate the arrhythmia and should be tried first. If ineffective, the management strategy is to use drugs to block the re-entrant pathway in the AV node. The most effective drugs are adenosine and the calcium channel blockers verapamil and diltiazem. Adenosine is the drug of choice because it is very short-acting and has a much less cardiac depressant action than calcium channel blockers. It is therefore always preferred to the latter drugs, particularly in patients with left ventricular dysfunction or heart failure (**12–14**). The drug is given as a bolus of 6 mg by intravenous injection. After 2 minutes, 12 mg may be repeated if necessary. The dose is reduced by 50 per cent if the drug is injected through a central venous line instead of a peripheral vein, or in patients receiving calcium channel blockers or dipyridamole (**15**). This is because adenosine has been reported to produce prolonged cardiac asystole when a standard dose is given through a CVP line (**15**). Adenosine terminates PAT in 90 to 100 per cent of cases within 2 to 3 minutes. It is contraindicated in patients with bronchial asthma and AV block.

Theophylline blocks adenosine receptors; adenosine may thus be ineffective in patients receiving theophylline. The side effects of adenosine are described in the Chapter on Antiarrhythmic Drugs.

In the rare instance when adenosine or calcium channel blockers fail to act, intravenous digoxin is used—0.25 mg intravenously repeated 6 hourly to a maximum digitalizing dose of 1 mg. In older patients who experience severe angina or in the presence of shock, a DC cardioversion or an overdrive cardiac pacing should be considered. Quinidine or procainamide given as stated earlier can also terminate this rhythm disturbance and should be used if the haemodynamic condition is stable, if adenosine or the calcium channel blockers are ineffective or contraindicated.

PAT due to a concealed accessory pathway is generally accompanied by a delayed P wave as retrograde depolarization through the accessory pathway is slower. The inverted P wave in leads II, III and aVF is observed on the T wave; a prolonged PR interval suggests the diagnosis. Treatment is identical to that described above for AV nodal re-entry tachycardia provided that the accessory pathway conducts the impulse only in a retrograde fashion. In a WPW syndrome however, the accessory or anomalous pathway can also conduct antegradely in a rapid manner. As will be discussed later, the administration of verapamil or digitalis can be dangerous in these patients.

Automatic Atrial Tachycardia

SVT due to enhanced automatic activity of an ectopic atrial focus is often related to drugs or to metabolic disturbances. A classic example is 'paroxysmal atrial tachycardia with block', which is caused by digitalis intoxication, but which also occurs in severe pulmonary disease and in advanced ischaemic heart disease. The atrial rate is generally between 150–220/minute, and the P wave morphology is abnormal. There is a varying degree of AV block. When atrial activity is very rapid there is a resemblance to atrial flutter, though atrial activity is best seen in the precordial leads rather than in Leads II, III and aVF.

Management Strategies

Discontinuation of digitalis (even if the serum digoxin levels are not unduly raised), and treatment of the underlying metabolic abnormalities is necessary. If inadvertently the arrhythmia and its relation to digitalis is missed, and digitalis is continued, lethal ventricular arrhythmias may result. An infusion of potassium in dextrose helps to terminate the arrhythmia even if digoxin levels

are normal. Beta-blockers and verapamil may help slow a fast ventricular rate.

Non-Paroxysmal AV Junctional Tachycardia

This form of SVT is associated with digitalis intoxication, but may also be observed after a myocardial infarction, in the post-operative period following open heart surgery, and in severe pulmonary disease. It generally does not produce significant haemodynamic changes and is then best ignored, as it converts to sinus rhythm spontaneously. Therapy of the underlying disease is the treatment of choice. The overuse of digitalis in atrial fibrillation leads to a complete AV block with the occurrence of a regular accelerated junctional rhythm at a rate of 70–100/minute. The significance of this rhythm disturbance under these circumstances, should be promptly recognized, and digitalis should be immediately stopped.

Wide Complex (QRS > 0.12 seconds) Tachyarrhythmias

These chiefly include ventricular tachycardia and torsade de pointes, which in fact is an unusual or peculiar form of ventricular tachycardia. Supraventricular tachycardias with delayed or aberrant conduction can also produce wide QRS complexes (> 0.12 seconds) which are difficult to distinguish from ventricular tachycardias. As a matter of principle it should be remembered that ventricular tachycardia probably causes more than 95 per cent of wide complex tachycardias in patients who have underlying cardiac disease (**16**). Therefore in an ICU setting a wide QRS complex should be taken as ventricular tachycardia unless proved otherwise.

There are a number of ECG features which help to distinguish ventricular tachycardia from supraventricular tachycardia with delayed or aberrant conduction (**17**) and these are tabled below (**see Table 7.5.1**).

The features of note are as follows:

(a) In a long rhythm strip the presence of fusion beats, capture beats, and/or AV dissociation in a wide QRS tachycardia, point to a ventricular tachycardia.

(b) In a 12 lead ECG, ventricular tachycardia is more likely if:

Table 7.5.1. Differentiating features between ventricular tachycardia and SVT with delayed or aberrant conduction

SVT with delayed or aberrant conduction	Ventricular tachycardia
* Slowing or termination by increase in vagal tone	* Fusion beats present
* Premature P waves present at onset	* Capture beats present
* PR interval < 100 msec	* AV dissociation present
* QRS duration usually < 120 msec	* QRS duration > 140 msec
* P and QRS rate and rhythm often linked, to suggest that ventricular activation depends on atrial discharge	* Left axis deviation often present
* QRS complexes— rSR' frequently seen in V$_1$	* QRS complexes—specific QRS patterns often seen in precordial leads (see text)

(i) in the presence of a RBBB pattern, the pattern in V_1 is monophasic. If it is biphasic, then R is taller than R'. Small R and large S waves or a QS pattern is present in V_6; (ii) in the presence of a LBBB pattern, the axis is to the right, the QRS is wider than 0.16 seconds, and V_6 shows a small q and a low amplitude R wave, or a QS pattern; (iii) QRS complexes are similar in V_1–V_6, either all positive or all negative.

Ventricular Tachycardia (VT)

This dangerous tachyarrhythmia is characterized by a series of three or more ventricular ectopic impulses at a rate of 100 or more beats/minute. Accelerated ventricular rhythm is defined as a ventricular rhythm occurring at 50–100 beats/minute. Ventricular tachycardia can be brief, subsiding within 30 seconds (non-sustained VT), or it can last for longer periods of time (sustained VT). The most frequent and the most likely cause of ventricular tachycardia is myocardial ischaemia or a recent myocardial infarction. Other organic heart diseases complicated by VT include aortic valve disease, cardiomyopathies and VT following coronary artery bypass surgery, particularly after aneurysmectomy or aneurysmorrhaphy of a ventricular aneurysm. In an ICU setting however, ventricular tachycardia can also occur in the absence of serious organic heart disease. It is important to look for potentially reversible factors which may initiate or perpetuate serious ventricular arrhythmias. Important reversible conditions causing sustained ventricular tachycardia have been listed below in **Table 7.5.2**.

Table 7.5.2. Potentially reversible causes of ventricular tachycardia

* Ischaemic heart disease
* Hypoxia/hypercapnia
* Acidosis
* Electrolyte abnormalities—hypokalaemia, hypocalcaemia, hypomagnesaemia
* Hyperthyroidism
* Excess of circulating catecholamines—endogenous/exogenous
* Drug toxicity—particularly digitalis
* Presence of intracardiac catheters

These factors include hypoxia, hypercapnia, hypoglycaemia, hypokalaemia, hypomagnesaemia, hypocalcaemia, excessive use of inotropes (catecholamines) or excessive endogenous catecholamine production, hyperthyroidism, drug toxicity (commonly produced by antiarrhythmic drugs), digitalis toxicity and the presence of intracardiac catheters.

The initial work-up should therefore include measurements of serum electrolytes, calcium, magnesium, arterial pH, blood gas analysis and cardiac enzymes. If the patient has an indwelling catheter e.g. a Swan-Ganz catheter or a central venous line, it is important to check with an X-ray that it does not lie within the right ventricle.

Management Strategies

(i) Non-sustained VT need not be treated unless associated with cardiac disease. In a critically ill patient with non-sustained VT, potentially reversible causes enumerated above, should be looked for and if present, corrected.

(ii) Sustained VT should always be treated. If the patient is hypotensive or haemodynamically unstable, he should be immediately cardioverted by a synchronized DC shock starting with 100 joules. If this is ineffective, 200 joules are used; if still ineffective, 300 or even 360 joules may be required for cardioversion. After conversion to sinus rhythm, a prophylactic lidocaine drip at a rate of 2–4 mg/minute is started.

(iii) If a patient with sustained VT is haemodynamically stable, lidocaine is used in a bolus dose of 1 mg/kg intravenously. 0.5–0.75 mg/kg may be repeated as an intravenous bolus dose within 10 minutes if the patient has not reverted to sinus rhythm. After reversion, a prophylactic lidocaine drip at a rate of 2–4 mg/minute is started.

(iv) If a patient with sustained VT fails to respond to full doses of lidocaine, it is important to re-evaluate the patient for factors which can potentiate the tachyrhythm. Hypokalaemia, hypoxia, myocardial ischaemia and metabolic acidosis if present should be promptly corrected. At times, 20–40 mEq potassium chloride in a 5 per cent dextrose infusion is useful and worth a try even if the serum K^+ is within the normal range. If the potentiating factors stated above are not present, or if sustained VT persists even after they are corrected, we would first prefer to attempt cardioversion with a synchronized DC shock before using further pharmacotherapy.

(v) Sustained VT not responding to the above regimen poses a serious threat to life, particularly if the ventricular rate is > 160 beats/minute, or if the patient is hypotensive and shows signs of increasing haemodynamic instability. The antiarrhythmic drugs used are intravenous amiodarone, or intravenous procainamide, or oral quinidine, provided the corrected QT interval is < 0.44 seconds. The corrected QT interval (QTc) is the QT interval usually measured in Lead II divided by the square root of the R-R interval. A QTc > 0.44 seconds is considered abnormal (**18**). We prefer the initial trial with amiodarone to quinidine or procainamide. The drug is given in a bolus dose of 300 mg intravenously over 10 minutes followed by a slow intravenous infusion of 1 to 1.2 g over 24 hours.

If amiodarone fails, we try oral quinidine 0.4 g 2 hourly for 4 doses or intravenous procainamide. When there is impending haemodynamic compromise, intravenous procainamide is preferred. It is given in a slow intravenous infusion of 5 mg/minute till cardioversion occurs. The total dose of procainamide should not exceed 1 g. If the QRS interval increases by more than 50 per cent or hypotension develops, procainamide should be stopped temporarily.

If the QTc interval is prolonged or even otherwise if amiodarone or procainamide fail, magnesium sulphate is given intravenously in a bolus dose of 2 g over 2 minutes. The dose is repeated if necessary in 10 minutes. If sinus rhythm is restored, magnesium sulphate is given in a slow infusion of 1 g/hour for 6 to 8 hours or even longer. Magnesium sulphate has proved effective in ventricular tachycardia refractory to lidocaine (**19**).

(vi) Other antiarrhythmic drugs that can be used are bretylium tosylate 5–10 mg/kg intravenously over 10–20 minutes, which can be repeated after an hour, or phenytoin sodium 250 mg intravenously over 10 minutes. 100 mg of the drug may be repeated every 15 minutes till a total dose of 500 mg is reached. A maintenance dose of 100 mg 8 hourly may be required. In our experience, both bretylium tosylate and phenytoin sodium have proved hopelessly ineffective at this stage and we rarely if ever use these drugs.

(vii) Failure to convert sustained VT by DC shock or by antiarrhythmic drugs necessitates a trial of programmed electrical stimulation of the ventricles, or overdriving the ventricles through a transvenous pacing catheter introduced into the right ventricle. In our experience, this method is rewarded with a 50 per cent success rate in patients whose VT is refractory to DC shock and conventional drugs. After conversion the pacing rate should be kept between 110–120/minute for prevention of further attacks. If VT recurs after a lapse of a few days, the possibility that the pacing catheter may itself be responsible for inducing ventricular tachycardia should be kept in mind. In such cases removal of the catheter solves the problem.

(viii) Prophylaxis after conversion to sinus rhythm is important. A lidocaine drip should be continued till such time as ventricular ectopics are by and large suppressed—this may generally take between 2–4 days. Subsequent prophylaxis may need to be continued with oral medication. Useful oral antiarrhythmic drugs for prophylaxis include quinidine 200 mg 6–8 hourly, pronestyl 500 mg 6–8 hourly, and amiodarone 200 mg 8 hourly.

A flow algorithm given below outlines the management strategies in sustained ventricular tachycardia (**Fig. 7.5.3**).

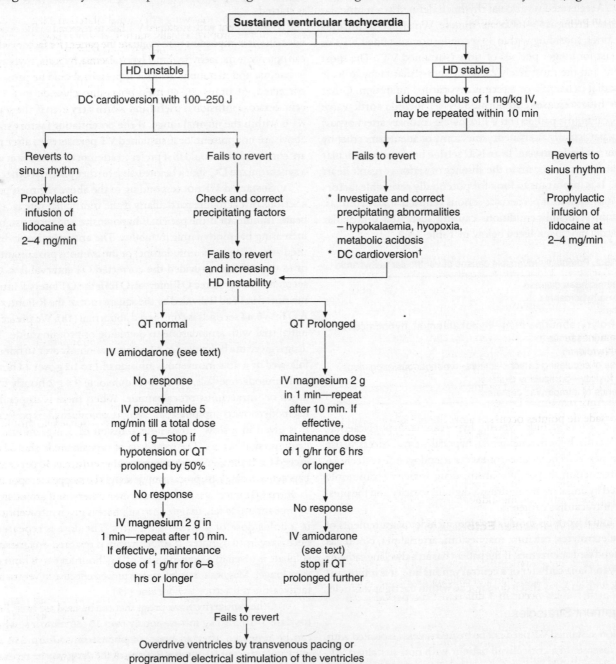

†A bolus of 300 mg IV amiodarone is often tried in many units before resorting to a DC shock.

Fig. 7.5.3. Algorithm for the management of sustained ventricular tachycardia.

Torsade de Pointes

This is a form of VT in which there are changes in the amplitude and polarity of the ventricular complexes after every 15–20 beats or even earlier. Torsade de Pointes is generally a self-limiting tachyarrhythmia but can rarely degenerate into ventricular fibrillation (20). It however often recurs and is associated or preceded by a prolonged QT interval (21). Hypokalaemia, hypomagnesaemia, hypocalcaemia, drugs like quinidine, procainamide, disopyramide, phenothiazines, haloperidol and tricyclic antidepressants are known to predispose to 'Torsade de Pointes' (Table 7.5.3). This arrhythmia occurs against a background of a prolonged QT interval and also in patients with myocardial ischaemia.

Table 7.5.3. Important causes of Torsade de Pointes

* Electrolyte disturbances—hypokalaemia, hypocalcaemia, hypomagnesaemia
* Drug-induced
  – antiarrhythmic drugs eg. quinidine, procainamide
  – phenothiazines
  – tricyclic antidepressants
* Miscellaneous causes
  – ischaemic heart disease
  – myocarditis
  – congenital disorders
  – organophosphorus poisoning

Management Strategies

(a) If the QT interval is prolonged, all offending drugs should be withdrawn. Hypokalaemia or hypomagnesaemia if present, should be corrected. Lidocaine is usually ineffective in torsade de pointes but may be tried; drugs which prolong the QT interval (e.g. quinidine or procainamide) are contraindicated. If the arrhythmia recurs, temporary pacing through a transvenous pacing catheter in the right ventricle at a rate of 120/minute may help. The aim here is to increase the heart rate and thereby shorten the QT interval. This can also be achieved by the use of intravenous isoproterenol, though ventricular pacing is generally preferred (see Chapter on Antiarrhythmic Drugs).

(b) If torsade de pointes occurs against the background of a normal QT interval, then therapy with quinidine or procainamide is safe and may be given.

(c) Magnesium sulphate (2 g intravenously over 1–2 minutes, followed by an infusion at 3–20 mg/minute), has been successful in the management of quinidine-induced torsade de pointes.

Management of Ventricular Ectopics in the ICU

Management of ventricular ectopics assumes importance in the presence of continuing myocardial ischaemia or soon after myocardial infarction. MacMohan and colleagues (22) stress that ventricular arrhythmias occur in 3 different time periods after myocardial infarction.

The first period begins within minutes of the onset of myocardial infarction and lasts for 2–6 hours. Most deaths following infarction occur in this time span. Ventricular ectopics in this period are dangerous as they often are forerunners of VT and ventricular fibrillation (VF).

The second period begins from 6–12 hours after infarction and persists for 72 hours. Ventricular ectopics are not as dangerous here as in the first period, but can still lead to VT and VF. Reperfusion arrhythmias following thrombolytic therapy occur in this time span. It is to be noted that over 50 per cent of patients who develop VF in the immediate post-infarction period do so without warning (23).

The third and final period occurs 3–7 days after myocardial infarction, and arrhythmias during this period tend to be benign except in individuals with ongoing ischaemia, or in those in whom the myocardial infarct extends further.

Lidocaine is the drug of choice for suppression of ventricular ectopics in the period following myocardial infarction. Many units also use lidocaine prophylactically, starting as early as possible after the onset of myocardial infarction (24). However there is no proof that prophylactic lidocaine in the immediate post-infarction period improves mortality (22). We prefer to use lidocaine for suppression and not as prophylaxis. A bolus dose of 50–75 mg intravenously, is followed by a maintenance dose of 2 mg/minute in patients with frequent ectopics, or when ventricular ectopics fall on the T wave, or when they occur late in diastole. Ventricular ectopics, not well controlled by lidocaine, are treated by using intravenous amiodarone in the dose stated earlier, or oral amiodarone 200 mg 8 hourly, or oral quinidine 200 mg 6 hourly or procainamide 500 mg 8 hourly.

Frequent ventricular ectopics in an ICU setting causing VT or VF can also occur in situations unrelated to ischaemic heart disease. These conditions are chiefly:

(i) Electrolyte abnormalities mainly hypokalaemia or hypomagnesaemia.

(ii) Hypoxia and hypercapnia.

(iii) Drugs, notably digitalis. The proarrhythmic effects of antiarrhythmic agents like procainamide should also be considered.

(iv) Both acidosis and alkalosis can induce ventricular ectopics. Respiratory alkalosis in particular can increase myocardial irritability, which when severe can lead to VT or VF.

All the above factors should first be corrected before using antiarrhythmic drugs. More often than not, ventricular ectopics seen in the ICU, when not related to myocardial ischaemia, should not be treated with antiarrhythmic agents.

Wide QRS Tachyarrhythmias Caused by Supraventricular Tachycardia with Delayed Conduction

Once a wide QRS is identified as being due to a SVT with delayed conduction either through the right or left bundle branch of His, management is exactly as for SVT. It however must be emphasized as a precautionary measure that one should not use intravenous verapamil in the management of wide QRS tachyrhythms. If the latter turns out to be a ventricular tachycardia, verapamil often produces a crash in the arterial blood pressure necessitating the use of vasopressors and electrical cardioversion.

Wide QRS Tachyrhythms due to SVT in the WPW Syndrome

Patients with WPW syndrome are predisposed to develop atrial flutter or fibrillation with a very fast ventricular rate when the anomalous pathway is capable of antegrade conduction. If the anomalous pathway has a short refractory period, it can conduct impulses in atrial flutter or fibrillation at a rate of up to 300 beats/minute. This can result in ventricular fibrillation and death. When antegrade conduction occurs through the anomalous pathway in atrial flutter or fibrillation, a wide, very rapid tachyrhythm closely resembling a ventricular tachycardia results. Patients with the presentation described above are haemodynamically in shock and should be immediately reverted by cardioversion.

It is important to note that in the WPW syndrome, the use of standard drugs for PAT (verapamil, digoxin, beta-blockers) may be dangerous in patients in whom rapid antegrade conduction through the anomalous pathway is possible. Digitalis shortens the refractory period of the anomalous pathways, and thereby enhances conduction through it. Verapamil and beta-blockers slow conduction in the AV node and thus indirectly promote antegrade conduction through the anomalous pathway. Digitalis and verapamil can markedly increase the ventricular rate in such patients with atrial flutter or fibrillation and cause ventricular fibrillation and death. Initial pharmacotherapy in a patient with a delta wave should either be quinidine or procainamide. As stated earlier, DC cardioversion is frequently necessary as an emergency measure.

Digitalis Induced Arrhythmias (25–28)

Digitalis induced arrhythmias are still fairly frequent in the ICU. They were even more frequent till about 5 years back because of larger oral and intravenous doses recommended at that time.

Every arrhythmia in the book can be produced by digitalis toxicity. Bradyrhythms include sinus bradycardia, SA block, AV block, wandering pacemaker, junctional and idioventricular rhythms. Tachyrhythms include ectopic beats, non-paroxysmal AV junctional tachycardia, PAT with block, ventricular tachycardia and ventricular fibrillation.

In a critically ill individual it is often difficult to determine whether an arrhythmia is related or not to digitalis. Estimating digoxin levels in blood is not necessarily of help. Therapeutic serum levels of digoxin are 0.8–2.0 ng/ml—yet toxicity is sometimes seen even when digoxin levels are within the therapeutic range. When there is doubt as to whether the arrhythmia is related to digitalis or not, it is best to omit the drug, and observe the result of drug withdrawal.

Digitalis toxicity is most likely to occur (i) in those extra sensitive to the drug, particularly in the very young and the old; (ii) when the drug is administered in high doses as recommended some years ago; (iii) in patients with associated hypokalaemia, hypomagnesaemia, hypocalcaemia; (iv) in patients with associated hypoxia.

Management

Digoxin should be stopped whenever in doubt. Diuretics like furosemide are withheld, and hypokalaemia and hypomagnesaemia if present, are corrected.

Bradyrhythms in Digoxin Toxicity

For a first degree block or a Wenckebach block the drug is stopped and intravenous atropine 0.25–0.5 mg given. For high grade SA or AV blocks temporary transvenous pacing is necessary. Potassium should not be given intravenously in high grade SA or AV blocks as both potassium and digitalis have a synergistic effect on the AV node, and cardiac arrest can result. An infusion of potassium chloride can however be used for PAT with block.

Tachyrhythms in Digoxin Toxicity

Potassium chloride 40–60 mEq in a dextrose infusion given over 2–4 hours is the treatment of choice in both supraventricular and ventricular tachycardias induced by digitalis. More potassium is needed in the presence of hypokalaemia. PAT with block due to digitalis is treated along the same lines.

For digitalis-induced ventricular tachycardias, a bolus of 100 mg lignocaine intravenously is followed by an intravenous potassium infusion. If the tachyrhythm persists, the drug of choice is dilantin sodium 100 mg intravenously every 5 minutes, till 500 mg have been administered. The most important and immediate side effect of dilantin is hypotension. If the ventricular tachycardia still persists, overdriving the ventricles through a transvenous pacing catheter may be successful. The danger of inducing ventricular fibrillation through mechanical stimulation by the pacing catheter, is however always present. Quinidine or procainamide should not be used as far as possible in digitalis induced ventricular tachycardia, as these drugs prolong intraventricular conduction and can cause fatal ventricular fibrillation in these patients.

If intravenous infusions of potassium chloride in dextrose do not succeed in reverting digitalis-induced SVT, the use of beta-blockers may help. Indian patients, in our experience, are often very sensitive to the use of intravenous propranolol. Intravenous esmolol is safer because of its very short half-life. Beta-blockers are also useful in suppressing digitalis-induced ventricular ectopics, but should be avoided in digitalis-induced ventricular tachycardia.

It is best to avoid synchronized DC shock in the management of digitalis-induced tachyrhythms for fear of inducing lethal ventricular fibrillation. This particularly holds true when digoxin levels are well above the therapeutic range. However in patients who are very ill with digitalis-induced ventricular tachycardia, and in whom drug therapy has failed, a synchronized DC shock may be given as a measure of desperation. The patient is pretreated with a bolus of 100 mg intravenous lidocaine followed by 100 mg intravenous dilantin sodium. The energy levels used should be lower than usual.

The recent introduction and use of digoxin-induced Fab to counter digitalis toxicity can be life-saving (29, 30). This preparation is a sheep antibody fragment which binds to digoxin and reverses the effects of the drug. The Fab-digoxin complexes are excreted in the urine. This digoxin antibody is very expensive and its use is restricted to life-threatening digitalis-induced arrhythmias. The dosage of Fab is dependent on serum digoxin levels, but in emergency situations, the maximum dose should be used. We have no experience with Fab in our unit.

Over the years we have slowly learnt to reduce digitalis toxicity by (i) using lesser loading doses; (ii) omitting the drug whenever digitalis toxicity is even suspect; (iii) avoiding the drug or using very small doses in the very old, or in the presence of significant renal insufficiency; (iv) reducing the dose of the drug by 50 per cent if quinidine is being simultaneously used; v) ensuring that the serum potassium, magnesium and calcium are within normal limits.

In fact, prevention of digitalis toxicity is far easier than the treatment of its toxic effects.

REFERENCES

1. Emergency Cardiac Care Committee and Subcommittees, American Heart Association. (1992). Guidelines for cardiopulmonary resuscitation and emergency cardiac care. JAMA. 268, 2199–2241.

2. Collier WW, Holt SE, Wellford LA. (1995). Narrow complex tachycardias. Emerg Med Clin North Am. 13, 925–954.

3. Guyton AC. (1981). The relationship of cardiac output and arterial pressure control. Circulation. 64, 1079–1088.

4. Keefe DL, Miura D, Somberg JC. (1986). Supraventricular tachyarrhythmias: their evaluation and therapy. Am Heart J. 11, 1150–1161.

5. Barnett JC, Touchon RC. (1989). Verapamil infusion with calcium pretreatment for acute control of supraventricular tachycardia. Crit Care Med. 17:S11.

6. Ferling J, Citron PD. (1983). Haemodynamic and myocardial performance characteristics after verapamil use in congestive heart failure. Am J Cardiol. 51, 1339–1345.

7. Walsh KA, Ezri MD, Denes P. (1986). Emergency treatment of tachyarrhythmias. Med Clin North Am. 70, 791–811.

8. Levine JH, Michael JR, Guarnieri T. (1985). Multifocal atrial tachycardia: A toxic effect of theophylline. Lancet. 1, 1216.

9. Iseri LT, Fairshter RD, Hardeman JL et al. (1985). Magnesium and potassium therapy in multifocal atrial tachycardia. Am Heart J. 110, 789–791.

10. Arsura EL, Solar M, Lefkin AS et al. (1987). Metoprolol in the treatment of multifocal atrial tachycardia. Crit Care Med. 15, 591–594.

11. Levine JH, Michael JR, Guarnieri T. (1985). Treatment of multifocal atrial tachycardia with verapamil. N Engl J Med. 312, 21–26.

12. Shen W-K, Kurachi Y. (1995). Mechanisms of adenosine-mediated actions on cellular and clinical cardiac electrophysiology. Mayo Clin Proc. 70, 274–291.

13. Ranklin AC, Brooks R, Ruskin JM, McGovern BA. (1992). Adenosine and the treatment of supraventricular tachycardia. Am J Med. 92, 655–664.

14. Chronister C. (1993). Clinical management of supraventricular tachycardia with adenosine. Am J Crit Care. 2, 41–47.

15. McCollam PL, Uber W, Van Bakel AB. (1993). Adenosine-related ventricular asystole. Ann Intern Med. 118, 315–316.

16. Akhtar M, Shenasa M, Jazayeri M et al. (1988). Wide QRS complex tachycardia. Ann Internal Med. 109, 905–912.

17. Olgin JE, Zipes DP. (2001). Specific Arrhythmias. In: Heart Disease— A Textbook of Cardiovascular Medicine (Eds Braunwald E, Zipes DP, Libby P). pp. 815–889. W B Saunders Company, Philadelphia, London, Toronto, Montreal, Sydney, Tokyo.

18. Garson A Jr. (1993). How to measure the QT interval: what is normal? Am J Cardiol. 72, 14B-16B.

19. Roden D. (1989). Magnesium treatment of ventricular arrhythmias. Am J Cardiol. 63, 43G-46G.

20. Stratmann HG, Kennedy HL. (1987). Torsade de pointes associated with drugs and toxins: Recognition and management. Am Heart J. 113, 1470–1482.

21. Vukmir RB. Torsades de pointes: a review. (1991). Am J Emerg Med. 9: 250–262.

22. MacMahon S, Collins R, Peto R et al. (1988). Effects of prophylactic lidocaine in suspected acute myocardial infarction. JAMA. 260, 1910–1916.

23. Ahmad S, Giles TD. (1988). Managing ventricular arrhythmias during acute MI. J Crit Illness. 3, 29–40.

24. Stamato NJ, Josephson ME. (1986). When and how to manage premature ventricular contractions. J Crit Illness. 1, 41–48.

25. Smith TW, Antman EM, Friedman PL et al. (1984,1985). Digitalis glycosides: Mechanisms and manifestations of toxicity. Prog Cardiovasc Dis. 26, 413,495. 27, 21.

26. Roden DM. (2001). Antiarrhythmic Drugs. In: The Pharmacologic Basis of Therapeutics (Eds Hardman JG, Limbird LE). pp. 933–970. McGraw-Hill, USA.

27. Fisch C, Knoebel SB. (1985). Digitalis cardiotoxicity. J Am Coll Cardiol. 5, 91A.

28. Moorman JR, Pritchett EC. (1985). The arrhythmias of digitalis intoxication. Arch Intern Med. 146, 1289.

29. Ochs HR, Smith TW. (1977). Reversal of advanced digitoxin toxicity and modification of pharmacokinetics by specific antibodies and Fab fragments. J Clin Invest. 60, 1303.

30. Hickey AR, Wenger TL, Carpenter VP et al. (1991). Digoxin immune Fab therapy in the treatment of digitalis intoxication—safety and efficacy. Results of an observational surveillance study. J Am Coll Cardiol. 17, 590.

Bradyrhythms and Heart Blocks in the ICU

Bradyrhythms in the intensive care unit may be harmless or may portend disaster. They are due to slowing of impulse formation, or a delay in impulse conduction through one or more areas of specialized conducting tissue that propagate the cardiac impulse. A bradyrhythm may be totally asymptomatic. Yet in patients with intrinsic heart disease or in ICU patients admitted for other serious problems, a marked fall in heart rate reduces the cardiac output. This is invariably so if the heart rate falls below 45/minute. A fall in cardiac output is certain to cause a further deterioration in an already seriously ill patient. The rate should be corrected before such a deterioration is clinically observed. Symptomatic brady-rhythms, whatever the aetiology, need immediate treatment (1).

A bradyrhythm is defined as a cardiac rhythm slower than 60/minute. Bradyrhythms are divided into two major categories:

(i) Disturbance in sinus impulse formation and conduction (sinus bradycardia, sinoatrial block, a Wenckebach block in the SA node, sinus arrest, the sick sinus syndrome).

(ii) Atrioventricular (AV) block. The term is applied to a delay in conduction in the AV node or in the infranodal conduction tissue. Delayed conduction in infranodal tissue is of far greater prognostic import compared to conduction delay within the AV node itself.

Sinus Bradycardia

In the ICU this condition is observed chiefly in the sick sinus syn-drome or in ischaemic heart disease, particularly after an acute inferior myocardial infarction. It can also occur in patients with no organic heart disease—chiefly due to increased intracranial tension, hypothyroidism, to hyperactive vagal reflexes and to drugs. An important example of increased vagal tone is in patients with tetanus. These patients when undergoing a tracheal suction, may show marked bradycardia that may culminate in cardiac arrest. The above mentioned problem is also occasionally observed in other critical illnesses. Numerous drugs can also produce sinus bradycardia (chiefly digitalis and beta-blockers).

The following problems can arise as a result of marked sinus bradycardia:

(i) A low output state—this may occur suddenly or over a period of time. A slow rate can also produce faintness or syncope.

(ii) A potentiation of ventricular ectopics—the unfortunate use of antiarrhythmic drugs in an attempt to suppress these ectopics, further slows the heart. Greater ectopic activity is then often ob-served, and this may lead to ventricular tachycardia or fibrillation. On the other hand, increasing the ventricular rate may abolish ventricular ectopics.

SA Block (2)

A second degree SA block is evident on the monitor or on a rhythm strip, as a long pause between two sinus impulses. A Wenckebach type of SA block is characterized by a progressive shortening of the PP intervals until a long pause occurs because of the blocked beat. A third degree SA block leads to atrial and ventricular standstill, and if this is sufficiently long, a nodal or ventricular escape rhythm is noticed. SA block occurs after excessive vagal stimulation, in inferior myocardial infarction, acute myocarditis or as a side effect or a toxic effect of drugs like digitalis, propranolol and other antiarrhythmic drugs. It also occurs as part of a sick sinus syndrome which may manifest as a bradyrhythm due to SA block or even an AV block. Bradytachyrhythms are also often observed with a sick sinus syndrome.

One of the most important causes of SA block (and later an AV block as well) in critically ill ICU patients is hyperkalaemia. Hyperkalaemia should always be thought of in a patient with a bradyrhythm. The P waves are absent and the QRS complexes are slow and wide, followed by tall T waves. A bundle branch block pattern (without preceding P waves) is sometimes observed. The possibility of hyperkalaemia is particularly important in patients with renal insufficiency, or in those on chronic dialysis.

Management

The following points should be noted:

(i) All drugs that slow the heart rate should be omitted.

(ii) If the bradyrhythm in a critically ill patient falls well below 50/minute, the rate should be increased by drugs. It does not matter whether the bradyrhythm is due to organic heart disease or occurs in other critical illnesses.

(iii) If the bradyrhythm produces a low output state or if an SA block produces faintness or syncope, or is complicated by ventricular ectopics, the basic heart rate should be increased with atropine or isoprenaline, or if need be, by transvenous cardiac pacing.

Atropine is administered slowly intravenously in a dose of 0.3–1 mg.

In an emergency, isoprenaline is given in an infusion of 1 mg in 500 ml dextrose. The infusion rate is initially kept at 1 µg to 4 µg/minute and is carefully increased till the desired effect on the heart rate is achieved. The patient should be carefully monitored for ectopics that may be induced by isoprenaline.

When a symptomatic bradyrhythm persists, or when it fails to respond to drugs, or when the use of drugs produces toxic effects (isoprenaline induced ventricular ectopics or tachycardia), transvenous pacing should be done. Many units would opt for transvenous pacing in symptomatic bradyrhythms or bradyrhythms which cause a low output state without taking recourse to drugs.

When severe persistent bradycardia occurs in acute inferior myocardial infarction and does not respond to atropine, a temporary transvenous pacing is the method of choice to increase the heart rate. Isoprenaline should be avoided in these circumstances, except as a temporary emergency measure; this drug increases myocardial oxygen consumption and thereby can cause an extension in the area of infarction.

If hyperkalaemia is strongly suspected as the cause of a SA block, a blood sample is quickly sent for serum K$^+$ estimation. 10–20 ml of 10 per cent calcium gluconate is given intravenously without waiting for the result. This is followed by a dextrose-insulin infusion as detailed in the Section on Fluid and Electrolyte Disturbances in the Critically Ill.

AV Block (3)

All forms of AV block can be either nodal or infranodal. Infranodal blocks can be intra-Hisian or infra-Hisian and are far more dangerous than nodal blocks.

A *First Degree AV Block* is characterized by a prolonged PR interval. It needs no treatment (4), except careful assessment whether drugs known to produce a first degree AV block can be reduced or omitted. Digitalis is the commonest cause of prolonged AV conduction. Other antiarrhythmic drugs can also do the same.

Second Degree AV Block of the Wenckebach Type (the block in most cases is nodal and not infranodal), is characterized by progressive prolongation of the PR interval with a progressive shortening of the RR interval, till a P wave is blocked at the AV node and does not produce a ventricular QRS complex. A Wenckebach type of AV block does not constitute a problem, except when it is a forerunner of a high grade block (5). This is typically observed in some patients with acute inferior myocardial infarction.

A Mobitz Type II AV Block is of ominous significance as the site of the block is infranodal. It is associated with a sudden block of the P wave occurring sporadically in an otherwise normal rhythm, or is characterized by a regular 2:1 or 3:1 block at the AV node. It often precedes a high grade or complete AV block and is at times a forerunner to sudden death.

The most important causes of second degree AV block are myocardial infarction, acute myocarditis and drugs—particularly digitalis, quinidine and procainamide.

Atropine may be used for a Wenckebach block. A Mobitz Type II block needs prompt transvenous pacing to forestall a possible catastrophe (4).

Complete or Third Degree AV Block (2) is characterized by a very slow ventricular rate of close to 30/min, with a total dissociation between the atria and the ventricles. All impulses reaching the AV node are blocked, and the ventricles beat from a focus within the AV node, or from a focus below the AV node. AV dissociation with a ventricular rate > 40/min cannot be called a complete AV block, though a high grade AV block obviously exists in these patients. Complete or third degree AV block in an ICU setting, is observed in acute myocardial infarction, or in drug toxicity, chiefly digitalis toxicity. Most antiarrhythmic drugs used to treat tachyrhythms can also produce a complete AV block as a toxic effect.

Patients with Leriche's disease or Lev's disease, which is characterized by fibrosis of the infranodal conducting tissue, may also find admission to the ICU due to syncopal spells, or to Stokes-Adams attacks occurring against a background of complete AV block. Rarely, acute myocarditis or calcific aortic stenosis may also be associated with a complete AV block.

Hyperkalaemia induces both SA block and AV block; the former invariably precedes the latter. Hyperkalaemia (serum K$^+$ > 6.5–7 mEq/l) also prolongs the intraventicular conduction, causing slow wide complexes.

Complete AV block with a slow ventricular rate needs emergency transvenous pacing in the ICU (4).

Complete or High Grade AV Block in Relation to Acute Myocardial Infarction. Acute inferior myocardial infarction often results in a Wenckebach block followed by a high grade, and rarely by a complete AV block. Transvenous pacing should be done for high grade AV blocks. The block almost always resolves within 7–12 days (6), with a return to sinus rhythm, when the pacing catheter is withdrawn.

Complete AV block in the presence of acute anterior myocardial infarction is of grave prognostic significance, and carries a high mortality (70–80 per cent) (7). This is because in all such instances there is extensive damage of the anterior wall, the septum, and the lateral wall with ischaemic destruction of conducting tissue below the AV node. This may include the Bundle of His, the branches of the His Bundle, and the Purkinje conducting fibres as well. As the block is infranodal, ventricular escape rhythms are much slower and more unstable, than in patients with heart block due to acute inferior myocardial infarction, where the high grade or complete AV block is nodal. The block in acute anterior myocardial infarction is often associated with pump failure, not only because of the marked bradyrhythm, but because of the extensive myocardial damage. Complete AV block in these patients might occur suddenly, or might be preceded by various combinations of blocks in the branches of the Bundle of His. These blocks include: (i) a right bundle branch block with a block in the anterosuperior division of the left bundle branch; (ii) a right bundle branch block with a block in the posteroinferior division of the left bundle branch; (iii) a left or right bundle branch block pattern; (iv) a bilateral bundle branch block, characterized either by a left or right bundle branch block pattern on the ECG, with a significantly prolonged PR interval; (v) a trifascicular block which causes an ECG pattern of a bifascicular block with a prolonged PR interval.

Complete AV block needs prompt transvenous pacing. There is a considerable difference of opinion as to which other combinations of blocks involving the Bundle of His, need to be paced in acute anterior myocardial infarction. We generally prophylactically pace patients with a bilateral bundle branch block or a trifascicular block. We do not pace those with a right bundle block together with a block in the anterosuperior division of the left bundle branch. We may occasionally pace patients with a right bundle branch block together with a block in the posteroinferior division of the left bundle branch. We do not generally pace a patient who develops an isolated right or left bundle branch block. There are however a number of units who would prophylactically pace all or most of these combinations of heart blocks in the His bundle conducting system that have been listed above.

REFERENCES

1. Myerburg RJ, Kloosterman EM, Castellanos A. (2001). Recognition, Clinical Assessment, and Management of Arrhythmias and Conduction Disturbances. In: Hurst's The Heart, 10th edn (Eds Valentin F, Alexander RW, O'Rourke RA). pp. 797–873. McGraw-Hill Inc, New York, London, Toronto.

2. Jeffrey EO, Zipes DP. (2001). Specific Arrhythmias: Diagnosis and Treatment. In: Heart Disease—A Textbook of Cardiovascular Medicine (Eds Braunwald E, Zipes DP, Libby P). pp. 815–889. WB Saunders Company, Philadelphia, London, Tokyo.

3. Denes P. (1987). Atrioventricular and intraventricular block. Circulation. 75 (Suppl III), III-19–III-25.

4. Dreifus LS, Fisch C, Griffin JC et al. (1991). Guidelines for implantation of cardiac pacemakers and and antiarrhythmic devices. J Am Coll Cardiol. 18, 1–13.

5. Strasberg B, Amat-y-Leon F, Dhingra RC et al. (1981). Natural history of chronic second degree atrioventricular nodal block. Circulation. 63, 1043–1049.

6. Rotman M, Wagner GS, Wallace AGP. (1972). Bradyarrhythmias in acute myocardial infarction. Circulation. 45, 703.

7. Kostuk WJ, Beanlands DS. (1970). Complete heart block associated with acute myocardial infarction. Am J Cardiol. 26, 380.

Antiarrhythmic Drugs Used in the ICU

General Considerations

It is important to be familiar with antiarrhythmic drugs used in the acute or emergency management of arrhythmias in the ICU. Antiarrhythmic drugs are double-edged weapons—they can effectively reverse an arrhythmia and salvage a potentially dangerous situation. At the same time they can themselves produce side effects which could be cardiac or non-cardiac. Remarkably enough, cardiac side effects include heart failure and induction of arrhythmias. In other words, antiarrhythmic agents could well produce the very problem which they are supposed to eradicate or suppress. Drug induced or drug aggravated cardiac arrhythmias (bioarrhythmias) are a major clinical problem. In one study, proarrhythmic events occurred in 6.9 per cent of 506 consecutive patients and in 3.4 per cent of 1268 drug trials for ventricular tachycardia (VT) and ventricular fibrillation (VF) (1). Factors predisposing to such proarrhythmias include the presence of left ventricular dysfunction, treatment with digitalis and diuretics, and a longer pre-treatment QT interval (2).

Antiarrhythmic drugs are therefore of help, but need to be used with caution. As a matter of principle it is wise not to use multiple antiarrhythmic drugs simultaneously. If more than one antiarrhythmic drug is being used, possible pharmacokinetic interactions between various drugs should be noted (see Table 7.7.1). It is also important to constantly bear in mind whether an arrhythmia one is treating may not have been actually caused or potentiated by the very drugs used to treat it. Finally, arrhythmias can be precipitated by factors such as hypoxia, hypercapnia, electrolyte and acid-base disturbances. Correction of these factors can restore sinus rhythm, and is far more important than the use of antiarrhythmic drugs.

This chapter gives a brief account of important commonly used

Table 7.7.1. Pharmacokinetic interactions of common antiarrhythmic drugs

Drugs	Clearance
Quinidine	Increased by phenytoin, phenobarbital, rifampicin Decreased by cimetidine, amiodarone
Lidocaine	Decreased by cimetidine, propranolol
Digoxin	Decreased by quinidine, verapamil, amiodarone Volume of distribution decreased by quinidine
Disopyramide	Increased by phenytoin, phenobarbital, rifampicin
Procainamide	Decreased by cimetidine, amiodarone

antiarrhythmic agents in the ICU. It is important to be perfectly familiar with a few important drugs and use them skillfully rather than grapple with a host of drugs. **Table 7.7.2** lists the commonly used antiarrhythmic drugs with their dosages, and major side effects.

Lidocaine (3–5)

Lidocaine is an extremely useful Class IB antiarrhythmic agent. It depresses depolarization and shortens repolarization in ventricular muscle fibres. It also depresses both normal and abnormal forms of automacity. It is only effective when given intravenously.

The drug is metabolized in the liver. It has a mean half-life of 1–2 hours in normal subjects, > 4 hours in patients with uncomplicated myocardial infarction, > 10 hours in patients with myocardial infarction and associated cardiac failure, and even longer in patients with cardiogenic shock. Severe hepatic dysfunction or reduced hepatic blood flow as in patients with cardiac failure or shock, can markedly reduce the metabolism of the drug in the liver. In patients with liver disease, or in those with cardiac failure with low-output states, the dose of the drug should be reduced by one-third to half.

Clinical Indications

Its main indication is the acute or emergency treatment of ventricular arrhythmias of diverse aetiology, but particularly those occurring in acute myocardial infarction and after open heart surgery. It is the drug of choice for suppression of ventricular ectopics, sustained ventricular tachycardia and symptomatic ventricular tachycardia. It should be administered to patients with pulseless ventricular tachycardia or ventricular fibrillation that is refractory to electrical countershocks and epinephrine. After ventricular tachycardia or ventricular fibrillation is terminated, it is advisable to use the drug in a slow intravenous infusion to prevent recurrences of dangerous ventricular arrhythmias. This is particularly imperative in patients with active myocardial ischaemia, hypokalaemia and myocardial dysfunction. Since most wide QRS complex tachyrhythms are presumed to be ventricular rather than supraventricular, lidocaine is the drug of choice in all wide-complex tachycardias of unknown origin (6). Lidocaine is of no effect in supraventricular arrhythmias, and in fact, may even accelerate

Table 7.7.2. Indications, doses, and main adverse effects of antiarrhythmic drugs commonly used in the ICU

Drug	Indications	Adverse Effects	Dose Loading	Dose Maintenance	Special Remarks
1. Lidocaine	Emergency treatment of ventricular arrhythmias of any aetiology, specially in AMI and after open heart surgery	CNS—dizziness, seizures confusion, coma; sinus node depression, aggravates LV dysfunction, myocardial depression and hypotension	1–2 mg/kg IV bolus, repeat 1/2 dose in 30 mins	1–2 mg/min infusion	—
2. Mexiletine	Treatment of ventricular arrhythmias when lidocaine ineffective	Dizziness, nystagmus, confusion, vomiting. CVS—bradycardia, hypotension, worsening of arrhythmia	100–150 mg IV bolus	2–4 mg/min infusion for first 3 hrs, then 0.5 mg/min; later 200 mg 8 hrly orally	—
3. Quinidine	Supraventricular and ventricular ectopics and tachycardias	Nausea, vomiting, diarrhoea CNS—tinnitus, hearing loss, visual disturbances; haemolytic anaemia, thrombocytopaenia, CVS—various blocks, Torsade de Pointes, myocardial depression	400 mg 2 hrly for 4–5 doses orally	200 mg 6 hrly orally	Elevates S.digoxin levels
4. Procainamide	Treatment of ventricular arrhythmias where lidocaine ineffective; treatment of atrial flutter/ fibrillation after AV conduction is blocked/slowed	Hypotension, various heart blocks, ventricular arrhythmias and myocardial depression	25–50 mg IV over 1 min, repeated every 5 mins to maximum of 1000 mg	2–6 mg/min infusion	Contraindicated in Torsade de Pointes where QT prolonged.
5. Amiodarone	Ventricular arrhythmias or SVT refractory to conventional drugs	Hypotension, worsens ventricular arrhythmias, can induce torsade de pointes, aggravates LVF; rise in liver enzymes	5 mg/kg IV over 20 mins	10 mg/kg/ day × 3–4 days	Dose reduced by 25–40% if digoxin being used.
6. Bretylium Tosylate	Refractory ventricular tachycardia	Hypotension	5 mg/kg IV over 30 mins	1–2 mg/min infusion	—
7. Esmolol	Emergency control of ventricular rate in atrial flutter, atrial fibrillation and SVT	Hypotension, heart block, bronchospasm, acute LVF	500 µg/kg/min over 1–2 mins	50–200 µg/ kg/min infusion	Side effects very transient
8. Verapamil	PAT, AV nodal entry or reciprocating tachycardias; to slow ventricular rate in atrial flutter/fibrillation	Hypotension, LVF, bradycardia, AV block	7.5–10 mg IV over 2–3 mins	0.005 mg/kg/min	Contraindicated in heart blocks, ventricular tachycardia, wide QRS complex tachycardias, hypotension, cardiogenic shock. Dose of digitalis should be reduced when verapamil is being used.
9. Adenosine	SVT when verapamil contraindicated (drug of choice for SVT)	Transient AV nodal block, flushing, dyspnoea	6–12 mg bolus IV, preferably in central vein		Smaller dose to be used in patients on dipyridamole
10. Digoxin	Atrial flutter/ fibrillation, SVT	Nausea, vomiting, visual disturbances, induces arrhythmias, particularly in presence of hypokalaemia, hypomagnesaemia and renal dysfunction	0.25 mg IV over 5 mins, repeated 4 hourly till digitalizing dose of 1–1.25 mg reached in 24 hrs	0.25 mg/ day	Dose should be reduced when using with quinidine and verapamil. Care to be taken when used with amiodarone

the ventricular response in patients with atrial fibrillation and the WPW syndrome.

Dosage

For multiple ventricular ectopics, sustained ventricular tachycardia, symptomatic ventricular tachycardia, as also for pulseless ventricular tachycardia or refractory ventricular fibrillation, an initial bolus of 1–1.5 mg/kg body weight is given intravenously at a rate of 30–50 mg/minute. A maintenance drip with an infusion rate of 1–4 mg/minute generally suffices to prevent recurrence. A blood lidocaine level of 1.5 to 6 mg/ml is an effective suppressive range.

If the initial bolus is ineffective, two or more boluses of 1 mg/kg can be given at 5 minute intervals. Patients who require higher doses of the drug, and higher plasma levels of lidocaine to revert to sinus rhythm, need a larger maintenance dose of 2–4 mg/minute. A maintenance drip is generally continued for 24–48 hours. Doses should be reduced by 50 per cent in patients with shock, heart failure or liver dysfunction and in patients older than 70 years.

Cardiac arrest victims may need only a single bolus of lidocaine. The drug can also be administered in patients with cardiac arrest through the endotracheal tube, using 2.5 times the intravenous dose. Once circulation has been restored after successful resuscitation from cardiac arrest, an intravenous infusion of 2 to 4 mg/minute of lidocaine should be given.

Adverse Effects

Side effects chiefly involve the central nervous system. These are dose-related effects, and are more frequently seen in the aged. Neurological toxicity includes dizziness, paraesthesia, confusion, delirium, drowsiness and even coma. Seizures may also occur. Sinus node depression may occur. The drug is remarkably free of haemodynamic effects, but in large doses and particularly in old patients with poor left ventricular function, the drug may further depress the myocardium, worsen failure and induce hypotension. Lidocaine can increase defibrillation thresholds and has been rarely reported to cause malignant hyperthermia (7, 8).

Quinidine (9–11)

This is a class I antiarrhythmic agent. It depresses depolarization and prolongs repolarization in the atria and the ventricles. It can facilitate AV conduction and prolongs the QT interval.

Twenty per cent of the drug is excreted by the kidneys, the remainder being metabolized by the liver. Plasma quinidine levels peak at about 90 minutes after oral administration of quinidine sulphate. Elimination half life is 5 to 8 hours after oral administration. The drug dosage should be reduced in patients with hepatic or renal disease and in those with poor hepatic blood flow (e.g. in cardiac failure and shock).

Indications

Quinidine is a useful antiarrhythmic agent for suppressing supraventricular and ventricular ectopic activity and also for suppressing and reverting both atrial and ventricular sustained tachyrhythms. It does this chiefly by increasing the refractory period of the atria and ventricles, and by suppressing atrial and ventricular ectopic activity. Prior to using quinidine for the conversion of atrial flutter or fibrillation to sinus rhythm, the ventricular rate should be first slowed by digitalis or verapamil or a beta-blocker. This is because if quinidine is used first, it can slow the atrial flutter rate from say 300 to 200/minute. This effect coupled with enhanced AV conduction (a vagolytic effect of the drug) may convert a 2:1 atrioventricular response to a 1:1 response, with a resulting increase in the ventricular rate.

Dosage

For conversion of both sustained supraventricular and ventricular tachyarrhythmias we prefer to use the drug orally—400 mg 2 hourly for 4 to 5 doses in our opinion being better than 400 mg 6 hourly, as this schedule leads to a more frequent reversion to sinus rhythm.

Quinidine can be given intravenously in an emergency situation e.g. a VT not responding to lidocaine, amiodarone or DC conversion. Quinidine gluconate is given in a dose of 10 mg/kg intravenously very slowly at a rate of 0.5 mg/kg/min, the blood pressure and ECG being constantly monitored.

Adverse Effects

The most common adverse effects include nausea, vomiting and diarrhoea. CNS disturbances include hearing loss, tinnitus, visual disturbances, confusion, delirium and psychosis. Hypersensitivity responses include haemolytic anaemia, thrombocytopaenia, fever and rash. Remarkably enough, in our Indian patients these adverse effects are uncommon, the drug being fairly well tolerated.

Its cardiovascular effects can indeed be dangerous and should therefore be very closely monitored. It can slow conduction and may produce an SA or AV block or a bundle branch block. Quinidine-induced cardiac toxicity can be treated with molar sodium lactate.

Quinidine may produce a QT prolongation and a torsade de pointes, a polymorphic ventricular tachyarrhythmia which can cause a syncopal attack and may even be fatal. Syncope is unrelated to plasma concentrations of quinidine or duration of therapy, though the majority suffer these episodes within the first 2 to 4 days. In these cases, the drug should be promptly omitted and hypokalaemia which is frequently present should be corrected. The drug of choice in a patient who has syncope from torsades de pointes is magnesium, given intravenously (2 g over 1 to 2 minutes followed by an infusion of 3 to 20 mg/minute) (12, 13). Drugs which do not prolong the QT interval like lidocaine or phenytoin may also be tried. Atrial or ventricular pacing may act by suppressing depolarization. If pacing is not available, isoproterenol may be used.

Quinidine may elevate serum digoxin levels by displacing digoxin from tissue receptors, and by decreasing both its total body clearance and volume of distribution.

Procainamide (5, 14)

This is an antiarrhythmic drug very similar to quinidine in its mode of action. It depresses depolarization and prolongs repolarization both in the atria and the ventricles, facilitates AV conduction through its vagolytic effect and prolongs the QT interval.

The drug is chiefly excreted through the kidneys though it is also partly metabolized by the liver. 15 per cent is metabolized to N-acetyl procainamide, which also has antiarrhythmic effects and is excreted by the kidneys. The drug's dosage should therefore be reduced in patients with a low-output state and in those with renal insufficiency. Renal clearance of procainamide is diminished by cimetidine.

Clinical Indications

The main indications for its use are:

(i) Emergency suppression of ventricular arrhythmias when lidocaine is ineffective.

(ii) Conversion of atrial flutter or fibrillation after digitalis or verapamil or beta-blockers have been first used to slow or block AV conduction.

Dosage

Most units in the West prefer procainamide to quinidine for the emergency treatment of ventricular arrhythmias in the ICU. Several intravenous regimes have been advocated. One regime is to give 25 to 50 mg of the drug intravenously over a one minute period. This is repeated every five minutes until the arrhythmia is controlled, or hypotension results, or the QT interval is prolonged by more than 50 per cent. Another regime is to give a slow infusion of the drug at a rate of 2 to 6 mg/minute with a careful monitoring of the blood pressure and ECG. It is wise not to exceed a total dose of 1000 mg. In less emergent situations, procainamide can be used orally—500 mg every 3–4 hours, the total daily dose being between 2 to 4 g.

Adverse Effects

Hypotension, which can be precipitous, is the most frequent side effect. Procainamide is a myocardial depressant and can worsen myocardial function in a patient with left ventricular disease. It can also induce ventricular arrhythmias by prolonging the QT interval. It can also suppress conduction in the SA node or the AV node or within the conduction system in the ventricles and can lead to various forms of heart block. The syndrome of systemic lupus erythematosus reported on prolonged oral administration of the drug does not occur following emergency administration of the drug.

Procainamide should never be used to treat torsade de pointes associated with a prolonged QT interval.

Amiodarone (15, 16)

This is a class III antiarrhythmic agent useful in the management of ventricular and supraventricular tachyrhythms in the ICU. It prolongs action potential duration and refractoriness and blocks the sodium channel. It also prolongs the QT interval but is less likely to induce torsade de pointes than quinidine, procainamide or disopyramide. It also has a depressant action on the myocardium and can produce a mild alpha and beta blockade.

The drug is lipid soluble and is metabolized by the liver. It is not excreted by the kidneys and the dose need not be reduced in patients with renal failure.

The onset of action after intravenous administration is generally within several hours (17). Oral medication takes 2 to 3 days or even 1 to 3 weeks to produce an effect and is therefore of no use in an emergency situation. Therapeutic serum levels range from 1 to 3.5 µg/ml.

Clinical Indications

Amiodarone can suppress a wide range of supraventricular and ventricular tachyarrhythmias (18). These include AV nodal re-entrant tachycardia, junctional tachycardia, atrial flutter, atrial fibrillation, ventricular tachycardia and ventricular fibrillation. Its efficacy is 60 to 80 per cent for most supraventricular tachycardias and 40 to 60 per cent for ventricular tachycardias (19). It has been shown to be superior to Class I antiarrhythmic agents in maintaining sinus rhythm in patients with recurrent atrial fibrillation. In the ICU, we use this drug for ventricular tachycardia resistant to lidocaine and use it frequently in the management of supraventricular arrhythmias occurring in a critical care setting.

Dosage

A loading dose of 5 mg/kg dose is given intravenously over 20 minutes; this is repeated after 30 minutes. This is then followed by a maintenance dose of 10 mg/kg/day for 3 to 4 days. We generally do not exceed a total dose of 1.2 g in 24 hours. The drug is administered in a 5 per cent dextrose infusion as it may precipitate in normal saline.

Adverse Effects

Amiodarone has significant potential toxicity. Cardiac side-effects include bradycardia, hypotension, aggravation of tachyarrhythmias in 1 to 2 per cent (20) and worsening of congestive heart failure in 2 per cent. The drug can prolong the QT interval and should not be given to patients with torsade de pointes.

Non-cardiac toxic effects chiefly involve the pulmonary and gastrointestinal systems. Pulmonary toxicity very rarely can begin acutely within 6 to 10 days of treatment in the ICU (21), but generally occurs after a few months of continuous oral therapy. It is characterized clinically by cough, breathlessness and crackles over the lungs on auscultation. The underlying pathology consists of areas of pulmonary consolidation with progressive respiratory failure. The pathogenesis is believed to be related to an immune-mediated hypersensitivity response of the lung to the drug. Amiodarone should be promptly stopped at the first sign of lung involvement.

The drug can also produce liver cell dysfunction with elevated liver enzymes, gastrointestinal disturbances and neurological dysfunction. Other potential toxic effects (e.g. corneal microdeposits and thyroid dysfunction) are not observed during use in critical care units.

In spite of its potential toxicity, the drug is indeed extremely useful in a critical care setting, for a variety of supraventricular and ventricular arrhythmias.

As far as possible, amiodarone should not be used in combination with quinidine or procainamide as it increases the serum level of these drugs. If digoxin is being used, the dose should be reduced by 25 to 40 per cent.

Bretylium Tosylate (22, 23)

This drug was introduced in the 1950s as an antihypertensive agent. Its sole indication is to counter ventricular tachyrhythms unresponsive to conventional therapy with lidocaine, procainamide or amiodarone.

The drug prolongs action potential duration and increases the refractory period of the atria and ventricles. It is excreted almost exclusively by the kidneys so that the drug is either avoided totally or its dose sharply reduced in patients with renal failure.

Dosage

The initial dose is 5 mg/kg given over 30 minutes; a maintenance drip with an infusion rate of 1 to 2 mg/minute is then continued. The drug should be omitted after 24 hours, particularly if an antiarrhythmic effect is not observed.

Adverse Effects

Hypotension is frequently observed; nausea and vomiting are also frequent side effects.

Esmolol (24, 25)

Esmolol is a short-acting cardioselective beta-blocker with a half-life of approximately 9 minutes after intravenous administration. It has an action similar to other beta-blockers—it chiefly prolongs AV conduction, slows the heart rate and reduces contractility. The action starts within 2 minutes of an intravenous loading dose. It is metabolized by red blood cell esterases and is rapidly inactivated so that complete recovery from its physiological effects occurs within 20 minutes after intravenous administration.

Its main indication is in the acute or emergency control of the ventricular rate in SVT, atrial flutter and atrial fibrillation.

Dosage

This drug is administered in a loading dose, an intravenous bolus of 500 μg/kg/minute being given over 1–2 minutes. A maintenance dose of 50–200 μg/kg/minute is then continued as a slow intravenous infusion.

Adverse Effects

These are the same as with other beta-blockers, only these effects if present disappear within 15–20 minutes. The drug therefore has a higher margin of safety compared to other beta-blockers, particularly in patients with left ventricular dysfunction. Even so, hypotension, heart block, bronchospasm and acute heart failure may be observed.

Verapamil

Verapamil is a class IV antiarrhythmic agent that blocks the slow calcium channel in cardiac muscle (26). It thereby reduces the plateau height of the action potential, shortens muscle action potential, and prolongs total Purkinje fibre action potential (27). In vivo, verapamil prolongs conduction time through the AV node and lengthens functional and effective refractory periods of the AV node. Like all calcium channel blockers the drug has a negative inotropic effect on ventricular contraction though this is not as marked as that observed with beta-blockers. Verapamil also produces significant peripheral vasodilatation; the resulting hypotension induces reflex sympathetic stimulation. The drug produces coronary vasodilatation and decreases myocardial oxygen demand.

The drug acts promptly on intravenous administration. AV nodal conduction delay occurs within a few minutes and is detectable for over 6 hours. The elimination half-life of verapamil is 3–7 hours, 30 per cent being metabolized in the liver, and 70 per cent being excreted by the kidneys (27).

Clinical Indications

The drug is extremely useful in the treatment of PAT, AV nodal entry or reciprocating tachycardia. It should be tried if simple vagal manoeuvres fail. However, most units prefer to administer intravenous adenosine as the drug of choice for the above mentioned supraventricular tachyrhythms. Even so, verapamil given intravenously terminates more than 90 per cent of episodes of supraventricular tachycardia. The drug is also used to slow the ventricular rate in atrial flutter and fibrillation. It can be used with digoxin for this purpose but should not be combined with beta-blockers.

Verapamil has no action on, and should not be used for ventricular tachycardias. As a general rule, intravenous verapamil should not be given in any wide QRS complex tachycardias. If the latter happens to be a ventricular tachycardia, haemodynamic collapse (severe hypotension and arrest) may occur.

Dosage

For emergency use in critical care units, 5 to 10 mg is given intravenously over 2 to 3 minutes, with close monitoring of the blood pressure and ECG. Slowing of the ventricular rate in atrial fibrillation may be maintained if necessary, by the oral use of the drug, or by a continuous infusion of the drug at a rate of 0.005 mg/kg/minute.

Adverse Effects

Hypotension, during or immediately after intravenous administration, can be marked. This effect can be reversed by intravenous calcium gluconate. Because of its negative inotropic action, the drug can further depress cardiac function and cardiac output in a patient with left ventricular dysfunction or in a patient with congestive cardiomyopathy. This adverse effect can be dangerous and at times fatal if the drug is administered to a patient already on beta-blockers (28). Bradycardia, AV block and asystole can also occur as dangerous side effects; they are more likely to occur when the drug is combined with beta-blockers.

Contraindications to the use of verapamil are sinus node dysfunction, AV block without a pacemaker in place, atrial fibrillation occurring against the background of a WPW syndrome with antegrade conduction over an accessory pathway. In the latter situation, verapamil can facilitate conduction through the accessory pathway with a marked rise in ventricular rate that may end with ventricular fibrillation and death. The drug is also contraindicated in ventricular tachycardias, all wide QRS complex tachycardias, in hypotensive states and in cardiogenic shock. It is generally contraindicated, as stated earlier, in a patient receiving beta blockers. Verapamil can decrease the excretion of digoxin by 30 per cent; the dose of the latter should therefore be reduced if it is to be used with verapamil.

Diltiazem

The mechanism of action of diltiazem is the same as verapamil. Intravenous diltiazem is effective in terminating paroxysmal supraventricular tachycardia (PSVT) and in controlling the ventricular rate in patients with atrial flutter and fibrillation. Diltiazem should not be used for ventricular tachycardia.

Dosage

An initial bolus of 0.25 mg/kg (20 mg in an average adult) is administered intravenously over 2 minutes. If satisfactory rate control in atrial flutter or fibrillation is not achieved, a further 20 mg is given over 2–3 minutes after a lapse of 15 minutes. The bolus dose is followed by an infusion at 5–15 mg/hour. The infusion should not exceed a period of 24 hours.

Adverse Effects

Adverse effects are as those observed with verapamil. The hypotensive and negative inotropic effects are however much less marked as compared to verapamil.

Verapamil and diltiazem are best avoided in patients with a sick sinus syndrome or AV block in the absence of a functioning pacemaker.

Adenosine

This is a comparatively new drug used to treat SVT (**29, 30**). It is administered intravenously and is an extremely effective antiarrhythmic agent. Adenosine interacts with A_1 receptors present on the extracellular surface of cardiac cells and activates K^+ channels. The increase in K^+ conductance shortens the atrial action potential duration, hyperpolarizes the membrane potential and decreases atrial contractility (**27**). It delays conduction and induces a block in the AV node.

Adenosine is removed from the system by washout, by enzymatic degradation to inosine, phosphorylation to AMP or by re-uptake into the cells (**27**). It has a very short elimination half-life of 1 to 6 seconds. It is worth noting that therapeutic concentrations of theophylline block the action of adenosine. Dipyridamole blocks re-uptake of adenosine and delays its clearance from the circulation; hence smaller doses of adenosine must be used in patients on dipyridamole. The onset of action of adenosine begins in less than 30 seconds and lasts for 1 to 2 minutes.

Clinical Use

This drug is used by many as the first choice to terminate acutely occuring SVT such as AV nodal or AV re-entry tachycardias (**31–**

33). It is particularly indicated when SVT occurs in patients with heart failure, hypotension, WPW syndrome or in patients receiving calcium channel blockers or beta-blockers.

Dosage

An intravenous dose of 6 mg is given by a rapid intravenous injection. After 2 minutes, a second dose of 10 mg may be administered in the same manner, if necessary. The dose should be reduced by 50 per cent if the injection is given through a central line or in patients on beta-blockers, calcium channel blockers or dipyridamole (see Chapter on Tachyarrhythmias). Conversion to sinus rhythm occurs in 90 to 100 per cent of cases.

Adverse Effects

Facial flushing, dizziness, nausea, dyspnoea and angina-like chest pain are observed quite frequently. Sinus bradycardia or a temporary AV block may occur. Cardiac asystole for a few seconds may be a worrying feature.

Digoxin

Digoxin is still very frequently used in the ICU both in the management of cardiac failure and in the control of supraventricular arrhythmias.

Digitalis has a significant inotropic action on the heart. It binds to and inhibits $Na^+ K^+$ ATPase resulting in an increased intracellular Na^+ which is exchanged for extracellular calcium (**34**). The increased availability of activated calcium to the contractile proteins of the myocardial cells results in enhanced contractility. The action of digoxin on $Na^+ K^+$ ATPase activity also alters the transmembrane potential of other cells affecting the refractory period, conduction velocity and excitability. Various cell types may be affected differently accounting for different effects on the atria, on the AV node and conducting tissues and on the ventricles. Digitalis (including digoxin) enhances the parasympathetic, and diminishes the sympathetic effects on the heart. It also acts as a peripheral vasoconstrictor (**35**).

The main action of digitalis glycosides in clinical practice is an inotropic action on the heart and a prolongation of AV conduction. The latter is due to varying degrees of block in the AV node. This effect is made use of in slowing the ventricular rate in atrial flutter and fibrillation, and in inhibiting re-entrant supraventricular tachycardia.

Pharmacokinetics

Digoxin is widely distributed in the tissues and the serum half-life is fairly long—36 to 48 hours. Intravenous digoxin acts within 1–2 hours of administration. Therapeutic blood levels of digoxin are between 0.8–2 ng/ml. Unfortunately, the drug has a relatively narrow therapeutic ratio, and toxicity may occur even when serum levels are within the therapeutic range. The drug is primarily cleared by the kidneys. Interactions between digoxin and other drugs are frequent. Impaired renal function and drug interactions which raise serum digoxin levels dangerously, contribute to the frequent occurrence of digitalis toxicity observed in the ICU.

Clinical Indications

These chiefly include:

(i) Cardiac failure—both left ventricular failure and congestive cardiac failure.

(ii) Supraventricular tachyarrhythmias—atrial flutter, atrial fibrillation and re-entrant supraventricular tachycardia.

Dosage

Emergency slowing of the ventricular rate in supraventricular tachyrhythms, or a quick inotropic action in left ventricular failure, necessitates intravenous administration of the drug. 0.25 mg (or in exceptional instances 0.5 mg) is given intravenously over 5 minutes. 0.25 mg is then repeated 4 to 6 hourly till a digitalizing dose of 1–1.25 mg is reached over a 24 hour period. It is wise not to exceed this dose, at least not in patients in our country. Patients with atrial flutter or fibrillation may require a larger dose of 1.5 or even 1.75 mg in 24 hours. A maintenance dose of 0.25 mg orally daily for 5 to 6 days in a week, generally suffices. In the presence of renal failure, the loading and maintenance doses need to be sharply reduced. Frequent digoxin levels may need to be done and digoxin levels should be kept below 2.0 ng/ml. In the elderly, intravenous digoxin should be given with caution. We prefer to give half the loading dose followed by a maintenance dose of 0.125 mg orally daily for 5 days in a week.

Toxic Effects

Digitalis is a toxic proarrhythmic drug particularly in the presence of hypokalaemia, hypomagnesaemia and renal insufficiency. The simultaneous use of quinidine alters the renal clearance and the volume of distribution of digoxin. In fact, therapeutic levels of quinidine may nearly double the serum concentration of digoxin. The dose of digoxin should be halved when using quinidine. Amiodarone and verapamil have similar but lesser effects on digoxin levels in the blood.

Digitalis-induced arrhythmias and their management have been discussed in an earlier chapter. Nausea, vomiting, and visual disturbances are also observed in patients in the ICU and may precede or accompany rhythm disturbances caused by digoxin.

Digoxin is contraindicated in the presence of AV block, in severe hypokalaemia or hyponatraemia, and in hypertrophic cardiomyopathy.

REFERENCES

1. Stanton MS, Prystowsky EN, Fineberg NS et al. (1989). Arrhythmogenic effects of antiarrhythmic drugs: A study of 506 patients treated for ventricular tachycardia or fibrillation. J Am Coll Cardiol. 14, 209.
2. Minardo JD, Heger JJ, Miles WM et al. (1988). Clinical characteristics of patients with ventricular fibrillation during antiarrhythmic drug therapy. N Engl J Med. 319, 257.
3. Lie KI, Wellens JH, van Capelle FJ et al. (1974). Lidocaine in the prevention of primary ventricular fibrillation. A double-blind, randomized study of 212 consecutive patients. N Engl J Med. 291, 1324–1326.
4. MacMohan S, Collins R, Peto R et al. (1988). Effects of prophylactic lidocaine in suspected acute myocardial infarction. JAMA. 260, 1910–1916.
5. Woosley RL. (2001). Antiarrhythmic Drugs. In: Hurst's The Heart (Eds Fuster V, Alexander RW, O'Rourke RA). pp. 899–924. McGraw-Hill Inc., New York, London, Toronto.
6. Akhtar M, Shenasa M, Jazayeri M, Caceres J et al. (1988). Wide QRS complex tachycardia: reappraisal of a common problem. Ann Intern Med. 109, 905–912.
7. Tatsukawa H, Okuda J, Kondoh M et al. (1992). Malignant hyperthermia caused by intravenous lidocaine for ventricular arrhythmia. Ann Intern Med. 31, 1069.
8. Echt DS, Gremillion ST, Lee JT et al. (1994). Effects of procainamide and lidocaine on defibrillation energy requirements in patients receiving implantable cardioverter defibrillator devices. J Cardiovasc Electrophysiol. 5, 752.
9. Bloomfield SS, Romhilt DW, Chou T-C et al. (1973). Natural history of cardiac arrhythmias and their prevention with quinidine in patients with acute coronary insufficiency. Circulation. 47, 967–973.
10. Carliner NH, Crouthamel WG, Fisher ML et al. (1979). Quinidine therapy in hospitalised patients with ventricular arrhythmias. Am Heart J. 98, 708–715.
11. Coplen SE, Antman EM, Berlin JA et al. (1990). Efficacy and safety of quinidine therapy for maintenance of sinus rhythms after cardioversion. A meta-analysis of randomized control trials. Circulation. 82, 1106–1114.
12. Bailie DS, Inoue H, Kaseda S et al. (1988). Magnesium suppresses early after depolarizations and ventricular tachyarrhythmias induced in dogs by cesium. Circulation. 77, 1395.
13. Tzivoni D, Banai S, Schuger C et al. (1988). Treatment of torsade de pointes with magnesium sulphate. Circulation. 77, 392.
14. Hoffman BF, Rosen MR, Wit AL. (1975). Electrophysiology and pharmacology of cardiac arrhythmias. VII. Cardiac effects of quinidine and procainamide. Am Heart J. 90, 117–122.
15. Graboys TB, Podrid PJ, Lown B. (1983). Efficacy of amiodarone for refractory supraventricular tachyarrhythmias. Am Heart J. 106, 870–876.
16. Mason JW. (1987). Amiodarone. N Engl J Med. 316, 455–466.
17. Ochi RP, Goldenberg IF, Almquist A et al. (1989). Intravenous amiodarone for the rapid treatment of life-threatening ventricular arrhythmias in critically ill patients with coronary artery disease. Am J Cardiol. 64, 599.
18. Weinberg BA, Miles WM, Klein LS et al. (1993). Five-year follow-up of 589 patients treated with amiodarone. Am Heart J. 125, 109.
19. Miller JM, Zipes DP. (2001). Management of Patients with Cardiac Arrhythmias. In: Heart Disease—A Textbook of Cardiovascular Medicine (Eds Braunwald E, Zipes DP, Libby P). pp. 700–774. WB Saunders Company, Philadelphia, London, Tokyo.
20. Hohnloser SH, Klingenheben T, Singh BN. (1994). Amiodarone-associated proarrhythmic effects: A review with special reference to torsades de pointes tachycardia. Ann Intern Med. 121, 529.
21. Ashrafian H, Patrick D. (2001). Is Amiodarone an underrecognized cause of Acute Respiratory Failure in the ICU? Chest. 120(1), 275–282.
22. Bacaner MB. (1986). Treatment of ventricular fibrillation and other acute arrhythmias with bretylium tosylate. Am J Cardiol. 21, 530–543.
23. Narang PK, Adir J, Josselson J, Yacobi A. (1980). Pharmacokinetics of bretylium in man after intravenous administration. J Pharmacokinet Biopharm. 8, 363–372.
24. Frishman WH, Murthy VS, Strom JA. (1988). Ultra-short acting beta-adrenergic blockers. Med Clin North Am. 72, 359–372.
25. Miura D, Frishman WH. (1991). Class II drugs. In: Basis and Clinical Electrophysiology and Pharmacology of the Heart (Eds Dangman DH, Miura D). pp. 665–676. Marcel Decker. New York.
26. Nademanee K, Singh DN. (1988). Control of cardiac arrhythmias by calcium antagonism. Ann NY Acad Sci. 522, 536.
27. Miller JM, Zipes DP. (2001). Management of the Patient with Cardiac

Arrhythmias. In: Heart Disease—A Textbook of Cardiovascular Medicine (Eds Braunwald E, Zipes DP, Libby P). pp. 700–774. W B Saunders Company, Philadelphia, London, Toronto, Montreal, Sydney, Tokyo.

28. Ferling J, Citron PD. (1983). Hemodynamic and myocardial performance characteristics after verapamil use in congestive heart failure. Am J Cardiol. 51, 1339–1345.

29. Bellardinelli L, Pelleg A. (1990). Cardiac electrophysiology and pharmacology of adenosine. J Cardiovasc Electrophysiol. 1, 327.

30. Homeister JW, Hoff PT, Fletcher DD. (1990). Combined adenosine and lidocaine administration limits myocardial reperfusion injury. Circulation. 82, 595.

31. Belhassen B, Glick A, Laniado S. (1988). Comparative clinical and electrophysiologic effects of adenosine triphosphate and verapamil on paroxysmal reciprocating junctional tachycardia. Circulation. 77, 795.

32. DiMarco JP, Miles W, Akhtar M et al. (1990). Adenosine for paroxysmal supraventricular tachycardia: dose ranging and comparison with verapamil. Ann Intern Med. 113, 104.

33. Ros SP, Fisher EA, Bell TJ. (1991). Adenosine in the emergency management of supraventricular tachycardia. Pediatr Emerg Care. 7, 222–223.

34. Smith TW. (1988). Digitalis: Mechanism of action and clinical use. N Engl J Med. 318, 358.

35. Longhurst JC, Ross J. (1985). Extracardiac and coronary vascular effects of digitalis. J Am Coll Cardiol. 5, 99A–105A.

CHAPTER 7.8

Hypertensive Crisis and Aortic Dissection in the ICU

Hypertensive Crisis

Hypertensive crisis generally occurs in patients who have a background of essential or accelerated hypertension. It may occasionally occur in patients who were previously normotensive. In patients with pre-existing hypertension, the blood pressure during a crisis can be very high—as high as, or even > 250 mm Hg systolic, and 120–130 mm Hg diastolic. In previously normotensive patients, a crisis may occur with a comparatively lesser rise in the blood pressure. A hypertensive crisis or emergency in a previously normotensive, or a very recently diagnosed hypertensive patient, suggests an acute glomerulonephritis, acute renovascular hypertension, toxaemia of pregnancy, a pheochromocytoma, or a drug reaction to a monoamino oxidase (MAO) inhibitor. Important pathologies underlying an acute crisis in known hypertensives are essential hypertension, chronic glomerulonephritis, chronic pyelonephritis, renovascular hypertension, and pheochromocytoma. Severe rebound hypertension causing an acute crisis, may be observed following sudden omission of antihypertensive drugs. This can occur following the withdrawal of any antihypertensive drug, but is most frequently observed following withdrawal of clonidine, particularly if the patient is or has recently been on beta-blockers.

Hypertensive emergencies often necessitate critical care. The danger caused by a sudden rise in blood pressure to high levels, is invariably related to a disturbance in structure and/or function of important organ systems—chiefly the CNS, the heart, aorta and coronary circulation, and the kidneys. Equally important is the potential hazard of a sudden increase in blood pressure in specific critical situations, such as in the peri-operative or immediate post-operative phases of intracranial surgery, open heart surgery or other vascular surgeries. Thus a sudden rise in blood pressure during or after intracranial surgery or following trauma to the head, is fraught with the risk of increasing cerebral oedema with all its attendant complications. A hypertensive crisis peri- or post-operatively following open heart surgery, subjects the heart to an unnecessary increase in afterload, and can trigger cardiac failure and pulmonary oedema. A rise in the blood pressure in the immediate post CABG phase, can also accentuate myocardial ischaemia, and can precipitate a myocardial infarction. The risk of increased bleeding

due to post-operative hypertension is also ever present, particularly following open heart surgery and vascular surgery.

Hypertensive crisis necessitating critical care, can be grouped as follows:

1. An acute hypertensive crisis causing acute structural damage and functional changes in organ systems. The organ systems most frequently involved are the central nervous system, the cardiovascular system, and the kidneys.

A. Central Nervous System—problems involving the central nervous system include hypertensive encephalopathy, cerebral haemorrhage, subarachnoid haemorrhage, stroke, or stroke in evolution.

B. Cardiovascular System—acute hypertensive crisis can precipitate unstable angina, myocardial infarction, aortic dissection, acute left ventricular failure.

C. Renal System—malignant hypertension with rapidly evolving renal destruction and failure, are the most dreaded features of severe accelerated hypertension.

2. Hypertension posing a potential hazard in specific critical situations.

A. After intracranial surgery (greater risk of cerebral oedema and bleeding).

B. After trauma to the head (same as above).

C. After open heart surgery (risk of myocardial infarction, acute heart failure, bleeding).

D. After vascular surgery (risk of bleeding).

E. After other major surgery (risk of bleeding, risk to sutures).

3. Eclampsia. This is a special situation in pregnancy where sudden increase in blood pressure is associated with seizures and albuminuria. There is a great risk of multiple organ dysfunction, particularly involving the CNS and kidneys.

4. Uncommon conditions causing a sudden dangerous rise in blood pressure.

A. Pheochromocytoma: This often causes paroxysmal hypertension. Even so, the commonest cause of paroxysmal hypertension in clinical practice, occurs against a background of mild essential hypertension.

B. Drug reactions in patients on MAO inhibitors.

Approach to a Hypertensive Emergency

The management of a hypertensive emergency, rests on quick assessment and immediate treatment. Quick assessment consists of a relevant history and physical examination. The urgency of the situation at times may demand measures to control the hypertensive crisis as the first and initial step. History taking and physical examination may then need to be delayed till this is achieved. The most important feature in the history is to determine whether the patient has had a background of hypertension, and if so, the duration of this hypertension. As mentioned earlier, if there is a history of long-standing hypertension, then the underlying aetiology is generally essential hypertension. The possible factors precipitating an acute crisis in a patient need to be carefully evaluated. Emotional stress, physical fatigue, excessive ingestion of salt, administration of corticosteroids, or the occurrence of secondary renovascular problems, are important causes of an acute crisis in these patients. Not uncommonly, no cause can be found for a precipitious rise in the blood pressure. The causes of an acute hypertensive crisis in normotensive patients have been mentioned earlier.

The physical examination in such an emergency should be brief, and is conditioned to an extent by the nature of the presenting illness. A brief CNS examination should include a rapid assessment of cognition and memory, of motor function, and of tendon and plantar reflexes. A quick examination of the cardiovascular system should include clinical assessment of heart size, presence of significant murmurs, and the presence or absence of signs of pulmonary congestion and cardiac failure. The carotid, brachial and femoral pulses should be palpated, and any inequality noted. Bruits over the carotids and the abdomen should also be looked out for. Unequal pulses against an appropriate background, should raise the possibility of diffuse atherosclerotic disease, or aortic dissection. A fundoscopic examination is mandatory in every case. A fundus examination will reveal the severity of hypertension (presence of exudates and haemorrhages), the duration of hypertension (sclerosed vessels with A-V nicking), and the presence of malignant hypertension as judged by papilloedema.

It is also important to assess priorities in management. Though control of hypertension is of great importance, the presence of continuous seizures should prompt the urgent use of antiepileptic drugs. Similarly, the use of aspirin or other anticoagulants in a patient with a stroke in evolution, should be delayed till such time as imaging studies have excluded a cerebral haemorrhage. In these patients one should rest content with lowering of the blood pressure, and the use of anti-oedema measures, if these are indicated.

Emergency laboratory investigations are of marginal help. A routine blood count, ESR and urine examination are always done. A chest X-ray, ECG, serum electrolytes, blood urea, creatinine and blood glucose, will help to further assess cardiac and renal functions in relation to a hypertensive crisis. Evidence of cardiac failure should warn the intensivist against the use of a beta-blocker. Special tests include imaging studies for CNS lesions, for a possible aortic dissection, and for kidney size. Echocardiography is of use in assessing wall motion abnormalities, ejection fraction and the presence of clots within the heart. There should be a protocol which allows a sequential work-up based on immediate priorities; these would depend on the nature of the crisis and its presenting features.

Initial Management of Hypertensive Emergencies

Before starting therapy for blood pressure control, it is necessary to decide how quickly the blood pressure in an individual patient needs to be lowered, and to what extent it should be lowered. In many cases it may be unwise or even positively harmful to lower the blood pressure to normal levels. In older people (over 60 years), even in the absence of a history of coronary or cerebrovascular disease, it is best not to lower the systolic blood pressure below 140–150 mm Hg. In patients with a history of cerebrovascular or ischaemic heart disease, it is even more important to avoid sharp reductions in blood pressure. A reading of 150/90–100 mm Hg is satisfactory till a more careful evaluation of the past history and present problem is done. On the other hand, in patients with dissection of the aorta, the systolic pressure should be rapidly reduced to 100–120 mm Hg. In paroxysmal hypertensive crisis induced by a pheochromocytoma or due to drug interactions in a patient on MAO inhibitors, the pressure can also be safely brought down to normal levels.

The speed at which the blood pressure needs to be lowered depends on the nature of the emergency or crisis. For example, hypertensive encephalopathy characterized by seizures or by mental obtundation and coma due to cerebral oedema, requires an urgent and rapid reduction in the blood pressure. Similarly a patient in acute pulmonary oedema with marked hypertension would benefit by a rapid reduction in blood pressure. On the other hand, in the presence of a stroke in evolution, or a myocardial infarction, it would be more beneficial if the blood pressure is reduced less rapidly, over a period of 2–4 hours. Rapid swings in blood pressure are dangerous in these patients.

The decision as to whether the patient requires parenteral therapy and the duration of this therapy, prior to starting oral medication, is also important. The ideal parenteral drug to reduce blood pressure in a hypertensive crisis should be quick acting, effective and rapidly reversible, should not exhibit tachyphylaxis and should have minimal side effects and no adverse effects on other organ systems. No drug fulfills all these criteria ideally. When the hypertensive crisis is acute and associated with seizures due to hypertensive encephalopathy, or with pulmonary oedema due to acute left ventricular failure, or with aortic dissection, the quickest way of reducing and controlling hypertension, is by the use of intravenous nitroprusside or diazoxide. We prefer to use intravenous nitroprusside in all patients with a life-threatening severe hypertensive crisis as it is easily available and we are familiar with its use.

Sodium Nitroprusside

This drug immediately lowers the blood pressure through a direct vasodilator action on the arteriolar, capillary and venous walls (1, 2). The drug action ceases within 3–5 minutes of stopping the drug. 50 mg of the drug are added to 500 ml of 5 per cent dextrose, so that 1 ml (60 microdrops) of this constituted solution contains 100 µg. The solution should be protected from light by wrapping it in a dark cloth; it should be freshly prepared and promptly used. Normally it is faint brown in colour and should not be used if the colour changes to dark brown.

Sodium nitroprusside is always given through a microdrip, the average dose being 2–3 µg/kg/min. It is best to start the infusion with a smaller dose of 0.25 µg/kg/min. A 60 kg patient would receive 15 µg/min, which would work out to 8–9 microdrops/min. The blood pressure is checked every half a minute, and if necessary one can increase the flow rate by 5 microdrops at 3–4 minute intervals. When the blood pressure shows a clear drop, close monitoring is necessary, as it can crash to unrecordable levels. Fortunately the effect of this drug is short-lived, so that the blood pressure starts to rise within a few minutes of stopping the drug. Occasionally protracted hypotension may result, which is countered by stopping the drug and if necessary, by the use of mephentermine or norepinephrine in a separate intravenous infusion. It is best not to continue intravenous nitroprusside for more than 72 hours as this drug is converted to thiocyanate. Cyanide poisoning (suspected when there is a sharp fall in the pH) can occur with prolonged excessive use. Nausea, abdominal pain, headache, mental confusion and other side effects are occasionally observed.

Diazoxide

This drug has an immediate potent anti-hypertensive effect due to a direct vasodilator action on the arterial wall. It is best given as a 50 mg intravenous bolus which is repeated at 5–10 minute intervals. This results in a safe, smooth reduction in blood pressure, without the sharp hypotension observed with larger bolus doses. Besides hypotension, other side effects include salt and water retention with development of congestive cardiac failure, and hyperglycaemia which often requires treatment, particularly in diabetic patients. Severe hypotension is countered by intravenous infusion of dopamine or norepinephrine.

We no longer use ganglionic blocking drugs like trimethaphan or pentolinium parenterally for urgent reduction in blood pressure.

Nitroglycerine

Nitroglycerine is predominantly a venodilator, in larger doses, it also produces arteriolar dilatation and reduces the blood pressure. An intravenous infusion of 50 to 100 µg/minute can be easily titrated because of its rapid and yet short action. The drug is however, much less potent than the other parenteral drugs. Its main use is to control a sudden rise of blood pressure in the peri-operative period and in hypertension associated with myocardial ischaemia or with acute left ventricular failure and pulmonary oedema.

Nifedipine

Nifedipine sublingually (squeezed from a punctured capsule) can sharply reduce pressure (3). It is best not to use more than 5 mg sublingually as the fall in blood pressure though temporary, may be otherwise dramatic and uncontrolled. Though anecdotal reports

of myocardial infarction and arrhythmias have been reported following sublingual nifedipine, we have never encountered problems when the drug is used in the dose stated above.

The sublingual use of nifedipine is a temporary expedient till other antihypertensive therapy is organized and put into effect.

Nicardipine Hydrochloride (4)

This drug is a calcium channel blocker which is available for intravenous use. We have no experience in its use. It is potent, has a rapid effect due to a direct vasodilatory action on vascular smooth muscle causing both a sharp lowering of blood pressure together with coronary vasodilatation. It is given as a loading infusion of 5–15 mg/hour, followed by a maintenance infusion of 3–8 mg/hour. Most experience with this drug is in the management of acute hypertension occurring peri-operatively or post-operatively in cardiac and non-cardiac surgery. Side effects are similar to those observed with other calcium channel blockers—flushing, headache, hypotension, nausea and vomiting.

Beta-blockers

Labetalol (a combined alpha and beta-blocker) can be used intravenously as a 20–80 mg bolus every 10 minutes, followed by a 2 mg/min infusion. Labetalol when given intravenously, has a predominant beta blocking effect and should not be used in patients with asthma, severe bradycardia or heart block. Beta-blockers should also be avoided in patients with cardiac dysfunction as they can precipitate cardiac failure. On the other hand, a beta-blocker preferably given orally together with intravenous nitroprusside, is an ideal combination to reduce and control blood pressure in aortic dissection. Propranolol reduces dv/dt in these patients and this is of advantage in aortic dissection. It is used as a 1–5 mg intravenous bolus, followed by an infusion at the rate of 3 mg/hr (see Subsection on Aortic Dissection).

Esmolol is a very rapid acting selective beta-blocker that is given intravenously for quick control of hypertension and tachycardia. Its mode of administration is given under Aortic Dissection.

Phentolamine

Phentolamine in a dose of 5–10 mg is given in a slow intravenous infusion in hypertensive crisis due to a pheochromocytoma. The drug blocks the alpha receptors and is ideally suited in this situation. It should be carefully titrated against the blood pressure response.

Once a satisfactory reduction in blood pressure has been achieved, oral medication is used to keep the blood pressure under control. These agents include beta blockers, calcium channel blockers, clonidine and angiotensin converting enzyme (ACE) inhibitors.

Table 7.8.1 lists the parenteral drugs used in the management of hypertensive emergencies.

Each emergency situation related to a hypertensive crisis will need other special treatment depending on the nature of the emergency. Intracerebral haemorrhage will require measures to counter cerebral oedema; acute pulmonary oedema will necessitate treatment for acute left ventricular failure.

Table 7.8.1. Parenteral drugs used in the management of hypertensive crisis

Drugs	Dose	Onset of Action	Duration of Action	Adverse Effects
Drugs with Rapid Action				
1. Sodium Nitroprusside	0.25–10 µg/kg/min as IV infusion	Immediate	1–3 mins	Hypotension, nausea, vomiting, muscle twitchings, cyanide poisoning with prolonged excessive use
2. Nitroglycerin	5–100 µg/min as IV infusion	2–5 mins	1–3 mins	Tachycardia, headache, flushing, vomiting, methaemoglobinaemia
3. Diazoxide	50 mg IV bolus repeated at 5–10 min intervals, or 15–30 mg/min IV infusion	1–2 mins	6–8 hrs	Hypotension, fluid retention, hyperglycaemia, tachycardia
4. Hydralazine	10–20 mg IV 10–50 mg IM	10–20 mins 20–30 mins	3–6 hrs	Tachycardia, flushing, headache, vomiting, precipitation of angina
5. Phentolamine	5–15 mg IV	1–2 mins	10–30 mins	Tachycardia, flushing
6. Trimethaphan	1–4 mg/min IV infusion	1–5 mins	5–10 mins	Orthostatic hypotension, bowel or bladder paresis, blurred vision, dry mouth
7. Esmolol	500 µg/kg/min for 4 mins; then 150–300 µg/kg/min IV	1–2 mins	8–10 mins	Hypotension
8. Labetalol	20–80 mg IV bolus every 10 mins; 2 mg/min IV infusion	5–10 mins	3–6 hrs	Vomiting, dizziness, nausea, postural hypotension, precipitation of cardiac failure
9. Propranolol	1–5 mg IV bolus; 3 mg/hr IV infusion	1–2 mins	3–6 hrs	Bronchospasm, hypotension
10. Nicardipine hydrochloride	5–15 mg/hr as a loading infusion; 3–8 mg/hr as a maintenance infusion IV	1–3 mins	15–40 mins	Hypotension, headache, flushing
11. Enalaprilat	0.625–1.25 mg IV bolus every 6 hours	10–15 mins	6–8 hrs	Hypotension, cough, hyperkalaemia, renal insufficiency
Slower Acting Drugs				
1. Reserpine	1 mg IV; 2–2.5 mg repeated after 4–6 hrs	2–4 hrs	Few weeks	Drowsiness, Parkinsonian-like rigidity, reactivation of peptic ulcer, nasal obstruction, bronchospasm
2. Alphamethyldopa	250–500 mg IV 6 hrly	1–3 hrs	90–120 mins	Drowsiness

Newer Drugs for Parenteral Use

Newer Drugs that can be parenterally administered in an acute hypertensive crisis are Fenoldopam and Enalaprilat.

Fenoldopam Mesylate (4)

Fenoldopam is a new parenteral drug which is a dopamine 1 receptor agonist and which lowers blood pressure by decreasing peripheral vascular resistance. It has a rapid onset of action (4 minutes) and a short duration of effect. Its efficacy in reducing acute hypertension is believed to be equivalent to that of nitroprusside. We have no experience with its use.

Enalaprilat (4)

Enalaprilat is a new intravenously administered angiotensin converting enzyme inhibitor. It acts by decreasing angiotensin II activity and decreasing aldosterone secretion. However, its efficacy is lower than that of other parenteral agents. The drug is administered as an intravenous bolus injection of 0.625–1.25 mg every 6 hours. Its onset of action is within 1 to 3 minutes and the duration of its effect is for 6 to 8 hours. Its side effects are common to other angiotensin converting enzyme inhibitors, which include renal dysfunction, hyperkalaemia, cough and severe hypotension. We again have no experience with its use.

Slower Acting Drugs

Alphamethyldopa

Alphamethyldopa can be given intravenously 250–500 mg 6 hourly, for a comparatively slower blood pressure reducing effect.

Reserpine

Reserpine is available in India and is given intially in a dose of 1 mg intravenously. If well tolerated, 2–2.5 mg is repeated after 4 hours. The drug can be repeated every 4–6 hours till the desired effect is obtained. Its main disadvantage is that it causes drowsiness and thus confuses the clinical picture. It also often causes a parkinsonian-like rigidity. Other side effects include activation of a peptic ulcer, distressing nasal obstruction, and bronchospasm resembling bronchial asthma.

Malignant Hypertension

Critical care is often needed in the presence of rapidly deteriorating renal function. This is often associated with other end-organ complications particularly in relation to the heart and the CNS. Unfortunately in many patients renal dysfunction continues to progress even after reasonable blood pressure control. Malignant-phase hypertension is invariably associated with a marked increase in renin activity, even when the underlying hypertension is 'essential'. Angiotension converting enzyme inhibitors are very effective as initial therapy for these patients. These drugs include captopril, enalapril, lisinopril and recent additions spirapril and cilazapril (5, 6). An ACE inhibitor often needs to be combined with other antihypertensives.

Hypertensive Crisis in Eclampsia

The diagnosis of eclampsia requires the presence of seizures, oedema, proteinuria and hypertension in pregnancy. It should be differentiated from preeclampsia wherein seizures are absent, and where a prompt reduction in the blood pressure may well prevent morbidity and transition to eclampsia. The antihypertensives best suited for the pregnant state include hydralazine and alphamethyldopa. 10–40 mg of hydralazine may be given orally or intramuscularly every 6 hours. The dose of alphamethyldopa has already been mentioned. Diazoxide may be used for a hypertensive crisis, but may cause a reduction in the placental flow. Our experience with other drugs in acute hypertensive states in pregnancy is limited. Magnesium sulphate administered intravenously is extremely useful for the control of seizures (7); it also has an antihypertensive effect. A loading dose of 4–6 g is given intravenously over 20–30 minutes. This is followed by doses of 1.5–3 g/hr intravenously. A plasma magnesium level of 4–6 mEq/l is considered to be within the therapeutic range. Once the seizures and hypertension are reasonably controlled, the foetus should be delivered.

REFERENCES

1. Kaplan NM. (2001). Systemic Hypertension: Therapy. In: Heart Disease. A Textbook of Cardiovascular Medicine. (Ed. Braunwald E). pp. 972–994. WB Saunders Company, Philadelphia, London, Toronto, Tokyo.

2. Brush JE Jr, Udelson JE, Bacharach SL et al. (1989). Comparative effects of verapamil and nitroprusside on left ventricular function in patients with hypertension. J Am Coll Cardiol. 14, 515.

3. Jaker M, Atkin S, Soto M et al. (1989). Oral nifedipine vs oral clonidine in the treatment of urgent hypertension. Arch Intern Med. 149, 260.

4. Zimmermen JL. (2000). Hypertensive Crises: Emergencies and Urgencies. In: Textbook of Critical Care (Eds Grenvik A, Ayres SM, Holbrook PR, Shoemaker WC). WB Saunders Company, Philadelphia, USA.

5. Gavras H. (1990). Angiotensin converting enzyme inhibition and its impact on cardiovascular disease. Circulation. 81, 381.

6. Black HR, Bakris GL, Elliott WJ. (2001). Hypertension: Epidemiology, Pathophysiology and Treatment. In: Hurst's The Heart, 10th edn (Eds Fuster V, Alexander RW, O'Rourke RA). pp. 1553–1604. McGraw-Hill Inc., New York, London, Toronto.

7. Pritchard JA, Cunningham FG, Pritchard SA. (1984). The Parkland Memorial Hospital Protocol for treatment of eclampsia. Evaluation of 245 cases. Am J Obstet Gynecol. 148, 951.

Dissection of the Aorta

Aortic dissection is a catastrophic emergency most frequently associated with hypertension. Dissection occurs through a tear in the intima, and this takes place either in the ascending aorta or at the beginning of the descending aorta, distal to the origin of the left subclavian. Blood dissects the aorta between the intima and the media for a varying length, with catastrophic results. The condition is more common in men than in women, and the mortality is over 50 per cent in the first 48 hours, and over 70 per cent within the first week. Rarely aortic dissection can occur in the absence of hypertension in patients with a congenital weakness in the aortic wall as in Marfan's syndrome, or in aortic cystic medionecrosis.

Classification

A classification of aortic dissections based on approach to therapy, delineates 3 types—Types A, B and C, which have been illustrated in **Fig. 7.8.1**.

A more current classification is that proposed by the Stanford group of workers (1). This classification delineates just two types—Type A and B. In Type A, the ascending aorta is involved, irrespective of the site of intimal tear. 15 per cent of tears in the transverse aorta and 5 per cent of tears in the descending aorta also involve the ascending aorta. In Type B, only the descending aorta beyond the left subclavian is involved. The risk of sudden death is highest in Type A as the dissection can cause tamponade, aortic insufficiency, congestive heart failure and coronary occlusion. Type B dissections carry less risk and therefore can be managed conservatively.

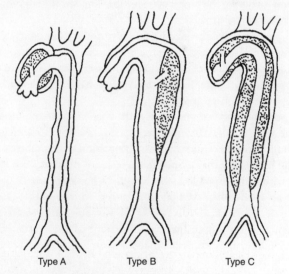

Type A   Type B   Type C

Fig. 7.8.1. Classification of aortic dissections.
Type A dissection: Dissection proximal to origin of left subclavian artery.
Type B dissection: Tear distal to origin of left subclavian artery with no involvement of the ascending aorta.
Type C dissection: Dissection extends both proximally and distally to origin of left subclavian artery.
The current standard classification recognizes two types—Type A when the ascending aorta is involved, irrespective of the site of tear; Type B, when only the descending aorta distal to the origin of the left subclavin artery is involved.

Clinical Features and Diagnosis (2–4)

Excruciating pain starting most often in the back is the presenting feature (5). The pain is also felt in the front of the chest and may radiate to the shoulders and the left arm, or to both arms. Invariably, the patient is admitted to the intensive care unit with a diagnosis of acute myocardial infarction. The correct diagnosis depends on a high index of suspicion. The clinical features of shock often accompany the agonising pain, but a noteworthy feature in a number of these patients is the persistence of hypertension in the presence of other shock-like features.

Clinical features that must be carefully searched for are:

(a) An inequality of pulses in the upper limbs, or the disappearance of the pulse in an upper limb or even a lower limb.

(b) The appearance of a rough systolic murmur at the base, or over one or both carotids.

(c) Pulsations over one or the other sternoclavicular joint.

(d) The development of a diastolic murmur of aortic incompetence. At times a soft systolic or even continuous murmur is heard over the middle of the back in extensive dissection of the thoracic aorta.

(e) Focal neurological signs, if dissection involves the carotid or vertebral arteries, with compression of the lumen of these vessels.

(f) The absence of classical ECG changes of myocardial infarction, and no rise in CK-MB or troponin levels in blood, in spite of severe pain compatible with myocardial infarction.

(g) Extremely wide radiation of pain which may be felt over the lower thoracic spine, the small of the back, in the abdomen, and even involving the lower extremities. This should suggest a possible extensive dissection.

A haemorrhagic left-sided pleural effusion, when associated with the clinical features of an acute myocardial infarction should also suggest the diagnosis of an aortic dissection. The pleural effusion is due to a slight leak of the dissection into the pleura, or at times due to pleural irritation.

About one-third of patients with dissection of the aorta present with manifestations of compromised flow to a major branch of the aorta. This is due to compression or thrombosis of the true lumen of a major branch as a result of pressure from the blood within the expanded false lumen. When the carotids and vertebrals are involved, the presentation is with a neurological deficit or a stroke; involvement of the subclavian causes ischaemia to the upper limb; involvement of the mesenteric artery results in intestinal ischaemia; involvement of a renal artery results in renal failure or hypertension and of the ilio-femoral vessels in lower limb ischaemia.

Sudden death can occur from rupture of the dissected aorta into the pleura, the pericardium (causing cardiac tamponade), the retroperitoneum or into the abdomen.

Investigations

An X-ray of the chest shows a widened mediastinum in 50 per cent of cases. A double contour of the arch at the start of the descending aorta, may occasionally suggest the diagnosis. A small left sided pleural effusion may occasionally be observed when the adventitia oozes red blood cells from the dissecting haematoma. A progressive widening of the mediastinal shadow strongly suggests the diagnosis.

Echocardiography, Trans-oesophageal echocardiography (with the probe within the oesophagus) is a very useful non-invasive method of demonstrating a dissection, and also of demonstrating the intimal flap which points to the site of the dissection (**6, 7**).

A CT scan (**8, 9**) *or an MRI* (**10**) of the thorax invariably proves a dissection, clearly demonstrating the double lumen in the aorta, and often pointing to the site or origin of the dissection.

Most surgeons before surgery prefer to have an anatomical display of the dissection through an aortography. This indeed is not required if all the necessary information is available through echocardiography and a CT or MRI of the chest. What is more, if the intimal flap has been sealed off (which may happen within a few days of the dissection), an aortogram may not be able to pick up the dissection. In such patients, if the diagnosis is highly suspect, it is mandatory to do a CT or MRI of the chest, if these investigations have not been done.

Management (Table 7.8.2) (11)

The patient under intensive care should be continuously monitored with regard to vital signs, ECG, relevant investigations on the blood, and serial X-rays of the chest. The blood pressure should be constantly monitored. The principles of management are:

(i) Complete bed rest.

(ii) Relief of pain with morphine, buprenorphine or pethidine. Small bolus doses (2–5 mg of morphine) should be given intravenously, and repeated as and when necessary.

(iii) Reduction of blood pressure. This is imperative in all hypertensive patients. The pressure should be quickly and sharply reduced to a systolic of about 100 mm Hg provided tissue perfusion is adequate. It should never exceed 120 mm Hg. In the rare instances when the patient is not hypertensive, the systolic blood pressure should be kept around 90 mm Hg. It is preferable to use intravenous infusions of nitroprusside to lower the blood pressure and to maintain it at the desired level. The method of infusion has already been described earlier. It is important to combine the use of nitroprusside with a beta-blocker. This is because sodium nitroprusside increases the dP/dT which is a measure of the velocity of left ventricular ejection. An increase in the velocity of left ventricular ejection is an undesired effect in aortic dissection, and can be countered by a beta-blocker which reduces dP/dT—an advantage in dissection. For an acute or rapid reduction in dP/dT, propranolol is given intravenously in a dose of 0.5–1 mg every 15

Table 7.8.2. Principles of management of aortic dissection

---

* Complete bed rest
* Relief of pain with morphine (2–4 mg IV), or buprenorphine (0.2–0.4 mg IV), or pethidine (75–100 mg IM)
* Quick reduction of blood pressure—In hypertensive patients systolic BP should be maintained between 100–120 mm Hg; in non-hypertensive patients, keep systolic BP around 90 mm Hg. A combination of IV nitroprusside + IV propranolol (0.5–1 mg every 15–30 mins till beta-blockade achieved), is commonly used
* Medical therapy continued with in the following cases:
  – In patients with uncomplicated Type B dissection (dissection distal to origin of left subclavian artery, with no involvement of the ascending aorta), who have responded well to medical therapy (relief of pain, control of BP), and are haemodynamically stable
  – In patients with stable, chronic dissection (2 weeks or more after onset)
  – Failure of opacification of double lumen on aortography
* Definitive surgical therapy for aortic dissection

---

to 30 minutes till satisfactory beta-blockade occurs. For the maintenance of beta-blockade in a stable dissection, propranolol is given orally in a dose 20–40 mg thrice daily.

Many units in the West prefer the use of labetalol to nitroprusside in control of hypertension in aortic dissection. The drug is a selective alpha-blocker and a non-selective beta-blocker, and thereby reduces dP/dT and the systolic blood pressure by beta-blockade and vasodilation. A bolus injection of 0.25 mg/kg is given intravenously over 2 minutes and repeated every 10 to 15 minutes. The drug can also be given through a continuous infusion at 1 to 2 mg/minute. Unfortunately, parenteral labetalol is not easily available in India.

Esmolol, a very short acting beta-1 selective receptor blocker is also very useful in the prompt control of acute hypertension in aortic dissection. It is given as an intravenous bolus in a dose of 500 µg/kg/minute over 11 minutes and then as an infusion of 150–300 µg/kg/minute. The infusion is titrated to keep the systolic blood pressure at 100 mm Hg.

If labetalol and esmolol are unavailable, sodium nitroprusside combined with propranolol or metoprolol are equally effective. In fact, we are more familiar with sodium nitroprusside than with other drugs.

Oral antihypertensives like alphamethyldopa, ACE inhibitors or calcium channel blockers may be used in addition, once the blood pressure has been urgently brought down to a desired level (about 100 mm Hg systolic) with intravenous parenteral therapy.

Patients who do not tolerate beta-blockade (patients with asthma, congestive heart failure and COPD) can be treated with trimethaphan, a ganglion blocking agent for a quick reduction in blood pressure. The drug is given in a dose of 1–2 mg/minute in a slow intravenous infusion for 24 to 48 hours. The head end of the bed is elevated to maximize the orthostatic hypotension the drug induces and the blood pressure is monitored and maintained around 100 mm Hg systolic. The use of trimethaphan is associated with rapid tachyphylaxis and with unpleasant side-effects due to ganglion blockade. We have little experience with the drug and continue to prefer the use of sodium nitroprusside.

Lowering the blood pressure produces dramatic relief in back and chest pain. Once the pain is relieved and the blood pressure lowered, the patient may be sent for a CT or a MRI of the chest, or if need be for an emergency aortography. An echocardiography can easily be done at the bedside. Oesophageal echocardiography as mentioned earlier, is of great help. It must be done expertly without causing a rise in the blood pressure during passage of the probe into the oesophagus.

Medical therapy is continued for a Type B tear—i.e. a tear distal to the origin of the left subclavian in which the ascending aorta is uninvolved, provided there is relief of pain, control of blood pressure and a stable clinical state. Other indications for medical therapy are a stable, chronic aneurysm (onset more than 2 weeks), failure of opacification of a double lumen on aortography, and the unavailability of surgical expertise.

The first requisite for surgical therapy is surgical expertise and experience with the problem. If this is available, the indications for surgery include a Type A dissection (dissection starting in and only involving the proximal aorta), Type C dissection (where dissection extends both proximal to the origin of the left subclavian, and also extends distal to it). Other indications for surgery are aortic insufficiency, impending rupture of the aneurysm (even in the Type B variety), a large haemorrhagic pleural effusion, cardiac tamponade, and inability to control pain or reduce hypertension with drug therapy. Indications for definitive surgical therapy are listed in **Table 7.8.3**. Surgical therapy involves resection and graft replacement. Successful medical or surgical therapy should be followed-up by the continued use of antihypertensive drugs which should include a beta-blocker.

Table 7.8.3. Indications for definitive surgical therapy in aortic dissection (surgical expertise and experience mandatory)

* Type A Dissection (dissection starting in proximal aorta)
* Type C Dissection (dissection extends both proximal and distal to origin of left subclavian artery)
* In presence of aortic insufficiency
* Impending rupture of aneurysm (even if Type B variety)
* Compromised blood flow to a major branch of the aorta.
* Large haemorrhagic pleural effusion
* Cardiac tamponade
* Failure to control hypertension/pain with medical therapy

REFERENCES

1. Austin JJ, Shragge BW. (1998). Aortic Dissection. In: Principles of Critical Care 2nd edn (Eds Hall JB, Schmidt, Wood LDH). pp. 483–496. McGraw-Hill Inc., New York.

2. Crawford ES. (1990). The diagnosis and management of aortic dissection. JAMA. 264, 2537–2541.

3. DeSanctis RW, Doroghazi RM, Austen WG et al. (1987). Aortic dissection. N Engl J Med. 317, 1060–1067.

4. Lindsay JL Jr. (2001). Diagnosis and Treatment of Diseases of the Aorta. In: Hurst's The Heart, 10th edn (Eds Fuster V, Alexander RW, O'Rourke RA). pp. 2375–2395. McGraw-Hill Inc., New York, London, Toronto.

5. Isselbacher EM. (2001). Diseases of the Aorta. In: Heart Disease—A Textbook of Cardiovascular Medicine (Eds Braunwald E, Zipes DP, Libby P). pp. 1422–1456. WB Saunders Company, Philadelphia, London, Tokyo.

6. Erbel R, Engberding R, Daniel W et al. (1989). Echocardiography in diagnosis of aortic dissection. Lancet. I, 457.

7. Adachi H, Kyo S, Takamoto S et al. (1990). Early diagnosis and surgical intervention of acute aortic dissection by transoesophageal color flow mapping. Circulation. 82(Suppl. IV), IV-19–IV-23.

8. Perez JE. (1983). Noninvasive Diagnosis: Computed Tomography and Ultrasound. In: Aortic Dissection (Eds Doroghazi RM, Slater EE). pp. 133. McGraw-Hill Book Company, New York.

9. Thorsen MK, San Dretto MA, Lawson TL et al. (1983). Dissecting aortic aneurysms: Accuracy of computed tomographic diagnosis. Radiology. 148, 773.

10. Amparo EG, Higgins CB, Hricak L et al. (1985). Aortic Dissection: Magnetic Resonance Imaging. Radiology. 155, 399.

11. Asfoura JY, Vidt DG. (1991). Acute aortic dissection. Chest. 99, 724–729.

Pulmonary Embolism

It is a general belief that pulmonary embolism (within or outside the ICU) is a rare entity in India. This is untrue. There is no good prospective study of its incidence in critically ill patients. Perhaps it is not as frequent as in the West, but is does occur, and it certainly is an important potential hazard or complication in patients being cared for in critical care settings.

The problems in pulmonary embolism in the intensive care unit are two-fold:

(i) It can occur as a complication in patients who are already critically ill with diverse medical and surgical problems. The manifestations may be subtle, and the diagnosis in these patients is difficult to make, and even more difficult to confirm. The usual modes of treatment in many of these critically ill patients are hazardous. The importance of being reasonably certain of the diagnosis, before starting potentially hazardous therapy is therefore evident.

(ii) Patients with pulmonary embolism may also present with acute cardiorespiratory failure. When this occurs against a background of recovery from recent surgery, the diagnosis is generally obvious, and the management well-defined. When acute cardiorespiratory failure due to pulmonary embolism occurs against a background unrelated to surgery, the diagnosis may be often missed with disastrous consequences.

Sources of Pulmonary Embolism

The two main sources of embolism are venous thrombosis in the lower limbs, and thrombi within the right atrium in patients with atrial fibrillation.

Conditions which lead to venous stasis, endothelial cell damage and a subclinical hypercoagulable state, predispose to venous thrombosis. Venous thrombi in the legs leading to thromboembolism, are most frequent in the popliteal veins above the knee, and in the femoral vein within the thigh. Rarely thrombi within the pelvic veins may also lead to pulmonary embolism. Deep vein thrombosis in the calves is common; generally these thrombi extend upwards into the popliteal veins before thromboembolism occurs.

Risk factors of venous thrombosis in the lower limbs include trauma to a limb, generalized trauma, immobilization of a limb, complete bed rest, sitting for long periods, as in air, train, or vehicular travel, congestive heart failure, recent surgery, pregnancy, pelvic disease and recent myocardial infarction. Femoral and popliteal vein thrombosis with thromboembolism are important complications of total hip or knee replacement surgery. Both, oral contraceptives and post-menopausal hormone replacement therapy, increase the risk of venous thromboembolism. Cancer promotes the production of procoagulant factors and is an important risk factor in venous thrombosis and thromboembolism. Occasionally, venous thrombi in the legs and thromboembolism is a manifestation of an occult cancer, in particular, cancer of the pancreas, ovary and a primary cancer of the liver. Any acute critical illness requiring intensive care may perhaps be associated with an increased incidence of venous thrombosis.

In patients who present with venous thrombosis with or without thromboembolism, and who have no risk factors, it is important to test for hypercoagulable states, either genetic or acquired. This is particularly important in young individuals, who present with repeated episodes of venous thrombosis or thromboembolism. Hypercoagulable states are induced by Factor V Leiden deficiency, Protein C, Protein S and antithrombin III deficiency, homocysteinaemia, and by anti-phospholipid antibodies.

Venous thrombosis in the upper limbs is generally not associated with pulmonary embolism. However if the patient has had a central venous line for many weeks, there is a small but definite risk of thrombus formation in the central vein, even if the central line has been changed periodically. Occasionally massive fatal pulmonary embolism resulting from such a thrombus may be seen.

Very rarely in the ICU, a catheter tip of a central venous line is sawed off by the bevel or the point of the large needle through which the catheter is introduced. This tip may travel to the lung and produce pulmonary embolism.

Fat embolism after fractures and crush injuries, air embolism following accidental injection of a large bolus of air into the systemic venous circulation, or tumor emboli particularly in hypernephromas, or from other tumor tissue gaining access to the venous circulation, may also be very rarely observed.

Physiopathology

The clinical features of pulmonary embolism are due to three possible physiopathological changes:

(i) Acute circulatory compromise due to an obstructed pulmonary circulation. This occurs with massive embolism, or when numerous thromboemboli block a large cross-section of the pulmonary circulation. This circulatory compromise is characterized by pulmonary hypertension, a right ventricular dilatation and dysfunction, right sided heart failure and a low cardiac output, which when marked leads to cardiogenic shock. The dilated right ventricle causes a septal shift to the left, resulting in underfilling of the left ventricle, a decreased systemic cardiac output and myocardial ischaemia from reduced coronary perfusion.

(ii) Gas exchange abnormalities generally characterized by a low PaO_2 with a lowered $PaCO_2$. High $\dot{V}/\dot{Q}$ areas are responsible for increased dead space ventilation. Tachypnoea and an increased minute ventilation allow a normal, and often a lower than normal $PaCO_2$ to be maintained. If the dead space is markedly increased, and the minute ventilation does not increase proportionately, the $PaCO_2$ may rise. The alveolar PCO_2 is characteristically slightly lower than the $PaCO_2$.

Normal arterial blood gases do not exclude pulmonary embolism. In fact, arterial hypoxaemia is generally never marked, except in massive embolism associated with a shock-like state. The PaO_2 is rarely < 55 mm Hg. A lowered PaO_2 is due to ventilation-perfusion mismatching resulting from atelectasis, and to redistribution of pulmonary blood flow, which causes a fall in the $\dot{V}/\dot{Q}$ ratio in areas of the lung that are unobstructed by pulmonary emboli.

(iii) Pulmonary infarction may occur, but is not commonly observed in pulmonary embolism. Patients with congestive heart failure are more prone to develop pulmonary infarction because of pre-existing raised pulmonary venous pressure.

The clinical manifestations of thromboembolism often appear to be far more serious than what is expected from the degree of vascular occlusion. In critically ill patients in the ICU, this could be due to two causes: (i) a poor pre-existing cardiopulmonary reserve; (ii) release of vasoactive and bronchoconstrictive mediators from platelets and perhaps from other sources, following embolism. This potentiates pulmonary hypertension, accentuates ventilation-perfusion disturbances, and adds to the already existing tachypnoea.

Clinical Presentation

The presentation in the ICU is varied. The clinical syndromes observed may be classified as follows:

(i) Sudden death.

(ii) Shock—with a low output hypotensive state. Severe chest pain (indistinguishable from the pain of acute myocardial infarction) may or may not be associated with the shock-like state.

(iii) Acute right heart failure—with increase in the central venous pressure, prominent 'a' waves in the jugular veins, and auscultatory evidence of pulmonary hypertension.

(iv) Acute respiratory failure—with dyspnoea, tachypnoea, and at times, cyanosis.

(v) Features of (ii), (iii), and (iv) are combined in massive embolism—various combinations are observed depending on the interval after acute embolism. Shock often predominates in the earliest phase, and is associated with a raised central venous pressure, hypotension and hypoxic respiratory failure. If recovery ensues, features of pulmonary hypertension become more evident.

(vi) Rarely massive pulmonary embolism causes acute pulmonary oedema, or overwhelming bronchoconstriction.

(vii) Less massive, frequent, multiple, small emboli in already critically ill patients, may show very subtle features. These include tachycardia, an increasingly unstable circulatory state, and supraventricular tachycardia. Tachypnoea (at times episodic), faintness or actual syncope, particularly on changing from the supine to the sitting posture, may also be observed. There may be an unexplained fall in the PaO_2, or an increase in an already existing hypoxia. Sometimes a rapid deterioration in the clinical state of a seriously ill individual, or a low grade fever, or a high ESR without apparent cause, or unexplained icterus may be related to silent pulmonary embolism. All these subtle features described above unfortunately lack specificity and sensitivity, and may well be due as much to the critical illness per se, as to a complicating pulmonary embolism.

(viii) Pulmonary infarction. Pulmonary infarction is not frequently observed. When it does occur, its significance should not be missed. Haemoptysis, pleural pain, an unexplained occurrence of a pleural effusion in a critically ill patient suggest embolism. One or more shadows within the lung, or other radiological features compatible with pulmonary embolism, should also prompt a correct clinical diagnosis.

Clinical evidence of accompanying venous thrombosis in the lower limbs is the strongest pointer to a possible pulmonary embolism, as the two are often associated. Amongst the significant features to be looked out for, are tenderness and swelling of the calf muscles, pain in the calf on dorsiflexion of the foot (Homan's sign), rise in the skin temperature of one limb, oedema of the leg or foot, and delayed cooling of an exposed lower limb (Provan's sign). One or more of these signs are positive in 50 per cent of patients with pulmonary embolism. *However, absence of clinical signs in no way excludes femoral, popliteal, or deep vein thrombosis.*

Investigations

The two easily performed non-invasive tests include a chest X-ray and an ECG. Both may however be non-contributory to a definite diagnosis. It is important however to know what exactly to look out for.

Radiologically the diagnostic sign of massive pulmonary embolism is characteristic blanching or the presence of an oligaemic zone within the affected lung, or part of the lung (Westermark's sign). A 'cut-off' in one of the larger vessels supplying an area of the lung may be observed. The affected vessel may be significantly enlarged proximal to the 'cut-off'. If pulmonary infarction occurs, one or more classically wedge-shaped shadows, with the base of the wedge resting on the pleura may be seen. A pleural effusion, linear atelectatic shadows, and unilateral elevation of a dome of the diaphragm may also be observed.

Though an X-ray chest may be unrevealing in over 50 per cent of cases, *a normal or near-normal X-ray in the presence of severe respiratory distress for which there is no other obvious cause, is strongly suggestive of pulmonary embolism. This is particularly so in a critical care setting or against a backdrop predisposing to thromboembolism.*

ECG changes may be transient, and may occur early in the natural history of pulmonary embolism. In patients with a pre-existing abnormal ECG, further changes are often impossible to interpret. ECG changes include:

(i) An S_1Q_3 pattern. aVF and Lead III may both show a QR pattern with elevation in the ST segment simulating an inferior wall infarction.

(ii) Clockwise rotation with an RS pattern or an rS pattern extending from V_1–V_6. A qR pattern may be seen in V_1 and V_4R.

(iii) T wave inversion may be seen in the right precordial leads—at times T wave inversions are present in all precordial leads.

(iv) Transient incomplete or complete right bundle branch block may be observed.

(v) A P pulmonale may be observed in Leads II, III and aVF.

(vi) A QRS axis in the frontal plane may shift sharply to the right to +100 degrees or more.

(vii) Supraventricular arrhythmias may occur—these include supraventricular tachycardia, atrial flutter and atrial fibrillation.

Three other features are worthy of note:

(i) None of these ECG changes may be present at a given time in documented pulmonary embolism.

(ii) Changes may be non-specific and of no diagnostic value.

(iii) The changes described above, when present are due to pulmonary hypertension, right heart strain, and myocardial ischaemia.

Plasma D-dimer ELISA

An abnormal rise in the ELISA-determined plasma D-dimer level in blood has more than 90 per cent sensitivity in the diagnosis of pulmonary embolism proven by lung scan or angiography (1, 2). The ELISA D-dimer test is extremely sensitive, so that a negative test for all practical purposes excludes pulmonary embolism. However, the test is not very specific; a rise in the ELISA D-dimer can easily occur in other systemic illnesses e.g. myocardial infarction, sepsis, and for a week after major surgery. The test is therefore, of particular use in patients with suspected pulmonary embolism who do not have co-existing systemic illnesses.

Arterial Blood Gases

These have been discussed earlier. Though moderate hypoxia may be observed, normal arterial blood gases do not exclude pulmonary embolism.

Venous Doppler Ultrasonography

The Doppler ultrasound is a fairly reliable test to pick up venous thrombi in the leg or thigh veins (3). The presence of deep vein thrombi in a patient suspected to have pulmonary embolism is an indication to treat the patient for pulmonary embolism. Unfortunately, the Doppler ultrasound is available only in a few well-equipped centres in our country. In critical care units that do not possess this facility, the diagnosis of venous thrombosis in critically ill patients is therefore necessarily clinical and clinical methods have well-marked limitations. Also, according to Hull

and colleagues (4), as many as 30 per cent of patients with pulmonary emboli do not show evidence of venous thrombosis. This may be because the Doppler ultrasound may fail to detect some venous thrombi or the thrombus may have been dislodged 'in toto', to constitute an embolus blocking part of the pulmonary circulation; there is then no evidence of venous thrombosis at the time of examination.

Radionuclide Lung Scan

It is impossible to perform this investigation in critically ill individuals in hospitals where nuclear scanning facilities are unavailable. Transport to distant centres is hazardous, and the risk often unacceptable. When facilities are available within a centre, a perfusion scan is of help (5). An abnormal scan (i.e. a perfusion defect), against a proper clinical background, is in itself suggestive of pulmonary embolism. To further enhance the diagnostic value of a perfusion scan, a ventilation scan is also ideally performed. One or more perfusion defects (particularly if large), without corresponding ventilation defects in the same area (mismatched ventilation-perfusion defects), strongly support the diagnosis of pulmonary embolism. On the other hand, a perfusion defect with a matched ventilation defect in the same area, is often due to other diseases, and does not support the diagnosis of pulmonary embolism.

The Prospective Investigation Of Pulmonary Embolism Diagnosis (PIOPED) multicentre study in the United States, compared results of lung scans with pulmonary angiography in patients with pulmonary embolism (6). Important criteria laid down by the PIOPED group for the diagnosis of pulmonary embolism on pulmonary scans are listed below in **Table 7.9.1**.

A high probability result in a ventilation-perfusion scan strongly points to a diagnosis of pulmonary embolism (87 per cent likelihood; 96 per cent if there is strong clinical suspicion). *A normal perfusion scan excludes, for all practical purposes, the diagnosis of pulmonary embolism.* Even so, the following points need to be

Table 7.9.1. Modified PIOPED criteria for lung scan interpretation **(6)**

1. High Probability
   * 2 or more large mismatched perfusion lung scan defects
      or
   * 2 or more moderate + 1 large mismatched perfusion lung scan defect
      or
   * 4 or more moderate mismatched perfusion lung scan defects
2. Intermediate Probability
   * Borderline high or borderline low
   * Not falling into high, low or normal categories
3. Low Probability
   * Non segmental perfusion defects only
      or
   * 1 moderate mismatched segmental perfusion defect with normal chest X-ray
      or
   * Any perfusion defect with a larger abnormality on chest X-ray
4. Normal
   * No perfusion defects
   * Perfusion outlines exactly the same as shape of lungs on chest X-ray

noted in relation to the diagnosis of this problem in critical care medicine.

(i) Only a few patients with suspected pulmonary embolism will show a high probability result. The majority will fall into intermediate or low probability result. A substantial number in these two categories will not actually have pulmonary embolism.

(ii) Studies reported in PIOPED are mostly in patients who were not critically ill. How does one interpret these results in patients who are critically ill in the ICU, and in whom pulmonary embolism is a further complication to the critical illness? This remains unanswered.

(iii) It is often impossible to shift such critically ill patients outside the ICU, even when facilities for nuclear scanning are available within the hospital.

The value of nuclear imaging in critically ill patients is thus limited. Interpretation and predictive value of findings of nuclear imaging in very ill patients with multiple problems, may not be comparable to results that have been obtained in less seriously ill patients.

Pulmonary Angiography

Before the results of the PIOPED multicentre study in the United States, pulmonary angiography was the only method of exclusively diagnosing pulmonary embolism. Even today, there are many who consider it the gold standard for diagnosis. This is an invasive test requiring placement of a catheter in the right ventricle or pulmonary artery in a critically ill individual. The angiographic signs of pulmonary embolism include 'cut-off' of an artery, intraluminal defects, and poor perfusion in the area supplied by the blocked vessel. We resort to pulmonary angiography increasingly infrequently in patients under critical care for reasons mentioned below.

Spiral Computed Pulmonary Angiography

In our opinion, this non-invasive test offers excellent imaging of the pulmonary vasculature. It has, by and large, replaced $\dot{V}/\dot{Q}$ scanning as a diagnostic modality for pulmonary embolism and has nearly (if not completely) eliminated the need for invasive pulmonary angiography. In an ongoing multicentre European trial, CT angiography was 88 per cent sensitive and 94 per cent specific in the diagnosis of pulmonary embolism (7). Again, inter-observer agreement was 74 per cent for CT angiography, 39 per cent for $\dot{V}/\dot{Q}$ scanning and 46 per cent for pulmonary angiography in this study.

The advantages of CT angiography when compared to $\dot{V}/\dot{Q}$ scanning and invasive pulmonary angiography are summarized below:

(i) CT angiography is non-invasive, convenient and can be performed safely and quickly in critically ill patients, particularly those in shock and/or in acute right heart failure.

(ii) Studies comparing CT angiography to $\dot{V}/\dot{Q}$ scanning suggest that CT angiography is a better test because of more frequent definitive confirmation of pulmonary emboli (8, 9).

(iii) In a critically ill individual, there is often a large differential diagnosis to pulmonary embolism. A CT angiography offers evidence of other causes as well as that of pulmonary embolism, which neither a V/Q scan nor invasive pulmonary angiography can provide.

(iv) Loud et al. (10) found that CT angiography of the legs and pelvis could be performed with the same contrast injection used to image the pulmonary vasculature. Detection of deep vein thrombosis in the femoro-popliteal veins was as accurate as with ultrasonography. This procedure could also detect clots in iliac, renal and caval veins which are ultrasonographically inaccessible.

The major limitation of CT angiography is its inability to diagnose subsegmental branch emboli. However, invasive pulmonary angiography also has significant limitations in detecting isolated subsegmental emboli (11). The only other major limitation of spiral computed pulmonary angiography is the need to use contrast material, precluding its use in patients with renal failure.

The role of invasive pulmonary angiography in the diagnosis of pulmonary embolism is now sharply reduced. We very rarely perform this procedure knowing full well that as a result some subsegmental pulmonary emboli will not be diagnosed. But is it necessary to accurately diagnose subsegmental emboli? Would this affect overall patient outcome? Data from three large studies (12–14) suggests that underdiagnosing subsegmental emboli by avoiding pulmonary angiography does not affect clinical outcomes of recurrent embolism or death. A clinical outcome approach is as safe as the PIOPED approach, less expensive, more convenient, less fraught with immediate risk to the patient, and more acceptable to the patient and the physician (15).

Approach to Diagnosis (Fig. 7.9.1)

1. The initial assessment of patients with suspected pulmonary embolism includes a history, clinical examination, ECG, X-ray chest and a careful assessment of the clinical background to determine the risk factors for venous thromboembolism.

2. We next do a rapid plasma D-dimer ELISA. If the X-ray chest and the D-dimer are both non-diagnostic, the diagnosis of pulmonary embolism is unlikely.

3. If either the X-ray chest is abnormal or the D-dimer is positive, a further work-up is warranted.

4. We now basically rely on two further tests—a Doppler ultrasound of the veins in the lower limbs and the pelvis, and a spiral CT angiography of the chest. If either one or the other is positive, the patient is treated for pulmonary embolism.

5. If however, both are negative or indeterminate, we have two options: (a) to perform a pulmonary angiography and treat only if pulmonary embolism is demonstrated; or (b) to decide the further course of action on clinical judgment.

Barring rare exceptions, we prefer the latter option. If we feel on clinical grounds that the probability of pulmonary embolism is high, that the patient's cardiac reserve is poor, or the patient is haemodynamically unstable, we would treat as pulmonary embolism. If on the other hand, clinical judgment dictates that the probability of pulmonary embolism in a given case is low or moderate and the patient is otherwise haemodynamically stable, we would prefer not to treat; we observe and pursue other causes

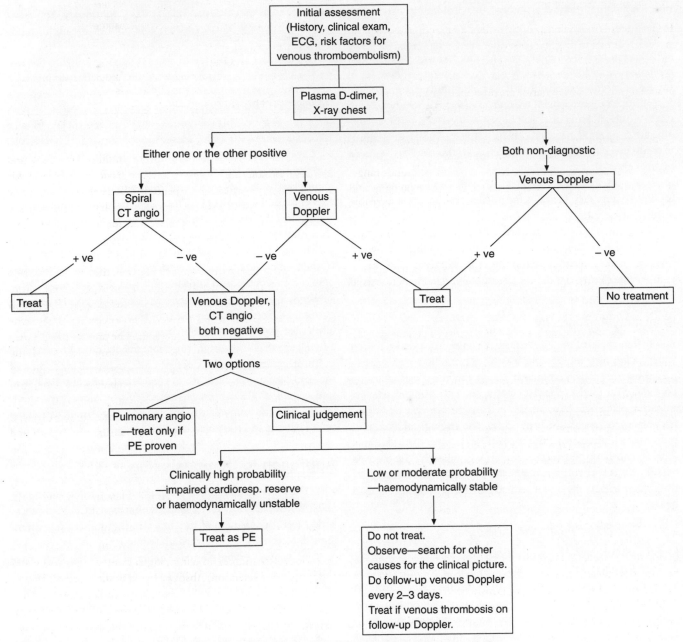

Fig. 7.9.1. Algorithm for a diagnostic work-up of pulmonary embolism.

that could result in a similar clinical picture. In the above-mentioned scenario, we would repeat the Doppler ultrasound of the pelvic and leg veins every two to three days and treat the patient as pulmonary embolism if a follow-up ultrasound detects venous thrombosis.

We fully realize that by sharply reducing invasive pulmonary angiographic studies in patients with non-diagnostic CT angiograms and normal venous Doppler ultrasound of the leg veins, we must be missing out on patients with subsegmental pulmonary emboli. But for reasons discussed earlier, this does not significantly alter patient outcome as judged from the occurrence of repeated pulmonary embolism or by death. We do not do $\dot{V}/\dot{Q}$ scans because we lack this facility and we would need to transfer critically ill people to another hospital for this purpose, and be-

cause there is sufficient evidence that spiral CT angiography can replace $\dot{V}/\dot{Q}$ scanning as an investigational mode in suspected pulmonary embolism.

Principles of Management

(i) Use of anticoagulants or the use of thrombolytic therapy for the purpose of dissolution of thrombi obstructing the pulmonary circulation. This therapy also helps in dissolution of thrombi in the leg veins, and prevents further embolization.

(ii) Cardiorespiratory support in patients with major or massive embolism.

(iii) Preventive measures.

(i) Use of Anticoagulants

Heparin forms the mainstay of treatment. Unfractionated heparin is started after the diagnosis is made. 5000–7500 units are given intravenously as a bolus dose, followed by a continuous microdrip infusion at the rate of 1000 units/hr (16). The dose is adjusted so as to keep the activated partial thromboplastin time (APTT) to about twice the normal value. Initially this is measured every 6 hours, and then once or twice daily.

It is important to ensure that the requisite rise in the APTT is quickly achieved, and constantly maintained. If the APTT done after the first 6 hours has not risen to the desired therapeutic range, the 24 hour dose of heparin is increased by 2000–4000 units, and the APTT is repeated after 6 hours. Conversely, if the APTT is > than the therapeutic range of 2.5 times the normal value, the 24 hour dose of heparin is reduced by 2000–4000 units, followed by a repeat APTT after 6 hours.

Proper heparinization leads to a decrease in the rate of further embolization to < 5 per cent. It is best to continue heparin in the above manner for 5–10 days. Warfarin is introduced only when the APTT is within the therapeutic range, starting with 5 mg daily and adjusting the dose so that the INR is maintained between 2.5 and 3. It is important to overlap heparin and warfarin for 5 to 7 days and not to start warfarin alone. This is because if warfarin is introduced in an active thrombotic state, there is a fall in Protein C and Protein S, with an increase in the thrombogenic potential. An overlap with heparin prevents this. Once a therapeutic INR is reached, heparin is omitted. We prefer to continue warfarin for a period of 6 months. Poor risk patients who are likely to develop venous thrombosis easily, as in those with congestive cardiac failure or those with rare hypercoagulable states, may require warfarin for a much longer period of time and in some cases indefinitely.

The most important complication of anticoagulants is bleeding. If the bleeding is moderate and is due to heparin, stopping the drug suffices as the APTT usually returns to normal after 6 to 8 hours. If the bleeding is excessive or life-threatening as in intracranial haemorrhage, protamine sulphate in a dose of 1 mg/100 units of heparin is administered intravenously over 5 to 10 minutes.

Rarely, heparin can cause thrombocytopaenia. This is an IgG antibody mediated disorder associated with a tendency to venous and even arterial thrombosis. It can be fatal and should be suspected if the platelet count drops below 100,000/mm³ or is less than 50 per cent of the baseline value while the patient is on heparin. The peak incidence is 4 to 14 days after starting heparin. The drug should be stopped; lepirudin or argatroban have antithrombotic activity and may need to be used to counter this severe drug effect of heparin (17).

Bleeding due to excessive anticoagulation with warfarin can be catastrophic. It can be countered by administering fresh frozen plasma intravenously. Vitamin K in a dose of 10 mg given intravenously, can reverse the warfarin effect in 12 to 24 hours. However, once this is achieved, patients are refractory to warfarin for up to 2 weeks, so that effective reinstitution of warfarin therapy is difficult.

Contraindications to the use of heparin are listed in **Table 7.9.2**.

Table 7.9.2. Contraindications to anticoagulant therapy

* Recent major surgery/ocular surgery/neurosurgery
* Diastolic BP > 110 mm Hg
* CNS haemorrhage
* Recent trauma/head injury
* Recent cerebrovascular accident/transient ischaemic attack
* GI bleeding or other haemorrhagic diathesis
* Concomitant hepatic/renal failure

Thrombolytic Therapy (18, 19)

Thrombolytic therapy effectively dissolves pulmonary emboli and reduces morbidity and mortality. It results in effective thrombolysis with excellent reperfusion in 90 per cent of patients. It is particularly useful against large, centrally located emboli in the pulmonary vessels. Thrombolytic therapy is also lytic for venous thrombosis or for any other thrombus which is the source of pulmonary embolism.

The classic indication for thrombolytic therapy is major or massive pulmonary embolism characterized by hypotension, cardiorespiratory failure with a shock-like state, syncope, and angiographic evidence of occlusion of 40 per cent or more of the pulmonary circulation. Thrombolysis is to be preferred to heparin under these circumstances, as it is more prompt in reversing the above haemodynamic abnormalities. There are many units in the world who use thrombolytic therapy in preference to heparin for less extensive pulmonary embolization.

We use either streptokinase or urokinase for thrombolysis. If streptokinase is used, a loading dose of 250,000 units is administered intravenously over 30–60 minutes. This is followed by an infusion at the rate of 100,000 units/hr for 24 hours (16). Urokinase is administered in a loading dose of 4400 units/kg over 10 minutes, followed by a maintenance infusion of 4400 units/kg/hr for 12 hours.

Bleeding is the main complication of thrombolytic therapy. To minimize the chances of this complication, important considerations include avoidance of non-essential invasive procedures, and proper patient selection. Absolute contraindications to thrombolytic therapy have been discussed in an earlier chapter. They include active bleeding pathologies, presence of an intracranial tumour or a recent cerebrovascular accident, and severe uncontrolled hypertension, with the diastolic blood pressure > 110 mm Hg. Relative contraindications include general surgical procedures within 5–7 days, liver or kidney failure, presence of a peptic ulcer, other bleeding diathesis, and pregnancy.

It is best to avoid invasive procedures during thrombolytic therapy, as the patient can bleed from the puncture sites. If a central line is to be inserted, it should be done prior to starting therapy. If a Swan-Ganz catheter is already in situ, the thrombolytic drug is administered through it. There is however no special advantage in giving the drug through a centrally placed catheter. Arterial punctures for blood gas analysis are best avoided during thrombolysis. If estimation of arterial pH and blood gases is imperative, the radial and not the femoral artery should be punctured.

Plasma fibrinogen levels may be estimated to monitor the lytic state, and the APTT is monitored for the eventual change over to heparin. The plasma fibrinogen levels often drop to 50 per cent of pre-treatment values during the streptokinase infusion. Once this fibrinolytic state is observed, the patient is continued on the scheduled therapy with the dose stated above. After completing the infusion, and after waiting for a further 4 hours, the APTT is tested. If this is elevated to 1.5–2 times the control, a heparin infusion is started at the rate of 1000 units/hr for 24 hours, and the APTT is maintained within the above range. If the APTT is > 2.5 times the control, it is advisable to wait for another 4 hours so as to allow the APTT to fall to within the therapeutic range. Once this occurs, the heparin infusion is commenced in the dose stated above. If the APTT is < 1.5 times the control, a bolus dose of heparin is first given, followed by a continuous heparin infusion at the rate of 1000 units/hr.

Heparin and streptokinase should not be used simultaneously as this can result in uncontrollable bleeding and death.

(ii) Cardiorespiratory Support

This is imperative in major or massive pulmonary embolism. Shock should be promptly treated. An intravenous infusion of isoproterenol (1–2 mg in 500 ml dextrose) is very useful as it dilates the pulmonary vasculature. If possible, the patient is monitored through a Swan-Ganz catheter, or at least through a central venous line. It is advisable to keep the CVP between 12–14 mm Hg in order to ensure an adequate right ventricular stroke volume. This is best achieved by infusing 500 ml Dextran or Haemaccel, which besides raising right atrial pressure, also expands the pulmonary vascular bed, and thereby reduces pulmonary vascular resistance. If the patient does not respond to isoproterenol, or has marked tachycardia to start with, it is best to use dobutamine as outlined in the Chapter on Cardiogenic Shock. Dopamine may need to be used in addition to dobutamine. The use of digoxin is disappointing, but it may be used in a dose of 0.25 mg intravenously to start with, and repeated 6 hourly till a digitalizing dose of 1 mg is given over 24 hours.

Oxygen is administered at 6–8 l/minute.

Ventilator support is invariably required in the presence of acute cardiorespiratory failure.

Morphine or pethidine is used for the relief of pain and/or restlessness.

Embolectomy (16). Embolectomy can be performed through catheter based strategies or through emergency surgical embolectomy with cardiopulmonary bypass. Catheter based strategies imply suction, or clot pulverization through a rotating catheter. Percutaneous rheolytic thrombectomy or balloon angioplasty has also been used to improve pulmonary arterial flow. Embolectomy is indicated under the following conditions:

(i) In patients who are in severe shock and would die unless offered prompt relief.

(ii) When more than 60 per cent of the pulmonary circulation is obstructed.

(iii) In patients who fail to respond to earlier mentioned therapy.

(iv) When thrombolytic therapy is contraindicated.

(v) Emergency surgery is indicated if catheter based strategies fail.

Results of embolectomy (catheter based and surgical) are better if performed before the onset of severe cardiogenic shock.

(iii) Preventive Measures

Prevention of venous thrombosis with the associated risk of pulmonary embolism, is a major objective in the management of critically ill patients in the ICU. These patients often form a high-risk group as a consequence of bed rest, serious infections or trauma. As mentioned at the very outset, though the frequency of venous thrombosis and pulmonary embolism is not as high as seen in intensive care units in Western countries, it is still significant. Surprisingly, the risk of venous thrombosis following total hip or knee replacements, or following surgery for a fractured hip, in our hospital and ICU is < 5 per cent, even in old, obese patients. This is in contrast to the 40–70 per cent risk of developing venous thrombosis after similar surgery in the West. The risk in other medical and surgical patients, in our opinion, is around 5 per cent—again less than in the West, where the risk is 15–20 per cent.

Prevention of venous thrombosis in high-risk patients reduces morbidity. High-risk patients include the old and obese, those who are poorly mobile or are confined to bed, patients with myocardial infarction or a stroke, or those with atrial fibrillation and congestive heart failure. Post-operative patients are also at high-risk, particularly after orthopaedic surgery (particularly hip replacement or hip fracture), gynaecological surgery and other major surgery. Low dose heparin 5000 units 12 hourly, is shown to be effective and safe in most groups. Low molecular weight heparin can be given in a dose of 3000 units subcutaneously, just once a day; it offers good prophylaxis, and is more convenient to administer. Occasionally, as after trauma, or following surgery on the brain or spinal cord, or in patients with an active peptic ulcer or other bleeding diathesis, even low dose heparin, or the use of low molecular weight heparin once daily, is contraindicated because of the risk of bleeding. In this group, prophylaxis through the use of firmly applied compression crepe bandages to both lower limbs, or pneumatic compression to the lower limbs is helpful.

Once venous thrombosis is detected, the patient should be heparinized with 5000 units of heparin given as a bolus intravenously, followed by a heparin infusion at the rate of 1000 units/hr for 24 hours, so that the APTT is maintained at 1.5 times the control. Heparin should be continued for 7 days, and subsequent anticoagulation is by warfarin as outlined earlier. We prefer to use warfarin for 6 months, and follow this up with aspirin 300 mg daily for a further 6 months or even longer. Patients with atrial fibrillation who have had an embolic episode, may need to be put on warfarin indefinitely. In older patients (above 75–80 years), or in non-compliant patients who are unlikely to keep a check on their prothrombin time, it is safer to use just aspirin for prophylaxis.

Secondary Prevention Through Interruption of the Inferior Vena Cava

This is achieved by the placement of a filter in the inferior vena cava generally below the renal veins (20). The procedure is done by a vascular surgeon or an interventional radiologist through the transvenous route. The filter stops emboli from the lower limb or pelvic veins from reaching the lungs. Specific indications for vena caval interruption include the following (**21**):

(a) Pulmonary embolism in patients in whom anticoagulants are absolutely contraindicated—as in the neurosurgical patient, or in those with active bleeding.

(b) Recurrent thromboembolism in spite of adequate anticoagulation.

(c) Patients who have survived a massive embolism, but who are haemodynamically unstable, and in whom the risk of a fresh embolism is ever present.

(d) Patients with septic pulmonary embolism from thrombi in the lower limbs or pelvis, who have shown an unsatisfactory response after 48 hours of antibiotic plus anticoagulant therapy.

(e) Prophylaxis in high risk patients, as in—

(i) extensive or progressive venous thrombosis;

(ii) in conjunction with catheter based or surgical pulmonary embolectomy;

(iii) in patients with active cancer with extensive venous thrombosis of the pelvic or leg veins.

Vena caval interruption in the last four groups should be accompanied by the use of intravenous heparin in the dosage recommended earlier.

REFERENCES

1. Bounameaux H, de Moerloose P, Perrier A et al. (1994). Plasma measurement of D-dimer as diagnostic aid in suspected venous thromboembolism: An overview. Thromb Haemost. 71, 1.
2. Goldhaeber SZ, Simons GR, Elliot CG et al. (1993). Quantitate plasma D-dimer levels among patients undergoing pulmonary angiography for suspected pulmonary embolism. JAMA. 270, 2819.
3. Sumner DS, Lamwith A. (1979). Reliability of Doppler ultrasound in the diagnosis of acute venous thrombosis both above and below the knee. Am J Surg. 138, 205–210.
4. Hull RD, Hirsh J, Carter CJ et al. (1983). Pulmonary angiography, ventilation lung scanning, and venography for clinically suspected pulmonary embolism with abnormal perfusion scans. Ann Intem Med. 98, 891–899.
5. Kelley MA, Carson JL, Palevsky HI, Schwartz JS.(1991). Diagnosing pulmonary embolism: New facts and strategies. Ann Intem Med. 114, 300.
6. The PIOPED Investigators. (1990). Value of the ventilation/perfusion scan in acute pulmonary embolism: Results of the prospective investigation of pulmonary embolism diagnosis (PIOPED). JAMA. 263, 2753–2759.
7. Holbert JM, Costello P, Federele MP. (1999). Role of spiral computed tomography in the diagnosis of pulmonary embolism in the emergency department. Ann Emerg Med. 33, 520–528.
8. Remy-Jardin M, Remy J, Deschildre F et al. (1996). Diagnosis of pulmonary embolism with spiral CT: comparison with pulmonary angiography and scintigraphy. Radiology. 200, 699–706.
9. Cross JJ, Kemp PM, Walsh CG et al. (1998). A randomized trial of spiral CT and ventilation perfusion scintigraphy for the diagnosis of pulmonary embolism. Clin Radiol. 53, 177–182.
10. Loud PA, Katz DS, Klippenstein DL et al. (2000). Combined CT venography and pulmonary angiography in suspected thromboembolic disease: diagnostic accuracy for deep venous evaluation. Am J Roentgenol. 174, 61–65.
11. Quinn MF, Lundell CJ, Klotz TA et al. (1987). Reliability of selective pulmonary arteriography in the diagnosis of pulmonary embolism. Am J Roentgenol. 149, 469–471.
12. Perrier A, Desmarias S, Miron MJ et al. (1999). Non-invasive diagnosis of venous thromboembolism in outpatients. Lancet. 353, 190–195.
13. Wells PS, Ginsberg JS, Anderson DR et al. (1998). Use of a clinical model for safe management of patients with suspected pulmonary embolism. Ann Intem Med. 129, 997–1005.
14. Hull RD, Raskob GE, Ginsberg JS et al. (1994). A non-invasive strategy for the treatment of patients with suspected pulmonary embolism. Arch Intem Med. 154, 289–297.
15. Wolfe TR, Hartsell SC. (2001). Pulmonary embolism: Making sense of the diagnostic evaluation. Ann Emerg Med. 37 (5), 504–514.
16. Goldhaber SZ. (2001). Pulmonary Embolism. In: Heart Disease—A Textbook of Cardiovascular Medicine (Eds Braunwald E, Zipes DP, Libby P). pp. 1886–1907. WB Saunders Company, Philadelphia, London, Tokyo.
17. Walenga JM, Frenkel EP, Bick RL. (2003). Heparin-induced thrombocytopenia, paradoxical thromboembolism, and other adverse effects of heparin-type therapy. Haematol Oncol Clin North Am. 17 (1), 259.
18. Goldhaber SZ. (1991) Thrombolysis for pulmonary embolism. Prog Cardiovas Dis. 34, 113–134
19. Tapson VF. (2001). Pulmonary Embolism. In Hurst's The Heart (Eds Fuster V, Alexander RW, O'Rourke RA). pp 1625–1643. McGraw-Hill Inc., New York, London, Toronto.
20. Grassi CJ, Goldhaber SZ. (1989). Interruption of the inferior vena cava for prevention of pulmonary embolism: Transvenous filter devices. Herz. 14, 182.
21. Girard P, Stern JB, Parent F. (2002). Medical Literature and Vena Cava Filters—So Far So Weak. Chest. 122, 963–967.

Respiratory Problems Requiring Critical Care

8.1 Acute Respiratory Failure in Adults

8.2 Oxygen Therapy

8.3 Airway Management

8.4 Acute Respiratory Crisis in Chronic Obstructive Pulmonary Disease (COPD)

8.5 Acute Lung Injury (ARDS)

8.6 Acute Severe Asthma

8.7 Community-Acquired Pneumonias Requiring Critical Care

8.8 Massive Haemoptysis

Acute Respiratory Failure in Adults

General Considerations

Acute respiratory failure is an important and frequently encountered problem in intensive care units all over the world. The usual or traditional definition of respiratory failure is the inability of the respiratory system to maintain the normal homeostasis of arterial blood gases, so that the oxygen tension in arterial blood (PaO_2) is < 60 mm Hg, and/or the carbon dioxide tension in arterial blood ($PaCO_2$) is 50 mm Hg or greater.

Respiratory failure may be acute or chronic depending on the onset and duration of the failure. An acute exacerbation may at times prevail over a background of chronic respiratory failure (acute on chronic failure).

Respiratory failure is mainly of two types. Type I or hypoxic respiratory failure is due to a failure of oxygenation with a PaO_2 < 60 mm Hg; Type II or hypercapnic respiratory failure (ventilatory failure) is due to hypoventilation and is characterized by a $PaCO_2$ > 50 mm Hg. Hypoxaemic and hypercapnic respiratory failure may both occur in the same patient. Some intensivists also consider Type III and Type IV failure (1).

Type III respiratory failure is that occurring peri-operatively and is largely due to basal atelectasis. Cardiothoracic surgery and/or major upper abdominal surgery splint the diaphragm and induce an abnormal mechanics of the abdominal muscles. These factors cause a fall in the functional residual capacity and an increase in the closing volume of the lungs. The end result is increasing atelectasis of the dependent alveoli, 'small lungs' with a high diaphragm, respiratory distress and hypoxaemia (1).

Type IV respiratory failure is that associated with shock—a poorly functioning circulatory system with a low cardiac output is the main cause of hypoxaemic failure in this situation. Both Type III and Type IV failure merely constitute hypoxaemic failure or both hypoxaemic and hypercapnic failure occurring against specific background conditions.

It is important to realize that the significance of the absolute value of arterial blood gas tensions varies from patient to patient. Thus a fall in arterial PaO_2 from 95 mm Hg to even 70 mm Hg can be of ominous significance in a young man with rapidly evolving acute respiratory failure due to acute poliomyelitis or to any acute neuromuscular disease. This is because (i) this fall constitutes a sharp or acute drop below the predicted range; (ii) ventilatory

failure due to acute poliomyelitis, acute neuromuscular disease, or to severe respiratory muscle fatigue from any cause, can produce a further precipitous fall in PaO_2 that can lead to death from severe hypoxia within a matter of a few hours or even minutes. Such a fall in PaO_2 does not necessarily occur in a graded or step-wise fashion. Under the above circumstances, to await a fall in PaO_2 to < 55–60 mm Hg before realizing the gravity of the situation, can prove dangerous. Abnormal arterial blood gas tensions in a patient should therefore be judged in perspective with the natural history of the problem producing such an abnormality. *Disaster should be anticipated, and if possible prevented; it should never be awaited.*

The above traditional definition of acute respiratory failure evolved when measurements of arterial pH and arterial blood gas tensions were first introduced into clinical medicine. This definition is useful in that (i) it focuses attention on abnormalities of gas exchange due to disturbances in lung function; (ii) it stresses the importance and need for a laboratory diagnosis of respiratory failure; (iii) it emphasizes the difficulty and often the impossibility of either diagnosing acute respiratory failure, or gauging its severity on clinical grounds. Yet, this traditional definition ignores the role of the cardiovascular system in gas exchange, and above all in oxygen transport to tissues. In a critical care setting, this is of particular concern. It is vital to look upon the circulatory and respiratory systems as a single interrelated unit whose purpose is to supply oxygen to the tissues.

A broad definition of respiration would be an exchange of oxygen and carbon dioxide between man and his environment (2). It can be divided into the following sequential steps:

(i) *Ventilation*—in which an exchange of oxygen and carbon dioxide occurs between the lungs and the atmosphere.

(ii) *Gas exchange*—this occurs across the alveolar-capillary membrane within the lungs, mixed venous blood being oxygenated, and carbon dioxide being removed during its transit through the lungs.

(iii) *Gas transport*—the transport of oxygenated arterial blood to the tissues, and of venous blood (with a high carbon dioxide content), to the lungs.

(iv) *Gas exchange within the tissues*—release of oxygen, oxygen uptake and utilization by the tissues, and release of carbon dioxide by the cells for transport back to the lungs.

In critical care medicine, it is a great advantage to look upon acute respiratory failure as an acute impairment of any one or more of the steps described above. We shall briefly consider (I) acute ventilatory failure; (II) acute failure in gas exchange or acute hypoxaemic failure; (III) a combination of (I) and (II); (IV) a failure of oxygen transport; (V) a failure of tissue oxygenation.

I. Acute Ventilatory Failure

Definition

Acute ventilatory failure occurs when alveolar ventilation cannot adequately remove the carbon dioxide produced by cell metabolism, via the lungs.

Relation between PaO₂ and PaCO₂ in Ventilatory Failure

Ventilatory failure always results in a rise in $PaCO_2$ and a fall in PaO_2, and as mentioned earlier is also termed hypercapnic respiratory failure. The relation between PaO_2 and $PaCO_2$ is defined by the alveolar gas equation

$$PAO_2 = PIO_2 - PaCO_2 \times \frac{1}{R}$$

where PAO_2 is the alveolar oxygen tension, PIO_2 the inspired oxygen tension corrected for water vapour, and R is the respiratory exchange ratio (see Section on Basic Cardiorespiratory Physiology in the ICU). Once the PAO_2 is calculated from the above equation, the PaO_2 can be determined if the alveolar-arterial oxygen gradient is known. In ventilatory failure due to CNS causes or due to neuromuscular disease, the alveolar-arterial gradient is normal (i.e. 10–20 mm Hg), so that the PaO_2 is 10–20 mm Hg less than the PAO_2. The oxygen-carbon dioxide diagram (**Fig. 8.1.1**) gives the value of PAO_2 and PaO_2 for any given value of $PaCO_2$. The arterial blood gas tensions of oxygen and carbon dioxide fall on this line in pure or isolated ventilatory failure.

Physiopathology of Ventilatory Failure

The carbon dioxide produced by tissue metabolism ($\dot{V}CO_2$) is removed by the lungs. Normally the alveolar carbon dioxide tension ($PACO_2$) and the arterial carbon dioxide tension ($PaCO_2$) are maintained around 40 mm Hg by adjusting alveolar ventilation to balance the $\dot{V}CO_2$. Thus an increase in the latter is met by a proportionate increase in alveolar ventilation. The relationship between $PACO_2$, $\dot{V}CO_2$ and alveolar ventilation, can be stated as follows:

$$PACO_2 = PaCO_2 = \frac{\dot{V}CO_2}{\dot{V}_A} \times \text{a constant (0.86)}$$

(see Chapter on Cardiorespiratory Physiology in the ICU).

$\dot{V}_A$ or the alveolar ventilation is the difference between minute ventilation ($\dot{V}_E$) and the physiological dead space ventilation ($\dot{V}_D$) within the lungs—i.e. the ventilation that does not participate in gas exchange. The above equation can thus be rewritten:

$$PACO_2 = PaCO_2 = \frac{\dot{V}CO_2}{\dot{V}_E - \dot{V}_D}$$

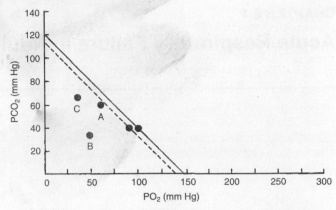

Fig. 8.1.1. O_2–CO_2 diagram. The continuous line represents the relation between alveolar PO_2 and alveolar PCO_2 with an RQ of 0.8 and when breathing air ($PIO_2 = 149$ mm Hg). The circle marked on this line represents the normal PAO_2 and $PACO_2$. The broken line represents the normal relation between PaO_2 and $PACO_2$ (or $PaCO_2$) when breathing air. It takes into consideration the slight venous admixture occuring in normal lungs so that the PaO_2 may be 10–15 mm less than PAO_2. The circle marked on the broken line represents the normal PaO_2 and PCO_2. Points A, B and C illustrate blood gas readings in different types of respiratory failure:

A. Ventilatory failure: $PaCO_2$ 60 mm Hg; PaO_2 65 mm Hg. The point falls on or is very close to the broken line.

B. Hypoxaemic failure: $PaCO_2$ 38 mm Hg; PaO_2 45 mm Hg. The point is markedly to the left of the broken line. The large alveolar-arterial gradient is chiefly due to a ventilation-perfusion imbalance and/or an increase in the true venous admixture.

C. Hypoxaemic and ventilatory failure: $PaCO_2$ 70 mm Hg; PaO_2 30 mm Hg. Note high $PaCO_2$ indicating ventilatory failure and PaO_2 less than what can be predicted from the $PaCO_2$ reading. The point is again to the left of the broken line. (from: Udwadia FE. 1979. Diagnosis and Management of Acute Respiratory Failure, OUP, Mumbai).

Thus a rise in $PaCO_2$ due to ventilatory or hypercapnic respiratory failure can occur under the following conditions: (i) A fall in $\dot{V}_A$ or alveolar ventilation—this could be due to (a) a fall in $\dot{V}_E$ or minute ventilation or to (b) a rise in physiological dead space ventilation ($\dot{V}_D$), without a concommitant increase in minute ventilation ($\dot{V}_E$). (ii) A rise in carbon dioxide production ($\dot{V}CO_2$) without a proportionate increase in alveolar ventilation ($\dot{V}_A$).

Important Causes of Acute Ventilatory or Hypercapnic Respiratory Failure in an Intensive Care Setting

(i) Hypoventilation in lungs which are normal to start with. This occurs in patients with a depressed ventilatory drive or in neuromuscular disease. A depressed ventilatory drive is observed in poisonings with narcotics, sedatives, antidepressants, coma from other causes, in head injuries, encephalitis, increased intracranial tension, and other pathologies depressing the respiratory centre. Important neuromuscular diseases causing hypoventilation include acute poliomyelitis, acute infective polyneuritis (Guillan Barré syndrome), tetanus, myasthenia gravis, botulism and snake bite poisoning. Other causes of respiratory muscle weakness and/or decreased respiratory muscle endurance include severe myopathy, amyotrophic lateral sclerosis, polymyositis, critical illness polyneuropathy / myopathy, malnutrition, severe electrolyte disturbances, notably hypokalaemia, hyperkalaemia, hypomagnesaemia, malnutrition, prolonged ventilator dependence, disorders of the phrenic nerve, respiratory muscle fatigue from any cause.

(ii) Rarely hypoventilation can occur following large airways obstruction. In an ICU setting, this is chiefly observed in tracheal or subglottic stenosis, when an artificial airway has been in place for many weeks, or has been incorrectly managed. Upper airways obstruction with hypoventilation can also occur in children with acute epiglottitis, in obstructive sleep apnoea, vocal cord paralysis, and foreign bodies including dentures, clots, secretions, soft tissue tumours or inflammation obstructing the upper airway.

(iii) Poor expansion of the thoracic cage with ventilatory failure can occur following trauma to the thorax (as in flail chest), in patients who are severely obese, or have marked kyphoscoliosis, or in those with well-marked pleural disease (as in bilateral pleural effusion or pneumothorax).

It is important to realize that in most of the above-mentioned conditions, the lungs are normal to start with. However, if hypoventilation is not promptly recognized and correctly managed (and this is most important in hypoventilating comatose patients), secretions accumulate within the large and small airways producing areas of atelectasis. As a result of secondary changes within the lungs, gas exchange due to ventilation-perfusion imbalance is further impaired.

(iv) Hypoventilation can also occur in lungs which are abnormal. This is most frequently seen in severe airways obstruction—either acute severe asthma, or an acute crisis in chronic bronchitis emphysema. In these patients hypoventilation is due to a decrease in $\dot{V}_E$, and/or an increase in physiological dead space. Extensive thromboembolic disease within the lungs can rarely produce a sufficient rise in dead space ventilation ($\dot{V}_D$), so as to cause a fall in alveolar ventilation. Severe late (almost terminal) stage restrictive disease can also be associated with hypoventilation and hypercapnic respiratory failure.

(v) Increase in carbon dioxide production, at times cannot be countered by an increase in alveolar ventilation. Marked increase in carbon dioxide production can occur in high fever, hypermetabolic critical illnesses, severe hyperthyroidism, frequent seizures, and uncontrolled tetanus. In patients with respiratory muscle fatigue, or in those with mechanical limitations to breathing (as in chronic bronchitis), alveolar ventilation cannot keep pace with carbon dioxide production, and hypercapnic respiratory failure is observed. Hyperalimentation with increased caloric intake through carbohydrates, or a high carbohydrate diet given by the enteral route also results in an increase in $\dot{V}CO_2$. An increase in $\dot{V}_A$ is imperative if this excess CO_2 is to be removed. In critically ill patients, carbon dioxide retention may occur as respiratory muscle fatigue may prevent a proportionate rise in alveolar ventilation (see Section on Nutritional Support in the Critically Ill Adult).

The important causes of hypercapnic respiratory failure in the ICU are listed in **Table 8.1.1.**

Table 8.1.1. Important causes of hypercapnic respiratory failure in the ICU

1. Patients with normal lungs to start with (decrease in $\dot{V}_E$)
   * Depressed ventilatory drive
     - Poisonings e.g. narcotics, antidepressants, sedatives
     - Head injury, encephalitis, increase in intracranial tension
   * Neuromuscular diseases
     - Acute poliomyelitis, acute infective polyneuritis, polymyositis, critical care neuropathy/myopathy, amyotropic lateral sclerosis
     - Tetanus, myasthenia gravis, botulism
     - Snake bite poisoning
     - Respiratory muscle weakness or fatigue from any cause
   * Large airways obstruction
     - Tracheal/subglottic stenosis, obstructive sleep apnoea, vocal cord paralysis, foreign bodies
   * Poor expansion of the thoracic cage (failure of the 'Bellows')
     - Trauma (flail chest), severe obesity, kyphoscoliosis, extensive eschar after burns, pleural effusion, pneumothorax
2. Patients with abnormal lungs (decrease in $\dot{V}_E$ and/or increase in $\dot{V}_D$)
   * Acute severe bronchial asthma
   * Acute crisis in chronic bronchitis, emphysema
   * Extensive thromboembolic disease
   * Severe terminal stage restrictive lung disease
3. Patients with increased production of CO_2
   * High fever, hypermetabolic critical illnesses
   * Frequent seizures, uncontrolled tetanus
   * Hyperalimentation with increased carbohydrate intake

II. Hypoxaemic Respiratory Failure

Acute hypoxaemic respiratory failure results from poor gas exchange of oxygen within the lungs leading to a low PaO_2. The $PaCO_2$ may be normal or even less than normal (**Fig. 8.1.1**).

Physiopathology

The normal alveolar ventilation ($\dot{V}_A$) is about 4–5 l, and the normal perfusion ($\dot{Q}$) around 5 l, the $\dot{V}_A/\dot{Q}$ ratio being approximately 0.8–1. Even in the normal lung, there are regional differences in ventilation perfusion ratios, but by and large the ventilation perfusion ratios are even and range from 0.8 to 1.2. For explanatory purposes, the lung can be compartmentalized into the following divisions:

(a) Alveoli with normal ventilation and perfusion—normal $\dot{V}/\dot{Q}$ ratios.

(b) Alveoli with increase in ventilation-perfusion ratios, the $\dot{V}/\dot{Q}$ ratios being > 1. The capillaries leaving these alveoli have a normal or slightly increased PaO_2 but a reduced $PaCO_2$.

(c) Alveoli with a decrease in ventilation-perfusion ratios; blood after perfusing these alveoli has a lowered PaO_2, and an increased $PaCO_2$. The lower the $\dot{V}/\dot{Q}$ ratio, the lower the PaO_2 of the blood leaving these alveoli.

(d) Alveoli that are ventilated, but have no perfusion. The $\dot{V}/\dot{Q}$ ratio is infinity, and such alveoli contribute significantly to increased physiological dead space.

(e) Alveoli which are atelectatic but continue to be perfused. These alveoli contribute to a right to left shunt within the lungs. The blood leaving the alveoli has the same PaO_2 as mixed venous blood i.e. 40 mm Hg.

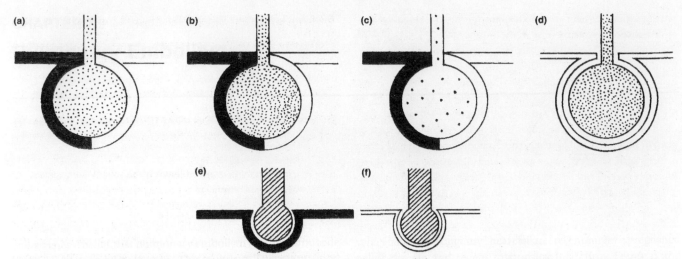

Fig 8.1.2. Various gas exchange units in the lung (a) Normal unit—alveoli with normal $\dot{V}/\dot{Q}$ ratios; (b) Hyperventilated unit—alveoli with increase in $\dot{V}/\dot{Q}$ ratios (> 1); (c) Hypoventilated unit—alveoli with decrease in $\dot{V}/\dot{Q}$ ratios; (d) Dead Space unit—alveoli are ventilated, but have no perfusion; (e) Shunt unit—alveoli are atelectatic but have good perfusion (f) Silent unit—alveoli are neither ventilated nor perfused (modified from Udwadia FE. 1979. Diagnosis and Management of Acute Respiratory Failure. OUP, Mumbai).

(f) Alveoli which are neither ventilated or perfused. These are 'resting' alveoli, and probably come into physiological action only when ventilatory or respiratory demands increase (**Fig. 8.1.2**).

Acute hypoxaemic respiratory failure occurs when: (a) there is a ventilation-perfusion mismatch characterized predominantly by low ventilation-perfusion ratios in the lungs; (b) there is a significant increase in the right to left shunt due to perfusion of atelectatic alveoli; (c) both the above factors are present; (d) there is a marked decrease in diffusion of oxygen across the alveolar capillary membrane.

(a) Low Ventilation-Perfusion ($\dot{V}/\dot{Q}$) Ratios

Alveoli which have a perfusion in excess of ventilation (i.e. low $\dot{V}_A/\dot{Q}$ ratios), will have a reduced PAO_2, and therefore a reduced PaO_2, as well as a reduced oxygen content of blood leaving the alveoli. When the poorly oxygenated blood mixes with the blood perfusing the alveoli that have $\dot{V}_A$ which is normal in proportion to the perfusion, or $\dot{V}_A$ even in excess of the perfusion, the resultant blood stream has a lower oxygen content, and a lowered PaO_2. Increased $\dot{V}/\dot{Q}$ ratios in some alveoli cannot therefore compensate for sharply lowered $\dot{V}/\dot{Q}$ ratios in other alveoli. After all, the oxygen saturation of arterial blood in the presence of normal $\dot{V}/\dot{Q}$ ratios is close to 100 per cent. A further increase in the $\dot{V}/\dot{Q}$ ratio may increase both the PAO_2 and the PaO_2, but because of the plateau-shape of the upper part of the oxygen-haemoglobin dissociation curve, there will be no appreciable increase in oxygen saturation or content of blood leaving such alveoli. This is illustrated in **Fig. 8.1.3**.

(b) Increase in Right to Left Shunt within the Lungs

A shunt refers to the proportion or fraction of venous blood that enters the systemic arteries without coming into contact with gas exchanging areas of the lungs. The present discussion is not concerned with right to left shunts in the heart or the larger vessels due to congenital defects or anomalies. Right to left shunts within

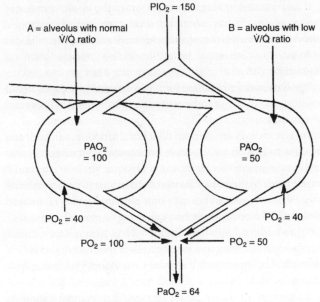

Fig. 8.1.3. The PaO_2 of blood leaving A (alveolus with normal $\dot{V}/\dot{Q}$ ratio) is normal; the PaO_2 of blood leaving B (alveolus with reduced $\dot{V}/\dot{Q}$ ratio) is reduced. When this poorly oxygenated blood mixes with well-oxygenated blood from alveoli with normal or high $\dot{V}/\dot{Q}$ ratios, the resultant PaO_2 is still lower than normal. This shows that increased $\dot{V}/\dot{Q}$ ratios in some alveoli cannot compensate for markedly lowered $\dot{V}/\dot{Q}$ ratios in other alveoli.

the lungs due to perfusion of atelectatic alveoli constitute the most important cause of refractory acute hypoxaemic respiratory failure. It is to be remembered that there is a small right to left shunt even in normal lungs. This is because of bronchial venous blood draining directly through pulmonary veins into the left atrium, and a small amount of coronary venous blood that drains via the thebesian veins directly into the left ventricle. The normal shunt averages not more than 5 per cent. In patients with a right to left shunt due to perfusion of atelectatic alveoli, the shunt fraction

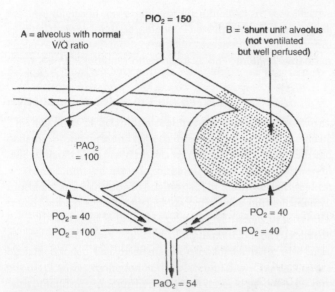

Fig. 8.1.4. The PaO$_2$ of blood leaving A (alveolus with normal V̇/Q̇ ratio is normal. The mixed venous blood perfusing B (shunt unit alveolus) is not oxygenated at all. When this blood mixes with well-oxygenated blood perfusing a normal alveolus, the resultant PaO$_2$ is still very low.

may be as high as 30–50 per cent. The higher the right to left shunt within the lungs, the greater the degree of hypoxaemia, and lower the PaO$_2$.

The effect of a right to left shunt within the lungs is illustrated in **Fig. 8.1.4**.

(c) Combination of Low V̇/Q̇ Ratios and Increased Shunt

Most lung diseases causing acute respiratory failure are characterized by a pathology in which there are areas of low V̇/Q̇ ratios, high V̇/Q̇ ratios, and increase in the right to left shunt. Patients in whom disturbance in gas exchange is predominantly due to an increase in the shunt have the gravest prognosis.

(d) Impairment in Diffusion of Oxygen

A diffusion **abnormality** does exist in several lung diseases, but it almost never is the chief cause of a low PaO$_2$ at rest. **All patients with diffusion** abnormalities have regional variations in compliance resulting in uneven and low ventilation-perfusion ratios.

Effect of an Increasing Inspired Oxygen Content (FIO$_2$) on V̇/Q̇ Abnormalities

Increase in the FIO$_2$ rapidly produces an increase in the PaO$_2$ and the oxygen content of blood leaving the alveoli with low V̇/Q̇ ratios. The hypoxaemia of acute respiratory failure in patients with low V̇/Q̇ ratios is thus easily corrected. The improvement in PaO$_2$ depends upon the degree of perfusion to areas with poor ventilation. Except where the V̇/Q̇ ratios are extremely low, a satisfactory PaO$_2$ of about 60 mm Hg, with an oxygen saturation of 90 per cent is achieved by using a FIO$_2$ of < 0.6. Even in alveoli with extremely low V̇/Q̇ ratios, as long as there is some ventilation present, an FIO$_2$ of 100 per cent will always produce a marked increase in the PaO$_2$ of blood leaving such alveoli. This is illustrated in **Fig. 8.1.5(a)**.

Effect of an Increased FIO$_2$ on the Shunt

It is obvious that the treatment of hypoxaemia due to a severe right to left shunt within the lungs is difficult, because increasing the FIO$_2$ improves the oxygen content to a very slight extent. The greater the shunt, the poorer the response in PaO$_2$ to a rise in FIO$_2$ (**Fig. 8.1.5(b)**). Fortunately, acute hypoxaemic respiratory failure solely due to a marked increase in the right to left shunt within the lungs is rare. Even in patients with severe acute respiratory distress syndrome (ARDS), though there are many areas of shunt which do not respond to an increase in FIO$_2$, there are some areas of V̇/Q̇ mismatch which respond to such an increase.

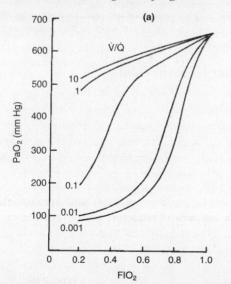
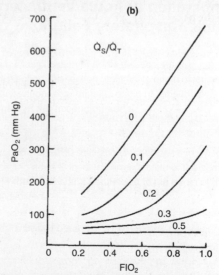

Fig 8.1.5. (a) PaO$_2$ improves with increasing FIO$_2$ in patients with a V̇/Q̇ mismatch. When the FIO$_2$ is increased to 1 (100%), the PaO$_2$ reaches 600 mm Hg even if the V̇/Q̇ ratio is very low. **(b)** Note that with increase in Q̇$_S$/Q̇$_T$ beyond 0.3, increasing the FIO$_2$ has little or no effect on the PaO$_2$ (from Albert RK, Physiology and Management of Failure of Arterial Oxygenation. 1988. In: Clinics in Critical Care Medicine, Cardiopulmonary Critical Care Management (Eds Fallat RJ, Luce JM) pp. 37–59. Elsevier, Inc.).

Clinical Problems Causing Acute Hypoxaemic Respiratory Failure

These can be broadly divided into three groups:

(i) Those characterized chiefly by airways obstruction causing uneven ventilation and $\dot{V}/\dot{Q}$ inequalities—an acute crisis in chronic bronchitis emphysema, and acute severe asthma are classic examples. In some of these patients there is an element of acute ventilatory failure in addition to hypoxaemic respiratory failure. This is due to mechanical limitations which prevent increased ventilatory demands from being adequately met, to alveolar hypoventilation consequent to a marked increase in physiological dead space ventilation, or to a diminished respiratory drive. One or more of these factors may contribute to an associated ventilatory failure.

(ii) Restrictive lung diseases. Examples of these include acute pulmonary oedema, acute pulmonary infections, acute lung injury (ARDS), and major atelectasis within the lungs.

(iii) Acute thromboembolic lung disease. This is characterized by $\dot{V}/\dot{Q}$ inequalities and increase in the dead space resulting in acute hypoxaemic respiratory failure.

The important causes of acute hypoxaemic respiratory failure are listed in **Table 8.1.2.**

Table 8.1.2. Important causes of acute hypoxaemic respiratory failure

* Obstructive airways disease
  – Acute crisis in chronic bronchitis emphysema
  – Acute severe bronchial asthma
* Restrictive lung disease
  – Acute pulmonary oedema
  – Acute pulmonary infection
  – Acute lung injury (ARDS)
  – Major pulmonary atelectasis
* Trauma to the chest
* Acute thromboembolic lung disease

III. A Combination of Acute Ventilatory and Hypoxaemic Respiratory Failure

This is seen in intensive care medicine in four groups of patients:

(a) Acute severe asthma.

(b) Acute on chronic respiratory failure due to a respiratory crisis in patients with chronic airways obstruction.

(c) Muscle fatigue involving muscles of respiration in patients with acute respiratory failure due to severe lung disease.

(d) Advanced or late stage interstitial lung disease.

IV. Failure of Oxygen Transport

A satisfactory gas exchange at the alveolar level must be accompanied by an adequate transport of oxygenated blood to the tissues. This requires an adequate cardiac output, a normal oxygen content of arterial blood and good tissue perfusion (see Section on Cardiorespiratory Physiology). A low output state, or shock from any cause can also indirectly lower the PaO_2 in the following ways:

(a) A low cardiac output results in increased oxygen extraction from the blood by the tissues. This leads to a fall in the mixed venous oxygen content ($P\bar{v}O_2$). The lowered $P\bar{v}O_2$ in the mixed venous blood reaching the alveoli will lead to a lowered PaO_2. This can be even more marked if the cardiac output falls in a patient who already has a right to left shunt within the lungs (**Fig. 8.1.6**).

(b) A low output state leads to a low pressure of perfused blood in the pulmonary vessels; perfusion is more in the dependent alveoli of the lungs. This results in an increase in the physiological dead space involving non-dependent alveoli, and to low $\dot{V}/\dot{Q}$ ratios within the dependent alveoli of the lungs, thereby contributing to a fall in PaO_2.

(c) Respiratory muscle fatigue is an important factor in low output states. Hypotension and shock lead to poor perfusion of respiratory muscles and quick, easy fatiguability. Respiratory muscle fatigue can cause hypoventilation, can increase ventilation-perfusion inequalities, and can thereby further reduce the PaO_2.

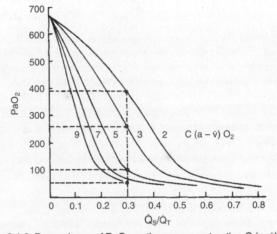

Fig. 8.1.6. Dependence of PaO_2 on the oxygen extraction C (a–v̄) O_2 and the shunt fraction. If the shunt fraction is 30%, the PaO_2 varies from 100 to 400 mm Hg, as the C (a–v̄) O_2 narrows. The patient may have a high PaO_2 if he has a high cardiac output and a decreased C (a–v̄) O_2 of 3, even if his shunt fraction is as high as 0.3. However if the patient's oxygen consumption increases without a corresponding increase in the cardiac output, the C (a–v̄) O_2 widens to 9, and the PaO_2 falls sharply to 50 mm Hg. (Source: as in Fig. 8.1.5).

Respiratory Muscle Fatigue

The importance and role of muscle fatigue in acute respiratory failure in critically ill patients, cannot be overemphasized and is best considered at this stage. As with other muscle groups in the body, excessive work performed by the muscles of respiration leads to fatigue (**1, 3**). Increasing fatigue results in increasingly poor function and hypoventilation; ultimately the patient literally stops breathing. Increasing respiratory fatigue explains the abrupt stoppage of breathing with resulting disaster, in patients with acute severe asthma, or in patients with a very low pulmonary compliance due to acute alveolar oedema. Difficulties in weaning patients off ventilator support are also frequently related to respiratory muscle fatigue brought on by the inability to cope with the work of breathing.

The second major factor predisposing to respiratory muscle fatigue is the gravity or critical nature of an illness. The more critically ill the patient, the easier and quicker does fatigue arise in respiratory muscles. Tachypnoea and an unstable circulation, hypotension with poor perfusion of the respiratory muscles, electrolyte disturbances, probably all play a role in muscle fatigue in these individuals.

The clinical recognition of respiratory muscle fatigue is difficult, and may occasionally be impossible to detect till the patient very nearly has a respiratory arrest. A voiced complaint by an ill patient that he or she is tired and cannot continue to breathe for long, should always be taken seriously, particularly in a patient with severe airways obstruction. Tachypnoea with a rate > 35/min, always predisposes to fatigue, particularly in obese individuals or very ill patients. Poor chest excursions, irregular breathing and above all apnoeic spells, all point to fatigued respiratory muscles. Respiratory alternans, in which intercostal muscle and diaphragmatic contractions alternate, is also observed at times. Fatigued muscles also occasionally cause a paradoxical respiratory movement, with the lower part of the chest and the upper abdomen being drawn in, instead of being pushed out during inspiration.

Objective measurements are also of use. As a rough guide, spontaneous breathing can be easily sustained if the effort involved in each spontaneous breath is less than one-third of the maximal respiratory effort that can be achieved (3–5). The maximum inspiratory pressure (MIP) is a good guide to the respiratory muscle power. A MIP of < 30 cm H_2O generally denotes muscle fatigue. Similarly a tidal volume (measured by a Wright's spirometer) of < 300 ml, or a vital capacity (VC) less than 3 times the tidal volume, suggests respiratory muscle fatigue under appropriate clinical conditions. A minute ventilation > 10–12 l/min is difficult to sustain indefinitely in critically ill individuals, and often ultimately leads to hypoventilation from respiratory muscle fatigue. The objective measurements stated above when judged against an appropriate clinical background can give only indirect evidence of probable respiratory muscle fatigue. It has to be admitted that unequivocal direct evidence of contractile fatigue has not yet been demonstrated. The major determinants of respiratory muscle fatigue are inspiratory muscle strength, mean inspiratory pressure and the duration of inspiration, which when combined form the tension time index (TTI) (6). However, interpretation of the TTI is difficult and often misleading (6). Recent work suggests that the magnetic stimulation of the phrenic nerve (a procedure far less painful than electrical stimulation) can detect diaphragmatic fatigue, and by measuring changes in the oesophageal twitch pressure, can also detect ribcage muscle fatigue (7, 8). Magnetic stimulation of the phrenic nerve is however a research procedure in our setting. *Medicine need not always be evidence based.* For the present we should act on the premise that respiratory muscles (particularly if they are weak) can, like other skeletal muscles experience fatigue if subjected to excessive work for a prolonged period of time.

The clinical features of respiratory muscle fatigue are listed in **Table 8.1.3**.

Respiratory muscle fatigue causing or contributing to acute respiratory failure should be managed by resting the respiratory muscles by mechanical ventilation. During the period of rest, the acutely depleted glycogen stores of the respiratory muscles are

Table 8.1.3. Features of respiratory muscle fatigue

* Complaint of fatigue in relation to breathing
* Respiratory rate > 35/min
* Poor chest excursions, irregular breathing, apnoeic spells
* Respiratory alternans, paradoxical respiratory movements
* MIP < 30 cm H_2O
* V_T < 300 ml; VC < 3 × V_T; MV > 10–12 l/min

replenished, and lactic acid and other metabolites associated with muscle fatigue are washed out (9–11). Aminophylline is believed to preserve muscle strength and contraction of the diaphragm; however it is doubtful if this drug has a clinical role in patients with severe respiratory muscle fatigue.

V. Failure of Oxygen Uptake

Despite good ventilation, normal exchange of blood gases at the alveolar level, and good oxygen transport, oxygen uptake may be deficient at the tissue level. The main purpose of the cardiorespiratory system is then defeated. Thus cyanide poisoning is characterized by an arrest of intracellular respiration due to the inactivation of an intracellular enzyme, cytochrome oxidase. The patient with cyanide poisoning has a normal PaO_2, SaO_2, CaO_2 and oxygen transport, but cannot utilize oxygen at the tissue level. Blood after perfusing tissues shows severe lactic acidosis and has a high $P\bar{v}O_2$ and $S\bar{v}O_2$. The patient literally dies of 'strangulation' or hypoxia at the tissue level.

The most important clinical problem associated with failure of oxygen uptake is septic shock, often associated with ARDS [this is discussed under Septic Shock and Acute Lung Injury (ARDS)]. To many physicians it may seem inappropriate to consider failure of oxygen uptake by tissues in acute respiratory failure. Yet in critical care medicine, it is ultimately the oxygen supply to, and oxygen uptake by tissues (in particular tissues of vital organs), which are of crucial importance. In the final analysis, acute cardiorespiratory failure is a failure to adequately oxygenate the tissues.

Clinical Features of Acute Respiratory Failure

In the presence of a background disease known to cause acute respiratory failure, the only sure way to diagnose the latter is by estimating the arterial blood gases. One should never rely only on clinical features to diagnose acute respiratory failure. Clinical features may however be present. These include the presence of disease known to cause acute respiratory failure, and the features associated with hypoxia and hypercapnia. Many, though not all patients also show respiratory distress.

Hypoxia

Hypoxia is the basic underlying feature in every patient with acute hypoxaemic respiratory failure. Increasing hypoxia depresses cell function, induces metabolic acidosis, and if marked and unrelieved leads to cellular death. It may be impossible to detect hypoxia on clinical grounds in critically ill patients. The only sure way of detecting hypoxia is by measuring the arterial PaO_2. The importance of this fact cannot be overemphasized.

The only pathognomonic manifestation of hypoxia is central cyanosis. Nevertheless, well marked arterial hypoxaemia may exist in the absence of clinical cyanosis, so that to await the development of cyanosis before diagnosing acute respiratory failure, is to court disaster. Cyanosis can only be clinically evident if the mean capillary concentration of reduced haemoglobin exceeds 5 g/dl. It is evident that a patient with severe anaemia (Hb < 7 g/dl), may die of severe arterial hypoxaemia before cyanosis can become clinically manifest. A hypermetabolic state with a hyperdynamic circulation characterized by a quick blood flow through the peripheries, also renders the clinical recognition of cyanosis difficult. The presence of anaemia together with a quickened circulatory flow therefore constitutes a formidable combination which prevents the clinical appearance of cyanosis in spite of marked hypoxia.

Mental confusion, restlessness, acute anxiety, are early manifestations of hypoxia. The ghastly pitfall of dubbing the anxiety and restlessness of early hypoxia in acute respiratory failure as 'functional', should be guarded against.

Compensatory Mechanisms Induced by Hypoxia

Hypoxia triggers compensatory mechanisms which are easily recognized, and are therefore of diagnostic value. The main compensatory mechanism is sympathetic stimulation which causes tachycardia and hypertension. Increase in the respiratory rate is another compensatory mechanism produced by stimulation of the chemoreceptors in the carotid body and aorta. Increase in respiratory rate will not occur if the respiratory centre is markedly depressed, or if there is weakness or paralysis of the respiratory muscles. However, tachycardia and hypertension are important signs of hypoxia. They should be sought for, and their significance recognized in situations that can lead to acute respiratory failure. These signs depend on the integrity of the sympathetic nervous system. In the old and feeble, in diabetics with a neuropathy involving the sympathetic nerves, or in patients who have received drugs affecting the autonomic nervous system, sympathetic response to hypoxia may be absent or feeble. With severe increasing hypoxia, the clinical hallmarks are progressive bradycardia, hypotension, lactic acid acidosis, arrhythmias, circulatory failure and death.

The myocardium has no oxygen reserve so that hypoxia depresses myocardial function, and increases ectopic irritability. Bradycardia and hypotension result from the direct depressant effect of hypoxia on the myocardium. Arrhythmias arise due to increased ectopic irritability. Atrial flutter and fibrillation are often observed; severe hypoxia ultimately results in ventricular tachycardia, fibrillation and arrest.

Hypercapnia

Hypercapnia may also be impossible to detect on clinical grounds. The $PaCO_2$ should therefore always be estimated in any disease which can conceivably produce carbon dioxide retention.

Carbon dioxide has a local depressant effect on the cardiovascular system. It thus produces generalized vasodilatation except in the pulmonary circulation. Generalized vasodilatation manifests as *cutaneous flushing, warmth, sweating, and a bounding pulse.*

The depressant effect of carbon dioxide on the central nervous system leads to confusion, disturbance in behaviour, a reversal in the sleep rhythm, and increasing drowsiness that may lead to deep coma (carbon dioxide narcosis). Carbon dioxide narcosis is an important metabolic cause of coma, and can be often missed if the $PaCO_2$ is not measured. Wing flap tremors of the outstretched hands are often observed with CO_2 retention. They are indistinguishable from those observed in hepatic failure. Wing flap tremors are not consistently present. At times, even a slight rise in the $PaCO_2$ induces wing flap tremors; at other times, a marked rise in $PaCO_2$ may not be associated with 'flaps'. However, increasing levels of $PaCO_2$ produce increasing disturbance of consciousness. Marked confusion and drowsiness occur by the time $PaCO_2$ rises to between 80–100 mm Hg, and the patient is generally unconscious when the $PaCO_2$ is well over 100 mm Hg. Coma in CO_2 narcosis is associated with loss of the deep reflexes, and urinary incontinence. The plantars are generally not elicitable or are flexor; rarely they may be extensor.

High levels of $PaCO_2$ can produce headache, muscle twitchings, seizures and papilloedema. The combination of drowsiness, headache and papilloedema closely simulate an intracranial tumour.

An increasing $PaCO_2$ stimulates the respiratory centre, producing an increase in the respiratory rate and tidal volume. Nevertheless, a depressed centre or a centre with a reduced or absent sensitivity to increasing $PaCO_2$, will not permit an increased respiratory drive to materialize.

Hypercapnia also produces a central stimulation of the sympathetic nervous system, resulting in tachycardia and hypertension. The pattern of symptoms in a patient will depend on the balance between the depressant action on the cardiovascular system, and the stimulant effects on the sympathetic nervous system.

Respiratory Distress or Dyspnoea

Many patients in acute respiratory failure are uncomfortably aware of a difficulty in breathing. This unpleasant awareness of respiration, and difficulty in breathing is termed dyspnoea. Dyspnoea is a subjective phenomenon, and its correlation with the degree of respiratory failure is difficult. In fact, breathlessness and respiratory failure are not synonymous. Many patients who are breathless, are not in respiratory failure, and a number of patients in respiratory failure are not breathless. Nevertheless, in a patient

Table 8.1.4. Important clinical features of hypoxia and hypercapnia

Hypoxia	Hypercapnia
* Cyanosis	* Flushing, warmth, sweating, bounding pulse
* Mental changes, restlessness, anxiety	* Headache, wing-flap tremors
* Tachycardia, hypertension	* Drowsiness, confusion, coma
* Rhythm disturbances	* Muscle twitching, seizures, papilloedema
* Metabolic acidosis	
* Bradycardia, hypotension, circulatory failure, when hypoxia is marked	

with chronic lung disease, increasing impairment of lung function and increasing respiratory failure, are invariably associated with increasing dyspnoea.

The important clinical features of hypoxia and hypercapnia are listed in **Table 8.1.4**.

An Elective Diagnostic Assessment in Acute Respiratory Failure (Table 8.1.5)

Acute respiratory failure may occur with a suddenness and severity that warrants immediate efforts towards resuscitation. Nevertheless, whenever time and the patient's condition permit, an elective diagnostic work-up is necessary. This is done with 3 objectives in mind:

(i) To establish the cause of acute respiratory failure.

(ii) To determine the nature of disturbance in respiratory physiology.

(iii) To estimate in so far as is possible, the tempo or the rate of progression of the disease, and the problems or complications likely to occur in the immediate or near future.

Table 8.1.5. Elective diagnostic assessment in acute respiratory failure

1. **Establish cause and estimate tempo or rate of progression of problem causing acute respiratory failure**
   * Detailed history e.g. of poisoning, of symptoms suggestive of important diseases causing acute respiratory failure
   * Physical examination
     – Check for features of hypoxia, hypercapnia, patency of airways
     – Meticulous examination of the cardiovascular and respiratory systems
   * Routine investigations
     – Arterial blood gas analysis
     – Other tests e.g. CBC, serum biochemistry, chest X-ray
   * Special investigations
     – Monitoring of central venous pressure
     – Monitoring of pulmonary artery pressures, cardiac output, and shunt fraction by use of the Swan-Ganz catheter

2. **Determine nature of disturbance in respiratory physiology**
   * Evaluate if ventilation is adequate
     – Hypoventilation if $PaCO_2$ > 48–50 mm Hg
     – Hyperventilation if $PaCO_2$ < 35 mm Hg
   * Evaluate the following possible physiological abnormalities underlying a low PaO_2
     – Hypoventilation
     – Mismatched $\dot{V}/\dot{Q}$ ratios
     – Increased right to left shunt within lungs
     – Impaired diffusion
   * Assess if there is increase in physiological dead space
   * Evaluate if work of breathing is increased
   * Check for evidence of respiratory muscle fatigue
   * Check if oxygen transport and tissue oxygenation are adequate

I. History

This is of great importance in evaluating the nature and tempo of the problem causing acute respiratory failure. Special stress should be laid on a history of poisoning, or of symptoms suggestive of important diseases known to cause acute respiratory failure— e.g. acute infective polyneuritis, acute poliomyelitis, intracranial and other central nervous system lesions, myasthenia gravis, and cardiopulmonary diseases.

II. Physical Examination

A thorough physical examination is mandatory. The following points are of special importance:

(a) An examination particularly oriented towards detection of clinical situations that lead to acute respiratory failure.

(b) A careful examination of the respiratory system. The importance of carefully counting the respiratory rate over a minute cannot be overemphasized. Polyphonic wheezes denote airways obstruction. The rhythm and pattern of breathing are also of importance. In ventilatory failure due to neuromuscular disease, the ability to hold the breath in inspiration and count numbers serially should be noted. Ordinarily one can easily count up to 30. Inability to count up to 20 or more, is a sure sign of marked neuromuscular weakness or of respiratory muscle fatigue. Crackles over the lungs point to pulmonary oedema or to interstitial lung disease. Tight airways obstruction need not be accompanied by an auscultatory wheeze, particularly in patients with a 'lazy' respiratory centre and with carbon dioxide retention. A forced expiratory effort may bring out a wheeze in such patients, provided they are not obtunded, and can follow commands.

(c) The cardiopulmonary system should be regarded as a single or interrelated unit, responsible for supplying oxygen to the tissues. A careful examination of the heart and the circulatory system is therefore as important as an examination of the respiratory system. The pulse, arterial blood pressure, central venous pressure, body temperature, moisture and colour of the skin, and colour of the mucosal surfaces and the nails are all of importance.

(d) Specific features of hypoxia and hypercapnia should be looked out for; their absence however, should never lull the clinician into a false sense of complacency.

III. Routine Investigations

Arterial blood gas analysis (pH, PaO_2, $PaCO_2$) is absolutely mandatory to confirm a clinical suspicion of acute respiratory failure, or for that matter, to establish a diagnosis even when no clinical suspicion of acute respiratory failure is entertained.

Other routine laboratory investigations include a complete blood count with a PCV, urine analysis, serum electrolytes, other relevant biochemical parameters, and a chest X-ray.

IV. Special Investigational Procedures

In difficult cases, e.g. in the management of acute lung injury (ARDS), or in severe fulminant tetanus, or in patients with acute respiratory failure and shock, special procedures are of use not only in the diagnostic evaluation, but also in the management. These investigational procedures include measurements of the central venous pressure through a central line, and of the arterial blood pressure through a cannula in the radial artery. A Swan-Ganz catheter may need to be inserted to measure the pulmonary artery pressure, the pulmonary capillary wedge pressure, and the cardiac output by the thermodilution technique. The Swan-Ganz catheter is also necessary to measure the mixed venous oxygen content, and thereby determine the shunt fraction or venous admixture within the lungs. Invasive procedures outlined above, should never be done routinely, but only in problem patients where further information is necessary not only for a complete evaluation, but also for management. Iatrogenic problems with invasive procedures can be significantly frequent and dangerous. *Every good critical care unit must be able to confidently state that the value of an invasive procedure undertaken in a given case clearly outweighs the potential iatrogenic hazards involved.* Fortunately, the high cost of the Swan-Ganz catheter, prohibits its frequent use in our country.

As mentioned earlier, the basic disturbance in respiratory physiology must be determined. The following standard questions should therefore be asked, and their answers determined.

(a) Is ventilation adequate? The only certain way to determine this is to measure the $PaCO_2$; a $PaCO_2 > 48$–50 mm Hg indicates hypoventilation, while a $PaCO_2 < 35$ mm Hg, hyperventilation.

(b) What is the physiological abnormality underlying a low PaO_2? A lowered PaO_2 is an essential feature of acute respiratory failure, and this could be due to:

(i) A reduced FIO_2, which could arise only at high altitudes.

(ii) Hypoventilation. If so, the decreased PaO_2 is related to the increased $PaCO_2$, as determined by the O_2–CO_2 diagram, or the alveolar-oxygen equation stated earlier. The alveolar-arterial gradient remains normal (between 10–20 mm Hg) in patients in whom a lowered PaO_2 is due to hypoventilation.

(iii) Mismatched ventilation-perfusion ratios. Unequal $\dot{V}/\dot{Q}$ ratios with an overall reduction in the ratio, produce a lowered PaO_2. When plotted on the O_2–CO_2 diagram, the point lies well to the left of the line representing the O_2–CO_2 relationship. The alveolar-arterial gradient is therefore increased (> 20 mm Hg).

Hypoxia due to mismatched $\dot{V}/\dot{Q}$ ratios is easily corrected by administering an increased FIO_2. Thus oxygen administered through nasal prongs or catheters, or via an orofacial mask at a rate of 4–6 l/min suffices to produce a substantial rise in the PaO_2, and a fall in the alveolar-arterial oxygen gradient. However if the $\dot{V}/\dot{Q}$ ratios are very low, a FIO_2 of 0.6 or more is necessary to produce a significant rise in the PaO_2. 100 per cent oxygen always abolishes hypoxia (and a low PaO_2) resulting from even the most severe ventilation-perfusion inequalities.

(iv) Increased right to left shunt within the lungs i.e. an increase in the true venous admixture. A significant right to left shunt is suspected clinically when even a high FIO_2 fails to result in a significant rise in the PaO_2. The exact degree of right to left shunt can be calculated by the shunt equation as follows:

$$\frac{\dot{Q}_S}{\dot{Q}_T} = \frac{CcO_2 - CaO_2}{CcO_2 - C\bar{v}O_2}$$

The $C\bar{v}O_2$ can be obtained by sampling the mixed venous blood through a Swan-Ganz catheter. The $\dot{Q}_S/\dot{Q}_T$ ratio determined on 20 per cent oxygen gives the overall physiological shunt i.e. the true venous admixture plus the shunt effect produced by alveoli with low ventilation-perfusion ratios. The $\dot{Q}_S/\dot{Q}_T$ ratio determined on 100 per cent oxygen inspired over 20 minutes, abolishes the shunt effect produced by alveoli with low ventilation-perfusion ratios, and gives a value of the true venous admixture, or the actual

right to left shunt due to perfusion of totally atelectatic alveoli.

The degree of true venous admixture can also be roughly estimated by noting the alveolar-arterial oxygen gradient when the patient is on 100 per cent oxygen for 20 minutes. If the alveolar-arterial gradient exceeds 100 mm Hg, it points to the presence of a right to left shunt. The greater the alveolar-arterial gradient on 100 per cent oxygen, the greater the degree of shunt (see Chapter on Basic Cardiorespiratory Physiology in the ICU).

(v) Impaired Diffusion. Though interstitial and alveolar disease might cause impaired oxygen diffusion across the alveolar capillary membrane, the contribution of this impairment to a lowered PaO_2 is not as important in clinical medicine as the effect of ventilation-perfusion inequalities. What is more, an increased FIO_2 can counter any fall in PaO_2 related to reduced oxygen diffusion.

It is extremely important to realize that a lowered PaO_2 could be due to, or influenced by factors other than an abnormal gas exchange within the lungs (**Table 8.1.6**). Factors unrelated to gas exchange which can lower the arterial PaO_2 include:

(1) A low $P\bar{v}O_2$ due to a lowered cardiac output, or to increased oxygen extraction by the peripheral tissues because of increased tissue metabolism.

(2) Severe anaemia. This is initially compensated by an increase in cardiac output. When this does not occur, or when the haemoglobin falls below 7 g/dl, there is a significant fall in the $P\bar{v}O_2$ and the mixed venous oxygen content, which ultimately causes a fall in the PaO_2.

Table 8.1.6. Causes of low PaO_2 unrelated to abnormal gas exchange within the lungs

---

* Low $P\bar{v}O_2$ due to decreased cardiac output, or increased oxygen extraction by peripheral tissues due to increased tissue metabolism
* Severe anaemia (Hb < 7 g/dl)
* Shift of oxygen dissociation curve to the left as in alkalosis, hypothermia, lowered $PaCO_2$, decreased 2,3—diphosphoglycerate in RBCs

---

(3) A shift in the oxygen dissociation curve to the left as in alkalosis, hypothermia, lowered $PaCO_2$, or a decrease in the 2,3-diphosphoglycerate in the red blood cells. A leftward shift of the oxygen dissociation curve leads to a fall in the PaO_2 for an equivalent degree of oxygen saturation, as compared to a normal oxygen dissociation curve. This is even more marked when there is a sudden shift of this curve from right to left (**Fig. 8.1.7**).

A clear evaluation of extrapulmonary factors is of great importance in critically ill patients, as it improves patient management and care.

(c) Is there an increase in the physiological dead space? An increase in the physiological dead space immediately points to uneven ventilation-perfusion ratios and to regional hyperinflation. An indirect method of assessing dead space is by determining the minute ventilation required to maintain a normal $PaCO_2$. The volume of ventilation exceeding the predicted value, is a measure of increased ventilatory requirements, and is generally due to an increase in the physiological dead space, provided that an increase in the $\dot{V}CO_2$ (i.e. CO_2 produced by tissue metabolism) can be excluded.

If the PCO_2 of mixed expired gas can be determined, then the

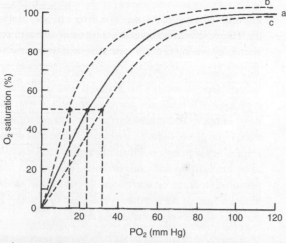

Fig 8.1.7. Normal oxygen-dissociation curve (**a**), and curves shifted to left (**b**), and right (**c**). Curve **b** indicates increased affinity for oxygen, while curve **c** denotes decreased affinity for oxygen. Note that for an equivalent degree of O_2 saturation, the PO_2 level falls with a leftward shift in the oxygen dissociation curve.

dead space volume (V_D), in relation to the tidal volume (V_T) is given by the following equation:

$$\frac{V_D}{V_T} = \frac{PaCO_2 - P_{\bar{E}}CO_2}{PaCO_2}$$

where $P_{\bar{E}}CO_2$ is the PCO_2 of mixed expired gas.

In patients on ventilator support, Levesque and Rosenberg (**12**) have devised a rapid and easy method of calculating dead space in relation to tidal volume. Assuming a normal V_D/V_T of 0.3, and a normal $PaCO_2$ of 40 mm Hg,

$$\frac{V_D}{V_T} = \frac{\dot{V}_M}{\dot{V}_E} \times \frac{P_aCO_2}{40} \times 0.3$$

where $\dot{V}_M$ is the measured minute ventilation, and $\dot{V}_E$ is the expected minute ventilation from a Radford nomogram.

(d) Is the work of breathing increased? Increased airways obstruction and/or a decrease in the compliance of the lungs or the thoracic wall, or both, result in an increased work of breathing. Though both can be gauged clinically, an exact estimation of airways resistance, and/or of pulmonary compliance in a critically ill patient with acute respiratory failure, is convenient only when the patient is on ventilator support. However peak flow readings in patients with obvious airways obstruction, particularly when serial readings are measured, are of considerable value in estimating the degree and progress of airways obstruction (see Chapter on Acute Severe Asthma).

(e) Is there evidence of respiratory muscle fatigue? Muscle fatigue is determined by the strength of the respiratory muscles and the load of breathing on respiration. Weak muscles and an increased load or work of breathing predispose to muscle fatigue. A clinical evaluation of muscle fatigue and simple bedside objective measurements to assess the possible presence and degree of respiratory muscle fatigue, have already been discussed earlier.

(f) Is oxygen transport satisfactory? An adequate cardiac output is necessary for oxygenated arterial blood to reach the tissues. Cardiac output can be clinically gauged by noting the pulse,

arterial blood pressure, skin temperature, urine output per hour, the presence or absence of lactic acid acidosis, and the presence or absence of dysfunction of major organ systems. In difficult problems, the cardiac output needs to be measured by the thermodilution technique. When the cardiac output is low, oxygen transport can be enhanced by measures to increase the cardiac output. This chiefly is through manipulation of factors that determine cardiac output, namely the preload, cardiac contractility, the afterload, and the rate and rhythm of the heart (see Section on Basic Cardiorespiratory Physiology in the Intensive Care Unit).

A normal haemoglobin is also necessary for an adequate oxygen content; a haemoglobin of 11 g/dl is generally aimed at in critically ill patients with acute respiratory failure.

(g) Is tissue oxygenation adequate? Good tissue oxygenation is the ultimate aim of restored cardiopulmonary function. There is a great deal more that we need to know about assessment of tissue oxygenation. An increase in lactate levels in the blood is a sure sign of poor tissue oxygenation. In septic shock and in ARDS, utilization of oxygen by the tissues may be inadequate even in the presence of a normal oxygen transport and supply.

Management of Acute Respiratory Failure (Table 8.1.7)

There are a number of diseases producing acute respiratory failure for which there is no specific cure. The patient then needs respiratory care and support till such time as the disease resolves. There are other diseases producing acute respiratory failure for which specific therapy is available. Prompt diagnosis and specific treatment in such instances can quickly reverse respiratory failure. The general principles involved in the management of acute respiratory failure include: (I) maintenance of a clear airway; (II) maintenance of adequate ventilation; (III) use of oxygen; (IV) treating the cause of acute respiratory failure, in so far as this is possible; (V) the use of mechanical ventilation when indicated— if the cause of acute respiratory failure cannot be treated, or if

Table 8.1.7. Management of acute respiratory failure

1. Maintenance of clear airway
   * Clear secretions
      - Liquefy secretions
      - Promote cough—good physiotherapy
      - Suctioning of secretions
      - Use of an airway—oropharyngeal airway, other airways, endotracheal intubation/ tracheostomy
2. Maintenance of adequate ventilation
   * Artificial ventilation with AMBU bag in emergency, till mechanical ventilator support is organized
   * Use of respiratory stimulants (in rare situations)
3. Use of oxygen
4. Treat cause of acute respiratory failure whenever possible
5. Use mechanical ventilator support if cause cannot be treated, or if patient hypoxic or hypercapnic despite above measures

despite treatment the patient is hypoxic or hypercapnic, ventilatory support is indicated.

I. Maintenance of a Clear Airway

Obstruction of the airways due to retained secretions, mucus plugs or foreign matter (invariably food particles), worsen respiratory failure. Secretions obstructing airways can lead to hypoventilation with a further fall in the PaO_2. Mucus plugs within airways contribute to uneven and poor distribution of inspired gas to the alveoli within the lungs, and also produce areas of atelectasis. Uneven ventilation accentuates $\dot{V}/\dot{Q}$ inequalities, whilst increasing areas of atelectasis worsen or produce a right to left shunt within the lungs. The net effect is increasing hypoxia and worsening respiratory failure. Undrained secretions or mucus plugs also form a nidus for infection, which may ultimately lead to pneumonia or bronchopneumonia. Maintaining a clear airway is therefore, vital. This is often lost sight of in a comatose patient who may have normal lungs to start with, but who develops a quickly worsening respiratory failure due to undrained secretions plugging the airways.

Methods to Clear Secretions

(a) *Liquefy Secretions.* Undrained secretions can dry and form crusts which obstruct the airways. Such crusted secretions can be removed only with great difficulty; therefore drying of secretions should be prevented, and their liquefaction promoted by:

(i) Proper hydration of the patient, if necessary with intravenous fluids. A severely ill, distressed, breathless patient generally does not drink enough water on his own.

(ii) Humidification of inspired gas. This is of utmost importance when the nasal and upper respiratory passages are bypassed, and the patient is breathing through an endotracheal or tracheostomy tube. Lack of humidification in such patients besides causing drying and crusting of secretions in the trachea, the large and the small airways, can also result in inspissated secretions that block the endotracheal or tracheostomy tube with disastrous consequences.

(iii) Use of N saline. We often instil N saline (2–5 ml at a time) through an endotracheal or tracheostomy tube, to help liquefy inspissated mucus secretions. This is particularly of value in patients with acute severe asthma on ventilator support.

Acetylcysteine is also a good liquefactant of inspissated mucus,

but is a strong irritant. It can produce severe bronchospasm even in a dose as small as 0.5 ml. The drug can also markedly increase the volume of secretions in the tracheobronchial tree, necessitating very frequent suction. We use this drug very rarely in our unit.

(b) *Promotion of Cough.* Cough, in a patient with acute respiratory failure should always be assisted and promoted, and never suppressed. When pain prevents cough (as after thoracic, open heart or upper abdominal surgery, or in crush injuries), analgesics need to be given, taking care to use a dose that does not produce respiratory depression. Physiotherapy is vital to enable secretions to be brought up and coughed out. The patient may need to be postured to drain his secretions. *In critically ill patients who retain secretions within the respiratory tract, good physiotherapy often spells the difference between survival and death.*

(c) *Removal of Secretions by Suction.* When secretions gather in the mouth and the upper respiratory passages, and the patient is too ill to spit or cough them out, frequent suction should be done to keep the upper airways patent, and to prevent the possibility of aspiration of the secretions into the lungs. Secretions around the larynx can be sucked with the aid of indirect laryngoscopy. Suction stimulates cough in an obtunded patient, and this is of added help. It is important never to roughly touch or 'hit' the tip of the catheter to the pharynx or larynx during suctioning, as this can traumatize the pharyngeal or laryngeal mucosa, induce bleeding and sloughing, and further worsen the problem of maintaining a clear airway. The tip of the suction catheter should lie on the posterior portion of the tongue, preferably not touching the pharynx during suctioning. The floor and sides of the mouth should be suctioned; the nasal cavity and the pharynx can also be conveniently suctioned through a catheter inserted through the nares.

(d) *Endotracheal Intubation* (also see Chapter on Airway Management). If the upper airway cannot be kept clear and open by the methods indicated above, or by the use of a simple oropharyngeal or nasopharyngeal airway, the patient should be intubated. Endotracheal intubation is an invaluable aid to maintain a clear airway as it allows easy access to secretions in the trachea and the large airways.

The main indication for endotracheal intubation is upper airways obstruction and the inability of the patient to handle upper respiratory secretions. The latter feature is frequently observed in unconscious patients, and is invariably so in comatose patients. It also occurs when the cough reflex is poor or the patient is just too ill or feeble to cough. Paralysis of the palate and pharynx will also prevent the patient from handling his upper respiratory secretions because of difficulty in swallowing. This could lead to aspiration of accumulated secretions, as also to aspiration of regurgitated stomach contents. The four common conditions in critical care medicine wherein an endotracheal tube serves to maintain an open airway, are poisonings by respiratory depressants, cerebrovascular accidents, coma from any cause and following major surgery. Endotracheal intubation is also indicated when the patient is to be put on mechanical ventilator support.

Suctioning of secretions through the endotracheal tube should be done with all aseptic precautions, and with the 'no-touch' technique as described in the section on tracheostomy. Humidification of inspired gas is absolutely essential. We ordinarily never keep an endotracheal tube in situ for more than 7–10 days, simply because the incidence of complications, chiefly subglottic oedema and narrowing, are significantly higher if the tube is kept for a longer period of time. If experience indicates that the nature of the disease causing acute respiratory failure is likely to last for over 10 days, we prefer to do an elective tracheostomy after first intubating the patient with an endotracheal tube. Tracheostomy has been discussed in a separate chapter.

II. Maintenance of Adequate Ventilation

(a) Artificial Ventilation

When respiration is feeble, or the patient is apnoeic, immediate resuscitation is aimed at ensuring adequate ventilation. Initially mouth to mouth respiration may be necessary, followed within seconds by a mask fitted to an AMBU or anaesthetic bag, fed with 100 per cent oxygen. This should be quickly followed by endotracheal intubation, mechanical ventilation being carried out either through an AMBU bag or by a mechanical ventilator.

(b) The Use of Respiratory Stimulants in Acute Respiratory Failure

The role of respiratory stimulants in acute respiratory failure in ICUs is very limited and to many non-existent. No respiratory stimulant acts specifically and solely on the respiratory centre; all such drugs in addition to stimulating the respiratory centre, also act as analeptics, in that they awaken the patient, and thereby enable him to ventilate and cough better. In fact, almost certainly the analeptic effect is clinically more important than the specific stimulating effect on the respiratory centre. Good physiotherapy should always be given during an analeptic phase, so that secretions within the lungs are mobilized, and either coughed up or removed through suction. Unfortunately, all respiratory stimulants and analeptics frequently produce vomiting as a side effect, and if the dose is large, or the drug is administered rapidly, localized twitchings or generalized seizures can result. If alveolar hypoventilation due to a depressed respiratory centre is sufficiently severe to produce well-marked hypoxia and hypercapnia, it is far better to use non-invasive ventilation or to intubate and ventilate the patient, rather than waste time in administering respiratory stimulants. We have stopped using respiratory stimulants in our unit.

Perhaps the only valid use of respiratory stimulants is (a) to tide over a critical period in a patient with acute respiratory failure, while he awaits transfer to an ICU; (b) in patients with hopelessly crippling COPD who on balance, are not given ventilator support. Respiratory stimulants could then be tried along with the other far more important conservative measures.

The respiratory stimulant with probably the least side effects is doxapram. It is given intravenously at a rate of 1–3 mg/min, and can be continued till a maximum dose of 600 mg is reached (13). The risk of seizures is low with doxapram. The infusion can however cause hypertension and cardiac arrhythmias as the drug can stimulate the release of epinephrine from the adrenals. It should therefore be avoided in hypertensive patients, and in those with ischaemic heart disease.

Doxapram is not easily available in India, and one has to therefore make do with nikethamide or prethcamide (micoren). Nikethamide is a potent respiratory stimulant and an analeptic when given intravenously in a dose of 0.5–2.5 g (2–10 ml), diluted in 10 ml dextrose, very slowly over 10–15 minutes. It produces hyperventilation starting within 30 seconds, and lasting for 5–7 minutes after completion of the injection. The drug may need to be repeated every 1–4 hours, or may be given as a slow intravenous infusion, the dosage being calculated from the hourly requirement for intermittent injections. Prethcamide has a slower and more prolonged action than nikethamide. The dose is 225–450 mg, and the drug is preferably given as a slow intravenous infusion.

III. Use of Oxygen

The prompt administration of oxygen is crucial in the management of acute respiratory failure. This is considered in a separate section.

IV. Treatment of the Cause of Acute Respiratory Failure Whenever Possible

Treatment is individualized depending upon the aetiological factor operating in a patient. The following examples are illustrative and worthy of mention:

(i) Treatment of infection This is the commonest cause that precipitates acute respiratory failure in patients with chronic lung disease. Infection can also occur later as a complication in the natural history of acute respiratory failure due to other causes.

(ii) Removal of air in a tension pneumothorax, and tapping of a massive unilateral pleural effusion or moderate sized bilateral effusions.

(iii) Removal of a foreign body obstructing the larynx, trachea, or a large bronchus.

(iv) Expanding an atelectatic lobe or lung with physiotherapy or bronchoscopic suction.

(v) Use of prostigmine in myasthenia gravis, and of antivenin in snake bite poisoning.

(vi) Use of naloxone in narcotic poisonings.

(vii) Use of nebulized beta-2 agonists, intravenous aminophylline, and oral or intravenous corticosteroids in acute severe asthma.

There are many situations where the cause of acute respiratory failure cannot be promptly treated. This particularly holds true for the numerous conditions which produce the acute respiratory distress syndrome, severe tetanus, severe head injuries and other CNS problems, and poisonings due to sedatives and tranquillizers. The doctor in charge of the ICU has then to rely on the general principles of management outlined above, till such time as the illness causing acute respiratory failure resolves over a period of time.

V. Mechanical Ventilation

When well-marked and in particular life-threatening hypoxia and/or hypercapnia are uncorrected by the general principles mentioned above, the patient needs mechanical ventilator support to aid in more effective gas exchange within the lungs. This is dealt with in a separate chapter.

REFERENCES

1. Wood LH. (1998). The Pathology and Differential Diagnosis of Acute Respiratory Failure. In: Principles of Critical Care (Eds Hall JB, Schmidt GA, Wood, LH). pp. 499–507. McGraw-Hill, New York.

2. Pierson DJ, Luce JM. (1988). Cardiopulmonary Components of Respiratory Failure. In: Clinics in Critical Care Medicine: Cardiopulmonary Critical Care Management (Eds Fallat RJ, Luce JM). pp. 1–9. Churchill Livingstone, New York, Edinburgh, London, Melbourne.

3. Roussos CS, Macklem PT. (1977). Diaphragmatic fatigue in man. J Appl Physiol. 43, 189–197.

4. Respiratory Muscle Fatigue Workshop Group. (1990). NHLBI Workshop Summary: Respiratory Muscle Fatigue. Am Rev Respir Dis. 142, 474–480.

5. Zocchi L, Fitting JW, Majani U et al. (1993). Effect of pressure and timing contraction on human rib cage muscle fatigue. Am Rev Respir Dis. 147, 857–864.

6. Laghi F. (2001). Hypoventilation and Respiratory Muscle Dysfunction. In: Critical Care Medicine (Eds Parillo JE, Dellinger RP). pp. 754–768. Mosby, USA.

7. Laghi F, Harrison M, Tobin MJ. (1996). Comparison of magnetic and electrical phrenic nerve stimulation in assessment of diaphragmatic contractility. J Appl Physiol. 80, 1731.

8. Similowski T, Straus C, Attali V et al. (1998). Cervical magnetic stimulation as a method to discriminate between diaphragm and ribcage muscle fatigue. J Appl Physiol. 84, 1692.

9. Manthous CA, Hall JB, Schmidt GA. (1993). The effect of assist-control ventilation and muscle relaxation on oxygen consumption in critically ill patients. Am Rev Respir Dis. 147, A881.

10. Ward ME, Magder SA, Hussain SNA. (1992). Oxygen delivery-independent effect of blood flow on diaphragm fatigue. Am Rev Respir Dis. 145, 1058–1063.

11. Viires N, Sillie G, Aubier A et al. (1983). Regional blood flow distribution in dogs during induced hypotension and low cardiac output: Spontaneous breathing versus artificial ventilation. J Clin Invest. 72, 935–947.

12. Levesque PR, Rosenberg H. (1976). Rapid bedside estimation of wasted ventilation. Anaesthesiology. 42, 98–100.

13. Martin RJ, Ballard RD. (1986). Respiratory stimulants. In: Drugs for the Respiratory System (Ed. Cherniak RM). pp. 191–212. Grune and Stratton, Orlando.

Oxygen Therapy

Oxygen is used as therapy in most critically ill patients under intensive care. It can be life-saving in acute respiratory failure, yet can be lethal if incorrectly used. Oxygen administration aims at increasing the PAO_2, and thereby the PaO_2 and the oxygen saturation of arterial blood. Except in some instances, it is enough to aim at a saturation of 90 per cent; an oxygen saturation < 90 per cent generally corresponds to a PaO_2 < 60 mm Hg, and denotes the presence of moderate hypoxia. A moderate degree of hypoxia disturbs normal cell metabolism and function; marked hypoxia results in cellular death. A PaO_2 < 20 mm Hg for a significant length of time generally produces brain death; yet a PaO_2 a little above 30 mm Hg probably maintains adequate cell function if the blood flow is adequate (1).

We have no means of accurately assessing cell function, and there is no doubt that the sensitivity of certain tissues (such as the brain and the heart) to oxygen lack is far greater as compared to other tissues (e.g. skin and muscle). It is possible that even minor degrees of hypoxia which are easily tolerated in a young healthy individual, might pose problems in critically ill individuals, or in those with a poor coronary circulation, or with impaired cerebral blood flow due to diffuse cerebrovascular disease. It is important to relieve hypoxia of even mild intensity in all such critically ill patients, and preferably aim at an oxygen saturation well over 90 per cent.

Indications for Oxygen Therapy

Hypoxia is the prime indication for oxygen administration. Dramatic relief with oxygen therapy is chiefly observed when arterial hypoxaemia (i.e. a low PaO_2) is due to a low PAO_2 or to ventilation-perfusion mismatch within the lungs. Relief of hypoxia in such patients often brings in its wake three other effects:

(i) Decrease in the work of breathing. Hypoxia often causes increased ventilatory work and relief of hypoxia is often followed by a decrease in the work of breathing.

(ii) Decrease in myocardial work. The heart and circulatory systems are frequently involved in compensatory responses to hypoxia; once the hypoxia is reversed, these compensatory responses abate and the work of the myocardium is reduced.

(iii) Improvement in cell function involving various organ systems of the body is a welcome aspect of adequate oxygenation to the tissues.

In an ICU setting, patients requiring oxygen fall into the following groups:

(a) *Decreased PaO_2 due to respiratory arrest, hypoventilation, or to disturbances in gas exchange.* These patients benefit the most by oxygen therapy. The following situations are included in this group:

(i) Cardiopulmonary or respiratory arrest. Administration of oxygen is of vital importance, but is of no avail unless the patient is simultaneously ventilated.

(ii) Anaesthetic error or accident.

(iii) Hypoventilation from any cause.

(iv) Respiratory diseases characterized by ventilation-perfusion mismatch, with or without impaired diffusion across the alveolar capillary membrane. These include severe chronic obstructive pulmonary disease (COPD), as also interstitial lung disease.

(v) Respiratory diseases associated with an increase in the right to left shunt within the lungs—as in ARDS, atelectasis, and pneumonia. As explained in the Chapter on Acute Respiratory Failure in Adults, oxygen administration by conventional methods easily increases the PaO_2, and relieves the hypoxia in patients with hypoventilation or ventilation-perfusion mismatch; however it fails to satisfactorily increase the PaO_2 and relieve hypoxia in those with a significant right to left shunt in the lungs.

(b) *Decreased oxygen content of arterial blood* (other than that caused by a decrease in PaO_2).

(i) Severe anaemia.

(ii) Carbon monoxide poisoning.

(iii) Methaemoglobinaemia and sulphaemoglobinaemia.

The use of high concentrations of inhaled oxygen is useful but very limited in its scope, as the PaO_2 is generally normal in this group; it is the oxygen content which is low.

(c) *Decreased transport of oxygen with impaired perfusion of tissues.*

(i) Shock from any cause.

(ii) Left ventricular failure.

(iii) Poor coronary perfusion, including extensive myocardial infarction.

(iv) Cardiac arrhythmias causing haemodynamic instability.

(v) Cardiac arrest.

A marked fall in the $P\bar{v}O_2$ due to a fall in the cardiac output leads to a fall in the PaO_2. Also many of these conditions produce an increase in the physiological dead space and a ventilation-perfusion mismatch. It is important to maximize both the PaO_2 (and the oxygen content), as also increase oxygen transport, through an increase in the cardiac output in these patients.

(d) *Poor uptake or utilization of oxygen by tissues.* This is seen in septic shock and in ARDS, and here again the PaO_2, the oxygen content, and the oxygen transport or delivery to the tissues must be maximized if cellular and organ function are to be well maintained.

Oxygen is not utilized by tissues in cyanide poisoning, as cyanide inactivates the enzyme cytochrome oxidase within the cells. A high FIO_2 is of marginal help; reversal of cyanide toxicity by suitable antidotes is of prime importance.

It is important to remember that oxygen helps in the relief of hypoxia. Even so, oxygen does not eradicate the root cause of hypoxia. It is therefore no substitute for adequate alveolar ventilation, neither does it solve the problem of $\dot{V}/\dot{Q}$ abnormalities, nor does it abolish a right to left shunt within the lungs. Again the oxygen content of blood is not only dependent on the PaO_2, but also on the haemoglobin concentration in the blood. The importance of an adequate cardiac output in ensuring good oxygen transport and the proper uptake and utilization of oxygen within the cells has already been stressed.

Important Considerations in Oxygen Administration

Two considerations should be kept in mind before starting oxygen therapy in a hypoxic patient:

(a) Does the patient have a normally sensitive respiratory centre, and a normal control over respiration? If so, he will tolerate high concentrations of oxygen (at flow rates of 6–8 l/min through a mask or nasal prongs), and the correction of his arterial hypoxaemia will not result in CO_2 retention. Such a patient has normal sensitivity of the respiratory centre to a rise in $PaCO_2$, except when the centre is temporarily but severely depressed by drugs. Uncontrolled oxygen therapy at high flow rates is safe in most pulmonary problems causing hypoxia. It is safe therefore to give high oxygen concentrations in severe interstitial lung disease, pneumonia, pulmonary oedema, atelectasis. Patients with acute hypoventilation from any cause, if treated with oxygen will have relief from hypoxia though hypercapnia will remain unchanged. Uncontrolled oxygen therapy will not however, increase the hypercapnia in these patients.

(b) Does the patient have an abnormal control over respiration, in that is the respiratory centre comparatively insensitive to increasing PCO_2, and is the respiratory drive significantly dependent on the hypoxic stimulus? If so, inhaling high concentrations of oxygen will produce a sharp increase in the PaO_2, but will thereby sharply reduce his respiratory drive. This will result in hypoventilation, and the comparative lack of sensitivity of the respiratory centre to increasing carbon dioxide tension will cause a dangerous rise in the $PaCO_2$. Such a patient may be pink through abolition of his arterial hypoxaemia, but he may become drowsy, obtunded or even comatose because of carbon dioxide narcosis.

The above situation chiefly occurs in many (but not all) patients with severe COPD. It may occasionally also be observed in chronic hypoventilation syndromes due to other causes. It must be mentioned at this juncture, that the traditional belief that patients with severe COPD have a respiratory centre insensitive to a rising PCO_2, and that uncontrolled oxygen therapy leads to hypercapnia by abolishing the hypoxic stimulus to breathe, is strongly disbelieved and disputed by many workers today. There is data to suggest that carbon dioxide retention following uncontrolled oxygen therapy is due to more than one factor, and may be contributed to by an increase in the $\dot{V}/\dot{Q}$ ratio with an increase in the dead space, rather than from the suppression of the hypoxic drive to breathe (2–4). Stradling (5) however persists with the old traditional belief of global hypoventilation induced by uncontrolled oxygen administration in these patients, with an additional contribution of the Haldane effect and only a minor contribtion by an increase in $\dot{V}/\dot{Q}$.

Fortunately, almost all patients with acute severe asthma who are hypoxic, tolerate and respond well to oxygen given at flow rates of 6–10 l/min. However a small minority, particularly in the older age group, do develop a sharp rise in $PaCO_2$ due to increasing hypoventilation, following the use of high flow rates of oxygen.

Oxygen should be given with caution in all patients with chronic airways obstruction and in other chronic hypoventilation syndromes. It should be administered in a *controlled concentration (of 24–30 per cent)*, as will be discussed below, and its effect on the patient should be carefully assessed. When in doubt as to the nature of the expected response to oxygen administration, it is wise to start with controlled oxygen therapy.

Methods of Oxygen Administration

I. Routine Oxygen Therapy using Low-flow Oxygen Administration Devices

A moderate rise of oxygen concentration in the alveoli suffices to relieve moderate hypoxia. An oxygen concentration of approximately 40 per cent may be achieved by using nasal catheters, nasal prongs, or simple orofacial masks, if the flow rate is maintained between 6–8 l/min. Patients cannot ordinarily tolerate flow rates higher than 6–8 l/min through the above-mentioned devices.

Nasal Catheters and Nasal Prongs

These are the simplest and most commonly used devices for oxygen administration. If a nasal catheter is used, its tip should be advanced to the fold of the soft palate, and then pulled back very slightly. If it is introduced too far, it can produce gaseous distension of the stomach, as oxygen finds its way into the stomach rather than into the lungs. Irritation of the nasal mucosa can be minimized by lubricating the catheter by xylocaine jelly. The catheter can be changed from one nostril to the other every 4 hours.

Most units prefer nasal prongs to nasal catheters. Nasal prongs (two short plastic prongs that fit into the external nares) (**Fig. 8.2.1**) offer the advantage of simplicity and comfort. An added advantage

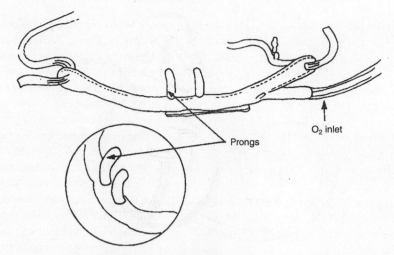

Fig. 8.2.1. Nasal prongs.

over an orofacial mask is that the administered oxygen does not have to be discontinued during eating, speaking or coughing.

When oxygen is administered through nasal prongs or a nasal catheter, at a flow rate of 1 l/min, the oxygen concentration is approximately 24 per cent. At flow rates of 6–8 l/min, the oxygen concentration approximates 40 per cent. Further increase in flow rates are poorly tolerated and produce very little additional increase in oxygen concentration.

The effect of a given flow of oxygen through a nasal catheter or prongs is dependent not only on the flow rate, but the tidal volume and minute ventilation of the patient. If the tidal volume and minute ventilation decrease, i.e. the patient hypoventilates, then the inspired oxygen concentration will rise. Precise regulation or control over inspired oxygen concentration is thus not possible with nasal prongs or catheter. Recently developed methods of administering supplemental oxygen include the use of reservoir cannulae, transtracheal oxygen delivery and pulsed oxygen delivery. Transtracheal oxygen delivery is effected via a small catheter inserted into the trachea at the base of the neck (**6**). It is totally unnecessary for ICU use though it has some benefits for patients on domiciliary oxygen therapy. Pulsed oxygen devices deliver oxygen only during inspiration. This conserves oxygen, yet provides a PaO$_2$ equivalent to that obtained with a continuous flow system through prongs or a face mask (**7**). We are unfamiliar with the use of pulsed oxygen delivery devices.

Face Mask (Fig. 8.2.2)

A simple oronasal plastic mask fed with oxygen at a flow rate of 6–10 l/min, is a frequently used method for administering oxygen. The oxygen fed directly into the mask (after humidification), displaces air and creates a small oxygen reservoir. During inspiration oxygen in the mask is inhaled; room air is also entrained through the ports and through the space between the face and the mask. The oxygen concentration of inspired gas is thus much < 100 per cent. The extent to which inspired oxygen concentration can increase, depends on the size of the mask (and therefore of the oxygen reservoir), and the flow rate of oxygen. Higher flow rates

are generally better tolerated through the use of a mask as compared to nasal prongs or catheters. At a flow rate of 6–10 l/min, an oxygen concentration of approximately 35–55 per cent can be achieved.

The face mask is less easy and less comfortable to wear than nasal prongs. The major disadvantage is that it has to be removed when the patient speaks, eats, drinks, coughs, or expectorates.

Face Mask with Reservoir Bag (Fig. 8.2.3)

The addition of a reservoir bag to the face mask increases the potential reservoir of oxygen, and allows a further increase in the concentration of inspired oxygen.

Inspired oxygen consists of oxygen from the reservoir bag of the face mask, together with some air entrained through the side ports and the small space between the mask and the skin of the face. During expiration, most of the exhaled gas passes out through the side ports, but some expired gas may return to the reservoir bag. This could lead to a fall in PO$_2$ and a rise in the PCO$_2$ in the reservoir bag, and should be avoided by a sufficiently high rate of oxygen flow to keep the bag washed out. Oxygen flow rates of 8–12 l/min are commonly used with this device, and can provide an inspired oxygen concentration between 50–80 per cent. The flow rate of oxygen must be so adjusted that the reservoir bag is not emptied by more than half during inspiration.

Face Mask with Reservoir Bag and Directional Valves (Fig. 8.2.4)

The entrainment of room air during inspiration can be almost completely prevented by covering the side ports with directional valves. Except for some air passing between the mask and the face, the entire volume of inspired gas consists of oxygen from the reservoir bag and the face mask. During exhalation, the side port directional valves open and air passes out from the mask into the atmosphere. The passage of expired air back into the reservoir bag can be prevented by a directional valve.

It is important that the flow rate of oxygen fed into the mask and reservoir bag with directional valves is in the range of 10–15

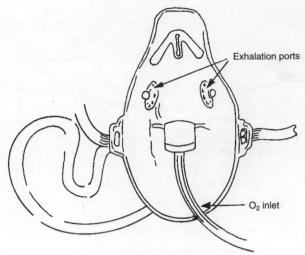

Fig. 8.2.2. Simple face mask.

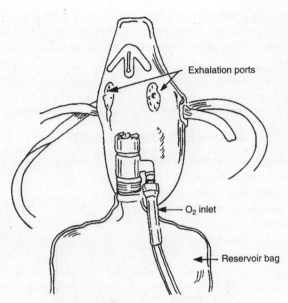

Fig. 8.2.3. Face mask with reservoir bag.

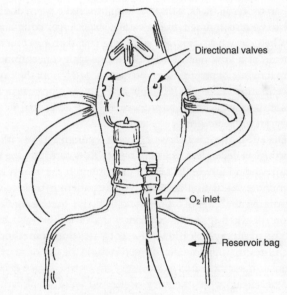

Fig. 8.2.4. Face mask with reservoir bag and directional valves.

l/min. The inspired oxygen concentrations can thereby be raised in such instances to as high as 90–95 per cent. It is also extremely important to ensure that there is no failure in oxygen supply nor a sharp fall in the flow rate, as breathing is dependent on oxygen fed into the mask-reservoir device. If the reservoir bag is inadvertently empty, asphyxia results. **Table 8.2.1** compares the oxygen flow (l/min) and oxygen concentrations (per cent) obtained by using low flow oxygen administration devices.

Table 8.2.1. Correlation between oxygen flow (l/min) and oxygen concentrations using low-flow oxygen administration devices

Device	O$_2$ Flow (l/min)	O$_2$ Concentration
Nasal cannula	approx. 6	approx. 40–45%
Facial mask	approx. 8	approx. 35–55%
Mask with reservoir	approx. 10	approx. 50–80%
Mask with reservoir plus directional valves	approx. 12	approx. 90–95%

II. Controlled Oxygen Therapy

Principles

Controlled oxygen therapy is necessary in all patients who show a hypercapnic response to unlimited or uncontrolled oxygen administration. In these patients (chiefly those with severe COPD), the inspired oxygen concentration is carefully controlled between 24–30 per cent.

The purpose of controlled oxygen therapy is to relieve dangerous hypoxia by producing an adequate increase in the PAO$_2$ and the PaO$_2$, and yet control and limit the associated rise of PaCO$_2$. This would also limit the fall in arterial pH due to respiratory acidosis.

In a severely hypoxic patient, the arterial point lies on the steep portion of the S-shaped oxygen dissociation curve. Thus even a small rise in the PaO$_2$ produces a significantly greater rise in the oxygen saturation of arterial blood. For example, an increase in

PaO_2 from 25–40 mm Hg will increase the oxygen saturation from 40–70 per cent. This increase in the oxygen saturation with increased availability of oxygen to tissues, could spell the difference between survival and death. In vitro, a rise of oxygen pressure in blood by 15 mm Hg can be brought about by an increase in oxygen concentration by 2 per cent, as 2 per cent of 760 mm Hg (atmospheric pressure) is equal to 15 mm Hg. In clinical practice, we deal with patients who have well marked ventilation-perfusion mismatch within their diseased lungs. Hence, an increase in inspired oxygen concentration of 4–10 per cent (giving an inspired oxygen concentration of 24–30 per cent) is generally necessary to bring about a similar rise in PaO_2. Even in patients who are totally insensitive to a rise in PCO_2, and whose respiratory drive is solely dependent on hypoxia, the maximal theoretical rise in PCO_2 is equal to the increase in PO_2 multiplied by the respiratory quotient (0.8). Thus an increase in the oxygen concentration of inspired gas by 3 per cent (i.e. from 21–24 per cent), would cause a rise in oxygen tension by 3 per cent of 760 mm Hg, i.e. 21 mm Hg. Therefore the maximal rise in PCO_2 would be $21 \times 0.8 = 17$ mm Hg. It needs to be pointed out that (i) hypoxic patients in the ICU have diseased lungs so that a greater increase in oxygen concentration is necessary to produce a desired increase in the PaO_2 than is estimated from in vitro calculations; (ii) it is rare for patients to lose all sensitivity to increasing PCO_2, and to be solely dependent on the hypoxic drive. Usually, sensitivity to increasing PCO_2 is impaired in varying degrees, but is not lost completely. Thus the rise in $PaCO_2$ is not often as high as is theoretically computed from a rise in PaO_2. For those who disagree with the concept that relief of hypoxia suppresses the hypoxic drive to breathe, the increase in PCO_2 on oxygen administration, can only be explained by increase in dead space with resulting alveolar hypoventilation.

It is best to start controlled oxygen therapy with an inspired oxygen concentration of 24 per cent. If a rise in $PaCO_2$ does not occur, or is less than 10 mm Hg, the inspired oxygen concentration is further increased to 28–30 per cent. The PaO_2, the rise in $PaCO_2$, the arterial pH, and the clinical state of the patient should be carefully monitored. A moderate rise in $PaCO_2$ by 20 mm Hg and a pH > 7.25 are permissible if dangerous hypoxia has been relieved.

Technique

The concentration of inspired oxygen is controlled by using high air flows with known oxygen enrichment. The principle underlying this technique is entrainment of air with constant-pressure jet mixing. High air flows allow the immediate space or environment around the patient's face to be so thoroughly flushed, that there is no rebreathing and no contamination with room air. In this manner, the concentration of inspired oxygen can be controlled to within 2 per cent.

Ventimask. This works on the Venturi principle and allows perfectly controlled oxygen administration. Oxygen is delivered to the mask through a nozzle, and the aperture of the nozzle is of set size so that as the oxygen is released through the aperture, it entrains a fixed portion of air through the side hole of the mask. Thus if an oxygen concentration of 24 per cent is desired, the aperture of the delivery nozzle is such that 1 l of oxygen/minute will entrain 20 l of air, and 2 l of oxygen/min will entrain 40 l of air. The entrainment ratio is 1:20, and is independent of the flow rate; the oxygen concentration of the inspired gas is thus independent of the flow rate.

Different ventimasks have different aperture size nozzles, and provide different but fixed oxygen concentrations. For example, a mask that is designed to provide an oxygen concentration of 28 per cent, will have a nozzle aperture that allows 1 l of oxygen delivered through the nozzle to entrain 10 l of air through the side holes i.e. a 1:10 entrainment ratio, which is again independent of the flow rate of oxygen.

As mentioned at the outset, the ventimask works on the Venturi principle, and the Venturi is fairly accurate at the recommended total flow of 40 l/min (i.e. 2 l of oxygen/min for a 24 per cent mask, and 4 l of oxygen/min for a 28 per cent mask). The gas flow around the patient's nose and mouth flushes the mask continuously, washing out the expired carbon dioxide, and ensuring that the patient only breathes the oxygen-air mixture provided to him.

The greatest advantage of the ventimask is that the oxygen concentration it provides is independent of the flow rate, and also independent of the patient's tidal volume and minute ventilation. It can be easily used by all nurses, and requires no special adjustment. Also, the concentration of oxygen delivered is not at the mercy of faulty flow meters or reducing valves. The disadvantage as with all oronasal masks, is that it has to be removed during coughing, eating, speaking, or drinking. In a seriously ill patient, removing the mask during feeds can cause a dangerous deterioration due to a sharp fall in the PaO_2 and worsening hypoxia. In severely hypoxic patients, the administration of oxygen should be continued, even when the patient is being fed, via nasal prongs at a flow rate of 1–2 l/min; this prevents the temporary but dangerous hypoxia.

Currently other commercially available high airflow systems have been designed to deliver oxygen concentrations varying from 24–50 per cent, using the same principle as the Venturi mask. A jet of oxygen from a wall or tank source is passed through a precisely designed (exact size) orifice, and this results in the entrainment of room air through the ports in the surrounding cylinder.

Nasal Prongs. Many ICUs in Mumbai and other large cities (leave aside smaller towns all over the country), do not use ventimasks or other high airflow oxygen-enriched delivery systems to provide controlled oxygen therapy. It is recommended that in the absence of these devices, nasal catheters or nasal prongs be used in an attempt to give controlled oxygen therapy. Oxygen at a flow rate of 1–2 l/min through nasal prongs or catheters is generally effective in providing controlled oxygen concentrations of 24–28 per cent in inspired gas. The flow rate should be initially kept at 1 l/min; if this is well tolerated, it is increased to 2 l/min. Measurements of the PaO_2 and the $PaCO_2$ are of help, and a close watch is kept on the patient, specially as regards his ventilation. If the patient has marked hypoventilation, administration of oxygen even at 1–2 l/minute can lead to an uncontrolled or higher than desired

Table 8.2.2. Effect of oxygen (administered through a nasal catheter at flow rate of 2 l/min) in relieving hypoxia without causing dangerous hypercapnia in 7 patients with obstructive airways disease

Patient	Before O$_2$ Therapy		After O$_2$ Therapy			
			4 hrs		24–36 hrs	
	PO$_2$	PCO$_2$	PO$_2$	PCO$_2$	PO$_2$	PCO$_2$
	(mm Hg)			(mm Hg)		
1	50	56	75	60	80	55
2	48	52	66	60	75	46
3	45	50	60	54	70	56
4	55	48	70	48	86	46
5	42	48	65	54	78	50
6	40	68	60	76	66	58
7	38	72	60	86	60	65

(From Udwadia FE. 1979. Acute Respiratory failure. Oxford University Press, Mumbai.)

concentration of oxygen. In such patients the flow rate should be reduced to < 1 l/min. Oxygen delivered through nasal prongs or catheters at low flow rates as stated above, is generally effective in relieving hypoxia without producing a dangerous rise in the PCO$_2$, even in patients whose respiratory drive is chiefly dependent on the hypoxic stimulus (**Table 8.2.2**).

III. Hyperbaric Oxygen

Hyperbaric oxygen is not administered in the ICU. Yet some critically ill patients under intensive care have to be transported to hyperbaric oxygen chambers in the same or distant hospitals to avail of this therapy. The administration of oxygen at higher than atmospheric pressure has certain advantages. When breathing air at atmospheric pressure, the oxygen in solution in plasma is 0.3 ml/dl; when breathing oxygen at a pressure of 2 atmospheres, it is 4.5 ml/dl. This is just a little less than the amount of oxygen taken up by tissues in unit time, and goes a long way in aiding jeopardized tissue perfusion, and relieving tissue hypoxia. The main use of hyperbaric oxygen is in the treatment of carbon monoxide poisoning. The dissolved oxygen relieves hypoxia, and the markedly increased oxygen tension helps the quick dissociation of carbon monoxide from carboxyhaemoglobin. Hyperbaric oxygen therapy is also useful in the management of sepsis secondary to wounds contaminated by anaerobic gas forming organisms, and in the treatment of wounds with a poor blood supply.

Delivery of Humidified Oxygen or Inspired Gas to Patients with an Endotracheal or Tracheostomy Tube

Tracheostomy Mask (Fig. 8.2.5)

This is a small soft plastic mask with a large opening for expiration, loosely positioned over a tracheostomy tube. Humidified oxygen is fed into the mask through an inlet, and expired gas escapes through the expiration port. The disadvantage is that patients also breathe in unheated and poorly humidified room air around the mask.

Briggs Adaptor (Fig. 8.2.6a)

This is a large bore T-piece adaptor fitted to the endotracheal tube. One limb of the T-tube delivers nebulized oxygen, while expired air leaves via the other limb. The usual T-tube used in our ICU at the Breach Candy Hospital, Mumbai is illustrated in **Fig. 8.2.6b**.

Highly humidified inspired air or gas mixtures are also administered to spontaneously breathing patients after extubation, or to spontaneously breathing patients who have thick tracheobronchial secretions. Devices used for this purpose include aerosol masks and face tents. An aerosol mask consists of a plastic face mask with a large exhalation port on either side. The mask is connected to a large bore delivery tube for the delivery of humidified oxygen or oxygen-air mixture.

A face tent (**Fig. 8.2.7**) is a plastic wrap-around face mask, which

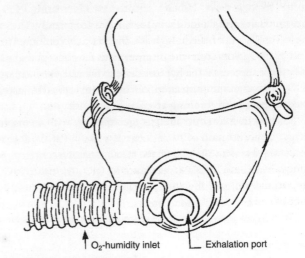

O$_2$-humidity inlet   Exhalation port

Fig. 8.2.5. Tracheostomy mask.

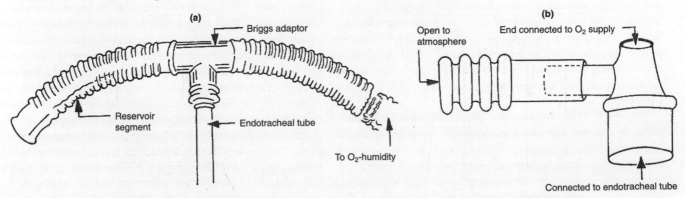

Fig. 8.2.6. (a) Briggs adaptor (T-piece fitted to an endotracheal tube). **(b)** Usual T-tube in our ICU.

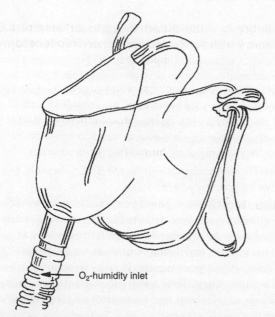

Fig. 8.2.7. Face tent.

fits loosely around the cheeks and chin. Humidified oxygen is fed from the bottom of the tent; expired air passes out through the open upper portion.

Humidification of Oxygen and Inspired Gas

Oxygen is dry and should always be humidified before administration. Ventilation of the lungs with dry gases produces heat loss, and moisture loss from the respiratory passages, and also alters pulmonary function (8). Heat loss causes a fall in body temperature and increases oxygen consumption. Moisture loss leads to drying or dehydration of the respiratory mucosa. The most important effect consequent to this drying is a reduced activity of the muco-ciliary escalator with sputum retention. Blocked airways from inspissated respiratory secretions result in ventilation-perfusion inequalities, and may lead to or accentuate hypoxia. Thus the importance of humidifying oxygen in inspired gas cannot be over-emphasized.

When oxygen is administered by nasal prongs, nasal catheters, or a facial mask, the upper respiratory passages, particularly the nose, will normally humidify the inspired gas. Even so, oxygen should preferably be humidified before administration. When upper respiratory passages are bypassed by an endotracheal or tracheostomy tube, humidification becomes absolutely mandatory.

It should be noted that even if room air or administered oxygen is saturated to 100 per cent with water vapour at room temperature, this saturation drops considerably when it comes into contact with respiratory passages whose normal temperature is 37°C. The fall in saturation is even greater if the body temperature is higher, as in patients running fever. Therefore to prevent drying of the respiratory mucosa either (i) the air or oxygen inspired by the patient should be saturated with water vapour at 37°C; or (ii) the inspired air or oxygen should be supersaturated by suspending water droplets in it at room temperature. When this supersaturated oxygen or air is warmed during its passage through the trachea, the suspended droplets vaporize and provide a humidity of well-nigh 100 per cent.

There are a number of techniques for humidification. All modern ventilators are provided with humidifiers with temperature control of the humidified gas delivered to the patient, as also with nebulizers which allow nebulization of inspired gas or nebulization of drugs into the respiratory tract.

Devices for the humidification of inspired gas or oxygen can be broadly divided into those that add water to gases, and those that retain water from expired gases (heat and moisture exchangers) (9).

(a) Devices Adding Water to Gases

(i) *Vaporizers (unheated)* (**Fig. 8.2.8**) A bubble humidifier is an example of an unheated vaporizer. When oxygen is moistened by bubbling it through a large surface of water, because of the heat loss by vaporization, the temperature of oxygen falls below the ambient temperature, at flow rates > 6 l/min. The cooled gas has sufficient moisture, but when it comes into contact with the warm respiratory mucosa, the water vapour saturation falls to 20–25 per cent. With nasal prongs or a face mask, this method suffices as warmth and humidification are supplied by the nose, mouth and pharynx. A bubble humidifier is however quite inadequate for humidification of oxygen or inspired gas in patients with an endotracheal tube or tracheostomy.

(ii) *Heated Vaporizers* (**Fig. 8.2.9**) (**10–12**) The Blower Humidifier

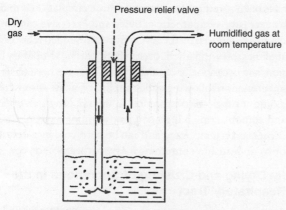

Fig. 8.2.8. A cold water humidifier.

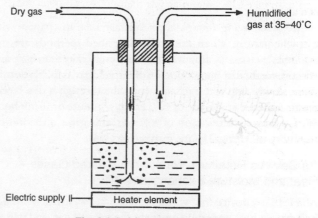

Fig. 8.2.9. A hot water humidifier.

devised by Spalding (13), is a good example of this type. Air or oxygen from a blower or a mechanical ventilator is passed over a surface of water thermostatically maintained at a temperature of 45–55°C. The inspired gas is 100 per cent saturated at this temperature, and the thermostat is set so that the air or oxygen is delivered to the patient at about 37°C. At this temperature, the inspired gas or oxygen is saturated to about 70–90 per cent. The blower humidifier tends to get overheated, and the temperature of inspired gas should therefore be frequently checked to prevent thermal injury to the respiratory passages. There is also a risk of bacterial colonization of the water in the reservoir, or in the delivery tubing (14, 15).

(iii) *Nebulizers.* Various nebulizers can be used to suspend water particles in inspired gas. The water droplets should be 1–10 μm in diameter. Larger droplets are of no use as they get deposited within the delivery tubes. Smaller droplets are stable and are not deposited in the respiratory tract. Nebulizers can be gas driven (**Fig. 8.2.10**), mechanically actuated (e.g. spin disc nebulizer), or ultrasonic (**9**).

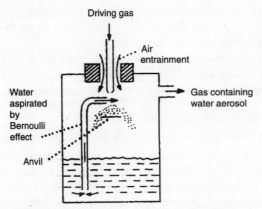

Fig. 8.2.10. A gas-driven nebulizing humidifier.

The main disadvantage of gas driven and mechanically actuated nebulizers, is the risk of microbiological contamination of the reservoir. This can be dangerous as microbes suspended in the aerosol can reach deep into the lungs, right upto the alveoli. Ultrasonic nebulizers are costly and can cause overhydration, as most devices can produce water well in excess of 250 g/m³, and some, over 1000 g/m³ (**9**). Bacterial contamination of the aerosol can also occur.

(iv) *A saline drip through the tracheostomy tube.* In a patient with a tracheostomy, when the above-described methods are not available because of financial or other constraints, an easy and effective method of humidification of inspired gas, is to drip normal saline slowly into the tracheostomy tube through a thin sterile plastic catheter, at the rate of 10–12 drops/minute or 16 ml/hour. With a minute ventilation of 8 l/min, this gives a theoretical humidity of 31 mg/l to the inspired gas (**16**).

(b) Devices Retaining Water from Expired Gases— Heat and Moisture Exchangers (HME)

An HME is a device that when connected to an artificial airway will extract heat and moisture from the expired gas, and will return this heat and moisture to the inspired gas during inspiration

(17, 18). Ideally a HME should retain at least 70 per cent of expired moisture. HME devices include Condenser Humidifiers, Hygroscopic Condenser Humidifiers and Hydrophobic Condenser Humidifiers (**9**). Filtration of inspired and expired gases can be provided by the associated use of heat and moisture exchanging filters.

HME devices have important advantages:

(i) Humidification is satisfactory with artificial airways (endotracheal or tracheostomy tubes).

(ii) The breathing circuit remains dry.

(iii) They are comparatively inexpensive, disposable, and do not require an external power source.

They cannot however provide very high levels of humidification, and ventilation can be obstructed if sputum is expectorated on the exchanger membrane. Some HME devices have a significant internal volume, and therefore increase the dead space. This is a disadvantage in a spontaneously breathing patient with a reduced tidal volume. These devices also produce a slight increase in the resistance to breathing, and when saturated with water vapour, result in a significant obstruction to airflow.

In conclusion, humidification of inspired gases is necessary for all critically ill patients receiving ventilatory support, for those breathing through a tracheostomy or endotracheal tube, and for those who have been breathing spontaneously, but have recently been extubated. The humidifier used should produce adequate saturation of the inspired gas or oxygen with water vapour. Heat and moisture exchangers have greater advantages as compared to hot water bath humidifiers. Bacterial colonization is a major risk and can result in nosocomial pneumonias. The use of filters that prevent bacterial or viral contamination of humidified inspired gas, helps to decrease the incidence of this complication.

Complications of Oxygen Therapy

(a) Progressive Hypercapnia

The danger of progressive hypercapnia, particularly after uncontrolled oxygen therapy in a number of patients with hypoxia due to chronic bronchitis, has already been discussed.

(b) Circulatory Depression

This is very rare, but has been occasionally observed in patients who have been severely hypoxic, and whose circulation is maintained by excessive sympathetic activity and excessive catecholamine discharge, induced by the severe hypoxia. Sudden relief of hypoxia abolishes this sympathetic overactivity, causing temporary hypotension, and occasionally circulatory collapse. We have observed this phenomenon following sudden relief of acute severe hypoxia in glottic or subglottic obstruction, after establishing an open airway and administering a high concentration of oxygen. Circulatory depression is temporary, and can be corrected by a volume load, or by an infusion containing a sympathomimetic agent.

(c) Drying and Crusting of Secretions in the Respiratory Tract

As stressed earlier, oxygen should always be humidified prior to administration. This is particularly imperative in patients with artificial airways. Unhumidified oxygen causes drying of secretions, and this can result in blockage of the bronchi by inspissated mucus. Partial or complete blockage of artificial airways (endotracheal or tracheostomy tube) by crusted secretions can have disastrous consequences.

(d) Danger of Oxygen Withdrawal

Moderate or severe hypoxia warrants continuous oxygen therapy till such time as the hypoxia is relieved. Some hypoxic, chronic bronchitics may become drowsy or disoriented even on controlled oxygen therapy. To discontinue oxygen in such a situation, is dangerous and wrong. If oxygen administration is stopped with the $PaCO_2$ markedly elevated, the PAO_2 (and consequently the PaO_2) falls to an even lower level than that prior to starting oxygen therapy. This is because the $PACO_2$ has risen to a higher level than that prevailing at the start of oxygen therapy. Such patients therefore have a worsening of their already severe hypoxic state. Intermittent oxygen therapy can be dangerous in a hypoxic patient, and is wrong on principle. It only serves to give periods of relief from hypoxia, followed by periods of worsening and often extreme hypoxia. Oxygen, if indicated, needs to be *given continuously* till hypoxia is relieved.

(e) Oxygen Toxicity

Lung Toxicity

High concentrations of oxygen over a prolonged period of time can produce changes in the lungs characterized by atelectasis, damage to the surfactant, interalveolar oedema, and interstitial thickening and fibrosis (19). It is generally accepted that oxygen concentrations up to 50 per cent are safe for long periods (19). We have used 60 per cent oxygen for weeks, and have observed that the patients have recovered without residual effects. We have also been forced to use 100 per cent oxygen in 2 patients (who would otherwise have died of hypoxia) for as long as 2 days, followed by 80–90 per cent oxygen for the next 4–7 days, and then 60–70 per cent oxygen for another week. Both patients survived without any significant residual damage to the lungs. This does not mean that very high oxygen concentrations should be used with abandon. It does however signify, that in our experience, the use of 100 per cent oxygen is not as lethal as is often made out to be.

The practical applications to be derived from experimental and clinical studies on oxygen toxicity are summarized below:

(i) For patients with chronic hypoxaemia (as in severe chronic airways obstruction), it is sufficient to use a concentration of oxygen that will correct dangerously low PaO_2 levels. A PaO_2 of even 50–55 mm Hg is generally adequate in these patients.

(ii) Positive end-expiratory pressure (PEEP) should be used during mechanical ventilation, if an inspired oxygen concentration > 50 per cent fails to relieve dangerous hypoxia. PEEP however, even in the above circumstances, should not be used in patients with chronic airways obstruction or emphysema.

(iii) In acute pulmonary problems with severe hypoxia, the oxygen concentration must be sufficient to allow an oxygen saturation of about 90 per cent. If in spite of the use of PEEP, oxygen concentrations of > 60–70 per cent are needed for several days to produce a satisfactory rise in PaO_2, it is wiser to choose to maintain a PaO_2 in the mild to moderate hypoxaemic range. This will allow the patient to make do with a lower oxygen concentration. The degree of hypoxia one allows will depend on the patient's tolerance to hypoxia, the age of the patient, and the ability or otherwise to increase oxygen transport to the tissues.

(iv) Life-threatening hypoxia must always be relieved, even if this requires the use of 100 per cent oxygen for prolonged periods of time. The fear and danger of possible oxygen toxicity is never an argument to allow a patient to irreversibly deteriorate and die of hypoxia.

(v) It is difficult, if not impossible, to detect signs of lung toxicity due to high oxygen concentrations in critically ill individuals with serious pulmonary problems. A fall in the compliance and the PaO_2 can occur due to very high oxygen concentrations, but we have found it impossible to ascertain in clinical practice, whether this is related to the disease, or is iatrogenic due to oxygen toxicity.

Retrolental Fibroplasia

This complication occurs in the neonatal period, and is related to high PaO_2 levels. If the inspired oxygen concentration is high enough to raise the PaO_2 to about 160 mm Hg even for a few hours, retrolental fibroplasia can occur. Therefore in neonates, PaO_2 levels should never exceed 100 mm Hg.

Cerebral Oxygen Toxicity

This is occasionally observed when oxygen is breathed at hyperbaric pressures above one atmosphere. The syndrome is chiefly characterized by epileptic fits and is termed the Paul Bert effect, after the individual who first described it (20).

REFERENCES

1. Eldridge F. (1966). Blood lactate and pyruvate in pulmonary insufficiency. New Engl J Med. 274, 878.

2. Aubier M, Murciano D, Fournier M et al. (1980). Central respiratory drive in acute respiratory failure of patients with chronic obstructive pulmonary disease. Am Rev Respir Dis. 122, 191–199.

3. Aubier M, Murciano D, Milic-Emeli J et al. (1980). Effects of the administration of O_2 on ventilation and blood gases in patients with chronic obstructive pulmonary disease during acute respiratory failure. Am Rev Respir Dis. 122, 747–754.

4. Sassoon CSH, Hassell KT, Mahutte CK. (1987). Hyperoxic-induced hypercapnia in stable chronic obstructive pulmonary disease. Am Rev Respir Dis. 135, 907–911.

5. Stradling JR. (1986). Hypercapnia during oxygen therapy in airways obstruction: A reappraisal. Thorax. 41, 897–902.

6. Scacci R. (1979). Air entrainment masks: Jet mixing is how they work; the Bernoulli and Venturi principles is how they don't. Respir Care. 24, 928.

7. Brooks CJ et al. (1986). Performance of a demand oxygen saver system during rest, exercise, and sleep in hypoxemic patients. Kansas City Pulmonary Clinic and Research Medical Centre, Kansas City, Missourie. Presented at the American Thorax Society.

8. Nolan DM. (1991). Problems of Inadequate Humidification. In: Problems in Respiratory Care. Recent Advances in Humidification (Eds Shelly MP, Branson RD, MacIntyre NR). 4(4), 413–417. JB Lippincott Company, Philadelphia.

9. St. John Gray H. (1991). Humidifiers. In: Problems in Respiratory Care. Recent Advances in Humidification (Eds Shelly MP, Branson RD, MacIntyre NR). 4(4), 423–434. JB Lippincott Company, Philadelphia.

10. Evaluation of humidifiers for medical use, Heated Humidifiers. Health Equipment Information. 1986. p. 151. Department of Health and Social Security.

11. Evaluation of heated humidifiers. Health Equipment Information, 1987. p. 177. Department of Health and Social Security.

12. Heated humidifiers. Health Devices. 1987. 16(7), 223. Emergency Care Research Institute.

13. Spalding JMK. (1956). Humidifiers for patients breathing spontaneously. Lancet. ii, 1140.

14. Redding PJ, McWalter PW. (1980). Pseudomonas fluorescence cross infection due to contaminated humidifier water. Br Med J. 281, 275.

15. Craven DE, Giularte TA, Make BJ. (1984). Contaminated condensate in mechanical ventilator circuit: a risk factor for nosocomial pneumonia. Am Rev Respir Dis. 129, 625–628.

16. Sara C. (1965). The management of patients with a tracheostomy. Med J Aust. i, 99–103.

17. Evaluation of heat and moisture exchangers. Health Equipment Information. 1987. p. 166. Department of Health and Social Security.

18. Heat and moisture exchangers. Health Devices. 1983. 12(7), 155. Emergency Care Research Institute.

19. Eubanks DH, Bone RC. (1990). Oxygen Analysers. In: Comprehensive Respiratory Care. A Learning System, 2nd edn. pp. 361–370. CV Mosby Company, Philadelphia, Toronto.

20. Fleney DC. (1990). Principles of Oxygen Therapy. In: Respiratory Medicine (Eds Brewis RAL, Gibson GJ, Geddes DM). pp. 370–384. Balliere Tindall, London, Sydney, Tokyo.

CHAPTER 8.3

Airway Management

Establishing the Airway

Nothing is more critical in emergency respiratory care than ensuring a patent airway and then maintaining it. An obstructed airway can lead to death within a few minutes. In patients with cardiac arrest, inability to secure a patent airway generally renders all efforts at cardiopulmonary resuscitation ineffective. In the West, airway care and management is entrusted to non-medical respiratory care therapists and the respiratory nurse specialists. In our country this responsibility is met by trained physicians and intensivists and by trained nurses in the ICU.

Upper Airways Obstruction

Upper airways obstruction may result from 'soft tissue' obstruction or from laryngeal obstruction.

'Soft tissue' obstruction is probably the commonest airway emergency. It results from the encroachment on the patency of the upper airway by soft tissues of the pharynx or by tissue in close relation to the pharynx. Upper airways obstruction is thus seen in comatose patients when the pharynx loses its tone, or in patients with lower cranial nerve palsies when the pharynx is paralysed. It also occurs in angioneurotic oedema, inflammation, retropharyngeal abscess and can be caused by bleeding and soft tissue tumours within that area. Foreign bodies, dentures, vomitus, blood clots, thick oropharyngeal secretions can also block the upper airway. The common factor underlying all these causes of upper airways obstruction is the absent or the markedly diminished patency between the base of the tongue and the pharyngeal wall.

Obstruction at the larynx can be caused by a bilateral vocal cord abductor palsy, by inflammatory or neoplastic lesions above or within the larynx or by laryngeal oedema. A foreign body or food (such as a piece of meat) may also obstruct the larynx and cause severe asphyxia and death.

Partial upper airways obstruction is characterized by noisy breathing, akin to snoring. Partial upper airways obstruction can be easily missed particularly in comatose patients who in addition often hypoventilate due to a depressed respiratory centre. Laryngeal or tracheal obstruction gives rise to a high pitched inspiratory sound termed 'stridor'.

Complete or almost complete airways obstruction results in marked inspiratory efforts with little or no movement of air into the lungs. There is severe retraction of the intercostal spaces, the sternum and epigastrium, together with strong contraction of the accessory muscles of respiration during inspiratory efforts. The patient, to start with, is extremely distressed, restless, anxious and becomes increasingly cyanosed. Tachycardia or a bradyrhythm is related to hypoxia. Death ensues if hypoxia is unrelieved.

Management

The treatment obviously is to relieve soft tissue obstruction by simple basic manoeuvres.

Neck Extension with Forward and Upward Chin Thrust

This should be the first manoeuvre to be attempted as it can promptly relieve mild to moderate obstruction by increasing the patency between the back of the tongue and the pharynx. The procedure is described in the Chapter on Cardiopulmonary resuscitation and Cerebral Preservation.

The Oropharyngeal Airway

This device is a conduit inserted along the top of the tongue until the teeth or gums limit its insertion. It is positioned between the base of the tongue and the pharynx (separating the two) thereby maintaining a patent airway. The airway should be inserted with its curve up initially and rotated into position when the end reaches the base of the tongue. It is designed to permit a suction catheter to pass through it, and allow suction of secretions in the pharynx and upper larynx.

An oropharyngeal airway is chiefly suited for comatose patients and that too for limited periods of time. As it rests at the base of the tongue, it stimulates the gag reflex, and can induce excessive salivation, vomiting and even laryngospasm in the conscious patient.

Nasopharyngeal Airway

The nasopharyngeal airway is a pliable plastic tube inserted (after lubrication) through the nares to follow the posterior wall curvature of the nasopharynx and oropharynx so that its tip rests on the base of the tongue, separating it from the pharyngeal wall. This airway is better tolerated than the oropharyngeal airway by the semiconscious and fully awake patient. It can prevent or relieve soft tissue upper airways obstruction and allows suctioning of the pharynx through a suction catheter passed through the airway. The nasopharyngeal airway can cause bleeding and airway trauma through pressure necrosis. Some advocate daily changing of the airway from one nare to the other to minimize trauma to the nasal passages. We very rarely use the nasopharyngeal airway in our unit.

Artificial Airways

If the above simple manoeuvres do not relieve upper airway obstruction or if the obstruction, to start with, is unlikely to be relieved by the oropharyngeal or nasopharyngeal airway, a more elaborate 'artificial airway' is established. An artificial airway is a conduit or tube inserted into the trachea bypassing the pharynx and larynx which no longer form part of the total airway. In essence, this means endotracheal intubation or a tracheostomy.

Indications

There are four indications for endotracheal intubation or tracheostomy.

1. To maintain an upper airway in the presence of obstruction to the pharynx or larynx. If the obstruction is such that it is technically impossible to do an endotracheal intubation one has no option other than to perform a tracheostomy.

2. To protect the airway in a patient whose protective mechanisms are poor.

The pharynx, vocal chords and the epiglottis play an important role in protecting the airway from aspiration of secretions, foreign matter, food or regurgitating gastric contents. The reflexes that normally protect the airways are: (i) the pharyngeal reflex, which normally includes the gag and swallowing reflexes; (ii) the laryngeal reflex, which is a vagal reflex, and is responsible for the apposition of the vocal cords, and closure of the epiglottis on stimulation of the larynx by secretions or by foreign matter; (iii) the tracheal reflex, which is a vagal reflex causing cough when the trachea is stimulated by some irritant or foreign matter; (iv) the carinal reflex, which is a vagal reflex causing cough on irritation of the carina.

The protective reflexes are generally obtunded from above downwards, irrespective of whether the cause of obtundation is due to drugs, disease or a deepening state of unconsciousness. When these reflexes return in a recovering patient, they recover from 'below' 'up'. The preservation of the pharyngeal reflex (gag reflex) therefore suggests preservation of the laryngeal and tracheal reflexes. However, the gag reflex is believed to be diminished or inelicitable in 10 per cent of the normal population. Therefore, absence of this reflex does not always indicate absence of other protective reflexes. Clinically, the inability to handle secretions in the upper airway and to swallow in a co-ordinated manner, denotes a loss of protective airway reflexes and necessitates the establishment of an artificial airway. In such patients, the artificial airway also seals the respiratory from the alimentary tract, thereby preventing aspiration of gastric contents into the tracheobronchial tree.

3. To facilitate suction of secretions (from within the tracheo-bronchial tree), which the patient is incapable of coughing up and expectorating. This could be because the secretions are copious, the cough reflex is poor, or the patient is just too feeble to cough and expectorate. Although it is possible to insert a suction catheter through the vocal cords for suctioning tracheal secretions, it is not advisable to do so except on rare occasions. Laryngeal oedema and obstruction, and precipitation of fatal arrhythmias in critically ill patients can occur following such attempts. The establishment of an artificial airway allows easy, safe and direct suctioning of the tracheobronchial tree.

4. It is mandatory that an artificial airway be established if ventilator support is required for an extended period of time. Non-invasive ventilation through an orofacial or nasal mask is advocated in special conditions but cannot be used for long periods of time.

The Disadvantages of Artificial Airways

The establishment and maintenance of an artificial airway (endotracheal intubation or tracheostomy) has its hazards and complications depending on the expertise with which it is established, the quality of after care, and the nature and degree of the critical illness in the patient. These complications are dealt with later. However, there are some inherent universal drawbacks of artificial airways which need to be considered.

1. An artificial airway bypasses the normal defence mechanisms which counter bacterial contamination of the airways. The airways and lungs are more prone to nosocomial infection.

2. An endotracheal tube removes the effectiveness of cough because the vocal cords are non-functional; a tracheostomy bypasses the cords.

3. An artificial airway prevents the patient from communicating vocally. This can be frustrating and frightening, and it is important, in a conscious patient, to provide a pad and a pen to help the patient communicate in writing.

4. In a conscious patient, there is often a feeling of a loss of dignity and a loss of control over one's self due to tubes which prevent the patient from speaking or breathing normally.

Establishing an Emergency Airway

An emergency airway is one that must be established immediately, with utmost urgency, as it involves a matter of life and death. The chief indications for an 'immediate' airway are:

(i) Severe life-threatening upper airways obstruction.

(ii) Cardiac or respiratory arrest—or impending cardiorespiratory arrest.

(iii) Fulminant pulmonary oedema.

The emergency airway of choice is an oral endotracheal intubation, with the aid of direct laryngoscopy. In an ICU or in any setting where the expertise and the necessary equipment is promptly available, oral endotracheal intubation can be performed in a matter of minutes. However, emergency endotracheal intubation may prove difficult even in experienced hands, and at times, may fail (see subsequent Section on Difficult Airway). In such circumstances, an alternative airway needs to be established urgently.

An emergency tracheostomy can be performed by an experienced surgeon in 15 minutes. A percutaneous tracheostomy can be carried out by an experienced intensivist or surgeon in perhaps even lesser time (see Chapter on Procedures in the ICU). If facilities for a tracheostomy are not immediately available, or if the emergency requires an airway to be established within a matter of minutes, a cricothyroidotomy with the insertion of a tube or conduit into the trachea may serve as a life-saving temporary emergency procedure. A cricothyroidotomy should be replaced with an appropriate airway as soon as possible. Nasotracheal intubation is an alternative for those used to this procedure, but it almost always lacks the speed of an oral laryngoscopic endotracheal intubation and is more often carried out as an elective procedure. Till such time as an emergency airway is ultimately secured, it is vital to continue to ventilate the patient with a bag-mask (AMBU) and to ensure that at least the upper airway (above the vocal cords) is patent (see Other Emergency Airways).

Technique of Oral Endotracheal Intubation

See Chapter on Procedures in the Intensive Care Unit

Technique of Nasotracheal Intubation

See Chapter on Procedures in the Intensive Care Unit

Technique of Cricothyroidotomy

See Chapter on Procedures in the Intensive Care Unit

Technique of Minitracheostomy (Percutaneous Tracheostomy)

See Chapter on Procedures in the Intensive Care Unit

Other Emergency Airways

The Laryngeal Mask Airway

The laryngeal mask airway (LMA) can secure the airway in an emergency, in a situation where endotracheal intubation fails, or in a situation where experienced personnel to intubate are unavailable. A properly placed LMA not only secures the airway, but allows ventilatory support and reduces the risk of gastric aspiration. A standard adult LMA consists of a 12 mm internal diameter tube fused at a 30° angle to an elliptical spoon shaped cuff with an inflatable rim (**Fig. 8.3.1(a)**). The cuff is soft and when inflated adapts to the shape of the larynx forming an airtight seal over it. The tube opens into the concavity of the cuff ellipse through a fenestrated aperture. The LMA should be placed with the patient placed in sniffing position—neck flexed and head extended. The cuff is deflated and lubricated prior to insertion. The patients mouth is opened and with the distal aperture of the cuff positioned anteriorly, the tip of the cuff is applied against the hard palate and advanced by the index finger of the right hand over the back of the tongue till it meets resistance when it abuts on the upper oesophageal sphincter. The cuff is inflated with 10 to 30 ml air

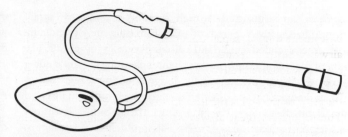

Fig. 8.3.1(a) Laryngeal Mask Airway.

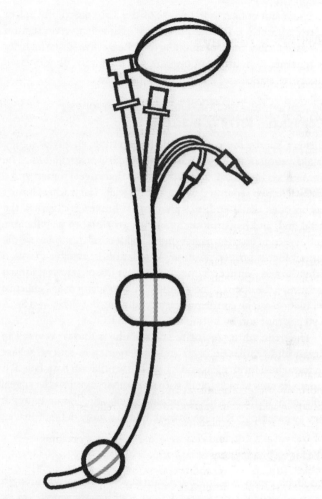

Fig. 8.3.1(b) Combitube.

so that the cuff centres on the laryngeal inlet. Studies show that the procedure is easily learnt by nurses and that adequate ventilation could be provided in 87 per cent of cases (**1**). Studies in mannequins suggest that the LMA decreased gastric distension compared to the AMBU and could be more easily placed than the combitube (**2**).

Intubating Laryngeal Mask Airway

The standard LMA can allow intubation through the aid of a fibreoptic bronchoscope. However, the size of the endotracheal tube that can be inserted through the LMA is necessarily small. The intubating LMA consists of an anatomically curved rigid tube with a metal guided handle and a distal silicone laryngeal cuff. The floor of the cuff aperture has an epiglottis elevating bar and guiding ramp which permits a specially designed endotracheal tube (8 mm in diameter) to be directed towards the glottis and inserted blindly into the trachea. The intubating LMA can be placed without moving the patient's head or neck. This is of definite advantage to patients who have sustained an injury to the cervical spine or to those who have an unstable cervical spine—situations where spinal flexion is best avoided.

The major concerns in the use of the LMA are: (i) the risk of gastric aspiration, (ii) the possibility of ineffective ventilation because of suboptimal positioning over the larynx, (iii) the inability to generate high inflation pressures in patients with increased airway resistance and a low lung compliance.

Oesophageal-Tracheal Double Lumen Airway (Combitube) (3) (Fig. 8.3.1(b))

This is a blindly inserted, double lumen tube, chiefly designed to aid ventilation during cardiopulmonary resuscitation. The combitube consists of two lumens—a pharyngeal lumen and a tracheal lumen separated by a partition wall. The tracheal lumen has an open distal end; the pharyngeal lumen is closed at the distal end, and has multiple openings proximal to its inflatable cuff. A second large ororpharyngeal balloon inflates to secure the combitube in proper position. Ventilation is possible through either lumen—either via the openings in the pharyngeal lumen or through the open tracheal lumen. Tube placement and effective ventilation can be confirmed by auscultating the chest, by a SaO_2 ≥ 90 per cent and by noting the end-tidal CO_2.

The main advantage of the combitube is that it provides an airway and ventilation in an acute emergency, in patients where endotracheal intubation and bag-mask ventilation have failed. It cannot be used in individuals with intact pharyngeal and laryngeal reflexes or in those with upper airways obstruction or an upper airway pathology. It is always a prelude to a more definite airway.

Difficult Airway

A difficult airway is a clinical situation in which an anaesthesiologist or an intensivist experiences difficulty with mask ventilation, or difficulty with tracheal intubation or both (4). Difficult mask ventilation implies an inability to maintain an O_2 saturation > 90 per cent using 100 per cent oxygen and positive pressure mask ventilation. Difficult intubations are those requiring three or more attempts using conventional laryngoscopy. In an ICU setting, a difficult to intubate airway may be apparent on a pre-intubation evaluation or becomes manifest only on attempted intubation. A markedly receding jaw, prominent incisors, macroglossia, soft tissue lesions obstructing the oropharynx or the entrance to the larynx, a rigid spine as in ankylosing spondylitis or a very anteriorly placed glottis can make intubation difficult or impossible.

Mallampati (5) assessed the ability to perform a direct laryngo-scopic endotracheal intubation by noting the degree of visibility of the faucial pillars and the uvula, with the patient seated, mouth wide open and the tongue fully protruded. Patients were classi-fied into three classes according to the difficulty experienced in intubation.

Class I—clearly visible fauces, uvula, with a wide oropharynx—easy intubation.

Class II—less clearly visible fauces and uvula, with a smaller opening of the oropharynx—intubation not as easy as in Class I.

Class III—poorly visible fauces, uvula with a small oropharynx, encroached upon by the above structures—intubation could prove difficult. This pre-intubation evaluation correlated with the laryn-goscopic visualization of the larynx—in Class I the larynx being well visualized and in Class III, the larynx being poorly visualized. Samsoon and Young (6) added a Class IV to Mallampati's classi-fication; Class IV is characterized by the inability to see the fauces, uvula and the oropharyngeal opening (patient seated, tongue pro-truded, mouth wide open). The vocal cords are not visualized on direct laryngoscopy, and intubation in these patients is generally unsuccessful.

In an emergency setting in the ICU, there is no time for elaborate pre-intubation evaluation. Patients requiring intubation are often hypoxic, restless, uncooperative and haemodynamically unstable. The simplest predictor of a likely successful intubation at the bedside in an emergency is the 'Rule of Threes'. If the intensivist can place three finger breadths (6 to 7 cm) between the upper and lower teeth, between the mandible and the hyoid bone and between the thyroid cartilage and the sternal notch, intubation is usually successful (7).

Difficult Intubation in the Critical Care Unit

It is important not to make several attempts at intubation as this traumatizes the pharynx, larynx and makes a subsequent successful intubation doubly difficult. Also, repeated attempts can render a hypoxic patient even more so, and often worsen haemodynamic instability. The management of failed endotracheal intubation attempts in a critical care setting should be considered under two heads.

I. Failed intubation attempts in patients in whom securing an airway and establishing effective ventilation is a matter of extreme urgency, a matter of life and death—e.g. cardiac arrest, respiratory arrest, extreme obstruction to the airway (Fig. 8.3.2).

The following emergency measures need to be followed:

1. Call for help

2. Continue bag-mask ventilation with 100 per cent oxygen. Two individuals can perform this more effectively than one. One individual ensures that the mask fits tightly over the nose and mouth, preventing any air leak; the other squeezes the AMBU bag fed with 100 per cent oxygen. The intensivist should note whether the bag-mask ventilation is effective, as judged by good breath sounds over both lungs and by an oxygen saturation ≥ 90 per cent. Difficulties in bag-mask ventilation are likely if any two of the following are present—age > 55 years, edentulous patient, obesity (body mass index > 26 kg/m^2), beard, history of snoring.

3. If a bag-mask ventilation fails or is ineffective, the situation is indeed very critical ('cannot intubate—cannot ventilate' scenario).

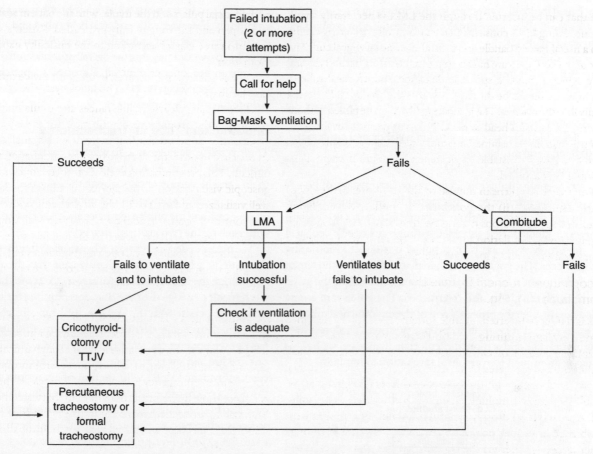

Fig. 8.3.2. Algorithm for the management of difficult airway and ventilation (in the ICU) in a life and death emergency.

Insert a laryngeal mask airway (LMA) or even better (if available), an intubating laryngeal mask airway (I-LMA) and ventilate the patient via this airway. If the intubating LMA is in place, attempt to intubate blindly using the specially designed endotracheal tube that goes with the I-LMA. Intubation (with a small sized endotracheal tube) can also be attempted through a plain LMA with the aid of a fibreoptic bronchoscope.

A combitube could be inserted into place instead of a LMA (by those who are more familiar with its use) in the hope of establishing effective ventilation. Effective ventilation is judged by an O_2 saturation ≥ 90 per cent and by measuring the end-tidal CO_2 through a capnograph.

If effective ventilation through a laryngeal mask airway or a combitube fails, and intubation via the LMA or via the I-LMA is unsuccessful, the quickest way of securing ventilation and preventing death from hypoxia, is by performing a cricothyroidotomy (see Chapter on Procedures in the ICU). A cricothyroidotomy should be promptly followed by an emergency percutaneous tracheostomy or by an emergency formal tracheostomy.

4. Even if either bag-mask ventilation or ventilation through a LMA or combitube is successful, a more permanent and secure artificial airway is mandatory if spontaneous effective breathing has not returned. This is achieved either by a percutaneous tracheostomy or a formal tracheostomy. In expert hands, this can be performed within 10 to 15 minutes.

5. If a pre-intubation clinical evaluation suggests that bag-mask ventilation or LMA ventilation cannot possibly be successful (as in extreme obstruction to the oropharynx, facial, neck injuries), proceed straight to a cricothyroidotomy, or a percutaneous tracheostomy, or a formal tracheostomy depending on the degree of urgency of the situation.

6. Transtracheal jet ventilation (TTJV) (8) is an alternative to a surgical airway in a 'cannot intubate–cannot ventilate' situation. After stabilizing the larynx, a 12 to 16 gauge catheter-over-needle (attached to a syringe partially filled with saline) is directed caudally through the cricothyroid membrane into the trachea. Tracheal entry is confirmed by aspiration of air bubbles. The catheter is now advanced (up to the hub), over the needle into the trachea with the aid of a small skin incision. The placement is confirmed by aspiration of air. The hub of the catheter is connected to a jet ventilation system. Care should be taken to stabilize the catheter and prevent any air leak at the incision site. We are not familiar with TTJV but it has been performed in all age groups and is the preferred surgical airway in children below 12 years. Airway obstruction below the larynx or complete upper airway obstruction can render expiration impossible and is a contraindication to TTJV. Complications with TTJV include subcutaneous emphysema, oesophageal puncture, bleeding, barotraumas. TTJV is an emergency measure and is continued only till such time as a definitive airway has been secured.

II. Failed intubation attempts in situations which are emergent but which still allow some time to the intensivist for establishing an airway (**Fig. 8.3.3**).

In the above circumstance, the intensivist should use one or more of the other intubation techniques:

(a) direct laryngoscopy with topical or local anaesthesia;

(b) use of a stylet, preferably a lighted one, to help guide the endotracheal tube into the trachea;

(c) a flexible fibreoptic scope to aid nasal or oral intubation;

(d) blind nasal intubation;

(e) intubation through a LMA;

(f) retrograde intubation (in very rare circumstances) (**9**)

Retrograde intubation is attempted by first puncturing the cricothyroid membrane with an 18-gauge introducer needle with catheter. A guide wire is threaded through the needle cephalad into the oropharynx and is then pulled out under vision using Magill forceps. The guide wire is then placed directly in the lumen of the endotracheal tube. The latter is then guided along the guide wire through the glottis into the trachea. The guide wire is now pulled out through the proximal end of the endotracheal tube and the endotracheal tube fixed in proper position. This procedure requires practice and is more difficult than it appears; we have as yet never attempted retrotracheal intubation in our unit.

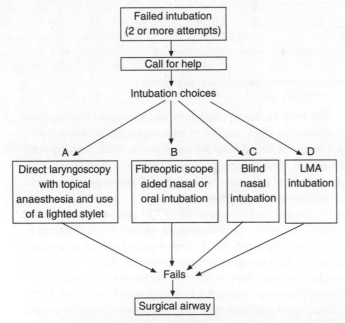

Fig. 8.3.3. Algorithm for the management of difficult airway and ventilation (in the ICU) in failed laryngoscopic attempts in less emergent situations.

Tracheostomy

A tracheostomy is, in our opinion, the most satisfactory artificial airway, particularly when the airway needs to be maintained for over 7 to 10 days. It completely bypasses the upper airway and the glottis, thus preventing any potential complications in that area. It causes less resistance to airflow (*vis à vis* the endotracheal tube), reduces dead space, allows easy and efficient suction of the tracheobronchial tree, and is easy to fix and stabilize. The conscious patient can eat freely, is not bothered by oropharyngeal secretions commonly observed with endotracheal tubes and tolerates the tracheostomy without undue discomfort. When performed by a skilled, experienced surgeon, the overall mortality (procedural with the tube in situ, or after removal) is around 1.5 per cent (range 0 per cent to 5 per cent) (**10, 11**). This holds even when the procedure is done in critically ill patients.

Endotracheal Tube vs Tracheostomy

There is still a controversy as to when to continue with an endotracheal tube and when to opt for a tracheostomy. The decision to do a tracheostomy or persist with the endotracheal tube rests on the intensivist's perception of optimal patient care, available nursing care and the unit's experience and record of complications with each of the two artificial airways.

We prefer to do an elective tracheostomy after first intubating the patient, whenever we are convinced that the disease will necessitate the use of an artificial airway for more than 7 days. If it is difficult to gauge the time duration required for the artificial airway, we persist with the endotracheal tube for about 7 to 10 days, and then change over to a tracheostomy. Probably each unit has its own preferences. We base our preferences on the fact that our unit has had few complications with tracheostomies, and that tracheobronchial toilet with suction of secretions is far easier through a tracheostomy than through an endotracheal tube. We have also noticed a significant incidence of subglottic oedema and stenosis whenever an endotracheal tube has been in place for more than 7 to 10 days, prompting us to switch to a tracheostomy if we feel that an artificial airway is required beyond that period of time. However, there are many units in the West which persist with an endotracheal tube for as long as 3 weeks without encountering significant complications.

Maintaining the Artificial Airway

It is not enough to establish and secure the airway. It is equally important to maintain, manage and care for the artificial airway, if the hazards and complications involving the use of artificial airways are to be minimized. This section initially describes the care of the tracheostomy; it then discusses artificial airway emergencies, followed by a brief mention of the other complications of tracheostomy. There then follows a description of the special features of endotracheal tube care and of complications peculiar to endotracheal intubation. The section ends with a brief description of the indications to extubate the patient.

Tracheostomy Care (Table 8.3.1)

A high tracheostomy is always preferable as it enables the tip of the tube to lie well above the carina. It is best to use the largest tube that can be comfortably accommodated by the trachea. Small tubes should be avoided as they tend to get blocked, and they offer resistance to airflow. This is particularly unwelcome in those patients with acute respiratory failure who have well marked airways obstruction, or who have a low compliance due to 'stiff lungs'. The tube should have an even inflated cuff. High residual

Table 8.3.1. Salient points in tracheostomy care

* Use sterile gloves for handling tracheostomy tube
* Care of cuff
  - Use minimal occluding volume for inflating cuff—minimal leak technique
  - Measure cuff pressure daily, and keep this within acceptable limits (14–24 cm H_2O)
  - Deflate cuff periodically, except when this is contraindicated for specific reasons
* Care over Suction of Secretions
  - Use 'no-touch' sterile technique
  - Pre-oxygenate (with high FIO_2) a haemodynamically unstable patient before suction
  - Do not suck for more than 10 seconds
  - Do not use a very large bore catheter for suction
  - If possible, suck through an adaptor so that ventilator support on high-flow oxygen is not interrupted
  - Stop suction if bradycardia or hypotension occur; Increase FIO_2 to 100 per cent for a short time
  - Liquefy viscid secretions; use physiotherapy
  - Humidify inspired gas
* Care of tracheostomy tube
  - Ensure that tube is central in position and does not tilt and slip into one bronchus
  - Ensure that tube does not get blocked
  - Change tube every 4–7 days
* Care of tracheostomy wound
  - use sterile dressing and antibiotic ointment
* Be alert to possible complications of tracheostomy (as listed in the text)

volume (low pressure) cuffs should be always used; high pressure cuffs have no place in modern respiratory care. Even when using high volume, low pressure cuffed tubes, the cuff pressure should be checked daily and kept within acceptable limits. Excessive cuff pressures can induce tracheal injury and subsequent stenosis, particularly if the tracheostomy has been in use over several days or weeks.

The following features are of great importance in tracheostomy care, and help in sharply reducing the incidence of complications in tracheostomy (**Table 8.3.1**):

(a) Use Sterile Gloves when Handling the Tracheostomy

Ensure that the tube is central in position and is not tilted at a sharp angle. The inspiratory blast from a ventilator during ventilator support is otherwise preferentially directed to the side of the tilt, resulting in uneven ventilation.

(b) Care over the Cuff

Keep the cuff inflated, but periodically deflate it to prevent undue pressure on the tracheal wall. The object of proper inflation is to push the minimal volume of air in the cuff, which will allow sealing of the airway—in other words, the aim is to use the minimal occluding volume, or as some prefer to term it—the minimal leak technique. This technique prevents undue pressure on the tracheal mucosa, and minimizes ischaemic necrosis of the mucosa (**12**). To achieve a minimal occluding volume within the cuff, inflate the cuff, and auscultate with a stethoscope over the larynx, so that no leak is heard. In patients on mechanical ventilator support, remove

small volumes of $^1/_4-^1/_2$ ml of air from the cuff until a small leak can be auscultated at the point of peak inflation pressure. In patients with spontaneous breathing, remove small increments of gas from the cuff till a small leak is audible with the stethoscope in early or mid-expiration. Once the minimal occluding volume is determined, the cuff volume should not be unnecessarily manipulated, unless the leak is too great to maintain appropriate airway pressure, or the peak inflation pressure has fallen significantly. Fortunately, small inexpensive pressure manometers are now available, so that cuff pressures as stated earlier, can be checked daily.

We periodically deflate the cuff though there are many units which do not advocate periodic deflation once the cuff has been inflated with the minimal leak technique. It is wiser to periodically deflate the cuff during prolonged ventilator support extending over many weeks or months, to relieve pressure on the tracheal mucosa for 10–15 minutes every 4–6 hours, provided that the increased leak following deflation allows adequate ventilation. In spontaneously breathing patients, we deflate the cuff for longer periods of time provided that there is no risk of aspiration. The cuff should always be kept inflated for a couple of hours after a patient has been fed, particularly if the feeding is through a nasogastric tube. Before deflating the cuff, the pharynx should be suctioned, to prevent accumulated secretions above the inflated cuff from being aspirated following deflation. The tracheobronchial tree should also be properly suctioned after deflation, so as to prevent any secretions above the cuff from trickling down into the tracheobronchial tree.

(c) Care over Suction of Secretions

(i) Suction of secretions should be done using sterile gloves, by a sterile catheter, held by sterile forceps. Sterile gloves are expensive and we have clearly proven that thorough scrubbing of the hands as in a surgical procedure, and use of the 'no-touch' technique through use of a sterile forceps, suffices. The procedure for suctioning is as follows: thoroughly pre-oxygenate the patient by using a high FIO_2, particularly if the patient is critically ill or haemodynamically unstable. Then introduce the catheter through the tracheostomy, well beyond the tip of the tracheostomy tube, using the 'no-touch' technique, and keeping the suction off. Apply suction while gently withdrawing the catheter, which is done with a slight rotating movement. This technique causes minimal trauma to the tracheal mucosa, and yet effectively suctions tracheobronchial secretions. Suctioning should not be carried out for more than 10–15 seconds. The catheter used for suction should not be too large, nor the force of suction too powerful, as this can result in a massive collapse of the lung. Nevertheless, adequate suction to remove secretions is necessary. In a critically ill, haemodynamically unstable patient, re-oxygenate with a high FIO_2, and allow the vital signs to return to baseline values before repeating the procedure. Suctioning should be repeated till the airway appears clear.

(ii) If possible, suction should be done through adaptors that allow tracheal suctioning without disconnecting the patient from the ventilator, or a high flow oxygen system. This reduces the severity of hypoxaemia during suctioning, and reduces the risk of cardiovascular complications (**13–17**).

(iii) The tracheobronchial tree is never free of secretions; in fact, there is something amiss if it is totally dry. Improper humidification of inspired gas is generally responsible for a dry tracheobronchial tree; drying and crusting of secretions often results in a partial blockage of the tracheostomy tube. On the other hand, routine suctioning at predetermined intervals is unwarranted. Suctioning should only be done as and when necessary.

(iv) Tracheobronchial secretions can be collected for culture in sterile 'traps' attached to the line of a suction catheter. Cultures should be done if secretions change colour, or are yellow or green in colour, particularly in the presence of fever and leucocytosis. Routine cultures done at periodic intervals are a waste of money, and do not help in management.

(v) Frequent, expertly given physiotherapy is vital in the drainage of secretions.

(vi) Normal saline or acetylcysteine help to liquefy viscid secretions, which can then be aspirated. We prefer normal saline, and only very rarely use acetylcysteine.

(vii) Adequate humidification of inspired gas or oxygen is mandatory, as it prevents drying and crusting of secretions.

Complications of Suctioning the Airways

The major complications are (i) cardiac arrest; (ii) arrhythmias; (iii) hypotension; (iv) massive lung collapse; (v) introduction of infection; and (vi) mechanical irritation of the tracheal mucosa. Ulceration of the mucosa can result from repeated powerful suctioning, when the catheter tip rests against the mucosal wall.

Cardiac arrest has been observed during or immediately after suctioning. It is more likely to occur in patients who are haemodynamically unstable, who have a low PaO_2 even while on ventilator support, or in those where the suctioning technique is faulty. Suctioning should not be continued for more than 10 seconds in critically ill patients, and prior oxygenation for 5–10 minutes (if necessary with 100 per cent oxygen) is mandatory in seriously ill cases. Cardiac arrest is generally due to acute hypoxaemia induced by suctioning which withdraws the oxygen rich gas from the tracheobronchial tree. In certain diseases, e.g. tetanus, cardiac arrest is triggered by a hyperactive vagal reflex.

Arrhythmias. Tachycardias or sudden bradyrhythms are frequent during suctioning in critically ill individuals. These could be due to hypoxia; bradycardia may occasionally be related to overactive vagal reflexes.

Hypotension results following a bradyrhythm induced by vagal stimulation, or is related to prolonged coughing during suctioning. Prolonged coughing interrupts ventilation, reduces venous return, and in conjunction with bradycardia can precipitate dangerous hypotension.

Massive lung collapse is likely to occur if a large bore suction catheter is inserted and a powerful suction force is applied. The large bore catheter prevents air from being entrained by the side of the catheter, and the associated powerful suction causes a lung collapse. Suction catheters should be no more than half the size of the tracheostomy tube, and a very powerful suction force should be avoided.

(d) Care of the Tracheostomy Tube

(i) Careless, unsterile methods of handling the tube are an important cause of infection of the tracheostomy wound or of the respiratory tract.

(ii) The greatest care should be taken to ensure that the tube is not blocked. Acute respiratory distress with a marked rise in peak inflation pressure and in dynamic compliance in a patient on ventilator support, should promptly suggest a blocked tube. When in doubt, it is always better to change the tube; in any case the tracheostomy tube should be changed every 4–5 days.

(iii) In a low tracheostomy, or in a patient with a short neck, ensure that the tube does not tilt and slip into one main bronchus (generally the right). The tube should be positioned so that it is well above the carina, and yet should be fixed so that it does not slip out.

(iv) Reinsertion of a tracheostomy tube may be difficult at times. A laryngoscope and an endotracheal tube must be kept at all times at the bedside of every patient with a tracheostomy.

(e) Care of the Tracheostomy Wound

Sterile dressing of the wound with the use of a topical antibiotic application or a spray containing neomycin is generally effective in keeping the wound clean. Heavy dressings should be avoided as otherwise the wound and the tube cannot be well observed.

Artificial Airway Emergencies (Fig. 8.3.4)

The three major emergencies associated both with tracheostomies and endotracheal tubes are:

(i) obstruction to the artificial airway;

(ii) inadvertent extubation;

(iii) cuff leaks.

(i) *Obstruction.* Partial or complete obstruction of the tube by crusted inspissated secretions is perhaps the commonest and most important complication. A blocked tube can be disastrous if undetected or detected too late. Prevention of blockage by proper care of the artificial airway is vital.

Obstruction at times is observed below the lower end of the artificial airway. This is generally due to an overdistended cuff herniating over the lower end and blocking it. Prompt deflation of the cuff rapidly relieves the obstruction. Obstruction also occurs when the trachea below the cuff is partially clogged by inspissated mucous—a problem invariably due to inadequate humidification of inspired gas.

An endotracheal tube may sometimes be obstructed by a kink; slight manipulation of the head and neck should then restore patency. The bevel of the artificial airway may occasionally abut against the tracheal wall, carina or even bronchus, producing partial obstruction. This is relieved by gentle manipulation of the tube.

When faced with a possible obstruction to an artificial airway: (a) attempt to pass a suction catheter through the tube and note its passage—whether easy or obstructed; (b) deflate the cuff; (c) gently manipulate the tube. If none of these measures are effective, then the tube is promptly removed. Also, whenever there is a doubt about the exact cause of respiratory distress, as an ample measure of safety, the tube should be promptly changed. It is worth bearing in mind that an important cause of severe respiratory distress which resembles a blocked tube is a tension pneumothorax. A cardinal rule in the ICU is that a patient with an artificial airway must always have a duplicate artificial airway as also intubation and ventilation equipment at his bedside.

(ii) *Inadvertent extubation.* This could prove disastrous if not urgently rectified in a patient on ventilator support who is paralyzed or heavily sedated. It abruptly cuts off ventilation, can produce serious surgical emphysema of the head, neck and chest as also mediastinal emphysema. If the endotracheal tube lies above the vocal cords serious gastric distension can occur.

(iii) *Cuff leaks.* Cuff leaks are the least dangerous of the three artificial airway emergencies. A cuff leak can generally be compensated for by merely increasing the tidal volume in a patient on ventilator support. If this does not provide adequate ventilation, the airway will need to be changed.

Other Complications of Tracheostomy (Fig. 8.3.4)

(a) *Ulceration with pressure necrosis of the trachea.* Pressure of an inflated cuff or the tip of the tracheostomy tube may result in ulceration with pressure necrosis. The incidence of this is increased by the presence of an associated infection or the use of corticosteroids. In rare instances, the trachea may be perforated, and there is serious danger of erosion of a large vein or even the inominate artery, with severe bleeding and death resulting from aspiration of blood into the lungs.

(b) *Tracheal bleeding.* Bleeding often occurs into and around the trachea, and within the wound in patients who have a bleeding tendency, particularly in the presence of hypoxia and hypercapnia. It takes the form of a capillary ooze, the main danger being of aspiration pneumonia and infection. Tracheal bleeding also occurs from pressure of the tube, specially when the tracheal mucosa has been rendered friable by repeated suction or infection. Exsanguinating bleeds are invariably due to perforation of a large vessel within the mediastinum.

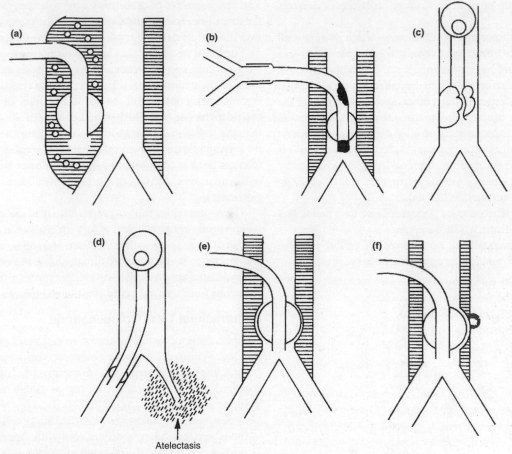

Atelectasis

Fig. 8.3.4. Complications of tracheostomy.
(a) Tube in pretracheal fascia—resulting in surgical emphysema of face and neck and sometimes of the mediastinum.
(b) Blocked tube.
(c) Overinflated cuff slipping over the end and blocking it.
(d) Tube slipping into right main bronchus, preventing ventilation to the left lung.
(e) Damage to trachea, either due to a very tight-fitting tube with an overinflated cuff, or injury to the posterior wall—end result, dilatation (as in the figure) or stricture.
(f) Erosion of the posterior wall of the trachea, and rarely erosion of the inominate artery.
(from Udwadia FE. (1979). Diagnosis and Management of Acute Respiratory Failure. OUP, Mumbai).

(c) *Respiratory nosocomial infection.* Infection is a serious and common complication. Prevention is by scrupulous asepsis during the performance of tracheostomy, and meticulous after-care of the tracheostomy. *Every single tracheal aspiration should be considered as an aseptic surgical procedure, and should be performed with meticulous attention to detail.* The mere growth of bacteria in tracheal aspirates is no evidence of active infection. Gram-negative organisms invariably grow from tracheal aspirates within a few days of a tracheostomy. The presence of fever, purulent secretions, leucocytosis and changing X-ray shadows determine the diagnosis of nosocomial infection (see Chapter on Nosocomial Pneumonia).

(d) *Mediastinal Emphysema.* This is invariably associated with surgical emphysema of the neck, and at times of the face and chest.

(e) *Tracheal stenosis* (**Fig. 8.3.5**). Tracheal stenosis is an important and dreaded complication of tracheostomy. It can occur anytime between 1 week to 2 years following tracheostomy. Post-extubation tracheal stenosis occurs at any one of the following three sites: (i) at the tracheostomy site, the incidence of this depends on the surgical technique; (ii) at the cuff site: this is the commonest site for stenosis; (iii) at the point where the tube tip irritates or damages the tracheal wall.

Conditions predisposing to tracheal stenosis include a high cuff pressure (**12, 18, 19**), prolonged ventilatory support over weeks or months (**20**), and haemodynamic instability with periods of poor perfusion which contribute to devitalization of the tracheal mucosa (**18, 21**). Infection of the trachea, undue movement of the tracheostomy tube, or a tube tilted to one side so that its end irritates and produces pressure necrosis of a localized area of tracheal mucosa, are all contributory factors (**18, 22, 23**). Some workers have incriminated toxicity from chemical irritation produced by the tube material as an aggravating factor, particularly following ethylene chloride sterilization (**22, 24**).

In over 1200 tracheostomies performed, we have had only 5 patients with significant tracheal stenosis.

(f) *Tracheal Dilatation.* This occurs over the area of pressure exerted by the cuff, and can be prevented by proper cuff care.

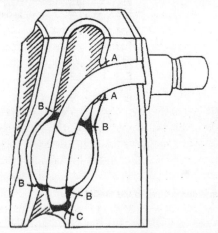

Fig. 8.3.5. Sites for occurrence of post-extubation tracheal stenosis.
A—site of tracheostomy
B—cuff site (commonest)
C—where tip irritates tracheal wall

(g) *Tracheomalacia.* A softening of the trachea may occur following tracheostomy. This leads to inspiratory collapse of the trachea with obstruction of the airway following extubation.

(h) *Cardiorespiratory Collapse.* The association of cardiorespiratory collapse has been observed by us immediately following tracheostomy performed to relieve severe upper airways obstruction. It is generally seen when the tracheostomy is done on a patient who is 'in extremis'. It does not occur if the airway has been first secured by an endotracheal tube, and the patient ventilated and oxygenated before doing a tracheostomy. Bendixen and his colleagues (**25**) believe that in patients with sudden severe airways obstruction, the hypoxia and hypercapnia produce a marked sympathetic stimulation with catecholamine liberation. If the sympathetic stimulus is suddenly removed, as after an emergency tracheostomy, then cardiovascular collapse may occur. In a similar fashion, if the respiratory drive produced by acute hypoxia and hypercapnia ceases, respiratory arrest can occur.

Care of Endotracheal Tube

The discussion on tracheostomy care also applies generally to the care of the endotracheal tube, particularly in relation to care over the cuff and care over suction of airway secretions.

There are just two other important points that need to be stressed. Frequent movement of head and neck, or sharp movement of the endotracheal tube (as when the attached ventilator is shifted from one side of the bed to the other or shifted from behind to the side of the bed) should be avoided. Reattachment of the tube to the ventilator should be done without swinging the tube up and down or from side to side. The tube rests with its fulcrum on the vocal cords and frequent movement of the tube is an important cause of damage to the vocal cords and the subglottic area.

The endotracheal tube is a foreign body in the upper airway. It often promotes a great deal of salivation which accumulates in the throat or settles on to the cuff. These secretions, often teeming with bacteria, can be aspirated into the lungs not only when the cuff is deflated but even otherwise. It is important to suction these secretions from the oral cavity at required intervals.

Endotracheal Tube Complications

Complications following the use of an endotracheal tube are in the main, common to those observed with a tracheostomy. Complications which are peculiar to endotracheal intubation (and observed after extubation) are laryngeal complications. These include the following:

(a) *Sore throat and hoarse voice.* Minimal damage to the epithelium of the pharynx and larynx occurs even with expert intubation. There is some degree of sloughing of the mucosa leading to a sore throat and hoarse voice. Hoarseness lasts for a day or two. Adequate humidity of the inspired gas helps in quick recovery.

(b) *Glottic oedema.* Glottic oedema is due to (i) trauma during intubation; (ii) poor maintenance of the tube; (iii) insertion of oversized tubes. Glottic oedema occurs in the submucosa of the vocal cords, but can also involve the submucosa of the epiglottis or the aryepiglottic folds. Inspiratory stridor and respiratory distress occur if more than half the glottic opening is narrowed. Inspiratory stridor occurring immediately after extubation is a source of worry, as extension of the oedema could cause increasingly dangerous narrowing of the glottic orifice.

Treatment consists of: (i) adequate humidification of inspired gas; (ii) intravenous administration of 10 mg dexamethasone to reduce inflammatory oedema; (iii) the application of a topical vasoconstrictor (2.25 per cent racemic epinephrine) through a nebulizer, if this drug is available.

If glottic oedema progresses and is unrelieved by the above measures, the patient may need reintubation or an elective tracheostomy.

(c) *Subglottic oedema.* Subglottic oedema after extubation is dangerous as it often obstructs the airway, and then necessitates either reintubation or an elective tracheostomy; we prefer the latter procedure under the above circumstance. It is more common in infants and children due to the small internal diameter of the larynx. The subglottic region is vulnerable to trauma because of the presence of loose submucosal connective tissue in that area, and because of the cricoid cartilage which encircles the larynx and prevents any external expansion.

Subglottic oedema may be assumed if post-extubation oedema does not respond to treatment within a day or two. It may be treated with intravenous dexamethasone for a few days, but if unresponsive, the definitive treatment is reintubation or preferably an elective tracheostomy.

(d) *Vocal cord ulceration, granuloma.* Hoarseness persists for over a week after extubation. The aetiology is trauma by the tube during intubation or during maintenance of the tube. Excessive movement of the tube or the head and neck, or excessive coughing can seriously damage the cords.

(e) *Vocal cord paralysis.* Unilateral recurrent laryngeal nerve palsy may result from surgery in the neck and upper chest. However, bilateral vocal cord palsy is a known complication of endotracheal intubation, the cause of which is uncertain.

(f) *Laryngeal web.* Necrosis of the glottic and subglottic area may heal with the formation of fibrous tissue that forms a web in the subglottic area. The web must obstruct two thirds or more of the opening below the cords to cause obstructive symptoms of stridor and respiratory distress. Laryngeal webs generally occur 4 to 5 days after extubation but have been reported to occur or manifest 2 months to 2 years post-extubation. The obstructing web is frequently visualized during reintubation. Aspiration through a suction catheter serves to remove the web, else it could obstruct the endotracheal tube or slip into a main bronchus. A tight subglottic obstructing membrane may need specific laser surgery to restore the patency of the subglottic airway.

Removal of the Tracheostomy Tube

The patient should be extubated when the reason for performing a tracheostomy to secure an artificial airway no longer exists. The patient should have normal protective reflexes that enable him to handle his upper respiratory secretions, and swallow well. He should be able to cough effectively, and breathe spontaneously without ventilator support (see Chapter on Mechanical Ventila-

tion). We have never encountered any difficulty in directly removing the tube and closing the tracheostomy orifice with a dressing. We have hardly ever found it necessary to change to smaller tubes or to fenestrated tubes, even in patients who have had a tracheostomy together with ventilator support for over 4–6 months. If the decision to remove the tracheostomy tube proves to be premature, the tube is promptly reinserted, till it is deemed fit to again extubate the patient. The tracheal stoma usually heals and closes within 3–7 days of extubation.

Endotracheal Tube Extubation

The tube is removed when the indications for its use cease to exist. The procedure must be explained to the patient so that cooperation is ensured. To start with, tracheal secretions are aspirated, followed by suction of secretions from the oropharynx and nasopharynx. It is preferable that the lungs are inflated completely so that the patient exhales or coughs as the tube is withdrawn from the larynx. This is achieved by asking the patient to take a deep breath and at the height of inspiration the cuff is deflated and the tube withdrawn from the larynx. Following extubation, oxygen is promptly administered at 2 to 4 l/minute. The airway should be carefully watched for obstruction, manifested by noisy breathing or stridor. The patient should not be left unattended till it is certain that he can function without the need for an artificial airway.

Special Considerations in Airway Management

Cervical Spine Injury

A patient with polytrauma, who requires intubation should be presumed to have a cervical spine injury. In the absence of severe maxillo-facial trauma or cerebrospinal rhinorrhoea a nasal intubation can be attempted. However, if urgent intubation is required as in the apnoeic or hypoxic patient, oral intubation should be done. During oral endotracheal intubation, a colleague or assistant should hold the neck in position, ensuring axial stability and preventing any flexion or anterior movement of the neck for fear of damaging the spinal cord.

Increased Intracranial Tension

Intubating patients with head injury who have a rise in intracranial pressure may be difficult for several reasons—change in mental state, difficulty in opening the mouth, associated facial trauma. Further rise in intracranial pressure should be avoided as far as possible during intubation. Also, cervical spine trauma should always be suspected in a patient with head injury. The anaesthetic agent used for intubating these patients should ideally preserve cerebral perfusion, and lower cerebral blood volume while maintaining haemodynamic stability. Thiopental offers neuroprotection but cerebral hypoperfusion may result from its depressant effect on the myocardium and because of peripheral vasodilatation. Etomidate is preferred in haemodynamically unstable patients. If a neuroparalytic agent needs to be used for intubation, vecuronium (0.25 mg/kg) or rocuronium (1.2 mg/kg) is to be preferred.

In patients with polytrauma including head injury with raised intracranial pressure, it may at times be impossible to perform a laryngoscopic endotracheal intubation. The airway may need to be secured by alternative means (see Difficult Airway).

REFERENCES

1. Stone BJ, Leach AB, Alexander CA et al. (1994). The use of the laryngeal mask by nurses during cardiopulmonary resuscitation: results of a multicentre trial. Anaethesia. 49, 3.

2. Doerges V, Sauer C, Ocker H et al. (1999). Airway management during cardiopulmonary resuscitation—a comparative study of bag-valve mask, laryngeal mask airway and combitube in a bench model. Resuscitation. 41, 63.

3. Frass M, Rodler S, Frenzer R et al. (1989). Esophageal tracheal combitube, endotracheal airway, and mask: comparison of ventilatory pressure curves. J Trauma. 29, 1476.

4. Mallampati SR. (1983). Clinical Signs to predict difficult tracheal intubations. Can Anaesth Soc J. 30, 316–318.

5. Mallampati SR, Gatt SP, Gugino LD et al. (1985). A clinical sign to predict difficult tracheal intubation: a prospective study. Can Anaesth Soc J. 32, 429–434.

6. Samsoon GLT, Young JRB. Difficult tracheal intubation: a retrospective study. Anaesthesia. 1987. 42, 487–490.

7. Watson CB. (1999). Prediction of difficult intubations. Resp Care. 44, 777–798.

8. Benumof JL, Scheller MS. (1989). The importance of transtracheal jet ventilation in the management of the difficult airway. Anaesthesiology. 71, 769.

9. Sanchez A, Pallares V. (1996). Retrograde intubation technique. In: Airway Management: principles and Practice (Ed. Benumof JL). pp. 320–341. Mosby, St Louis.

10. Stauffer JL, Olson DE, Petty TL. (1981). Complications and consequence of endotracheal intubation and tracheostomy: a prospective study of 150 critically ill adult patients. Am J Med. 70, 65.

11. Marsh HM, Gillespie DJ, Baumgartner AE. (1989). Timing of tracheostomy in the critically ill patient. Chest. 96, 190.

12. Off D, Braun SR, Tompkins B et al. (1983). Efficacy of the minimal leak technique of cuff inflation in maintaining proper intracuff pressures for patients with cuffed artificial airways. Respir Care. 28, 1115.

13. Belling D, Kelley RR, Simon R. (1978). The use of the swivel adaptor aperture during suctioning to prevent hypoxemia in the mechanically ventilated patient. Heart Lung. 7, 320.

14. Bodai BI. (1982). A means of suctioning without cardiopulmonary depression. Heart Lung. 11, 172.

15. Brown SE, Stansbury DW, Merrill EJ et al. (1983). Prevention of suctioning related arterial oxygen desaturation: comparison of off ventilator and on ventilator suctioning. Chest. 83, 621.

16. Cabol L, Devaskar S, Siassi B et al. (1979). New endotracheal tube adaptor reducing cardiopulmonary effects of suctioning. Crit Care Med. 7, 552.

17. Zmora E, Merritt TA. (1980). Use of a side hole endotracheal tube adaptor for tracheal aspiration. Am J Dis Child. 134, 250.

18. Stauffer GL, Olson DE, Petty TL. (1981). Complications and consequences of endotracheal intubation and tracheostomy. A prospective study of 150 critically ill adult patients. Am J Med. 70, 65.

19. Cooper JD et al. (1969). The evaluation of tracheal injury due to ventilatory assistance through cuffed tubes. Ann Surg. 169, 334.

20. Kastanow W, Mire RE, Perez AM et al. (1983). Laryngotracheal injury due to endotracheal intubation: incidence, evolution, and predisposing factors. A prospective long-term study. Crit Care Med. 11, 362.

21. Asas AS. (1975). Complications of tracheostomy and long-term intubation: A follow-up study. Acta Anesthesiol Scand. 19, 127.

22. Geffin B et al. (1971). Stenosis following tracheostomy for respiratory care. JAMA. 216, 1984.

23. Pearson FG et al. (1968). A prospective study of tracheal injury complicating tracheostomy with cuffed tubes. Ann Otol Rhinol Laryngol. 77, 1.

24. Shapiro BA, Kacmarek RM, Cane RD, Peruzzi WT, Hauptman D. (1991). Laryngeal and Tracheal Complications of Artificial Airways. In: Clinical Application of Respiratory care, 4th edn. pp. 195–205. Mosby Year Book, Boston, Chicago, London, Toronto.

25. Bendixen HH, Egbert LD, Hedley-Whyte J, Laver MB, Pontoppidan H. (1965). In: Respiratory Care. CV Mosby, St. Louis.

Acute Respiratory Crisis in Chronic Obstructive Pulmonary Disease (COPD)

Acute respiratory crisis occurring in patients with chronic airways obstruction is an important and frequent problem encountered in ICUs in most parts of the world (1–3). This chapter briefly deals with the precipitating factors, recognition, and management principles in acute respiratory crisis in patients with chronic obstructive pulmonary disease. Respiratory crisis in these patients is often in the form of acute respiratory failure occuring against a background of a pre-existing chronic respiratory failure. A crisis of acute respiratory failure may also be triggered by various precipitating factors in patients with well marked COPD, who under basal conditions are not in respiratory failure.

Precipitating Factors

Various precipitating factors produce acute respiratory failure in patients with chronic airways obstruction (**Table 8.4.1**).

The single most important precipitating factor is an acute infection causing an exacerbation of bronchitis, or a pneumonia. Bronchial infection causes increasing airways obstruction from bronchoconstriction, mucosal oedema and inflammation and increased secretions. The commonest organisms encountered in our unit during an acute exacerbation are the Streptococcus pneumoniae and the Haemophilus influenzae. Moraxella catarrhalis and Staphylococcus have been isolated with an increasing incidence over the last five years. In elderly patients, Gram-negative infections chiefly due to Klebsiella or Pseudomonas are observed. In the West,

Table 8.4.1. Precipitating factors for acute respiratory failure in patients with COPD

* Acute infection, causing exacerbation of bronchitis or pneumonia
* Noncompliance with prescribed drugs
* Use of respiratory depressant drugs and sedatives
* Post-operative
* Pneumothorax, pleural effusion from any cause
* Atelectasis of one or more segments of a lung
* Trauma (fractures e.g. fracture femur or fracture of a rib)
* Acute infections outside the respiratory system
* Pulmonary thromboembolism
* Associated left ventricular failure with pulmonary oedema
* Sputum retention from any cause
* Blood loss

respiratory viruses are associated with 30 per cent of exacerbations with or without superadded bacterial infection (4). Atypical bacteria, mostly Chlamydia pneumoniae, account for 10 per cent of acute exacerbations (5). The role of viral infections, Chlamydia and Mycoplasmal infections in acute exacerbations of COPD in India is not known.

The next most important precipitating factor is the use of sedatives and respiratory depressants in patients with chronic bronchitis and emphysema. Morphine can be lethal; pethidine, diazepam, barbiturates and other tranquillizers are also dangerous, and often tip the patient into an acute respiratory crisis.

Acute respiratory failure occurs as an important post-operative complication in patients with chronic bronchitis or emphysema. This is due to several factors, including the depressant effects of anaesthesia, and the use of sedatives and narcotics for insomnia and pain. Suppression of cough due to pain, or by drugs, or because the patient is critically ill, leads to sputum retention, and worsens respiratory failure.

Environmental factors play an important role in acute exacerbations of COPD. In Mumbai, the sharp rise in incidence of acute respiratory crisis in the months of December, January, February are partly related to weather conditions causing a thick layer of polluted air to hang low over the city till mid-afternoon. Increased levels of ozone and fine particulate air pollutants particularly in dense vehicular traffic can also precipitate an acute crisis.

The complication of even a shallow pneumothorax, pleural effusion or a small patch of pneumonia or atelectasis in a patient with severe chronic bronchitis, emphysema, can also cause acute respiratory failure. These complications may often be impossible to detect on clinical examination.

Acute respiratory failure may be triggered in chronic bronchitis by acute congestive heart failure, pulmonary thromboembolism, sleep disordered breathing, trauma, blood loss, fractures, prolonged recumbency, or acute infections not involving the respiratory tract. Pulmonary thromboembolism can be easily missed. When suspected, a Doppler study of the leg veins for deep vein thrombosis, followed if necessary by an HRCT pulmonary angiography is warranted.

It is important to search for and identify precipitating factors in patients admitted to the ICU for an acute respiratory crisis in COPD.

It is only then that management becomes more meaningful and more likely to meet with success.

Pathogenesis

The physiopathology underlying a worsening crisis in COPD consists of: (a) increase in ventilation-perfusion ($\dot{V}/\dot{Q}$) mismatch leading to hypoxaemia; (b) a decrease in minute ventilation or an increase in dead space or both combined together, so that there is a fall in alveolar ventilation with a rise in $PaCO_2$.

If $\dot{V}/\dot{Q}$ mismatch is alone present the patient is hypoxaemic; if $\dot{V}/\dot{Q}$ mismatch is associated with alveolar hypoventilation, the patient is both hypoxaemic and hypercapnic.

Severe airflow obstruction (due to spasm, mucosal oedema, inflammation or secretions) results in air-trapping, a reduced chest wall compliance and dynamic hyperinflation (i.e. the development of increasing intrinsic or auto-PEEP). The latter feature necessitates an increased work load on the inspiratory muscles to generate the increased negative intrapleural pressure required to initiate inspiratory airflow. The inspiratory muscles lengthen consequent to increased air-trapping, so that their optimal length-tension relationship is exceeded. They therefore work at a mechanical disadvantage. The diaphragm too is far less effective in aiding inspiration than in normal subjects. The combination of increased work of breathing, reduced mechanical efficiency and capability of respiratory muscles, together with dynamic hyperinflation can lead to disastrous consequences—progressive respiratory muscle fatigue, increasing alveolar hypoventilation and even respiratory arrest (6–9).

Dynamic hyperinflation (increasing auto-PEEP) results in compression of the capillaries, worsening pulmonary hypertension and right heart strain and failure. Pulmonary vasoconstriction, chiefly due to hypoxia, but also due to hypercapnia further increases pulmonary hypertension. Right ventricular strain may cause a shift of the interventricular septum to the left, thereby reducing diastolic filling of the left ventricle and compromising left ventricular function. Haemodynamic instability and compromise result.

Diagnosis

An acute exacerbation of COPD generally includes a combination of the following features: increasing dyspnoea, purulent sputum, increased quantity of sputum. An increased respiratory rate and tachycardia are commonly observed, together with the clinical signs of airways obstruction (prolonged expiration, polyphonic rhonchi, use of accessory muscles of respiration and often an over-inflated chest). Acute respiratory failure results when the PaO_2 falls well below 60 mm Hg and/or the $PaCO_2$ is greater than 48 to 50 mm Hg. Patients with severe COPD who are in a stable state, may however show a $PaO_2 < 60$ mm Hg and a $PaCO_2 > 50$ mm Hg. An exact assessment of the degree of respiratory compromise in an acute exacerbation can only be assessed if blood gas studies during a stable state are available.

The difficulty arises in hypercapnic individuals who appear to have a 'lazy' respiratory centre, and who do not demonstrate the usual respiratory distress. Due to hypoventilation and very tight airways obstruction, auscultation may not reveal any wheeze, unless the patient is made to perform a forced expiratory manoeuvre. Warm peripheries and flapping tremors are not always evident with hypercapnia. What is more, flaps are sometimes observed with a very mild to moderate rise in the $PaCO_2$, but may be absent with a marked rise in $PaCO_2$. Drowsiness, confusion, apathy and cyanosis are all important pointers to the gravity of the situation. Carbon dioxide retention is an important cause of metabolic coma, and could be missed unless the $PaCO_2$ is measured.

Blood Gas Patterns in Chronic Bronchitis Emphysema

Not all patients with chronic bronchitis emphysema retain carbon dioxide. Our experience over many years suggests that there are three blood gas profiles prevalent in our country, in patients with severe chronic airways obstruction:

(i) A lowered PaO_2 and a raised $PaCO_2$ even under basal or optimal conditions. This profile is observed in about 40–50 per cent of patients. In an acute crisis there is a significant change in the baseline values. The PaO_2 is further lowered, generally to < 55 mm Hg and often to as low as 30 mm Hg, and the $PaCO_2$ is sharply increased. Whereas under basal or optimal conditions the pH is generally normal (in spite of hypercapnia) because of bicarbonate retention by the kidneys, in an acute crisis the further sharp rise in the PCO_2 produces a fall in pH due to respiratory acidosis and acidaemia. In acute respiratory acidosis the pH is expected to drop by 0.08 for every 10 mm rise in PCO_2. It is extremely important from both the prognostic and management point of view, to consider not only the severity of hypoxia and hypercapnia, but the degree of acidaemia as judged by pH values in patients with COPD who develop acute on chronic respiratory failure. The lower the pH, the worse the prognosis.

(ii) A lowered PaO_2 with a normal $PaCO_2$ under basal or optimal conditions. However during an acute crisis (as following an acute infection), there is hypoxia (< 60 mm Hg) and definite hypercapnia (> 48–50 mm Hg). The $PaCO_2$ may show a further progressive rise if uncontrolled oxygen therapy is given. The propensity to alveolar hypoventilation in this group of patients, is thus only evident during an acute crisis. Once the crisis is weathered, the $PaCO_2$ returns to normal levels. This pattern is observed in about 30–40 per cent of patients.

(iii) A lowered PaO_2 with a normal or low $PaCO_2$. Here the $PaCO_2$ does not rise during an acute crisis or following the 'uncontrolled' use of oxygen at > 2 l/min. This pattern is seen in < 20 per cent of patients. The $PaCO_2$ in these patients may remain normal almost up to the end. A rise may be observed only in the terminal stages.

The marked rise in the $PaCO_2$ often observed in the first two profiles could be due to the following factors:

(i) An abnormal control over respiration with a comparative lack of sensitivity of the respiratory centre to increasing $PaCO_2$. This has now been disputed by some workers. It is however a point which is both difficult to prove or disprove. In clinical practice, the 'lazy' undistressed, unhurried respiration seen in some of these patients in spite of severe hypoxia and hypercapnia, does suggest a 'lazy' centre.

(ii) An inability of the 'bellows' or the thoracic pump (the respiratory muscles and thoracic cage) to increase ventilation. In patients with COPD, the 'load' against which respiratory muscles work is significantly increased due to increased airways resistance and increased elastance. The cause of an increased elastic load is 'air trapping' within the lungs, also termed dynamic overinflation. This results in the occurrence of a positive end-expiratory pressure within the lungs (auto-PEEP), with the patient having to breathe with greater difficulty at larger lung volumes. The presence of auto-PEEP and hyperinflation causes the inspiratory muscles to operate at a disadvantageous portion of their force-length relationship, predisposing to muscle fatigue. A slight increment in respiratory load (further increase in airways resistance and/or elastance), or a slight decrement in muscle strength, precipitates increasing fatigue, resulting in hypoventilation, progressive hypoxia and hypercapnia.

Both these factors are probably of equal importance. There may be different subsets of patients where one or the other factor may play a dominant role.

Investigations

Investigations should include a total blood count and PCV, arterial pH and blood gas analysis, serum electrolytes, sputum examination for Gram's stain and culture sensitivity tests, and a chest X-ray. An elective detailed diagnostic work-up has been detailed in the Chapter on Acute Respiratory Failure. In particular, the degree of airways obstruction should be assessed by measuring the peak expiratory flow rate, the FVC and the FEV_1, if at all possible. An ECG may show the presence of right ventricular or right atrial hypertrophy, demonstrating the presence of chronic cor pulmonale; it could also reveal associated left heart disease.

Management (Table 8.4.2)

The objectives of management are:

1. To improve ventilation, correct $\dot{V}/\dot{Q}$ abnormalities in so far as this is possible, increase the PaO_2, correct a lowered pH,

Table 8.4.2. Management of acute respiratory crisis in patients with COPD

---

1. Improve ventilation, correct ventilation-perfusion mismatch, and correct severe hypoxia
   * Controlled oxygen therapy (24–30% oxygen)
   * Treat infection with antibiotics
   * Relieve airways obstruction—nebulize salbutamol 4 hrly, ipratropium bromide 12 hrly
   * Use corticosteroids
   * Physiotherapy to drain secretions and prevent sputum retention
   * Mechanical ventilator support when so indicated
   * Cardiovascular support when necessary
2. Treat complications encountered during acute respiratory failure
   * Correct fluid and electrolyte disturbances
   * Manage cardiac complications e.g. arrhythmias, right-sided heart failure, and pulmonary thromboembolism
   * Treat GI bleeds
   * Drain even a shallow pneumothorax

---

and reduce the $PaCO_2$. *Relief of dangerous hypoxia is the* prime objective.

2. Recognize and treat complications that occur in the course of acute respiratory failure, or those that are produced iatrogenically by measures used to treat the acute crisis.

Management Strategy (10, 11)

The fundamental measures include the use of controlled oxygen therapy, the treatment of infection with antibiotics, the recognition and management of any other precipitating factor, the use of bronchodilators and corticosteroids to help relieve airways obstruction, and physiotherapy to help drain secretions and prevent sputum retention.

About seventy per cent of patients will show a satisfactory response with the above treatment. The remaining however demonstrate significant and often progressive rise in the $PaCO_2$, with a dangerous fall in arterial pH and with increasing symptoms of carbon dioxide narcosis even on controlled oxygen therapy. Previously, we used to add respiratory stimulants (doxapram 0.5–4 mg/min in an infusion) to this regime to help tide patients over a critical period, and allow time for the antibiotics, bronchodilators, corticosteroids and physiotherapy to act. Today however, we prefer to electively ventilate these patients till such time as lung function improves to a point which will allow spontaneous ventilation, with satisfactory PaO_2, pH and $PaCO_2$ levels. The selection of patients for ventilatory support requires experience and expertise, and is often difficult.

Details of Management

(i) Antibiotics and the Recognition and Treatment of Precipitating Factors (12)

Antibiotics play a vital role, as control of infection leads to improvement in lung function, and reverses acute respiratory failure. We now prefer amoxicillin or amoxicillin + clavulanic acid to cover Gram-positive infections, and gentamicin or ciprofloxacin for Gram-negative ones. Change in antibiotic cover may be necessary if the clinical features of infection persist, and if sputum cultures and antibiotic sensitivity reports suggest an alternative choice of antibiotics.

Precipitating factors such as even a shallow pneumothorax, pleural effusion, pulmonary embolism, pulmonary oedema should be recognized and promptly treated.

(ii) Bronchodilators (13–15)

These are very similar to those used in acute severe asthma. 5 mg salbutamol in 4 ml N saline is nebulized 4 hourly or more frequently to start with; the frequency is then reduced as improvement occurs.

Ipratropium bromide 0.5 mg 12 hourly is also nebulized routinely in these patients (14).

If a patient has been on long-term use of theophylline, it is best not to use more than 0.5–0.75 g of intravenous aminophylline in a slow drip given over 24 hours. Serum levels of theophylline help in adjusting the dosage.

(iii) Corticosteroids (13)

Most units use oral or intravenous corticosteroids in patients with acute on chronic respiratory failure due to airways obstruction. Prednisolone 40–60 mg orally, or intravenous hydrocortisone 200 mg 8 hourly, is used till improvement occurs. The dose is then gradually tapered off over 8 to 15 days and inhaled corticosteroids, budecort 1 mg nebulized 12 hourly substituted.

(iv) Physiotherapy (13, 16)

Many patients have excess of respiratory secretions which they are unable to clear. Physiotherapy chiefly consists of liquefying viscid secretions with steam inhalation, the use of nebulization, deep breathing, and promotion of effective coughing. Chest percussion can be harmful and should not be done as it is often followed by a fall in the oxygen saturation. Postural drainage is also avoided except in patients who have well marked associated bronchiectasis with plenty of foul retained sputum. Patients with COPD tend to hypoventilate and retain secretions specially during sleep at night. It is important to wake the patient at night, help him to deep breathe, cough and expectorate.

(v) Controlled Oxygen Therapy (17, 18)

Patients admitted to the ICU with moderate to severe hypoxaemia ($PaO_2 < 50$–55 mm Hg) always need oxygen, and are at a risk of death from hypoxia. *It should therefore be a rule to administer oxygen immediately, and as the very first measure, to any acutely ill patient with chronic airways obstruction.* As explained in the Chapter on Oxygen Therapy, uncontrolled oxygen can however be lethal in these patients; its administration should therefore be 'controlled' and carefully supervised. Intensive care is of crucial importance for survival (10, 11). The objective is to increase the low PaO_2 to a safe level (PaO_2 of 60 mm Hg suffices), without the arterial pH falling below 7.25. *The severity of the acidosis is a better prognostic guide in these patients, than the absolute PCO_2 levels.*

The response to controlled oxygen therapy (starting with an inspired oxygen content of 24 per cent, (and increasing to 26 per cent or even 28–30 per cent if dangerous hypoxia is unrelieved), falls into the following three patterns (19):

(a) Relief of hypoxaemia, with a fall in the $PaCO_2$ and an overall clinical improvement.

(b) Relief of hypoxaemia, but an initial increase in the $PaCO_2$ with a further fall in arterial pH to not less than 7.25. The $PaCO_2$ then steadies at a higher level, or returns to pretreatment levels. After a couple of days, the $PaCO_2$ generally falls below pretreatment levels. The initial rise in $PaCO_2$ with a fall in arterial pH, is usually observed during the first night after starting oxygen therapy, and is associated with increasing drowsiness, dullness, confusion and apathy. Thereafter, there is a gradual fall in the $PaCO_2$ to pretreatment or even lower levels and a return of pH towards normal, occurring *pari passu* with clinical improvement.

(c) Relief of hypoxaemia, but a rapid, progressive, marked increase in the $PaCO_2$ with an increasing respiratory acidosis (pH < 7.25). This response is to be expected if oxygen is administered in an uncontrolled manner, using high oxygen concentrations. It can however also occur with carefully controlled and supervised oxygen therapy (O_2 concentration between 24–28 per cent). The severe respiratory acidosis and the marked rise in the $PaCO_2$ can prove lethal in these patients.

Unfortunately, it is generally the severely hypoxic patient with a fairly high $PaCO_2$ to start with, who is more prone to develop a progressively increasing, dangerously high $PaCO_2$ with a dangerously low arterial pH (< 7.2). When pretreatment $PaCO_2$ values range between 65–70 mm Hg, there is a permissible margin of safety for a further rise in $PaCO_2$ by 20–25 mm Hg, after starting oxygen therapy. If however the initial pretreatment $PaCO_2$ values are well over 75–80 mm Hg and arterial pH already lowered to 7.25 or less, a further abrupt rise by 30 mm Hg in the $PaCO_2$ and a further lowering of arterial pH, within a few hours of starting oxygen therapy, can prove dangerous, and at times fatal. Yet, the prime objective is to relieve dangerous hypoxia, for which oxygen is vital.

(vi) Non-invasive Mechanical Ventilation

Some patients fail to improve or even worsen after adequate treatment described above. Thus, even on controlled oxygen therapy (and measures described earlier), though hypoxia may improve, the $PaCO_2$ rises sharply with a dangerous fall in pH (< 7.25). At times even the hypoxia is unrelieved. These patients require mechanical ventilation. Ventilator support could be of two types—non-invasive and invasive. About 40 per cent of patients admitted to our ICU with acute respiratory failure in COPD require mechanical ventilator support. Non-invasive positive-pressure ventilation (NPPV) has been proven useful in several studies of acute respiratory failure caused by an exacerbation of COPD (20, 21). A recent study showed that the use of NPPV was associated with a lesser risk of nosocomial infection, less antibiotic use and a lower mortality when compared to patients equally ill but who did not receive NPPV (21).

NPPV has the ability to increase alveolar ventilation, rest muscles of respiration, reduce work of breathing and prevent muscle fatigue. Potential benefits include an increase in tidal volume, a fall in respiratory rate, improved oxygenation, a fall in $PaCO_2$ and greater patient comfort. When these benefits occur, they do so within a few hours of initiating NPPV. Perhaps the most important advantage of NPPV in an acute crisis of COPD is that it obviates the need for endotracheal intubation and invasive mechanical ventilation which is far more inconvenient to the patient, and has more risks—particularly the risk of nosocomial infection.

Having said this, it is our considered opinion that many patients admitted to ICUs in this country for an acute exacerbation of COPD are offered NPPV when ventilatory support is not required—i.e. these patients would have recovered on conservative measures outlined above. Also, many such patients are offered NPPV when they in fact needed prompt intubation and invasive ventilator support.

The indications in our unit for initiating NPPV in an acute crisis of COPD are:

(i) Respiratory rate > 30/minute.

(ii) Respiratory distress due to moderate or severe dyspnoea.

(iii) pH ≤ 7.30 and/or a $PaCO_2$ > 60 mm Hg, provided these values fail to improve or worsen after a trial of 6 to 8 hours (or even earlier) of conservative measures.

We initiate NPPV earlier than what we used to do five years ago.

Non-invasive mechanical ventilation should not be used as the mode of ventilatory support if the patient is obtunded, breathes poorly or irregularly, is unable to protect the airway, has copious respiratory secretions, and has a risk of aspirating gastric contents. We also prefer to intubate and ventilate those whose PaO_2 < 45 mm Hg and who are admitted with a pH < 7.20. Patients who show an acute rise of $PaCO_2$ of > 70 mm Hg are often obtunded, and in our opinion, are more effectively managed by endotracheal intubation and invasive ventilator support. Endotracheal intubation and ventilation should obviously be also resorted to when NPPV fails to prove of benefit within 6 to 10 hours of its initiation, or even earlier if the patient worsens on this mode of support.

Implementation of NPPV—NPPV can be offered through either a light fitting face mask or a nasal mask. Each has its own advantages (see chapter on Mechanical Ventilation in the Critically Ill). We prefer the face mask in patients with severe respiratory failure. A wide variety of ventilatory modes can be used in NPPV. We prefer the BiPAP mode because it allows for good gas exchange and effectively reduces both the work of breathing and patient distress. Pressure support ventilation (PSV) is perhaps an equally useful mode and is generally better tolerated than the assist-control mode. In a BiPAP mode, to start with, the inspiratory pressure (IP) is kept at 8 to 10 cm above the end-expiratory pressure (EP), so that if the EP is 5 to 7 cm H_2O, the IP is 12 to 15 cm H_2O. The pressure can then be adjusted to allow for effective alveolar ventilation and good gas exchange.

If the PSV mode is used for NPPV, the inspiratory pressure support to start with is kept at 15 to 20 cm H_2O. A small PEEP of 4 to 5 cm H_2O may be of help in patients who have a large auto-PEEP as it helps reduce inspiratory effort to generate inspiratory airflow in these patients.

Weaning from NPPV is accomplished by progressively decreasing the level of inspiratory pressure support if the PSV mode is used, or by allowing the patient to be intermittently off NPPV for increasing lengths of time.

(vii) Intubation and Mechanical Ventilation

Patients who show a sharp progressive rise in the $PaCO_2$ with a pH < 7.2 on controlled oxygen therapy, or those whose dangerous hypoxia stands unrelieved on conservative therapy or NPPV, are best intubated and put on mechanical ventilator support. Selection of cases for this mode of treatment is difficult. It would be disastrous for a patient and his family if after starting mechanical ventilation, it becomes impossible to wean the patient off ventilator support. In our opinion, the best indication whether to opt for invasive ventilator support or not, is the activity and state of health of the patient under basal conditions. If the patient's activity was hopelessly poor under basal conditions to start with (i.e. he was more or less confined to his bed due to poor respiratory reserve), it is unwise to opt for invasive ventilator support, and the family should be advised accordingly. If he was reasonably active prior

to the crisis that brought him to the ICU, he should be offered ventilator support.

Endotracheal intubation in patients showing poor response to antibiotics, bronchodilators, physiotherapy and controlled oxygen therapy, offers two advantages. It allows proper access for suctioning of respiratory secretions, and it allows mechanical ventilator support.

Mechanical ventilation (see Chapter on Mechanical Ventilation) is difficult in patients with chronic airways obstruction. We prefer and recommend the assist/control mode in patients with severe acute respiratory failure so that total support and appropriate choice of ventilator settings can be provided. Sedation and rarely neuromuscular paralysis may be necessary for effective respiratory support. As recovery proceeds or in patients who are not very ill, pressure support ventilation may be used. The principles for successful ventilation are outlined below (**Table 8.4.3**).

Table 8.4.3. Principles of mechanical ventilation in patients with COPD and acute respiratory crisis

Ventilator Settings	Objectives
* Low tidal volumes of 300–400 ml with MV < 5–6 l/min	* Prevents overinflation * Prevents further increase in auto-PEEP * Decreases peak inflation pressure * Reduces risk of barotrauma
* Flow rate 40–60 l/min	
* I:E ratio of 1:2 or 1:3	* Allows good distribution of inspired gas, allows time for expiration
* FIO_2 of 50–70%	* Allows quick correction of hypoxia
* Sedate or use pancuronium	* Allows machine to take over, and prevents clashing with the machine

Note: (i) Lower $PaCO_2$ very gradually over 24 hours or even longer to 50 mm Hg—a PaO_2 of 60 mm Hg suffices

(ii) If weaning is difficult, use pressure support ventilation

(a) Small tidal volumes of 300–400 ml are used with minute ventilation not exceeding 5–6 l/min. The FIO_2 is increased to 50 or 60 per cent so that dangerous hypoxia is quickly corrected. It is unnecessary to aim for an oxygen saturation > 90 per cent. The low tidal volumes prevent overinflation, and prevent a further increase in auto-PEEP which is invariably present in these patients (see Chapter on Mechanical Ventilation in the Critically Ill). Low tidal volumes also lead to lower peak inflation pressures. This is a great advantage, as high peak pressures if transmitted to the intrapleural space, cause a sharp reduction in the venous return and the cardiac output, and can produce sudden severe hypotension. In fact, hypotension should be carefully looked out for, particularly after starting ventilation. A fall in the arterial pressure should prompt one to further reduce the inflation pressure by further reducing the tidal volume. The blood pressure should also be raised by volume expansion or by using inotropic support. Once the patient is on mechanical ventilation with the hypoxia corrected by a high FIO_2, an increase in $PaCO_2$ need not be feared. Under these circumstances death usually does not occur due to a high $PaCO_2$.

Sensitivity. The optimal triggering threshold is difficult in an acute COPD crisis in the presence of dynamic hyperinflation (i.e. auto-PEEP). This is because the patient has to generate a negative pressure at least equal to the level of auto-PEEP before interfacing with the pre-set sensitivity on the ventilator. If the auto-PEEP is high, the required inspiratory effort (before reaching trigger sensitivity) to initiate airflow is significant and this can lead to patient-ventilator dyssynchrony. Yet if the trigger sensitivity is kept very low, the ventilator could be triggered very frequently and inappropriately.

(b) Ventilator requirements are so adjusted so as to bring down the raised $PaCO_2$ level very slowly over 24–48 hours. It is generally unnecessary to reduce the $PaCO_2$ to < 50 mm Hg unless the basal $PaCO_2$ levels were normal. A sudden drop in the $PaCO_2$ is dangerous as it causes a sudden shift from respiratory acidaemia to metabolic alkalosis and alkalaemia. This can precipitate dangerous arrhythmias and cause sudden death.

(c) The flow rates used in such patients are usually between 40–60 l/min, and the inspiration:expiration ratio is initially set at 1:3.

(d) Patients should not be allowed to clash with the machine; they can be safely given pancuronium, or sedated once they are put on ventilator support.

(e) Mechanical ventilator support is generally necessary for a period of 3–7 days. The maximum period over which we have used ventilator support, and then finally succeeded in weaning the patient, has been 6 weeks. An elective tracheostomy is preferred if ventilator support needs to be extended for more than 7 days, or if the patient has thick copious secretions which cannot be easily suctioned through the endotracheal tube.

(f) Weaning is generally carried out by the traditional methods outlined in the Chapter on Mechanical Ventilation in the Critically Ill. We have used intermittent mandatory ventilation, and pressure support ventilation, but have never been totally convinced of their absolute necessity. The patient is taken off ventilator support when he can maintain an adequate gas exchange on his own. This generally happens when infection has been controlled, airways obstruction has decreased, and $\dot{V}/\dot{Q}$ abnormalities have been significantly rectified.

(g) Older patients with ischaemic heart disease often need careful cardiovascular support. The presence of associated left ventricular failure with pulmonary oedema, together with generalized water retention is not uncommon in these patients. *It is indeed remarkable how good ventilator support with improvement in blood gases initiates a diuresis in these patients, even though earlier use of large doses of furosemide was ineffective.* Correction of severe hypoxia and hypercapnia are probably responsible for the improved cardiac function and diuresis.

(h) Expert nursing, humidification of inspired oxygen and persistence with the regime outlined earlier, are all essentials of good respiratory care in these patients.

Our mortality in patients with acute respiratory failure in COPD who require invasive ventilator support is about 20 per cent.

Treatment of Complications during Acute Respiratory Failure

Complications (**Table 8.4.4**) frequently met with are discussed below:

Table 8.4.4. Common complications encountered during acute respiratory failure in patients with COPD

1. Pulmonary infection—this may trigger the crisis or complicate a crisis
2. Fluid, electrolyte and acid-base disturbances—respiratory acidosis with hypokalaemic metabolic alkalosis being the commonest Severe water logging can occur due to salt and water retention
3. Cardiac arrhythmias
4. Right-sided heart failure
5. Hypotension if there is marked auto-PEEP
6. Pneumothorax
7. Complications due to mechanical ventilation
8. Gastrointestinal bleeds
9. Pulmonary thromboembolism
10. Mental depression

(i) *Fluid and Electrolyte Disturbances.* The commonest disturbance is a respiratory acidosis often associated with a hypokalaemic metabolic alkalosis. Many patients have a potassium deficit, particularly if corticosteroids, beta-2 agonists, theophylline and diuretics have been used. Severe potassium loss should be corrected by a slow intravenous infusion of 20–60 mEq of potassium chloride in dextrose.

(ii) *Cardiac Arrhythmias* (**22**). These are frequently observed in these patients. Supraventricular tachycardia, multifocal atrial tachycardia and atrial fibrillation are common; AV dissociation and multiple ventricular extrasystoles may also occur. The mortality rate is significantly higher in patients having arrhythmias.

(iii) *Haemodynamic Instability.* Patients with COPD often suffer from pulmonary hypertension. An acute exacerbation of COPD worsens pulmonary hypertension due to hypoxic vasoconstriction, dynamic hyperinflation or the presence of auto-PEEP during mechanical ventilation. A sharp increase in pulmonary artery pressure leads to severe right ventricular dysfunction, right-sided heart failure, with a fall in both systolic and mean arterial blood pressure (**23**). An intravenous fluid challenge expands the intravascular pulmonary bed and improves right ventricular pump function. It should be the initial step in the management of hypotension and haemodynamic instability in an acute crisis of COPD. If the haemodynamic state fails to improve, we prefer to use inotropic support with dobutamine. Ventilator adjustments to reduce dynamic hyperinflation and auto-PEEP are also often necessary.

In older individuals, associated left heart disease with poor left ventricular function may complicate the issue. Inotropic support is again often necessary in the presence of hypotension and pulmonary oedema. Severe hypoxia needs urgent correction as it worsens myocardial dysfunction.

(iv) *Pulmonary thromboembolism* is an important complication, which should be promptly recognized and treated with intravenous heparin. Severe polycythaemia may contribute to thromboembolism. If the haematocrit reads over 60 per cent, small frequent phlebotomies may be performed, provided there is no shock or hypotension. The haematocrit reading is preferably kept below 50 per cent.

(v) *Pneumothorax* can trigger an acute respiratory crisis in a patient with chronic airways disease, or may complicate its natural history. Pneumothorax can be iatrogenic due to insertion of central lines, or due to barotrauma from mechanical ventilation. It can be missed on clinical examination and should always be considered as a possible cause for sudden deterioration in a patient, or if there is poor response to therapy. An X-ray chest is mandatory; the diagnosis however can still be missed if the portable chest X-ray is of poor quality.

(vi) Gastrointestinal bleeds and other iatrogenic problems during mechanical ventilation need to be recognized and treated along conventional lines.

(vii) Nosocomial infections should be guarded against in the ICU, and when present, promptly treated.

(viii) Severe depression and a feeling of hopeless despair are frequent in these patients; this is particularly so when acute respiratory failure occurs time and again in patients with chronic airways obstruction, necessitating frequent admission to an ICU. Good, efficient and sympathetic nursing is of great help.

REFERENCES

1. Derenne JP, Fleury B, Pariente R. (1988). Acute respiratory failure of chronic obstructive pulmonary disease. Am Rev Respir Dis. 138, 1006.

2. Schmidt GA, Hall JB. (1989). Acute on chronic respiratory failure: Assessment and management of patients with COPD in the emergent setting. JAMA. 261, 3444.

3. Curtis RJ, Hudson LD. (1994). Emergent assessment and management of acute respiratory failure in COPD. Clinics in Chest Medicine. 15(3), 481–500.

4. Sethi S. (2000). Infectious etiology of acute exacerbations of chronic bronchitis. Chest. 117, 380S.

5. Blasi F, Legnani D, Lombardo VM et al. (1993). Chlamydia pneumoniae infection in acute exacerbations of COPD. Eur Respir J. 6, 19.

6. Tantucci C, Grassi V. (1999). Flow limitation: an overview. Chest. 116, 488.

7. Stubbing DG, Penegelly LD, Morse JLC. (1980). Pulmonary mechanics during exercise in subjects with chronic air-flow obstruction. J Appl Physiol. 49, 511.

8. Smith TC, Marini JJ. (1988). Impact of PEEP on lung mechanics and work of breathing in severe airflow obstruction. J Appl Physiol. 65, 1488.

9. Tobin MJ, Perez W, Guenther SM et al. (1986). The pattern of breathing during successful and unsuccessful trial of weaning during mechanical ventilation. Am Rev Respir Dis. 134, 111.

10. Roger RM, Weiler C, Ruppenthal B. (1972). Impact of the respiratory care unit on survival of patients with acute respiratory failure. Chest. 62, 94.

11. Petty TL, Lakshminarayan S, Sahn SA et al. (1975). Intensive respiratory care unit: Review of 10 years' experience. JAMA. 233, 34.

12. Anthonisen NR, Manfreda J, Warren CPW et al. (1987). Antibiotic therapy in exacerbations of chronic obstructive pulmonary disease. Ann Intern Med. 106, 196.

13. Grippi MA. (1998). Respiratory Failure: An Overview. In: Fishman's Pulmonary Diseases and Disorders (Ed. Fishman AP). pp. 2525–2536. McGraw-Hill Book Company, New York, Paris, London, Toronto.

14. Schmidt GA, Hall JB. (1999). Acute on Chronic Respiratory Failure. In: Principles of Critical Care (Eds Hall JB, Schmidt GA, Wood LDH). pp. 565–578. McGraw-Hill Inc., Philadelphia, London, Toronto.

15. Fernanadez A, Lazaro A, Garcia A et al. (1990). Bronchodilators in patients with chronic obstructive pulmonary disease on mechanical ventilation. Am Rev Respir Dis. 141, 164–168.

16. Wollmer P, Ursing K, Midgren B et al. (1985). Inefficiency of chest percussion in the physical therapy of chronic bronchitis. Eur J Resp Dis. 66, 233.

17. Shapiro BA, Kacmarek RM, Cane RD et al. (1991). Obstructive Pulmonary Disease. In: Clinical Application of Respiratory Care, 4th edn. pp. 414–425. Mosby Year Book, Boston, Chicago, London, Toronto.

18. Schmidt GA, Hall JB. (1989). Oxygen therapy and hypoxic drive to breathe: Is there danger in the patient with COPD? Intensive and Crit Care Dig. 8, 124.

19. Udwadia FE. (1979). Chronic Obstructive Airways Disease. In: Diagnosis and Management of Acute Respiratory Failure. pp. 261–278. Oxford University Press. London, New York, Delhi.

20. Brochard L, Mancebo J, Wysocki M et al. (1995). Noninvasive ventilation for acute exacerbations of chronic obstructive pulmonary disease. N Engl J Med. 333, 817.

21. Girou E, Schortgen F, Delclaux C et al. (2000). Association of noninvasive ventilation with nososcomial infections and survival in critically ill patients. JAMA. 284, 2361.

22. Incalzi RA, Pistelli R, Fuso L et al. (1990). Cardiac arrhythmias and left ventricular function in respiratory failure from chronic obstructive pulmonary disease. Chest. 97, 1092.

23. Vizza CD, Lynch JP, Ochoa LL et al. (1998). Right and left ventricular dysfunction in patients with severe pulmonary disease. Chest. 113, 576.

Acute Lung Injury (ARDS)

Contributed by Dr F.E. Udwadia with Dr Z.F. Udwadia, MD, FRCP (London), MNAMS, FCCP (USA). Consultant Physician, P D Hinduja National Hospital, and Parsee General Hospital, Mumbai.

General Considerations

The Acute Respiratory Distress Syndrome (ARDS) is an important condition characterized by severe hypoxaemic respiratory failure, necessitating prolonged intensive care and ventilator support in ICUs all over the world.

The first description of what probably was ARDS was given by Osler in his textbook of Medicine in 1927. He wrote of 'uncontrolled septicaemia leading to pulmonary oedema' and went on to describe the clinical features and autopsy findings very nearly as we know them today (1). In 1967, Ashbaugh, Bigelow and Petty reported in the Lancet the occurrence of non-cardiogenic pulmonary oedema and acute respiratory failure in a number of diverse pathologies not directly involving the lungs (2). They termed this condition the adult respiratory distress syndrome. Semantically speaking, this was an unfortunate term. The syndrome can occur at all ages and is not related in its pathogenesis and pathology to the respiratory distress syndrome of the newborn. Also, the connotation of 'respiratory distress' is both vague and common to numerous other unrelated pathologies in cardiorespiratory medicine. Semantic confusion would have been avoided if from the very outset the condition had been termed Acute Lung Injury. Since 1967, the syndrome has been reported from many countries, including India (3). The precipitating factors have been recognized and the pathology of the lung has been elucidated. However, the pathogenesis after more than 30 years of research remains unclear and the mortality in spite of expert intensive care, even today is as high as 30–60 per cent.

Definition and Concept

The existing clinical definition of acute lung injury (ARDS) is characterized by (i) an antecedent history of a precipitating condition; (ii) respiratory distress and refractory hypoxaemia not responding satisfactorily to supplemental oxygen and invariably necessitating the use of mechanical ventilatory support; (iii) radiographic evidence of newly evolving bilateral pulmonary infiltrates; (iv) pulmonary artery occlusion pressure (PAOP) < 18 mm Hg in the presence of a normal colloid oncotic pressure.

The physiological changes underlying the above clinical definition include a reduced functional residual capacity (FRC), stiff lungs (reduced pulmonary compliance), increased ventilation-perfusion inequalities, an increase in the right to left shunt within the lungs, and an increase in the extravascular water content of the lungs with, as already mentioned, a normal pulmonary capillary wedge pressure. The underlying pathological abnormality is damage to the alveolar capillary membrane with increased capillary permeability, leading to oedema, inflammation and subsequent fibrosis.

Recently an American–European Consensus Conference has clinically defined and distinguished between acute lung injury (ALI) and acute respiratory distress syndrome (ARDS), so as to avoid semantic confusion (4).

The American–European Consensus Definition of Acute Lung Injury (ALI) and Acute Respiratory Distress Syndrome (ARDS) is as follows:

Acute Lung Injury (ALI)	Acute Respiratory Distress Syndrome (ARDS)
1. Acute onset respiratory failure	1. Acute onset respiratory failure.
2. Bilateral chest infiltrates on frontal radiographs	2. Bilateral chest infiltrates on frontal radiographs
3. Absence of elevated left heart filling pressure (PAOP < 18 mm Hg)	3. Absence of elevated left heart filling pressures (PAOP < 18 mm Hg)
4. $PaO_2 / FIO_2 < 300$	4. $PaO_2 / FIO_2 < 200$

According to this Consensus Conference acute lung injury when mild to moderate is termed acute lung injury and when severe is termed the acute respiratory distress syndrome, the degree of severity of injury being assessed by the PaO_2/FIO_2 ratio. To us it seems illogical that the same clinical entity should be given separate names depending on whether it is mild to moderate or severe.

There are certain further points to be considered for a balanced perspective of the syndrome.

1. It is important to exclude cardiogenic pulmonary oedema before diagnosing ALI or ARDS. However, this can generally be done on a clinical assessment. Measurement of the PAOP through a Swan-Ganz catheter is not mandatory (as suggested in

the definition) and is required only in the rare instances where cardiogenic pulmonary oedema cannot be clinically excluded.

2. Though ALI and ARDS signify non-cardiogenic pulmonary oedema, patients with a background of left ventricular dysfunction and raised left heart pressures may suffer from sepsis and then evolve into ALI and ARDS.

3. The concept of ALI and ARDS stated above is narrow in its perspective. An expanded concept should include not only the severity of acute lung injury (5) but also the background factor causing or precipitating the syndrome and most importantly, the associated or evolving dysfunction of other organ systems. Most investigators consider ALI and ARDS as merely one facet of the multiple organ dysfunction syndrome (6).

Aetiology

A variety of clinical disorders can lead to ALI and ARDS. These may directly involve the lung (direct injury), or may involve the lung indirectly (indirect injury). Our experience on ARDS with regard to aetiology, and mortality in relation to each aetiological factor is summarized in **Table 8.5.1**.

In 187 patients of ARDS treated till the end of 2002 in one of our intensive care units, 'direct injury' was the aetiological factor in 67 patients (35.83 per cent); 'indirect injury' was the causative factor in 68 patients (40.72 per cent); 52 patients (27.81 per cent) developed ARDS due to fulminant infections and problems peculiar to the tropical and developing countries of the world— for convenience these 52 patients were categorized under ARDS due to tropical problems. The first two groups of patients for convenience were categorized under non-tropical problems i.e. problems more or less common to the whole world (**Table 8.5.1**).

Important causes of direct injury were acute pulmonary infections (chiefly bacterial or viral), aspiration of gastric contents, trauma to the chest with lung contusions, inhalation of toxic fumes, pulmonary vasculitis and near-drowning.

Indirect injury to the lung from non-respiratory causes was observed in 40.72 per cent of cases. Sepsis was the most important indirect or non-respiratory cause of acute lung injury (19.25 per cent of patients) (**Fig. 8.5.1**). In sepsis, ALI and ARDS form merely one facet of the multiple organ dysfunction syndrome. The incidence of ALI in severe sepsis or septic shock is over 25 per cent (7). Sepsis not only initiates acute lung injury but also perpetuates it. It should also be noted that even when acute lung injury is caused by a direct injury or insult to the lung, sepsis may subsequently supervene as a major complication (8), and can worsen both the lung injury and multiple organ dysfunction.

In our experience (as also in the West), when sepsis *causes* acute lung injury, the source of sepsis is most frequently intra-abdominal. On the other hand, when sepsis is a supervening complication in a patient suffering from acute lung injury due to any other aetiology, the source of sepsis is most frequently within the lung itself.

Other important causes of indirect injuries causing ARDS in our intensive care unit include the following—major extra-thoracic trauma, shock from any aetiology, acute pancreatitis, burns, poisonings—in particular organophosphorus poisoning, disseminated

Table 8.5.1. The aetiology of ARDS as observed in our unit with observed mortality for each aetiological factor. Note the difference in mortality between ARDS (and MODS) in 'tropical problems' and 'non-tropical problems'.

Severe Acute Lung Injury Data	Total	Expired	Mortality
Total no. of patients	187	91	49%
Patients with tropical problems	52	14	27%
Patients with non-tropical problems	135	77	57%
Patients with non-tropical problems (n=135)			
1. Direct Injury			
Acute pulmonary infection	33	23	70%
Aspiration pneumonia	18	11	61%
Direct trauma	7	2	29%
Noxious fumes	5	0	0%
Pulmonary vasculitis	4	0	0%
Total	67	36	54%
2. Indirect Injury			
Severe sepsis	36	24	67%
Pancreatitis	9	5	56%
Burns	4	3	75%
Extrathoracic injury	4	0	0%
Poisoning	2	0	0%
Miscellaneous	13	8	62%
Total	68	41	60%
Patients with tropical problems			
Tetanus	9	4	44%
OP poisoning	10	1	10%
Cerebral malaria	10	3	30%
Gram-negative septicaemia from contaminated food	5	0	0%
Miliary / Disseminated haematogenous tuberculosis	8	3	38%
Amoebiasis	5	2	40%
Salmonella infections	3	0	0%
Rabies	1	1	100%
Leptospirosis	1	0	0%
Total	52	14	27%

intravascular coagulopathy, following cardiopulmonary bypass, miscellaneous causes (e.g. multiple blood transfusions, eclampsia, amniotic fluid embolism, hepatic dysfunction, hepatorenal failure, Steven-Johnson syndrome).

Tropical Infections and Problems

It is pertinent and important to briefly outline tropical problems causing ALI and ARDS. These, in our experience, include fulminant Pl. falciparum infections (**Fig. 8.5.2**), severe tetanus (**Fig. 8.5.3**), severe typhoid and salmonella infections, fulminant Gram-negative infections following ingestion of contaminated food, acute miliary tuberculosis and acute disseminated haematogenous tuberculosis (**Fig. 8.5.4**), fulminant amoebic infections of the liver and large bowel, fulminant leptospirosis, haemorrhagic fevers and rabies. Severe organophosphorus poisoning is the most frequently encountered poisoning causing ARDS in Western India. In the north, Aluminium Phosphide poisoning (added generally for the preservation of food grains) is an important cause of severe ARDS which invariably ends fatally. Fulminant tropical infections (except

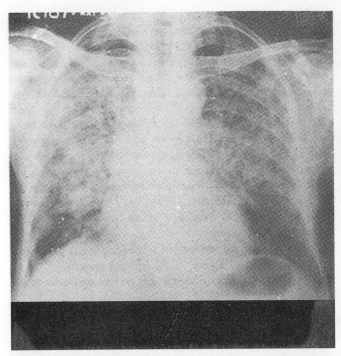

Fig. 8.5.1. Acute Lung Injury in patient *SS* who developed septic peritonitis following a caesarian section.

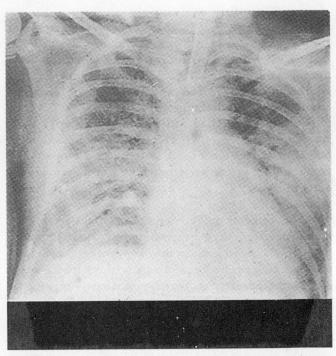

Fig. 8.5.2. Acute lung injury in patient *SP* with fulminant Pl. falciparum infection.

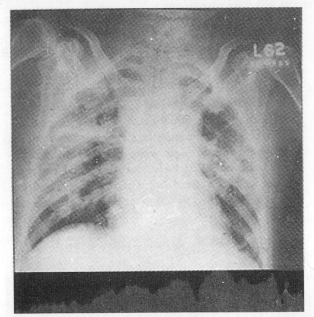

Fig. 8.5.3. Acute lung injury in patient *AM* with very severe (Grade IV) tetanus.

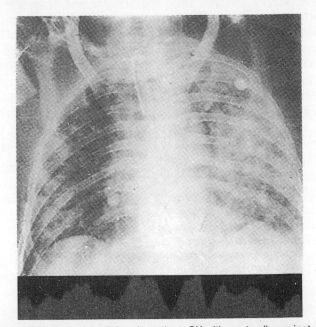

Fig. 8.5.4. Acute lung injury in patient *CK* with acute disseminated haematogenous tuberculosis. This patient presented with pyrexia of unknown origin (PUO), and rapidly deteriorated, developing acute lung injury and multiple organ failure. A fibreoptic bronchoscopy with bronchoalveolar lavage was done and demonstrated the presence of acid-fast bacilli.

for rabies), have been discussed in the Chapter on Fever and Acute Infections in a Critical Care Setting. Each of these tropical problems can lead not only to acute lung injury, but to progressive multiple organ failure and death. The most important of these causes are fulminant Pl. falciparum infections, tetanus, acute miliary tuberculosis, acute haematogenous disseminated tuberculosis, leptospiral infections and fulminant B typhosus and salmonella infections.

The following clinical forms of acute lung injury have been noted in relation to severe Pl. falciparum malaria:

(i) Acute pulmonary oedema due to hyperpyrexia (temperature > 107°F).

(ii) Progressive bilateral shadowing within the lungs characterized physiologically by marked ventilation-perfusion inequalities, but by only a slight increase in the right to left shunt within the lungs—recovery is possible with good management.

(iii) Progressive bilateral fluffy shadows characterized physiologically by a marked increase in the right to left shunt—recovery is unlikely.

(iv) ARDS caused by disseminated intravascular coagulopathy complicating falciparum infection.

(v) ARDS due to aspiration of gastric contents in obtunded patients.

The time from the original insult (direct or indirect), to the development of full-blown acute lung injury has been studied in many large series. In Petty's original group it ranged from 1 to 96 hours. In a comprehensive, recent epidemiological study, 80 per cent of patients had developed acute lung injury within 48 hours of the initial insult, and 90 per cent by 80 hours (7). This latent period offers a window of opportunity for therapeutic interventions, when effective blockers of the inflammatory process can be identified. Indeed, today there is a massive search for circulating markers of acute lung injury which can be identified in the serum or bronchoalveolar lavage fluid (9).

Pathology

The basic pathological feature is damage to the alveolar capillary membrane, which results in early interstitial and alveolar oedema and alveolar atelectasis. Three overlapping phases are observed:

(i) Exudative phase in which there is an alveolar exudate with hyaline membrane formation along the alveolar ducts and within the alveoli.

(ii) Proliferative phase in which there is a proliferation of inflammatory cells, lymphocytes and type 2 pneumocytes. Organization of the inflammatory exudate, combined with damage to the surfactant leads to obliteration of air spaces, atelectatic alveoli and a poorly compliant lung.

(iii) Fibrotic phase which follows soon upon the proliferative phase, and is characterized by fibroblasts laying down fibrous tissue that strangles alveoli, and further reduces pulmonary compliance (10).

Severe lung injury distorts the pulmonary vasculature. Distortion with remodelling of the vasculature is due to fibrous tissue formation, thromboembolism, and increased muscularization with thickening and intimal fibrosis of the larger arteries. Thrombi may be present in the microcirculation and in the larger vessels. They may form in situ, or may have an embolic source. The end-result is an obstructed, distorted pulmonary circulation with increased pulmonary vascular resistance, causing pulmonary hypertension.

Pathogenesis (11)

The pathogenesis of ALI continues to remain unclear. Even so, current research allows a better comprehension of what transpires in this syndrome at the cellular and molecular level. Research into molecular genetics in the eighties has revealed a complex network of interacting factors at the cellular level. No longer is there a simplistic illusion that any single mediator of acute lung injury exists; therefore a corresponding therapeutic 'magic bullet' is also an illusion. Indeed it is clear that the cascade of mediators is far more complex than we thought, and many of yesterday's putative mediators are in reality modulators and regulators that fine-tune the inflammatory cascade, rather than cause it (12). **Fig. 8.5.5** illustrates the steps in the pathogenesis of acute lung injury and organ failure.

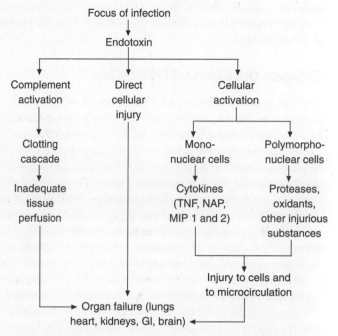

Fig. 8.5.5. Pathogenesis of acute lung injury and organ failure.

Role of Cytokines, Neutrophils and the Coagulation System

Cytokines which are cell derived peptide compounds, are the main mediators. Recombinant cDNA technology has permitted identification of the existence, structure and function of several cytokines. The cytokine on which most attention is currently focussed is the tumour necrosis factor (TNF). This cytokine has a molecular weight of 17 kD and is released from macrophages in response to Gram-negative bacterial endotoxin. TNF is one of the main mediators of the septic state (13). After injection of endotoxin into animals or humans, TNF can be detected in the serum, the levels peaking at 2 hours (14). When TNF is infused into the sheep model, acute lung injury is produced (15). Three other cytokines of importance mediating inflammatory response, include neutrophil activating peptide (NAP), interleukin-8 and macrophage inflammatory proteins (MIP 1 and 2). The neutrophil plays a vital role in the inflammatory response and TNF is the chief mediator that promotes adherence of the neutrophils to the vascular endothelium and together with interleukin-8 causes and enhances neutrophil activation. The primed neutrophils degranulate releasing proteases, reactive oxygen species, leukotrienes, all harmful to lung structure and function. The lipid mediators and platelet activating factor also enhance inflammation.

The activation of the coagulation and complement systems promotes coagulation and decreases fibrinolysis. Endothelial damage results in pulmonary oedema with a disturbance in pulmonary microcirculation. The end result is increasing respiratory failure with an increasing poverty of gas exchange often leading to death. As mentioned earlier, changes in the lung often form just one facet of similar changes in other organs of the body.

There is a complex, poorly understood interaction at the molecular and cellular level as the syndrome continues to evolve. This interaction and interrelation will continue to be the subject of future research.

Oxygen Uptake and Utilization

Acute lung injury is believed by a number of workers to be a multisystem disease, the changes occurring in the pulmonary endothelium being a reflection of a more generalized pan-endothelial disorder affecting the entire microcirculation (16). The lung involvement manifests early, and is more readily apparent than endothelial damage in other organs. The gas exchange abnormalities that originate in the lung result in diminished oxygen delivery to other organs, and this amplifies dysfunction in other non-pulmonary organs. In addition, some investigators are of the opinion that a defect in peripheral tissue oxygen uptake and utilization is central to the pathogenesis of acute lung injury (16).

In normal subjects oxygen consumption ($\dot{V}O_2$) is dependent on tissue demand for oxygen and not on oxygen delivery ($\dot{D}O_2$). Thus oxygen uptake ($\dot{V}O_2$) is maintained at a constant value over a wide range of oxygen delivery ($\dot{D}O_2$) (Fig. 8.5.6). This is accomplished by means of local compensatory mechanisms that include increase in oxygen extraction, and increase in the cross sectional area of perfused capillaries within an individual organ (recruitable oxygen reserve). Once these local compensations are exhausted,

further reduction in oxygen delivery is accompanied by reduction in oxygen uptake. The oxygen delivery below which oxygen uptake begins to fall, is termed the critical threshold ($\dot{D}O_2$ crit.), and it signifies the $\dot{D}O_2$ below which oxygen supply and demand are unbalanced. Initial studies of patients with ARDS suggested that the $\dot{V}O_2$ and $\dot{D}O_2$ relation was altered (17). It was postulated that oxygen uptake was dependent on oxygen delivery at all levels of oxygen delivery, including delivery levels that were normally more than sufficient to meet tissue metabolic demands (i.e. above $\dot{D}O_2$ crit.) (Fig. 8.5.6). This signified that there was an oxygen supply-demand imbalance, adding up to a covert oxygen debt (17). However, recent studies do not demonstrate a correlation between oxygen uptake and oxygen delivery in patients with ARDS and sepsis (18). The earlier studies which showed abnormal dependence of oxygen consumption on oxygen delivery were probably flawed by methodical problems. Also, in many studies of oxygen delivery the interpretation of results can be potentially vitiated by the problem of mathematical coupling of shared measurement error (18).

The equations generally used to calculate oxygen consumption ($\dot{V}O_2$) and oxygen delivery ($\dot{D}O_2$) share many variables (see Chapter 3.1). Hence errors in the measurement of any one of these variables will result in similar directional errors in oxygen delivery and oxygen consumption calculations. This could result in an artefactual relationship between oxygen consumption and oxygen delivery caused by the coupling of shared measurement errors rather than to an actual presence of a pathological dependence of oxygen consumption on oxygen delivery.

The above problem can be avoided if oxygen consumption and oxygen delivery are determined by separate techniques. When this is done, oxygen consumption in ARDS and sepsis is not dependent on oxygen delivery, until just prior to death, at an oxygen delivery less than 4 ml O_2/kg/minute—a condition easily detected by the clinical features of shock (19).

Alterations in Cardiopulmonary Physiology

The pulmonary oedema, atelectasis, proliferation of inflammatory cells and increasing fibrosis occurring as a result of 'injury', produce a fall in the total lung capacity (TLC) and FRC by 50 per cent. The low lung recoil pressure at FRC leads to early closure of the small airways, with further alveolar collapse, necessitating high inflation pressures to expand or re-inflate the lungs. The physiological consequences are an increase in the right to left shunt within the lungs due to perfusion of atelectatic alveoli, increased ventilation-perfusion inequalities, increase in dead space, and increasingly non-compliant or stiff lungs. 'Injury' as stressed earlier, may be mild, moderate or severe. Of equal importance is the fact that even in severe injury, the lungs are not evenly or homogenously affected. Computerized tomography has demonstrated a three zone model of the lung—healthy alveoli, diseased alveoli which cannot be recruited, and damaged alveoli which continue to be recruitable.

Severe lung injury is sooner or later associated with increasing pulmonary hypertension. The latter is due to hypoxia and to an obstructed, distorted pulmonary circulation. The resultant increase in right ventricular afterload can not only lead to right heart failure,

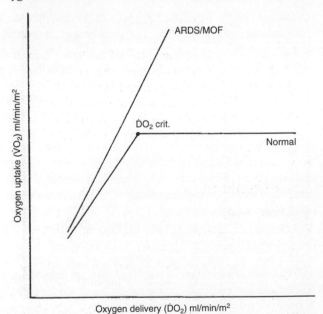

Fig. 8.5.6. Relationship between oxygen uptake and delivery in patients with ARDS/MOF and in normal subjects.

but also cause a shift of the septum to the left. The septal shift can significantly reduce left ventricular filling and stroke volume.

Myocardial dysfunction is an important feature of acute lung injury. It is contributed to by a circulating myocardial depressant factor (probably the same as TNF) in patients with sepsis. A significant fall in cardiac output is frequently observed in these patients particularly when the mean pulmonary artery pressure exceeds 35 mm Hg. A fall in cardiac output, particularly when combined with a low oxygen tension in arterial blood, can cause a significant reduction in oxygen transport to the tissues. A decreased oxygen transport in association with a possible abnormality of oxygen uptake by the tissues, so frequently observed in acute lung injury, invariably spells disaster.

Clinical Features

Against a background of one of the aetiologies mentioned earlier, the patient with ARDS presents with rapidly worsening dyspnoea and restlessness. On examination such a patient has tachycardia, tachypnoea, and increasing hypoxaemia despite supplemental oxygen. Auscultation reveals scattered crackles and occasionally a wheeze. The condition may evolve rapidly over a few hours, or may take a few days to reach its maximum intensity. Respiratory distress is obvious, and the accessory muscles of respiration are active. Cyanosis may occur, but is not always evident in spite of severe hypoxaemia.

In the early stages, a slight but disproportionate tachypnoea may be the only warning sign of early acute lung injury, and in an appropriate setting this must never be ignored, even in the absence of auscultatory crackles, and with a normal chest X-ray. An important warning diagnostic feature in the early phase, is a slight fall in the PaO_2 and an increased alveolar-arterial oxygen gradient.

As the respiratory failure worsens, one or more other organ systems may show signs of dysfunction and failure. This is in keeping with the current concept that acute lung injury is a multi-system disease, with the changes in the pulmonary endothelium mirroring widespread endothelial damage in other organs.

Complications

Death is uncommon from severe refractory hypoxia, provided the patient receives good ventilator support. In our unit it occurs in not more than 7–10 per cent of patients.

Nosocomial Pneumonia

This is an extremely important complication. The incidence of this complication in severe acute lung injury (ARDS) varies in different units, and in our ICU is about 15 per cent. The incidence increases with the length of time on ventilator support, and in our experience, is most marked when acute lung injury is due to severe abdominal sepsis. It is less than 10 per cent in our unit when acute lung injury is caused by a direct insult—e.g. inhalation of noxious fumes, near-drowning, chest trauma, even when ventilator support is prolonged for weeks.

The various factors predisposing to nosocomial pneumonia have been discussed in another chapter. The lung injury per se, together with the ventilatory effects of high inflation pressures, high tidal volumes, high FIO_2, and the prolonged use of PEEP, also probably impair local immune and other defence mechanisms within the lung, and predispose to iatrogenic infection and sepsis. Background illnesses which impair immune function, and malnutrition, either present before the acute lung injury or occurring during the evolution of the syndrome, are other important predisposing factors. Colonization of the upper respiratory tract and of the gastrointestinal tract by Gram-negative organisms, remains an important source of infection.

The diagnosis of nosocomial pneumonia is difficult in the presence of shadows caused by atelectasis and oedema. We have missed a good-sized lung abscess causing an empyema in a patient with ARDS due to severe tetanus, the diagnosis being apparent only at autopsy. The choice of antibiotics in the management of nosocomial pneumonia is often empiric. The problem has been discussed at length in the Section on Fever and Acute Infections in a Critical Care Setting.

Multiple Organ Dysfunction

The better and more intensive the care offered to the patient, and hence the longer he is kept alive, the more often is the complication of multiple organ dysfunction observed. It occurs early and most frequently when sepsis is the cause of acute lung injury. It can however complicate the course of acute lung injury from any cause.

In our experience, renal dysfunction occurs in 30–40 per cent of patients, cardiovascular dysfunction necessitating inotropic support in 50–70 per cent of patients, and liver cell dysfunction occurs in about 50 per cent of patients. Complications and dysfunction involving the gastrointestinal tract are observed in 20–30 per cent of patients. There is an obvious interrelation between various organ systems, so that impairment of one organ system induces, amplifies and modulates impairment in other organ systems.

Translocation of bacteria from the lumen of the gut to the lymphatics, peritoneal cavity and even the bloodstream, plays an important role in perpetuating the inflammatory cascade that underlies multiple organ dysfunction. This is observed when the protective barrier normally provided by the wall of the gut is breached. The problem is markedly worsened in the presence of associated liver cell dysfunction. In fact when acute lung injury occurs against the background of liver cell failure, death invariably results.

Investigations

(i) Chest X-ray

The chest radiograph shows interstitial oedema in the early stages, and full-blown pulmonary oedema in established cases. The pulmonary oedema usually causes bilaterally symmetrical shadowing, but the shadowing may initially be predominantly unilateral, depending on the position of the patient. The absence of cardiomegaly, Kerley's lines and vascular redistribution towards the upper lobes, help distinguish the pattern from cardiogenic pulmonary oedema. The absence of lobar consolidation helps differentiate it from infection. Having said this, cardiac failure, pneumonia and pulmonary emboli may all cause diagnostic confusion. ARDS does not necessarily involve both lungs symmetrically; one lung may be considerably more involved than the other. This adds to the problem of effective ventilation.

(ii) Arterial Blood Gases

Blood gas estimation is essential in the initial diagnosis and subsequent monitoring of acute lung injury. In the initial stages, varying degrees of hypoxia are seen with hypocapnia. In late stages, hypercapnia may be seen. The pH disturbances range from respiratory alkalosis in the initial stages, to respiratory acidosis and metabolic acidosis in the later stages. The hypoxia is refractory to supplemental oxygen indicating that in addition to ventilation-perfusion mismatch, increased right to left shunt and dead space ventilation also play major roles.

(iii) Haemodynamic Measurements

The insertion of a Swan-Ganz catheter is not essential for the diagnosis of acute lung injury; however it may on occasion be the only way to conclusively distinguish acute lung injury from cardiogenic pulmonary oedema. Insertion of a Swan-Ganz catheter may also prove invaluable in the management of an individual patient. Much has been written concerning the wisdom of invasive monitoring in such patients, and there are some who feel that this technology may itself contribute to poor patient outcome. We now use the Swan-Ganz catheter infrequently. A Swan-Ganz catheter should only be inserted by doctors familiar with its use, to obtain specific answers to specific diagnostic or therapeutic dilemmas—for example assessing the adequacy of volume resuscitation, for titrating inotropic support, for assessing left ventricular dysfunction, degree of intrapulmonary shunting, or assessing adequacy of oxygen delivery in problem patients.

Pulmonary oedema with pulmonary wedge pressure < 18 mm Hg in the presence of a normal colloid oncotic pressure, is diagnostic of acute lung injury (ARDS). It should be noted that estimations of wedge pressure may be affected by the position of the catheter tip (which should be below the left atrium in Zone 3 lung), and the presence or absence of PEEP. All patients ill enough to require a Swan-Ganz catheter, are ill enough to require at least 10 cm H_2O of PEEP. In critically ill hypoxaemic patients, it may not be wise to switch off PEEP even whilst the necessary haemodynamic measurements are being made. Some authors have advocated subtracting 50 per cent of the PEEP value from the measured wedge pressure, but a study by Teboul and associates (20) suggested that PEEP did not affect the correlation between wedge pressure and left ventricular end-diastolic measurements, even in patients with severe acute lung injury. To avoid iatrogenic complications, we prefer to remove a Swan-Ganz catheter within three days.

(iv) Pulmonary Compliance

Lung compliance is usually decreased to < 30 ml/cm H_2O. Compliance can easily be measured in patients on mechanical ventilator support.

(v) Routine Tests

Tests for evidence of other organ dysfunction—e.g. renal, hepatic, haematological parameters, should be done.

(vi) Full Bacteriological Screen

This should include blood culture, cultures of tracheal aspirates, and in some patients with nosocomial pneumonia, culture of broncho-alveolar lavage fluid or culture of protected brush samples obtained bronchoscopically, to determine the nature of the infecting organism. Cultures of urine and other body secretions and discharges are often necessary.

Prognosis

Four factors determine prognosis in acute lung injury:
  (i) Severity of the lung injury
 (ii) Nature and severity of the precipitating factor
(iii) Presence and degree of dysfunction of other organ systems
(iv) Background or associated disease

In our experience, prognosis depends less on the severity of acute lung injury and more on the other three factors listed above. Uncontrollable sepsis, particularly uncontrollable intra-abdominal sepsis, has a hopeless prognosis with a 100 per cent mortality. Severe sepsis even when controlled, can set into motion a chain of events that may carry a mortality of > 60 per cent. Prognosis is worse in the presence of septic shock. On the other hand, direct injury to the lungs as in drowning, inhalation of noxious fumes, mild to moderate aspiration of gastric contents, in our experience, has a mortality of < 20 per cent, provided there is no nosocomial infection and no other major complication. Severe nosocomial pneumonia occurring in ARDS has a mortality of about 30 per cent.

In the West, the reported mortality for single organ failure is 15–30 per cent, for two organ failure it is 45–55 per cent, and for three or more organ failure lasting for more than four days > 85 per cent (**21**). In our experience we have found this true only for Gram-negative sepsis. These figures are unnecessarily pessimistic and are not true when multiple organ failure complicates fulminant Pl. falciparum infection, fulminant **tetanus** and other severe tropical infections. Fulminant tetanus with excellent intensive care has a mortality of less than 10 per cent, and in fulminant Pl. falciparum infection the mortality even with severe prolonged multiple organ dysfunction is below 30 per cent. The subject has been further discussed in the Chapter on Multiple Organ Dysfunction Syndrome.

Management

Despite the many recent advances in intensive care, acute lung injury continues to carry an overall mortality of 30–60 per cent. As mentioned earlier, patients with acute lung injury and ARDS do not usually die of respiratory failure (only 16 per cent of all deaths in one large series were due to refractory hypoxaemia and hypercapnia). The majority of patients die of sepsis and multiple organ failure (**22**). The following management principles apply:

I. Treatment of the Underlying Condition

This should be identified promptly and treated aggressively. As mentioned earlier, sepsis is the usual trigger and should be treated with appropriate antibiotics and surgical drainage if necessary. Prompt surgery for abdominal sepsis is mandatory. Specific therapy for fulminant tropical problems causing ARDS should be immediate—in particular the use of quinine for severe Plasmodium falciparum infections.

II. Respiratory Support

This forms the cornerstone in the management of ALI and ARDS. Yet it needs to be stressed that mechanical ventilation is purely supportive, allowing the lungs time to recover from the acute insult. Mechanical ventilation in patients with severe acute lung injury (ARDS) presents complex problems and difficulties. To be effective, the intensivist must be aware of the changes in cardiorespiratory physiopathology, the interaction between the heart and the lungs, the importance not only of effective gas exchange but of efficient oxygen transport, the dangers and complications of ventilator support.

Initiating Ventilator Support

There are two important indications for initiating ventilator support in this syndrome. The first is progressive hypoxaemia not responding to oxygen inhalation; the second is a marked, unsustainable increase in the work of breathing, as when the respiratory rate is > 35 to 40/minute and the minute ventilation exceeds 12 l/minute. A lowered lung compliance adds even more to the work of breathing. Under the above circumstances, it is best to electively intubate and initiate ventilatory support even if the PaO_2 is greater than 60 mm Hg on supplemental oxygen. Elective intubation and ventilatory support is also preferred in the presence of haemodynamic instability and if for any reason the patient is unable to maintain and protect the airway (**Table 8.5.2**).

Table 8.5.2. Indications for endotracheal intubation and mechanical ventilation

---

* Refractory hypoxaemia unresponsive to supplemental oxygen
* Excessive work of breathing
  – respiratory rate > 35 / min
  – minute ventilation > 12 l / min
* Haemodynamic instability
* Inability to protect airway
* Anticipated rapid clinical deterioration

Non-invasive Ventilator Support

Severe acute lung injury (ARDS) always needs intubation and mechanical ventilation. A very small subset of patients with mild acute lung injury may however be adequately oxygenated with the help of continuous positive airway pressure (CPAP) or by the use of a BiPAP ventilator, using a tight fitting face mask. CPAP levels are usually kept between 10–12 cm H_2O. In order to maintain intrathoracic pressure at the required level of CPAP throughout the respiratory cycle, high gas flows in excess of 70 l/min are required (**16**). With a BiPAP machine, reasonable initial ventilator settings

are EPAP of 7 to 10 cm H_2O and IPAP of around 15 cm, the settings being adjusted both for patient comfort and for providing and maintaining an SaO_2 of greater than 90 per cent. Non-invasive mechanical ventilation in patients with mild acute lung injury recruits collapsed alveoli, increases the functional residual capacity (FRC) and lung compliance, thereby unloading the respiratory muscles and reducing the work of breathing. A good response to non-invasive positive pressure ventilation is generally observed within 30 minutes of its initiation and is characterized by improved oxygen saturation, a fall in respiratory rate and less patient distress. An inability to maintain SaO_2 to ≥ 90 per cent or the presence of haemodynamic instability, or a worsening clinical state are indications for intubation and mechanical ventilation.

Dangers of Endotracheal Intubation in ALI and ARDS

The major danger during intubation is a severe increase in hypoxia, in an individual who is already hypoxic to start with. Haemodynamic instability and the danger of gastric aspiration form additional risks during intubation.

Endotracheal intubation should therefore be performed by an expert, preferably with the patient awake, using mild sedation with a benzodiapine or a narcotic. In an acute crisis, succinylcholine along with intravenous propofol may be used.

Changing of the endotracheal tube in a patient with ARDS following rupture of the cuff, or due to obstruction of the tube is also risky. A sudden loss of PEEP during this procedure may cause rapid desaturation with dangerous sequelae.

Principles of Mechanical Ventilation

The basic tenet as always, is to maintain adequate oxygenation and ventilation while minimizing complications. The last several years have seen the evolution of two fundamental concepts in the ventilatory support of patients with ARDS. First, is the prevention of over-distension of the alveoli by limiting tidal volume or the inspiratory pressure. Second, is to choose a level of positive end-expiratory pressure (PEEP) which is sufficiently high to prevent derecruitment of the alveoli at end expiration. The fundamental concepts that guide ventilator support in ARDS are these two lung-protection goals. Avoidance of oxygen toxicity to the lungs and prevention of haemodynamic instability of the cardiovascular system are two other important conditions guiding ventilator support in these patients.

Limiting Tidal Volume. Large tidal volumes (10–15 ml/kg) in patients with ARDS are dangerous (**23**). It is now increasingly believed that over-distension of alveoli in these patients can cause an amplification of the already existing lung injury (volutrauma), presumably by increasing oedema and pulmonary cytokine production (**24**). In addition to 'volutrauma', high intra-alveolar and inspiratory pressures can lead to an increased incidence of barotrauma. The concept of barotrauma is not new, but its spectrum includes not just pneumothorax, but also pneumomediastinum, interstitial emphysema, subcutaneous emphysema, and pulmonary haemorrhage (**25**). Hence, to avoid overdistension of the alveoli and undue increase in intra-alveolar pressure, the tidal volume in patients with ARDS is limited to 6–8 ml/kg to start with.

It is then adjusted downwards as necessary so as to keep the plateau pressure (P plat) below 30 cm H_2O. Alternatively, if a pressure-cycled mode is being used the peak inspiratory pressure should not be more than 30 cm H_2O. A frequent consequence of a limitation of the tidal volume in the above manner, is a rise in the $PaCO_2$ to above 40 mm Hg. The $PaCO_2$ is allowed to rise—a condition called permissive hypercapnia, which is discussed later.

Recently, the ARDS network trial (26) proved that patients treated with a low tidal volume of 6 ml/kg had a reduced mortality of 22 per cent compared with patients treated with a tidal volume of 12 ml/kg. This difference in mortality was related to a greater reduction in IL-6 levels in patients with low tidal volumes (27). Rainieri and co-workers (27) have also shown lower levels of TNF, IL-1, IL-6, and IL-8 in the broncho-alveolar lavage fluid of patients treated with the 'lung protective' ventilatory strategies, when compared to patients treated with the more conventional ventilatory techniques.

The Use of PEEP

PEEP has been discussed fully in the Chapter on Mechanical Ventilation.

PEEP is not a new ventilatory strategy but a mainstay of oxygenation in ALI and ARDS ever since the original description of the syndrome. Its mode of action in promoting oxygenation has been known for several years. It acts by recruiting collapsed alveoli, restoring FRC to normal, and thus increasing compliance (28). It also causes redistribution of lung water within the alveolar space, improving $\dot{V}/\dot{Q}$ mismatch and decreasing the shunt and venous admixture. By improving oxygenation, PEEP allows the oxygen concentration delivered to the patient to be reduced, thus decreasing the chances of oxygen toxicity, which in itself can worsen lung injury.

Of recent interest, is the likelihood that PEEP, if properly adjusted, also prevents further lung injury during mechanical ventilation of patients with ARDS. How does it do so? The concertina effect of opening of the alveoli during the inspiratory phase of mechanical ventilation, followed by well-nigh total closure of alveoli during the expiratory derecruitment, generates strong shear forces that worsen and perpetuate lung injury. Choosing the exact level of PEEP that can prevent the derecruitment of alveoli during mechanical ventilation is a difficult but an important 'lung protection' goal in patients with ALI and ARDS. One can do so by plotting a pressure volume curve in a given patient (**Fig. 8.5.7**), noting the lower inflection point, the upper inflection point and adjusting the PEEP level a little above the lower inflection point. Most intensivists do not routinely perform pressure volume curves but choose a minimum PEEP that is likely to prevent derecruitment of alveoli. This level in many, though not in all, patients is generally between 10–12 cm H_2O. Remarkably enough, this approach is similar in effect to the use of the least PEEP that provides adequate oxygenation on an $FIO_2 < 0.6$, because most patients with ARDS will need a PEEP of at least 10 cm H_2O for adequate oxygenation.

PEEP can cause important complications during mechanical ventilation. These complications and the various other methods

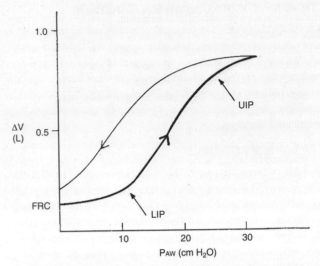

Fig. 8.5.7. Pressure-Volume curve in ARDS. To start with, there is not much change in volume with increasing airway pressure. At the Lower Inflation Pressure level, volume suddenly increases disproportionately to the rise in pressure signifying opening of atelectatic alveoli. The LIP is generally around 10 cm H_2O. At the upper inflation point the curve flattens—further pressure would lead to alveolar overdistension. To prevent repeated opening and closure of alveoli, ventilation should occur beyond the LIP. Hence, PEEP is usually adjusted between 10 to 15 cm H_2O.
LIP = Lower inspiratory pressure
UIP = Upper inspiratory pressure
ΔV = Change in volume

of adjusting PEEP, have been discussed in the Chapter on Mechanical Ventilation to which the reader is referred.

Ventilator Modes (also see Chapter on Mechanical Ventilation)

There are a large number of ventilatory modes offered by currently available ventilators. Whichever mode one uses, the focus should be on preventing alveolar overdistension, preventing derecruitment, avoiding oxygen toxicity and minimizing cardiovascular instability. The intensivist should be thoroughly familiar with a few common modes rather than attempt to know all available modes. Adequate ventilatory support in ARDS can almost always be offered by the basic and conventional volume-cycled modes and the pressure-cycled modes. Many units also use inverse ratio ventilation which is either volume-controlled or pressure-controlled. The use of prone posture ventilation is also frequently adopted in most ICUs to help improve poor oxygenation, whatever the ventilatory mode in use. Finally, permissive hypercapnia is a frequently adopted policy in the ventilatory management of ARDS. The above commonly used modes and strategies are briefly discussed below.

The unconventional and investigational modes include open lung ventilation, airway pressure release ventilation, proportional assist ventilation, high frequency ventilation, extracorporeal membrane oxygenation (ECMO), ECMO + CO_2 removal (ECMCO$_2$R), intravascular oxygen device (IVOX). Open lung ventilation is now being increasingly used by many units to ventilate patients with acute respiratory failure, in particular patients with ARDS.

Therefore, it can hardly be termed unconventional. The principles of this mode are considered later in this chapter. The detailed procedure or application of the open lung concept is considered in the Chapter on Mechanical Ventilation. The other unconventional and investigational modes listed above are briefly touched upon in the Chapter on Mechanical Ventilation.

Volume-cycled Modes. The assist/control mode in our opinion, should be the first choice in most ICUs. Its advantages include the delivery of a fixed tidal volume, the easy determination of respiratory mechanics and its operational simplicity. Volutrauma is prevented by using small tidal volumes of 4 to 8 ml/kg so as not to exceed a peak plateau pressure of 30 cm H_2O. Sedation, with or without induced neuromuscular paralysis, is generally necessary for efficient ventilatory support. The use of intermittent mandatory ventilatory support in severe lung injury, in our opinion, is not advocated (see Chapter on Mechanical Ventilation). Typical initial ventilator settings in the assist-control mode are given in **Table 8.5.3**.

Table 8.5.3. Initial ventilatory settings

Mode	Assist/Control
VT	7 ml/kg
RR	18–20
MV	8.5 l/min
I/E ratio	1:2 to 1:3
PEEP	10 cm H_2O
FIO$_2$	1

Mode	Pressure-control
PIP	30 cm H_2O
PEEP	10 cm H_2O
RR	15
FIO$_2$	1
I/E ratio	1:2 to 1:3

Mode	Pressure-control inverse ratio ventilation

All settings as in pressure-control but I/E ratio varying from 1:1 to 2:1.

Mode	Pressure-support
PIP	30 cm H_2O
PEEP	10 cm H_2O
RR	Governed by patient
FIO$_2$	1

Once the patient is stabilized (generally within 10 to 20 minutes), the ventilatory settings are tailored to the individual patient guided by pulse oximetry (SaO$_2$ > 90%), arterial blood gases, patient comfort. Lung protection goals are always kept in mind even if this leads to hypercapnia.

Pressure-cycled Modes. These include the pressure-control mode (PCV) and pressure-support mode. The intensivist sets both the peak inspiratory pressure which should not exceed 30 cm H_2O and also sets a suitable positive end expiratory pressure. Severe lung injury is best ventilated using the pressure control mode. The pressure-support mode (PSV) may be given a try in mild acute lung injury. The difference in flow profile between the assist/control mode and the pressure-control mode can be exploited to the benefit of the patient. Thus, lesser peak inspiratory pressures are required to produce an equivalent tidal volume in the pressure control mode when compared to the assist control mode, thereby reducing the risk of barotrauma. Pressure control modes are often uncomfortable and invariably necessitate sedation with or without induced neuromuscular paralysis. Typical initial ventilator settings for PCV and PSV are given in **Table 8.5.3**.

Inverse Ratio Ventilation

The usual inspiration-expiration ratio on ventilatory support varies from 1:2 to 1:3. This can be changed to 1:1 or even inversed to 1.5:1 or 2:1. Inverse-ratio ventilation (IRV) can be volume-controlled (VC-IRV) or pressure-controlled (PC-IRV) so that inspiratory time exceeds expiratory time. The inspiratory time can be prolonged in the VC-IRV mode by lowering the inspiratory flow rate, introducing an end-inspiratory plateau or by using a decelerating flow profile. In the PC-IRV mode, the inspiratory time is prolonged by adjusting the inspiratory-expiratory (I:E) ratio to 1:1, 1.5:1 or even 2:1. We always prefer PC-IRV to VC-IRV as the latter often results in high peak pressures by stacking mandatory breaths one on top of the other (**29**). This has the potential for reducing oxygen transport through reduction of the cardiac output.

The advantages attributed to PC-IRV compared to assist-control mode for a similar tidal volume are: (a) a lower peak pressure due to the low end-inspiratory flow rate; (b) a higher mean alveolar pressure; (c) an increased tendency to cause auto-PEEP. The benefits that are supposed to accrue are improved oxygenation, less chances of barotrauma and a reduction in the shear stresses during ventilatory support. Improved oxygenation is chiefly related to enhanced alveolar recruitment as a consequence of increased gas exchange time, and to auto-PEEP (**29**). It could also be due to high mean alveolar pressure and a more efficient mixing of alveolar gas and airways gas (**30**). Nevertheless, increased mean alveolar pressure and increasing auto-PEEP could well reduce cardiac output and oxygen transport. Again, the influence of IRV on barotrauma is uncertain. High mean alveolar pressures and high auto-PEEP could perhaps contribute to barotrauma, just as reduced peak pressures tend to prevent it. The majority of patients (though not all) who are switched over to PC-IRV have a significant improvement in oxygenation (**29**). The improvement is often dramatic, occurring within a few hours of switching to PC-IRV. Unfortunately, this improvement in oxygenation does not necessarily last and one may need to again switch to a mode which best suits the patient. Another important disadvantage of PC-IRV is that it is an uncomfortable mode of ventilation and patients need to be sedated heavily and often paralysed. In a study of 20 patients with severe ARDS who were switched from VC-IRV to PC-IRV, Wang (**31**) has reported that early PC-IRV in severe ARDS improves oxygenation, decreases high PEEP or PIP and results in the improvement of patient outcome. Initial ventilatory settings in PC-IRV are given in **Table 8.5.3**.

Use of Prone Posture (32)

It was not until an original report by Piehl and Brown in 1976, that the benefits of a switch from the supine to the prone position was appreciated (**33**). The improvement in oxygenation may be dramatic occurring soon after the patients are made prone. In their initial series, 5 patients of Piehl and Brown with acute lung injury showed a mean rise in PaO$_2$ of 47 mm Hg.

The generally accepted explanation for improved oxygenation in the prone position is improved perfusion to less damaged portions of the lung. The disadvantages of this method are the great difficulty in nursing such patients in the prone posture, the danger of disconnection of life supporting lines, of obstruction to the airway, the occurrence of facial dependent oedema and even pressure sores. Even so, the prone position should be utilized when conventional modes of ventilator support do not result in adequate oxygenation. It has been suggested that improvement with prone posture ventilation may be more significant if it is used early in patients with a large shunt (34).

Permissive Hypercapnia

When patients with ARDS are ventilated with the lung protection goal of low tidal volumes and pressure limited ventilation, alveolar hypoventilation frequently occurs, causing a rise in PaCO$_2$ to 60 to 70 mm Hg or even more (35). Increasing PaCO$_2$ with respiratory acidosis can have potential adverse physiological effects such as arrhythmias, cardiovascular and central nervous system depression. However, these effects are not generally encountered in clinical practice. In fact, high PaCO$_2$ levels seem to be very well tolerated in adequately sedated patients. Perhaps this is related to efficient compensatory mechanisms that tend to maintain intracellular pH at reasonable levels. The intensivist must balance the risk of increasing PaCO$_2$ levels and respiratory acidosis, against the risk of increasing alveolar overdistension which can worsen already existing lung injury. Most clinicians and intensivists favour permissive hypercapnia to the injurious effects of overdistended alveoli and high inspiratory inflation pressures. The PaCO$_2$ in permissive hypercapnia should preferably be allowed to rise slowly at the rate of 10 mm Hg/hr. Some use intravenous sodium bicarbonate to counter respiratory acidosis below a pH of 7.25. This may temporarily correct the pH but could add substantially to the CO$_2$ that needs to be excreted by the patient via the lungs. Intravenous sodium bicarbonate could also lead to volume overload and potassium depletion in critically ill patients who already have an increase in intrapulmonary extravascular water content. Once lung injury improves, ventilation is slowly increased, the PaCO$_2$ being slowly brought down to prevent a swing to metabolic alkalosis. Since increased PaCO$_2$ and respiratory acidosis raise intracranial pressure, permissive hypercapnia should be avoided as a ventilatory strategy in patients with head injury, cerebral oedema and space occupying lesions.

Stabilizing the Patient

The initial ventilator settings have been discussed earlier. Once the patient is stabilized, the FIO$_2$ is generally lowered to less than 60 per cent. Ventilator settings may need adjustment both for better oxygenation and patient comfort. The flow rate in particular may need adjustment in the volume control / assist control mode. The goals of lung protection should always be kept in mind. PEEP might require upward or downward adjustments. A PEEP over 15 cm H$_2$O is unwise and often causes barotrauma. A PEEP below 5 cm

is likely to be ineffective. The occurrence of auto-PEEP is to be always anticipated particularly with the pressure controlled inverse ratio ventilatory mode. The effects of PEEP and positive pressure ventilation on the heart and circulation should be carefully looked out for and the PEEP accordingly adjusted.

Management of ARDS is not just the management of mechanical ventilatory support. Efficient gas exchange is not enough; oxygen transport (dependent on cardiac output and Hb concentration) is equally important and the interrelation between the heart and lung should always be kept in mind. Finally, ARDS more often than not, is one aspect of a multiple organ dysfunction syndrome. Overall critical care, good nutrition and support of all organ systems is necessary for survival.

The Open Lung Concept

The open lung concept though described first by Lachmann in 1977 has been adopted as a ventilatory strategy for ARDS only in the last decade (36). Gattinoni and co-workers (37) showed that patients with ARDS had multiple areas of atelectasis chiefly in the dependent lung regions, due to reduced volume of the aerated lung. The ventilatory strategy of an open lung, opens up the atelectatic areas and keeps them open. Thereby the cyclic shear forces of alveolar opening and closing are minimized and optimal gas exchange is achieved (PaO$_2$ > 450 mm Hg on an FIO$_2$ of 1). The 'open lung' procedure is always attempted using pressure controlled ventilation with an I:E ratio of 1:1 to 2:1. To start with PEEP is applied at 15 to 20 cm H$_2$O in patients with ARDS, and the lung is opened with slow progressive increase (by 2 cm at a time) in the peak inspiratory pressure up to 40–60 cm H$_2$O. The 'opening pressure' is the peak inspiratory pressure at which the lung is 'opened'. The success of recruitment of closed alveoli is gauged either by noting the sudden sharp increase in PaO$_2$ > 450 mm Hg when the lung fully 'opens up' or by the proportional increase in tidal volume following increase in the peak inspiratory pressure. The peak inspiratory pressure and PEEP are now adjusted to the lowest pressure which keeps the lung open. This lowest pressure is realized when the tidal volumes are stable and the arterial blood gases continue to show a high constant PaO$_2$. The ideal pressure is generally 15 to 30 cm H$_2$O less than the required recruitment 'opening' peak pressure. After opening the lung and finding the lowest pressure to keep it open, the resultant pressure amplitude is minimized and gas exchange maximized. The ventilatory strategy described above enables a reduction in FIO$_2$ and protects the lung from further injury. It is possible that an open lung is less likely to produce cytokines injurious to itself as also to other organ systems.

The procedure of the open lung ventilatory strategy is further detailed in the Chapter on Mechanical Ventilation.

The open lung strategy, if adopted, should preferably be put to use in the first 24 to 48 hours of mechanical ventilation in ARDS. Amato and co-workers (38) showed a reduced mortality in ARDS patients using the open lung ventilatory strategy as compared to ARDS patients on conventional modes. A number of critical care units use the open lung concept strategy as their first choice in ARDS. However, the open lung strategy requires experience, close attention to ventilator settings and extra care. There is a learning curve in the application of this strategy and at least in our unit, we still are on that curve and have yet to achieve familiarity with this ventilatory mode.

III. Other Measures

Fluid Balance

It is important not to overhydrate the patient as this worsens pulmonary oedema. In established acute lung injury we would prefer to keep the filling pressures of the left ventricle on the lower side of normal (pulmonary capillary wedge pressure < 12 mm Hg), provided perfusion of vital organs remains satisfactory. At times the filling pressure may need to be raised to provide an increase in cardiac output and in oxygen transport. The advantage of increased oxygen transport may unfortunately be associated with the disadvantage of increased pulmonary oedema. Furosemide may be necessary to adjust preload to desired levels, and to maintain an adequate urine output.

Circulatory Support

It is important to ensure adequate oxygen transport or delivery to the tissues. Oxygen transport or delivery ($\dot{D}O_2$) is not only dependent on an adequate PaO_2, but is also dependent on cardiac output and the haemoglobin concentration. The Hb concentration should be kept around 11 g/dl with a haematocrit of 33–36 per cent. Inotropic support should be given even in patients with moderate lung injury. Dobutamine is preferred if the cardiac output is low as it does not induce tachycardia. If the systolic blood pressure is < 90 mm Hg, or if the systemic vascular resistance is low, dopamine is to be preferred. The use of inotropes is on the same lines as outlined in the Chapter on Cardiogenic Shock.

Supramaximal oxygen transport (cardiac index > 4.5 l/min/m^2 and oxygen delivery above 600 ml/min/m^2), was earlier thought to reduce oxygen debt in the tissues, prevent hypoxic injury and organ system failure. This is however by no means certain, and there are a number of conflicting studies that support or refute this suggestion (**39–44**). It is possible that increasing oxygen delivery to supramaximal levels reduces mortality in just a subgroup of patients, such as high risk surgical patients. In our experience, supramaximal oxygen delivery does not reduce mortality in acute lung injury. Volume loading patients with acute lung injury to maintain pulmonary capillary wedge pressure (PCWP) at upper normal limits (15–18 mm Hg) in an attempt to raise the cardiac output, invariably does harm by potentiating the lung injury. In fact it is generally very difficult or impossible to achieve supramaximal oxygen transport in these patients. We would prefer, in acute lung injury, to keep the PCWP to not > 10–12 mm Hg, and to increase the cardiac output with dobutamine or dopamine. The dose of inotropes should be titrated to a point where there is definite clinical improvement with regard to skin temperature, capillary refill, urine output, mentation, mean and systolic arterial blood pressure. The arterial pH and serum lactate levels should return to within normal limits. Very high doses of inotropes (including dobutamine) given with a view to provide supramaximal transport, may perhaps do more harm than good (**44**).

Haemodynamic measurements through a pulmonary artery catheter may help in adjusting fluid balance and in titrating inotropic support in difficult problem cases. If haemodynamic measurements are decided upon, they are best done early in the natural history of the syndrome so that management aimed at adequate oxygen transport, is quickly achieved.

Support to Other Organ Systems

All organ systems often need support, in particular the kidneys. A dopaminergic dose of dopamine (2–3 μg/kg/min) is often used to help maintain a good urine output. Ultrafiltration or dialysis may be necessary to treat volume overload or renal failure.

Nutritional Support

Good nutrition is vital, particularly when acute lung injury is due to excessively catabolic states as in fulminant tetanus, burns or severe sepsis. Severely catabolic states require a caloric intake of 3000 or more calories/day, and this could lead to excessive fluid intake in a clinical situation which often necessitates fluid restriction. Under these circumstances, nutritional requirements are sacrificed on a short-term basis to allow fluid restriction. The alternative is to remove additional water by the use of loop diuretics if renal function is good, or by the use of ultrafiltration if renal function is impaired. Enteral feeding is always to be preferred. In the presence of ileus, abdominal sepsis, parenteral feeding becomes necessary.

IV. Treatment of Complications

These can involve any organ system; they should be promptly diagnosed and treated. Iatrogenic sepsis and nosocomial pneumonias are of ominous significance. They have been discussed in another chapter. Complications related to ventilator support are dealt with in the Chapter on Mechanical Ventilation.

V. Role of Corticosteroids in ARDS

Corticosteroids do not prevent ARDS, nor do they alter the outcome when given in the early phase of its natural history. In Bone's study of 382 patients with sepsis and ARDS, those with impaired renal function had a higher mortality when given steroids, compared to a control group given placebo (**45**). Yet Meduri and co-workers (**46**) in 1994, reported in a study of 20 patients, that intravenous methyl prednisolone instituted 7 days after the onset of ARDS helped recovery and improved survival. We agree with this experience and use 40 mg methyl prednisolone (in the late stage of unresolved ARDS) intravenously 6 hourly till such time as the patient is off ventilator support. Methyl prednisolone is then tapered off over the next two to three weeks. Steroids in the late stage of ARDS probably exert a beneficial effect on the fibroproliferative stage of the lung pathology. Steroids may be tried only if there is no evidence of infection, and in particular, no evidence of nosocomial pneumonia. A larger randomized study on the use of steroids in late ARDS is necessary and is long overdue.

VI. Use of Activated Protein C

(See Chapter on Septic Shock)

In a large study on 1690 patients, Bernard, Vincent and colleagues

(47) showed that the use of activated protein C in sepsis significantly reduced mortality from 31 per cent in the control group to 25 per cent in the treated group. The drug is therefore indicated when sepsis is the cause of ARDS as is so frequently the case.

VII. Pharmaceutical Measures (48, 49)

A great deal of research continues to be concentrated on pharmacological measures that could reduce or counter the inflammatory cascade that initiates and perpetuates injury to the lung and other organ systems. Except for the benefit conferred by the use of activated protein C in patients with ARDS due to severe sepsis and the possible though not completely proven benefit of corticosteroids in late ARDS, none of these measures have shown to be effective.

Anti-endotoxin immunotherapy, using monoclonal antibodies against the J5 strain of E. coli held promise a decade ago. However, large scale clinical trials with monoclonal antibodies failed to demonstrate any benefit in sepsis or ARDS.

Though the role of cytokines in sepsis and ARDS has been well understood, the use of antagonists to cytokines has not proved to be useful. Anti-TNF antibodies, soluble TNF receptors and exogenous IL-Ira have been the subject of human trials in sepsis, without providing consistent results.

The use of cyclo-oxygenase inhibitors (Ibuprofen), antioxidants (superoxide dismutase, glutathione, N-Acetyl cysteine), eicosanoids (prostaglandin E_1, ketoconazole), remains of unproven benefit. Surfactant replacement, nitric oxide inhalation, platelet activating factor antagonists, pentoxifylline, and antiprotease have all been tried without avail. Perhaps some of these drugs may prove useful in small subsets of patients. None of these drugs can be recommended in the treatment of ARDS at this stage.

Immunonutrition has attracted attention in recent years. Immune enhancing diets are low in carbohydrate, high in fat and have in addition supplements of fatty acids—e.g. linoleic acid. These diets are believed to modulate the inflammatory response and improve outcome. Other supplements thought to be of benefit include arginine, glutamine, nucleotides, and omega-fatty acids. Results in trials with immunomodulating diets have been conflicting, though several studies have reported reduced infection rates in critically ill patients treated with enteral immune-enhanced feeds (50, 51).

REFERENCES

1. Osler W. (1927). The Principles and Practice of Medicine, 10th edn D Appleton, New York.
2. Ashbaugh DG, Bigelow DB, Petty TL et al. (1967). Acute respiratory distress in adults. Lancet. 2, 319–323.
3. Udwadia FE. (1979). Acute Pulmonary Injury. In: Diagnosis and Management of Acute Respiratory Failure. pp. 293–331. Oxford University Press. New Delhi, New York.
4. Bernard GR, Artigas A, Brigham KL et al. (1994). The American-European Consensus Conference on ARDS. Am J Respir Crit Care Med. 149: 818–824.
5. Murray MF, Mathay MA, Luce JM et al. (1988). Pulmonary perspectives: An expanded definition of the adult respiratory distress syndrome. Am Rev Respir Dis. 138, 720–723.
6. Fulkerson WJ, MacIntyre N, Stamler J et al. (1996). Pathogenesis and treatment of the adult respiratory distress syndrome. Arch Intern Med. 156, 99.
7. Fowler AA, Hamman RF, Good JT et al. (1983). Adult respiratory distress syndrome: Risk with common predispositions. Ann Intern Med. 99, 293–298.
8. Niederman MS, Fein AM. (1990). Sepsis syndrome, the adult respiratory distress syndrome and nosocomial pneumonia. In: Clinics in Chest Medicine (Eds Wiedmann HP, Mathay MA, Mathay RA). 11(4), pp. 633–656. W B Saunders Company, Philadelphia.
9. Petty TL. (1994). The acute respiratory distress syndrome: Historic perspective. Chest. 105(3), 445–475.
10. Tomashefski JF Jr. (2000). Pulmonary pathology of acute respiratory distress syndrome. Clin Chest Med. 21(3): 435–466.
11. Kunkel SL, Standiford T, Caldwell C et al. (1999). Cytokine induced mechanisms of acute lung injury leading to ARDS. In: Acute Respiratory Distress Syndrome (Eds Russel JA, Walley KR). pp. 63–99. Cambridge University Press, Cambridge, UK.
12. Rinaldo JE, Christmas JW. (1990). Mechanisms and mediators of the adult respiratory distress syndrome. In: Clinics in Chest Medicine (Eds Wiedmann HP, Mathay MA, Mathay RA). 11(4), pp. 621–632. W B Saunders Company, Philadelphia.
13. Mathison JC, Wolfson D, Ulewith RJ. (1988). Participation of tumor necrosis factor in the mediation of gram-negative bacterial lipopolysaccharide-induced injury in rabbits. J Clin Invest. 81, 1925–1937.
14. Michie HR, Marogue KR, Spriggs DR et al. (1988). Detection of circulating tumor necrosis factor after endotoxin administration. N Engl J Med. 318, 1481–1486.
15. Wheeler AP, Hardie WD, Brigham KL et al. (1989). Effect of cyclooxygenase inhibition on tumor necrosis factor induced lung injury in sheep. Cytokine. 1, 134.
16. Macnaughton PD, Evans TW. (1991). Adult respiratory distress syndrome. In: Recent Advances in Respiratory Medicine (Ed. Mitchell DM). 5, pp. 1–21. Churchill Livingstone, London.
17. Danek ST, Lynch JP, Weg JG et al. (1980). The dependence of oxygen uptake on oxygen delivery in the adult respiratory distress syndrome. Am Rev Respir Dis. 122, 387–395.
18. Ronco JJ, Phang PT, Walley KR et al. (1991). Oxygen consumption is independent of changes in oxygen delivery in severe adult respiratory distress syndrome. Am Rev Respir Dis. 143, 1267–1273.
19. Ronco JJ, Jenwick JC, Tweedlae MG et al. (1993). Identification of the critical oxygen delivery for anaerobic metabolism in critically ill septic and non-septic humans. JAMA. 270, 1724–1730.
20. Teboul JL, Zapol WM, Brun-Buisson C et al. (1989). A comparison of pulmonary artery occlusion pressure and left ventricular end-diastolic pressure during mechanical ventilation with PEEP in patients with severe ARDS. Anaesthesiology. 70, 261–266.
21. Knaus WA, Draper EA, Wagner DP et al. (1985). Prognosis in acute organ system failure: the role of failure. Ann Surg. 202, 685–693.
22. Montgomery AB, Stager MA, Carrino C et al. (1985). Causes of mortality in patients with the adult respiratory distress syndrome. Am Rev Respir Dis. 132, 485–489.
23. Marini JJ, Kelsen SG. (1992). Re-targeting ventilatory objectives in adult respiratory distress syndrome. Am Rev Respir Dis. 146, 2–3.
24. Tremblay L, Valenza F, Ribeiro SP et al. (1997). Injurious ventilatory strategies increase cytokinesand c-fos m-RNA expression in an isolated rat lung model. J Clin Invest. 99, 944–952.
25. Marini JJ. (1990). Lung mechanics in the adult respiratory distress syndrome. In: Clinics in Chest Medicine (Eds Wiedmann HP, Mathay MA, Mathay RA). 11(4), pp. 673–690. W B Saunders Company, Philadelphia.

26. The ARDS Network. (2000). Ventilation with lower tidal volumes as compared with traditional tidal volumes for acute lung injury and the acute respiratory distress syndrome. N Engl J Med. 342, 1301–1308.

27. Ranieri VM, Suter PM, Tortorella C et al. (1999). Effect of mechanical ventilation on inflammatory mediators in patients with acute respiratory distress syndrome: A randomized controlled trial. JAMA. 282, 54–61.

28. Katz JA, Ozanne M, Zinn SE et al. (1981). Time course and mechanisms of lung volume increase with PEEP in acute pulmonary failure. Anaesthesiology. 54, 16.

29. Stoller JM, Kacmarek RM. (1990). Ventilatory strategies in the management of the adult respiratory distress syndrome. In: Clinics in Chest Medicine (Eds Wiedmann HP, Mathay MA, Mathay RA). 11(4), pp. 755–772. W B Saunders Company, Philadelphia.

30. Armstrong BW, Macintyre NR. (1995). Pressure-controlled, inverse ratio ventilation that avoids air trapping in the adult respiratory distress syndrome. Crit Care Med. 23, 279–285.

31. Wang SH. (2002). The outcome of early pressure-controlled inverse ratio ventilation on patients with severe acute respiratory distress syndrome in surgical intensive care units. Am J Surg. 183 (2), 151–155

32. Pappert D, Rossaint R, Slama K et al. (1994). Influence of positioning on ventilation-perfusion relationships in severe adult respiratory distress syndrome. Chest. 106, 1511–1516.

33. Piehl M, Brown R. (1976). Use of extreme position changes in acute respiratory failure. Crit Care Med. 4, 13–14.

34. Lee DL. (2002). Prone-position ventilation induces sustained improvement in oxygenation in patients with acute respiratory distress syndrome who have a large shunt. Crit Care Med. 30(7), 1446–1452.

35. Hickling KG, Walsh J, Henderson S et al. (1994). Low mortality rate in adult respiratory distress syndrome using low-volume, pressure-limited ventilation with permissive hypercapnia: a prospective study. Crit Care Med. 22, 1568–1578.

36. Lachmann B. (1992). Open up the lung and keep it open. Intensive Care Med. 118, 319–321.

37. Gattinoni L, Pesenti A, Torresin A et al. (1986). Adult respiratory distress syndrome profiles by computed tomography. J Thorac Imaging. 1, 25–30.

38. Amato MB, Barbas CS, Medeiros DM et al. (1995). Beneficial effects of the "open lung approach" with low distending pressures in acute respiratory distress syndrome: A prospective randomized study on mechanical ventilation. Am J Respir Crit Care Med. 152, 1835–1846.

39. Shoemaker WC, Appel PL, Kram HB et al. (1988). Prospective trial of supranormal values of survivors as therapeutic goals in high risk patients. Chest. 94, 1176–1186.

40. Shoemaker WC, Appel PL, Kram HB. (1992). Role of oxygen debt in the development of organ failure, sepsis, and death in high-risk surgical patients. Chest. 102, 208–215.

41. Bone RC, Slotman G, Maunder R et al. (1989). Randomized double-blind multicenter study of prostaglandin E1 in patients with adult respiratory distress syndrome. Chest. 96, 114–119.

42. Tuchschmidt J, Fried J, Swinney R, Sharma OP. (1989). Early hemodynamic correlates of survival in patients with septic shock. Crit Care Med. 17, 719–723.

43. Gutierrez G, Palizas F, Doglio G et al. (1992). Gastric intramucosal pH as a therapeutic index of tissue oxygenation in critically ill patients. Lancet. 339, 195–199.

44. Hayes MA, Timmins AC, Yau EHS et al. (1994). Elevation of systemic oxygen delivery in the treatment of critically ill patients. N Engl J Med. 330(24), 1717–1722.

45. Bone RC, Fisher CJ, Clenner TP et al. (1987). A controlled clinical trial of high-dose methylprednisolone in the treatment of severe sepsis and septic shock. N Engl J Med. 317, 653–658.

46. Meduri GU, Chinn A. (1994). Fibroproliferation in late ARDS: Pathophysiology, clinical and laboratory manifestations, and response to corticosteroid rescue treatment. Chest. 105(3), 127S-129S.

47. Bernard GR, Vincent JL, Laterre PF et al. (2001). Efficacy and safety of recombinant human activated protein C in severe sepsis. N Engl J Med. 842, 699–709.

48. Bernard GR. (1999). ARDS: Innovative Therapy. In: Acute Respiratory Distress Syndrome (Eds Russel JA, Walley KR). pp. 233–50. Cambridge University Press, Cambridge, UK.

49. Vincent JL. (2002). New Management Strategies in ARDS. Crit Care Clin. 18(1), 69–78.

50. Bowler RH, Cerra FB, Bershadsky B et al. (1995). Early enteral administration of a formula (Impact) supplemented with arginine, nucleotides, and fish oil in intensive care unit patients: Results of a multicenter, prospective, randomized clinical trial. Crit Care Med 23, 436–449.

51. Galban C, Montejo JC, Mesejo A et al. (2000). An immune-enhancing enteral diet reduces mortality rate and episodes of bacteremia in septic intensive care unit patients. Crit Care Med. 28, 643–648.

Acute Severe Asthma

Contributed by Dr Zarir F. Udwadia, MD, FRCP (London), MNAMS, FCCP (USA), Consultant Physician, PD Hinduja National Hospital, Breach Candy Hospital and Parsee General Hospital, Mumbai.

Acute severe asthma is characterized by a severe asthmatic attack unrelieved by the repeated use of aerosolized bronchodilators. It is a medical emergency that spells danger and should never be underestimated. Considering that asthma is a widely prevalent disease with incidence rates in the West of around 10 per cent in school children, and around 4–5 per cent in adults, deaths from asthma are relatively rare (1). What is of more significance is that despite asthma being by definition a reversible disease, deaths still occur with predictable frequency. Data from this country is not available, but in the UK 2000–4000 people die of asthma every year. There is no evidence that the death rate is declining, in fact, most recent studies show that it is on the increase. This increase in death rate applies to every age group and is rising by approximately 4.5 per cent per annum in the 5–34 year age group (2). An asthma death is always cause for introspection because it generally affects previously healthy young adults with no background of other illness. It becomes even more poignant when one reviews the asthma death-audits available. Most of these studies clearly show that up to 80 per cent of all asthma deaths are related to lapses on the part of the patient and the doctor, and are thus potentially preventable (3). Education of the public and the medical profession is essential in preventing many of these deaths. Some of the patient and doctor related factors that may contribute to asthma deaths are tabulated in **Table 8.6.1** (4).

Pathophysiology of an Acute Severe Asthma Attack

The airway obstruction in asthma is widespread but uneven in its distribution. It is caused by a combination of thick tenacious mucus-plugging of the smaller airways, bronchial mucosal inflammation and oedema, and smooth muscle spasm. The more severe an asthma attack, the greater the tendency to closure of the airways at higher than normal lung volumes. The increase in lung volumes raises the static transpulmonary pressure and results in an increased outward radial traction on the airways that attempts to keep them open. The airway obstruction is reflected in falling peak expiratory flow (PEF) and forced expiratory volume in one second (FEV$_1$), whilst the increasing lung volume is recognized clinically and radiologically by a hyperinflated chest,

Table 8.6.1. Points emerging from asthma death studies 1968–1987 **(4)**

I. Patient-related Factors
(a) Most patients dying from asthma have a long history of asthma
(b) Most have had multiple admissions
(c) Patient compliance is poor
(d) Patients accustomed to a degree of disability
(e) Patients unable to gauge severity of an attack
(f) Underuse of peak flow meters
(g) Poor control for days/weeks prior to fatal attack

II. Doctor-related Factors
(a) Doctors underestimate severity of the attack
(b) Objective measurements (PEF, ABG) not made
(c) Underuse of steroids
(d) Underuse of beta-agonists
(e) Overuse of beta-agonists
(f) Injudicious use of sedatives
(g) Beta-blockers always contraindicated
(h) Theophylline levels not monitored

and physiologically by a markedly increased residual volume (RV), functional residual capacity (FRC), total lung capacity (TLC), and RV/TLC. During recovery hyperinflation may resolve with a fall in TLC occurring before there is much increase in FEV$_1$ or PEF.

The combination of advanced airway obstruction and hyperinflation results in markedly increased work of breathing. The extreme dyspnoea experienced by an asthmatic is a reflection of the difficulty experienced in breathing at high lung volumes for prolonged periods of time. The work of breathing during a severe attack of asthma is estimated at 5–25 times that done by normal adults at rest (5).

The gas exchange abnormalities and the hypoxaemia in asthma are a consequence of ventilation-perfusion imbalance. The degree of hypoxaemia correlates with the severity of airways obstruction and hence the number of low $\dot{V}/\dot{Q}$ units. Flenley observed that a PaO$_2$ below 60 mm Hg was usually associated with a FEV$_1$ of < 0.5 l (6). In some lung units the airway obstruction may be complete (e.g. airways in that area completely blocked off by mucus plugs) and then a right to left shunt ($\dot{Q}_S/\dot{Q}_T$) may contribute to the hypoxaemia.

In a mild attack or the initial phase of a severe attack the primary gas exchange problem is hypoxaemia accompanied by hypocapnia. The latter reflects the increased alveolar ventilation induced by hypoxia and anxiety. As the attack evolves and airway obstruction worsens, the $PaCO_2$ starts to rise. Whilst the incidence of hypercapnia is low, prompt identification is critical because of the frequent need for mechanical ventilation at this stage. Respiratory acidosis and lactic acidosis are also grave prognostic signs (7).

Clinical Features

The *onset* of an acute severe asthma attack can be dramatic, for example in the atopic patient suddenly exposed to high concentrations of a provocating allergen, or in a patient markedly sensitive to aspirin. Such a patient may have a catastrophically sudden attack with extreme chest tightness and inability to breathe. More often the acute attack may have been building up over several hours, days or even weeks before the patient is hospitalized. A study by Bellany and Collins revealed that 50 per cent of patients dying of asthma in hospital had been waking up for 5 nights a week, in the week prior to death and as many as 35 per cent had been waking up that often in the previous month (8). Clearly an intensification of their treatment at this stage (for example with a short oral course of steroids) might have prevented the fatal attack.

A *history* of wheeze at night, bad enough to wake the patient up, must always be elicited. Worsening of exertional dyspnoea and increasing requirement of inhaled beta-agonists with less relief after each puff, are also pointers to severe attack. The longer the delay in initiating effective therapy, and the more protracted the attack, the worse the prognosis in acute severe asthma.

On examination, the patient is distressed and able to speak in short sentences only. He gasps for breath, each breath being accompanied by loud wheezing and sometimes uncontrollable coughing. He is unable to lie flat and usually sits upright or leans forward struggling to breathe. A respiratory rate of 30/minute or more is a bad prognostic sign. On auscultation of the chest most patients have loud, widespread inspiratory and expiratory rhonchi, but the occasional patient with severe asthma has a silent chest with hardly any audible breath sounds or rhonchi. A silent chest is another grave prognostic sign and denotes obstruction so severe that there is hardly any air-flow. Accessory muscles of respiration are in active use as the patient struggles to overcome the airway obstruction by sternocleidomastoid contraction and intercostal

Table 8.6.2. Features of a severe attack of asthma (4)

* Inability to complete sentence in one breath
* Disturbance in level of consciousness
* Respiratory rate ≥ 30/min
* Silent chest
* Cyanosis
* Respiratory muscle fatigue
* Tachycardia ≥ 110/min
* Systolic paradox ≥ 15 mm Hg
* Peak expiratory flow (PEF) ≤ 30 per cent of predicted or known best
* PaO_2 < 60 mm Hg despite supplemental oxygen at 60 per cent FIO_2
* $PaCO_2$ which is normal or high, and rising

Note: Not all these features are necessarily present in a patient.

retraction. Cyanosis may be difficult to detect but when present denotes a severe and dangerous attack. Tachycardia is always present and may be worsened by the medication the patient has already taken or received to ward off the attack. A pulse rate over 110/minute denotes a severe attack. The presence of a significant pulsus paradoxus has been shown to reflect lung hyperinflation combined with wide fluctuations in intrathoracic pressure, and when more than 15 mm Hg, reflects a severe attack (**Table 8.6.2**).

Differential Diagnosis

The axiom 'all that wheezes is not asthma' must never be forgotten. Some of the asthma masqueraders are cases of acute left ventricular failure (cardiac asthma), tracheal or large airway obstruction, bronchiolitis, pulmonary eosinophilia, pulmonary embolism, sarcoidosis, carcinoid syndrome, angioneurotic oedema, laryngeal spasm (vocal cord spasm), and factitious asthma. In a child admitted to the ICU for a first episode of 'asthma', the possibility of a foreign body obstructing the airway should always be entertained.

Monitoring

(i) Peak Flow Rate (PFR)

This is the most essential but least frequently performed monitoring test. Peak flow meters are cheap, easily available and portable, and should be present in every doctor's office, casualty department, hospital ward and ICU. Even in a very tachypnoeic patient a peak flow manoeuvre can be performed at the bedside (unlike a FEV_1 manoeuvre), and gives objective evidence of the severity of an asthmatic attack. The peak flow must be measured on admission to the ICU; a PFR < *30 per cent* of the predicted normal or known best, signifies a severe attack. Thereafter peak flow is measured 1 hour after initiating treatment, and twice a day throughout hospital stay, ideally pre- and post-nebulization. Serial peak flow charting gives a good idea of improvement or worsening of the acute attack (4).

(ii) Arterial Blood Gases

Every patient admitted to the ICU for acute severe asthma should have arterial pH and blood gases estimated on admission. Markers of a severe attack are a PaO_2 < 60 mm Hg, a normal or rising $PaCO_2$ and a respiratory or metabolic acidosis.

(iii) Chest Radiography

The usual finding is hyperinflated lungs. The chest X-ray may on occasion show an unexpected pneumothorax or pneumomediastinum. A complicating consolidation or collapse secondary to mucus plugging or allergic bronchopulmonary aspergillosis may also be detected. Co-existing cardiac failure may also be picked up.

(iv) Haematology

A leucocytosis with neutrophilia is a pointer to infection as a possible trigger of the asthma attack. A marked eosinophilia may be a pointer to one of the pulmonary eosinophilia syndromes.

(v) Sputum analysis

Sputum eosinophilia may give the sputum of an asthmatic a purulent appearance. Hence a Gram's stain and culture should be performed if bacterial infection is suspected.

(vi) Electrolytes

Up to 10 per cent of hospitalized asthmatics may have hypokalaemia, which in turn increases the risk of potentially fatal arrhythmias (4). The hypokalaemia is usually related to beta-agonist and steroid use.

Treatment of an Acute Severe Asthma Attack (Table 8.6.3)

(i) Oxygen

The majority of asthmatics hospitalized for asthma have hypoxaemia of varying degrees of severity at the time of admission. Death when it occurs during an acute asthma attack is almost always a consequence of hypoxaemia. Oxygen should be started as promptly as possible. Unlike in patients with COPD there is little risk of suppression of ventilatory drive, hence oxygen should be given at high flow rates. The oxygen should be well humidified to minimize bronchial irritation and drying of secretions. Since the main cause of hypoxia in asthma is $\dot{V}/\dot{Q}$ mismatch, inspired oxygen concentrations of 35–50 per cent are usually adequate and will reverse the hypoxaemia. An oximeter is invaluable in detecting the improvement or deterioration in oxygen saturation as the attack evolves, and repeated arterial punctures are often unnecessary.

Table 8.6.3. Management of acute severe asthma

1. Oxygen—high flow rates, well humidified
2. Nebulized beta-agonists—salbutamol or terbutaline 5 mg in 3 ml N saline; repeat every 1–2 hours initially
3. Steroids—intravenous hydrocortisone 200 mg 8 hrly initially
4. Intravenous beta-agonists—salbutamol infusion 10 µg/min or terbutaline infusion 5 µg/min, if nebulized beta-agonists do not give relief
5. Aminophylline—loading dose 6 mg/kg body weight in 20 ml of 5 per cent dextrose intravenously over 20 minutes; subsequent infusion 0.6–0.9 mg/kg/hr via an infusion pump
6. Ipratropium—nebulized in a dose of 500 µg every 6 hours
7. Adrenaline—0.5 ml of 1:1000 solution subcutaneously*; repeat to a maximum of 2 ml
8. Ventilatory support (when indicated)

Note: Monitor oxygen saturation, peak flow rates. Always take chest X-ray on admission, or if there is sudden worsening to exclude a pneumothorax.
* Use when nebulization not available and inhaled beta-agonists have failed. Avoid in patients with ischaemic heart disease, hypertension; in elderly patients monitor use carefully.

(ii) Nebulized Beta-agonists

Nebulized beta-agonists are the mainstay of treatment of acute severe asthma. By the time a patient with severe asthma is hospitalized, metred-dose inhalers will be ineffective because the hyperinflated asthmatic will be too breathless to effectively use his inhaler. These limitations may be overcome by the use of the compressor-driven nebulizer, in which drug delivery is less dependent on a co-ordinated breathing pattern, and the more prolonged period of administration permits delivery of a larger total dose. Nebulized salbutamol or terbutaline in a dose of 5 mg diluted with 2–3 ml of normal saline must be given promptly. The dose can be repeated every hour initially (watching for excessive tachycardia), and then every 2–4 hours once the patient shows a good response. Theoretically, nebulizers driven by air can worsen hypoxaemia if they improve ventilation (by reducing bronchospasm) to a lung unit that is not being perfused, hence they should ideally be driven by oxygen mains, or if driven by a compressor the patient should simultaneously receive supplemental nasal oxygen. An oxygen cylinder will not suffice to generate the 6–8 l of gas flow necessary to effectively drive most nebulizers.

(iii) Intravenous Beta-agonists

In severe asthma with extensive small airway mucus plugging, nebulized medication may not be able to reach the affected airways. Hence the addition of intravenous beta-agonists or aminophylline is recommended in all severe asthma attacks. When given by this route, beta-agonists have a rapid onset of action, but have a high rate of adverse effects, especially tremors and tachycardia, and must be carefully monitored. Salbutamol is given as an intravenous infusion at 10 µg/min, and terbutaline as an infusion at 5 µg/min.

(iv) Steroids

Every patient requiring critical care for acute asthma, should promptly receive systemic steroid therapy. With the realization that asthma is an inflammatory airway disease, the role of steroids in the treatment of acute asthma has been established beyond doubt. Failure to administer systemic corticosteroids has been cited as a preventable risk factor for death, during an exacerbation of asthma (4).

Though no study has conclusively shown the benefit of any particular type of steroid over the other, or established any particular optimal dose of steroid, the following generalizations can be made:

(a) Steroids must be administered early, ideally by the patient himself as soon as his peak flow drops below a pre-specified level (usually < 50 per cent of best). If this has not been done, they should be administered as soon as the patient is hospitalized, because they take about 6 hours to act. Available data suggests that a clear benefit from corticosteroids is unlikely to be noticed in the first 6 hours of administration, but may become evident after 6–12 hours of the initial dose.

(b) In the hospitalized asthmatic who does not have a very severe attack and is not vomiting, oral prednisolone in a dose of 40–60 mg given promptly and then repeated daily, may be as effective as intravenously administered steroids.

(c) In the critically ill asthmatic admitted to an ICU, steroids should be given intravenously in an initial dose of 200 mg of hydrocortisone every 6–8 hours.

(d) There is no evidence that giving much larger doses significantly speeds up or improves the response. There is on the other hand, the real risk of precipitating an acute steroid myopathy if mega-doses are used initially.

(e) Complications following a short duration, moderately high-dose course of steroids appear to be minimal even when this has to be continued for 7–14 days.

(v) Aminophylline

Intravenous aminophylline should be started in all severely ill asthmatics admitted to the ICU, especially those who have failed to respond to nebulized beta-agonist and steroids alone.

In patients who are not on oral theophylline preparations at the time of admission, a loading dose of 6 mg/kg body weight diluted in 20 ml of 5 per cent dextrose is given slowly intravenously over 20–30 minutes. The loading dose is increased in smokers (× 1.5) and reduced in patients with pneumonia or cardiac failure (× 0.4), and those with severe hypoxia (× 0.8). The loading dose is best omitted in patients on any form of oral theophylline. Following the loading dose, an infusion is set up at a rate of 0.6 to 0.9 mg/kg/hour ideally by an infusion pump. The plasma concentration of theophylline must be monitored and maintained within the therapeutic range of 10–20 μg/ml. The bronchodilator effect of theophylline increases when the serum concentrations are maintained at the upper end of the therapeutic range. However adverse effects also increase and are common at serum concentrations greater than 25 μg/ml. These adverse effects include nausea, vomiting, diarrhoea, headache, insomnia, hypotension, cardiac arrhythmias, convulsions and death. Unquestionably some of the deaths from asthma in most asthma death-audits are linked to theophylline toxicity; hence the drug must be used with the utmost caution, monitoring levels whenever facilities to do so exist. A number of disease states (liver disease, cardiac failure, pneumonia and hypoxaemia) and drugs (macrolides and most quinolones) affect theophylline clearance and doses need to be adjusted carefully, and blood levels monitored frequently in these settings.

(vi) Adrenaline

Subcutaneous adrenaline is a potent bronchodilator but has the potential to cause cardiac toxicity especially is elderly patients and those with hypertension and pre-existing ischaemic disease. Many patients with catastrophic asthma are given pre-loaded syringes which they can self-administer at the first sign of a severe attack. The usual dose is 0.5 ml of a 1:1000 solution given subcutaneously. It may be cautiously repeated if the patient is being monitored in an ICU, to a maximum of 2 ml. With the availability, and the ready ease with which nebulized beta-agonists can be administered, adrenaline is now much less frequently used.

(vii) Hydration

Many asthamatics are dehydrated during an acute attack because of reduced oral intake and excessive sweating. Adequate hydration with oral and intravenous fluids is essential. As mentioned earlier oxygen must be well humidified. The efficacy of mucolytics and expectorants is unproven and these are best avoided during an acute attack. Therapeutic bronchial lavage via a bronchoscope in patients on ventilators in an attempt to remove thick mucous plugs,

can cause significant desaturation and other complications, and cannot be routinely recommended.

(viii) Ipratropium Bromide

Nebulized ipratropium bromide in a dose of 500 μg every 6 hours has some bronchodilator effect, though it is not as potent a bronchodilator as salbutamol. When these two agents are combined there may be an additive bronchodilator effect. An advantage of ipratropium is that unlike nebulized salbutamol it does not cause any tachycardia.

(ix) Antibiotics

Routine administration of antibiotics is not recommended. Though infection is a common trigger, such infections are usually viral.

(x) Magnesium sulfate

Several studies now show convincingly, that 2 g of $MgSO_4$ in adults, given as a 20 minute IV infusion undoubtedly improves pulmonary function when used as an adjunct to standard therapy (9). Some studies have shown a trend towards female asthmatics and more severe asthmatics responding better to $MgSO_4$. Because it is a safe and cheap form of therapy it is worth considering in all refractory cases. A recent study looked at the bronchodilating effects of $MgSO_4$ given via the nebulized route and found that an isotonic solution of nebulized $MgSO_4$ was a useful adjuvant to salbutamol in the treatment of severe asthma in adults (10).

Subsequent Monitoring

In addition to subjective improvement in symptoms and signs, objective monitoring of peak flow and oxygen saturation is the best way of assessing the progress of an acute asthma attack. Peak flows are recorded and charted throughout the patient's stay in the ICU. In the initial days they remain low and morning dips are severe. However as the asthma stabilizes, the amplitude of these variations gradually decreases, and the peak flow gradually approaches the patient's best or predicted normal (4).

The PaO_2 returns to normal more slowly than the peak flow and one is often surprised to find some degree of hypoxia persisting for several days after the patient seems to have recovered from an acute attack. Serial measurements of oxygen saturation (SaO_2) are much easier than serial arterial blood gas measurements.

Once subjective and objective improvement occurs, treatment can be gradually scaled down. Intravenous aminophylline is stopped and oral theophylline substituted, intravenous steroids are converted to oral steroids, and nebulized beta-agonists can be replaced by metered dose inhalers. This is the ideal opportunity to teach the patient more about asthma, instruct him about correct inhaler techniques, and give him a self management plan based on home peak flow recordings.

The patient is usually discharged when he is free of symptoms and peak flows have returned to predicted normal or best, without any of the major diurnal swings that characterize persisting bronchial hyper-reactivity. The first few weeks after discharge from hospital following a severe attack, are an unstable period and recurrent attacks and re-hospitalization are not uncommon (11).

The patient must have clear, written instructions on his discharge card telling him what to do in case of worsening symptoms. Follow-up in the OPD should ideally be within two weeks after discharge.

Complications of Acute Severe Asthma

The complications of asthma can be divided into those due to the disease itself, and those associated with treatment of the disease. In the former category we include barotrauma, and all its manifestations like subcutaneous emphysema, interstitial emphysema, pneumomediastinum, pneumothorax and pneumoperitoneum. Collapse, usually of the right middle lobe, is another well known complication. Arrhythmias are well recognized complications of hypoxia during an acute attack, and of beta-agonists and theophylline. Hypokalaemia too can result from asthma-induced respiratory alkalosis, and from beta-agonists and steroids used in the treatment of asthma. The side effects of large doses of steroids are too well known to enumerate. Acute gastrointestinal bleeds and hypokalaemia are the two complications most frequently encountered. Two rarer acute side effects are paradoxical bronchoconstriction that has been reported after intravenous hydrocortisone, methyl prednisolone and even inhaled beclomethasone and budesonide, and acute proximal and distal myopathy in patients receiving large doses of intravenous hydrocortisone (4). Beta-agonists induce tremors, arrhythmias and hypokalaemia when given by the intravenous or nebulized route. The side effects of aminophylline and the special complications that may arise as a consequence of mechanical ventilation, are discussed elsewhere in this chapter.

Ventilatory Support in Acute Severe Asthma (Table 8.6.4)

Despite all the above measures, a small proportion of patients with acute severe asthma (fortunately no more than 1–2 per cent of all hospitalized asthamatics) will continue to deteriorate and eventually require mechanical ventilation. It must be remembered that even in this select group of asthmatics mechanical ventilation is not

Table 8.6.4. Mechanical ventilation in acute severe asthma

I. Indications
* Cardiorespiratory arrest with apnoea or near-apnoea
* Deterioration in the level of consciousness
* Increasing respiratory muscle fatigue
* Worsening hypoxaemia despite high oxygen concentrations
* Hypercapnia with rising $PaCO_2$ on serial blood gas estimation

II. Settings
* Low tidal volumes
* Low respiratory rates
* Low minute ventilation ('permissive hypercapnia')
* Prolonged expiratory time

III. Guard Against
* Dynamic hyperinflation (see text)
* High airway pressures
* Hypotension
* Pneumothorax

---

therapeutic, but only supportive until bronchodilators and steroids take effect.

Indications for Commencing Ventilatory Support

1. Cardiac or respiratory arrest with apnoea or near-apnoea.
2. Deteriorating level of consciousness with inability to protect the airway.
3. Increasing respiratory muscle fatigue.
4. Cyanosis or worsening hypoxia ($PaO_2 < 60$ mm Hg) despite maximal oxygen concentrations via face mask (i.e. FIO_2 of 60 per cent).
5. Hypercapnia with serial arterial blood gas measurements showing a rising $PaCO_2$. It must be stressed that the arterial blood gas values alone should never dictate when ventilatory support should commence. Each patient should be evaluated individually; the trends of serial blood gases viewed in context with the clinical condition, are far more informative than a single blood gas report viewed in isolation.

Hazards in Ventilating Asthmatics

Even before details of ventilatory support in severe asthma are discussed, it would be prudent to point out that mechanical ventilation though unquestionably life-saving, is potentially hazardous and can be directly responsible for significant morbidity and mortality. Death rates in ventilated asthmatics vary from 0–38 per cent in different series, and in a recent review of patients ventilated over a nine year period in an excellent ICU in the USA, at least one major complication occurred in each and every patient with an overall mortality rate of 22 per cent (12). Clearly this form of treatment is potentially fraught with danger.

The dynamics of the respiratory system in asthmatics are different from that observed in respiratory failure due to other pathologies. There is little doubt that attempting to ventilate patients with asthma in a manner akin to that used for other lung pathologies, has contributed to the high morbidity and mortality in asthmatics. Even with conservative tidal volumes of 500 ml, rates of 12–15/minute and I/E ratios prolonged to 1:3 to allow adequate time for expiration, the high airway resistance in most severe asthmatics results in the generation of peak airway pressures of 50–60 mm Hg, and the potential for gas trapping and dynamic hyperinflation. Dynamic hyperinflation occurs when a machine pre-set breath is delivered before the previous expiration is complete, so that the volume of elastic equilibrium is not reached before the next inspiration starts (13). This results in a positive alveolar pressure persisting at the end of expiration, a phenomenon called occult, intrinsic or auto-PEEP. The degree of auto-PEEP is directly proportional to tidal volume, and inversely related to the expiratory cycle length. Dynamic hyperinflation must be assiduously guarded against when ventilating patients with severe asthma. It can be clinically assessed by direct auscultation (making sure expiration is complete before the next breath is delivered), or by placing a measure-tape around the patient's chest at the level of the nipples, and actually noting the increasing chest girth with each breath if dynamic hyperinflation is occurring. The most accurate method is to actually measure the amount of auto-PEEP by measuring the pressure deflection when the expiratory tubing is clamped off at the end of expiration (end-expiratory occlusion method). This method should be routinely used to assess the severity of dynamic hyperinflation in any ventilated asthmatic. Another monitor of the severity of dynamic hyperinflation is serial measurements of plateau pressure (P plat). Attempts should be made to keep P plat below 30 cm H_2O.

The two major complications encountered during mechanical ventilation are directly linked to dynamic hyperinflation. These are barotrauma, and circulatory depression with hypotension. Branthwaite in a review on mechanical ventilation in acute severe asthma, stresses that 'avoiding death from either tension pneumothorax or acute right heart failure remains the cardinal objective' whilst ventilating severe asthmatics (14). Barotrauma includes not just pneumothorax, but also interstitial emphysema, pneumomediastinum, subcutaneous emphysema, pneumoperitoneum and tension lung cyst. In a series of 21 episodes of mechanical ventilation for acute severe asthma, pneumothorax occurred in 33 per cent, and was associated with decreased survival (15). Most episodes of pneumothorax occurred in patients with peak airway pressures exceeding 55 mm H_2O. Hypotension occurred in about 25 per cent of patients in this series. It is caused by high mean intrathoracic pressures impairing venous return and resulting in a fall in cardiac output. The problem may be aggravated by hypovolaemia, and by the use of drugs like morphine and diazepam that increase venous capacitance. It can be minimized by maintaining adequate intravascular fluid volume and by shortening the inspiratory phase of ventilation. Hypotension that occurs during the course of mechanical ventilation of severe asthma, should always be attributed to excess dynamic hyperinflation until proven otherwise. A brief trial of apnoea (30–45 seconds) is usually diagnostic: when hypotension is due to excessive dynamic hyperinflation, a period of apnoea serves to increase venous return and raise the blood pressure. A favourable response to a trial of apnoea should lead to a reduction of the respiratory rate, and increased intravenous fluid administration. If on the other hand, a brief trial of apnoea and a fluid challenge fail to promptly improve the blood pressure, then a mechanism other than dynamic hyperinflation is likely. The possibilities then include most ominously, a tension pneumothorax or myocardial depression (16). Other complications include pneumonia, atelectasis, arrhythmias, sepsis, and complications related to airway management.

Ventilatory Strategies

1. Intubation

This should be performed deftly and expeditiously by an expert. Intubation of the critically ill asthmatic involves considerable risk. Many patients have increased bronchospasm and laryngeal spasm during attempted intubation, and hence thorough local anaesthetic spray of the pharynx and larynx is important. The patient must be pre-oxygenated, and care taken to avoid gastric aspiration. A large diameter endotracheal tube (ideally ≥ to 8 mm) must be used to mimimize airway resistance and facilitate suction. Sedation before intubation is obtained with a small intravenous dose of diazepam (5–10 mg), and if paralysis is needed, pancuronium or vecuronium will suffice.

2. Controlled Hypoventilation in Acute Severe Asthma

In an attempt to counter the problems posed by traditional ventilation in asthma, Darioli and Perret introduced the concept of 'controlled hypoventilation' in 1984 (17). Realizing that high peak airway pressures were to be avoided at any cost, they set a limit of 30 cm H_2O pressure on the peak inspiratory pressure (Ppk), and achieved this by reducing tidal volume, respiratory rate, minute ventilation and inspiratory flows. This deliberate hypoventilation resulted in $PaCO_2$ levels up to 60–70 mm Hg which were accepted and tolerated by most patients without complication. Arterial pH was maintained with intravenous sodium bicarbonate if necessary. An adequate oxygen saturation was maintained by increasing the FIO_2 as necessary. Using this strategy in 34 episodes of mechanical ventilation in 26 asthmatic patients, all survived. Equally important, there was no barotrauma in any of their patients. Hypotension, though it occurred in 45 per cent of their cases, was usually transient.

3. Care of the Ventilated Asthmatic

These patients should be kept well sedated with intravenous diazepam, and if necessary paralyzed with pancuronium or vecuronium. Sedatives like morphine and meperidine, and paralyzing agents like d-tubocurarine and gallamine, have histamine-releasing properties and are hence best avoided. Any paralyzing agent used must be cautiously administered. Simultaneous administration of pancuronium with aminophylline may cause serious arrhythmias, and *simultaneous administration of pancuronium with steroids, has been implicated recently in prolonged residual muscle paralysis and weakness.*

Adequate hydration is essential and small doses of normal saline may be instilled down the endotracheal tube in an attempt to liquefy viscid bronchial secretions. Suction must be done efficiently with meticulous care taken to ensure full aseptic precautions.

As mentioned earlier, complicating barotrauma, hypotension and dynamic hyperinflation must be guarded against by frequent checks of auto-PEEP.

4. Weaning

Most patients do not require prolonged periods of ventilatory support, and once bronchospasm has settled and the asthma attack is felt to have resolved on clinical grounds, weaning may be attempted. Most patients can be easily and successfully weaned. Some units prefer to switch to the pressure support ventilatory mode during the weaning process. Difficulty in weaning may be encountered in patients with respiratory muscle weakness from hypokalaemia, hypophosphataemia, excessive use of steroids, and long term use of neuromuscular blocking drugs.

5. Unconventional Therapies

Many anecdotal case studies have reported on the use of various anaesthetic agents, both intravenous and by inhalation, in the therapy of refractory bronchospasm in the ventilated asthmatic.

The drugs used include halothane, ether, isoflurane, enflurane, thiopental, ketamine and droperidol (15). Heliox (an oxygen-helium mixture) has been tried in eight randomized trials to date and in the occasional patient with acute severe asthma or brittle asthma can result in dramatic improvement (18). There have also been reports of extracorporeal membrane oxygenation (ECMO) succeeding when all conventional forms of therapy have failed.

REFERENCES

1. Tatterfield AE. (1994). Asthma—where now? In: Current Medicine 4. (Ed. Lawson DH). pp. 29–49.

2. Burney PGJ. (1986). Asthma mortality in England and Wales: Evidence for a further increase, 1974–1984. Lancet. ii,323–326.

3. British Thoracic Association. (1982). Death from asthma in two regions of England. Br Med J. 285, 1251–1254.

4. Harrison BDW. (1990). Acute severe asthma. In: Respiratory Medicine (Eds Brewis RAL, Gibson GJ, Geddes DM). pp. 674–690. Baillere Tindall.

5. Wells RE Jr. (1959). Mechanics of respiration in bronchial asthma. Am J Med. 26, 384.

6. Flenley DC. (1971). Blood gas tensions in severe asthma. Proc R Soc Med. 64, 1149.

7. Sybert A, Weiss EB. (1985). Status asthmaticus. In: Bronchial Asthma. (Eds Weiss EB, Segal MS, Stein M). pp. 808–842. Little, Brown and Company.

8. Bellany D, Collins JV. (1979). Acute asthma in adults. Thorax. 34, 36.

9. Sydow M, Crozier TA, Zielman S et al. (1993). High dose intravenous magnesium sulphate in the management of life threatening status asthmaticus. Intensive Care Med. 19, 467–471

10. Hughes R, Goldkorn A, Masoli M et al. (2003) Use of isotonic nebulised magnesium sulfate as an adjunct to salbutamol in treatment of severe asthma in adults. Lancet. 361, 2114–2117.

11. Udwadia ZF, Harrison BDWH. (1990). An attempt to determine the optimal duration of hospital stay following a severe attack of asthma. Journal of the Royal College of Physicians of London. 24, 112–114.

12. Mansel JK, Stogner SW, Petrini MF et al. (1990). Mechanical ventilation in patients with acute severe asthma. The Am J Med. 89, 42–48.

13. Sim KM, Keogh BF. (1994). Ventilation in severe acute asthma: is there safety in numbers? Thorax. 49, 297–299.

14. Branthwaite MA. (1990). An update on mechanical ventilation for severe acute asthma. Clin Int Care. 1, 4–6.

15. Scoggin CH, Sahn SA, Petty TL. (1977). Status asthmaticus: A nine year experience. JAMA. 238, 1158–1162.

16. Leatherman J. (1994). Life threatening asthma. In: Clinics in Chest Medicine (Ed. Ingbar DH). 15 (3), pp. 453–479. WB Saunders Company, Philadelphia.

17. Darioli R, Perret C. (1984). Mechanical controlled hypoventilation in status asthmaticus. Am Rev Respir Dis. 129, 385–387.

18. Kass JE. (2003). Heliox Redux. Chest. 123, 673–676.

Community-acquired Pneumonias Requiring Critical Care

Contributed by Dr Zarir F. Udwadia MD, MNAMS, FRCP (London), FCCP (USA) Consultant Physician, PD Hinduja National Hospital, Breach Candy Hospital and Parsee General Hospital, Mumbai with Dr F.E. Udwadia.

Pneumonias can be classified into community-acquired pneumonias, nosocomial pneumonias, pneumonias occurring in the immunocompromised host, and aspiration pneumonias. This chapter deals with community-acquired pneumonias requiring critical care (1–3).

Community-acquired pneumonias (CAP) are an important cause for hospital admissions. Most pneumonias are managed in the general wards of the hospital. Critical care for community-acquired pneumonias may however be necessary under the following circumstances (**Table 8.7.1**):

(i) When pneumonia occurs in the very young and the old.

(ii) When it is complicated by acute respiratory failure or shock.

(iii) When a community-acquired pneumonia leads to ARDS.

(iv) When pneumonia in rare instances is complicated by spread of infection to other organs or systems, notably the pericardium, the meninges or the brain.

(v) When it exists as a complication of another serious illness for which the patient is hospitalized—e.g. a cerebrovascular accident, diabetic ketosis or head injury.

(vi) When it is the result of a fulminant viral or bacterial infection. Fulminant influenzal pneumonia can cause death within 48 hours. Fulminant bacterial infections due to virulent strains of the pneumococcus, H. influenzae, or Gram-negative bacilli carry a forbidding mortality in spite of good care and appropriate management. Infections by rare virulent organisms like Y. pestis and anthrax can cause fulminant infections and quick death. The tubercle bacillus on occasion can cause extensive acute

consolidation resulting in a life-threatening illness; the diagnosis is missed if this possibility is not kept in mind.

(vii) When community-acquired pneumonia occurs in an immunocompromised host as in a patient with leukaemia, malignancy or AIDS, or in a patient who has recently received radiation or is on corticosteroids or cytotoxic drugs. Pneumonias in the immunocompromised patient have been discussed in the Chapter on the Immunocompromised Patient.

Aetiology

There is a paucity of data on the aetiology of CAP from developing countries in general and India in particular. The high cost of routinely performing microbiological and serological tests in all patients with CAP is probably the main reason for this. Moreover, the cost effectiveness of making such an exact microbiological diagnosis of CAP remains debatable even in the West. Empirical antibiotics, started promptly, according to guidelines would be the preferred approach, but guidelines from the West cannot be blindly transposed to India without some idea of local epidemiology. A recent prospective study of 100 adult patients hospitalized in two major Mumbai hospitals was the first attempt to determine the aetiology of CAP in this country (4). Despite an array of costly laboratory tests being performed, no organism could be detected in 42 per cent of patients. 23 per cent of patients had Strep. pneumoniae isolated, whilst 'atypicals' accounted for 19 per cent of cases (Chlamydia 11 per cent, Mycoplasma 5 per cent and Legionella 3 per cent). H. influenzae and M. cattarrhalis accounted for 9 per cent and 6 per cent of cases respectively whilst Gram-negatives accounted for only 5 per cent of all cases. These findings and the overall ranking of pathogens are remarkably similar to data from most Western series (5).

Community-acquired pneumonias occurring against a background of chronic lung disease can produce critical illnesses and often precipitate respiratory failure. Acute on chronic respiratory failure is most frequently observed when acute pneumonia occurs in a patient with chronic bronchitis or in a patient with bronchiectasis. Pneumonia in these patients is most often due to the pneumococcus, H. influenzae, or Gram-negative organisms (6).

Table 8.7.1. Indications for critical care in community-acquired pneumonia

* At extremes of age
* When complicated by acute respiratory failure or shock
* When followed by ARDS
* When complicated by spread of infection to other organs or systems e.g. the brain, meninges or pericardium
* When pneumonia occurs as a complication of another serious illness e.g. head injury, cerebrovascular accident
* When the aetiology is a fulminant viral or bacterial infection
* When it occurs in an immunocompromised host

Pathogenesis

This varies with the infecting organism. Aspiration of organisms resident in the nasopharynx is responsible for pneumococcal pneumonia, as also for pneumonia caused by other Gram-positive and Gram-negative organisms. Viral infections are generally due to inhalation of infected droplets from other patients. Inhalation of water droplets contaminated with Legionella produce a Legionella infection (7). Haematogenous infection from a distant source of sepsis can also produce pneumonia. Staphylococcal pneumonias and Gram-negative pneumonias are occasionally caused by haematogenous infection (8).

Clinical Features

Fever, prostration, respiratory distress, cough with signs of consolidation over a lobe and a polymorphonuclear leucocytosis are the classic features of pneumonia. Signs of consolidation include an impaired percussion note, bronchial breathing and respiratory crackles over the involved lobe. None of these signs may be evident if the pneumonia is close to the hilum or is centrally placed within a lobe. Inspiratory crackles localized to a lobe should be looked out for carefully in a suspected case. This may be the only physical finding in the chest in a fulminant pneumonia. An X-ray chest is of course diagnostic. The shadow produced by a consolidation may not be always evident in the very early stage of the natural history of pneumonia. The British Thoracic Society in 1987 identified 3 core features that could easily be checked at admission and which were of great prognostic value (9). They were: (i) Respiratory rate > 30/min; (ii) Diastolic BP < 60mm Hg; and (iii) Blood urea > 7 mmol/l. Patients with 2 or more of these core features had a 21 times higher risk of death. Besides, this simple bedside rule had a sensitivity of 88 per cent, specificity of 79 per cent and a high negative predictive value of 99 per cent. Other features of grave prognostic import were mental confusion or obtundation, hypoxia (PaO_2 < 55 mm Hg) and the presence of metabolic acidosis (pH ≤ 7.2). Pointers to the severity of pneumonia are listed in **Table 8.7.2**.

Table 8.7.2. Pointers to severity of community-acquired pneumonia

* Age > 60 years
* Associated with pre-existing serious illness
* Respiratory rate > 30/minute
* Systolic blood pressure < 80–90 mm Hg
* Mental confusion
* WBC count < 4000/mm^3
* PaO_2 < 55 mm Hg on oxygen; $PaCO_2$ > 48–50 mm Hg
* Metabolic acidosis pH ≤ 7.2
* Chest X-ray shows multilobe or spreading shadows
* Spread of infection to pericardium or meninges
* Multiple organ dysfunction syndrome present

There are a few important variations in the clinical picture described above (**Table 8.7.3**).

(i) In some pneumonias, non-respiratory symptoms predominate and confuse the picture. A lower lobe pneumonia may present with acute abdominal pain and may mimic an acute abdomen. A

Table 8.7.3. Unusual presentations of acute life-threatening community-acquired pneumonias

* Predominance of non-respiratory symptoms e.g. acute abdominal pain in case of lower lobe pneumonia
* Subtle manifestations (tachycardia, increased respiratory rate, mental confusion, rapid clinical deterioration) seen sometimes in old, debilitated patients
* Acute delirium, confusion, disorientation
* Multisystem involvement (hepatitis, diarrhoea, hypotension, SIADH, renal involvement) mainly in Legionella pneumonia; can also occur in other pneumonias
* Atypical manifestations in Mycoplasma pneumonia
* Acute respiratory distress, inspiratory crackles similar to the acute form of interstitial pulmonary fibrosis, bilateral pulmonary shadows, with rapid progression to acute respiratory failure, is a rare manifestation of tuberculous pneumonia

wrong diagnosis of acute appendicitis or acute hepatitis is not infrequently made, particularly in children and young adults.

(ii) Life-threatening community-acquired pneumonias in old debilitated patients, may present with subtle manifestations. Tachycardia, an increased respiratory rate, mental confusion, and a rapid deterioration in the clinical state leading to death, may be observed.

(iii) Acute delirium, with confusion and disorientation may occur with any acute pneumonia. It also specially occurs with Legionella infection. Multisystem involvement can occur with any pneumonia but again is often present early with acute Legionella infection. Hepatitis, diarrhoea, hyponatraemia, SIADH, and renal involvement occurring in a patient with consolidation should suggest the diagnosis of a Legionella infection (6).

(iv) The commonest atypical pneumonia is probably a Mycoplasmal infection. Acute Myocoplasmal infection (like Legionella infection) can also rarely cause multisystem involvement. Cold agglutinins are positive in about 50 per cent of patients with Mycoplasmal pneumonia (10).

(v) Acute tuberculous pneumonia can present with bizarre manifestations. An unusual presentation is that of acute respiratory distress, bilateral shadows in the lungs with inspiratory crackles indistinguishable from those seen in interstitial pulmonary fibrosis (**Fig. 8.7.1**). There is cough but no sputum for examination. The patient can progress to quick acute respiratory failure with a low PaO_2 (< 60 mm Hg), even on supplemental oxygen. The diagnosis is impossible without an examination of bronchoalveolar lavage samples which show acid fast bacilli, or without an open lung biopsy. The latter shows tubercles on histopathological examination, and acid fast bacilli on appropriate staining of tissue sections.

(vi) Acute viral infections can at times be fulminant, as in severe influenza. Recently the epidemic of Severe Acute Respiratory Syndrome (SARS) was proven to be due to a new human coronavirus. The epidemic originated in China and spread not only to all of South East Asia but also to North America, Australia and parts of Europe. It was characterized by fever, myalgia, progressive dyspnoea, diffuse pulmonary shadowing and hypoxaemic respiratory failure often resulting in death (11). The overall mortality was 10 per cent; for those admitted to the ICU it ranged from 10 to 38 per cent. Treatment consisted of ventilator

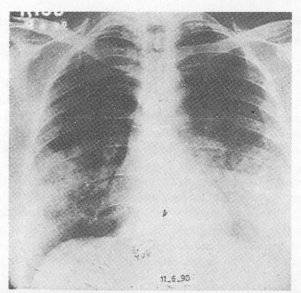

Fig. 8.7.1. Acute tuberculous pneumonia causing acute respiratory failure. Patient *PA* presented with fever (spiking upto 104°F) and clinical features suggestive of acute interstitial pulmonary fibrosis (Hamman-Rich syndrome). She developed respiratory distress with marked hypoxia (PaO_2 < 45 mm Hg on supplemental oxygen) and had to be mechanically ventilated. The diagnosis of acute tuberculous pneumonia was reached only after an open lung biopsy showed tubercles on histopathological examination, and acid-fast bacilli on staining the tissue section.

support and the use of zidovudine, corticosteroids and antibiotics.

Still more recently the bird flu virus was shown to infect human beings in South East Asia resulting in a few deaths from hypoxaemic respiratory failure.

Complications (Table 8.7.4)

The most important complication is acute respiratory failure. There is often a large shunt from right to left in a pneumonia, particularly when more than one lobe is involved. This leads to a marked fall in the PaO_2 even when the patient is on oxygen at 4–6 l/min. Acute respiratory failure can also occur because of the evolution of the acute respiratory distress syndrome following upon a fulminant lobar pneumonia (**Fig. 8.7.2**). Multiple shadows in both lungs, with a large right to left shunt following a lobar consolidation, is now invariably thought to be due to acute lung injury (ARDS), and not to spreading infection in the lungs.

Table 8.7.4. Complications of acute life-threatening community-acquired pneumonia

* Acute respiratory failure
* Acute Lung Injury (ARDS)
* Sepsis Syndrome/MODS
* Acute circulatory failure
* Spread of infection to contiguous areas or haematogenous spread e.g. empyema, acute meningitis, cerebral abscess, acute pericarditis
* Acute left ventricular failure/acute myocarditis
* Acute abdominal distension—acute dilatation of the stomach, ileus
* Femoral vein thrombosis

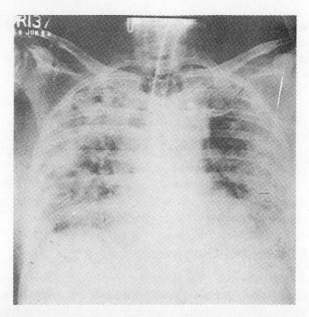

Fig. 8.7.2. Acute lung injury in patient *PM* with fulminant lobar pneumonia. This elderly lady presented with high fever and right upper lobe pneumonia, which rapidly evolved into severe acute lung injury necessitating mechanical ventilation and the use of PEEP.

Acute life-threatening pneumonia is a source of sepsis. All the complications of the sepsis syndrome may be observed. These include hypotension, septic shock, and tissue hypoperfusion with metabolic acidosis culminating in multiple organ failure.

Spread of infection to contiguous areas, or haematogenous spread, may rarely add to the gravity of the illness. Empyema is the commonest of these complications. It may be tucked away posteriorly in the paravertebral gutter and can be missed on a chest X-ray. It is clearly demonstrated on a CT of the chest. It may be responsible for the sepsis syndrome after the consolidation in the lung has resolved clinically and radiologically.

Acute purulent pericarditis is now a very rare complication. It is lethal if undiagnosed and not promptly treated. As little as 300 ml of pus in the pericardium can cause death from cardiac tamponade in a child. The diagnosis should be suspected when there is a sudden clinical deterioration in a patient with acute pneumonia—particularly in the presence of shock with a raised central venous pressure.

Acute pyogenic meningitis may be the presenting feature of an underlying lobar pneumonia. Neck stiffness and a positive Kernig's sign may however be present in acute lobar pneumonia even without acute meningitis. This is more frequently observed with upper lobe pneumonia in young adults. A lumbar puncture is always mandatory as it is the only certain way of distinguishing meningism from meningitis.

A sharp deterioration in the clinical state with confusion, delirium, and severe prostration may also occur when infection from the lungs spreads haematogenously to produce one or more cerebral abscesses. Localizing signs may be present. A CT scan is invaluable in confirming the clinical diagnosis.

Acute left ventricular failure is rare except in patients with pre-existing left ventricular disease. Acute myocarditis can and does however occur in some patients with acute influenza. It is characterized by tachycardia, hypotension, cardiac dilatation and a diastolic gallop. It may progress to an increasingly severe low output state and death from cardiogenic shock.

In the older age group, we have admitted to the ICU patients severely ill with acute pneumonia presenting with marked abdominal distension. Acute dilatation of the stomach is particularly dangerous as it compounds respiratory difficulties. Ileus may also occur due to toxaemia.

Femoral vein thrombosis is occasionally observed in patients critically ill with pneumonia. Sudden death in acute pneumonia could well be related to pulmonary embolism.

Differential Diagnosis

A large pulmonary infarct is an important differential diagnosis of acute lobar pneumonia. The distinction at times is difficult. Acute extrinsic allergic alveolitis or acute cryptogenic fibrosing alveolitis may produce bilateral lower lobe shadows with increasing hypoxia. Acute eosinophilic pneumonia should be suspected on the fairly typical radiological features (peripheral shadows in both lung fields). Acute consolidation due to a vasculitis (e.g. Wegener's) may be indistinguishable from consolidation due to an infection. Finally an acute life-threatening pneumonia may occur as a presenting feature of bronchial obstruction produced by a tumour or a foreign body. Aspiration of betel nut *(supari)* can cause a life-threatening acute necrotizing pneumonia.

Investigations

The diagnosis is made on the basis of clinical features and an X-ray of the chest which shows one or more areas of consolidation.

Radiological Abnormalities

Generally speaking it is impossible to determine the aetiology from the nature of the radiological shadowing. Homogenous shadows, lobar or segmental in distribution, are more often seen in bacterial pneumonias. Diffuse patchy shadows occur more frequently in atypical pneumonias (e.g. mycoplasmal or viral pneumonias). The latter however also can produce homogenous shadows indistinguishable from bacterial pneumonia. The development of ARDS is recognized by bilateral fluffy shadows, with increasing hypoxia.

Hilar adenopathy is observed in tuberculous pneumonia in children and in young adults. Rarely it may also occur with mycoplasmal infection.

Pleural effusion is common and when present, a diagnostic tap is helpful in determining the causative organism responsible for pneumonia.

Microbiological Tests

The nature of the infecting organism can only be determined by specific microbiological tests. Sputum samples should be quickly collected whenever possible, but antibiotic therapy should be started without awaiting results. Blood cultures are also sent prior to starting treatment. A positive blood culture is rare in our set-up, but when present, identifies the pathogen with certainty.

Sputum examination in our opinion, has a low sensitivity but a high specificity, if positive. A Gram's stain and a culture should be done. It is important to first ascertain the adequacy of the sample. If under low power the sputum sample shows more than 25 neutrophils and less than 10 epithelial cells, it signifies a satisfactory sample, which is worth staining and worth culturing. Such a specimen is minimally contaminated by oropharyngeal flora. The presence of just one kind of organism in large numbers on Gram's stain of a suitable sputum specimen, is very significant. This finding provides a good guide for initial antibiotic therapy.

Positive sputum cultures should not be viewed as sacrosanct in arriving at an aetiological diagnosis. The culture may not necessarily reflect the aetiology of infection deep within the lung. Washing or diluting the sputum may help by encouraging only bacteria present in large numbers to grow on culture. We feel that if repeated cultures grow the same organism, the results are generally significant. Sputum cultures are generally negative, or may only grow commensals if the patient has received an antibiotic before admission to the ICU. Most patients have received one or more courses of antibiotics in the community before their eventual hospitalization.

If pleural fluid is present it should be aspirated, and sent to the laboratory for Gram's stain and culture. Organisms seen on Gram's stain, or grown on culture of the pleural fluid point to the aetiological agent responsible for pneumonia.

A positive diagnosis of pneumococcal pneumonia can be made more frequently by testing for pneumococcal polysaccharide capsular antigen in sputum (12), blood, urine and pleural fluid, by counter immunoelectrophoresis, coagglutination and latex agglutination (13–15).

The diagnosis of acute viral, mycoplasmal, other atypical pneumonias and Legionella infection is made by serological methods which identify antibodies in the blood at the start of the illness, and again 10–14 days later. There generally has to be a four-fold rise of the antibody titer for the test to be considered as positive (6). This is obviously of no use in the management of life-threatening infections by these agents. Specific IgM antibody detection can however aid early diagnosis of Legionella or mycoplasmal infection. Legionella antigen, if detected in the urine points to a legionella infection. It is unfortunate that these tests are unavailable except in a few microbiological laboratories in this country. The cost of some of these specialized serological tests is also high and a deterrent to routine use of these tests.

In patients who are seriously ill, who have not responded to initial therapy, and in whom an aetiological diagnosis is therefore important for management, secretions from the lower respiratory tract should be obtained through fibreoptic bronchoscopy using protected brushes (16–19), and through bronchoalveolar lavage (20–23). Material obtained by these methods should be appropriately stained and cultured, and subjected if necessary to special tests stated above.

A *CT guided biopsy* of the area of lung consolidation may also be necessary to arrive at a diagnosis. In difficult cases, one may

Table 8.7.5. Diagnostic value of investigations in community-acquired pneumonia

Tests	Remarks
Microbiological	
Sputum—Gram's stain/ culture	– Check if sample satisfactory
	– Collect sputum prior to starting antibiotics
	– Oropharyngeal contamination may be present
	– Low sensitivity (10%), high specificity (70–80%) if positive
	– Washing/diluting sample helpful
Blood Culture	– Should be done prior to starting antibiotics
	– Positive cultures rare in our set-up, but when present, identify the pathogen
Pleural Fluid— Gram's stain/culture	– If positive, useful in establishing aetiological agent
Serological	
Antigen Detection;	
Pneumococcal (blood, urine)	– Mainly useful for pneumococcal infection
Legionella (urine)	– Accurate means of diagnosing Legionella infection
Cold Agglutinins	– Positive in over 50% of patients with mycoplasmal pneumonia
Antibody detection:	
Anti-mycoplasma Anti-chlamydia Anti-influenzae	– Help in diagnosis of Mycoplasma, Chlamydia, and viral pneumonias.
Invasive Tests	
Examination of secretions obtained from protected brush biopsies, broncho-alveolar lavage, or CT guided biopsy of lesion	– Should be done in serious illness not responding to initial empiric antibiotic therapy
	– Helps in aetiological diagnosis
Open lung biopsy	– Helps in diagnosis in the above situation if BAL, protected brush smears and CT guided biopsies are negative

have to resort to open lung biopsy. This is particularly necessary in life-threatening acute respiratory infections which have not responded to an empiric regime of antibiotics. Through *open lung biopsy* we have stumbled frequently on bizarre manifestations of acute pulmonary tuberculosis and acute vasculitis—conditions which require a different approach in management.

The diagnostic value of the various investigations done for community-acquired pneumonias is listed in **Table 8.7.5**.

General Investigations

Leucocytosis > 15,000/mm³ is generally present in bacterial infections. In patients with atypical pneumonias due to viral or mycoplasmal infections, the white blood cell count is usually normal. Severe leucocytosis (WBC > 30,000/mm³) or marked leucopaenia (WBC < 4000/mm³) is a poor prognostic sign.

The PaO_2 is often low and in severe cases may be less than 50 mm Hg, even when the patient is receiving oxygen at a flow rate of 6–10 l/min. Hypocapnia is usual and this results in respiratory alkalosis. In critically ill patients, overall alveolar hypoventilation ultimately prevails, and the $PaCO_2$ shows a progressive rise. A sudden deterioration in the clinical state is characterized by increasing hypoxia, hypercapnia, and a combination of respiratory-cum-metabolic acidosis.

Abnormal liver functions are frequently present, particularly a mildly raised serum transaminase and slightly elevated serum bilirubin. Hypokalaemia and hypoalbuminaemia may be observed. Inappropriate secretion of the antidiuretic hormone may cause well marked hyponatraemia. This is more commonly observed in Legionella infections, but can also occur with other pneumonias.

A raised blood urea, proteinuria and haematuria may also occur. Investigations in critically ill patients should include an assessment of function of various organ systems.

Management

Use of Antibiotics (See **Table 13.4.1**)

Antibiotics must be started promptly, empirically, and by the parental route in all hospitalized patients with CAP. If possible sputum and blood culture should be sent off prior to initiating therapy. The pneumococcus must always be covered as must H. influenzae and atypical bacteria. Antibiotic choice must be governed by knowledge of local epidemiology and resistance patterns of prevailing organisms. More epidemiological studies from different parts of the country will help physicians to choose the initial antibiotic regime. The following are the authors' antibiotic recommendations based on the results of an epidemiological study from Mumbai (4):

1. If the patient is ill but not in the ICU. We would recommend co-amoxyclav or ceftriaxone in full intravenous doses plus either a quinolone or a macrolide intravenously. This combination would effectively cover the pneumococcus, H. influenzae, M. catarrhalis, Mycoplasma, Chlamydiae and Legionella.

2. If the patient fails to respond or is ill enough to be in the ICU. We would in addition add on an antibiotic with Gram-negative (specifically anti-pseudomonal) cover. In the Mumbai series, though Gram-negatives were rarely responsible for CAP (5 per cent overall), their numbers rose in ICU patients (Pseudomonas 2 out of 19, Klebsiella 2 out of 19). An anti-pseudomonal antibiotic like ceftazidime or ticarcillin should be considered in this critically ill group of patients where failing to cover a Gram-negative pathogen could make the difference between life and death.

3. Specific situations. If staphylococcal infection is strongly suspected on clinical or radiological grounds, intravenous cloxacillin can be added. If there is a strong suspicion of MRSA, vancomycin should be added. If the history suggests aspiration is a possibility, metronidazole should be used.

If over 48 hours, the patient has not improved, and if sputum is unavailable for examination, or is noncontributory to the diagnosis, it is important to make an exact aetiological diagnosis. Examination of bronchoalveolar lavage material, or of material obtained by protected brush biopsy through a fibreoptic bronchoscope may help. In desperate situations, a CT guided biopsy or an open lung biopsy may be necessary. It is important to be bold and establish an early diagnosis in patients who are critically ill and who do not respond to a wide cover of multiple antibiotics. Yet boldness must be tempered with good sense. The decision as to whether a patient will stand an invasive diagnostic procedure, and whether he is likely to benefit from it or not, is a matter of judgement based on experience and expertise.

Management in the ICU

The patient in the ICU should be carefully monitored with regard to his vital signs and his oxygen saturation. An increasing respiratory rate, a falling blood pressure, and increasing hypoxia in spite of oxygen therapy, are warning signs of impending cardiorespiratory failure. We use ventilatory support if the respiratory rate is > 36–40/min, if there are signs of respiratory muscle fatigue, if the PaO_2 is < 55 mm Hg on oxygen, or if the $PaCO_2$ is > 50 mm Hg. We also use ventilator support in the presence of circulatory failure as evinced by hypotension, metabolic acidosis and other features of a low output state. Nearly 58 per cent to 85 per cent of patients with severe CAP require ventilatory assistance. There may be special ventilatory needs in severe CAP, particularly if extensive unilateral involvement is present. Patient positioning may be a simple and effective way of improving oxygenation if unilateral lobar pneumonia is present. By positioning the pneumonic lung up and the non-involved lung down, gravity can increase perfusion to the dependent noninvolved lung, optimizing matching between ventilation and perfusion and thus improving oxygenation (24). We generally initiate ventilator support in the volume control mode. If however peak inflation pressures are high, we prefer the pressure control mode using a pressure control limit of not > 30 cm H_2O. Positive end expiratory pressure (PEEP) is adjusted to optimize oxygenation. Sedation and induced muscle paralysis may be necessary for efficient ventilator support.

Non-invasive ventilation has been tried but with limited success in this critically ill group of patients but if the patient continues to deteriorate despite a short trial, intubation and mechanical ventilation should not be delayed. Patients may require ventilatory support for several weeks.

Fluid and electrolyte balance should be carefully maintained, and support to multiple organ systems is often necessary in fulminant infections. Inotropic support needs to be used in patients who are hypotensive.

REFERENCES

1. Marrie TJ, Durant H, Yates L. (1989). Community-acquired pneumonia requiring hospitalization: 5-year prospective study. Rev Infect Dis. 11, 586.
2. Research Committee of the British Thoracic Society and the Public Health Service. (1987). Community-acquired pneumonia in adults in British hospitals in 1982–1983: A survey of etiology, mortality, prognostic factors, and outcome. Q J Med. 62, 195.
3. Pachon J, Prados MD, Capote F et al. (1990). Severe community-acquired pneumonia: Etiology, prognosis and treatment. Am Rev Respir Dis. 142, 369.
4. Udwadia ZF, Doshi A et al. (2003). Etiology of community acquired pneumonia in India. Eur J Resp Dis. 544s.
5. Fang GD, Fine M, Orloff J et al. (1990). New and emerging etiologies for community-acquired pneumonia with implications for therapy. A prospective multicenter study of 359 cases. Medicine. 69, 307–316.
6. Johnson CC, Finegold SM. (1994). Pyogenic Bacterial Pneumonia, Lung Abscess, and Empyema. In: Textbook of Respiratory Medicine, 2nd edn (Eds Murray JF, Nadel JA). pp. 1036–1093. W B Saunders Company, Philadelphia, London, Toronto.
7. Broome CV, Fraser DW. (1979). Epidemiologic aspects of legionellosis. Epidemiol Rev. 1, 1–16.
8. Bruce Light R. (1992). Pneumonia. In: Principles of Critical Care (Eds Hall JB, Schmidt GA, Wood LDH). pp. 1249–1274. McGraw-Hill Inc., New York, London, Toronto.
9. Macfarlane JT (1987). Community acquired pneumonia. Br J Dis Chest. 81, 116–121.
10. Murray HW, Masur H, Senterfit LB, Roberts RB. (1975). The protean manifestations of Mycoplasma pneumoniae infection in adults. Am J Med. 58, 229–242.
11. Manocha S. (2003). Severe acute respiratory syndrome (SARS): a critcal care perspective. Crit Care Med. 31(11), 2684–2692.
12. Perlino CA. (1984). Laboratory diagnosis of pneumonia due to Streptococcus pneumoniae. J Infect Dis. 150,139–144.
13. Edwards EA, Coonrod JD. (1980). Coagglutination and counterimmunoelectrophoresis for detection of pneumococcal antigens in sputum of pneumonia patients. J Clin Microbiol. 11, 488–491.
14. Guzzetta P, Toews GB, Robertson KJ, Pierce AK. (1983). Rapid diagnosis of community-acquired bacterial pneumonia. Am Rev Respir Dis. 128, 461–464.
15. Schmidt RE, Anhalt JP, Wold AD et al. (1979). Sputum counterimmunoelectrophoresis in the diagnosis of pneumococcal pneumonia. Am Rev Respir Dis. 119, 345–348.
16. Chastre J, Viau F, Brun P et al. (1984). Prospective evaluation of the protected specimen brush for the diagnosis of pulmonary infections in ventilated patients. Am Rev Respir Dis. 130, 924.
17. Faling J. (1982). A tale of two brushes. Chest. 79, 155–156.
18. Teague RB, Wallace RJ, Awe RJ. (1981). The use of quantitative sterile brush culture and gram stain analysis in the diagnosis of lower respiratory tract infection. Chest. 79, 157–161.
19. Wimberley NW, Bass JB, Boyd BW et al. (1982). Use of a bronchoscopic protected catheter brush for the diagnosis of pulmonary infections. Chest. 81, 556–562.
20. Kahn FW, Jones JM. (1988). Analysis of bronchoalveolar lavage specimens from immunocompromised patients with a protocol applicable in the microbiology laboratory. J Clin Microbiol. 26, 1150–1155.
21. Helmers RA, Hunninghake GW. (1989). Bronchoalveolar lavage in the nonimmunocompromised patient. Chest. 96, 1184–1190.
22. Thorpe J, Baugham R, Frame PT et al. (1987). Broncholaveolar lavage for diagnosing acute bacterial pneumonia. J Infect Dis. 155, 855.
23. Khan FW, Jones JM. (1987). Diagnosing bacterial respiratory infections by bronchoalveolar lavage. J Infect Dis. 155, 862.
24. Remolina C, Khan AU et al. (1981). Positional hypoxemia in unilateral lung disease. N Engl J Med. 304, 523–526.

Massive Haemoptysis

Haemoptysis is the expectoration of blood, the source of bleeding being below the vocal cords, either from the tracheobronchial tree, or the lungs. In most cases, haemoptysis though frightening to the patient is self-limiting, and requires no treatment other than sedation and rest. In a few instances haemoptysis may be massive and life-threatening, and requires intensive care and emergency management. There is no generally accepted definition as to what constitutes massive haemoptysis. Various reports in literature use different criteria—haemoptysis varying in range from 100 ml/24 hours to 1000 ml over a period of several days (1–3). Most critical care units would consider the loss of 600 ml or more of coughed blood in 24 hours to constitute massive haemoptysis. From the practical point of view, haemoptysis should be considered massive when it is life threatening. This can be due to exsanguination, or to the risk of asphyxiation following aspiration or retention of blood within the lungs. Thus the risk of death from haemoptysis has been shown to be related to the amount of blood expectorated, the rate of bleeding, the quantity of blood retained within the lungs, and the underlying pulmonary reserve, regardless of the aetiology of bleeding (2–4). The rate of bleeding is of crucial importance. Crocco and co-workers (5), in a classic study in 1968 showed that haemoptysis of 600 ml blood in less than 4 hours was associated with a mortality of 71 per cent, compared to 22 per cent if the same blood loss was within 4–16 hours and 5 per cent if this loss occurred from 16 to 48 hours.

Blood Supply to the Lungs

The lungs have two relatively independent sources of blood supply—the pulmonary circulation and the bronchial circulation, so that bleeding with resultant haemoptysis can occur from either of these two vascular beds, or from both.

The pulmonary circulation arising from the right ventricle and the pulmonary artery, is a low pressure, high volume conduit which arborizes into fine capillaries around the alveoli, mediating gas exchange.

The bronchial circulation is a part of the systemic vascular bed and serves as a nutritional source for the structural elements of the lung. There are usually one or two bronchial arteries per lung, arising from the aorta and less commonly from the intercostal arteries. In a small percentage of individuals, the anterior spinal artery originates from the bronchial artery. The bronchial circulation has a systemic blood pressure, and factors which regulate and control systemic arterial flow and pressure, will equally influence blood flow and blood pressure within the bronchial vessels. The bronchial vessels anastomose freely with each other in the peribronchial space, and also penetrate the bronchial wall to form an extensive submucous plexus.

Beyond the terminal bronchioles, the bronchial vessels anastomose quite extensively with the precapillary pulmonary arterioles and the pulmonary veins. This anastomosis is often exaggerated in some lung pathologies, as for example in bronchiectasis, and plays an important role in severe bleeding that occasionally occurs in diseased lungs. The bronchial arteries also become hyperplastic and tortuous in many conditions causing haemoptysis. As these arteries are associated with the airways and are under systemic pressure, they have a propensity to bleed profusely in diseases involving the airways. Generally speaking, bleeding (and haemoptysis) due to erosion or rupture of bronchial vessels is brisker and more profuse, compared to bleeding due to erosion or rupture of pulmonary vessels.

This chapter now considers the common causes, clinical features, approach to diagnosis and management of life-threatening haemoptysis.

Important Causes of Life-threatening Haemoptysis (Table 8.8.1)

(i) Tuberculosis

Tuberculosis still remains the most important and most frequent cause of massive haemoptysis in India and other developing countries. Haemoptysis may occur in active tuberculous infection of the lung, or may be a sequel to burnt-out disease. Most patients with active tuberculosis who have severe haemoptysis, have cavitative lung disease with acid-fast bacilli present in the sputum. There are several mechanisms of massive haemoptysis in tuberculosis. These include:

(a) Bronchiolar ulceration with necrosis and rupture of the underlying bronchial vessels in tuberculous pneumonia. Rupture

Table 8.8.1. Important causes of life-threatening haemoptysis

* Tuberculosis—can cause massive haemoptysis due to several mechanisms:
  - bronchial ulceration with necrosis and rupture of underlying bronchial vessels, or rupture of pulmonary vessels due to alveolar necrosis in tuberculous pneumonia
  - rupture of aneurysmal portion of a branch of the pulmonary artery (Rasmussen's aneurysm) in cavitative tuberculosis
  - erosion of bronchial arteries by pressure of a calcified hilar lymph node on a bronchus
  - due to bronchiectasis occurring as a sequel to tuberculosis
  - formation of a mycetoma in chronic tuberculous cavities
* Bronchiectasis
* Lung abscess
* Mitral stenosis
* Mycetomas
* Bronchogenic carcinoma or other tumors
* Iatrogenic haemoptysis—following bronchoscopy, Swan-Ganz catheterization or transthoracic needle biopsy
* Intra-alveolar haemorrhage—autoimmune disorders, pulmonary vasculitis, Wegener's granulomatosis, Goodpastures syndrome, bleeding disorders, acute pancreatitis.
* Vascular anomalies—arteriovenous malformations
* Cryptogenic haemoptysis

of pulmonary capillaries due to alveolar necrosis may also be an associated feature.

(b) Rupture of an aneurysmal portion of a branch of the pulmonary artery in cavitative tuberculosis. Rupture of a Rasmussen aneurysm is a well-accepted cause of massive haemoptysis in either active tuberculosis, or in patients with prior infection. Pulmonary arteries traversing thick-walled cavities develop aneurysmal dilatations due to local inflammation of the vessel wall. These aneurysms herniate and project into the cavity lumen. Sudden transient increase in pulmonary artery pressure, or continued inflammation of the vessel wall can cause rupture of the aneurysm with profuse haemorrhage and haemoptysis.

(c) A healed calcified lymph node at or near the hilum can press on a bronchus, and erode through a bronchial vessel into the lumen of the airway, resulting in massive haemoptysis. The patient may cough up this calcified node in the form of a broncholith. This may immediately precede haemoptysis, or occur during a bout of haemoptysis.

(d) Massive haemoptysis can occur due to bronchiectasis which often occurs as a sequel to tuberculosis. Bleeding occurs due to erosion of tortuous, enlarged bronchial vessels, and a profuse anastomosis between the bronchial and pulmonary circulation.

(e) Chronic tuberculous cavities often predispose to the formation of aspergillomas. The latter can produce profuse bleeding.

(ii) Bronchiectasis

Bronchiectasis is often associated with bronchial artery hypertrophy, expansion of the peribronchial and submucosal bronchial arterial network, and increased anastomosis between the bronchial and pulmonary circulations. Massive bleeding can originate from hypertrophied bronchial arteries (under high systemic pressure), or from the submucosal vascular plexus in the bronchiectatic segments.

(iii) Mitral Stenosis

Before the era of valvulotomy and mitral valve replacement, massive haemoptysis occurred in 9–18 per cent of patients with mitral stenosis (5). Severe haemoptysis is generally due to rupture of engorged, tortuous, dilated varicose bronchial veins, that result as a consequence of an elevated left atrial pressure and passive pulmonary hypertension. In these patients massive haemoptysis may be precipitated by respiratory infection, by a bout of coughing, or by an increase in intravascular volume, as seen in pregnancy.

(iv) Lung Abscess

Massive bleeding occurs in 20–50 per cent of lung abscess patients with haemoptysis (7). It is related to necrotizing inflammation of the lung parenchyma eroding bronchial and pulmonary vessels.

(v) Mycetomas

Mycetomas are fungal balls occurring in patients with pre-existing cavitary lung disease. They are most frequently seen in tuberculous cavities, but have been reported in cavitary disease secondary to sarcoidosis, lung abscess, cavitary carcinoma, bronchiectasis, bullous emphysema, and pulmonary infarction. The most frequent mycetoma is an aspergilloma. The cause of massive bleeding in a mycetoma is disputed. Vascular injury by aspergillus-associated endotoxin, aspergillus-related proteolytic activity, and a Type III related hypersensitivity reaction have all been postulated (8).

(vi) Bronchogenic Carcinoma and Other Tumours

These very rarely cause massive or life-threatening haemoptysis.

(vii) Iatrogenic Haemoptysis

This is a potential complication of bronchoscopy, transthoracic needle biopsy, or the use of a Swan-Ganz catheter.

Rupture of the pulmonary artery is the most catastrophic complication following the use of the Swan-Ganz catheter; it carries a mortality of 50 per cent due to massive pulmonary haemorrhage (9). This complication is more frequently observed in patients with pulmonary hypertension.

(viii) Intra-alveolar Haemorrhage

Intra-alveolar haemorrhage is observed in pulmonary vasculitis, autoimmune diseases, Goodpasture's syndrome, Wegener's granulomatosis, bleeding disorders, acute infections and many other idiopathic systemic disorders. Whatever the aetiology, the presenting features are haemoptysis, alveolar infiltrates on chest X-ray, dyspnoea and hypoxaemia. The degree of haemoptysis need not always be a guide to the severity of intra-alveolar haemorrhage.

(ix) Vascular Anomalies

Arteriovenous malformations may rarely cause massive fatal haemoptysis.

(x) Cryptogenic Haemoptysis

About 15 per cent of patients with massive haemoptysis even after extensive investigation, have no detectable cause of their haemoptysis, and are labelled as cryptogenic haemoptysis. Patients with massive cryptogenic bleeds generally stop bleeding spontaneously, and require only supportive care (**10**). A periodic follow-up is mandatory in these patients.

Clinical Features

The clinical features of massive haemoptysis are related to: (i) aspiration of blood into the lungs which can cause hypoxaemic respiratory failure due to interference with gas exchange; (ii) effects of blood loss. Lethal haemoptysis more often than not kills because of aspiration of blood into the lungs, the patient literally drowning in his own blood, rather than dying because of blood loss.

Clinical examination may occasionally reveal focal signs pointing to the site of the bleed. Auscultation of the heart, specifically for the tell-tale murmur of mitral valve disease should always be done.

Diagnosis and Management (Fig. 8.8.1)

The immediate diagnostic step in a patient admitted to the ICU for massive haemoptysis, is to determine whether the source of bleeding is from the upper GI tract or from the respiratory tract. A thorough history, clinical examination, and examination of the material coughed up, generally suffice. The blood in haemoptysis is bright red, frothy and alkaline. Once the intensity of haemoptysis lessens, the patient often continues to cough up sputum mixed with blood or coughs up 'blobs' of bright red blood. In some instances, both bronchoscopy and an upper GI scopy are necessary to ascertain the source of the bleed. It is to be remembered that in severe haemoptysis, a patient may swallow large quantities of blood. Haematemesis (if he vomits) and malaena may then follow. Similarly, a patient with severe haematemesis may aspirate blood into the lungs, and this may result in cough with expectoration of blood. Blood in the mouth can also come from the sinuses, the nasal passage and the upper airway i.e. the pharynx and from above the vocal cords. Upper airway bleeding can be easily missed if not carefully sought.

The next step in diagnosis is to determine whether the bleeding is from the right or left lung—i.e. to lateralize the bleed and also if possible to determine the lobe or the segment of a lobe from which the blood arises. Diagnostic steps may also reveal the aetiology of the bleed. A baseline history, physical examination and a chest X-ray are mandatory. Focal signs over a lobe or a lung may well lateralize the bleed; similarly a chest X-ray may point to the lung or even the lobe involved. However, in our experience, in a truly massive haemoptysis it is frequently impossible to localize the lung or the lobe from which bleeding has occurred either on clinical examination or on a chest X-ray. This is because aspiration of blood into both lungs can result in diffuse or false localizing

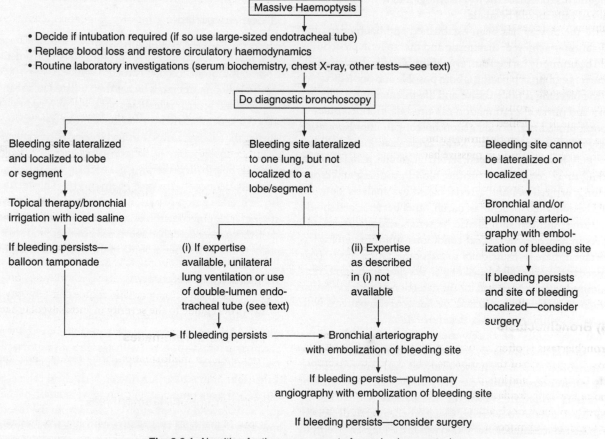

Fig. 8.8.1. Algorithm for the management of massive haemoptysis.

signs, and similarly an X-ray of the chest may show shadows related to aspiration of blood, rather than to the pathology causing the bleed.

Routine use of CT chest in massive haemoptysis is usually unrewarding. Aspirated blood often obscures the underlying lesion, or may result in a misleading mass-like effect. CT of the chest may detect arteriovenous aneurysms, cavitative lung disease not apparent on a plain X-ray of the chest, and bronchiectasis. Haponik et al. (11) noted that a CT of the chest did not obviate the need for bronchoscopy in any patient. They also noted that an X-ray chest and bronchoscopy provided all the information necessary for diagnosis and management in 94 per cent of patients (11).

Immediate priorities. The immediate priorities in the management of a truly massive haemoptysis are to maintain and protect a clear airway and to stabilize the haemodynamic state. These priorities should be established even before initiating diagnostic steps to determine the cause and site of the bleed. It should be decided whether the patient needs to be intubated for protection of the airway, proper suctioning, for maintaining adequate oxygenation and gas exchange, and for protection against sudden cardiorespiratory arrest. If intubation is decided upon, a large sized (no. 8) endotracheal tube should be used. This facilitates easy suction and permits bronchoscopic evaluation through the large endotracheal tube.

Resuscitation. A volume load with either colloids or crystalloids may be immediately necessary to restore blood volume, and arrangements to replace the lost haemoglobin with whole blood or packed cells should be made.

Once the airway has been established and haemodynamic stabilization is achieved, diagnostic and therapeutic procedures should be promptly carried out, even if the bleeding has lessened, as recurrence of brisk bleeding is both possible and unpredictable.

If the bleeding is not massive and life-threatening, a detailed history and physical examination can precede more considered diagnostic procedures, including bronchoscopy. Routine laboratory investigations include a chest X-ray, urine examination, blood count, PCV, blood urea nitrogen, serum creatinine, platelet count, bleeding time, coagulation profile, blood grouping and crossmatching, arterial pH and arterial blood gas analysis. Sputum should be examined for acid-fast bacilli, other bacteria, and should be cultured. Sputum should also be sent for fungal stains and cultures in appropriate clinical conditions. Sputum cytology is important if there is suspicion of a carcinoma. Other special tests may need to be performed depending on the clinical situation. Tests for autoimmune diseases, and for the detection of antiglomerular basement membrane antibodies, are necessary in patients with haemoptysis and intra-alveolar haemorrhage.

Vital signs should be closely monitored in the ICU, and the patient should be sufficiently sedated with morphine, 5–7.5 mg subcutaneously or 2 mg intravenously, or with buprenorphine 0.2 mg intravenously, to allay anxiety, restlessness, and to prevent unnecessary coughing. However, the patient should not be oversedated, and the cough reflex should not be unduly depressed; this can lead to accumulation of blood within the lungs, with serious impairment of gas exchange.

Localization of the Site of Bleeding and Therapeutic Measures to Stop Bleeding

Bronchoscopy

Early bronchoscopy is advocated preferably during active bleeding, with three specific objectives—to determine from which lung the bleeding occurs, to determine the site (i.e. the lobe or segment) of the bleed, and if possible, to determine the cause or pathology. In patients with lateralized or localized bleeding detected on bronchoscopy, the following therapeutic bronchoscopic procedures may help to stop the bleeding.

(i) *Topical Therapy.* Topical thrombin and fibrinogen-thrombin solutions have been successfully used to stop bleeding in massive haemoptysis (12). The bleeding may stop permanently or temporarily. This procedure allows time for further evaluation and future planned elective therapy if necessary. Topical epinephrine (1:20,000) has been used to treat haemoptysis secondary to transbronchial biopsy, but its efficacy in massive haemoptysis has not been proven (13). It would be perfectly justifiable to apply epinephrine over visibly bleeding lesions.

(ii) *Bronchial Irrigation.* Conlan et al. (14, 15) in a study in South Africa used endobronchial irrigation and lavage with iced saline to arrest bleeding in 23 patients with massive haemoptysis. 50 ml aliquots of iced saline arrested the bleeding in all patients, and the average volume of irrigation fluid required per patient was 500 ml (15). The iced saline presumably acts by inducing localized vasoconstriction with stoppage of bleeding.

Balloon Tamponade

Endobronchial balloon tamponade has successfully arrested bleeding in massive haemoptysis for prolonged periods of time (16). A fibreoptic bronchoscope is used to guide a 4 Fr 100 cm long Fogarty balloon catheter, which is then inflated in a segmental or subsegmental bronchus leading to the site of bleeding (17). The balloon is kept inflated for 24–48 hours. If bleeding has stopped on deflating the balloon, and no further bleeding occurs after 6–8 hours of further observation, the balloon can be removed. Balloon tamponade is helpful in preserving gas exchange in the nonbleeding lung in patients with massive haemoptysis. This technique can also be used as a stop-gap measure to support the patient before arteriographic embolization or surgical resection. Balloon tamponade in the manner described above, can however produce ischaemic mucosal injury, and pneumonia in the obstructed segment.

Unilateral Lung Ventilation

If bronchoscopy can only lateralize the lung from which bleeding occurs without exactly localizing the bleeding segment or lobe, a modified balloon tamponade technique may be employed (3, 18). The patient is first intubated with a large bore endotracheal tube. The bleeding site is lateralized by a flexible or rigid bronchoscope. If the right lung is bleeding, the endotracheal tube is advanced into the left main bronchus, permitting ventilation of the left lung only, and preventing aspiration of blood from the bleeding right lung into the left side (**Fig. 8.8.2a**). If the left lung is bleeding, a Fogarty balloon catheter is passed on the outside of the endotra-

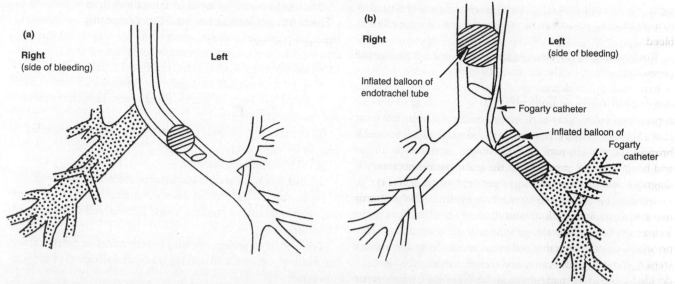

Fig. 8.8.2. Unilateral lung ventilation using endotracheal balloon tamponade. (a) In bleeding from the right lung, an endotracheal tube advanced into the left main bronchus permits selective ventilation of the left lung and prevents spill-over of blood from the right into the left lung. (b) In bleeding from the left lung, a Fogarty balloon catheter is passed on the outside of the endotracheal tube to a point below its lower end. After guiding the Fogarty catheter into the left main bronchus, the balloon is inflated. The right lung is thus ventilated by the endotracheal tube, and bleeding from the left side is prevented from spilling into the right lung (modified from Winter SM, Ingbar DI. 1988. Massive Haemoptysis: Pathogenesis and Management. J Intens Care Med. 3:171, Springer-Verlag, NY).

cheal tube, to a point below the lower end of the endotracheal tube. Through a fibreoptic bronchoscope passed via the endotracheal tube, the tip of the Fogarty balloon catheter is now guided into the left main bronchus, and the balloon is then inflated. The fibreoptic bronchoscope is now removed. The endotracheal tube now serves to ventilate the right lung, and blood from the bleeding left lung is prevented from being aspirated into the right lung (**Fig. 8.8.2b**). Selective intubation of the right lung carries the danger of occluding the right upper lobe bronchus orifice (18).

Unilateral ventilation is often unsuccessful in maintaining satisfactory gas exchange, particularly if aspiration of blood has already occurred into the non-bleeding lung.

Double-Lumen Endotracheal Tubes

In very selected situations, separation of the two lungs can be achieved by double lumen endotracheal tubes (**Fig. 8.8.3**). These tubes are often extremely difficult to place, and need an experienced and skilled anaesthetist. There is danger of the tube getting blocked by secretions and clotted blood. It is often impossible to pass a fibreoptic bronchoscope through the small lumen to verify the position of the tube. If successfully placed, both lungs can be ventilated independently, and aspiration of blood from one lung to the other is prevented. The patient often needs to be paralyzed to allow efficient ventilation. Other complications include dislodgement of the tube, and tracheobronchial rupture from use of too large a tube, or overinflation of the balloon.

Positioning of the patient. A patient with massive haemoptysis should be positioned with the bleeding lung down so as to confine the blood to that lung and prevent aspiration into the other. Once an airway is established, patient position is controversial. Blood could clot in the dependent lung and in the airways of that lung

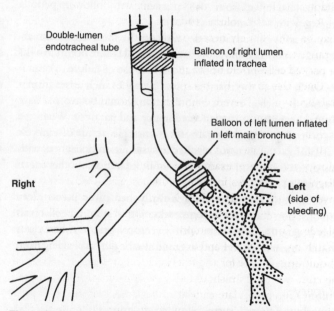

Fig. 8.8.3. Schematic representation of proper placement of a left-sided double lumen endotracheal tube. The inflated balloon in the trachea allows ventilation of the right lung. The inflated balloon in the left main bronchus prevents spill-over from left into right side. Source as in Fig. 8.8.2.

causing a permanent atelectasis. If bleeding is from the pulmonary circulation, placing the bleeding lobe or lung higher would, through gravity, perhaps lessen bleeding by creating Zone I conditions in which alveolar pressure is higher than the pulmonary artery pressure.

In very brisk bleeds a bronchoscopic evaluation often fails to lateralize the side of the bleed. This happens when the briskness of bleeding outstrips or is faster than what can be removed by suction, so that vision through the bronchoscope is obscured. A rigid bronchoscope may then be of greater value, as more efficient suction is possible through it. Even so, bronchoscopy at times fails to be of diagnostic help, and is unable to lateralize and localize the site of bleed.

Arteriography and Embolotherapy

We have no experience with either unilateral ventilation or double lumen endotracheal tubes in the management of massive haemoptysis. Therefore if bronchoscopic examination allows identification of the site of the bleed, and if the bleed cannot be controlled by topical methods used via the bronchoscope, we go immediately for arteriography. Arteriography is also promptly done if bronchoscopy fails to lateralize the bleed and localize its site. Initially bronchial arteriography is done. It should be noted that non-bronchial systemic collateral vessels from the axillary, subclavian and internal mammary arteries can also feed into diseased areas of the lung, and be responsible for massive haemoptysis. Once the bleeding site is identified by arteriography, embolotherapy is performed at the same sitting. The bleeding should stop; if it persists the pulmonary arteries are examined angiographically, and if a bleeding site is determined, embolotherapy is performed to stop the bleed. Successful long-term control of bleeding after embolization ranges from 70–88 per cent, with follow-up periods ranging from 1–60 months (**19–21**).

Successful embolization depends on the interventional radiologist's experience and expertise. Technical failure occurs in 4–13 per cent of attempted embolizations because of failure to cannulate the artery. If the anterior spinal artery branch arises from a bleeding bronchial artery, embolization should be avoided as it could otherwise cause spinal cord injury and paralysis. When the position of the tip of the catheter is unstable, reflux of embolic material into the aorta has resulted in systemic embolization, with dangerous complications due to embolic infarction of other organ systems (**22, 23**).

Recurrent haemoptysis generally indicates incomplete embolization due to incomplete evaluation of systemic collaterals seen frequently in patients with mycetoma and in tuberculous disease. Recurrent haemoptysis could also be due to bleeding from the pulmonary vessels.

Surgery

Surgery is indicated in the following situations:

(i) In uncontrolled massive haemoptysis when the site of bleeding has been lateralized, and preferably localized to a segment or lobe.

(ii) When embolization is not available or feasible, or when the patient continues to bleed in spite of embolization. The site of bleeding needs to be established by diagnostic bronchoscopy.

(iii) When bleeding from a known site within a lung is associated with persistent haemodynamic instability and respiratory compromise.

(iv) As definitive therapy in patients whose haemoptysis has stopped or has markedly reduced, and who are haemodynamically stable.

We would prefer to avoid immediate definitive surgery in patients whose bleeding has ceased spontaneously, or following bronchoscopic procedures, except under exceptional circumstances. Elective surgery is perhaps best planned at a later date when the patient's condition has improved significantly.

Surgery is contraindicated under the following circumstances:

(i) In the presence of well-marked arterial hypoxaemia and carbon dioxide retention.

(ii) In patients with poor pulmonary reserve with dyspnoea at rest, or on slight exertion.

(iii) In bilateral lung disease.

(iv) Inability to lateralize and localize the site of bleeding.

(v) In patients with diffuse disease as in multiple arteriovenous aneurysms or malformations, cystic fibrosis and non-localized bronchiectasis.

(vi) In patients with pulmonary hypertension—a mean pulmonary artery pressure > 30 mm Hg is a contraindication to surgical resection.

If surgery is decided upon, a few basic investigations need to be done to assess the risk and fitness for surgery. Bedside spirometry to measure the FVC and FEV_1, quantitative ventilation-perfusion scanning may be used to predict the cardiac output and the ventilation directed towards the portion of lung that is to be resected. The post-operative FEV_1 can be predicted from the above information. A predicted post-operative FEV_1 of < 800 ml contraindicates surgery because of the high risk of persistent severe post-operative respiratory failure.

Post-operative complications are common, and include the necessity for prolonged ventilatory support, bronchopleural fistula, infection and recurrent pulmonary haemorrhage. The overall mortality ranges from 10–50 per cent. Active bleeding at the time of surgery is associated with a greater degree of morbidity and mortality, probably related to an increased risk of aspiration. As far as possible, surgery if decided upon, should be done in between episodes of bleeding in massive haemoptysis, as this significantly reduces morbidity and mortality.

Better techniques in bronchial vessel embolization (**24**) and in other non-surgical bronchoscopic therapeutic procedures, have reduced the need for emergency surgery in the management of massive haemoptysis.

REFERENCES

1. Jones DK, Davies RJ. (1990). Massive haemoptysis: Medical management will usually arrest the bleeding. BMJ. 300, 889–890.

2. Stoller JK. (1992). Diagnosis and management of massive haemoptysis: A review. Respir Care. 37, 564–581.

3. Winter SM, Ingbar DH. (1988). Massive shock: Pathogenesis and management. J Inten Care Med. 3, 171–188.

4. Corey R, Hla KM. (1987). Major and massive haemoptysis. Reassessment of conservative management. Am J Med Sci. 294, 301–309.

5. Crocco JA, Rooney JJ, Fankushen DS et al. (1968). Massive haemoptysis. Arch Intern Med. 121, 495.

6. Hodes RM. (1992). Haemoptysis in rheumatic heart disease. Trop Geogr Med. 44, 328–330.

7. Thoms NW, Puro HE, Arbulu A. (1972). Life-threatening haemoptysis in primary lung abscess. Ann Thorac Surg. 14, 347–358.

8. Cahill BC, Ingbar DH. (1994). Massive Haemoptysis—Assessment and Management. Clinics in Chest Medicine. 15(1), 147–168.

9. Ermakov S, Hoyt JW. (1992). Pulmonary artery catheterization. Crit Care Clin. 8, 773–806.

10. Pursel SE, Lindskog GE. (1961). Haemoptysis: A clinical evaluation of 105 patients examined consecutively on a thoracic surgical service. Am Rev Respir Dis. 84, 329–336.

11. Haponik EF, Britt EJ, Smith PL et al. (1987). Computed chest tomography in the evaluation of haemoptysis: Impact on diagnosis and treatment. Chest. 91, 80–85.

12. Tsukamoto T, Sasaki H, Nakamura H. (1989). Treatment of haemoptysis patients by thrombin and fibrinogen-thrombin therapy using a fiberoptic bronchoscope. Chest. 96, 473–476.

13. Zavala DC. (1976). Pulmonary haemorrhage in fiberoptic transbronchial biopsy. Chest. 70, 584–588.

14. Conlan AA, Hurwitz SS. (1980). Management of massive haemoptysis with the rigid bronchoscope and cold saline lavage. Thorax. 35, 901–904.

15. Conlan AA, Hurwitz SS, Krige L et al. (1983). Massive haemoptysis: Review of 123 cases. J Thorac Cardiovasc Surg. 85, 120–124.

16. Feloney JP, Balchum OJ. (1978). Repeated massive haemoptysis: Successful control using multiple balloon-tipped catheters for endobronchial tamponade. Chest. 74, 683–685.

17. Gottlieb LS, Hillberg R. (1975). Endobronchial tamponade therapy for intractable haemoptysis. Chest. 67, 482–483.

18. Benumof JL, Alfrey DD. (1990). Anesthesia for thoracic surgery. In: Anesthesia, 3rd edn (Ed. Miller RD). p. 1517. Churchill Livingstone, New York.

19. Katoh O, Kishikawa T, Yamada H et al. (1990). Recurrent bleeding after arterial embolization in patients with haemoptysis. Chest. 97, 541–546.

20. Keller FS, Rosch J, Loflin TG et al. (1987). Nonbronchial systemic collateral arteries: Significance in percutaneous embolotherapy for haemoptysis. Radiology. 164, 687–692.

21. Nath H. (1990). When does bronchial arterial embolization fail to control haemoptysis? Chest. 97, 515–516.

22. Remy J, Arnaud A, Fardou H et al. (1977). Treatment of haemoptysis by embolization of bronchial arteries. Radiology. 122, 33–37.

23. Uflacker R, Kaemmerer A, Picon PD et al. (1985). Bronchial artery embolization in the management of haemoptysis: Technical aspects and long-term results. Radiology. 157, 637–644.

24. Tanaka N, Yamakado K, Murashima S et al. (1997). Superselective bronchial artery embolization for hemoptysis with a coaxial microcatheter system. J Vasc Interv Radiol. 8, 65.

SECTION 9

Mechanical Ventilation in the Critically Ill

Mechanical Ventilation in the Critically Ill

General Considerations

Ventilator support to any critically ill individual requires expertise and round-the-clock supervision and care. Life in many such patients is totally dependent on the efficient working of a machine. A mechanical failure, accidental disconnection of the machine from the patient, or a sudden obstruction of the airway, are all potential disasters which can lead to sudden death or brain damage from protracted hypoxia. A patient on mechanical ventilator support must therefore never be left unattended even for a minute. Thus the optimal and safe use of mechanical ventilation is only possible in intensive care units. Yet in many district hospitals in India and other developing countries, critical care units are mere apologies for what they ought to be, or are altogether non-existent. In the absence of a full-fledged ICU, the next best option is to use ventilator support in a patient who needs it, in a special or even a general ward, provided that the medical registrar and nurses are well-trained in ventilator management. We managed to do this at one of the large public teaching hospitals in Mumbai, and salvaged a number of very ill patients who would otherwise have died. The need for all medical registrars (at least in the large hospitals of this and other developing countries) to be familiar with the use of mechanical ventilators is thus imperative. It is the duty of the medical and administrative staff of such hospitals to provide basic facilities, and train a team of doctors and nurses who can manage critically ill patients on ventilator support, even in the absence of well-equipped ICUs.

This chapter first deals briefly with the physiological principles and basic concepts underlying mechanical ventilation. It then proceeds to discuss the indications and criteria for ventilator support, types of ventilators for intermittent positive pressure ventilation (IPPV) and the management of ventilatory support. This is followed by a description of the different modes of ventilator support, and the use of positive end-expiratory pressure (PEEP) as an adjunct. Then comes a section on the complications of mechanical ventilation. The chapter ends with a discussion on weaning from ventilator support, and with a procedure designed for trouble-shooting in ventilated patients.

Physiological Principles

The physiological effects of mechanical ventilation are listed in **Table 9.1.1**.

Table 9.1.1. Important physiological effects of mechanical ventilation

1. Venous Filling and Cardiac Output
   - Reduces venous return and right atrial filling with fall in CO during inspiration; this is compensated by increase in peripheral venous tone
   - Degree of circulatory tolerance to mechanical ventilation dependent on:
     * Degree to which positive airway and alveolar pressures are transmitted to intrathoracic structures and vessels during inspiration
     * Integrity of vascular reflexes
     * Normal circulating blood volume
2. Pulmonary Circulation
   - Pulmonary capillary blood flow impaired during inspiration due to increased alveolar pressures
   - Marked increase in PVR with pulmonary hypertension and right ventricular strain seen with high inflation pressures; this can cause a sharp fall in LV filling and CO
3. Other Effects of Positive Intrapleural and High Alveolar Pressures
   - CNS Effects:
     * Increased intracerebral venous pressure
     * Decreased CSF absorption and increased CSF volume and pressure
   - Increased vasopressin secretion, decreased urine flow, increased fluid retention
   - Barotrauma/Volutrauma

Venous Filling and Cardiac Output

Mechanical intermittent positive pressure ventilation involves a considerable deviation from the normal physiological act of spontaneous respiration. In normal respiration, the intrapleural pressure becomes increasingly negative during inspiration, and this not only helps to fill air into the lungs, but also promotes the return of venous blood into the right atrium. In contrast, mechanical intermittent positive pressure ventilation uses a positive pressure to inflate the alveoli during inspiration. This positive pressure is partially transmitted to the intrapleural space so that the intrapleural pressure is positive during inspiration. This reduces the pressure gradient between the venous system and the right atrium, and consequently reduces the venous return and right atrial filling, with a resultant fall in the cardiac output. It is only in the quiescent part of the expiratory phase that the negative intrapleural pressure in both positive pressure ventilatory support, as well as in spontaneous respiration is about the same. It is during this quiescent expiratory phase that maximal filling of the right heart occurs in patients on ventilatory support.

The fall in right atrial filling and cardiac output, anticipated during the inspiratory phase of positive pressure ventilatory support, is generally compensated for by an increase in peripheral venous tone. This increase restores the venous pressure gradient between the periphery and the right atrium, thereby ensuring adequate right atrial filling, and a normal cardiac output. The compensatory mechanism described above may however not be complete or perfect. The degree of circulatory tolerance to mechanical ventilation is dependent on the following factors:

(i) The degree to which positive airway and alveolar pressures during inspiration are transmitted to intrathoracic structures and intrathoracic veins. The higher the inspiratory inflation pressures, the higher the intrathoracic intrapleural pressure. An increase in the compliance of the lungs as in emphysema, will cause an increase in the lung volumes during inspiration, and will facilitate transmission of positive pressure to the intrapleural space. The longer the time duration for which the lung is kept inflated, the · greater the effects on venous filling and cardiac output. The use of positive end-expiratory pressure (PEEP) as an adjunct to ventilatory support, though often well tolerated, has the same effect. Transmission of this positive pressure to intrathoracic structures and the intrapleural space can effectively reduce venous return and cardiac output, particularly when high levels of PEEP are used.

(ii) The integrity of the vascular reflexes. An increase in peripheral venous tone offsets the tendency to reduced venous filling and reduced cardiac output during the inspiratory phase of mechanical ventilation. This increase in venous tone may not occur if the autonomic nervous system is abnormal, as in some patients with infective polyneuritis or cervical cord compression, in poisoning with barbiturates or other sedatives, in diabetics, in old debilitated patients, and in patients on drugs which block sympathetic activity. A significant fall in cardiac output may occur under these circumstances.

(iii) A normal circulatory blood volume. Hypovolaemia from any cause exaggerates the tendency to reduced atrial filling and reduced cardiac output in patients on mechanical ventilation. In these patients, restoration of the blood volume by infusions of crystalloids, colloids or blood transfusions, restores the cardiac output to normal.

Deleterious effects on circulation are most frequently observed at the initiation, and in the early phase of mechanical ventilation. Once circulatory adaptation to mechanical ventilation has occurred, even significant changes in the ventilatory pattern do not adversely affect the cardiac output. Thus a significant increase in the tidal volume or in airway pressure in patients well adjusted to ventilatory support, does not generally cause a fall in cardiac output. An important exception to this observation is in patients with emphysema. A large increase in tidal volume in these cases invariably results in a sharp fall in cardiac output due to 2 factors: (i) a marked rise in the intrapleural pressure during inspiration due to the combination of increased compliance of the lungs and a non-compliant chest wall; (ii) air-trapping at the end of expiration leads to a persistently positive intrapleural pressure with a further fall in venous return during expiration.

Pulmonary Circulation

During the inspiratory phase of mechanical ventilator support, the positive pressure within the alveoli can impair pulmonary capillary flow. The higher the alveolar pressure, the greater the alveolar distension, and greater the resistance to blood flow through the pulmonary capillary circulation. This imposes a burden on the right heart and can result in right ventricular failure. Even modestly raised alveolar pressures can impair pulmonary circulation and precipitate right heart failure in patients on the verge of decompensation (1).

Pulmonary vascular resistance (PVR) has been shown to be closely related to lung volumes. Pontoppidan and co-workers (2) observed in post-operative thoracic surgical patients, that when lung volumes were below normal, switching of these patients from spontaneous respiration to mechanical ventilation, produced a fall in pulmonary vascular resistance. If however the initial lung volumes were close to the normal functional residual capacity (FRC) or above it, further increase in lung volumes led to increased pulmonary vascular resistance.

A marked increase in the PVR with pulmonary hypertension is most commonly seen with high inflation pressures (and high alveolar pressures and volumes) in compliant lungs. This can lead to severe right heart strain and failure with a sharp fall in cardiac output. The systolic overload to the right ventricle distends it, and pushes the septum to the left, thereby distorting and reducing the left ventricular cavity. This further reduces left ventricular filling and cardiac output.

It must be stressed that in critically ill patients on ventilator support, numerous other factors also play a role in increasing the PVR. These include hypoxia, acidosis, pulmonary oedema, thrombi or emboli within the lungs, other neurohormonal mechanisms, and changes in pulmonary vasculature as observed in septic shock and in acute lung injury. More often than not, these factors play a greater role in increasing the PVR in critically ill patients with acute respiratory failure, as compared to the effects of mechanical ventilatory support.

Finally, pulmonary blood flow in mechanically ventilated patients is influenced not only by intra-alveolar pressure, but also by pulmonary artery pressure. An increase in the physiological dead space can result from increased positive pressure with overdistension of the alveoli, and/or to fall in pulmonary artery pressure. In shock or hypovolaemic states with a fall in pulmonary artery pressure, perfusion is chiefly distributed to the dependent parts of the lung, the physiological dead space is increased, and the V_D/V_T ratio may be as high as 0.7. Increasing the tidal volume or minute ventilation will compensate only to some extent, since part of this increase would be still directed to unperfused alveoli.

The correct solution to this problem would be to increase the circulating volume and the pulmonary artery pressure, thereby increasing the volume and pressure of the blood perfusing the ventilated alveoli.

In the practical management of a patient on ventilator support, it is important to remember that a disturbance in gas exchange may be due as much to a disturbance in pulmonary circulation, as to a disturbance or defect in ventilation.

Effects of Increased Positive Pressure on the Left Ventricle

An increase in the intrapleural and intrathoracic pressure during the inspiratory phase of mechanical ventilatory support decreases the transmural pressure across the ventricular wall during systole. This really amounts to a reduction in afterload, and should therefore increase left ventricular stroke output, as long as left ventricular filling is maintained. Obviously this effect on cardiac output is contrary to that produced by reduced venous filling of the right heart, and a possible reduction in output related to increased pulmonary peripheral vascular resistance.

The overall effect on cardiac output produced by increased positive airway and alveolar pressure during mechanical ventilator support will depend on whether the reduction in venous return to the right heart, and the effects of increased PVR due to compression of pulmonary capillaries, outbalance the reduced systolic afterload on the left ventricle. A markedly positive intrathoracic pressure is more likely to produce a fall in cardiac output not only due to right heart strain and reduced output, but because of poor filling of the left ventricle due to reasons discussed earlier.

Other Effects of Increased Airway Pressure

CNS Effects. Attention has been drawn to the possible effects of mechanical ventilation on intracranial pressure, particularly with the use of PEEP. Increasingly high intrapleural pressures can be transmitted to the intervertebral foramina and can result in a decrease in cerebral blood flow, and an increase in the CSF pressure. Increased levels of PEEP are also presumed to increase pressure on the vertebral and jugular venous plexus. These vessels are important for the drainage of venous cerebral blood. Obstruction to venous outflow leads to an increase in intracerebral venous pressure, a decrease in CSF absorption, and a subsequent increase in CSF volume and pressure. These changes may be subtle, yet may be of practical significance in patients with intracranial disease or injury (3).

Water Retention, Urine Flow and Vasopressin Secretion. Intermittent positive pressure ventilation is reported to decrease urine flow and increase vasopressin secretion (4, 5). Increased vasopressin secretion is thought to be related to reduced activity of the left atrial osmoreceptors consequent to a raised mean airway pressure which reduces intrathoracic blood volume. There is a tendency to fluid retention particularly in the early days of mechanical ventilation. This effect is more pronounced when high levels of PEEP are used; the tendency to fluid retention reduces with time.

Barotrauma and volutrauma. The higher the airway and alveolar pressures, the greater the chances of barotrauma—a dangerous

hazard in patients on ventilator support. Large tidal volumes also cause trauma to the alveoli (volutrauma). These aspects are dealt with in another part of this chapter and in the Chapter on Acute Lung Injury and ARDS.

Indications for Mechanical Ventilation (Table 9.1.2)

In many ICUs in this city and this country, there is yet a certain hesitation and trepidation observed regarding the use of mechanical ventilation in patients who need ventilator support. In other words, mechanical ventilation is started much later than what ought to have been in the natural history of a disease requiring ventilatory support. The other equally common misconception and error is to be in a tearing hurry to remove ventilator support in a critically ill patient. Such a premature withdrawal of ventilator support is love's labour lost—the patient regressing from near recovery to a critical state, which again necessitates the use of the ventilator.

Indications for mechanical ventilation are discussed below.

A. Established Acute Respiratory Failure

Early ventilator support is now initiated by all good units in patients with acute respiratory failure. The criteria and timing for initiating support depend on the aetiological agent producing acute respiratory failure, and above all, on the rate at which respiratory function is observed to deteriorate. Different diseases producing acute respiratory failure present their own special problems with

Table 9.1.2. Indications for mechanical ventilation

A. Established Acute Respiratory Failure
  – Primary ventilatory failure where lungs are normal to start with e.g. poisonings that depress the CNS, CNS and neuromuscular disorders (poliomyelitis, infective polyneuritis, myasthenia), snake bites, severe tetanus
  – Hypoventilating comatose patients
  – Acute pulmonary diseases e.g. fulminant pneumonia, acute lung injury (ARDS)
  – Fulminant pulmonary oedema
  – Major or massive pulmonary embolism
  – Major or massive atelectasis
  – Patients with COPD in acute crisis, unresponsive to conventional therapy
  – Patients with acute severe asthma unresponsive to conventional therapy
  – Patients with severe respiratory muscle fatigue

B. Incipient Respiratory Failure
  – Patients with excessive ventilatory demands
  – Obese patients who have undergone upper abdominal surgery, or poor risk surgical patients
  – Patients with acute/fulminant parenchymal lung disease with rapidly progressive impairment of pulmonary function and reserve
  – Respiratory muscle fatigue in critical illnesses

C. Low-Output States—Shock of any Aetiology

D. Purposeful Hyperventilation
  – To decrease intracranial tension in patients with head injury associated with increased intracranial tension
  – To reduce cerebral oedema after CPR or massive CVA

---

regard to initiating mechanical ventilation, to technicalities in maintaining ventilation, and to difficulties in weaning the patient from ventilator support. It is therefore best from the practical point of view to consider the indications in acute respiratory failure, with reference to the different groups of diseases frequently encountered in the ICU.

(i) Ventilator Support in Primary Ventilatory Failure

The commonest indication for mechanical ventilation is acute primary failure of ventilation. Ventilatory failure occurs commonly in poisonings that depress the CNS, in acute inflammatory and other diseases involving the central nervous system, in some patients with head injury, increased intracranial tension, poliomyelitis, acute infective polyneuritis, and myasthenia gravis. Severe tetanus is an important cause of ventilatory failure in India. Neuromuscular paralysis following a krait or cobra bite is particularly common in South India. The lungs are normal to start with, but changes within the lungs (chiefly increasing widespread atelectasis), almost always occur if treatment is delayed. In many patients with neuromuscular disease, deterioration can occur suddenly, almost precipitously, with disastrous consequences. It is therefore wise to start early ventilatory support in these patients.

(ii) Ventilator Support in a Hypoventilating Comatose Patient

Deep coma is an indication for securing the airways with an endotracheal tube or a tracheostomy. Hypoventilation in such patients may be due to depressed respiratory drive or to secretions causing obstructed airways or patchy atelectasis. Hypoxia and hypercapnia resulting from hypoventilation may further impair the conscious state, which in turn may further depress ventilation. Unless the patient is clearly hyperventilating, a deeply comatose patient is safer on mechanical ventilation.

(iii) Ventilator Support in Acute Pulmonary Disease

These patients are hypoxic due to hypoxaemic acute respiratory failure. Typical examples are in acute lung injury (ARDS), and fulminant pneumonia. Patients with acute pulmonary disease are difficult to ventilate. They have a strong respiratory drive, are often severely hypoxic, and 'fight' the ventilator. An inability to maintain a PaO_2 of > 60 mm Hg whilst on oxygen at a flow rate of 6–8 l/min, is an indication for initiating ventilator support. Other criteria for starting mechanical ventilation in these patients are dealt with later.

(iv) Ventilator Support in Fulminant Pulmonary Oedema

Acute pulmonary oedema, if fulminant, literally chokes the patient at the level of the alveoli. Mechanical ventilation is life saving not only because it allows the maintenance of an adequate PaO_2, but perhaps because the high inflation pressures used to ventilate the lungs reduces the transudation of fluid from the alveolar capillaries into the alveoli. Ventilator support buys time during which diuretics like furosemide have a chance to act, and other corrective measures to treat the underlying cause of acute pulmonary oedema may be profitably undertaken.

(v) Ventilator Support in Acute Thromboembolic Lung Disease

Ventilator support is indicated if the PaO_2 is < 60 mm Hg on supplemental oxygen, particularly in the presence of shock.

(vi) Ventilator Support in Acute on Chronic Respiratory Failure in Patients with Chronic Airways Obstruction

Many patients in this group are used to a low $PaO_2 < 65$ mm Hg, and a high $PaCO_2 > 50$–60 mm Hg. Ventilator support should not be used unless all other modalities of treatment have been of no avail, clinical deterioration is evident, and there is a further deterioration in the arterial blood gases and arterial pH. In such patients ventilatory support is fraught with difficulty, and requires experience and expertise.

(vii) Ventilator Support in Acute Severe Asthma

Acute severe asthma is probably one of the most difficult problems for effective mechanical ventilation. Yet ventilator support is lifesaving in those cases of acute severe asthma not responding to corticosteroids, nebulized bronchodilators and other medical therapy. The indications for using ventilator support in such patients are discussed separately.

(viii) Ventilator Support In Patients with Severe Muscle Fatigue

Severe muscle fatigue (involving the muscles of respiration), is an increasingly recognized and important cause of hypoventilation and respiratory failure. Muscle fatigue can occur in patients with primary neuromuscular disease involving the respiratory muscles. It occurs much more frequently in lung disease and in any condition (not necessarily involving the lungs), where ventilatory demands are excessive. The timing of initiating ventilator support in these patients is a matter of fine judgment. Altered blood gases or feeble ventilatory efforts are of course an immediate indication. Irregular breathing patterns, or the presence of a respiratory paradox in which the abdominal muscles move inwards rather than outwards during inspiration, point to excessive muscle fatigue. Respiratory alternans is characterized by alternate excursions involving the diaphragm and the intercostals, and is also a pointer to muscle fatigue. Another important pointer to impending disaster is the presence of apnoeic spells which are often forerunners of prolonged respiratory arrest. It is better to ventilate such patients even if the arterial blood gases are not significantly distorted, rather than wait for disaster to occur.

Factors which precipitate and contribute to respiratory muscle fatigue are hypoperfusion of the muscles, hypoxia, electrolyte and acid-base disturbances, poor nutrition as in alcoholics or those with chronic liver or renal diseases, and in old, feeble, debilitated patients (**6**).

B. Incipient Respiratory Failure

Mechanical ventilation is increasingly being used in patients in whom some degree of respiratory failure is anticipated. Perhaps the most important group comprises patients who have to meet increased ventilatory demands, and who therefore sooner or later show evidence of respiratory muscle fatigue. This is typically seen in acute severe asthma, but can occur in numerous medical and surgical problems. It is difficult for a seriously ill patient to sustain a ventilatory rate of > 35–40/min or a minute ventilation >10–12 l/min for any prolonged period of time without increasing muscle fatigue and the danger of impending sudden respiratory failure.

There is a special category of surgical patients who frequently require ventilator support for impending or insidious respiratory failure. These are obese individuals who have undergone upper abdominal surgery. This often leads to 'fixed' or 'splinted' domes of the diaphragm resulting in a loss of volume in both lower lobes. These patients are markedly tachypnoeic particularly in the presence of fever and infection; their minute ventilation is often as high as 12–15 l/min, and their respiratory rates between 35–45/min. They maintain their arterial blood gases within the normal range for some length of time, but not uncommonly these patients go into sudden respiratory failure, deteriorate sharply, and pose problems in emergency intubation and ventilation. A quick anticipation of worsening problems calls for early intubation and ventilator support before such a disaster occurs.

Other susceptible patients in whom hypoventilation is a likely sequel include poor risk surgical patients whose recovery from surgery or trauma is hindered by obesity, chronic lung disease, old age, debility, and electrolyte imbalance. In all these patients post-operative ventilatory support is merely an extension of surgical care in the operation theatre. They may require mechanical ventilation for a period varying from a few hours to a few days, and are weaned off ventilator support when they can maintain adequate gas exchange on spontaneous breathing.

Similarly in acute or fulminant parenchymal lung disease where the tempo of impairment of respiratory reserve and respiratory function is very rapid, it is best to anticipate events in advance to allow for elective intubation and ventilatory support.

C. Low-output States and Septic Shock

Ventilator support is now always indicated in low cardiac output states as in cardiogenic shock, or for that matter in shock from any aetiology. It is often used in septic shock, at times quite early in the natural history, when the march of events signifies a rapidly evolving dangerous clinical state. In shock from any cause, and in low-output states of any aetiology (e.g. in advanced liver cell failure or multiorgan failure), tissue perfusion is inadequate in relation to tissue oxygen needs. Also, a low cardiac output is generally associated with a low $P\bar{v}O_2$, which in turn is responsible for a low PaO_2. Shock of any aetiology which results in low pulmonary artery pressure and diminished perfusion of the lungs leads to an increase both in the V_D/V_T ratio, as well as to a $\dot{V}/\dot{Q}$ imbalance. Ventilator support helps in 2 ways: (i) with an increase in FIO_2 (if need be to 70–80 per cent), the PaO_2 increases, and therefore both the arterial oxygenation and the arterial oxygen content rise; (ii) the muscles of respiration are rested once the ventilator takes over the function of ventilation. This prevents incipient respiratory failure from progressing to frank ventilatory failure, and even ventilatory arrest. In patients who breathe excessively, the oxygen

cost of breathing is considerably increased. At rest, the normal work of breathing accounts for 2–3 per cent of total oxygen consumption (7). This can increase in acute respiratory failure to as high as 35–40 per cent (8). In low-output states, resting the overworked respiratory muscles through mechanical ventilation sharply reduces the oxygen cost of breathing and allows more oxygen to be diverted to vital organs starved of their oxygen supply. However in critically ill patients it is equally important to control fever, shivering, constant movement and restlessness, as these can all contribute to increased oxygen consumption, and thereby reduce the already meagre available oxygen supply to the vital organs.

D. Mechanical Ventilation for the Specific Purpose of Hyperventilation

A comparatively rare indication for mechanical ventilation is to hyperventilate patients with head injury, when associated with increased intracranial pressure. Hyperventilating these patients reduces the $PaCO_2$ which leads to reduction in the cerebral blood flow, and hence in the intracranial pressure. Hyperventilation is generally combined with sedation and muscle paralysis to prevent coughing and clashing with the ventilator, as these could lead to a rise in intracranial pressure. Clinicians often prefer to manage unconscious neurological and neurosurgical patients with increased intracranial pressure, with controlled mechanical hyperventilation. The same approach to counter cerebral oedema is sometimes used following resuscitation after a cardiopulmonary arrest, or in patients with cerebral oedema consequent to a massive cerebrovascular accident. However the efficacy of hyperventilation in all the above-mentioned situations is temporary (generally not exceeding 48 hours) and debatable.

Table 9.1.3 lists clinical problems requiring mechanical ventilator support in 1569 patients admitted to our intensive care unit at the Breach Candy Hospital, Mumbai. Patients requiring ventilator support for less than 2 days have been excluded. Almost all patients included in this study required ventilatory support for over 7 days; many required ventilator support for over 6 weeks, and some for over 3 months. The maximum duration of ventilator support provided was 8 months.

Objective Criteria for Initiating Ventilator Support in Adults

The criteria enumerated in **Table 9.1.4** are mere guidelines, and not sacrosanct rules. It is crucial to take the clinical picture, the evolution of the disease in a given patient, and the trend and rate of change in the parameters outlined below, into consideration.

The parameters given in **Table 9.1.4** apply to patients in ventilatory failure, and to respiratory failure occurring with acute lung disease; they are not applicable to patients with chronic obstructive airways disease. These patients even under normal or basal conditions may have a PaO_2 of 60 mm Hg, and a $PaCO_2$ between 55–60 mm Hg. They are used to hypoxia and hypercapnia, and tolerate both rather well. Criteria for ventilator support in acute severe asthma need special consideration, and are dealt with in a separate chapter (see Chapter on Acute Severe Asthma).

Table 9.1.3. Clinical problems requiring mechanical ventilator support in 1569 patients studied at the Breach Candy Hospital, Mumbai

Groups	No. of Patients (n)	Mortality (%)
1. Acute Lung Injury (ARDS)	173	47
(ARDS due to tropical problems)	(56)[a]	(32)
2. Neuromuscular	80	9
3. CNS	254	62
– CVA	173	61
– Head Injury	29	69
– Meningitis/encephalitis	29	69
– Others	23	52
4. Severe Sepsis/Septic Shock[b]	126	81
5. Post-operative	417	26
– Cardiac (mainly CABG)	168	21
– Chest (non-cardiac)	33	18
– Abdominal	74	35
– Others (including renal transplant)	49	41
6. Tropical Problems	109	11
– Fulminant Tetanus	36	6
– Organophosphorus poisoning	23	4
– Cerebral malaria	19	21
– Acute Gram-negative septicaemia from ingestion of contaminated food	8	0
– Miliary/disseminated haematogenous tuberculosis	6	16
– Fulminant amoebiasis	9	33
– Salmonella infections	5	0
– Rabies	1	100
– Dengue	2	0
7. Metabolic Disorders (including metabolic coma)	58	72
8. Airways obstruction[c]	131	37
9. Fulminant Pneumonias	76	64
10. Cardiovascular Problems (mainly cardiogenic shock and low-output states)	85	56
11. Poisoning (excluding organophosphorus poisoning)	26	15
12. Flail chest	9	0
13. Miscellaneous	25	28

[a]These 56 patients developed acute lung injury secondary to Tropical problems, and are also included in Group 6.
[b]Chiefly severe intra-abdominal sepsis
[c]No deaths in over 20 patients ventilated for acute severe asthma in the last 5 years.

Table 9.1.4 Criteria for initiating ventilator support in adults

* Respiratory rate > 35/min
* VC < 10–15 ml/kg
* MV > 10–12 l/min over a prolonged period
* Maximum Inspiratory Force < – 20 cm H_2O
* PaO_2 < 60 mm Hg on nasal oxygen at 6–8 l/min and/or $PaCO_2$ > 55 mm Hg
* Alveolar-arterial oxygen gradient > 300–350 mm Hg on FIO_2 of 1
* V_D/V_T > 0.6
* Visible excessive work of breathing in critically ill or debilitated patients
* Clinical evidence of respiratory muscle fatigue
  – Poor chest excursions
  – Tachypnoea
  – Respiratory muscle paradox, 'respiratory alternans'
  – Apnoeic spells

Types of Ventilators for Intermittent Positive Pressure Ventilation

Ventilators in intensive care units are either volume-cycled or pressure-cycled or time-cycled.

A volume-cycled i.e. a volume-targeted ventilator, delivers a preset volume and continues to do so regardless of a change in the patient's airway resistance or lung compliance.

A pressure-cycled i.e. a pressure-targeted ventilator, cycles to expiration after a specified preset pressure has been attained. Thus, gas flows into the lungs until a preset pressure limit is reached. The volume delivered will therefore change if the airway resistance and/or the lung compliance change.

In a time-cycled ventilator, the inspiratory phase ends when a predetermined time has elapsed. This time remains fixed, and is controlled by a timing mechanism within the ventilator, which is unaffected by conditions in the patient's lungs.

Volume-targeted ventilatory support is more flexible, easier to learn, and easier to manage than pressure-targeted or time-cycled ventilator support. All modern ventilators are capable of delivering an adequate minute ventilation and of varying the oxygen concentration (FIO_2) from 25–100 per cent.

Most modern ventilators incorporate within a single unit, mechanisms that allow either volume-targeted or pressure-targeted ventilatory support, the use of positive end-expiratory pressure (PEEP), and the choice of several modes of ventilator support, detailed later. Adjustment of minute ventilation, respiratory rates, flow rates, inspiratory-expiratory ratios are also possible. The ventilator is fitted with a series of alarms for better patient care, and can be fitted with modules that can monitor and display lung mechanics (compliance, airway resistance, waveforms, flow-volume loops) and the end-tidal PCO_2.

Comparison between Volume-controlled (Volume-targeted) and Pressure-controlled (Pressure-targeted) Ventilation

A comparison is tabled below:

	Volume-targeted	Pressure-targeted
Rate	Set or variable	Set or variable
Tidal volume (V_T)	Set	Variable
Peak Airway Pressure	Variable	Set
Peak Alveolar Pressure	Variable	Set
Peak Flow	Set	Variable
I:E Ratio	Variable	Set

From the clinical viewpoint, neither volume-targeted, nor pressure-targeted ventilation offers a distinct advantage with regard to gas exchange, haemodynamic stability, and pulmonary mechanics.

The major advantage of volume-targeted ventilatory support is its ease of application, and the provision of a fixed tidal volume in spite of changing airway resistance or pulmonary compliance.

The main advantage of pressure-cycled or pressure-targeted ventilation is that gas is delivered at a fixed preset pressure; if there

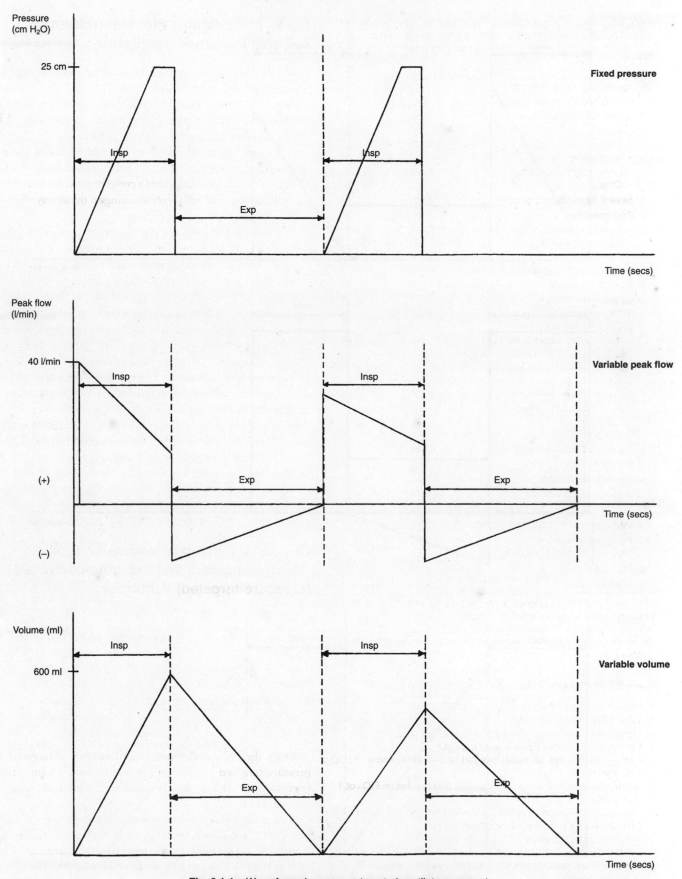

Fig. 9.1.1a. Wave forms in pressure-targeted ventilatory support

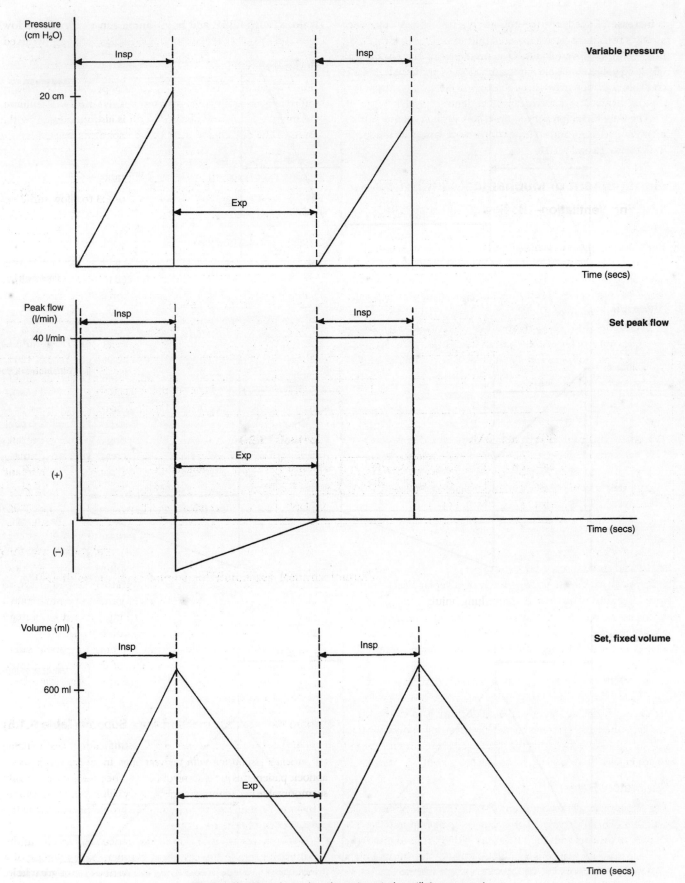

Fig. 9.1.1b. Wave forms in volume-targeted ventilatory support

is increased impedance to ventilation (either due to increased airways resistance or to a lowered pulmonary compliance), the tidal volume delivered falls. Overstretching of the alveoli with resulting volutrauma and barotrauma is thus prevented. Pressure control ventilation may also be able to provide the high inspiratory flow demands of some critically ill patients.

The wave forms (pressure vs time, flow vs time, volume vs time) in pressure control and volume control ventilation are illustrated in **Figs. 9.1.1a** and **9.1.1b**.

Management of Mechanical Ventilation

Initiating Ventilation—Basics of Initial Ventilator Set-up

There are a number of ventilator modes available to help ventilate a patient. We generally initiate ventilator support with volume-controlled or volume-targeted ventilation using the assist-control mode. In assist-control ventilation, the patient triggers the inspiration by a spontaneous effort which is enhanced by the ventilator. In this mode, if for some reason the patient fails to trigger the machine, the machine takes over, initiates inspiration and takes over full ventilatory support. Most patients with different respiratory problems can be adequately ventilated by the volume-targeted, assist-control mode.

Tidal Volume (V_T)

The tidal volume for an individual patient should be set between 5–12 ml/kg body weight. Selection of tidal volume in a given patient is influenced by the nature of the disease, the approximate minute ventilation requirement, pulmonary compliance, airway resistance, airway pressure, PaO_2 and $PaCO_2$.

Very low tidal volumes result in atelectasis, hypoventilation, hypoxaemia. On the other hand, very high tidal volumes can cause respiratory alkalosis, decrease cardiac output by reducing venous return and predispose to both barotrauma and volutrauma. There is definite evidence that overstretch of alveolar walls through very large tidal volumes can induce lung 'injury'.

In patients with normal lungs to start with (as in neuromuscular disease causing respiratory failure, CNS disease, coma, poisoning, and immediate post-operative conditions), the tidal volume is set at 10 ml/kg.

In patients whose lungs are stiff because of abnormal respiratory mechanics (as in acute lung injury, pneumonia) tidal volumes are set at 5–8 ml/kg. A convenient algorithm is to start with 10 ml/kg, stabilize the patient and then progressively reduce the tidal volume to 5–8 ml/kg so that the plateau pressure does not exceed 30 cm H_2O.

Respiratory Rate

The rate is generally set between 10–14 breaths per minute, if the patient is clinically stable. Higher rates may be required (20–25/minute) in patients with stiff lungs (e.g. ARDS), so as to match the machine to the spontaneous breathing pattern of the patient. Lower rates may be necessary in COPD patients where minute ventilation needs to be restricted. If the respiratory rate is too high, respiratory

alkalosis, auto-PEEP and barotrauma can result. If too low, hypoventilation, hypoxaemia and patient discomfort are observed.

Minute Ventilation

Minute ventilation is set according to the approximate ventilatory requirements of a patient and to start with is set at 5–10 l/minute. The minute ventilation decided upon is also influenced by the nature of the disease and the altered respiratory mechanics, for which ventilatory support is offered.

Inspiration : Expiration Ratio (I:E Ratio)

The I:E ratio to start with, is set at 1:2 or 1:3 to allow sufficient time for expiration.

Oxygen Concentration

If the patient is hypoxic, the FIO_2 to start with should be 1.0. After 15 to 20 minutes, this is gradually reduced to a level which allows a $PaO_2 \geq 60$ mm Hg, and an O_2 saturation ≥ 90 per cent.

Inspiratory Flow Rate

The inspiratory flow rate is usually set at 40–60 l/minute in volume-targeted ventilation. This can be increased to 60–100 l/min in patients with high inspiratory demands. However, higher inspiratory flow rates would cause an increase in the peak inspiratory pressure. Lower flow rates can be used to decrease peak inspiratory pressure in patients who to start with have high peak inspiratory pressures (as in ARDS). Lowering inspiratory flow rates would increase inspiratory time, but decrease expiratory time—this could lead to air trapping, auto-PEEP, patient discomfort and barotrauma.

PEEP

PEEP may need to be used if the O_2 saturation is < 90 per cent on an FIO_2 of 0.6 (see Section on PEEP).

It needs to be stressed that the tidal volume, respiratory rate, minute ventilation, I:E ratio and inspiratory flow rates are so adjusted as to enable good exchange of gases and yet maintain a plateau pressure ≤ 30 cm H_2O. This lung protection strategy minimizes the risk of barotrauma and volutrauma.

All alarms on the ventilator provided both for patient safety and as indicators of proper functioning of the ventilator should be activated—in particular, the high pressure, low pressure alarm and the apnoea alarm.

Problems at Initiation of Ventilator Support (Table 9.1.5)

(A) The major and the commonest problem is difficulty in synchronizing the patient's respiration with the ventilator. In an unconscious or apnoeic patient this presents no difficulty. The problem is also easily surmountable in patients with respiratory failure due to poisoning, neuromuscular disease or to other CNS problems. The following points are helpful in management:

(i) Allay anxiety and fright in the patient by explaining the situation in a gentle and confident manner, and by the use of a tranquilliser. Diazepam, 5 to 10 mg intravenously, is of great help.

(ii) The commonest cause of difficulty in synchronizing is an

Table 9.1.5. Common problems encountered during initiation of ventilator support

A. Difficulty in synchronizing patient's respiration with the ventilator
   – Reassure patient and use tranquillizers (diazepam 5–10 mg IV)
   – Use adequate alveolar minute ventilation to maintain $PaCO_2$ at 35–40 mm Hg
   – Use high FIO_2 temporarily to ensure there is no hypoxia
   – Increase TV and RR beyond patient's spontaneous rate. Once patient is taken over by machine, settings gradually lowered to desired values
   – Recognize and treat other factors contributing to 'clash' between machine and patient
   – If in spite of above measures asynchrony between patient and machine persists (as in patients with severe parenchymal disease producing stiff lungs), depress respiration by 2–4 mg IV morphine, or induce neuromuscular paralysis by 4 mg IV bolus of pancuronium
B. Other Problems
   – Malposition of endotracheal tube
   – Aspiration of stomach contents
   – Hypotension

inadequate alveolar minute ventilation. The minute ventilation selected should result in a $PaCO_2$ between 35–40 mm Hg. Ordinarily a tidal volume of 10 ml/kg with a respiratory rate of 12–15/min is adequate. However, many patients with lung disease require higher minute ventilations than that stated above.

(iii) If the patient continuously clashes with what appear to be reasonable ventilator settings, it is advisable to proceed as follows:

(a) Use a high FIO_2 temporarily to ensure that there is no hypoxia—this can be easily checked by noting the oxygen saturation on the pulse oxymeter.

(b) If a very strong respiratory drive is responsible for asynchrony between the patient and the machine, the tidal volume is increased, and the respiratory rate increased to well beyond the patient's spontaneous rate. Once the patient is taken over by the machine, the settings are gradually lowered and modified to the desired values. Generally, if alveolar ventilation is adequate, and if other causes contributing to restlessness and increased respiratory drive are looked into and taken care of, the patient does not fight the machine and is relaxed. The only way to determine whether the alveolar ventilation is adequate is by monitoring the $PaCO_2$. A $PaCO_2 > 45$ mm Hg denotes alveolar hypoventilation; that < 35 mm Hg, alveolar hyperventilation. Hyperventilation in the initial stages reduces the respiratory drive and helps the machine to take over. Once this is achieved minute ventilation is adjusted so that the $PaCO_2$ is maintained around 35 mm Hg, and preferably not < 30 mm Hg.

(c) In tachypnoeic patients with a strong respiratory drive, the patient's inspiratory flow rate is generally higher than the usual 40–60 l/min set on the machine. Increasing the inspiratory flow rate appropriately, or decreasing the inspiration:expiration ratio, prevents 'clashing' and allows smoother ventilatory support in these patients.

(d) Manual control of ventilation by using 100 per cent oxygen for 5 minutes is a useful method for abolishing the patient's respiratory effort, by ensuring oxygenation, and proper alveolar ventilation.

(e) Besides a strong respiratory drive chiefly related to altered mechanics of the lungs, there are other contributory factors which increase the degree of 'clash' between the machine and the patient. These may be present at the very outset, or may evolve during the critical care of a patient. They are briefly discussed later, and should be recognized and treated for more efficient ventilator support.

(iv) Asynchrony between the machine and the patient may persist however in spite of appropriate ventilator settings, the use of corrective measures, and despite all attempts to match the machine to the patient. This generally happens in patients with severe parenchymal lung disease producing very stiff lungs, tachypnoea and severe hypoxia. In many of these patients the spontaneous respiratory rate is > 40 per minute. It is unwise to even attempt to 'match' the machine to this spontaneous respiratory rate. What is more, these patients are critically ill, often with multiorgan failure and cardiovascular instability. It is important that the respiratory muscles are rested in such circumstances. Effective ventilation can be achieved only by depressing respiration, or by inducing neuromuscular paralysis. The respiration can be depressed by the use of 2–4 mg morphine, or 0.2–0.4 mg buprenorphine intravenously, repeated as and when necessary. This can be alternated with 10 mg intravenous diazepam. The main disadvantage of morphine is hypotension, which should be countered by vasopressors or by a volume load. In patients where morphine is unsuitable or ineffective, particularly in ventilating patients with severe lung injury, or in patients with severe tetanus, it is necessary to use intravenous pancuronium (or a similar curare-like agent) to induce neuromuscular paralysis and thereby abolish or sharply reduce spontaneous ventilatory support. 4 mg pancuronium is given as an intravenous bolus and repeated as and when necessary to allow smooth takeover by the machine. It is unwise and often unnecessary to produce total paralysis with curare-like drugs (see Subsection on Tetanus).

B. *Other important problems* occurring within the first few minutes or hours of initiating ventilator support are (i) malposition of the airway; (ii) aspiration of stomach contents; (iii) hypotension. These are dealt with at length under complications of ventilator support.

Objectives of Ventilator Support (9)

1. Regulate gas exchange
2. To overcome mechanical problems
3. Increase lung volumes—particularly in conditions in which the FRC is reduced.

1. *Regulate gas exchange*
Oxygenation

(i) Most patients requiring ventilator support have uneven ventilation and disturbed ventilation-perfusion ratios. Only a small minority on ventilator support can be adequately oxygenated with room air or 20 per cent oxygen; most require an increased concentration of oxygen in the inspired air.

(ii) It is best to use an inspired oxygen concentration (FIO_2) sufficient to maintain an O_2 saturation ≥ 90 per cent and a PaO_2 ≥ 60 mm Hg. In severe lung disease, high oxygen concentrations are necessary; oxygen concentrations > 70 per cent for a prolonged period are a hazard as they contribute to lung injury. In very severe lung injury, a FIO_2 of 100 per cent may be necessary to prevent death from hypoxia. If this is indeed so, 100 per cent oxygen should be used, notwithstanding the fear of oxygen toxicity.

(iii) Use of positive end-expiratory pressure (PEEP). PEEP is indicated when the $PaO_2 < 60$ mm Hg despite inspired oxygen concentrations exceeding 50 per cent.

Carbon Dioxide Elimination and Regulation

The physiological dead space in patients with lung disease is often increased. The increase in dead space in relation to tidal volume may in fact be so large, that in some patients on ventilators 50–70 per cent or even more of the tidal volume becomes dead space ventilation. It is therefore important to note the following points:

(i) It is impossible to predict the ventilation requirements of patients on ventilatory support as most patients have an increase in physiological dead space. Their ventilation requirements are invariably in considerable excess of that predicted by standard nomograms.

(ii) The only certain way to ensure adequate ventilation is to measure the $PaCO_2$ and to adjust volume exchange so that the $PaCO_2$ is close to normal.

(iii) It needs to be re-stressed that a disturbance in ventilatory exchange may be as much to a fault in the pulmonary circulation as to a fall in alveolar ventilation.

(iv) Ventilator support can also be manipulated so as to purposely induce hyperventilation (with a low $PaCO_2$) in patients with raised intracranial pressure, or to purposely settle for hypoventilation (permissive hypercapnia) in certain clinical situations (ARDS and airways obstruction).

2. Overcome mechanical problems

Mechanical ventilation is of use to rest fatigued respiratory muscles, to overcome the abnormal mechanics of the thoracic cage in flail chest and to prevent or treat atelectasis.

3. Increase in lung volumes in patients who have a low FRC (both during end-inspiration and during end-expiration through PEEP), improves ventilation-perfusion ratios and reduces the right to left shunt within the lungs.

Summary of Ventilatory Patterns in Different Groups of Respiratory Diseases Requiring Ventilator Support

These have been discussed at length in separate chapters. For convenience the relevant points are summarized below.

(i) In patients with normal lungs: Tidal volumes of 10 ml/kg with respiratory rates between 10–14/min, a flow rate of 40–60 l/min, and an I:E ratio of 1:2 to 1:3 are recommended.

(ii) Patients with trauma to the chest wall causing a flail chest, and often haematoma or injury to the lung: These patients may need controlled ventilation for which sedation or neuromuscular paralysis becomes necessary. Tidal volumes of 10–12 ml/kg, with a respiratory rate between 12–14/min are recommended. The minute ventilation is adjusted to maintain a $PaCO_2$ between 30–40 mm Hg.

(iii) Acute hypoxaemic respiratory failure due to severe lung disease e.g. acute lung injury (ARDS), pneumonia: The principle is to avoid as far as possible high inflation pressures and to use small tidal volumes of 5–8 ml/kg. In mild to moderately severe cases, smaller tidal volumes of 6–8 ml/kg with a higher respiratory rate of 20–25/min are used to match the patient's breathing pattern. The inspiratory flow rates are adjusted to between 40–60 l/min. An increased FIO_2 and the use of PEEP are necessary. If adequate or efficient ventilation is not possible, particularly so in severely hypoxic, tachypnoeic, critically ill individuals, heavy sedation or even muscle paralysis with controlled ventilation becomes necessary, the principle again being not to exceed a plateau pressure of 30 cm H_2O as far as possible, even if this entails a rise in $PaCO_2$ (permissive hypercapnia). If pressure-controlled or pressure-targeted ventilator support is given to these patients, the peak inspiratory pressure should as far as possible not exceed 30 cm H_2O. PEEP is used in all patients. Inverse ratio ventilator support is often tried when gas exchange remains unsatisfactory with the usual volume-targeted or pressure-targeted ventilatory support (see Chapter on Acute Lung Injury and ARDS and the subsequent Section in this chapter on Modes of Ventilator Support).

(iv) Acute on chronic respiratory failure in patients with chronic airways obstruction: Small tidal volumes of 5–7 ml/kg with a respiratory rate and minute ventilation enough to allow a $PaCO_2$ between 45–55 mm Hg are adequate. These patients are used to a high $PaCO_2$ and it is unwise to aim at a $PaCO_2$ of 40 mm Hg, as their $PaCO_2$ even under ordinary conditions is significantly elevated. Sedation or induced paralysis is often necessary for ventilator support to be effectively maintained. We use moderately low inspiratory flow rates (50 l/min), an I:E ratio of 1:2 to 1:3, and avoid high inflation pressures by using a low tidal volume. Hypoxia is countered by an appropriate increase in the FIO_2.

(v) Acute severe asthma: These patients also require low tidal volumes (350–400 ml), and a comparatively low minute ventilation (often < 5 l/min) to prevent hyperinflation of the lungs. A rise in $PaCO_2$ does not matter as long as hypoxia is relieved by an appropriate increase in the FIO_2. Ventilation in these patients can at times prove extremely difficult.

Details of management of patients in groups (iii), (iv) and (v) are dealt with in separate chapters of the book. Lung protection strategies (outlined in the Chapter on Acute Lung Injury and ARDS) should always be kept in mind in the management of mechanical ventilator support.

Guidelines in Practical Management (Table 9.1.6)

It is constant practice that allows the intensivist to adjust ventilatory requirements to the need of each individual patient. The following guidelines are useful in managing a patient on ventilator support:

(i) A flow chart of vital signs, PaO_2, $PaCO_2$, pH of arterial blood, other relevant parameters of gas exchange and lung mechanics, haemodynamic parameters and oxygenation calculations is essential (**Figs. 9.1.2 a** and **b**). Ventilator settings should be charted— these include tidal volume, minute ventilation, respiratory rate, peak inflation pressure and compliance.

Both the peak and plateau (static) pressures (**Fig. 9.1.3**) should be noted and charted—the difference between the peak and plateau

Table 9.1.6. Guidelines in practical management of patients on ventilator support

* Maintain flow chart of vital signs, PaO_2, $PaCO_2$ and pH of arterial blood
* Chart ventilator settings—V_T, MV, RR, Peak and Plateau Pressures, Compliance (static and dynamic)
* Maintain normal oxygenation (in most patients PaO_2 of 60–70 mm Hg suffices); maintain $PaCO_2$ between 35–40 mm Hg—permissive hypercapnia in selected cases
* Monitor alveolar-arterial oxygen gradient on 100 per cent oxygen and PaO_2/FIO_2 ratio
* Monitor V_D/V_T and shunt fraction ($\dot{Q}_S/\dot{Q}_T$) in selected patients
* Prevent gross alveolar hyperventilation ($PaCO_2 < 25$ mm Hg)
* Avoid oxygen toxicity by using least FIO_2 that allows adequate PaO_2 (60–70 mm Hg); use PEEP only when indicated
* Maintain normal circulatory volume, good pump function, normal BP and adequate Hb concentration
* Humidification of inspired gas, frequent aseptic suction of tracheo-bronchial secretions, and frequent good physiotherapy necessary
* Support other organ systems

pressures being the pressure used to overcome airways or flow resistance. If flow is measured, airway resistance (Raw) can be calculated thus—

$$Raw = \frac{\text{Peak Pressure} - \text{Plateau Pressure}}{\text{Flow}}$$

A sharp sudden rise in peak pressure can be due to a blocked endotracheal or tracheostomy tube, airways obstruction from spasm or mucous, pulmonary oedema, pneumonia, atelectasis or a pneumothorax. If there is a marked increase in the difference between the peak and plateau pressures, the rise in peak pressure is due to obstruction to airflow. If on the other hand, there is no increase in the difference between the peak and plateau pressures due to the latter being also elevated, the rise in peak pressure is due to a fall in pulmonary compliance. This fall is due to atelectasis, pneumonia, pulmonary oedema, pulmonary infarction, or to a pneumothorax.

A fall in compliance should be promptly recognized. In pressure preset ventilators, a fall in compliance will pass unnoticed unless the tidal volume is frequently checked. A chest X-ray will help in identifying gross pulmonary pathology which is responsible for the fall in static compliance—these include pulmonary oedema, pneumonia and pneumothorax.

(ii) The alveolar-arterial oxygen gradient on 100 per cent oxygen is noted and followed-up as and when required. The PaO_2/FIO_2 ratio is a very useful index of the alveolar-arterial gradient, and can be easily charted (see Chapter on Respiratory Monitoring).

The V_D/V_T ratio and the shunt fraction ($\dot{Q}_S/\dot{Q}_T$) in the lungs can also be measured and calculated as and when necessary. The above measurements are indicators of the presence and degree of disturbance in respiratory physiology and gas exchange.

(iii) Moderate alveolar hyperventilation does not matter, but gross hyperventilation with a $PaCO_2 < 25$ mm Hg can be dangerous.

(iv) The ventilator requirements of a critically ill patient may change from time to time. Patterns of ventilation are thus not necessarily constant even for one particular patient with respiratory failure.

		Time	
		8 am	8 pm
Vital Signs	Pulse/min		
	BP (mm Hg)		
	Temperature (°F): Axillary		
	Rectal		
	Clinical Signs		
Ventilator Settings	FIO_2 (%)		
	Tidal Volume (ml)		
	Respiratory Rate (breaths/min)		
	Inspiratory Flow Rate (l/min)		
	I : E Ratio		
	Minute Ventilation (l)		
	Inflation Pressure (cm H_2O)		
	– Peak Pressure		
	– Pause Pressure		
	Compliance (ml/cm H_2O)		
	– Dynamic		
	– Static		
	PEEP (cm H_2O)		
	Auto-PEEP (cm H_2O)		
Blood Gases	PaO_2 (mm Hg)		
	$PaCO_2$ (mm Hg)		
	pH		
	Actual Bicarbonate (mEq/l)		
	Standard Bicarbonate (mEq/l)		
Gas Exchange Parameters	PaO_2/FIO_2		
	V_D/V_T		
	$\dot{Q}_S/\dot{Q}_T$ (%)		
	Alveolar-Arterial Oxygen Gradient on 100% Oxygen (mm Hg)		

Fig. 9.1.2 a. Chart of vital signs, arterial blood gas analysis, ventilator settings and other parameters of gas exchange and lung mechanics.

		Time	Values
Haemodynamic Parameters	RAP (mm Hg)		
	PAP (mm Hg)		
	PCWP (mm Hg)		
	CO (l/min); CI (l/min/m²)		
	SV (ml)		
	SVRI (dynes-sec/cm⁵-m²)		
	PVRI (dynes-sec/cm⁵-m²)		
	LVSWI (g-m/m²)		
	RVSWI (g-m/m²)		
Oxygenation Calculations	CaO_2 (ml/dl)		
	$C\bar{v}O_2$ (ml/dl)		
	O_2AVI (ml/min/m²)		
	$\dot{V}O_2I$ (ml/min/m²)		
	O_2ER (%)		

Fig. 9.1.2 b. Chart of haemodynamic parameters and oxygenation calculations.

(v) Avoid oxygen toxicity by using the least FIO_2 that allows an adequate PaO_2 (60–70 mm Hg). However one should never compromise on using a FIO_2 of even 100 per cent if the patient is in danger of death from severe hypoxia. In clinical practice, a patient

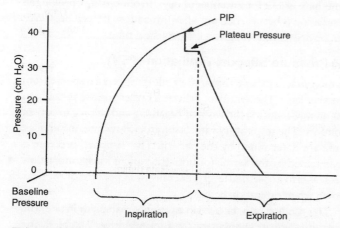

Fig. 9.1.3. The airway pressures (peak and plateau) during a positive pressure breath. Pressure rises during inspiration to peak inspiratory pressure (PIP). With a breath hold, the plateau pressure can be measured. Pressures fall back to baseline during expiration (from Pilbeam SP. 1992. Mechanical Ventilation, Physiological and Clinical Applications. Mosby Year Book, MO).

hardly ever dies of hypercapnia; death is generally due to hypoxia.

(vi) When tidal volumes of 10 ml/kg are used for ventilation, periodic hyperinflation with 'sighs' are unnecessary. These may however be needed when smaller tidal volumes are used. 'Sighs' are contraindicated in patients with airways obstruction.

(vii) Hypovolaemia contributes to poor gas exchange, and accentuates or precipitates hypotension in patients on mechanical ventilation. It is therefore important to ensure normal circulatory volume, good pump function, a normal blood pressure and an adequate haemoglobin concentration.

(viii) Humidification of inspired gas, aseptic suction of secretions through the tracheobronchial tree at frequent intervals, and good chest physiotherapy are all vitally important. Good physiotherapy often spells the difference between life and death in critically ill patients on ventilator support.

(ix) Efficiently carried out mechanical ventilation can only ensure a satisfactory gas exchange. More often than not, a critically ill patient on ventilator support in the intensive care unit has numerous other complications that pose potential hazards to life. Circulatory failure, renal dysfunction, gastrointestinal bleeding, acid-base disturbances, overwhelming sepsis, and in our country, a poor nutritional state, singly or in combination with other factors, can be dangerous enough to cause death. Therefore to concentrate solely on the correct and efficient working of a machine and on a single aspect of deranged physiology, constitutes bad medicine. An overall perspective should never be lost sight of in the management of a critically ill patient.

Modes of Intermittent Positive Ventilator Support and the Use of PEEP

(i) Controlled Mode (CMV)

In CMV, the ventilator completely controls the patient's ventilation, delivering a set tidal volume (or a preset peak pressure) at a set frequency. It is indicated in individuals who are apnoeic, or in those with respiratory muscle paralysis. It is also indicated in patients who are heavily sedated or those paralysed with neuromuscular agents so that ventilatory support is mandatory—a classic example of this situation is fulminant tetanus. Patients receiving CMV cannot increase their minute ventilation ($\dot{V}_E$) voluntarily; their ventilator needs should therefore be closely monitored, and changing needs should be met by suitable adjustments on the machine.

(ii) Assist/Control Mode (A/C)

This is the most commonly used mode. The machine delivers a preset volume (or pressure) in response to a patient initiated breath. To prevent the patient from being totally dependent on 'triggered' breaths, a backup minimum respiratory rate is set. The requisite minute ventilation can then be provided even if for some reason or the other the patient fails to trigger the machine. The main advantage of this mode is that the patient can increase his $\dot{V}_E$ by increasing his respiratory rate. The disadvantages include the production of respiratory alkalosis and of dynamic hyperinflation (particularly in COPD patients), if the machine is triggered too frequently, and the possibility of asynchrony between the ventilator and the patient. Initial ventilator settings are a $\dot{V}_E$ of 8–12 l/min, respiratory rate at 10–14/min, a sensitivity of –2 cm usually. If the patient triggers the machine too frequently, the sensitivity is set at –2 to –6 cm and the patient is sedated to reduce his respiratory drive.

(iii) Synchronized Intermittent Mandatory Ventilation (SIMV)

In this mode, the ventilator delivers synchronized breaths at a set rate at either a preset tidal volume (V_T) or a preset pressure, in addition to allowing the patient to breathe spontaneously. The tidal volume and rate are determined by the patient. If for any reason, the patient does not breathe for a predetermined period, a machine breath is delivered. SIMV can be used with pressure support for spontaneous breaths. PEEP can be introduced in this mode, in which case the machine breaths will be combined with PEEP and the spontaneous ones with continuous positive airways pressure (CPAP).

The advantages claimed for the SIMV mode are as follows:

(i) Decreased asynchrony with the machine and less sedation requirements.

(ii) Less chances of hyperventilation as compared to the A/C mode.

(iii) Greater patient comfort.

(iv) Continued use of respiratory muscles, which is believed to prevent respiratory muscle dysfunction.

(v) Reduced mean airway pressure even with the simultaneous use of PEEP, because many respiratory cycles are related to spontaneous breaths. This minimizes the cardiovascular effects of mechanical ventilation and is less likely to cause a fall in cardiac output or in arterial blood pressure.

We, however, feel that the advantages ascribed to SIMV with or without PEEP are theoretical, and that except in occasional instances, most patients are more comfortably and more satisfactorily ventilated with the assist/control mode of ventilator support. In fact, the more ill the patient, the greater the necessity to rest the respiratory muscles rather than exercise them. The $\dot{V}O_2$ by overworked respiratory muscles can be as high as 15–40 per cent of the total oxygen consumption and this is certainly undesirable. The SIMV mode cannot also respond to changes in the patient's condition, and therefore needs close monitoring.

The chief uses of this mode in our opinion are stated below:

(i) In patients who develop hypotension while on the A/C mode or CMV mode with PEEP. The use of SIMV in such patients is associated with a lower mean airway pressure and this may restore cardiovascular stability.

(ii) In patients on the A/C mode who develop respiratory alkalosis. This can be countered by either sedation or by changing to the SIMV mode.

(iii) To prevent auto-PEEP in certain situations.

(iv) In patients with respiratory failure and a bronchopleural fistula. In this situation, one would desire the lowest mean airway pressure that does not adversely affect ventilation and gas exchange, yet allows the bronchopleural fistula to heal and get sealed. Low tidal volumes with increased respiratory rates to allow for adequate minute ventilation, the avoidance of PEEP, and the use of the SIMV mode may be ideally suited to these patients. This should be combined with lowest effective chest drainage tube suction.

(v) For weaning purposes.

Initial Setting

Settings to deliver a $\dot{V}_E$ of 6–10 l/min or a preset pressure (sufficient to allow a $\dot{V}_E$ of 6–10 l/min) with 10–12 mandatory breaths.

(iv) Continuous Positive Airways Pressure (CPAP)

This is a mode of spontaneous breathing in which the airway pressure is maintained at levels greater than the ambient pressure throughout the entire respiratory cycle. A positive end-expiratory pressure may be added as an adjunct to CPAP. All modern volume ventilators incorporate CPAP as a ventilatory mode. The ventilator does not provide any machine generated breaths, but its humidification and alarm systems are available for use. Special CPAP systems without a ventilator are also available.

Mask CPAP

A light, translucent, well-fitting mask with an adjustable seal is most frequently used for CPAP. CPAP can also be given through nasal pillows, which are short silicone tubes fitted into a plastic shell device, which is inserted into the nares. The main indication for the use of CPAP through a nasal mask or through a nasal pillow, is to provide an alternative to intubation, and to alleviate the need for invasive ventilatory support. It has been reported to be useful in the following conditions:

(i) Mild to moderate acute lung injury (10–12).

(ii) In the treatment of cardiopulmonary oedema (13).

(iii) In post-operative states to prevent or treat atelectasis.

Complications with mask CPAP include aspiration, gastric dilatation, and facial necrosis from prolonged pressure of a tight-fitting mask. Ideally it should be used for 6–12 hours, though some units have used it for a number of days. In our opinion, prolonged ventilation is best carried out after intubation. If need be, CPAP can be delivered through an endotracheal tube.

(v) Pressure Support Ventilation (PSV)

In this mode, a patient's inspiratory effort triggers a response from the ventilator. The ventilator delivers a preset positive pressure to the airway, reducing the work of breathing and helping in patient comfort. The respiratory rate, inspiratory flow rate, inspiratory time are determined by the patient. The 'support' pressure is maintained by the ventilator until the patient's inspiratory flow decreases to a specified level (generally to 25 per cent of the peak flow), when expiration begins.

This mode cannot be used in an apnoeic patient or in one who lacks an adequate spontaneous respiratory drive. We chiefly use it in selected COPD patients and as a weaning procedure.

Initial Setting

Set a pressure support of 10–20 cm H_2O ensuring a V_T of 10 ml/kg. The pressure support is gradually decreased to 5 cm H_2O provided the tidal volume is maintained close to 10 ml/kg. Once this occurs, the patient can be weaned and allowed to breathe spontaneously.

(vi) Inverse Ratio Ventilation (IRV)

Inverse ratio ventilation can be volume-targeted or pressure-targeted. Whereas the normal I:E ratio is 1:2 to 1:3, in inverse ratio ventilation the I:E ratio is $\geq$ 1 i.e. I:E ratio is 1:1, 1.5:1, or 2:1. This is used in patients with ALI, ARDS, pneumonia, atelectasis, who show refractory hypoxaemia (O_2 saturation < 90 per cent on an $FIO_2 \geq$ 60 per cent on assist/control mode in spite of suitable PEEP). In volume-controlled inverse ratio ventilation (VC-IRV), the inverse ratio of inspiration: expiration is achieved by lowering inspiratory flow rate (and thereby lengthening inspiration) or by introducing a suitable end-inspiratory pause. The tidal volume is lowered sufficiently so as not to exceed a plateau pressure of 30 cm H_2O. In pressure-controlled IRV (PC-IRV), the I:E ratio is set to the desired level. The peak pressure should preferably not exceed 30 cm H_2O, or at most 35 cm H_2O.

PEEP is used with both VC-IRV and PC-IRV.

The advantages of IRV are better relief of hypoxaemia and promotion of lung protection strategy that reduces the risk of both barotrauma and volutrauma.

The details of pressure-targeted and volume-targeted IRV have been discussed in the Chapter on Acute Lung Injury and ARDS.

(vii) Permissive Hypercapnia

This approach has been discussed in the Chapter on ALI and ARDS and also in Acute Crisis in Chronic Airways Obstruction and in Acute Severe Asthma.

The principle behind this approach is to protect the lung from both volutrauma and barotrauma when using either volume-targeted or pressure-targeted ventilatory support. Small tidal volumes (5–7 ml/kg) are used in certain groups of patients in volume-targeted ventilatory support, so that plateau pressures do

Table 9.1.7. Advantages and disadvantages of some commonly used modes of positive pressure ventilatory support

Mode	Advantages	Disadvantages
1. Controlled Mode Ventilation (CMV) – Either volume-targeted or pressure-targeted	Complete control over ventilatory function with guaranteed V_E or peak pressure; May be used with heavy sedation and muscle paralysis	Ventilator cannot respond to patient's ventilatory needs; Requires close monitoring; Requires heavy sedation or paralysis Can cause hyperventilation Rarely used since advent of assist/control mode
2. Assist/Control Mode (A/C) – Preset volume or preset pressure delivered in response to patient initiated breath; Backup respiratory rate set to ensure minimal respiratory rate	Ventilator can respond to patient's changing ventilatory needs; Patient can thus increase V_E by increasing respiratory rate; Less work required to increase V_E	Patient-ventilator asynchrony Hyperventilation if patient overtriggers Dynamic hyperinflation (in COPD patients can occur)
3. Synchronized Intermittent Mandatory Ventilation (SIMV) – May be volume-targeted or pressure-targeted Machine delivers synchronized breaths at preset V_T or pressure and rate; it also allows patient to breathe spontaneously at his own V_T and rate; May be combined with pressure support during spontaneous breaths	Decreases 'clash' between patient and machine and decreases requirement of sedation; Less chance of hyperventilation Minimizes cardiovascular effects of mechanical ventilation with PEEP; Prevents respiratory muscle fatigue Greater patient comfort Used as a weaning mode	Cannot respond to patient's ventilatory needs Increased oxygen consumption Can increase work of breathing Comment: No clear advantage over assist/control mode, except in a few special circumstances
4. Pressure Support – Ventilator delivers a preset level of positive pressure when patient initiates a breath	Decreases work of breathing with minimal cardiovascular compromise; Patient determines own respiratory rate, inspiratory time, inspiratory flow rate, V_T; Improves patient comfort Helps in weaning	Can only be used if there is adequate spontaneous respiratory drive; Unsuitable if changing airway resistance or lung compliance; Unsuitable for severe acute respiratory failure
5. Inverse Ratio Ventilation – Volume controlled or pressure controlled with an I:E ratio ranging from 1:1 to 2:1	Improves recruitment of poorly compliant alveoli through prolongation of inspiratory time—thereby improves oxygenation; When properly used, reduces risk of both barotrauma and volutrauma; PC-IPV probably more effective than VC-IPV—unstable alveoli remain open at lower PIP	Decreased expiratory time can lead to increasing auto-PEEP; High auto-PEEP can cause barotrauma; can induce hypotension and cardiovascular compromise; sedation and paralysis often required; In VC-IRV peak inspiratory pressures may fluctuate; In PC-IRV tidal volume may vary

Note: All the above modes can be combined with use of PEEP.

not exceed 30 cm H_2O. When pressure-targeted ventilator support is used, peak pressures are generally set to not more than 30, or at most 35 cm H_2O. This lung protection strategy can lead to hypoventilation and thereby hypercapnia. The hypercapnia is generally well tolerated by the patient and is permissible as an offshoot of the lung protection strategy stated above.

Use of PEEP (14–20)

The use of positive end-expiratory pressure (PEEP) is a valuable adjunct to every mode of volume-targeted ventilatory support and to every mode of pressure-targeted ventilator support. The effects of PEEP are listed in **Table 9.1.8**.

Indications for use of PEEP

PEEP is indicated in patients with severe hypoxaemic respiratory failure who have poorly compliant lungs and a large degree of ventilation-perfusion mismatch, so that hypoxia ($PaO_2 < 60$–65 mm Hg) persists despite using a FIO_2 of 60 per cent or more to ventilate the lungs. It is invariably indicated in patients with acute lung injury, or severe pneumonia, or pulmonary oedema who require ventilatory support. The use of PEEP in these patients increases

Table 9.1.8. Physiological effects and complications of PEEP

A. Physiological Effects

1. On Lungs
* Opening up of fluid-filled atelectatic alveoli, with increase in FRC and TLC
* Decrease in shunt causing increase in PaO_2
* Increase in $\dot{V}_A/\dot{Q}$ units
* Increase in dead space and V_D/V_T ratio
* Increase in compliance up to a point; later fall in compliance

2. On Heart
* Decrease in cardiac output; this can decrease shunt, and thereby increase PaO_2. Thus rise in PaO_2 may also result from a fall in cardiac output, and not necessarily from improvement in lung function

B. Complications
* Barotrauma—pneumothorax, pneumomediastinum, interstitial emphysema
* Fall in cardiac output—hypotension, poor oxygen transport with inadequate tissue perfusion
* Fall in PaO_2 due to overdistension of compliant alveoli, and increase in $\dot{V}/\dot{Q}$ abnormalities
* Increase in intracranial pressure
* Water retention

the PaO_2 and allows a reduction in the FIO_2, thus reducing the risk of oxygen toxicity.

Mode of Action

Acute interstitial oedema and alveolar injury is associated with a fall in compliance, a reduced functional residual capacity (FRC), and increased resistance to inflation of the lungs. Above all, there is a ventilation-perfusion ($\dot{V}/\dot{Q}$) mismatch in which many atelectatic alveoli continue to be well perfused, leading thereby to an increase in the true venous admixture or the right to left shunt within the lungs. PEEP restores the FRC, which in turn improves compliance (**Fig. 9.1.4**). Atelectatic alveoli open up partially or completely with PEEP, so that $\dot{V}/\dot{Q}$ mismatch is reduced or even abolished, and the shunt fraction within the lungs is decreased. This in turn leads to better gas exchange, and a rise in the PaO_2. The FIO_2 can then be safely reduced. PEEP might also be of help in conserving surfactant, the activity of which is secondarily impaired in patients with acute lung injury (21). A correctly adjusted PEEP prevents the poorly compliant alveoli from collapsing or 'closing' during expiration, thereby reducing shear forces acting on the alveolar walls. PEEP therefore plays an important role in the lung protection strategy during ventilator support.

Selection of the Degree of PEEP Used

A variety of methods have been used to determine the optimal level of PEEP. In busy intensive care units, the simplest, safest and most practical method is to use the lowest level of PEEP which maintains the PaO_2 equal to or > 60 mm Hg, on a FIO_2 equal to or < 0.6 (**22**).

Other methods of selecting an optimum level of PEEP include the following (**14, 23**):

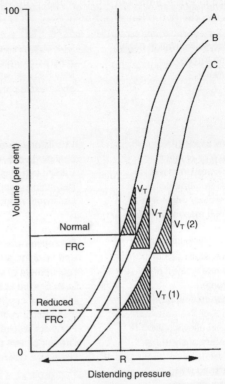

Fig. 9.1.4. Effect of Positive End-expiratory pressure on Functional Residual Capacity (FRC) in patients with reduced compliance e.g. acute lung injury. Curve A represents a normal pressure-volume curve, wherein a relatively small distending pressure is required to achieve a given tidal volume (V_T). Curve C represents a pressure-volume curve in a patient with reduced compliance (as in acute lung injury) with decreased FRC. This is a more flattened curve and requires a greater distending pressure to achieve the same V_T (1). With the addition of PEEP, the FRC may be improved along the same abnormal compliance curve (2), or would shift to curve B, so that lesser distending pressures are required to achieve the same V_T, but the absolute value of the distending pressure is still greater than that required for curve A.

(i) Optimal Oxygenation

It is wrong to aim at an ever increasing PaO_2 by increasing the levels of PEEP. A high PEEP can cause an increasing rise in the PaO_2 and yet can result in a sharp drop in the cardiac output. This fall in cardiac output further reduces oxygen transport to the tissues, in spite of the increase in the PaO_2; this can have disastrous consequences.

(ii) Maximal Oxygen Transport

Adjusting the PEEP so as to obtain a maximal oxygen transport (i.e. the product of arterial oxygen content and the cardiac output), takes the PaO_2, the haemoglobin and the cardiac output into consideration. Nevertheless frequent measurements of cardiac output often pose problems in critically ill individuals.

(iii) Best Compliance

With the use of PEEP, the reduced FRC increases, and the compliance increases up to a point. If static compliance is measured with a graded increase in PEEP, a level of PEEP which produces an optimal increase in the compliance can be arrived at. Further increase in PEEP beyond this point now leads to a fall in static compliance pointing to over-distension of the alveoli. An optimal compliance produced by a particular level of PEEP in any particular patient, is generally associated with an optimal rise in the PaO_2.

(iv) Lowest $\dot{Q}_S/\dot{Q}_T$

As long as the level of PEEP does not significantly reduce the cardiac output, the optimal level of PEEP correlates with the lowest level of $\dot{Q}_S/\dot{Q}_T$. Many workers aim at reducing the shunt fraction to 15 per cent, or aim at a PaO_2/FIO_2 ratio of 300 or more (**24**).

(v) Lowest V_D/V_T and Lowest $PaCO_2$–$PETCO_2$

The lowest V_D/V_T ratio and the lowest $PaCO_2$–$PETCO_2$ gradient are other parameters used by some workers to arrive at an optimal PEEP setting.

Complications of PEEP

The three major complications are barotrauma, a fall in cardiac output, and at times a fall instead of the expected rise in PaO_2. PEEP used over a number of days, can result in an increase in intracranial tension, and to an increase in water retention, and a decrease in renal and portal blood flow.

(i) Barotrauma

The risk of barotrauma depends on the end-inspiratory airway pressure and regional overinflation of parts of the lung. End-inspiratory pressure is a function of the tidal volume, the FRC, the inspiratory flow rate, the total compliance of the lungs, and the level of PEEP used. High tidal volumes, high inspiratory flow rates and high levels of PEEP, in association with a reduced FRC and compliance, potentiate the risk of barotrauma. Even in severely diseased lungs, there are some regional areas which are more compliant than others. With high levels of PEEP, these alveoli get enlarged and overdistended, and have a lower recoil pressure than the smaller, poorly compliant alveoli. High alveolar pressures in such distended alveoli predispose to rupture. On the other hand, the smaller, poorly compliant alveoli have a larger recoil pressure, and can therefore withstand high alveolar pressures and are less liable to rupture.

Alveolar rupture can lead to interstitial emphysema, pneumothorax (**Fig. 9.1.5**), mediastinal emphysema, and surgical emphysema of the soft tissues which may involve the neck, face and trunk. Pneumothorax on high levels of PEEP is a disaster which often leads to death.

(ii) Fall in Cardiac Output

High levels of inflation pressure and PEEP are transmitted to the pleural space. The rise in the intrapleural and intrathoracic pressures leads to a fall in the venous return to the right heart, and a poor filling of the left heart due to a decrease in the transmural pressure across the left ventricular wall. Overinflation of the alveoli also increases the pulmonary vascular resistance with right heart strain, which further reduces the cardiac output. Also, right ventricular strain produces a shift of the interventricular septum to the left, thereby distorting and diminishing the size of the left ventricular cavity, and further impairing left ventricular filling and cardiac output. A sharp fall in the cardiac output leads to hypotension, poor oxygen transport, and inadequate tissue perfusion. A volume load together with dopamine support may be necessary in some patients to restore the cardiac output and oxygen transport to desired levels.

(iii) Fall in PaO_2

A paradoxical fall in the PaO_2 is sometimes observed with PEEP. This occurs when there are regional areas of normally compliant or overcompliant lung in patients with hypoxemic respiratory failure due to parenchymal lung disease. Overdistension of compliant alveoli leads to a decrease in the blood flow to these alveoli, and a shift of blood flow to the non-ventilated, non-compliant areas of the lung. This causes a further increase in the shunt and a fall in the PaO_2. Ventilatory settings and PEEP levels should be adjusted to allow less distension of the compliant alveoli, and better distribution of inspired gas to the poorly compliant portions of the lungs.

Practical Guidelines for the use of PEEP (Table 9.1.9)

(i) PEEP basically helps to counter hypoxia in acute hypoxaemic respiratory failure due to acute lung injury, ARDS, atelectasis, pneumonia, acute pulmonary oedema. It does not alter the natural history of acute lung injury, pneumonia or other acute lung pathologies necessitating ventilator support.

(ii) In our opinion, PEEP should not be used as a preventive measure. It has not been proven to be useful under these conditions,

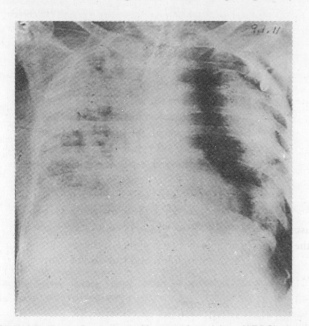

Fig. 9.1.5. X-ray of a patient with acute lung injury (ARDS) showing barotrauma caused by the use of PEEP.

Table 9.1.9. Practical guidelines for the use of PEEP

* PEEP only helps to counter hypoxia in acute hypoxemic respiratory failure due to lung injury; it does not alter the natural history of acute lung pathologies requiring ventilator support
* PEEP should not be used as a preventive measure, except after open heart surgery to prevent mediastinal bleeding
* It is not indicated if conventional ventilator support with FIO_2 of 50–60 per cent maintains PaO_2 > 60–65 mm Hg
* Start with PEEP levels of +5 cm H_2O, gauge effect, and then increase; do not exceed levels of +15 cm H_2O in Indian patients as barotrauma invariably results
* Use the lowest PEEP that allows a PaO_2 of 60 mm Hg on a FIO_2 < 0.6. Ascertain that the rise in PaO_2 following the use of PEEP is not associated with a fall in CO as this will lead to poor oxygen transport and poor tissue oxygenation
* If hypotension or decrease in CO is associated with use of PEEP, the PEEP level should be reduced, or even discontinued. The BP and CO are raised with volume load and/or inotropic support, and PEEP may then be better tolerated
* PEEP may rarely cause a fall in PaO_2—it then needs to be reduced, or even discontinued
* PEEP should be gradually tapered off, before discontinuing ventilator support

except perhaps after open-heart surgery to prevent mediastinal bleeding.

(iii) Except in patients with acute respiratory failure due to acute restrictive lung disease (ARDS, pneumonia, pulmonary oedema), PEEP should not be used if conventional ventilatory support on 50 per cent FIO_2 produces a PaO_2 > 60–65 mm Hg. In our experience these patients do perfectly well without PEEP.

(iv) To start with, the level of PEEP should be set at +5 cm H_2O, and its effect should be first gauged before a step-wise increase is made. A PEEP higher than +15 cm H_2O should not be used as far as possible in Indian patients. We have almost always found that barotrauma (pneumothorax) occurs at levels > +10 to + 15 cm H_2O. This is probably because Indians have smaller lung volumes as compared to people in the West. In our opinion, higher levels of PEEP (>15 cm H_2O) are not effective in improving the mortality or morbidity of acute lung disease. This has been our experience over the last 30 years.

(v) It is not enough to just aim for an increased PaO_2 on a comparatively lower FIO_2 following the use of PEEP. Good oxygen transport is crucial, and for this an adequate cardiac output is necessary. Pulse rate, arterial blood pressure, mentation, skin temperature, urine output and pH of arterial blood should be monitored for a possible fall in cardiac output induced by high levels of PEEP. In difficult situations the cardiac output may need to be measured by the thermodilution technique.

(vi) If hypotension or a sharp fall in cardiac output occurs following the use of PEEP, its level should be reduced. At times it may even have to be discontinued, as the patient may be unable to tolerate levels even as low as 5 cm of PEEP. An attempt to raise the blood pressure and cardiac output through a judicious use of volume load and/or dopamine support may be tried. If the patient responds to the above measures, PEEP can then be continued.

(vii) A sharp fall instead of the expected rise in PaO_2 is invariably related to overdistension of the compliant alveoli, producing an increase in the $\dot{V}/\dot{Q}$ mismatch. This overinflation of parts of the lung (generally the upper lobes), can be detected on a chest X-ray. Ventilator settings should be readjusted so that the high peak inflation pressures are significantly reduced. In some patients PEEP may even have to be discontinued.

(viii) A fall in the venous admixture (i.e. a decrease in the right to left shunt within the lungs), and a rise in the PaO_2 while on PEEP can be due to 2 factors: (a) Improvement in lung function and mechanics, this being the effect one desires or aims at; (b) a fall in the cardiac output. This is an undesirable effect as the rise in PaO_2 is not due to improved lung function, but to deterioration in circulatory haemodynamics which ultimately is responsible for reduced oxygen transport. Clinical judgment aided if necessary by measurements of cardiac output, can distinguish one effect from the other.

(ix) PEEP should be withdrawn slowly. It is unwise to withdraw ventilator support completely and abruptly without the patient being first taken off PEEP for a sufficient length of time.

Newer and Less Frequently Used Modes of Ventilator Support

Open Lung Concept

The 'Open lung concept' is being increasingly used in ALI and ARDS and in post-operative atelectasis (see Chapter on ALI, ARDS). The principle behind this concept is to 'open' the lung and keep it 'open' with the least changes in pressure so as to minimize alveolar shear forces. This serves to improve gas exchange and serves as a lung protection mechanism by avoiding the concertina-like opening of the alveoli during inspiration and their collapse and closure during expiration.

Sequential settings in a patient with ARDS on whom the open lung concept is used are given below.

I. *Use pressure control* and set upper pressure limit to 50 cm H_2O. Set PEEP at 10–15 cm H_2O. Set pressure control level above PEEP to a value which gives a V_T of 10–15 ml/kg. Set respiratory rate at 15/min. Inspiratory time 50 per cent or I:E 1:1.

II. *Determine opening pressure*. Raise peak inspiratory pressure step-wise by 2 cm H_2O at a time, allowing 10–15 breaths at each step-wise increase, till the lung is fully 'open'. This generally requires a rise in the peak inspiratory pressure to 40–60 cm H_2O. The features that signify a fully 'open' lung are a sudden and sustained jump of the PaO_2, so that the PaO_2/FIO_2 > 400, and also the sharp disproportionate increase in tidal volume in relation to the step-wise increase in peak pressure.

III. *Determine closing pressure* of the lung. Decrease peak inspiratory pressure step-wise by 2 cm H_2O, allowing a few breaths for each setting to enable a stabilized reading. The 'closing pressure' is that pressure at which the alveoli collapse or close. This is signified by an abrupt fall in the high PaO_2 and a sharp decline in tidal volume. Note 'closing pressure'.

IV. *Reopen the lung fully* by repeating the steps outlined in II.

V. *Keep the lung open*. Slowly, step-wise, reduce the peak inspiratory pressure once more to a level which is 1–2 cm above the

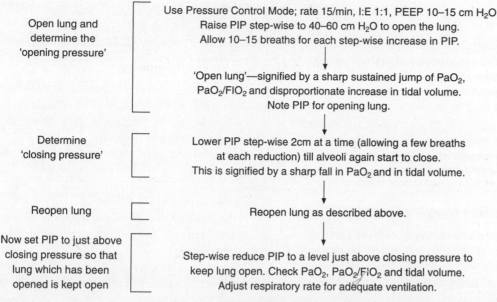

Open lung and determine the 'opening pressure'	Use Pressure Control Mode; rate 15/min, I:E 1:1, PEEP 10–15 cm H$_2$O Raise PIP step-wise to 40–60 cm H$_2$O to open the lung. Allow 10–15 breaths for each step-wise increase in PIP.
	'Open lung'—signified by a sharp sustained jump of PaO$_2$, PaO$_2$/FIO$_2$ and disproportionate increase in tidal volume. Note PIP for opening lung.
Determine 'closing pressure'	Lower PIP step-wise 2cm at a time (allowing a few breaths at each reduction) till alveoli again start to close. This is signified by a sharp fall in PaO$_2$ and in tidal volume.
Reopen lung	Reopen lung as described above.
Now set PIP to just above closing pressure so that lung which has been opened is kept open	Step-wise reduce PIP to a level just above closing pressure to keep lung open. Check PaO$_2$, PaO$_2$/FIO$_2$ and tidal volume. Adjust respiratory rate for adequate ventilation.

Fig. 9.1.6. Open lung procedure.

closing pressure. Now the lung has been opened and is being *kept open*. The tidal volume should remain stable, and the arterial blood gases good and constant.

PEEP is generally set at 10–15 cm H$_2$O. Some units prefer to set PEEP at higher levels of 15–25 cm H$_2$O. It is however, not known if this high PEEP is necessary. Therefore the same procedure as described above to determine ideal peak inspiratory pressure is now performed to find the lowest level of PEEP. After once again opening the lung, the peak inspiratory pressure and the PEEP are adjusted to just above closing pressures, so that the lungs remain 'open'.

Avoid unnecessary ventilatory disconnects, or changes in ventilator settings. If ventilator disconnects occur or there is a change in lung condition to suggest further atelectasis, the whole procedure described above to reopen lung and keep it open is repeated.

Fig. 9.1.6 describes the step-wise open lung procedure.

Airway Pressure Release Ventilation (APRV)

This ventilatory mode comprises CPAP that is intermittently released to allow a brief expiratory interval. The advantage is a lower mean alveolar pressure as compared to that during positive pressure ventilation. It has been used in patients with ARDS, and post-operatively in some patients, and has been found to be effective in providing adequate oxygenation (25–28).

Proportional Assist Ventilation

Proportional assist ventilation is a new ventilatory mode intended only for spontaneously breathing patients. It attempts to normalize the relationship between the patient's inspiratory effort and the resultant ventilatory response. The ventilator adjusts pressured inspiration depending on patient effort, modulating the patient's breathing pattern and overall ventilation (29, 30). Greater patient comfort with lower peak pressures are observed,

and ventilation is adjusted to the patient's breathing pattern and requirements. The ability to sense every inspiratory effort breath by breath, and adjust ventilatory support accordingly may prove to be of great advantage. This new mode holds out considerable hope for the future.

High Frequency Ventilation (HFV) (31)

Several modes of HFV have been employed. The basic feature in common is the use of tidal volumes which are smaller than the dead space volume (32, 33). Gas exchange does not occur through convection as in conventional ventilatory modes, but by molecular diffusion, non-convective mixing, and by other mechanisms. The two important modes of HFV are high frequency oscillatory ventilation, and high frequency jet ventilation. The advantages claimed for HFV include a decreased risk of barotrauma, and efficient gas exchange. This mode is believed to be best suited for healing of bronchopleural fistulae. Controlled trials however have shown no distinct benefit with this mode as compared to other conventional modes. The risk of complications is also significant (34, 35).

Differential Lung Ventilation

Patients in respiratory failure due to severe asymmetrical lung disease may fail to be adequately ventilated by conventional ventilatory modes. In such patients adequate gas exchange can be provided by differential lung ventilation.

Clinical examples include patients with bronchopleural fistulae, unilateral trauma, scoliosis, or marked asymmetrical degree of parenchymal inflammatory disease in each lung (one lung being grossly affected, and the other only slightly so). When there is a large difference in compliance, resistance, or both parameters between the two lungs, a larger proportion of each tidal breath (using conventional ventilatory modes), is distributed to the comparatively unaffected lung. This results in a mismatching of ventilation and perfusion, an increase in the shunt, and poor gas exchange.

The initiation of differential lung ventilation requires the patient to be intubated with a double lumen endotracheal tube (Carlen, Robert-Shaw, Univent, or Bronchocath). Different tidal volumes, flow rates, minute ventilation, and if necessary even PEEP, are set for each lung. Differential lung ventilation can be through two asynchronous ventilators each with its own circuit and its own settings (36), or through two synchronized ventilators which deliver tidal breaths to both lungs through two independent circuits. The tidal volumes, FIO_2 and other ventilatory settings for each lung are independently adjustable (37, 38).

Extracorporeal Membrane Oxygenation (ECMO)

The prohibitive cost and laborious technique of ECMO preclude its use in most critical care settings. In fact, a large multicentre trial using ECMO in patients with acute lung injury, showed that there was no reduction in mortality in the ECMO treated group; rather there was a significantly greater incidence of complications in this group of patients (39). Hence till such time as ECMO is shown to significantly improve survival, it cannot be recommended for routine use.

Table 9.1.10. Newer modes of ventilatory support

* Open Lung Concept (see **Fig. 9.1.6**)
* Airway Pressure Release Ventilation—used in patients with ARDS; mean alveolar pressure is lower as compared to that during positive pressure ventilation
* Proportional Assist Ventilation—This ventilatory mode senses degree of inspiratory effort breath by breath, and adjusts ventilatory support accordingly
* High Frequency Ventilation—Expensive, with no proven advantage
* Differential Lung Ventilation—Used in patients with asymmetrical lung disease, bronchopleural fistula, unilateral trauma, scoliosis; tidal volumes, FIO_2 and other ventilatory settings are adjusted independently for each lung

Non-invasive Positive Pressure Ventilation (40, 41)

A number of critical care units attempt, in suitable patients, to offer ventilatory support through a nasal mask or through a fitting orofacial mask rather than through an endotracheal tube. The major advantage of NIPPV is the reduced incidence of nosocomial pneumonia and of other complications associated with endotracheal intubation.

The use of NIPPV has been standard therapy in patients with obstructive sleep apnoea (42, 43) and in many patients with central sleep apnoea (44). Other indications for NIPPV in acute respiratory failure are as follows:

(i) Acute crisis in chronic airways obstruction. This is dealt with at length in the Chapter on Acute Crisis in Chronic Airways Obstruction.

(ii) In some patients with mild to moderate cardiogenic or non-cardiogenic pulmonary oedema. The more severe forms need intubation and ventilatory support.

(iii) Community acquired pneumonia with acute respiratory failure.

(iv) In AIDS with pneumocystis carinii infection or with other forms of disseminated pulmonary infection.

(v) Hypercapnic respiratory failure due to progressive chronic airways obstruction, or due to the obesity hypoventilation syndrome.

(vi) Post-operative respiratory failure (chiefly due to atelectasis).

It is obvious that if NIPPV fails to effect efficient gas exchange, or cannot be tolerated by the patient, prompt intubation with ventilator support becomes necessary.

NIPPV is contraindicated under the following conditions:

(i) In patients with a respiratory arrest or need for immediate intubation.

(ii) Inability to protect the airway.

(iii) In the presence of copious respiratory secretions.

(iv) Haemodynamic instability or persistent hypotension (systolic < 90 mm Hg).

(v) Occurrence of dangerous or persistent arrhythmia.

(vi) Inability to cooperate or tolerate either the nasal or facial mask.

(vii) In the presence of facial injuries.

NIPPV is also occasionally used after extubation in patients with marginal weaning criteria. NIPPV offers a transition from intubation to spontaneous breathing.

Different modes of ventilator support have been used with NIPPV. These include volume assist/control, pressure control, pressure support and the CPAP modes.

The major danger with NIPPV is the risk of aspiration of gastric contents. It is best not to exceed positive inspiratory peak pressures of 20–25 cm H_2O as gastric dilatation with fear of aspiration can become a major problem. The setting should allow a tidal volume of 7–10 ml/kg.

Bilevel pressure ventilators (BiPAP machine) should generally be used for long term or chronic application of NIPPV as in patients with obstructive sleep apnoea or patients with chronic hypercapnic respiratory failure due to COPD. The expiratory positive airway pressure (EPAP) is set at 3–8 cm H_2O and the inspiratory airway pressure (IPAP) to +10 to +20 cm H_2O to provide effective ventilation. A backup assist rate should be set during sleep.

Complications of Mechanical Ventilation (45–48) (Table 9.1.11)

(i) Alveolar Hyperventilation

A $PaCO_2$ of < 20 mm Hg can be dangerous. Respiratory alkalosis results in cramps, tetany, reduced cerebral blood flow, and hypotension. Electrolyte disturbances characterized by a sudden shift of potassium from the extracellular to the cellular compartment can trigger dangerous arrhythmias like ventricular tachycardia, or ventricular fibrillation. Prolonged alveolar hyperventilation makes weaning difficult as the respiratory centre gets used to a low arterial carbon dioxide tension, and cannot tolerate a rise of $PaCO_2$ to even normal levels.

Table 9.1.11. Common complications encountered during mechanical ventilation

* Alveolar hyperventilation resulting in $PaCO_2 < 25$ mm Hg. This causes respiratory alkalosis (with decreased cerebral blood flow, tetany, hypotension), shift in K^+ from extracellular to cellular compartment causing arrhythmias, difficulties in weaning
* Atelectasis—segmental, lobar or massive/ diffuse airspace collapse
* Uneven compliances in different areas of the lung resulting in uneven distribution of inspired gas and difficulty in mechanical ventilation
* Occurrence of auto-PEEP
* Nosocomial infection
* Hypotension—Initially ventilator-related due to high inflation pressures; later, usually unrelated to ventilator support
* Barotrauma/Volutrauma—pneumothorax, pneumomediastinum, interstitial emphysema, damage to alveolar walls
* 'Clashing' with the machine
* GI complications—paralytic ileus, gastric dilatation, GI bleeds
* Water retention

(ii) Atelectasis

This may be of two kinds: (a) segmental, lobar, or even massive; (b) diffuse airspace collapse or atelectasis.

Lobar or massive atelectasis is easy to detect clinically as well as on X-ray. It produces distress with a rise in the static compliance (a rise in both peak and plateau pressures is observed). A slipping of the endotracheal tube into the right main bronchus is an important cause of collapse of part or whole of the left lung.

Diffuse airspace atelectasis is characterized by a collapse of very many scattered alveoli in both lungs, so that both the clinical examination, and the chest X-ray are essentially normal. It is at times observed when tidal volumes < 10 ml/kg are used to ventilate the lungs. The use of tidal volumes of 10–12 ml/kg is the best prophylactic measure for this complication. Diffuse airspace atelectasis is suspected when there is a fall in the compliance, with an increase in the alveolar-arterial oxygen gradient, and a normal chest X-ray. When due to an increase in the water content of the lungs, the condition can be corrected by the prompt use of a diuretic like furosemide.

(iii) Uneven Compliances within Different Areas of the Lung

These produce uneven distribution of inspired gas. When some areas of the lung are normal or overcompliant, while others show a marked decrease in compliance, the problem in mechanical ventilation is immense. Inspired gas overventilates the compliant lung, and often fails to 'open' or ventilate the stiff or non-compliant parts of the lung. Overdistension of the compliant areas leads to increase in the physiological dead space, increasing Zone I conditions especially when large tidal volumes are used. The capillary perfusion in these areas is severely diminished, with blood being shunted to the less compliant, poorly ventilated areas. This produces an increased right-to-left shunt with a fall in the PaO_2. Lower tidal volumes with a judicious adjustment of PEEP is necessary, but the difficulties in providing adequate gas exchange are not always solved.

(iv) Auto-PEEP (Fig. 9.1.7)

An increase in positive end-expiratory pressure occasionally occurs in patients on mechanical ventilation (auto-PEEP), even when PEEP is not used as an adjunct to ventilator support. Auto-PEEP (occult PEEP, intrinsic PEEP) is defined as an unintentional PEEP that occurs when a new inspiratory breath is delivered before expiration has ended in patients on ventilator support. A progressively increasing auto-PEEP results in a 'dynamic hyperinflation' of the lung, which is merely another expression for increasing air-trapping within the lung. Auto-PEEP and dynamic hyperinflation are most commonly seen in patients with COPD, where narrowed obstructed airways lead to prolonged expiration and air trapping. Other factors that predispose to the occurrence of auto-PEEP are (a) $\dot{V}_E$ equal to or > 10 l/min; (b) patients > 60 years of age; (c) use of a small-sized endotracheal tube; (d) increase in V_T specially in patients with COPD; (e) increase in compliance; (f) increase in respiratory rate with increase in risk of air trapping, particularly when inspiratory time equals expiratory time; (g) reduced inspiratory flow with shorter expiratory time.

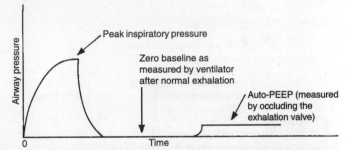

Fig. 9.1.7. Measurement of auto-PEEP. Following normal exhalation, the manometer reads zero pressure. By closing the exhalation valve, the manometer needle rises and measures the level of auto-PEEP. (Source: as in Fig. 9.1.3).

Measurement of Auto-PEEP (Fig. 9.1.8)

During normal mechanical ventilation, the auto-PEEP present in the patient's lungs at end-expiration is not registered on the ventilator manometer, as in most ventilators pressures during exhalation are measured internally on the inspiratory side of the machine. Also normally, the expiratory valve is open to the atmosphere during exhalation. Auto-PEEP can be measured by occluding the expiratory limb of the circuit just before the next positive pressure breath. When the exhalation valve is occluded, the manometer measures the pressure in the patient's airway as the pressure equilibrates with the circuit. This method of measuring auto-PEEP requires a quiet patient on controlled ventilation.

Some ventilators like the Siemens Servo 900C and the Ohmeda Advent have end-expiration pause buttons or controls. They are microprocessor ventilators that can time the closing of the exhalation valve. They close this valve just before the next positive breath is due, delay the next breath, and then measure the pressure in the circuit.

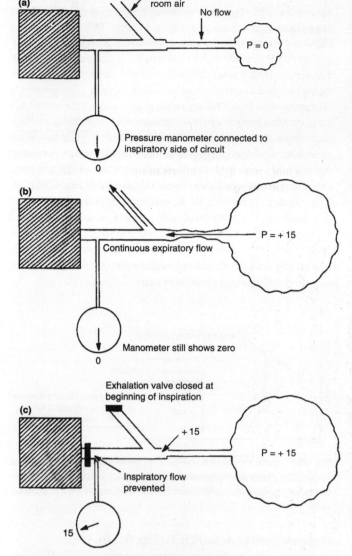

Fig. 9.1.8. A mechanical ventilator connected to a lung under normal conditions and when auto-PEEP is present.
(a) Ventilator system during normal exhalation with no air trapping, no auto-PEEP, and with the manometer reading zero.
(b) During exhalation with auto-PEEP present, the manometer still reads zero (ambient) because the exhalation valve is open to room air but there is 15 cm H_2O of air trapped in the lung.
(c) When the exhalation valve is closed and inspiratory flow stopped at end-exhalation and prior to the next breath, a manometer will be able to read the approximate auto-PEEP level in the lungs and circuit (Source: as in Fig. 9.1.3).

Effects of Auto-PEEP

Effects of auto-PEEP are the same as those of PEEP used on purpose as an adjunct to ventilatory support. Deleterious effects include barotrauma, hypotension and a fall in PaO_2.

Methods of Reducing Auto-PEEP

Auto-PEEP can be reduced by the use of (a) higher inspiratory flow rates, thereby shortening the inspiratory time and allowing longer time for expiration; (b) increased expiratory time by using smaller V_T and reduced respiratory rates; (c) low resistance exhalation valves and large bore endotracheal tubes to reduce air trapping; (d) low compressible volume ventilator patient circuit.

It must be mentioned that the occurrence of auto-PEEP is not confined to patients on ventilator support. It is frequently observed in spontaneously breathing patients who have severe airways obstruction that leads to air-trapping.

(v) Infection

Nosocomial infection is an important complication and the following preventive measures are enumerated below:

(a) Cleanliness in the patient's room with scrupulous attention to avoiding cross-infection. Washing hands prior to examining the patient is important.

(b) Care of the tracheostomy wound—spraying the wound with an antibiotic spray is useful.

(c) Aseptic suction of secretions through the tracheostomy / endotracheal tube—this should be done as often as is necessary.

(d) Meticulous attention to prevention of atelectasis by physiotherapy and postural drainage. Prompt treatment of atelectasis and diffuse airspace collapse is mandatory.

(e) Frequent sterilization of humidifiers, tubings is essential.

(f) Tracheostomy tubes should be changed every four days under aseptic conditions.

(g) Proper nutrition, oxygenation, and perfusion should be well maintained, so as to increase resistance to infection.

In patients on ventilator support, growth of Gram-negative organisms (chiefly pseudomonas strains and klebsiella) is frequently observed on culture of tracheal secretions. A positive culture by itself does not indicate infection, and does not warrant treatment (see Chapter on Nosocomial Pneumonia).

(vi) Hypotension

This is an important complication of mechanical ventilation. When it occurs soon after initiating ventilation, it is very likely to be related to the effects of the ventilator. In the presence of high inflation pressures, the use of PEEP, or in patients with overcompliant lungs as seen in emphysema, there may be a marked rise in intrapleural pressure. This reduces venous return and cardiac filling and induces a fall in blood pressure. Hypotension is often marked in hypovolaemic patients. The treatment in such patients is to reduce inflation pressures, reduce or go off PEEP totally (if this has been used), and give a volume load to expand the circulating volume. Hypotension can also result from barotrauma— e.g. a pneumothorax induced by ventilator support. This may occur at the time of initiation of ventilator support or at a later period.

When hypotension occurs later during mechanical ventilation (the patient having been haemodynamically stable for several days), the cause is generally unrelated to the ventilator. Severe hypoxia and hypocapnia should be looked out for, as they can induce a fall in blood pressure. If the blood gases are normal, hypotension may be due to shock, blood loss, fluid or electrolyte imbalance, sepsis, metabolic acidosis or poor pump function. Only if all these factors have been excluded, should the possibility of a ventilator-induced hypotension be considered.

(vii) Barotrauma and Volume Trauma

Barotrauma and volume trauma (volutrauma) are the most important and dreaded complications of mechanical ventilation. Probably both high inflation pressures and high tidal volumes, particularly when PEEP is also used, contribute to barotrauma. It is generally the more compliant parts of the lungs, and not the poorly compliant areas, that are susceptible to barotrauma. Barotrauma classically takes the form of pneumothorax—tension pneumothorax occurs when high tidal volumes are used with high inflation pressures. Unless promptly recognized, it causes cardio-respiratory collapse and death. Interstitial emphysema, mediastinal emphysema, and surgical emphysema of the soft tissues of the neck, spreading upwards to the face and downwards to the chest, may occur in the absence of pneumothorax.

A more subtle form of trauma to the alveolar walls can be caused by high tidal volumes (volume trauma or 'volutrauma'). High tidal volumes are as important in producing alveolar damage as high alveolar pressures. The over-stretched alveolar walls are damaged, so that alveoli (even those which were reasonably normal), are now thickened, distorted, and poorly compliant—thus adding to the overall stiffness and poor compliance of the lungs, and setting off a vicious cycle, which perpetuates respiratory failure to a point of no return. Over-stretch of alveoli with high tidal volumes is also believed to result in the production of cytokines that further injure the lung and perhaps also increase injury to other organs. The 'opening' and 'closing' of poorly compliant alveoli during inspiration and expiration results in shear forces that induce further lung injury (see Chapter on Acute Lung Injury and ARDS).

(viii) Clashing with the Machine

This can occur at any time during mechanical ventilation, though it is most commonly observed during initiation of ventilator support. Clashing or fighting with the machine can be due to several causes (**Table 9.1.12**), and each should be carefully evaluated prior to taking any decision on the management of the patient.

(a) Alveolar hypoventilation as stated earlier, is an important cause—if present, it should be corrected by increasing the minute ventilation.

(b) Obstructed tracheostomy/endotracheal tube or obstructed airways due to bronchospasm or mucus plugging is an important cause of distress, leading to a 'clash' with the machine. A rise in peak pressure, with a fall in the dynamic compliance and a marked difference between the peak and pause pressures should point to the above cause.

(c) Atelectasis, pneumonia, and pneumothorax are very important causes of a clash with the machine. Distress and high peak pressures with a fall in the compliance are observed.

(d) Blood loss (as in bleeding within the GI tract), shock from any cause, electrolyte imbalance, metabolic acidosis, high fever, pain, a distended bladder or colon, or a dilated stomach are other causes that aggravate difficulties in synchronization with the machine.

Table 9.1.12. Important causes of patient clashing with the machine

* Alveolar hypoventilation
* Hypoxia
* Obstructed tracheostomy / endotracheal tube or obstructed airways due to bronchospasm or mucus plugging
* Atelectasis / pneumonia / pneumothorax / pulmonary embolism
* Major blood loss (as in GI bleeds), shock of any aetiology, sepsis, fluid or electrolyte imbalance, metabolic acidosis, high fever, severe pain, dilatation of stomach, distended bladder or colon
* Strong respiratory drive due to altered mechanics within diseased lungs

(e) A strong respiratory drive due to altered mechanics within diseased lungs may defy all efforts to match the machine to the patient. It is in this group that controlled ventilation after inducing neuromuscular paralysis, or after depressing respiration with intravenous diazepam or morphine is mandatory.

(ix) Gastrointestinal Complications

Gastric dilatation and paralytic ileus are observed at times, particularly at the start of mechanical ventilation. The cause is obscure. Treatment is through gastric aspiration via a nasogastric tube, stopping all oral feeds, and using intravenous fluids till such time as gut motility returns. The maintenance of fluid and electrolyte balance in such patients is precarious. Hypokalaemia tends to aggravate the ileus, and needs to be carefully corrected by potassium replacement through intravenous infusions. Oral feeds are resumed once the gut motility returns.

Gastrointestinal bleeding occasionally occurs as a complication in patients on ventilator support. This is due to acute erosive gastroduodenitis in critically ill patients, particularly in those receiving corticosteroids. GI bleeding is particularly common in patients with acute on chronic respiratory failure secondary to infection in patients with chronic bronchitis. These patients generally have a well-marked acidosis. Antacids and H_2-receptor antagonists, or sucralfate reduce gastric acidity, and thereby help stop bleeding. At times, laser therapy or endoscopic cauterization of bleeding points may be necessary. The blood loss should be replaced by transfusions.

(x) Water Retention

Patients on prolonged ventilator support may retain water even in the clinical absence of left heart failure, or of a rise in venous pressure. Increase in the water content of the lungs may cause some degree of pulmonary oedema. This produces impaired gas exchange, and fluffy shadows in the lung on a chest X-ray. The problem is managed by restricting fluids to 1000 ml in 24 hours, and by the use of diuretics like furosemide.

Complications during mechanical ventilation observed in our study of 1569 patients are listed below in **Table 9.1.13**.

Weaning from Ventilator Support

There are a number of patients who are electively intubated and mechanically ventilated for brief periods of time for reasons other than respiratory failure. These include those ventilated briefly after major surgery as an extension of intra-operative and

Table 9.1.13. Common complications observed in our study of 1569 patients on mechanical ventilator support at the Breach Candy Hospital, Mumbai

Complications	No. of Patients
1. Related to Ventilator Support Directly or Indirectly	
(a) Weaning Problems	58
(b) Respiratory Infection	108
(c) Atelectasis	86
(d) Pneumothorax	
– Unilateral	46
– Bilateral	8
(e) Surgical Emphysema	27
(f) Severe Tachycardia due to PEEP	26
(g) Hypotension due to PEEP	27
(h) Empyema	2
2. Related to Tracheostomy or Endotracheal Tube	
(a) Blocked Endotracheal/Tracheostomy Tube	26
(b) Delayed Wound Healing	14
(c) Laryngeal Oedema	9
(d) Tracheo-oesophageal Fistula	4
(e) Accidental Removal of Tracheostomy Tube	13
(f) Right Bronchus Intubation	13
(g) Subglottic or Tracheal Stenosis	16
(h) Bleeding from Tracheostomy Site	25
(i) Haemorrhage following Perforation of Innominate Artery	4
(j) Dislodgement of Tooth in Right Bronchus	1

post-operative surgical care, or those intubated for airway protection. An abrupt termination of ventilator support and often quick extubation is generally possible in such patients, if the following criteria are satisfied.

(i) The patient is awake, alert and can breathe well spontaneously. He should have a good 'blast' through the endotracheal tube, and if need be, his tidal volume can be checked by connecting a spirometer to the endotracheal tube.

(ii) The clinical reason for ventilatory support no longer exists, or has resolved.

(iii) The airways are free of secretions through proper suction or spontaneous coughing, and the patient is capable of protecting the airways from aspiration.

(iv) The patient's chest X-ray is normal, and shows no atelectasis or pulmonary shadowing.

(v) In patients ventilated after open heart surgery or following major surgical procedures, the arterial blood gases and arterial pH should be normal or near normal, both during ventilator support, and after discontinuing support.

(vi) The patient should remain under intensive care so that respiratory care can be continued in the form of humidification of inspired gas, nebulization therapy, physiotherapy, and if necessary, reintroduction of ventilator support.

The weaning parameters stated below are generally not required to be followed in these patients. When however post-operative pulmonary complications produce respiratory failure, or the presence of infection, bleeding or other complications lead to an increasingly critical state, the decision to wean is necessarily delayed. Clinical considerations together with the respiratory parameters discussed below, help to decide the appropriate time to commence weaning from ventilatory support in these patients.

Patients who require ventilator support for long periods of time, extending for a week or even months, are not easy to wean. Prolonged mechanical ventilation is often necessary in severe or fulminant tetanus, severe acute lung injury, acute infective polyneuritis and poliomyelitis. The decision to wean such patients from ventilator support should first and foremost be a clinical one, based on clinical considerations. Parameters for weaning are useful, but they should support or supplement a clinical decision, and never be used as a substitute for it.

Clinical Considerations of Weaning (Table 9.1.14)

(i) As a general principle, mechanical ventilatory support can only be withdrawn when the reasons for initiating it are no longer present. This usually means that the underlying disease, whether it involves the lungs or not, has been cured or has markedly improved.

(ii) It is important that the patient on ventilator support maintains normal arterial blood gases at a FIO_2 of 0.4, before withdrawal of ventilator support is even contemplated. An important exception to this is in patients with chronic airways obstruction who are being ventilated for acute on chronic respiratory failure. These patients are used to a PaO_2 of around 60 mm Hg and to a high $PaCO_2$, even under 'normal' conditions.

(iii) The lungs should be free of infection, atelectasis or oedema, as far as possible. Airways obstruction, either from mucus plugging or bronchospasm should be relieved as best as possible, as it significantly increases the work of breathing.

(iv) Disturbances in acid-base balance should be corrected before weaning is commenced. Metabolic acidosis can increase the work of breathing significantly, while alkalosis can result in mental obtundation, and depress respiration.

(v) A clinical judgment should be made whether the patient in the immediate future can withstand or cope with the demands imposed by the work of breathing. The general nutritional state

Table 9.1.14. Clinical considerations for weaning patient from ventilator support

* Mechanical ventilator support should be withdrawn only when the underlying disorder (pulmonary or extra-pulmonary) has completely resolved, or has improved markedly
* Patient should maintain normal arterial blood gases on FIO_2 of 0.4 (except in patients with COPD whose basal $PaCO_2$ values are raised, and PaO_2 is around 60 mm Hg)
* There should be no significant pulmonary infection, pulmonary oedema, atelectasis or airways obstruction
* Acid-base and electrolyte disturbances should be corrected prior to weaning
* The patient should generally be alert, cooperative and mentally prepared to be weaned; he must be haemodynamically stable and preferably off inotropic support
* General nutritional state and neuromuscular status must be clinically assessed as to whether patient can cope with the work of breathing
* In presence of high fever, seizures, gastric dilatation, paralytic ileus, GI bleeds, hepatic or acute renal failure, weaning should not be attempted
* On T-tube breathing, there should be no significant change in pulse rate, BP, no tachypnoea or respiratory distress, should maintain normal blood gases and a tidal volume of 5–7 ml/kg

and the neuromuscular status should be given careful consideration. Poor nutrition, electrolyte abnormalities, hypomagnesaemia and hypophosphataemia lead to difficulties in weaning. Severely catabolic states like tetanus result in marked weight loss and loss of muscle mass in spite of providing a large caloric and protein intake. High carbohydrate diets lead to an increase in carbon dioxide production with increasing demands on ventilation, particularly in debilitated individuals, or in those with pre-existing lung disease. In such patients, less carbohydrates and more fats should be used for nutrition.

Patients with severe liver cell dysfunction, chronic renal failure, chronic alcoholics, and those who have weathered a prolonged critical illness, often pose great difficulties in weaning, chiefly because of their poor nutritional state, and their inability to cope with the work of breathing.

(vi) Haemodynamic stability, particularly in critically ill patients, is necessary before weaning can be commenced. As far as possible it is best to await the withdrawal of inotropic support before attempting to wean a seriously ill patient off ventilator support.

(vii) Ventilator support should be continued and weaning delayed in the presence of high fever, seizures, or when complications such as gastric dilatation, ileus, GI bleeding, or acute renal failure exist.

(viii) The patient should be awake, alert and cooperative, though there are exceptions to this consideration. The patient should also be prepared, indoctrinated and motivated to go off the ventilator.

Objective Respiratory Parameters for Weaning (Table 9.1.15)

The objective criteria used to supplement the clinical decision to wean a patient are a respiratory rate < 30/min, a $\dot{V}_E$ preferably < or equal to 8 l/min, and not > 10 l/min, a V_T of at least 5–7 ml/kg, a VC of at least 800 –1000 ml, and a maximum inspiratory force > –20 cm H_2O. The arterial pH should be between 7.35–7.45, the PaO_2 between 75–100 mm Hg on a FIO_2 of 0.4, and the $PaCO_2$ should be normal, except in patients with chronic airways obstruction who are used to a higher $PaCO_2$. The finer niceties that may need to be looked into are a V_D/V_T ratio which should be < 0.6, and the alveolar-arterial gradient which should be < 250 on a FIO_2 of 1.

Weaning is not possible if the peak or the plateau pressures are high. The static compliance should preferably be equal to or > 30 ml/cm H_2O, and the airway resistance should not be significantly increased. PEEP should be withdrawn before starting to wean the patient off ventilator support.

Probably the simplest bedside test to assess the feasibility of weaning is to note the respiratory rate after removing the ventilator. Rapid (> 30 breaths/min) shallow (V_T < 300 ml) breathing, is a clear indication for continuing ventilator support. An attempt has been made to compute a weaning index to predict whether attempts at weaning will be successful or not. This weaning index incorporates the efficiency of gas exchange, along with determination of load and neuromuscular competence (**49**). It is the product of a modified pressure-time index and a factor derived from the minute ventilation required to maintain an arterial $PaCO_2$

Table 9.1.15. Objective respiratory parameters for weaning

1. Ventilatory Parameters
   * RR < 30/minute
   * $\dot{V}_E$ < 8 l/minute, and not > 10 l/minute
   * V_T of minimum 5–7 ml/kg
   * VC of minimum 800–1000 ml
   * Maximum Inspiratory Force > –20 cm H_2O
   * V_D/V_T < 0.6
   * Alveolar-arterial oxygen gradient on FIO_2 of 1 < 250 mm Hg
2. Arterial Blood Gases
   * pH 7.35–7.45
   * PaO_2 70–100 mm Hg on FIO_2 of 0.4
   * $PaCO_2$ 35–45 mm Hg

of 40 mm Hg. We feel that the use of such indices is confusing and unnecessary. Clinical considerations, simple bedside procedures and monitoring of arterial blood gases almost always suffice.

Method of Weaning or Withdrawal of Ventilatory Support

It matters little whether weaning is performed with IMV at progressively lower rates, with the PS mode, or with a T-piece. We prefer the T-piece and have always managed to wean patients successfully even after months on ventilator support. Weaning requires to be very gradual in patients who have been on mechanical ventilation for prolonged periods of time, in those who have had a prolonged critical illness, and in those with muscle weakness or a poor nutritional state. It should start with just 15–30 minutes off the ventilator. The period is slowly but progressively increased under constant supervision, to reach a stage where the patient is off the ventilator for longer periods, than on it. In the next stage, the patient is weaned off all support during the day, but is kept on the ventilator at night. Finally, the patient is weaned off ventilator support at night as well.

Parameters to watch during the weaning process include the pulse rate, blood pressure, the respiratory rate and signs of respiratory muscle fatigue. Tachypnoea > 30/min during weaning, points to fatigue of the respiratory muscles, and weaning should be delayed or slowed down. Arterial blood gases should be satisfactory while the patient is off ventilator support. A fall in oxygen saturation to < 90 per cent (as judged by pulse oximetry), or a rise in $PaCO_2$ to > 45 mm Hg whilst off ventilator support, are clear warnings that weaning should be slower.

Another method of weaning is to give a single daily trial of spontaneous breathing through a T-tube. This trial is carried out under close observation. If the patient can sustain spontaneous ventilation for 60 minutes without distress (a satisfactory respiratory rate, pulse, blood pressure, tidal volume), the patient can be extubated. If the patient shows features of distress, he or she is placed back on assist/control mode of ventilator support for the next 24 hours. The patient is reassessed the next day for another trial of spontaneous breathing. In a recent study (**50**) two-thirds of patients who were on ventilator support for about 7 days, could be extubated by the above technique; without being 'weaned' in the strict sense of the word. It is doubtful if this technique would prove equally successful in patients who have been critically ill on ventilator support for several weeks or months.

Patients with chronic bronchitis who are under intensive care for an acute respiratory crisis, are often used to higher $PaCO_2$ levels ranging between 45–60 mm Hg. During weaning, these patients should be given controlled oxygen therapy at 1–2 l/min to provide an oxygen saturation of not more than 90 per cent. Uncontrolled oxygen therapy can lead to progressive hypercapnia. Ventilator support may need to be restarted under these circumstances.

Some centres prefer to wean patients by using the IMV mode. The mandatory breaths in this mode are progressively decreased till almost all the breaths are spontaneous. This convinces and reassures the patient that ventilatory support can be dispensed with. Pressure support ventilation is also used at times as a mode to wean patients, particularly those with chronic airways obstruction. To start with, a pressure support of 20 cm or more is introduced. The pressure support is then reduced gradually, with a watch on the tidal volume and respiratory rate. If a patient can breathe comfortably with a good tidal volume when pressure support is down to 5 cm H_2O, spontaneous breathing through a T-tube is generally possible. Patients being weaned with this mode should be very carefully monitored—atelectasis, increased secretions or bronchospasm can result in low tidal volumes with disastrous consequences.

Two controlled prospective studies (**50, 51**) recently compared the efficacy of different weaning methods in 'difficult to wean' ventilator dependent patients. In both studies IMV was noted to delay weaning. In one study (**50**), a single daily trial of spontaneous breathing through a T-tube was responsible for a two-fold increase in successful weaning and extubation compared to the use of pressure support. In the second trial pressure support was found to be superior to T-tube trials (**51**).

Experience with more than 1000 patients has convinced us that T-tube weaning is almost always successful, even in the most difficult cases. The IMV and PSV modes are indeed very rarely necessary; if handled ineptly these modes can aggravate rather than solve problems during the weaning process.

Trouble-shooting in Patients on Ventilator Support (Table 9.1.16)

Patients on mechanical ventilation are at times prone to catastrophic problems. Acute respiratory distress in a patient previously stable on ventilator support is a matter of grave concern, and the problem needs to be promptly evaluated and corrected.

The present discussion deals briefly with acute respiratory distress associated with high pressure alarms, low pressure alarms, and to sudden worsening in oxygenation and hypercapnia. In a desperate crisis with a struggling patient, one should always re-move the ventilator and start manual bag ventilation with 100 per cent oxygen. This manoeuvre takes care of any ventilator mal-function, and provides the physician with direct assessment of respiratory system mechanics. If resistance to manual ventilation is clearly excessive and the patient is severely hypoxic, the airway (endotracheal/tracheostomy tube) should be changed immediately.

Table 9.1.16. Methods for trouble-shooting in ventilated patients

A. Tidal Volume Significantly Below Preset Volume
  (i) Partial or complete disconnection of patient from ventilator
  (ii) Malfunction of the exhaled V_T spirometer
  (iii) Leak in breathing circuit
  (iv) Poor or absent seal at endotracheal or tracheostomy tube
  (v) Malfunctioning ventilator
Check connection of ventilator to patient's airway—if discrepancy between preset V_T and measured $V_T > 20\%$, or if clinical deterioration in patient's status—
  (i) Disconnect patient from ventilator and 'handbag' patient manually
  (ii) If leak persists—endotracheal/tracheostomy tube at fault—check cuff
  (iii) If leak positional due to tracheal dilatation—reposition tube
  (iv) If leak still persists—change airway
  (v) If leak not present on manual ventilation, then fault in ventilator, ventilator breathing circuit, or in exhaled V_T spirometer—change ventilator

B. Low Pressure Alarm
  (i) Partial or complete disconnection of patient from ventilator
  (ii) Bronchopleural fistula
  (iii) Leak in system
    (a) On manual ventilation, if resistance to ventilation is normal—leak in ventilator or its tubings
    (b) If resistance markedly reduced—cuff leak likely
Use same protocol as with low V_T states

C. High Pressure Alarm*
  (i) Obstruction to endotracheal/tracheostomy tube
  (ii) Increased secretions in airways, bronchospasm
  (iii) Decreased compliance—pneumothorax, atelectasis, pulmonary oedema, consolidation
  (iv) 'Clash' or asynchrony with the machine
In (i) catheter cannot be easily introduced through airway; ventilation with manual bag difficult
Plateau pressure near normal, whilst peak pressure high
Treatment—Change tube even if in doubt
In (ii) auscultatory wheezes present
Plateau pressure near normal; peak pressure high
Treatment—Suck secretions, use bronchodilators, nebulize with salbutamol
In (iii) clinical examination (percussion and auscultation) suggests diagnosis
Plateau and peak pressures both markedly elevated. Chest X-ray confirms diagnosis
Treatment
  – Underwater seal drainage for pneumothorax
  – Expand atelectasis with physiotherapy or suction through a fibreoptic bronchoscope
  – Use diuretics for pulmonary oedema
In (iv) Check if any of the above are responsible for asynchrony
Check for other factors causing asynchrony, and correct them
Only then paralyze with pancuronium or sedate so that the machine takes over. Then evaluate again, checking both the peak and plateau pressures

D. Oxygen Alarm
  (i) Check FIO_2
  (ii) Check pressure source

*In an acute crisis (a) handbag with 100% oxygen; (b) change tube; (c) check quickly for pneumothorax, massive atelectasis, and severe pulmonary oedema. Treat accordingly.

In such a crisis, where every minute matters, it is preferable to change an airway unnecessarily, rather than persist with an almost totally blocked, unchanged airway.

Hypoxaemia

If the patient's blood gases show a sudden deterioration in the PaO_2, one should promptly raise the FIO_2 sufficiently so as to maintain the oxygen saturation at 90 per cent. This measure is however only a temporary expedient. The important causes of hypoxaemia are given in **Table 9.1.17**. The aetiology of hypoxaemia should be determined, and treated.

Table 9.1.17. Important causes of a low PaO_2 in a ventilated patient

* Hypoventilation—$PaCO_2$ is raised
* V̇/Q̇ mismatch due to airways obstruction, pulmonary oedema, atelectasis, infection, increase in dead space, pulmonary embolism—increasing the FIO_2 easily corrects the hypoxaemia
* Increase in right to left shunt due to increasing lung injury, atelectasis, pulmonary oedema, consolidation—increased alveolar-arterial oxygen gradient on FIO_2 of 1
* Related to low $P\bar{v}O_2$
  Causes of a low $P\bar{v}O_2$ are:
  (i) Low cardiac output
  (ii) Low haemoglobin
  (iii) Increased oxygen consumption by tissues
* Severe alkalosis with a marked shift of the oxygen dissociation curve to the left

Hypercapnia

Hypercapnia could be due to a fall in minute ventilation, increased carbon dioxide production (as in fever, restlessness, increased metabolism), or increase in dead space (as in pulmonary embolism, hypovolaemia, PEEP). Hypercapnia due to a fall in minute ventilation or to increased carbon dioxide production, can be easily corrected by increasing the minute ventilation. However increase in dead space as a possible aetiology of hypercapnia should be kept in mind, as increasing the minute ventilation in such a situation can paradoxically decrease alveolar ventilation, as increase in tidal volume or respiratory rate may at times increase the dead space.

REFERENCES

1. Mushin WW, Rendell-Baker L, Thompson PW et al. (1969). In Automatic Ventilation of the Lungs, 2nd edn Blackwell Scientific Publications, Oxford and Edinburgh.

2. Pontoppidan H, Geffin B, Lowenstein E. (1972). Acute respiratory failure in the adult. (Third of three parts). N Engl J Med. 287, 799.

3. Segal BJ, Johnston RP, Donovan DJ et al. (1987). Mechanical Ventilation. In: Respiratory Intensive Care (Eds MacDonnel KF, Fahey PJ, Segal MS). pp. 131–170. Little, Brown and Company, Boston, Toronto.

4. Khambotta HJ, Baratz RA. (1972). IPPB and plasma ZDHG and urine flow in conscious man. J Appl Physiol. 33, 362.

5. Sladen A, Laver MB, Pontoppidan H. (1968). Pulmonary complication and water retention in prolonged mechanical ventilation. N Engl J Med. 279, 484.

6. Pontoppidan H, Geffin B, Lowenstein E. (1972). Acute respiratory failure in the adult. (Second of three parts). N Engl J Med. 287, 743.

7. Comroe JH Jr., Forster RE II, Du Bois AB et al. (1962). In: The Lung: clinical physiology and pulmonary function tests (2nd edn). p. 194. Year Book Medical Publishers, Chicago.

8. Kirby RR, Banner MJ, Downs JB. (1990). In: Clinical Applications of Ventilatory Support. Churchill Livingstone Inc., New York.

9. Shutsky AS. (1993). Mechanical Ventilation: ACCP Consensus Conference. Chest 104, 1833–1835.

10. Covelli HD, Weled BJ, Beekman JF. (1982). Efficacy of continuous positive airway pressure administered by face mask. Chest. 81, 147.

11. Greenbaum DM, Miller JE, Eross B et al. (1976). Continuous positive airway pressure without tracheal intubation in spontaneously breathing patients. Chest. 96, 615.

12. Smith RA, Kirby RR, Gooding JM et al. (1980). Continuous positive airway pressure (CPAP) by face mask. Crit Care Med. 8, 43.

13. Rasanen J et al. (1984). Continuous positive airway pressure by face mask in acute cardiogenic pulmonary edema. A randomized study. Crit Care Med. 12, A235.

14. Pilbeam SP. (1992). Improving Oxygenation: Positive End-Expiratory Pressure, Continuous Positive Airway Pressure, and Inverse Ratio Ventilation. In: Mechanical Ventilation—Physiological and Clinical Applications, 2nd edn (Eds Pilbeam SP, Marshall DK, Tryboski J). pp. 363–427. Mosby Year Book Inc., London, Chicago, Toronto, Sydney.

15. Ranieri VM, Eissa NT, Corbeil C et al. (1991). Effects of PEEP on alveolar recruitment and gas exchange in patients with the adult respiratory distress syndrome. Am Rev Respir Dis. 144, 544–551.

16. Benito S, LeMaire F. (1990). Pulmonary pressure-volume relationships in acute respiratory distress syndrome in adults: Role of positive end-expiratory pressure. J Crit Care. 5, 27–34.

17. Fessler HE, Brower RG, Wise RA et al. (1991). Effects of PEEP on the gradient for venous return. Am Rev Respir Dis. 143, 19–24.

18. Valta P, Takala J, Eissa NT et al. (1993). Does alveolar recruitment occur with positive end-expiratory pressure in adult respiratory distress patients? J Crit Care. 8, 34–43.

19. Marini JJ. (1990). Lung mechanics in the adult respiratory distress syndrome: Recent conceptual advances and implications for management. Chest. 11, 673.

20. Tyler DC. (1983). Positive end-expiratory pressure: A review. Crit Care Med. 11, 300–307.

21. Webb HH, Tierney DF. (1974). Experimental pulmonary edema due to intermittent positive-pressure ventilation with high inflation pressures: Protection by positive end-expiratory pressures. Am Rev Respir Dis. 110, 556.

22. Hall JB, Schmidt GA, Wood LDH. (1994). Acute Hypoxemic Respiratory Failure. In: Textbook of Respiratory Medicine, 2nd edn (Eds Murray JF, Nadel JA). pp. 2589–2613. WB Saunders Company. London, Montreal, Tokyo.

23. Kirby RR. (1988). Best PEEP: Issues and choices in the selection and monitoring of PEEP levels. Respir Care. 33, 569–580.

24. Gallagher T, Civetta JM, Kirby RR. (1978). Terminology update: Optimal PEEP. Crit Care Med. 6, 323.

25. Downs JB, Stock MC. (1987). Airway pressure release ventilation: A new concept in ventilatory support. Crit Care Med. 15, 459–461.

26. Rasanen J, Cane RD, Downs JB et al. (1991). Airway pressure release ventilation during acute lung injury: A prospective multicentre trial. Crit Care Med. 19, 1234–1241.

27. Cane RD, Peruzzi WT, Shapiro BA. (1991). Airway pressure release ventilation in severe acute respiratory failure. Chest. 100, 460–463.

28. Garner W, Downs JB, Stock MC et al. (1988). Airway pressure release ventilation (APRV): A human trial. Chest. 94, 779–781.

29. Younes M. (1992). Proportional assist ventilation, a new approach to ventilatory support: Theory. Am Rev Respir Dis. 145, 114–120.

30. Younes M, Puddy A, Roberts D et al. (1992). Proportional assist ventilation: Results of an initial clinical trial. Am Rev Respir Dis. 145, 121–129.

31. Ferguson ND, Stewart TE. (2002). New therapies for adults with acute

lung injury: High-frequency oscillatory ventilation. Crit Care Clin. 18(1), 91–106.

32. Froese AB, Bryan AC. (1987). High frequency ventilation. Am Rev Respir Dis. 135, 1363–1374.

33. Drazen JM, Kamm RD, Slutsky AS. (1984). High frequency ventilation. Physiol Rev. 64, 505–543.

34. MacIntyre NR, Follett JV, Dietz JL et al. (1986). Jet ventilation at 100 breaths per minute in adult respiratory failure. Am Rev Respir Dis. 134, 897–901.

35. Borg UR, Stoklosa JC, Siegel JH et al. (1989). Prospective evaluation of combined high-frequency ventilation in post-traumatic patients with adult respiratory distress syndrome refractory to optimized conventional ventilatory management. Crit Care Med. 17, 1129–1141.

36. Hillman KM, Barber JD. (1980). Asynchronous independent lung ventilation. Crit Care Med. 8, 390.

37. Parish JM, Gracey DR, Southorn PA et al. (1984). Differential mechanical ventilation in respiratory failure due to severe unilateral lung disease. Mayo Clin Proc. 59, 822.

38. Gallagher TJ, Banner NJ, Smith AA. (1980). Simplified method of independent lung ventilation. Crit Care Med. 8, 396.

39. Zapol WM, Snider MT, Hill JD et al. (1979). Extracorporeal membrane oxygenation in severe acute respiratory failure. JAMA. 242, 2193–2196.

40. Phillipson EA. (1994). Sleep Disorders. In: Textbook of Respiratory Medicine, 2nd edn (Eds Murray JF, Nadel JA). pp. 2301–2324. WB Saunders Company, London, Montreal, Tokyo.

41. Goldstein RS, Avendano MA, DeRosie JA et al. (1991). Influence of non-invasive positive pressure ventilation on inspiratory muscles. Chest. 99, 408–415.

42. Hoffstein V, Viner S, Mateika S et al. (1992). Treatment of obstructive sleep apnoea with nasal continuous positive airway pressure: Patient compliance, perception of benefits and side effects. Am Rev Respir Dis. 145, 841–845.

43. Sanders MH, Kern N. (1990). Obstructive sleep apnoea treated by independently adjusted inspiratory and expiratory positive airway pressures via nasal mask. Chest. 98, 317–324.

44. Issa FG, Sullivan CE. (1986). Reversal of central sleep apnoea using nasal CPAP. Chest. 90, 165–171.

45. Griebel JA, Piantadosi CA. (1991). Hemodynamics and Complications of Mechanical Ventilation. In: Problems in Respiratory Care. Complications of Mechanical Ventilation (Eds Fulkerson WJ, MacIntyre NR). pp. 25–35. JB Lippincott Co., Philadelphia.

46. Tapson VF, Fulkerson WJ. (1991). Infectious Complications of Mechanical Ventilation. In: Problems in Respiratory Care. Complications of Mechanical Ventilation (Eds Fulkerson WJ, MacIntyre NR). pp. 100–117. JB Lippincott Co., Philadelphia.

47. Pilbeam SP. (1992). Effects and Complications of Mechanical Ventilation. In: Mechanical Ventilation—Physiological and Clinical Applications, 2nd edn (Eds Pilbeam SP, Marshall DK, Tryboski J). pp. 215–278. Mosby Year Book Inc., London, Chicago, Toronto, Sydney.

48. Samuelson WM, Fulkerson WJ. (1991). Barotrauma in mechanical ventilation. In: Problems in Respiratory Care. Complications of Mechanical Ventilation (Eds Fulkerson WJ, MacIntyre NR). pp. 52–67. JB Lippincott Co., Philadelphia.

49. Jabour ER, Rabil DM, Truwit JD et al. (1991). Evaluation of a new weaning index based on ventilatory endurance and the efficiency of gas exchange. Am Rev Respir Dis. 144, 531–537.

50. Esteban A, Frutos F, Tobin MJ et al. (1995). A comparison of four methods of weaning patients from mechanical ventilation. N Engl J Med. 332, 345–50.

51. Brochard L, Rauss A, Benito S et al. (1994). Comparison of three methods of gradual withdrawal from ventilatory support during weaning from mechanical ventilation. Am J Respir Crit Care Med. 150, 896–903.

Fluid and Electrolyte Disturbances in the Critically Ill

SECTION 16

Fluid and Electrolyte Disturbances in the
Critically Ill

CHAPTER 10.1

Fluid and Electrolyte Disturbances in the Critically Ill

Disturbances in fluid and electrolyte balance are frequently observed in critically ill patients under intensive care. They occur in a wide spectrum of diseases, are not confined to any particular field of medicine, and are common following burns, trauma and major surgery. An essential prerequisite for the management of fluid and electrolyte disturbances in the critically ill is the knowledge of the basic physiology which regulates fluid and electrolyte balance. The kidneys play a crucial role in this balance and are of paramount importance in maintaining the homeostasis of the milieu interior in relation to water and electrolytes. They conserve sodium and water through several mechanism. Hormonal mechanisms acting via the kidneys include the effects of the antidiuretic hormone, the renin-angiotensin system, aldosterone and the natriuretic hormone. The brief description that follows outlines the volume and composition (in relation to fluid and electrolytes) of various body compartments. This description serves as a background against which disturbances in fluid and electrolyte balance in the critically ill, are better understood. The reader should refer to a standard textbook for a more detailed analysis on the physiology of this important subject (1, 2).

Total Body Water

Water constitutes about 60 per cent (range between 50–70 per cent) of the total body weight in young adult males, and about 50 per cent in young adult females. Since fat contains less water, the lean individual has a greater proportion of water to body weight as compared to the obese person. The lower percentage of total body water in females corresponds to a smaller muscle mass and increased quantity of adipose tissue as compared to the males. In newborn infants the proportion of body water in relation to weight is as high as 70–80 per cent. At 1 year of age the body water averages 65 per cent of the body weight and remains so all through childhood. The proportion of the water content of the body to total body weight declines with age; in elderly individuals it averages 52 per cent in males and 47 per cent in females (3).

The water content of the body is divided into three functional compartments. Water within the cells (i.e. the intracellular compartment) constitutes 30–40 per cent of the body weight. The extracellular water (i.e. in the extracellular compartment) represents 20 per cent of the body weight and is further divided into the intravascular fluid or plasma (5 per cent of body weight), and the interstitial extracellular fluid (15 per cent of body weight). This is illustrated in **Fig. 10.1.1**.

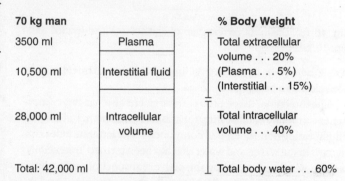

Fig. 10.1.1. Functional compartments of body fluids (from Tom Shires G et al. 1989. Fluid electrolyte and nutritional management of the surgical patient. In: Principles of Surgery, 5th edn, Eds Schwartz SI et al., pp. 69–103, McGraw-Hill Inc., NY, with permission).

Intracellular Fluid

This is determined after subtracting the measured extracellular fluid from the measured total body water.

The chemical composition of the intracellular fluid is as shown in **Fig. 10.1.2**. Potassium (K^+) and magnesium (Mg^{++}) are the principal cations, whilst phosphate (HPO_4^{---}), sulphate (SO_4^{--}) and proteins are the principal anions within the intracellular fluid. The cations and anions roughly approximate at 200 mEq/l each.

Extracellular Fluid

As mentioned earlier, this constitutes 20 per cent of the body weight—5 per cent as plasma volume in the vascular compartment, and 15 per cent as interstitial (extravascular and extracellular) fluid.

The normal composition of extracellular fluid is illustrated in **Fig. 10.1.3**. Sodium (Na^+) is the principal cation and chlorides (Cl^-) and bicarbonates (HCO_3^-) are the principal anions. There are minor differences in the ionic composition between the plasma in the vascular compartment and the interstitial tissue fluid, related to differences in protein concentration of these two compartments. For practical considerations however, the composition of these

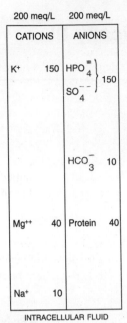

Fig. 10.1.2. Chemical composition of intracellular fluid (source as in Fig. 10.1.1.).

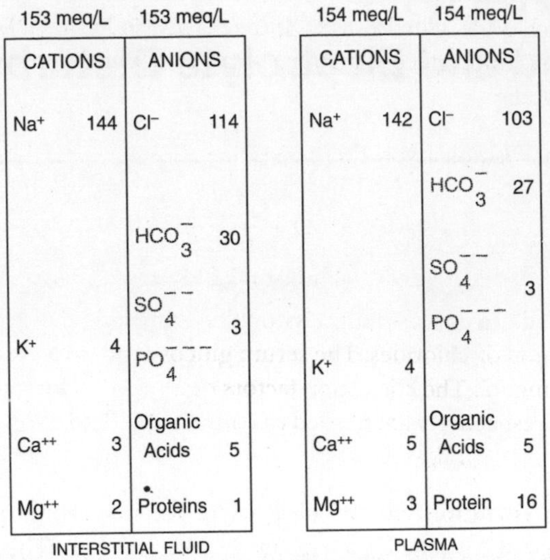

	153 meq/L	153 meq/L		154 meq/L	154 meq/L	
	CATIONS	**ANIONS**		**CATIONS**	**ANIONS**	
	Na⁺ 144	Cl⁻ 114		Na⁺ 142	Cl⁻ 103	

Fig. 10.1.3. Chemical composition of extracellular fluid (interstitial fluid and plasma) (source as in Fig. 10.1.1.).

two subdivisions of the extracellular fluid compartment may be considered to be equal.

The interstitial tissue fluid compartment also has two components—a rapidly equilibrating functional component, and a slowly equilibrating non-functional component. The latter includes connective tissue water, and water that has been termed 'transcellular water', which is formed by the active transport of extracellular water across epithelial cells. Normally this constitutes 15 ml/kg body weight, and is chiefly distributed between the gastrointestinal lumen, cerebrospinal fluid, biliary fluid and the lymphatics in the ratio of 7:3:2:3 respectively (1). In disease states large quantities of transcellular water with electrolytes lie 'sequestrated' within the body. Thus in intestinal obstruction, 10–20 litres may be sequestrated within the gut, and a similar quantity may lie sequestrated in ascites resulting from several causes. This sequestrated transcellular water, in disease, constitutes a loss of total body water and can assume very significant proportions.

Basic Concepts of Osmotic Activity

The osmotic activity of a solute is a measure of its concentration in fluid, and is measured in milliosmoles (mOsm).

Osmolarity is the osmotic activity per volume of the solution (solute + solvent). Osmolality is the term used for expressing osmotic activity per volume of the solvent (water). In biological fluids the volume of water is far greater than the number of electrolyte particles. There is little difference between osmolarity and osmolality, so that the two terms can be used synonymously in clinical medicine.

The differences in ionic composition of fluid within the intracellular and extracellular compartments are maintained by the semipermeable cell membrane. Although the total osmotic pressure of a fluid is the sum of the partial pressures of each of the

solutes in the fluid, the *effective osmotic pressure* is dependent on those solutes which do not pass through the semipermeable membrane. The proteins in the plasma which do not pass through the capillary membrane in the vascular compartment are thus responsible for the effective osmotic pressure between the vascular and interstitial fluid compartments. This is referred to as the *colloid oncotic pressure*. The effective osmotic pressure between the extracellular interstitial fluid and the intracellular fluid compartments is chiefly exerted by sodium which is the principal cation in the extracellular fluid and which does not ordinarily traverse the cell membrane. Glucose (or any other solute or substance) which does not easily traverse the cell membrane, also contributes to the effective osmotic pressure of the extracellular fluid compartment.

It is important to restress that cell membranes are easily and completely permeable to water, so that the effective osmotic pressure in the intra- and extracellular fluid compartments is equal. Therefore an increase in the effective osmotic pressure of the extracellular fluid compartment brought about by an increase in its sodium concentration would cause a transfer of water from within the cells to the outside so that osmotic equilibrium is re-established. Similarly a decrease in sodium concentration in the extracellular fluid compartment leads to transfer of water from the extracellular compartment into the intracellular compartment till osmotic equilibrium is re-established. Loss of extracellular fluid volume without change in sodium concentration will not however result in transfer or shift of water from the intracellular compartment.

Measurement of Plasma Osmolality

Plasma osmolality can be measured in the clinical laboratory using the freezing point of water. The temperature at which water in a plasma sample freezes when placed in a refrigerated bath, is converted directly into osmolality (one osmole solution freezes at −1.80°C). This is termed the freezing point depression method for determining osmolality. Plasma osmolality measures between 285–305 mOsmoles/kg H₂O.

Plasma osmolality can also be calculated by using the

concentrations of the major solutes in the extracellular fluid—sodium, chloride, glucose, urea. If the plasma sodium is taken as 140 mEq/l, blood glucose as 90 mg/dl and blood urea nitrogen as 14 mg/dl, then

$$\text{Plasma Osmolality} = 2 \times [\text{Na}] + \frac{[\text{Glucose}]}{18} + \frac{[\text{NPN}]}{2.8}$$

$$= 2 \times 140 + \frac{90}{18} + \frac{14}{2.8}$$

$$= 290 \text{ mOsm/kg H}_2\text{O}$$

The sodium concentration is doubled to include the osmotic contribution of chlorides. The serum glucose and urea are measured in mg/dl. The correction factors of 18 and 2.8 for glucose and urea respectively are needed to convert mg/dl to mOsm/kg H$_2$O.

Plasma Tonicity

The effective osmolality or plasma tonicity is obtained by removing urea from this equation, as urea passes freely across the cell membrane and therefore does not contribute to osmotic activity of the extracellular fluid compartment.

$$\text{Plasma Tonicity} = 2 \times [\text{Na}] + \frac{[\text{Glucose}]}{18}$$

$$= 2 \times 140 + \frac{90}{18}$$

$$= 285 \text{ mOsm/kg H}_2\text{O}$$

Urea contributes very little to the total extracellular solute pool in normal individuals, there being very little difference between plasma tonicity and osmolality. However in severe azotaemia due to renal failure, the difference between osmolality and tonicity increases significantly. Hyperosmolality without any increase in tonicity produces no shift of water across cell membranes.

Osmolal Gap

The difference between the measured and calculated plasma osmolality is due to the presence of unmeasured solutes (e.g. Ca^{++}, Mg^{++}, proteins etc.) in the osmolality equation stated above. This difference constitutes the osmolal gap and measures about 10 mEq/l or less (4–6). If this osmolal gap is high, and the calculated osmolality is within the normal range, it signifies an accumulation of abnormal osmotically active solutes in the plasma. These could include poisons like ethanol, methyl alcohol, or osmotically active solutes like mannitol or toxins that accumulate in renal failure. A high osmolal gap in the presence of a low calculated osmolality generally signifies a decrease in the aqueous phase of plasma caused by hyperproteinaemia or hyperlipidaemia.

Normal Fluid and Electrolyte Exchange

The internal environment with regard to fluid and electrolytes is kept stable and within a physiological range by the function of the kidneys, skin, lungs and gastrointestinal tract. This stability or constancy may be compromised by disease, trauma, surgery or by a pathology directly involving one or more of these organs.

Water Balance

The normal individual has an intake of 2000–2500 ml of water/day as is shown in **Table 10.1.1**. Daily water loss includes 1000–1500 ml in urine, and 500–700 ml as insensible loss through the skin and lungs. A patient deprived of all fluid intake must pass 500–800 ml urine to excrete products of catabolism; he also continues to lose 500–700 ml as insensible water loss. The latter is increased in fever, hypermetabolic states and during hyperventilation. Loss through sweating (which is separate from insensible water loss through the skin), can be excessive in hot humid climes. Loss of water from the lungs may be as high as 1.5 l/day in the presence of hyperventilation and an unhumidified tracheostomy. Normal water exchange is illustrated in **Table 10.1.1**.

Table 10.1.1. Water exchange in a 70 kg adult

Routes	Average volume (ml/24 hrs)	Minimal (ml/24 hrs)	Maximal (ml/24 hrs)
1. Water Gain			
Sensible:			
– Oral fluids	800–1500	0	1500/hr
– Solid foods	500–700	0	1500
Insensible:			
– Water of oxidation	250	125	800
– Water of solution	0	0	500
2. Water Loss			
Sensible:			
– Urine	800–1500	300	1400/hr*
– Intestinal	0–250	0	2500/hr
– Sweat	0	0	4000/hr
Insensible:			
– Lungs and skin	600	600	1500

*In diabetes insipidus.
Source as in Fig. 10.1.1.

Salt Balance

The salt intake of a normal individual varies from 40–120 mEq of sodium chloride. Excess salt is excreted by the kidneys. When salt intake is reduced, or extrarenal salt loss markedly increases, the normal kidney reduces salt excretion to as low as 1 mEq/day within a matter of 24 hours. The fluid lost in sweat is hypotonic, the sodium content varying from 15 mEq/l in acclimatized individuals, to 60 mEq/l in unacclimatized individuals.

The volume and concentration of gastrointestinal secretions are shown in **Table 10.1.2**. Fluid loss from the gastrointestinal tract as seen from the above table is either isotonic or hypotonic, and these losses should be replaced by isotonic saline. Sequestration of extracellular fluid in the gut, peritoneum, or tissue spaces also represents isotonic losses of salt and water.

Approach to Problems in Fluid and Electrolyte Imbalance

The conventional and easy method of evaluating disturbances in fluid and electrolyte balance is the frequent measurement of the concentration of serum electrolytes. It is crucial to remember that intracellular and extracellular electrolytes are normally constant,

Table 10.1.2. Composition of gastrointestinal secretions (range of values in parentheses)

Secretion	Volume (ml/24 hrs)	Na (mEq/l)	K (mEq/l)	Cl (mEq/l)	HCO₃ (mEq/l)
Salivary	1500 (500–2000)	10 (2–10)	26 (20–30)	10 (8–18)	30
Stomach	1500 (100–4000)	60 (9–116)	10 (0–32)	130 (8–154)	
Duodenum	(100–2000)	140	5	80	
Ileum	3000 (100–9000)	140 (80–150)	5 (2–8)	104 (43–137)	30
Colon		60	30	40	
Pancreas	(100–800)	140 (113–185)	5 (3–7)	75 (54–95)	115
Bile	(50–800)	145 (131–164)	5 (3–12)	100 (89–180)	35

Source as in Fig. 10.1.1.

and that major shifts in and out of 'compartments' can occur in disease with minimal changes in serum electrolytes. Again, it is very rare in clinical practice to have a disturbance confined to sodium balance per se; disturbances in water balance invariably accompany the latter. In fact, changes in plasma sodium concentration often are a pointer to disturbances in water balance. Finally, gross loss of sodium, potassium and water may exist in the body without any alteration in the plasma concentration of these electrolytes, if the fluid and electrolyte losses are in the same proportion as normally exist in extracellular fluid and plasma (ie. if the fluid loss is isotonic with plasma).

An evaluation of fluid and electrolyte changes in disease demands a consideration of (i) the electrolyte concentration in plasma; (ii) the volume of its distribution in the body; (iii) the rate and quantity of water and electrolyte loss out of the body (as in vomiting and diarrhoea) vis-à-vis the intake of water and electrolytes; (iv) the movement of electrolytes and water in and out of each compartment; (v) the possible sequestration of electrolytes and water within the body (as in ascites and intestinal obstruction), which represents a loss of extracellular fluid.

Nature of Fluid Changes in the Body (2)

These disorders are best categorized as follows:

(a) *Disturbances of Volume.* If isotonic fluid is lost from, or added to the body fluids, only a change in the volume of the extracellular fluid is observed. A loss of intestinal secretions thus leads to a loss of isotonic fluid and to a depletion of fluid within the extracellular compartment. As sodium, chloride and water that is lost is isotonic with plasma, the plasma concentration of sodium chloride remains unchanged. Fluid will not be transferred from the intracellular to the extracellular compartment as long as the osmolarity of the two remains the same. Addition of isotonic solution to the body fluids will result in a volume excess within the extracellular fluid compartment. However, the concentrations of sodium and chloride in plasma remain unchanged, and there is no shift of water between the intracellular and extracellular fluid compartments.

(b) *Disturbances in Concentration* which produce a change in osmotic activity of the extracellular fluid (and the plasma). If water alone is lost from or added to the extracellular fluid, the concentration of osmotically active solutes in this compartment will change. Sodium is the most important osmotically active ion in the extracellular fluid. If the sodium concentration in the extracellular fluid falls, water will pass into the intracellular compartment till the osmolarity of both compartments is again equalized. If sodium concentration in the plasma rises, osmotic activity of the extracellular fluid compartment is increased, and water passes from the intracellular to the extracellular compartment so that osmotic equality between the two compartments is re-established.

(c) *Disturbances in Volume and Concentration.* Volume and concentration abnormalities may both arise because of disease or from inappropriate parenteral fluid replacement therapy. A classic example is the association of a volume deficit together with a fall in serum sodium concentration that results from a massive loss of gastrointestinal fluid (causing a volume deficit), where fluid replacement is only through water (producing a fall in sodium concentration).

(d) *Disturbances in Composition.* Concentrations of ions other than sodium can be altered within the extracellular fluid compartment without much change in the effective osmotic activity of the extracellular fluid. This produces a compositional change which may be comparatively small when it involves an electrolyte like potassium, and yet has disastrous consequences (e.g. a rise in serum K^+ from 4 to 8 mEq/l), if not promptly corrected. Compositional changes also involve disturbances in acid-base balance.

A combination of any of the disturbances stated above is often present in a critically ill patient.

This chapter now briefly describes volume changes, and then proceeds to describe disturbances in sodium concentration (hyponatraemia and hypernatraemia). It then describes compositional abnormalities characterized by changes in plasma potassium, calcium, magnesium and phosphate levels. The compositional changes characterized by acid-base disturbances are dealt with in a separate section.

Volume Changes

Volume deficit or excess is diagnosed by clinical examination. It is to be stressed that a severe volume deficit may exist with a normal, low or even high serum sodium level.

Volume Deficit

Extracellular fluid volume deficit with a decreased volume within the effective intravascular compartment characteristically occurs in vomiting, diarrhoea, intestinal fistulae, nasogastric suction, and in fluid loss following burns.

Other important causes include sequestration of fluid in soft tissue injuries and infections, intra-abdominal or retroperitoneal infection, peritonitis, and sequestration of fluid within the gut in ileus or in intestinal obstruction.

Renal salt and water loss can occur because of diuretics, renal disease or to adrenal insufficiency.

In the ICU patient, the causes listed above are generally obvious. Less obvious causes include an unsuspected inadequate fluid intake, or fluid loss through excessive sweating as in high fever, hot humid temperatures, and in diseases like tetanus. The extent of volume changes during haemodialysis, haemofiltration, and fluid loss from surgical incisions and wounds may also be underestimated.

Clinical Features

Early features of hypovolaemia include tachycardia and postural hypotension (difference of 10–20 mm Hg in systolic arterial blood pressure between the supine and sitting postures). With increasing volume deficit and hypovolaemia, there is increasing tachycardia, hypotension, collapsed peripheral and central veins with a lowered central venous pressure, and a lowered pulmonary capillary wedge pressure. The skin is cold and clammy, and the urine output is decreased. The urinary sodium is < 10 mEq/l except in patients whose hypovolaemia is related to salt and water loss via the kidneys (the urinary sodium in these patients is normal or increased).

Mental changes include anxiety, restlessness, followed by apathy, and dullness that may progress to drowsiness and coma. Poor tissue perfusion leads to accumulation of lactic acid with lactic acid acidosis. Multiple organ failure ultimately results from prolonged uncorrected hypovolaemic shock.

Management

The first principle is to restore circulating volume through infusion of intravenous fluids. Once this is satisfactorily achieved, disturbances in electrolytes and acid-base balance if present need to be rectified. This is dealt with at length in subsequent subsections.

Volume Excess

In the ICU patient volume excess is often iatrogenic when the fluid intake has consistently exceeded the output. Excessive intravenous infusions of saline, and blood transfusions are important causes of hypervolaemia. Renal insufficiency, congestive heart failure,

liver disease and other causes of sodium retention or excessive sodium administration can all produce increase in extracellular fluid content and hypervolaemia.

A hypervolaemic state is manifested by oedema, and still later by ascites and pleural effusion. The neck veins are full, and pulmonary congestion may be obvious on clinical examination. If cardiac function is normal, the circulation is hyperdynamic with tachycardia, a warm skin, a bounding pulse with an increase in the systolic pressure and the pulse pressure. The central venous pressure is raised beyond 12 mm Hg, and the pulmonary capillary wedge pressure is often > 20 mm Hg in the presence of pulmonary oedema.

In cases of moderate volume excess, salt restriction, restriction of fluid intake and the use of furosemide as a diuretic, will correct the problem. Fulminant pulmonary oedema secondary to overhydration from overtransfusion of blood or fluids, is more appropriately dealt with by phlebotomy in stages, so that the pulmonary capillary wedge pressure is reduced below 15 mm Hg.

It is worth remembering that in certain disease states there may be an increase in the volume in the extracellular compartment, associated with a decrease in the effective circulating blood volume. Advanced congestive heart failure and cirrhosis of the liver are classic examples of salt and water retention producing an increase in the extracellular volume, yet being terminally associated with a failing circulation. Suboptimal filling of the vascular space can occur due to a loss of fluid into other spaces as is seen in hypoalbuminaemia, portal hypertension, and increased vascular permeability to solute and water.

Hyponatraemia (7)

Hyponatraemia is characterized by a serum sodium below 135 mEq/l. Severe hyponatraemia (Na < 120 mEq/l) is fraught with danger and should be promptly treated. Hyponatraemia is common in critical care medicine and is observed in diverse medical and surgical problems. The incidence in our intensive care unit patients is about 10–15 per cent. Anderson et al. (8) observed it in 1 per cent of a hospital population, whilst Chung and associates (9) noted its occurrence in 4–5 per cent of post-operative patients.

Hyponatraemia *always signifies an excess of water relative to sodium in the extracellular (and intravascular) compartment*. A pseudohyponatraemia may be observed in patients with extreme elevation of serum lipids or proteins, which causes an increase in plasma volume with consequent reduction in plasma sodium concentration. However this increase in volume is in the non-aqueous phase, while the sodium is contained in the aqueous phase of plasma. Therefore in these patients, hyponatraemia is not associated with excess of water relative to sodium.

True hyponatraemia (excess water in relation to sodium) can occur with a low, a normal or an expanded extracellular volume. It is important to make this assessment from the clinical background and the aetiology responsible for hyponatraemia. Hyponatraemia may occur acutely or may be slowly progressive or chronic. Acute hyponatraemia from any cause, when marked, is life-threatening, and should be promptly evaluated and treated.

The causes of hyponatraemia are considered below:

(a) True salt and water depletion—as in vomiting and diarrhoea, particularly when fluid loss is partially replaced by dextrose or hypotonic solutions without adequate replacement of sodium and other electrolytes. The important causes of fluid and electrolyte loss have already been enumerated in the earlier Subsection on Volume Deficit. Hyponatraemia due to loss of both fluid and electrolytes is associated with a contracted or low extracellular volume. The presence of a low intravascular volume is evident on clinical examination. Hyponatraemia related to vomiting, diarrhoea or loss of intestinal fluid is associated with a low urinary sodium (< 20 mEq/l); that associated with sodium loss in the urine through diuresis or an adrenocortical insufficiency is associated with increased urinary sodium (> 20 mEq/l).

(b) Dilutional hyponatraemia secondary to chronic heart failure, chronic liver or renal disease. These patients have an expanded extracellular volume, an increase in the total sodium content of the body, and are often waterlogged. The urinary sodium is < 20 mEq/l in cardiac failure and in liver cell dysfunction, while it is often > 20 mEq/l in chronic renal disease.

(c) Primary dilutional hyponatraemia is generally evident from the history e.g. overloading in acute renal failure, excessive infusions of 5 per cent dextrose in post-operative patients, and compulsive water drinking in patients with diabetes insipidus who are on pitressin. Here again hyponatraemia is associated with an increase in the intravascular volume and in the volume of the interstitial tissue compartment. In milder cases with this form of hyponatraemia, clinical examination may not suggest an expanded extracellular volume, as about 5 litres of excess water need to be retained to produce definite pitting oedema in an average sized adult. The urine osmolality in these patients is decreased, and is always < 100 mOsmoles/kg H_2O, with a urinary sodium < 10 mEq/l. The decreased urine osmolality distinguishes the above condition from the syndrome of inappropriate secretion of antidiuretic hormone (SIADH) described below.

(d) Syndrome of inappropriate secretion of antidiuretic hormone (SIADH). In critical care medicine this is most frequently observed after major surgery, probably due to a sustained nonosmotic release of vasopressin that occurs during 'stress'. This problem is compounded when the surgeon tries to increase the low urine output by intravenous infusions of large quantities of dextrose. SIADH is generally associated with a normal extracellular volume. Oedema (with an inference of an expanded extracellular volume) occurs in SIADH only when water retention exceeds 5 litres. This syndrome can be confidently diagnosed by an inappropriately concentrated urine (urine osmolality > 100 mOsmoles/kg H_2O) even after infusions of normal saline, and by a urinary sodium excretion > 20 mEq/l in the face of a hypotonic plasma (plasma osmolality < 290 mOsmoles/l) (10). The important causes of SIADH seen in critical care medicine are given in Table 10.1.3.

(e) Essential Hyponatraemia (sickle cell syndrome). This is observed in terminal stages of cardiac and liver cell failure, as also in the terminal stages of tuberculosis, malignancy, or other chronic illnesses.

Table 10.1.3. Important causes of SIADH

* Malignancies
  - Pharyngeal
  - Genitourinary
  - Pancreas
  - Lymphomas
* Pulmonary Disorders
  - Bronchogenic carcinoma/Mesothelioma
  - Fulminant pneumonia
  - Pneumothorax
  - Positive pressure ventilation
  - Acute severe asthma
* CNS Disorders
  - Infections (abscess, meningitis, encephalitis)
  - Trauma/intracranial haemorrhage
  - Brain tumours
  - Multiple sclerosis
  - Acute psychosis
* Drugs
  - Chlorpropamide
  - Carbamazepine
  - Clofibrate
  - Narcotic-analgesics/NSAID
  - Isoproterenol
  - Nicotine
  - Antimitotic drugs

It is important not only to diagnose hyponatraemia, but to determine its aetiology and to determine from the clinical background whether it is associated with a contracted, increased, or normal extracellular volume. The evaluation and approach to a hyponatraemic patient is illustrated in **Fig. 10.1.4**.

Clinical Features

The clinical picture of hyponatraemia, when there is both a true salt and water depletion, is invariably dominated by features of fluid loss which result in a reduced or contracted extracellular and intravascular volume. Dehydration and hypovolaemic shock of varying degrees result (see Chapter on Hypovolaemic Shock and the Subsection on Volume Deficit).

Salt depletion per se produces thirst, severe cramps in the legs, and later in the thighs and abdomen. Potassium depletion is also invariably present as an associated feature, and features of hypokalaemia are therefore also often seen (see Subsection on Hypokalaemia). Fluid and electrolyte loss is also often associated with acid-base disturbances—metabolic alkalosis in vomiting, and metabolic acidosis in diarrhoea. Lactic acid acidosis occurs with increasing impairment of tissue perfusion.

Symptoms due to hyponatraemia depend on its severity and the rate at which it evolves. Symptoms generally occur with a serum sodium < 125 mEq/l and are chiefly due to water intoxication with oedema of the brain cells. Patients may be lethargic, confused, stuporous or even comatose. In severe or rapidly evolving hyponatraemia with serum Na < 110 mEq/l, seizures and coma occur due to brain oedema. The clinical picture at times, particularly in older patients, simulates a brain stem infarction or a subarachnoid haemorrhage with neck stiffness, stiffness of the limbs and coma. In a few cases, the diagnosis first becomes apparent on a CSF examination which shows a very low chloride content.

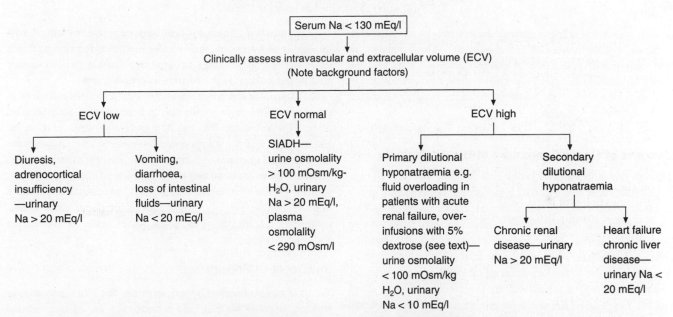

Fig. 10.1.4. Algorithm for approach to hyponatraemia.

Management

Hyponatraemia due to Salt and Water Loss

In hyponatraemia *due to both salt and water loss* causing a decreased intravascular volume, dehydration and hypovolaemia are corrected by infusions of N saline (see Chapter on Hypovolaemic Shock). As explained earlier, the flow rate is quicker through a large sized catheter inserted in a peripheral vein. A central venous line helps to monitor the CVP and should be inserted if the patient is in shock. In severe shock the simultaneous use of colloidal solutions (dextran or haemaccel) should be started to produce a more rapid expansion of the vascular compartment.

The total quantity of intravenous fluid depends on the degree of shock, the clinical history, an estimation of the rate and volume of fluid loss by carefully maintaining the output chart, and by the response to therapy. Thus in a patient with a violent gastrointestinal infection such as cholera, the fluid loss may amount to 500–1,500 ml/hour, and death results if the volume is not adequately replaced. Often in patients with a profuse fluid and electrolyte loss, 10–12 litres may need to be infused in the first 24 hours. The CVP should be maintained between 7–10 cm H_2O. Rapid infusions in patients with left heart disease or renal insufficiency can however trigger pulmonary oedema even with a normal CVP. Clinical auscultation of the lung bases for basal crackles and a chest X-ray for pulmonary congestion aid in diagnosing this complication, and help in controlling the administration of intravenous fluids.

We invariably go by clinical considerations (this includes CVP monitoring) in adjusting the quantity, quality and rate of intravenous administration of infusions in hyponatraemia associated with fluid and sodium loss. This is notwithstanding the formulae which are given to help evaluate the degree of salt and water loss in different situations. Hyponatraemia due to fluid and sodium loss is generally associated with hypokalaemia and often associated with acid-base disturbances which need to be corrected (see Subsection on Hypokalaemia and Section on Acid-Base Disturbances in the Critically Ill).

Severe Symptomatic Hyponatraemia (serum Na < 115 mEq/l)

Severe symptomatic hyponatraemia with serum sodium < 115 mEq/l deserves urgent correction as the mortality exceeds 50 per cent (**11**). Management is guided by the clinical background. It is important to clinically assess whether hyponatraemia is associated with a low extracellular volume (ECV), a normal or near normal ECV or an increased ECV.

Severe hyponatraemia with a Low ECV. Hypertonic 3 per cent saline is infused till the serum Na increases to about 125 mEq/l. The amount of sodium needed can be determined by estimating the sodium deficit.

Sodium Deficit = TBW × (125—serum Na of patient)
   (mEq)   (in mEq/l)

The total body water (TBW) is taken as 60 per cent of body weight, which in a 70 kg male amounts to 42 litres. It is to be noted (for reasons given below), that it is best not to increase serum sodium to more than 125 or at the most 130 mEq/l by the use of hypertonic saline.

Once the sodium deficit is calculated, the volume of 3 per cent hypertonic saline to be infused is easy to determine as 1 ml of 3 per cent hypertonic saline is equivalent to 1 mEq of sodium, 500 ml thereby roughly providing 500 mEq of sodium.

As mentioned earlier, volume replacement with isotonic saline to restore both vascular volume and the volume in the interstitial tissue compartment, should be of prime importance in these patients.

Severe Hyponatraemia with a Normal or Near Normal ECV. This is best treated with restriction of water intake to 700 ml and the use of diuresis with furosemide. This is then followed by the use of isotonic saline. In severely symptomatic cases (and this is rare), hypertonic saline as described above may be administered.

Severe Hyponatraemia with an Expanded ECV. These patients are best treated with restriction of water intake to 700 ml and the use of furosemide diuresis. Hypertonic saline infusions invariably do harm to these patients. Water excess can be roughly estimated by the following equation:

$$\text{Water Excess} = \text{TBW} \times (125 \ / \ \text{Current Plasma Sodium}) - 1$$

Dangers of Rapid Correction of Hyponatraemia

Though symptomatic hyponatraemia carries a mortality of over 50 per cent, rapid correction of hyponatraemia can in itself result in the dangerous complication of central pontine myelinolysis. This is a demyelinating brain stem lesion which can lead to permanent neurological deficit. It produces pupillary and ocular changes, coma, a decerebrate state, and can be fatal (**10**). Present evidence suggests that the lesion is produced by rapid correction of hyponatraemia, only if serum sodium is restored to normal levels (**10, 12**). As a practical solution in patients with severe hyponatraemia who are severely symptomatic, the rate of infusion of 3 per cent saline should be adjusted so that serum sodium is not raised by more than 1–2 mEq/hour (**10**). The end-point in serum sodium correction should not exceed 125 mEq/l. Alcoholics and malnourished patients are at greater risk of developing central pontine myelinolysis (**10**) so that the precautions stated above assume even greater importance.

Hypernatraemia

Hypernatraemia exists when the serum sodium is in excess of 145 mEq/l. It means that there is an excess of sodium relative to water in the extracellular and vascular compartments. Hypernatraemia, as is explained later, is invariably due to a massive depletion of water which relatively exceeds the depletion of sodium. In other words, most patients with hypernatraemia are hypovolaemic with a contracted extracellular volume. The increased osmolality in the extracellular fluid causes a shift of water from the intracellular to the extracellular compartment. Water loss from plasma is to an extent 'buffered'. Massive loss of water is therefore necessary for significant hypernatraemia to occur. The intracellular dehydration caused by hypernatraemia chiefly affects the function of the brain cells as will be discussed later.

Hypernatraemia observed in the ICU is (i) chiefly due to excessive loss of water relative to sodium; (ii) occasionally it is due to very inadequate water intake in comatose or obtunded patients treated at home, or in old patients who are not looked after, or in those in whom thirst is either deficient or unsatisfied; (iii) rarely it is iatrogenic and induced by excessive intravenous infusions of sodium bicarbonate (following cardiac arrest or to correct metabolic acidosis), or intravenous infusions of hypertonic saline used to correct hyponatraemia.

(a) Water Loss

(i) Through the gastrointestinal tract—gastric secretions are hypotonic to plasma; rarely unreplaced losses can lead to a hypernatraemic, hypovolaemic state.

(ii) Loss in hot climes can occur from excessive sweating. Large quantities of hypotonic fluid can be lost from the skin and to a lesser degree from the lungs. In burns involving a large body surface area, hypernatraemia is a common complication.

(iii) Loss of water from the kidneys in quantities sufficient to cause hypernatraemia, occurs only in 2 conditions—uncontrolled diabetes where water loss can be significantly greater than the sodium loss, and the solute diuresis observed after intravenous mannitol and in uraemic patients. Tube feeding in unconscious patients with feeds containing a high protein and low water content, can also produce hypernatraemia in ICU patients. The products of protein catabolism following the use of such feeds, act as solutes producing a solute diuresis, more water being excreted than sodium.

(b) Excess of Sodium

We have rarely observed hypernatraemia due to increased body sodium, because we carefully monitor the use of intravenous sodium bicarbonate, and use hypertonic saline only for the correction of acute symptomatic hyponatraemia. When hypernatraemia is due to an overall increase in the sodium content of the body, hypervolaemia and an expanded extracellular compartment are always accompanying features.

Clinical Features

The clinical features produced by hypernatraemia involve CNS dysfunction due to intracellular dehydration. To some extent the intracellular dehydration within the brain cells is reduced by a build-up of osmotically active solutes within the cells. Marked hypernatraemia however results in a shift of water from the brain cells. This could cause petechial, intracerebral, subarachnoid or subdural bleeds, resulting in neurological deficits, and an obtunded or even comatose state.

A flow chart for the evaluation and management of a hypernatraemic patient in the ICU is shown in **Fig. 10.1.5**.

Management

Hyperosmolar states (exactly like hypo-osmolar states), need gradual correction.

Hypovolaemic hypernatraemia (the commonest form) is treated by first restoring volume by intravenous infusions, preferably of isotonic saline. It should be noted that hypovolaemia though present, is not as marked as in hyponatraemic states. This is probably because the hypertonicity within the plasma continues to draw fluid from the intracellular and interstitial tissue compartments, thereby preserving the blood volume to an extent. Once volume replacement is adequate (and this can be roughly gauged clinically), the water deficit relative to sodium is corrected. Hypotonic (eg. half-strength saline) infusions are often advocated. However as gradual correction is the aim of treatment, N saline may be more suitable when plasma Na is > 165 mEq/l. It is wise to take at least 72 hours to correct the water deficit, only about one-third of the excess of sodium concentration being reduced in the first 8 hours. Overenthusiastic infusion of hypotonic

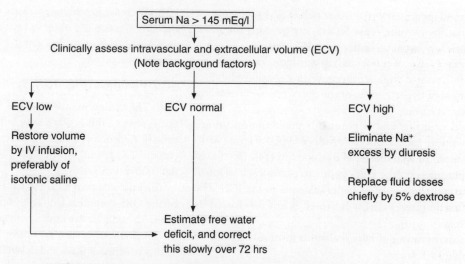

Fig. 10.1.5. Algorithm for management of hypernatraemia.

solutions can lead to a rebound cerebral oedema in place of the previous dehydration of nerve cells. Sudden shifts of water also enhance the tendency to cerebral haemorrhage. We have observed one patient who developed central pontine myelinolysis during correction of a hypernatraemic state.

It is difficult to determine the exact free water deficit in hypernatraemic patients. A method which gives a rough estimate of free water deficit and which serves as a guide to fluid replacement is illustrated below.

For example, a 70 kg man has a serum sodium of 170 mmoles/l which needs to be lowered to 140 mmoles/l. The total body water is taken as 60 per cent of the body weight, which in a 70 kg individual amounts to 42 litres. To reduce the plasma sodium, this volume needs to be increased to 170/140 × 42. This equals 51 litres, which means that a positive balance of 9 litres is required. A slow replacement with isotonic saline, or both isotonic and hypotonic saline infusions over 4 days should restore plasma osmolality safely to normal limits. Infusions to correct hypernatraemia should be monitored both clinically and by estimating the plasma electrolyte levels.

Hypervolaemic hypernatraemia is rarely encountered and is due to excessive infusion of sodium containing fluids, chiefly sodium bicarbonate. When due to infusions of sodium bicarbonate, if the bicarbonate solution contains 1 mEq sodium/ml, then the excess of sodium due to sodium bicarbonate can be calculated thus (**13**):

Sodium Excess (mEq) =
  0.6 × wt (kg) × (Patient's Serum Na −140)

The sodium excess is removed via the urine by diuresis, and the sodium concentration in the urine will give an approximate idea of the volume of urine required to be passed to eliminate the excess sodium. Thus a sodium excess of 500 mEq with a urine sodium of 100 mEq/l, would necessitate a urine output of 5 l to excrete the excess sodium.

$$\frac{\text{Volume of Urine to}}{\text{Excrete Excess Sodium}} = \frac{\text{Excess Na (mEq)}}{\text{Urinary Na (mEq/l)}}$$

Volume loss in the urine needs to be replaced mainly by 5 per cent

dextrose, else the excretion of hypotonic urine will cause a further rise in serum sodium.

Hyperosmolar Non-Ketotic Diabetic States

Hyperosmolar hypernatraemic non-ketotic diabetic coma is dealt with as a separate entity in another chapter.

Hyperkalaemia

Hyperkalaemia exists when the serum potassium (K^+) is above 5.5 mEq/l. Hyperkalemia is a dangerous, potentially fatal condition. A rise of K^+ above 7 mEq/l is life-threatening and values above 10 mEq/l are incompatible with life.

Hyperkalaemia in an ICU setting is due to:

(a) Release of K^+ from cells following injury—crush injuries, trauma, ischaemic injury due to acute severe peripheral vascular disease are all conditions causing hyperkalaemia.

(b) Uncontrolled diabetes even if associated with an overall K^+ deficit in the body, may be associated with hyperkalaemia due to shift of K^+ from the cells into the interstitial tissue and vascular compartments.

(c) Metabolic acidosis causes a shift of H^+ ions into cells, and a shift of K^+ ions out of the cells into the interstitial tissue compartment. Respiratory acidosis has little or no effect on serum K^+. Lactic acid acidosis has a lesser effect on cellular shifts in K^+ when compared to the acidosis of renal failure.

(d) Excessive K^+ intake particularly in patients with mild renal insufficiency, has in our experience produced dangerous rise in serum K^+ in critically ill patients. The routine, unchecked use of high concentrations of KCl orally in patients on a small dose of furosemide, is dangerous and reprehensible, particularly in elderly patients with impaired renal function.

(e) Hyperkalaemia is frequent when there is reduced renal excretion of K^+. This occurs in an ICU setting chiefly in patients with renal failure. Ordinarily the glomerular filtration rate should be as low as 10 ml/min, or the urine output < 1 l/24 hours for the serum K^+ to rise (**14**). Acute renal failure, acute on chronic renal failure and the ingestion of a diet rich in K⁺ by patients on haemodialysis for chronic renal failure, are perhaps the most frequent causes of hyperkalaemia in an ICU setting.

An important cause of moderately severe hyperkalaemia in an ICU setting is the use of angiotensin converting enzyme inhibitors in the treatment of hypertension, or the use of potassium-sparing diuretics like aldactone.

Interstitial nephritis and hyporenic hypoaldosteronism are comparatively rare causes, but can produce hyperkalaemia without the presence of marked renal dysfunction (14). Decreased potassium excretion via the kidneys due to adrenocortical insufficiency is also a rare cause of hyperkalaemia in the ICU. The clinical picture in these patients however, is not dominated by hyperkalaemia.

The important causes of hyperkalaemia in an ICU setting are listed in **Table 10.1.4**.

Table 10.1.4. Important causes of hyperkalaemia in an ICU setting

* Crush injuries, trauma, ischaemic injury due to acute, severe peripheral vascular disease
* Uncontrolled diabetes mellitus
* Metabolic acidosis
* Excessive potassium intake, particularly in patients with renal insufficiency, or in those on haemodialysis
* Acute renal failure, or acute on chronic renal failure
* Use of angiotensin converting enzyme inhibitors in the treatment of hypertension, or of potassium-sparing diuretics like aldactone
* Rarer causes—interstitial nephritis, hyporenic hypoaldosteronism, adrenocortical insufficiency

Clinical Features

The clinical features of hyperkalaemia are characterized by muscle weakness and conduction disturbances. Muscle weakness is associated with hypotonia, areflexia, and may proceed to flaccid quadriparesis.

Bradycardia, junctional rhythms, various degrees of heart block and hypotension are observed with increasing K⁺ levels. Death usually occurs from cardiac arrest. Electromechanical dissociation may be observed.

ECG Features (Fig. 10.1.6)

(i) The earliest manifestation of hyperkalaemia is a peaking of the T waves—this is often seen when the serum K⁺ exceeds 5.5 mEq/l. Absence of peaked T waves may be due to the fact that earlier ECG tracings (when the patient was stable), might have flat or inverted T waves.

(ii) A rise in serum K⁺ above 6 mEq/l often results in a widening of the QRS complex. Unlike a bundle branch block, all parts of the QRS complex are equally affected.

(iii) A rise of serum K⁺ above 7 mEq/l is usually associated with a widened P wave and delayed AV conduction. Occasionally this is accompanied by an elevation of the RS-T junction and a coving of the RS-T segment resembling changes seen in myocardial infarction. This is promptly corrected when the hyperkalaemia is treated by dialysis.

(iv) When the serum K⁺ is between 7.5–8 mEq/l, the P wave disappears, pointing to cessation of atrial contraction. A junctional, and later an idioventricular rhythm is observed. The QRS complex terminally resembles wide sine waves. Death occurs from ventricular fibrillation or cardiac arrest.

Diagnosis

Diagnosis depends on clinical suspicion and the recognition of clinical and ECG features of hyperkalaemia. It is confirmed by a rise in serum K⁺. A false or pseudohyperkalaemia may be observed if blood is haemolysed after collection. Excessive leucocytosis (> 750,000/mm³) and thrombocytosis (> 1 million/mm³) can also produce a hyperkalaemia due to K⁺ release from

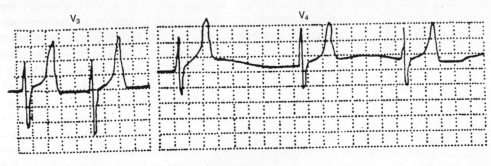

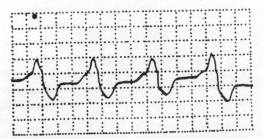

Fig. 10.1.6. ECG changes in hyperkalaemia. Note the slow idionodal rhythm with tall peaked T waves progressing to an idioventricular rhythm with marked widening of the QRS complex. Note also the absence of P waves.

clotted blood. An unclotted blood sample will give the true serum K$^+$ value. As with all laboratory investigations, a rise in serum K$^+$ should be correlated with the clinical picture; when in doubt, it is best to repeat the test.

Management

Hyperkalaemia should be treated on an emergency footing; it is even more dangerous than hypokalaemia. Therapy is always indicated when serum K$^+$ is > 6 mEq/l, even in the absence of ECG changes, as death can occur in these patients (15). The following methods are used to reduce the serum K$^+$ levels:

(i) *Intravenous calcium gluconate* is the emergency drug of choice when serum K$^+$ levels are > 7 mEq/l, or if there is evidence of wide QRS complexes, AV block or absent P waves on an ECG. 10–20 ml of 10 per cent calcium gluconate is given as a bolus over 3–5 minutes, and can be repeated after 5–10 minutes if the ECG remains unchanged after the first injection. Calcium directly antagonizes the effect of K$^+$ by increasing the membrane threshold, improving conduction, and increasing the force of myocardial contraction. Its effect is temporary and lasts for about 30 minutes. Other measures therefore need to be taken after this emergency treatment has been given. Intravenous calcium can produce cardiotoxicity in patients on digitalis—if administered to fully digitalized patients, it is diluted in 100 ml N saline, and given over 30 minutes. Patients with severe hypotension, and those showing an idioventricular rhythm with very wide QRS complexes, may fail to respond to intravenous calcium. Emergency transvenous pacing should then be tried; this may help to buy time for drugs to act.

(ii) *An insulin-dextrose infusion* will cause a quick shift of K$^+$ from the vascular and interstitial tissue compartments into the cells. 500 ml of 20 per cent dextrose to which is added 20 units of actrapid insulin, is given as an infusion over one hour. Hypoglycaemia should be watched out for, and if present should be corrected by supplemental glucose. An insulin-glucose infusion can be expected to reduce serum K$^+$ by 1–2 mEq, and can be repeated after a few hours.

(iii) *An intravenous infusion of sodium bicarbonate* (50–75 ml of a 7.5 per cent solution), given over 10 minutes. Bicarbonate acts by *shifting K$^+$ from the extracellular to the cellular compartment*. In our opinion it is a useful drug, though it may not always be very effective (16). Repeated use of intravenous bicarbonate can however aggravate intracellular acidosis and lactic acid production. Intracellular acidosis can result from increased CO_2 production following the use of intravenous bicarbonate. The CO_2 diffuses into the cells and combines with H_2O to form H_2CO_3. A significant increase in H_2CO_3 within the cells may be incompletely buffered, resulting in intracellular acidosis. Bicarbonate can also bind calcium, so if calcium gluconate has already been used, intravenous bicarbonate should be given at least 30–60 minutes later. Though some workers hesitate to use bicarbonate because of its possible side effects, we routinely use it to treat hyperkalaemia, with satisfactory results.

(iv) *Intravenous furosemide* in a dose of 40–100 mg should be used to promote excretion of K$^+$ via the urine. This method of course is of no use in patients with renal failure.

(v) *The use of sodium polystyrene sulfonate resin (Kayexalate)* can cause potassium to be excreted in large quantities via the gut. Polystyrene sulphonate is a cation exchange resin which binds K$^+$. However for each mEq of K$^+$ removed, 2–3 mEq of Na$^+$ are retained. A sodium overload can therefore occur with frequent use, particularly in the presence of cardiac or renal insufficiency. It can be given orally or as a retention enema. The oral dose of Kayexalate is 30 g in 50 ml of 20 per cent sorbitol. The rectal dose is 50 g in 200 ml as a retention enema.

(vi) *Dialysis* is the most effective method of reducing serum K$^+$ when other methods fail, particularly so in the presence of renal failure. Haemodialysis is preferred as it is quicker; however, peritoneal dialysis though slower, can also serve the same purpose.

Hypokalaemia

The serum potassium is normally maintained between 4–5 mEq/l. A fall in serum K$^+$ to below 3.5 mEq/l is termed hypokalaemia. A serum K$^+$ level below 2.5 mEq/l is fraught with danger to life. It is being increasingly realized that severe hypokalaemia is an important cause of death in critically ill individuals. This danger often goes unrecognized with disastrous consequences.

It has already been emphasized that the major quantity of K$^+$ within the body is in the intracellular compartment. The total quantity of K$^+$ in the body is roughly 50 mEq/kg body weight—i.e. 3500 mEq in a 70 kg adult. Of this, less than 2 per cent, i.e. less than 70 mEq is within the extracellular compartment (15, 17). The large gradient of K$^+$ between the intra- and extracellular compartments is due to the activity of the sodium-potassium membrane pump, which actively keeps the potassium within the cellular compartment. Transfer of K$^+$ from the intracellular to the extracellular compartment (including the vascular compartment) and vice versa, occurs frequently in various disease processes. The reasons or mechanisms underlying these shifts are not always clearly understood. It is obvious therefore that the serum K$^+$ does not necessarily reflect changes in total body K$^+$. In fact, the latter may well be significantly depleted with a normal serum K$^+$. This is evident if the patient has lost water and K$^+$ in the same concentration as in plasma. Even if the loss of K$^+$ exceeds that of water, serum K$^+$ may be normal in spite of significant body deficit because of shift of K$^+$ from the cells to the extracellular compartment. Similarly, a raised serum K$^+$ may occasionally exist with normal or even depleted body stores of K$^+$. This is illustrated in diabetic ketoacidosis where the serum K$^+$ can be high even though the total body K$^+$ is depleted. When diabetic acidosis is corrected, potassium from the plasma and the extracellular compartment moves into the cells, and the body deficit of potassium is now correctly represented by a low serum K$^+$ concentration.

However, a low serum K$^+$ invariably indicates depletion of K$^+$ in the body—in fact, a decrease in serum K$^+$ is a late finding in K$^+$ depletion. Thus even a slight decrease in serum K$^+$ is of import and needs to be corrected.

The aetiology of hypokalaemia in an ICU setting is due to either loss of K$^+$ from the body, or a poor intake of K$^+$, so that a state of negative balance exists, or is due to shifts of K$^+$ from the extracellular and vascular compartments into the cells.

(i) Loss of K⁺

This is generally due to vomiting, nasogastric suction, pancreatic or intestinal fistulae, intestinal obstruction and burns.

Loss of K^+ can also occur through the urine—the commonest cause being diuretic therapy in which adequate K^+ replacement has not been taken care of. The urinary K^+ loss in these patients is > 30 mEq/l. Another important cause of increased urinary loss of K^+ with resulting hypokalaemia, is the use of corticosteroids; the larger the dose used, the greater the K^+ loss.

(ii) Transcellular Shifts

The most important cause of hypokalaemia due to shifts of K^+ from the extracellular compartment into the cells, is metabolic alkalosis. In this condition, homeostasis induces shift of the H^+ ion from the cells to the plasma to restore pH to normalcy; in exchange, K^+ shifts from the vascular and interstitial tissue compartments into the cells. Beta-2 agonists when given systemically in severe asthma, particularly when combined with theophylline, can induce a modest fall in serum K^+ through transcellular shifts of K^+.

Diagnosis

The clinical diagnosis rests on the following factors:

(i) A high index of suspicion of hypokalaemia in any critically ill individual where the clinical background suggests a potassium deficit.

(ii) Recognition of clinical features of hypokalaemia. At times these are obvious and easily discernible, but unfortunately sometimes they are difficult to detect particularly in critically ill or in obtunded patients.

(iii) Electrocardiographic features suggestive of hypokalaemia. In the final analysis hypokalaemia can be confirmed only by the estimation of serum K^+ by a flame photometer. It would be a truism to state that every critically ill individual under intensive care will need a serum K^+ estimation to determine the presence or otherwise of changes in this electrolyte.

Hypokalaemia produces a disturbance in neuromuscular, muscular, and cardiac function. At times, only cardiac dysfunction is observed; at other times the clinical features are dominated by neuromuscular or muscular dysfunction. Occasionally, both neuromuscular and cardiac dysfunction may be observed. Long-standing K^+ deficits with hypokalaemia can also produce a nephropathy characterized chiefly by inability to concentrate the urine. This feature however, is hardly ever observed in patients under critical care.

Cardiac Dysfunction

This is the most dreaded feature of severe hypokalaemia. The most important effect of hypokalaemia on the heart is the propensity to cardiac arrhythmias. The commonest and earliest abnormalities are ventricular ectopic beats. In ill individuals, the occurrence of such ectopics against a background of a possible potassium deficit should always lead one to suspect hypokalaemia. The premature ventricular ectopics may lead to paroxysmal ventricular tachycardia, ventricular fibrillation and sudden death. Paroxysmal ventricular tachycardia may also occur without warning ectopics. In fact, sudden death due to ventricular fibrillation may be the sole catastrophic manifestation of a hypokalaemic state.

Many arrhythmias observed during digitalis administration are triggered or worsened by hypokalaemia resulting from the associated use of diuretics. Paroxysmal atrial tachycardia with block and interference dissociation are two important rhythm disturbances most frequently observed under the above circumstances. The occurrence of these arrhythmias in a patient on digitalis and diuretics should promptly point to underlying hypokalaemia.

Marked hypokalaemia can also induce hypotension, which is due to a lowered cardiac output and perhaps to poor sympathetic tone related to poor functioning of sympathetic nerve endings.

Neuromuscular and Muscular Dysfunction

Asthenia and apathy are often the earliest symptoms. Whenever the degree of asthenia is more than what is expected in a particular illness, the possibility of hypokalaemia should be entertained. The tendon reflexes are sluggish and may be totally absent. Muscle weakness may progress to flaccid paralysis. In severe hypokalaemia, the muscles of respiration are involved so that the patient hypoventilates; rarely, the muscles of deglutition may also be affected.

Abdominal distension due to mild ileus and urinary retention are at times the sole presenting features of hypokalaemia. In severe cases, a complete paralytic ileus with fluid levels seen on an abdominal X-ray results, closely mimicking an acute abdomen. Following major surgery, hypokalaemia is an important cause of delay in return of peristalsis.

ECG Features

In our experience, ECG changes may be occasionally observed even with a normal serum K^+ when total body K^+ is markedly depleted. ECG changes frequently (but not necessarily always) appear when the serum K^+ is < 2.5 mEq/l. The following ECG changes may be observed: (i) Flattening of T waves with ST depression of > 0.5 mm; (ii) Prominent U waves, frequently best observed in the precordial leads; (iii) Occurrence of various arrhythmias as noted earlier.

It is important to realize that ECG changes are non-specific and unreliable—their absence in no way negates the suspicion of hypokalaemia aroused on clinical grounds.

Management

This consists in replacement of K^+ to restore serum potassium levels within the normal range. Whenever possible, it is best to give KCl orally, 1 g thrice daily. Some patients vomit with oral medication, and an important, dangerous side effect following the use of oral potassium tablets, is the occurrence of acute duodenal ulceration with haemorrhage and perforation.

If the serum K^+ is < 3 mEq/l, and certainly if < 2.5 mEq/l, the intravenous route of administering potassium is to be preferred. Attempts have been made to formulate the K^+ deficit depending on the levels of serum K^+ in plasma. Stanaszek and Romankiewicz (**18**) are of the opinion that each 1 mEq/l decrease in serum K^+

from 4 to 2 mEq/l represents a 10 per cent decrease in total body potassium. This does not apply to serum K⁺ levels < 2 mEq/l, as the relationship between serum and total body potassium is no longer linear in this range (**15**). The estimated potassium deficit for a 70 kg adult vis-à-vis the serum K⁺ levels is as follows: for a s. K⁺ of 3.0 mEq/dl, the K⁺ deficit is 350 mEq constituting about 10 per cent of total K⁺; for a s. K⁺ of 2.5 mEq/dl, the K⁺ deficit is 470 mEq or about 15 per cent of the total K⁺; for a s. K⁺ of 2.0 mEq/dl, the K⁺ deficit is 700 mEq or about 20 per cent of the body K⁺. These estimates are based on a total body potassium of 50 mEq/kg lean body weight (**19**), but to my mind, can never even be reasonably accurate. The purpose of the exercise is to stress in general the magnitude and importance of the problem, and to emphasize the urgency in restoring K⁺ deficit.

Ordinarily with a K⁺ level of 2.5 mEq/l or less, or if muscle weakness, arrhythmias, or cardiac dysfunction are present, we prefer to give 80–120 mEq of KCl in a dextrose infusion over 24 hours. Replacement is of course adjusted by frequent monitoring of serum K⁺ levels. We find this method to be safe and effective. Occasionally large quantities need to be given at more rapid rates to restore low K⁺ levels in the presence of ongoing potassium loss.

The recommended dose for a quicker restoration of serum K⁺ levels is 0.7 mEq/kg lean body weight of KCl in a dextrose infusion given over 2 hours (**15**). This dose should not increase the K⁺ by more than 1–1.5 mEq/l, unless there is metabolic acidosis or renal impairment.

When hypokalaemia is below 2 mEq/l, or in the presence of multiple ventricular ectopics or ventricular tachycardia, 60–80 mEq of KCl in a dextrose infusion can be given over 2 hours under carefully monitored conditions.

Certain important features should be kept in mind regarding the intravenous administration of KCl.

(i) Intravenous potassium should not be administered, or administered very slowly and with great care, in patients with renal insufficiency or metabolic acidosis.

(ii) Intravenous potassium should not be given through a central vein in high concentrations or at a rate exceeding 40 mEq in 2 hours, as it can result in dangerous, life-threatening cardiac toxicity. When infusing high doses, the use of two separate peripheral veins minimizes the risk of thrombophlebitis, and reduces the pain experienced due to chemical irritation of the venous wall.

(iii) Magnesium depletion promotes potassium loss in the urine and impairs movement of K⁺ from the cellular into the vascular compartment. The reason for this is not clear. From the practical point of view, if serum K⁺ levels are difficult to raise, then the possibility of magnesium depletion should be entertained, and the magnesium deficit should be corrected. This generally allows for a quick restoration of serum K⁺ levels to the normal range.

Calcium and Phosphorus

The description of disturbances in calcium and phosphorus balance given below is chiefly with reference to critically ill patients under intensive care. Almost always, changes in serum calcium or phosphorus in an ICU setting, serve as markers of the severity of the illness, and do not in themselves pose major clinical problems nor do they present difficulties in management.

The normal 'total' serum calcium is 8.5 to 10.2 mg/dl. About 50 per cent of this calcium is bound to serum proteins, chiefly to albumin. An additional 5–10 per cent is in combination with anions like bicarbonate, and the remaining is in the free or ionised form. The ionized form is the physiologically active component of calcium, and measures 4.8–7 mg/dl. It is to be noted that laboratory tests indicate the total serum calcium levels, and not the active ionized calcium level. The total serum calcium level does not always reflect the level of ionized calcium. Thus a decrease in serum proteins, and in particular of serum albumin, leads to a decrease in the protein-bound fraction and in the total calcium, even though the ionized calcium remains unchanged. A hypocalcaemia may be wrongly diagnosed under these circumstances. In hypoalbuminaemic states, a correction factor that increases the total calcium by 0.75 mg/dl for each 1 g/dl decrease in serum albumin below 3.5 g/dl, gives a more correct picture of serum calcium levels (**20**). Ion specific electrodes can however directly measure ionic calcium, allowing a very accurate quantification of the physiologically active calcium in the serum (**20**). Unfortunately, only few reference laboratories can measure ionic calcium levels in the blood.

In an ICU setting, the most common causes of lowered serum calcium levels are related to hypoalbuminaemia. If these are excluded, then low serum calcium levels (i.e. low ionized calcium levels) are invariably related to the following causes:

(i) *Alkalosis*. An increase in the pH promotes binding of calcium to albumin (even though albumin levels are unchanged), and reduces ionic serum calcium; the total serum calcium however remains unchanged. Both metabolic and respiratory alkalosis can produce a fall in ionic serum calcium.

(ii) *Sepsis*. Hypocalcaemia is observed at times in sepsis. This could be due to a respiratory alkalosis produced by increased ventilation commonly observed in these patients, as also due to efflux of calcium across a disrupted, damaged microcirculation (**21**).

(iii) *Hypomagnesaemia*. Depletion of magnesium inhibits parathormone secretion and reduces the response of the end organ to parathormone, resulting in hypocalcaemia. Hypocalcaemia due to magnesium depletion is difficult to correct, as the infused calcium is excreted via the urine due to diminished action of the parathyroid hormone. Once the magnesium deficiency is corrected, serum calcium is quickly restored to normal. In the presence of normal renal function and in the absence of hypoalbuminaemia, sepsis or alkalosis, a persistently low serum calcium in an ICU setting should always suggest the strong possibility of an associated magnesium deficiency. The combined presence of hypokalaemia in the above situation strengthens the diagnosis of hypomagnesaemia even if the serum Mg⁺⁺ levels are normal.

(iv) *Renal Failure*. The serum calcium in renal failure may be normal, low, or increased depending on the nature of metabolic abnormality induced in a given patient (**22**).

(v) *Pancreatitis*. A low serum calcium is invariably present in severe pancreatitis, and it serves as a marker for the severity and prognosis of the disease.

Other causes of hypocalcaemia in an ICU setting include burns, massive blood transfusions, following cardiopulmonary bypass and in fat embolism. In massive blood transfusions the citrate preservative in banked blood binds calcium, whilst in fat embolism the circulating free fatty acids bind calcium causing hypocalcaemia.

The common causes of hypocalcaemia are given in **Table 10.1.5.**

Table 10.1.5. Common causes of hypocalcaemia in an ICU setting

* Related to hypoalbuminaemia (commonest cause)
* Metabolic or respiratory alkalosis
* Sepsis
* Hypomagnesaemia
* Renal failure
* Pancreatitis
* Other causes—burns, massive blood transfusions, following cardiopulmonary bypass, and in fat embolism

Clinical Features

Hypocalcaemia can cause tetany (carpopedal spasm), and neuromuscular excitability which in severe cases can manifest with seizures.

Hypotension, vasodilatation, and a prolonged QT interval are also observed in severe hypocalcaemia.

In an ICU setting, clinical features resulting from hypocalcaemia are rarely observed. The hypocalcaemia in critically ill patients as already mentioned, often draws attention to the nature and severity of the underlying illness, and at times is of prognostic value.

Management

Mild asymptomatic hypocalcaemia requires no specific treatment. Well-marked hypocalcaemia and symptomatic hypocalcaemia are treated with intravenous calcium gluconate, 10 ml being given very slowly over 10 minutes and repeated if necessary. A maintenance drip of 10 ml calcium gluconate in 100–200 ml 5 per cent dextrose saline given over 2–3 hours can then be administered.

Hypercalcaemia

Hypercalcaemia is a dangerous metabolic disturbance; serum calcium levels > 14 mg per cent can cause death if not promptly recognized and treated. There are many causes of hypercalcaemia, the important ones being listed in **Table 10.1.6.**

The two most frequent causes we have encountered in the

Table 10.1.6. Important causes of hypercalcaemia

* Primary hyperparathyroidism
* Metastatic carcinoma
* Sarcoidosis
* Myelomatosis
* Vitamin D intoxication
* Milk-alkali syndrome
* Ectopic parathyroid hormone producing tumours
* Hyperthyroidism
* Adrenal insufficiency
* Dysproteinaemia
* Myxoedema
* Osteoporosis following prolonged immobilization

ICU are hypercalcaemia due to hyperparathyroidism, and that secondary to malignant disease.

The clinical features of hypercalcaemia are varied, often misleading the physician with a wrong diagnosis. Drowsiness and mental apathy may simulate a stroke. Changes in mental state may lead to a wrong diagnosis of depression. Ileus, urinary retention, excessive muscular weakness and increasing renal failure are some of the other manifestations of an underlying hypercalcaemia.

Management

Hypercalcaemia > 13 mg/dl or hypercalcaemia associated with symptoms needs prompt treatment.

(i) *Volume Load + Furosemide.* Hypercalcaemia leads to increased excretion of calcium in the urine, with a resulting osmotic diuresis. Hypovolaemia with marked haemoconcentration of the blood results. Multiple infusions of normal saline to increase the circulating volume produce a natriuresis which in itself promotes excretion of calcium, and results in lowering of serum calcium levels (**23, 24**). It is preferable to combine a volume load (N saline infusion) with intravenous furosemide 40–60 mg given every 2–4 hours. The volume lost in the urine should be promptly replaced with N saline so that the 'intake' matches the 'output'. The strategy is to aim at a larger output of urine, and yet replace it with an equivalent large 'input' of N saline. Potassium replacements will also be necessary as diuresis progresses. Care must be taken to ensure that elderly patients or those with poor left ventricular function are not overhydrated, and pushed into pulmonary oedema.

(ii) *Calcitonin.* This drug can reduce serum calcium by inhibiting bone resorption. Salmon calcitonin is rapid acting but expensive; it can effectively reduce the serum calcium within 2–3 hours (**25**). It is administered subcutaneously or intramuscularly in a dose of 4 mg/kg every 12 hours for 2 doses. The dose can be doubled if the desired effect on serum calcium is not obtained within 2 days.

(iii) *Mithramycin.* This is an antimitotic drug which reduces serum calcium by inhibiting bone resorption. It is slower acting (24–36 hours to act) than calcitonin; the latter is therefore preferred for emergency use. It is given in a dose of 25 μg/kg preferably in an infusion over 6 hours, and can be repeated after 2–3 days (**25**). The risk of bone marrow depression is small as the dose used is less than that used in neoplastic diseases.

Calcitonin and mithramycin are often unavailable in developing countries.

(iv) *Dialysis.* Haemodialysis in particular, can effectively and quickly reduce serum calcium levels. It should be tried if other methods are ineffective. If saline diuresis is not possible as in patients with renal failure, haemodialysis is the only effective therapy for severe hypercalcaemia.

Phosphorus

The normal serum phosphate level is between 3–4.5 mg/dl. There is a slight diurnal variation in serum phosphate levels, the latter being lower in the mornings and higher at night (**26**). Phosphorus is chiefly an intracellular ion and less than 1 per cent is located in the extracellular fluid compartment (**26**).

Hypophosphataemia is uncommonly met with in patients

under critical care, or for that matter even in patients admitted to the general wards of a hospital (**27**).

King et al. (**27**) noted the following important causes of severe hypophosphataemia in a hospital population (**Table 10.1.7**):

(i) *Dextrose Infusions*. This is probably the most important cause of hypophosphataemia (**26–29**). Phosphate levels were observed to fall within a few hours of intravenous dextrose infusions particularly in alcoholics and debilitated patients. Increasingly low phosphate levels were also observed by the tenth day of starting total parenteral nutrition (**30**). Hypophosphataemia associated with dextrose infusions is related to transport of glucose and phosphorus into the liver and skeletal muscle through insulin action. The phosphorus within the cells is used as a co-factor for glycolysis. In adequately nourished patients infusions of intravenous dextrose do not affect phosphate levels, but in malnourished individuals, a sharp fall in the phosphate levels to < 0.5 mg/dl may occur within a few days.

(ii) *Nutritional Recovery Syndrome* (**27**). Overzealous feeding, in particular with a high carbohydrate intake in malnourished patients results in an illness characterized by lethargy, weakness, diarrhoea and multiple electrolyte abnormalities which include a low phosphate level. Death can also result. This is the reason why feeds should be gradually increased in malnourished or very ill individuals.

(iii) *Use of Aluminum Hydroxide as an Antacid*. Aluminium hydroxide when used as an antacid binds phosphate in the bowel and produces phosphate depletion. Aludrox and Digene are the two commonest antacids used in India, and unfortunately most critically ill patients seem to be receiving these drugs.

(iv) *Sepsis*. Hypophosphataemia has been reported in sepsis (**28**), and can occur early in the natural history of sepsis. The mechanism leading to hypophosphataemia in sepsis is however unknown (**31**).

(v) *Diabetic Ketoacidosis*. Glycosuria in diabetic ketoacidosis produces a loss of phosphate in the urine leading to a depletion in the phosphorus content of the body. The serum phosphate level however may be normal because of the transfer of phosphates from the intracellular compartment to the extracellular one. During therapy with insulin the phosphate from the vascular and interstitial tissue compartment returns into the cells and a marked fall in plasma phosphate levels is observed. Nevertheless, specific replacement of phosphorus does not seem to improve the outcome of diabetic ketoacidosis (**32**).

(vi) *Respiratory Alkalosis*. This is an important cause of hypophosphataemia (**26**). The increase of pH within the cells promotes glycosis and this induces the influx of phosphorus into the cellular compartment. Hypophosphataemia can thus occur in patients who are being overventilated whilst on ventilator support.

Table 10.1.7. Common causes of hypophosphataemia

* Dextrose infusions
* Nutritional recovery syndrome
* Use of aluminum hydroxide as antacid
* Sepsis
* Diabetic ketoacidosis
* Respiratory alkalosis

Clinical Features

Even well-marked hypophosphataemia is often silent (**27**). Low phosphate levels are associated with depleted stores of 2,3-diphosphoglycerate within the red blood cells, causing a leftward shift of the oxyhaemoglobin dissociation curve (**26**). As a consequence, oxygen bound to haemoglobin is less easily released to tissues.

Very low phosphate levels have been rarely reported to cause haemolysis (**27**). Hypophosphataemia reduces cardiac contractility and when severe and chronic, has been reported to cause cardiomyopathy (**29**).

The only convincing clinical feature of hypophosphataemia in my opinion, is the occurrence of proximal muscle weakness resembling a myopathy. We observed it in a patient who was taking excessive doses of aluminum hydroxide. The muscle weakness was associated with very low phosphate levels. Complete recovery ensued on stopping the antacid and on increasing the oral phosphate intake.

Management

Phosphate levels < 1 mg/dl require intravenous replacement even when no obvious clinical disorder is evident. The recommended solution for use contains sodium phosphate (3 mM phosphorus per ml), potassium phosphate (3 mM phosphorus per ml), and neutral sodium phosphate (0.09 mM phosphorus per ml). When the serum phosphate level is < 0.5 mg/dl, the dose recommended is 0.5 mM/kg over 4 hours. When the serum phosphate level is between 0.5–1 mg/dl, the dose recommended is 0.2 mM/kg over 4 hours (**33, 34**). Rapid infusion has been known to produce hypotension (**34**). Hypophosphataemia is often associated with hypokalaemia, hypocalcaemia and hypomagnesaemia. These electrolytes should be monitored, and if necessary, also replaced.

Hyperphosphataemia

Hyperphosphataemia is chiefly observed in renal failure when the glomerular filtration rate drops below 25 ml/minute (**26**). Widespread cellular necrosis as in patients with tumour lysis or rhabdomyolysis, is also associated with hyperphosphataemia due to release of phosphate from damaged or destroyed cells. Diabetic ketoacidosis may be associated with a rise in serum phosphate even though body phosphates are depleted.

Management of hyperphosphataemia is directed towards the underlying cause. Aluminum hydroxide orally is often used in chronic renal failure to bind phosphates within the gut and thereby reduce the degree of hyperphosphataemia.

The Magnesium Ion

Increasing attention has been given to this ion in the last 10 years. Magnesium (Mg^{++}) has a significant presence (second only to K^+) as an intracellular cation (**35**). It is an essential co-factor in enzymatic reactions involving adenosine triphosphate, and as part of the membrane pump it helps to maintain electrical excitability in nerves and muscles (**35**). The recommended daily intake of magnesium is 6–10 mg/kg/day (**36**) and the normal serum magnesium concentration is 1.5–2 mEq/l.

How important is the ion in critical care medicine? The difficulty in answering this query in critically ill patients stems from the fact that the magnesium ion is not uniformly distributed in body fluids. Only 0.3 per cent of the body magnesium is in the serum and as much as 50 per cent is within the bones (**35**). The magnesium distribution in adults is shown below in **Table 10.1.8**. Hence changes (in particular deficiencies) in body magnesium are unlikely to be reflected in the serum Mg^{++} levels, which can be normal in both Mg^{++} deficiency or excess (**36**). How then does one authenticate clinical features attributable to magnesium deficiency? And how does one gauge the true prevalence of Mg^{++} insufficiency in critically ill patients? There are a number of specialists in critical care medicine who feel that magnesium depletion is very frequent in an ICU population chiefly due to the lack of daily supplements, and the frequent use of diuretics in these patients.

Table 10.1.8. Magnesium distribution in adults

Tissue	Content (mmoles)	Total Body Mg (%)
Serum	2.6	0.3
RBCs	5	0.5
Soft Tissue	193	19.3
Muscle	270	27.0
Bone	530	53.0

From Elin RJ. Magnesium Metabolism in Health and Disease. Disease-A-Month, 1988. 34, 173, Elsevier.

The important causes of Mg^{++} deficiency include (**37**):

(i) Diuretics, in particular furosemide, which blocks reabsorption of Mg^{++} through the loop of Henle, causing an increased excretion of Mg^{++} in the urine (**38**).

(ii) Alcoholism which induces magnesium depletion chiefly through increased excretion of the ion in the urine. Magnesium deficiency may become manifest soon after ethanol withdrawal (**35**).

(iii) Diarrhoea which causes loss of the ion, as secretions within the lower GI tract are rich in Mg^{++}.

(iv) Aminoglycosides which act by reducing reabsorption of Mg^{++} in the renal tubules.

(v) Reduced intake in critically ill individuals in the presence of abnormal losses of this ion.

Clinical Features

The clinical diagnosis of Mg^{++} deficiency, to my mind, leaves much to be desired. Colleagues interested in this field diagnose Mg^{++} deficiency even with normal levels of serum Mg^{++}. The clinical situations suggestive of Mg^{++} deficiency include:

(i) Presence of other electrolyte abnormalities—in particular hypokalaemia, hyponatraemia, hypocalcaemia and hypophosphataemia (**39**). Of all these, the association between hypokalaemia and hypomagnesaemia is now fairly well established. Refractory hypokalaemia, at least in some patients, may be due to an associated hypomagnesaemia. Repletion of Mg^{++} in such patients leads to a rapid correction of the K^+ deficit (**35, 39, 40**).

(ii) Intractable arrhythmias have been dubiously ascribed to Mg^{++} deficiency. It is true that intravenous magnesium is occasionally an effective antiarrhythmic agent when other antiarrhythmic drugs have failed (**41**). But this could well be related to the specific antiarrhythmic effect of the ion, rather than to a true deficiency.

(iii) Arrhythmias in myocardial infarction—magnesium infusions have been reported to reduce the incidence of arrhythmias in acute myocardial infarction (**42–44**) and hypomagnesaemia can enhance calcium entry into vascular smooth muscle of the coronaries, and initiate vascular spasm (**41, 44**). The role of hypomagnesaemia in relation to the clinical aspect described above, in my opinion, remains debatable.

(iv) Muscle weakness has been occasionally reported with hypomagnesaemia (**46**), but here again the evidence is unconvincing. Neuromuscular excitability with a positive Chvostek's or Trousseau's sign has also been reported. Seizures have also been noted to be a feature of severe hypomagnesaemia (**37**).

In our opinion, the clinical features of import with reference to hypomagnesaemia, are the presence of hypokalaemia and cardiac arrhythmias in a setting where Mg^{++} loss through the urine or the gut, is likely to be increased.

Magnesium Replacement

In patients with symptomatic Mg^{++} depletion and normal renal function, magnesium sulphate is given at the rate of 1 mEq/kg for the first 24 hours, and then at 0.5 mEq/kg for the next 3 days (**47**). Magnesium sulphate is available as a 10 per cent or a 50 per cent solution. 5 ml of the 10 per cent or 1 ml of the 50 per cent solution will provide 4 mEq of elemental magnesium. The 50 per cent solution must be diluted before use.

In the presence of life-threatening hypomagnesaemia causing cardiac arrhythmias or seizures, 4 ml of a 50 per cent solution of magnesium sulphate is infused over 2 minutes. This is followed by 10 ml of 50 per cent magnesium sulphate in 500 ml of N saline over the next 6 hours. 12 hourly infusions of 10 ml of 50 per cent magnesium sulphate are then recommended for the next 5 days.

Magnesium administration should always be monitored by serum magnesium levels (**42**). Great care needs to be taken in administering magnesium intravenously in patients with renal insufficiency (**35, 47**). The dose stated above is preferably halved, and given over double the time.

Hypermagnesaemia

Hypermagnesaemia generally occurs in patients with chronic renal failure who are administered magnesium-containing antacids orally over prolonged periods of time (**37**). Diabetic ketoacidosis complicating renal failure induces magnesium transport from the intracellular to the extracellular compartment, and can raise serum Mg^{++} levels.

The most important clinical feature of hypermagnesaemia is hypotension which is observed when Mg^{++} levels exceed 3–5 mEq/l. The hypotension does not respond to the usual measures. Complete heart block is observed with serum Mg^{++} levels of 7.5

mEq/l; respiratory depression and mental obtundation progressing to coma occur with serum Mg^{++} levels of 10 mEq/l (**37**).

Treatment

Magnesium levels can be lowered and magnesium induced hypotension best countered by administering 20 ml of 10 per cent calcium gluconate intravenously. Magnesium excretion in the urine can be induced by the use of intravenous furosemide. If renal function permits, a volume load should precede the use of furosemide. Haemodialysis can effectively lower elevated serum magnesium levels, and is the treatment of choice in patients with severe renal failure.

REFERENCES

1. Shoemaker WC. (1989). Fluids and Electrolytes in the Acutely Ill Adult: Pansystemic Illness. In: Textbook of Critical Care, 2nd edn (Eds Shoemaker WC, Ayres S, Grenvik A, Holbrook PR, Leigh Thompson W). pp. 1128–1152. WB Saunders Company, Philadelphia, London, Tokyo.

2. Hammes M, Brennan S, Lederer ED. (1998). Severe electrolyte disturbances. In: Principles of Critical Care (Eds Hall JB, Schmidt GA, Wood LDH). pp. 1153–68. McGraw-Hill Inc., New York, London, Toronto.

3. Tom Shires G, Canizaro PC, Tom Shires G III et al. (1989). Fluid, Electrolyte, and Nutritional Management of the Surgical Patient. In: Principles of Surgery, 5th edn (Eds Schwartz SI, Tom Shires G, Spencer FC). pp. 69–103. McGraw-Hill Book Company, New York, London, Toronto.

4. Geheb M. (1987). Clinical approach to the hyperosmolar patient. Crit Care Clin. 5, 797–815.

5. Sterns RH. (2003). Fluid, Electrolyte, and Acid-Base Disturbances. J Am Soc Nephrol. 2(1): 1–33.

6. Wilson WC. (2001). Clinical approach to acid-base analysis: Importance of the anion gap. Anesthesiology Clinics of North America. 19(4): 907–912.

7. Lee CT. (2000). Hyponatraemia in the emergency department. Am J Emerg Med. 18(3): 264–8.

8. Anderson RJ, Chung HM, Klug R et al. (1985). Hyponatremia: A prospective analysis of its epidemiology and the pathogenic role of vasopressin. Ann Intern Med. 102, 164–168.

9. Chung HM, Klug R, Schrier RW et al. (1985). Post-operative hyponatremia. A prospective study. Arch. Intern Med. 146, 333–336.

10. Ayus JC, Krothapalli RK, Arieff AI. (1985). Changing concepts in treatment of severe symptomatic hyponatremia. Am J Med. 78, 897–902.

11. Arieff AI. (1988). Osmotic failure: Physiology and strategies for treatment. Hosp Pract. 22, 131–152.

12. Dubois GD, Arieff AI. (1984). Symptomatic hyponatremia: The case for rapid correction. In: Controversies in Nephrology and Hypertension (Ed. Narins RG). pp. 393–407. Churchill-Livingstone, New York.

13. Marino PL. (1998). Hypertonic and Hypotonic Syndromes—Fluid and Electrolyte Disorders. In: The ICU Book. pp. 631–646. Williams and Wilkins, USA.

14. Williams ME, Rosa RM. (1988). Hyperkalemia: Disorder of internal and external balance. J Intensive Care Med. 3, 52–64.

15. Smith JD, Bia MJ, DeFronzo RA. (1985). Clinical disorders of potassium metabolism. In: Fluid, Electrolyte and Acid-Base Disorders (Eds Arieff AI, DeFronzo RA). pp. 413–509. Churchill-Livingstone, New York.

16. Blumberg A, Weidmann P, Shaw S et al. (1988). Effect of various therapeutic approaches on plasma potassium and major regulating factors in terminal renal failure. Am J Med. 85, 507–512.

17. Brown RS. (1986). External potassium homeostasis. Kidney Int. 30, 116–127.

18. Stanaszek WF, Romankiewicz JA. (1985). Current approaches to management of potassium deficiency. Drug Intell Clin Pharm. 19, 176–184.

19. Rimmer JM, Horn JF, Gennari FJ. (1987). Hyperkalemia as a complication of drug therapy. Arch Intern Med. 147, 867–869.

20. Kassirer JP, Hricik DE, Cohen JJ. (1989). Repairing body fluids. pp. 73–99. WB Saunders, Philadelphia.

21. Zaloga GP, Chernow B. (1987). The multifactorial basis for hypocalcemia during sepsis. Studies of the parathyroid hormone—Vitamin D axis. Ann Intern Med. 107, 36–41.

22. Nowbar S, Anderson RJ. (2003). Acute Renal Failure. In: Current Therapy in Critical Care Medicine (Eds Parrillo JE, Dellinger RP). pp. 1133–1157. Mosby, USA.

23. Baker JR, Wray HL. (1982). Early management of hypercalcemia crisis: case report and literature review. Milit Med. 147, 756–760.

24. Hosking DJ, Cowley A, Bucknall CA. (1981). Rehydration in the treatment of severe hypercalcemia. QJ Med. 22, 473–481.

25. Roswell RH. (1987). Severe hypercalcemia: causes & specific therapy. J Crit Illness. 2, 14–21.

26. Yu GC, Lee DB. (1987). Clinical disorders of phosphorus metabolism. West J Med. 147, 564–576.

27. King AL, Sica DA, Miller G et al. (1987). Severe hypophosphatemia in a general hospital population. South Med J. 80, 831–835.

28. Halevy J, Bulvik S. (1988). Severe hypophosphatemia in hospitalised patients. Arch Intern Med. 148, 153–155.

29. Janson C, Birnbaum , Baker FJ. (1983). Hypophosphatemia. Ann Emerg Med. 12, 107–116.

30. Knochel JP. (1977). The pathophysiological and clinical characteristics of severe hypophosphatemia. Arch Intern Med. 137, 203–220.

31. Shoenfeld Y, Hager S, Berliner S et al. (1982). Hypophosphatemia as a diagnostic aid in sepsis. NY State Med J. 82, 163–165.

32. Desai TK, Carlson RW, Geheb MA. (1987). Hypocalcemia and hypophosphatemia in acutely ill patients. Crit Care Clin. 5, 927–941.

33. Lentz RD, Brown DM, Kjellstrand CM. (1978). Treatment of severe hypophosphatemia. Ann Intern Med. 89, 941–944.

34. Kingston M, Al-Siba MB. (1985). Treatment of severe hypophosphatemia. Crit Care Med. 13, 16–18.

35. Elin RJ. (1988). Magnesium metabolism in health and disease. Disease-A-Month, Apr. 34, 173.

36. Reinhart RA. (1988). Magnesium metabolism. A review with special reference to the relationship between intracelluar content and serum levels. Arch Intern Med. 148, 2415–2420.

37. Marino PL. (1998). Magnesium—Fluid and Electrolyte Disorders. In: The ICU Book. pp. 660–672. Lippincott, Williams and Wilkins, USA.

38. Ryan MP. (1987). Diuretics and potassium/magnesium depletion. Am J Med. 82(3A), 38–47.

39. Whang RA, Oei TO, Aikawa JK et al. (1984). Predictors of clinical hypomagnesemia. Arch Intern Med. 144, 1794–1796.

40. Whang RA. (1987). Magnesium deficiency: Pathogenesis, prevalence and clinical implications. Am J Med. 82(3A), 24–29.

41. Iseri LT. (1984). Magnesium in coronary artery disease. Drugs. 28 (Suppl 1), 151–160.

42. Iseri LT, Freed J, Bures AR. (1975). Magnesium deficiency and cardiac disorders. Am J Med. 58, 837–846.

43. Abraham AS, Rosenmann D, Kramer M et al. (1987). Magnesium in the prevention of lethal arrhythmias in acute myocardial infarction. Arch Intern Med. 147, 753–755.

44. Rasmussen HS, Suenson M, McNair P et al. (1987). Magnesium infusion reduces the incidence of arrhythmias in acute myocardial infarction. A double blind placebo-controlled study. Clin Cardiol. 10, 351–356.

45. Iseri LT, French JH. (1984). Magnesium: Nature's physiologic calcium blocker. Am Heart J. 108, 188–193.

46. Molloy DW, Dhingra S, Solven F et al. (1984). Hypomagnesemia and respiratory muscle power. Am Rev Respir Dis. 129, 497–498.

47. Oster JR, Epstein M. (1988). Management of magnesium depletion. Am J Nephrol. 8, 349–354.

Acid-Base Disturbances in the Critically Ill

Acid-Base Disturbances in the Critically Ill

General Considerations

The maintenance of normal acid-base balance (pH 7.35–7.45) in the blood is of crucial importance and is a vital homeostatic function of the body. Any variation from the normal constitutes an emergency in that a significant change in the H^+ ion concentration of the plasma or the extracellular fluid is incompatible with life; a pH $\leq$ 7, or a pH $\geq$ 7.8 spells imminent danger and death.

Acid-base disturbances occur very frequently in patients who are critically ill. They may dominate the clinical picture as in severe diabetic ketoacidosis or in renal failure. The diagnosis and importance of acid-base changes in these patients is obvious and is quickly appreciated. However more often than not a change in the acid-base equilibrium occurs surreptitiously against the background of a critical illness. The manifestations of an altered acid-base homeostasis in such patients are often subtle, virtually impossible to clinically detect, and are often masked by the clinical features of the illness. There are no barriers to these disturbances; they are encountered in all fields and all specialities of medicine and surgery. Not uncommonly, the realization that sudden clinical deterioration or death in a particular patient may have been related to acid-base disturbances dawns on the physician a trifle too late. An early diagnosis of a change in acid-base equilibrium demands a sharp clinical acumen, a grasp of the physiopathology underlying these changes, and an intelligent interpretation of laboratory data.

No satisfactory assessment of the presence and degree of acid-base disturbances can be made without measuring the pH of the blood by the pH electrode. It is imperative that the importance of pH and acid-base measurements through a blood gas machine using the Astrup technique is universally recognized in all developing countries. Today, though many critical care units in the large metropolitan cities of India provide this very necessary facility, most critical care units in smaller cities lack this basic amenity. It is also unfortunate that many doctors dealing with critical care medicine are unable to correctly appreciate the results provided by this technique. Most students and doctors are taught to interpret arterial blood gases and acid-base disturbances by rule of the thumb or by reference to standard charts and graphs which allow a prompt solution for the basic problem. This may be satisfactory—but only

to a point. Correct interpretation of blood gases and acid-base disturbances necessitates a familiarity with basic physiology in this field. Then only can altered physiology in a critically ill individual be better understood. Intelligent and in-depth interpretation leads to a more rational management of the patient as a whole.

This chapter first outlines the elementary basics necessary for satisfactory clinical interpretation. It then deals with the clinical description, the laboratory interpretation and assessment, and the treatment of these disturbances.

Basic Concepts

(a) Concept of an Acid

An acid is a potential H^+ ion or proton donor. Conversely a base is a potential proton acceptor.

The strength of an acid (HA) is measured by the extent to which it dissociates in an aqueous solution.

$$HA \rightleftarrows [H^+] + [A^-]$$

When the above reaction is in equilibrium, for a strong acid $[H^+] + [A^-]$ will be in a greater concentration than HA in the undissociated form. Also, at equilibrium, the product of the concentration on one side of the equation will bear a constant relationship to the product of concentration on the other.

$$Ka\,[HA] = [H^+]\,[A^-]$$

$$Ka = \frac{[H^+]\,[A^-]}{[HA]}$$

where Ka is the acid dissociation constant. Strong acids have a high Ka. Similar equations would apply to the dissociation of a base.

(b) Concept of pH

The acidity of an aqueous solution is measured by its hydrogen (H^+) ion concentration or activity. The H^+ activity is expressed as pH. This terminology was introduced to simplify expression of a wide range of H ions found in various fluids within the body. A quantification of H ions in various fluids in moles, would have been cumbersome and difficult. The notation pH is the negative logarithm of H ion concentration. This allows a large range of H^+ concentrations to be simply expressed and measured. Thus

$$pH = \log \frac{1}{[H^+]}$$
$$= -\log 10\,[H^+]$$
$$= \text{negative exponent of an expression of } [H^+]$$
to the power 10.

Thus a pH of $7.4 = [H^+] \times 10^{-7.4}$.

The normal H ion concentration of blood is 40 nanomoles/l or 40×10^{-9} moles/l. This is equivalent to a pH of 7.4. Changes in acid-base balance can be looked upon either as changes in the H ion concentration or as changes in pH. **Table 11.1** given below shows the H ion concentration in relation to the corresponding pH values.

Table 11.1. Correlation between H ion concentration and pH values

H ion concentration (nmoles/l)	pH
10	8.00
20	7.70
30	7.52
40	7.40
50	7.30
60	7.22
70	7.15
80	7.10
90	7.05
100	7.00

(c) The Henderson-Hasselbalch Equation

In the earlier section on the Concept of an Acid, it has been noted that

$$Ka = \frac{[H^+][A^-]}{[HA]}$$

If we wish to express H ion concentration (H^+) as pH ($\log 1/H$) we may rewrite the above equation thus:

$$[H^+] = Ka\,\frac{[HA]}{[A^-]}$$

Taking reciprocals,

$$\frac{1}{[H^+]} = \frac{1}{Ka} \times \frac{[A^-]}{[HA]}$$

Taking logs,

$$\log\frac{1}{[H^+]} = \log\frac{1}{Ka} + \log\frac{[A^-]}{[HA]}$$

i.e. $pH = pKa + \log \dfrac{[A^-]}{[HA]}$

where pKa is the negative logarithm of the dissociation constant Ka. The above is the Henderson-Hasselbalch Equation.

(d) Buffers

Buffers are substances which react with an acid or base and thereby minimize changes in pH. The metabolic processes within the body add a daily load of H ions to the body. These H ions if not properly dealt with within the body would produce a disastrous rise in H ion concentration, and a catastrophic fall in the pH. The homeostasis of acid-base balance however remains unchanged because of the buffering systems within the body and due to the role of the kidneys.

The main buffer systems of the body are:

(i) Haemoglobin and to a much lesser extent organic phosphates within the red blood cells.

(ii) Bicarbonates and inorganic phosphates within the blood.

(iii) Plasma Proteins.

(iv) Tissue Proteins.

(v) Minerals (phosphates, carbonates) within the bones.

It is only possible in this book to deal with the bicarbonate-carbonic acid buffer systems. The reader is referred to a standard textbook on Physiology for a more thorough understanding of the subject.

The bicarbonate-carbonic acid reaction is important in regulating acid-base balance. It constitutes a weak buffer system which can be used as a measure or reflection of all acid-base reactions within the body, because buffer systems are in dynamic equilibrium, and carbon dioxide diffuses freely across all tissues and membranes. Also, these chemical reactions occur very rapidly.

The CO_2 produced by tissue metabolism diffuses into plasma and the red blood cells. The enzyme carbonic anhydrase within the RBCs catalyses the formation of carbonic acid.

$$H_2O + CO_2 = H_2CO_3$$

The carbonic acid within the RBCs is dissociated thus:

$$H_2CO_3 \rightarrow H^+ + HCO_3^-$$

The bicarbonate within the RBCs diffuses out into the plasma, while the H ions are mopped up by the haemoglobin which acts as a buffer base. The loss of one ion from the cell has to be compensated by the entry of an equivalent ion. Thus chloride ions (Cl^-) from the plasma enter the red blood cells in place of the bicarbonate ions which have diffused out into the plasma.

When the blood reaches the lungs, the chloride shift is reversed and bicarbonate enters the red blood cells. The bicarbonate within the RBCs breaks down into H_2O and CO_2. The CO_2 diffuses out through the capillaries into the alveoli, and is washed out into the outside air.

The bicarbonate-carbonic reaction can be looked at from another angle as regards the role it plays in controlling acid-base balance. Thus when H^+ enters tissue fluids

$$H^+ + HCO_3^- \rightarrow H_2CO_3 \rightarrow CO_2 + H_2O$$

The CO_2 is rapidly washed out via the lungs leading to a rapid control of H ion production, but of course at the expense of a fall in $[HCO_3^-]$.

The Henderson-Hasselbalch equation for the bicarbonate-carbonic acid reaction aptly illustrates the role played by this reaction in regulating acid-base balance.

$$pH = pK + \log \frac{HCO_3}{H_2CO_3}$$

$$= 6.1 + \log \frac{HCO_3}{H_2CO_3}$$

$$= 6.1 + \log \frac{HCO_3}{0.03 \times PCO_2}$$

where 0.03 is the solubility of CO_2 in plasma, and PCO_2 the partial pressure of CO_2 in plasma.

If instead of pH one considers the H ion concentration, then the following modification of the Henderson-Hasselbalch equation can be used.

$$[H^+] = 24 \times \frac{PCO_2}{HCO_3} \text{ nanomoles/l}$$

Normally, $[H^+] = 24 \times 40/24 = 40$ nanomoles/l (pH 7.4).

The Henderson-Hasselbalch equation expresses the relationship between 3 reactants—H^+, HCO_3^- and PCO_2, and can be used as an expression of acid-base balance within the body.

Role of the Kidneys in Acid-Base Balance

The kidneys play an important and crucial role in H ion regulation. They do so in the following ways:

(i) Regulating excretion and reabsorption of bicarbonate (HCO_3^-). Bicarbonate is filtered by the glomerulus, the quantity of bicarbonate in the filtrate being dependent on the plasma bicarbonate, and the glomerular filtration rate. The bicarbonate is then dealt with as follows:

(a) Reabsorption of bicarbonate in the proximal renal tubules at a rate which is dependent on the PCO_2. The higher the PCO_2, the greater the degree of bicarbonate reabsorption; the lower the PCO_2, the lesser the degree of reabsorption of bicarbonate, and the greater its excretion. This enables respiratory acidosis (due to a high $PaCO_2$) to be compensated through retention of bicarbonate, and respiratory alkalosis (due to a low PaO_2) to be compensated by an increased excretion of bicarbonate (see Subsections on Respiratory Acidosis and Respiratory Alkalosis).

(b) In metabolic acidosis, H ions are excreted into the urine. The enzyme carbonic anhydrase catalyses the reaction

$$H^+ + HCO_3^- \rightarrow H_2CO_3 \rightarrow H_2O + CO_2.$$

The CO_2 is reabsorbed and is excreted into the lungs. This is an important means by which the pH is controlled.

(ii) Use of Buffering Systems. H ions can be mopped up by phosphate buffers, thus tending to increase the pH, while at the same time conserving bicarbonate.

Thus under the influence of carbonic anhydrase,

$$H^+ + HCO_3^- = H_2CO_3 \text{ (in the tubular cells)}$$
$$H_2CO_3 \rightarrow HCO_3^- + H^+$$

The bicarbonate ion is reabsorbed. The H ion is mopped up by $NaHPO_4$ thus:

$$H + NaHPO_4 \rightarrow NaH_2PO_4$$

which is excreted via the urine.

(iii) Formation of ammonia. NH_4^+ is formed in the tubular cells by conversion of glutamine to glutamate. Thus,

CONH$_2$		COO$^-$
|		|
(CH$_2$)$_2$		(CH$_2$)$_2$
|	$+ H_2O \rightleftarrows NH_4^+$	|
CHNH$_3$$^+$		CHNH$_3$$^+$
|		|
COO$^-$		COO$^-$
GLUTAMINE		GLUTAMATE

NH_4^+ combines with chloride and is excreted via the urine, the reaction being controlled by the enzyme glutaminase. NH_4 excretion to be fully operative takes time. It is however an extremely important mechanism for pH control, as excretion of ammonia allows the excretion of a significantly large quantity of H ions via the kidney.

(iv) Reabsorption of Sodium. The active reabsorption of sodium from the filtrate into tubule cells causes a potential gradient across the cell membrane. The positively charged H ion within the tubule cell thus passes across the membrane into the filtrate, and is buffered within the filtrate by a phosphate buffer.

$$H + NaHPO_4 \rightarrow NaH_2PO_4$$

In summary, the kidneys help to maintain acid-base balance in the following ways:

(i) Retention of bicarbonate when the PCO_2 increases.

(ii) Excretion of bicarbonate when the PCO_2 falls.

(iii) Reabsorption of bicarbonate when there is accumulation of H ions in the blood.

(iv) Excretion of titratable acid and NH_4 to counter an increase of H ions in the blood.

(v) Excretion of H ions when there is a primary loss of bicarbonate.

(vi) Increased bicarbonate excretion in the urine, together with a loss of K^+ in the urine, when there is a primary increase in plasma bicarbonate.

Disturbances in Acid-Base Balance: Terminology

Terms used: acidaemia, alkalaemia, acidosis, alkalosis.

The normal pH of arterial blood is maintained within the range of 7.35 to 7.45.

Acidaemia exists when the pH of arterial blood is below the normal range i.e. less than 7.35.

Alkalaemia is the state in which pH of arterial blood is above the normal range i.e. greater than 7.45.

Acidosis is an abnormal state leading to an increase in the acid in the body.

Alkalosis is an abnormal state leading to a fall in acid or an increase in the alkali in the body.

When acidosis induces compensatory changes in the body so that pH remains within the normal range, it is termed compensatory acidosis. When acidosis produces a fall in pH below 7.35, it is termed uncompensated acidosis. Uncompensated acidosis and acidaemia are thus synonymous.

Similarly, alkalosis can be compensated or uncompensated, and alkalaemia is synonymous with the latter.

Acidosis and alkalosis (as also acidaemia and alkalaemia) may result from primary respiratory or metabolic disturbances so that we have respiratory acidosis and metabolic acidosis, as also respiratory alkalosis and metabolic alkalosis.

Respiratory acidosis and respiratory acidaemia (uncompensated respiratory acidosis) result from alveolar hypoventilation which leads to hypercapnia.

Respiratory alkalosis and respiratory alkalaemia (uncompensated respiratory alkalosis) result from alveolar hyperventilation which causes hypocapnia.

Metabolic acidosis and metabolic acidaemia are caused by either accumulation of acid or loss of base from the body.

Metabolic alkalosis and metabolic alkalaemia are due to accumulation of base or loss of acid from the body.

Mixed acid-base disturbances are caused by a combination of respiratory and metabolic factors.

Laboratory Diagnosis of Disturbances in Acid-Base Equilibrium

A suspicion of possible acid-base disturbances should always be entertained in each and every patient with a critical illness. Disturbances in acid-base equilibrium can also occur under some reasonably well-defined clinical conditions. Thus in an unconscious hyperpnoeic patient, the possible diagnosis of diabetes or uraemia should be established by relevant blood and urine tests, and in suspected aspirin poisoning, the acetyl salicylic acid levels in the blood confirm the diagnosis. Such investigations help in two ways; they point to the possible nature of the acid-base disturbance, and they direct attention to the root cause of such a disturbance, which proves invaluable in the management of the patient.

Estimation of Serum Electrolytes

This is mandatory in every patient with acid-base disturbances, as electrolyte abnormalities are frequently seen and are often inseparable from changes in acid-base balance. Thus hyperkalaemia is frequently seen in metabolic acidosis, and hypokalaemia and hypochloraemia are commonly observed in metabolic alkalosis.

Interpretation of pH and Acid-Base Measurements by the Astrup Technique

In this technique, the pH and PCO_2 of the blood are measured by a sensitive instrument (radiometer). The values of standard bicarbonate, actual bicarbonate, CO_2 content, and base excess or deficit are then read from a standard nomogram. These concepts are briefly explained below.

The standard bicarbonate is the bicarbonate content in the plasma of blood which has been equilibrated at a PCO_2 of 40 mm Hg, as also with oxygen so as to saturate it with oxygen. The standard bicarbonate is a measure of the non-respiratory bicarbonate. It is the most active, mobile, rapidly reacting fraction

of the total buffer potential, and its rate of excretion and retention is governed by the kidneys. A fall in the standard bicarbonate therefore indicates a metabolic acidosis; conversely a rise in the standard bicarbonate indicates a metabolic alkalosis. A normal standard bicarbonate indicates metabolic equilibrium.

The actual bicarbonate content is the bicarbonate concentration in mEq or mmoles/l in the plasma. It is not directly estimated; its value is derived from a nomogram in the Astrup technique, or from the CO_2 content of blood which can be estimated by the Van Slyke Apparatus.

The CO_2 content of plasma is the actual bicarbonate content + dissolved CO_2. As stated above, it can be estimated by gasometry (Van Slyke Apparatus), or is derived from a nomogram if the pH and $PaCO_2$ are known.

Base excess defines the presence in blood of excess or deficit of base, the physiological range being ± 2.3 mEq/l. It denotes the amount of strong acid or base per litre of blood, which has been added as a consequence of a metabolic disturbance. It is an *in vitro* concept, and is again derived from a nomogram if the pH and $PaCO_2$ are known.

Some of the terms described above are apt to prove confusing to the resident working in critical care medicine. For purposes of simplification, acid-base changes are best interpreted by a consideration of the Henderson-Hasselbalch equation:

$$pH = pK + \log \frac{HCO_3}{PCO_2 \times 0.03}$$

In other words, pH is the 'balance' between the respiratory parameter represented by $PaCO_2$, and the metabolic parameter represented by bicarbonate. This is most simply illustrated in **Fig. 11.1.1**.

A primary change in the respiratory parameter ($PaCO_2$) disturbs the 'balance' illustrated in **Fig. 11.1.1** to produce respiratory acid-base disturbances; a primary change in the metabolic parameter (bicarbonate) disturbs the balance and produces metabolic acid-base disturbances.

A rise in $PaCO_2$ primarily due to alveolar hypoventilation causes respiratory acidosis, and when this acidosis lowers the pH to < 7.35, respiratory acidaemia results. A fall in $PaCO_2$ produced by hyperventilation induces respiratory alkalosis and if the pH rises to > 7.45, respiratory alkalaemia results.

Homeostasis demands that primary changes in $PaCO_2$ lead to secondary changes in the plasma bicarbonate, so that the pH is kept within the normal range as far as possible. An acute rise in $PaCO_2$ (due to sudden hypoventilation following poisoning or a near respiratory arrest), will lead to a very small rise in the plasma bicarbonate (see Subsection on bicarbonate-carbonic acid reaction). The degree of retention of plasma bicarbonate is just 0.1 mmole or 0.1 mEq per 1 mm Hg rise in $PaCO_2$. The standard bicarbonate will remain unchanged. This can produce a gross imbalance between the respiratory and metabolic parameters, and can lead to a sharp and dangerous fall in pH. This is illustrated in **Fig. 11.1.2**.

On the other hand, a slow or chronic rise in $PaCO_2$ (so frequently observed in patients with chronic airways obstruction) allows renal compensation to come into play. The kidneys retain bicarbonate—3–4 mEq or mmoles/l being retained for every 10 mm Hg rise in

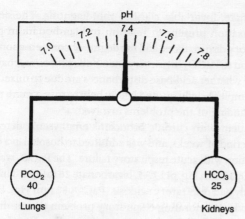

Fig. 11.1.1. Normal acid-base balance.

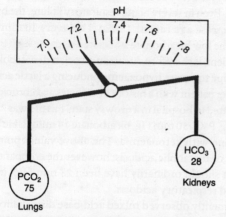

Fig. 11.1.2. Uncompensated respiratory acidosis and acidaemia.

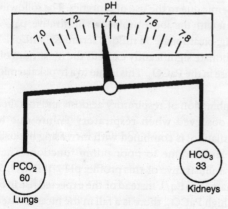

Fig. 11.1.3. Compensated respiratory acidosis.

PaCO$_2$. Significant bicarbonate retention thus compensates for the chronic rise in PaCO$_2$, and helps to preserve the 'balance'. Retention of bicarbonate by the kidneys takes time; it probably starts 4–6 hours after the rise in PaCO$_2$, and is complete after 2–3 days. Compensation however can only occur up to a point—a rise in PaCO$_2$ > 65 mm Hg is generally associated with a fall in pH below normal in spite of bicarbonate retention. The degree of rise in bicarbonate enables one to determine whether in a given patient the respiratory acidosis is acute or chronic. Uncompensated respiratory acidosis (respiratory acidaemia) and compensated

respiratory acidosis are illustrated in **Figs. 11.1.2** and **11.1.3**, respectively.

Comparison of degrees of rise in bicarbonate *in vivo* due to acute and chronic rise in PaCO$_2$ is illustrated in **Fig. 11.1.4**.

A fall in PaCO$_2$ primarily due to alveolar hyperventilation leads to a compensatory fall in plasma bicarbonate, the degree of fall approximating 0.1–0.3 mmoles/l for 1 mm Hg fall in PaCO$_2$. Acid-base balance in acute, uncompensated respiratory alkalosis is illustrated in **Fig. 11.1.5**.

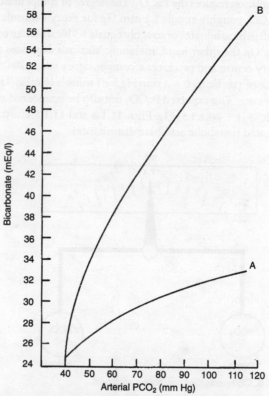

Fig. 11.1.4. Comparison curves showing rise in bicarbonate levels *in vivo* with chronic and acute hypercapnia. A = rise in acute hypercapnia. B = rise in chronic hypercapnia; the curve in this case is higher and steeper than that in acute hypercapnia, because of retention of bicarbonate by the kidney.

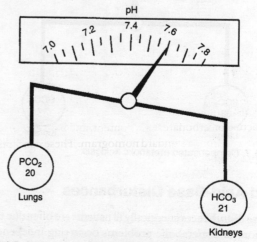

Fig. 11.1.5. Acute uncompensated respiratory alkalosis.

When primary metabolic problems produce a fall in bicarbonate, metabolic acidosis results. When the pH falls to < 7.35, metabolic acidaemia results.

Metabolic alkalosis results following retention of bicarbonate due to metabolic causes; metabolic alkalaemia ensues when the pH rises to > 7.45.

Primary metabolic changes in bicarbonate result in secondary changes in $PaCO_2$, thus minimizing changes in the pH. Thus metabolic acidosis stimulates the respiratory centre, and the resulting hyperventilation reduces the $PaCO_2$. The degree of compensatory fall in $PaCO_2$ roughly equals 1.2 mm Hg for every 1 mmole or mEq/l fall in bicarbonate (or roughly equals 1.5 bicarbonate content + 8). On the other hand, metabolic alkalosis depresses the respiratory centre and produces a compensatory rise in $PaCO_2$, the degree of rise being 0.6–1 mm Hg for 1 mmole or mEq/l rise in bicarbonate. The expected $PaCO_2$ can also be considered as = $0.7 \times [\,HCO_3^-\,] + 20(\pm 1.5)$ (1). **Figs. 11.1.6** and **11.1.7** illustrate compensated metabolic acid-base disturbances.

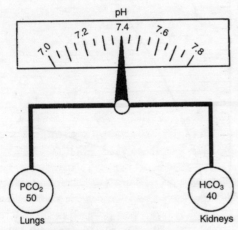

Fig. 11.1.6. Compensated metabolic alkalosis.

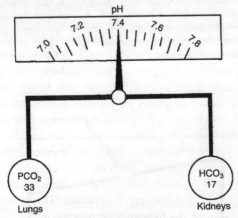

Fig. 11.1.7. Compensated metabolic acidosis.

Mixed Acid-Base Disturbances

Acid-base disturbances in critically ill patients are often due to both respiratory and metabolic problems occurring independently. A consideration of the clinical picture, the pH, $PaCO_2$ and

bicarbonate, invariably clarifies the diagnosis. The degree of compensation present in relation to bicarbonate in primary respiratory disturbances, and the degree of compensation present in relation to $PaCO_2$ in primary metabolic problems, enables one to judge whether acid-base disturbances are due to mixed causes. The examples briefly quoted below help to give a more practical understanding of the problems involved.

A patient with chronic bronchitis emphysema deteriorated over a period of weeks, and was admitted to hospital in a critically ill condition with acute respiratory failure. The $PaCO_2$ was 82 mm Hg, PaO_2 34 mm Hg, pH 7.15, bicarbonate 26 mEq/l. This patient obviously had respiratory acidosis ($PaCO_2$ 82 mm Hg). However in a slowly deteriorating respiratory problem the rise in $PaCO_2$ should have been offset by a rise in plasma bicarbonate at a rate of 4 mEq/l for every 10 mm Hg rise in $PaCO_2$ i.e. approximately 40 mEq/l. Even in severe acute respiratory failure, the bicarbonate should increase at a rate of 1 mEq/l for every 10 mm Hg rise in $PaCO_2$. The low bicarbonate associated with the high $PaCO_2$ seen in this patient, is therefore due to an associated metabolic acidosis, possibly due to severe hypoxaemia inducing a lactic acid acidosis.

Another patient with a history of diabetes and chronic bronchitis was admitted to hospital in a drowsy state. His pH was 7.21, $PaCO_2$ 42 mm Hg, PaO_2 50 mm Hg, bicarbonate 14 mEq/l. He had ketosis in the urine with ketonaemia. The above values pointed to the presence of metabolic acidosis; however the comparatively high $PaCO_2$ (it should ordinarily have been 28 mm Hg), indicates an associated respiratory acidosis.

A frequently observed mixed acid-base disturbance in critical care units is a combination of respiratory acidosis and metabolic alkalosis in patients with chronic airways obstruction, who are hypokalaemic due to the use of diuretics. The following example in a patient with the above problem is illustrative: pH 7.44; $PaCO_2$ 60 mm Hg; bicarbonate 38 mEq/l; serum K^+ 3mEq/l. The rise in the bicarbonate significantly exceeds the maximum of 0.4 mEq/ mm Hg rise in the $PaCO_2$. This is due to a hypokalaemic metabolic alkalosis.

A combination of respiratory acidosis and metabolic acidosis is often observed when respiratory failure due to alveolar hypoventilation, is combined with increasing hypoxia and poor tissue perfusion due to poor pump function. The following example is illustrative of this profile: pH 7.1; $PaCO_2$ 55 mm Hg; bicarbonate 15 mEq/l. Instead of the expected rise in bicarbonate due to a high $PaCO_2$, there is a fall in the bicarbonate because of metabolic lactic acid acidosis induced by hypotension and poor tissue perfusion in a patient with respiratory failure.

A combination of respiratory alkalosis and metabolic alkalosis is at times observed in hepatic failure. The latter causes tachypnoea with respiratory alkalosis. If there is associated vomiting, or there is aspiration of gastric contents through a nasogastric tube, the loss of H ions, K^+ and chloride leads to an associated metabolic alkalosis. The following example is illustrative: pH 7.61; $PaCO_2$ 25 mm Hg; bicarbonate 34 mEq/l.

A combination of respiratory alkalosis and metabolic acidosis may occur in septic shock and also in terminal acute liver cell failure. Both these conditions can cause tachypnoea with respiratory alkalosis. The metabolic (lactic acid) acidosis is related to shock and poor tissue perfusion. The same combination is often observed in patients who are hyperventilated on mechanical ventilation (with resulting respiratory alkalosis), and who are hypotensive from shock or poor pump function (which causes lactic acid acidosis).

Renal failure with excessive vomiting, or with a loss of gastric secretions from nasogastric aspiration, can result in a combination of metabolic acidosis and metabolic alkalosis, with the pH well within the normal range.

Arterial pH of blood gases and bicarbonate levels should always be interpreted with reference to the history, clinical findings, and other investigations in every individual problem. Occasionally, the complexity of an acid-base disturbance is only apparent on a follow-up of the patient.

Clinical Features and Management of Acid-Base Disturbances

Metabolic Acidosis

The diagnosis of metabolic acidosis rests on a clinical awareness of its presence in situations where it is a recognized complication. It should always be suspected in severe uncontrolled diabetes, in acute or chronic renal failure, in poisoning with acids, aspirin, or methyl alcohol, and in patients who have a continuing loss of bicarbonate (as in diarrhoea, or intestinal or pancreatic fistulae). Severe hypoxia, particularly when associated with poor tissue perfusion, is an important cause of metabolic acidosis due to accumulation of lactic acid. Poor tissue perfusion may be localized as in peripheral vascular disease, or generalized due to poor pump function, or to shock from any cause. Metabolic acidosis can also occur after cardiac arrest—the longer the period required for resuscitation, the greater the chances of increasing metabolic acidosis.

Metabolic acidosis is often divided into 2 groups—one group with a normal anion gap, and another group with a high anion gap. The group with a normal anion gap is characterized by loss of bicarbonate. This results in a replacement of chloride for the lost bicarbonate to preserve electrical neutrality, and the increase in serum chloride causes a hyperchloraemic metabolic acidosis. The group with the high anion gap is characterized by the addition of a fixed acid e.g. lactic acid. The common causes of metabolic acidosis are summarized in **Table 11.1.2**.

Table 11.1.2. Common causes of metabolic acidosis

1. Normal Anion Gap
   * Diarrhoea
   * Intestinal or pancreatic fistulae
   * Renal tubular acidosis
   * As compensation for respiratory alkalosis
   * Ureterosigmoidostomy
   * Infusion with fluids having high chloride content
2. High Anion Gap
   * Lactic acidosis
   * Ketoacidosis (alcoholics, diabetics)
   * Renal failure
   * Poisonings (salicylates, acids, methyl alcohol, ethylene glycol)

Anion Gap

It is assumed that the negatively charged anions and the positively charged cations are equal for purposes of electrical neutrality (2). If so, then the unmeasured anions and unmeasured cations can be determined using the serum chloride (Cl^-), bicarbonate (HCO_3^-) and sodium (Na^+). The difference between the unmeasured anions and cations in the serum is termed the anion gap, and is equal to $(Na^+) - ([Cl^-] + [HCO_3^-])$. The normal anion gap is 12–15 mEq/l (2, 3). An increase of over 15 mEq/l in the anion gap is generally considered to be abnormal.

The serum anion gap is illustrated below in detail in **Table 11.1.3**.

Table 11.1.3. The serum anion gap

Unmeasured Anions in Serum		Unmeasured Cations in Serum	
Proteins	15 mEq/l	K^+	4.5 mEq/l
Organic acids	5 mEq/l	Ca^{++}	5.0 mEq/l
PO_4^{---}	2 mEq/l	Mg^{++}	1.5 mEq/l
SO_4^{--}	1 mEq/l		
Total	23 mEq/l		11 mEq/l
The anion gap = 12 mEq/l			

$$Unmeasured\ Anions + ([Cl^-] + [HCO_3^-])$$
$$= (Na^+) + Unmeasured\ Cations.$$

Thus,

Unmeasured Anions – Unmeasured Cations (which constitute the anion gap) $= (Na^+) - ([Cl^-] + [HCO_3^-])$.

When a fixed acid like lactic acid donates an H^+ ion to the serum, the bicarbonate decreases by 1 mEq/l for every 1 mEq/l of H^+ ion added. The anion gap will increase by a similar amount. On the other hand, when bicarbonate is lost from the body (either through stools or intestinal fistulae), the chloride ion replaces it so that the anion gap is unchanged.

A fall (i.e. a reduction) in the anion gap in critical care medicine is chiefly observed in patients with a low albumin. This is because serum albumin constitutes about half (11 mEq) of the unmeasured anion pool of 23 mEq/l. Hence a decrease in serum albumin by 50 per cent should produce a 25 per cent decrease in the total unmeasured anionic pool. Assuming that the serum electrolytes and bicarbonate remain unchanged, a 50 per cent reduction in serum albumin will decrease the anion gap by 5–6 mEq/l (3).

Therefore in the presence of significant hypoalbuminaemia (e.g. reduction in albumin by 50 per cent) an anion gap of 12 mEq/l should really read 18 mEq/l, and this constitutes a mild but definite high anion gap metabolic acidosis. This is important simply because of the frequency of hypoalbuminaemia in patients in critical care units.

Other causes of reduced anion gap include paraproteinaemias, an increase in unmeasured cations (Ca^{++}, K^+, Mg^{++}), and hyponatraemia. The reason for a reduced anion gap in hyponatraemia is unclear. In dilutional hyponatraemia the extra water in serum should decrease serum chloride as much as serum sodium, leaving the anion gap unchanged. However, this is not necessarily the case; the chloride ion does not show an equivalent reduction as the sodium in many cases of hyponatraemia. Perhaps unmeasured cations like Ca^{++} and Mg^{++} may increase in the serum during hyponatraemia, and the chloride remains comparatively elevated to provide electrical neutrality (2).

Clinical Features

The clinical features of metabolic acidosis include:

(i) Hyperventilation due to stimulation of the respiratory centre. This is first characterized by an increase in the depth of breathing, followed by an increase in the rate.

(ii) An obtunded mental state—drowsiness progressing to deep coma.

The smell of ketones in the breath points to diabetic ketoacidosis, whilst an ammoniacal smell in the breath is observed in uraemic ketoacidosis.

(iii) The only manifestation of metabolic acidosis may be a progressive deterioration in the clinical state of a critically ill individual. Metabolic acidosis impairs the function of most organs of the body, particulary the heart. This can be slow, insiduous and unsuspected; if the acidosis remains uncorrected it can lead to irreversible organ dysfunction and ultimately to death. Hence the importance of measuring the arterial pH and blood gases in every critically ill patient.

Lactic Acid Acidosis

This deserves special consideration as it is fairly frequent yet an often missed entity in critically ill patients in the ICU.

Lactic acid is a product of glucose metabolism. It is produced at an average rate of 1 mEq/kg/hour (4, 5), the serum lactate levels being ≤ 2 mEq/l. Exercise can raise the serum lactate levels to 4 mEq/l (5). The lactate is metabolized by the liver and is used for gluconeogenesis or for energy production.

Aetiology

The most common cause of lactic acid acidosis in ICU patients is shock, in particular cardiogenic shock, and septic shock. Sepsis can produce lactic acid acidosis in the absence of hypotension or the other clinical features of shock. This is due to the fact that oxygen supply is not commensurate with the increased demand for oxygen by the tissues (see Section on Shock). Multiple organ failure is also frequently associated with lactic acid acidosis—this is chiefly related to poor pump function, and to liver cell dysfunction. The rise of serum lactate in these conditions is due to the increased production of lactic acid, and decreased clearance of lactate by the liver. The latter may well be related to poor liver function consequent to hypoperfusion of the liver observed in shock.

Other important causes of lactic acid acidosis in the ICU are:

(i) *Hypoxia*. A low PaO_2 by itself may not induce a significant rise in serum lactate (6). In most patients with a low PaO_2, it is the associated presence of a low cardiac output that is responsible for a rise in lactic acid.

(ii) *Severe anaemia* (Hb < 5 g/dl) if not adequately compensated for by a hyperdynamic circulatory state can also lead to an increase in lactic acid levels in the blood.

(iii) *Severe liver cell dysfunction*, particularly when associated with hypotension or shock can lead to lactic acid acidosis (7).

Rare causes of lactic acid acidosis in the ICU include:

(i) *Thiamine deficiency*. This causes lactic acidosis by reducing the mitochondrial oxidation of pyruvate (8). The conversion of pyruvate to acetyl-coenzyme A is blocked by the lack of thiamine, and the pyruvate is converted to lactate. In critically ill patients, particularly in those with prolonged illnesses and with poor nutrition, thiamine deficiency must be suspected when the other more common causes of lactic acid acidosis do not seem to be responsible. A quick reversal of acidosis following thiamine injections points to the diagnosis of lactic acidosis due to thiamine deficiency (8).

(ii) *Alkalosis*. Increased serum lactate levels have been reported with severe metabolic alkalosis and respiratory alkalosis (6, 9). This is probably due to extra production of lactate due to increased activity of pH dependent enzymes involving the glycolytic pathway. Severe alkalosis with pH > 7.6 is generally necessary for a rise in lactate levels, as a modest increase in lactate production is ordinarily metabolized by the liver, unless liver cell function is deranged, or there is associated hypoperfusion of the liver due to a poor circulatory state.

(iii) *D-Lactic Acid Acidosis*. The usual lactate produced in the body is a levo-isomer. The dextro-isomer is produced by bacterial fermentation of glucose in the colon. B-fragilis, other anaerobes, and Gram-negative organisms within the gut are also capable of inducing the formation of D-lactic acid (10). D-lactic acid acidosis is most frequently reported following small bowel resection and following jejunoileostomy for the treatment of severe obesity (11, 12). The condition should therefore be suspected in a patient with an ill-explained metabolic acidosis with a high anion gap, particularly if there is a history of small bowel surgery or persistent diarrhoea. A standard assay of lactate would not detect lactic acid, as it only measures the levo form of lactate. Special assays for D-lactic acid can only be done in highly specialized reference laboratories.

(iv) *Drugs*. Rarely the use of epinephrine and nitroprusside in the ICU may induce a lactic acid acidosis. The important causes of lactic acid acidosis in an ICU setting are listed in **Table 11.1.4**.

Table 11.1.4. Important causes of lactic acid acidosis in an ICU setting

---
* Shock of any aetiology, particularly cardiogenic or septic shock
* Hypoxia, specially when associated with a low cardiac output
* Severe uncorrected anaemia (Hb < 5 g/dl)
* Marked liver cell dysfunction, particularly when associated with shock or hypotension
* Thiamine deficiency
* Severe respiratory or metabolic alkalosis
* D-lactic acid acidosis often seen following small bowel resection or jejunoileostomy done for severe obesity
* Drugs e.g. epinephrine or nitroprusside

Diagnosis

Lactic acid acidosis should be suspected whenever metabolic acidosis is associated with an increased anion gap.

The Anion Gap. The anion gap in lactic acidosis is often

> 30 mEq/l. Even in patients with renal failure an anion gap > 30 mEq/l should prompt one to suspect an additional lactic acidosis.

Estimation of lactate levels may vary in samples of arterial and venous blood. The venous blood lactate is higher because it represents lactate production, while arterial blood lactate is lower as it probably represents effect of both production and hepatic clearance. In patients with a Swan-Ganz catheter in situ, samples from the pulmonary artery are probably more representative of blood lactate levels. There is a good correlation in lactate levels in blood drawn from the pulmonary artery, and that drawn from arterial blood (13).

Treatment

In the final analysis, treatment should be directed towards the cause. In emergency situations it is vital to temporarily correct a severe acidosis and then deal with its root cause, otherwise death may result. It is wrong to await results of laboratory investigations in desperate situations where the clinical picture obviously points to severe metabolic acidosis. In such situations, acidosis is corrected by administering 75–100 ml of 7.5 per cent sodium bicarbonate as a bolus dose. Further administration is guided by laboratory reports.

Ordinarily a pH of 7.25 or less deserves prompt correction. The amount of bicarbonate in mEq required to correct metabolic acidosis is given by either of the 2 formulae given below:

(i) Sodium bicarbonate to be given =
Body wt (kg) × 0.3 × base deficit

(ii) Sodium bicarbonate deficit =
0.5 × wt (kg) × (desired HCO_3 – serum HCO_3)

The usual recommendation is to give one half of the HCO_3 deficit as an intravenous bolus, and to replace the remaining deficit over the next 4–6 hours. It is best not to be over-reliant on formulae but to administer sodium bicarbonate at a frequency and dose which keep the arterial pH above 7.3.

In the presence of an associated respiratory acidosis it is important to first correct the respiratory acidosis, and then tackle the metabolic acidosis. Sodium bicarbonate given intravenously to a patient with respiratory acidosis induces further CO_2 production and this could further increase the degree of respiratory acidosis. When the pH is very low in combined respiratory and metabolic acidosis, measures to correct both can be undertaken simultaneously.

There is some degree of controversy on when to use sodium bicarbonate for the correction of metabolic acidosis. This is because $NaHCO_3$ can produce undesirable effects which include hyperosmolarity, fluid overload due to large quantities of sodium in the $NaHCO_3$, hypokalaemia, hypocalcaemia, and increased serum lactate levels (14, 15). At times hypotension and a reduced cardiac output have been observed, probably due to calcium binding by the bicarbonate (14). It is also obvious that an ongoing metabolic acidosis will remain uncorrected as soon as the administration of $NaHCO_3$ is stopped or reduced, simply because the cause of acidosis remains uncorrected. Theoretically, the CO_2 produced by the administration of HCO_3 may partly diffuse into the red blood cells and combine with the water to form carbonic acid, thus adding to the H ion load. In practice however, we have rarely encountered

problems with the administration of sodium bicarbonate. The most frequent side effects to be looked out for are hyperosmolarity, hypokalaemia, hypocalcaemia and fluid overload. These can all be corrected by timely measures. We feel that this controversy in the use of $NaHCO_3$ is unnecessary, and that its advantages far outweigh the possible drawbacks. Its use is particularly gratifying when poor pump function is associated with metabolic acidosis. A restoration of pH towards normal leads to improved pump function, increase in systemic blood pressure and improved perfusion to the tissues.

Metabolic Alkalosis

The suspicion of this acid-base disturbance rests on an awareness of its likely occurrence in certain pathological conditions. Metabolic alkalosis is very frequently encountered in patients under critical care, as the four most important causes are vomiting (or nasogastric aspiration), the use of diuretics, the use of corticosteroids, and hypokalaemia—all these factors being very frequently encountered in critical care medicine (16, 17). Galla and Luke (18) report an associated mortality of 40 per cent when the arterial pH rises above 7.55. It is probably the gravity of the underlying illness which contributes to this mortality. Marino (19) rightly points out that the danger with metabolic alkalosis is due to its ability to sustain itself in spite of correcting the underlying aetiological factor. This is attributed to chloride depletion which limits bicarbonate excretion in the urine by promoting its reabsorption, and reducing its secretion into the renal tubules.

Aetiology

(i) Vomiting or nasogastric suction is an important cause of metabolic alkalosis. Gastric juice contains 50–100 mEq/l of H ions so that loss of gastric contents leads to significant H ion loss. There is also an associated loss of chloride, sodium, and potassium, as well as volume depletion due to water loss.

(ii) Diuretics, in particular furosemide, produce alkalosis chiefly through the loss of chlorides and potassium via the urine. Chloride follows sodium and water during diuresis; the chloride that is not reabsorbed is replaced by bicarbonate. The increased bicarbonate reabsorption maintains or enhances the alkalosis. Increased K^+ loss in the urine leads to an increase in the H ion secretion into the distal tubules, probably in an attempt to reabsorb K^+, and replace it with H ions in the tubular fluid (18). Magnesium is also lost in the urine during diuresis and this promotes K^+ loss through mechanisms not clearly understood. A decrease in extracellular volume probably contributes to alkalosis by increasing the concentration of bicarbonate in the serum. A decrease in circulating volume also stimulates aldosterone release, and promotes the loss of K^+ and H ions in the distal tubule. Thus the importance of correcting the Na^+, K^+ and Cl^- loss as well as replenishing volume in management is self-evident.

(iii) Administration of excess alkali either orally or through intravenous use promotes metabolic alkalosis. This is particularly observed when renal dysfunction prevents excretion of bicarbonate, or when there are associated electrolyte abnormalities (e.g. chloride depletion), which interfere with bicarbonate excretion by the kidneys. Over enthusiastic use of intravenous sodium bicarbonate for the correction of metabolic acidosis can produce a dangerous swing to metabolic alkalosis. Massive blood transfusions (due to citrate in the blood), are also reported to cause a significant metabolic alkalosis (**20**).

(iv) Metabolic alkalosis occurs during corticosteroid therapy, in patients with adrenocortical hyperfunction, in aldosteronism, and it almost always complicates a well-marked hypokalaemia.

The common causes of metabolic alkalosis are given in **Table 11.1.5**.

Table 11.1.5. Common causes of metabolic alkalosis

* Vomiting/Nasogastric aspiration; hypokalaemia
* Use of diuretics, particularly furosemide
* Excessive administration of alkali (orally or IV), particularly in the presence of associated renal dysfunction or electrolyte abnormality
* During corticosteroid therapy in patients with adrenocortical hyperfunction, aldosteronism, specially in the presence of well-marked hypokalaemia

Clinical Features

It is remarkable how silent metabolic alkalosis can be. Severe alkalosis (serum bicarbonate > 40 mEq/l and pH > 7.6) can cause mental obtundation, seizures, cardiac dysfunction and cardiac arrhythmias. Ventilation may be depressed (so that the $PaCO_2$ is secondarily raised), but this is not always the case. Marino (**19**) believes that the infrequency or lack of hypoventilation in metabolic alkalosis is related to the baseline activity of the peripheral chemoreceptors, through which metabolic acid-base disorders chiefly exert their effect on ventilation. Under normal conditions the peripheral chemoreceptors have a low activity with a low 'input' from the chemoreceptors to the brainstem respiratory centres. There is thus very little scope for alkalosis to further inhibit activity. On the other hand, acidosis stimulates these receptors, resulting in an increased 'input' from the receptors to the respiratory centres, and thus causing hyperventilation.

It is also worth noting that a metabolic alkalosis shifts the oxygen dissociation curve to the left, thus reducing delivery of oxygen to the tissues. In a critically ill patient who already has a low PaO_2, a sudden shift of the oxygen dissociation curve can precipitate a further sharp fall in the PaO_2 and $P\bar{v}O_2$. If pump function is poor and the patient already has a low $P\bar{v}O_2$ (due to a low cardiac output), then the further fall in $P\bar{v}O_2$ can have disastrous consequences.

Management

This is directed to the underlying aetiology. Almost always (particularly in ICU patients), metabolic alkalosis is 'chloride responsive', and the chloride should be replaced in the form of N saline. This also permits adequate replenishment of fluid loss. Hypokalaemia also needs to be corrected by an infusion of KCl (20–40 mEq or more) in a dextrose infusion. It is important to note that uncorrected hypokalaemia can perpetuate metabolic alkalosis. In patients with mineralocorticoid excess, aldactone helps to correct the hypokalaemia and restore acid-base balance. When magnesium levels are depleted, magnesium should be replaced, thus allowing for easier correction of hypokalaemia.

The volume of 0.9 per cent saline necessary for correction of metabolic alkalosis can generally be gauged by clinical assessment of the degree of fluid loss, and the degree of electrolyte disturbances. The formula given below (**19**) is often used for estimating the chloride deficit.

$$\text{Chloride Deficit} = 0.27 \times \text{wt (kg)} \times (100 - \text{present Cl in mEq/l})$$
$$\text{Volume of saline to be administered (l)} = \text{Cl deficit}/154^*$$
$$(^*\text{the chloride present in 1 l N saline} = 154 \text{ mEq}).$$

Clinical judgement should never be replaced by didactic formulae and we prefer to rely on the former rather than on the latter.

The Use of Hydrochloric Acid

We have never found it necessary to use hydrochloric acid to correct metabolic alkalosis. It may however be used in rare instances where saline and potassium replacement are ineffective in correcting a severe metabolic alkalosis. The amount of HCl required is determined by the H ion deficit (**19**).

$$H^+ \text{ deficit (mEq)} = 0.5 \times \text{wt (kg)} \times (\text{present HCO}_3 - \text{desired HCO}_3)$$
$$\text{Volume (l) of 0.1N HCl} = H^+ \text{ deficit}/100^*$$
$$\text{Volume (l) of 0.25N HCl} = H^+ \text{ deficit}/250^*$$
$$\text{Infusion rate} = 0.2 \text{ mEq/kg/hour}$$
$$(^*\text{mEq of H ion per litre of solution}).$$

It is perhaps best to use a 0.1N HCl solution. However when volume needs to be restricted, 0.25N HCl may be preferred. The infusion is best given through a central line, as if given peripherally it can cause a thrombophlebitis. Though we have never used an intravenous HCl solution for metabolic alkalosis, it has been proven to be safe and effective (**21–23**).

Other chloride-containing acids such as ammonium chloride solutions and arginine hydrochloride have been used to correct metabolic alkalosis, but are best avoided. Arginine hydrochloride can cause severe hypokalaemia in patients with renal dysfunction. Ammonium chloride can result in high ammonia levels with possible toxic effects particularly in patients with liver cell dysfunction.

Haemofiltration

Continuous arteriovenous haemofiltration is valuable in the management of severe metabolic alkalosis with markedly increased extracellular volume. A reduction of water content through continuous haemofiltration should be combined with judicious administration of normal saline and potassium in dextrose. The water loss through ultrafiltration should be greater than the fluids infused, so as to correct the increase in extracellular volume.

Respiratory Acidosis

This is due to a rise in the $PaCO_2$ of arterial blood; it complicates acute and chronic respiratory failure. The clinical features, diagnosis and management have been dealt with in an earlier chapter (see Chapter on Acute Respiratory Failure in Adults).

Respiratory Alkalosis

This results from alveolar hyperventilation with a fall in the arterial $PaCO_2$, and in the carbonic acid content of plasma. It is common in hysterical or functional states, and in patients who are overventilated whilst on ventilator support. It can also occur because of hyperventilation produced by brain stem lesions. The recognition and diagnosis of respiratory alkalosis in patients on mechanical ventilation has been dealt with separately (see Chapter on Mechanical Ventilation in the Critically Ill).

REFERENCES

1. Javeheri S, Kazemi H. (1987). Metabolic alkalosis and hypoventilation in humans. Am Rev Respir Dis. 136, 1011–1016.

2. Emmet M, Narins RG. (1977). Clinical use of the anion gap. Medicine. 56, 38–54.

3. Oh MS, Carroll HS. (1977). The anion gap. N Engl J Med. 297, 814–817.

4. Kruse JA, Carlson RW. (1987). Lactate metabolism. Crit Care Clin. 3, 725–746.

5. Mizock BA. (1989). Lactic acidosis. Disease-A-Month. 35, 237–300.

6. Eldridge F. (1966). Blood lactate and pyruvate in pulmonary insufficiency. N Engl J Med. 274, 878–882.

7. Kruse JA, Zaidi SAJ, Carlson RW. (1987). Significance of blood lactate levels in critically ill patients with liver disease. Am J Med. 83, 77–82.

8. Campbell CH. (1984). The severe lactic acidosis of thiamine deficiency: Acute pernicious or fulminating beriberi. Lancet. 1, 446–449.

9. Bersin RM, Arieff AI. (1988). Primary lactic alkalosis. Am J Med. 85, 867–871.

10. Smith SM, Eng RHK, Buccini F. (1986). Use of D-lactic acid measurements in the diagnosis of bacterial infections. J Infect Dis. 154, 658–664.

11. Stolberg L, Rolfe R, Giflin N et al. (1982). D-lactic acidosis due to abnormal gut flora. N Engl J Med. 306, 1344–1348.

12. Dahlquist NR, Perrault J, Callaway CW et al. (1984). D-lactic acidosis and encephalopathy after jejunoileostomy: Response to overfeeding and to fasting in humans. Mayo Clin Proc. 59, 141–145.

13. Weil MH, Michaels S, Rackow EC. (1987). Comparison of blood lactate concentrations in central venous, pulmonary artery and arterial blood. Crit Care Med. 15, 489–490.

14. Graf H, Arieff AI. (1986). The use of sodium bicarbonate in the therapy of organic acidosis. Intensive Care Med. 12, 286–288.

15. Stacpoole PW. (1986). Lactic Acidosis. The case against bicarbonate therapy. Ann Intern Med. 105, 276–279.

16. Rimmer JM, Gennari FJ. (1987). Metabolic alkalosis. J Intensive Care Med. 2, 137–150.

17. Riley LJ, Ilson BE, Narins RG. (1987). Acute Metabolic Acid-Base Disturbances. Crit Care Clin. 3, 699–724.

18. Galla JH, Luke RG. (1987 Oct). Pathophysiology of metabolic alkalosis. Hosp Pract. 95–118.

19. Marino PL. (1998). Metabolic Alkalosis: Acid-Base Disorders. In: The ICU Book. pp. 608–616. Lippincott, Williams and Wilkins, USA.

20. Driscoll DF, Bistrian BR, Jenkins RL. (1987). Development of metabolic alkalosis after massive blood transfusion during orthotopic liver transplantation. Crit Care Med. 15, 905–908.

21. Williams DB, Lyons JH. (1980). Treatment of severe metabolic alkalosis with intravenous infusion of hydrochloric acid. Surg Gynecol Obstet. 150, 315–321.

22. Brimioulle S, Vincent JL, Dufaye P et al. (1985). Hydrochloric acid infusion for treatment of metabolic alkalosis: Effects on acid-base balance and oxygenation. Crit Care Med. 13, 738–742.

23. Duncan DA. (1984). Use of intravenous hydrochloric acid for the treatment of metabolic alkalosis in renal or hepatic failure. Int Med Spec. 5, 56–63.

Nutritional Support in the Critically Ill Adult

CHAPTER 12.1

Nutritional Support in the Critically Ill Adult

General Considerations

Good nutrition is often vital for survival in a critical illness. In poor developing countries many illnesses unfold against the background of malnutrition. The chances of a patient succumbing to a critical illness, increase with the degree of malnourishment present prior to the illness. A critically ill patient is often hypercatabolic from infection, injury and sepsis. Specific or multiple organ failure compounds the issue. These patients have an increase in energy requirements, and because of metabolic abnormalities have problems in the handling of energy substrates provided to them. Clinically they rapidly lose body weight, and in particular show a marked loss in the lean body mass. Nutritional support is therefore vital in the management of any critical illness. The more prolonged and more catabolic (or hypermetabolic) the illness, the greater the need and importance of nutritional support for survival.

In the large public and municipal hospitals of our country, in my opinion, over 50 per cent patients suffer from protein or calorie malnutrition. The cause of malnutrition in affluent groups is related to background disease, and occasionally to fads and fancies in eating habits. During the course of a critical illness, a loss of lean muscle mass of 10 per cent is significant, a loss of 20 per cent is critical, and a loss of 30 per cent or more is generally lethal (1). In a critical illness, absence of adequate nutritional support leads to a form of starvation. Skeletal muscle is therefore soon catabolized for gluconeogenesis and energy. Additional endogenous nutritional support is provided by important proteins synthesized by metabolically active tissue. These proteins have a rapid turnover and include liver enzyme proteins, renal tubular emzymes and proteins formed in the gastrointestinal mucosa (1). Endogenously derived nutritional support enables a critically ill individual to adapt to the stress of a critical illness, and provides the patient with an additional source of energy. The adaptation however is of benefit only in mild to moderate, short-lasting illnesses. In a severely catabolic long-lasting critical illness, the above response becomes 'maladaptive', and may well contribute to failure of individual or multiple organ systems, and thus be responsible for both increased morbidity and mortality.

Principles of Nutritional Management in the Critically Ill

The principles of nutritional support in the critically ill have evolved over the last 15–20 years. These are briefly enumerated below:

(i) Enteral nutrition (use of the gut for nutrition) has more advantages compared to parenteral nutrition (nutrients administered intravenously). The latter should therefore be offered only if the gut does not work, and hence cannot be used. When it is possible to provide even part of nutritional support via the gut, one should do so; parenteral nutrition is then used as a supplement to feeding via the gut. As a corollary to this principle, the importance of maintaining the structural and functional integrity of the gut, cannot be overstressed.

(ii) Conventional parenteral or enteral nutritional support has not been shown to produce an anabolic effect in malnourished critically ill patients. For example, patients with fulminant Grade IV tetanus (one of the most catabolic of all diseases), even if they survive, lose a great deal of body weight and lean muscle mass in spite of excellent nutritional support (3000 calories, with over 100 g proteins). The objective of parenteral nutrition in a critical illness, is therefore to blunt or reduce the effects of hypercatabolism.

Till the early nineties it used to be felt that the nutritional requirements of highly catabolic critical illnesses should be met by an increasing and excessive supply of calories. Patients in critical care units thus often received over 3500–4500 calories/day. Today this concept has been revised, and nutritional support is devised to provide a caloric intake of only 1500–2100 calories/day to most critically ill patients in the ICU. Only exceptional problems require a larger caloric intake. This revision is related to 2 observations: (a) Excessive caloric intake as already mentioned, does not prevent weight loss or loss of lean muscle mass. (b) Overzealous calorie administration contributes to a number of deleterious side-effects. These include hyperglycaemia, excessive carbon dioxide production, overhydration with peripheral and pulmonary oedema, hepatic dysfunction with steatosis and an increased incidence of non-catheter-related infections.

(iii) Most critical care units would prefer to initiate nutritional support early rather than late in the natural history of a critical illness. This is based on the logic that it is perhaps easier to prevent or reduce the complications of starvation, than to treat them after they have occurred. Early nutritional, and in particular early parenteral nutritional support, may however be overdone. Cost in our country is an important factor, and parenteral nutrition is extremely costly. The use of pre-operative parenteral nutrition in patients with mild malnutrition is of doubtful efficacy and may not result in any overall benefit. On the other hand, nutritional supplementation prior to surgery in severely malnourished patients, clearly reduces the incidence of post-operative complications (2).

(iv) Nutritional support should always be individualized both with regard to the appropriate mode of administration, and the nutritional requirements of each patient. This will depend on the nature of the disease and the nutritional state of the patient.

A little of 'this' added to a little of 'that' does not constitute good nutritional support; it only constitutes bad medicine.

(v) Nutritional support to a patient should be monitored with regard to the adequacy of the nutritional regime, response to treatment and possible side effects.

Clinical Effects of Nutritional Deprivation

The deleterious clinical effects of poor or absent nutrition include wound dehiscence, poor healing, breakdown of surgical anastomosis, and poor immune response to infection. Poor host resistance has been related to a deficiency in proteins and in essential aminoacids. Complicating sepsis or infection is thus an important feature in patients who have received poor nutritional support.

Non-specific effects are also observed in the central nervous system. These include apathy, drowsiness, and inability to clear secretions in the upper respiratory tract. The cause of these effects is unclear. They may be related to diminished energy supply to the brain, resulting in impaired function, or to toxic effects produced by the accumulation of products from the breakdown of muscle protein. Starvation produces an alteration in the aminoacid profile, and this may in turn affect the neurotransmitter profile within the brain, and thereby alter central nervous function.

The effect of nutritional deprivation is chiefly on lean muscle mass. More and more muscle is used for neoglucogenesis. Ultimately, even the intercostals, the diaphragm and the upper abdominals are compromised, and there is insufficient muscle mass to perform the work of breathing. This is one reason why it is difficult to wean patients after a very prolonged period of ventilator support. In some instances the muscles are so atrophic that even with hyperalimentation, muscle mass does not increase sufficiently for the patient to breathe on his own.

Berk is of the opinion that starvation in the presence of sepsis can contribute to multiple organ dysfunction and failure, particularly of the liver and kidneys (1). It was pointed out earlier that rapidly turning over proteins (such as enzymatic proteins produced by liver cells and kidney tubules), are used for gluconeogenesis to provide energy in patients with poor nutrition. It has been postulated that a significant contribution to hepatic and renal dysfunction may be due to cannibalization of important functional elements for gluconeogenesis (1).

Metabolic Effects of Nutritional Deprivation in 'Injury'

(Sepsis, Trauma, Catabolic Critical Illnesses)

The energy consumption pattern following 'injury' is altered, an increased proportion of energy (caloric) needs being derived from protein breakdown, rather than from the utilization of carbohydrates and fats. The requirement for an increased protein intake in these circumstances is obvious. The reason for altered utilization of energy substrates is due to glucose intolerance that develops as a response to hypercatabolic critical illnesses. Thus during stress, the maximal oxidation rate of glucose is only marginally increased to 3–5 mg/kg/min. The reasons for glucose intolerance include elevated levels of catecholamines and other catabolic hormones, increased glucagon levels with a high glucagon-insulin ratio, and a poor uptake and utilization of glucose by tissues, in particular by the liver. In fact, there exists a state of 'insulin resistance' during the 'stress' produced by a critical illness. The inability to take up and utilize glucose, has been thought to be related to both receptor and post-receptor defects in tissue cells. Post-receptor alterations in glucose metabolism may involve steps responsible for glucose uptake (transport and phosphorylation), glycogenolysis, glycolysis or oxidation. If exogenous glucose is not supplied (as in starvation), muscle, brain and other tissues will use for energy, glucose derived from muscle protein breakdown (gluconeogenesis), or ketone bodies derived from free fatty acids liberated by lipolysis. In addition, muscle is capable of using the branched-chain aminoacids (leucine, valine and isoleucine) for energy directly, without the intervention of glucose.

In the metabolic pattern produced by 'injury' (e.g. sepsis, severe trauma), in addition to glucose intolerance, there is an inability of the liver to manufacture ketone bodies, and an impairment in the utilization of fatty acids for energy. There is thus a marked increase in the breakdown of lean body mass to meet increased energy needs, and to provide the necessary calories for function of vital organ systems.

The association of fever, tissue damage, blood, plasma and protein loss, compound the metabolic problems in critically ill patients. Additional metabolic requirements secondary to the increased work of breathing may deprive important organ systems of necessary energy substrates, the latter being partially diverted to muscles of respiration. Fever significantly adds to caloric needs. Each degree of fever causes a 10–13 per cent increase in oxygen consumption (1), necessitating an increase in calorie requirement.

Timing for Nutritional Support

Theoretically speaking, any critically ill patient who is unable to take adequate nutrition, should promptly receive nutritional support. There are however important points to consider before initiating nutritional support, and in particular parenteral nutritional support.

(i) Nutritional deprivation, in an illness lasting for a few days, is not likely to produce problems or complications. The number of days that a patient can withstand inadequate nutrition depends on age, previous nutritional status, previous state of health, and the presence of sepsis or trauma. An adult under 60 years of age, and in a previously good nutritional state, will withstand 14 days of poor nutrition in a moderately catabolic illness, without demonstrating a measurable defect. For patients between 60–70 years, this tolerance drops to 10 days, and for those > 70 years, to less than 7 days (1). *Nevertheless, one does not await the effects of starvation before starting nutritional support.*

(ii) The excessive cost of parenteral nutrition precludes its unnecessary use during short periods of inadequate nutrition in a critical illness.

(iii) Nutritional support, and in particular parenteral nutritional support, has inherent risks and can cause dangerous iatrogenic complications. These risks may well outbalance the risk of poor nutrition that is anticipated to last just under a week.

(iv) For improved outcomes, *current recommendations advocate early nutritional support in patients critically ill in the ICU.* Our policy is to initiate support promptly if enteral feeds are feasible. If enteral feeds are not feasible, or provide only a portion of the patient's nutritional requirements, we initiate parenteral nutrition within 3 to 7 days depending on the severity of the catabolic nature of the illness.

(v) *In an acute, hypercatabolic critical illness, stabilization of haemodynamics, and correction of fluid, electrolyte and acid-base balance take precedence over nutrition. The latter can be started once the patient is reasonably stable in relation to his vital parameters.*

Objectives of Nutritional Support

A recent consensus conference held by the American College of Chest Physicians defined the objectives of nutritional support in critically ill patients as follows: (i) provide support consistent with the patient's medical problem, nutritional state and available route for nutrient administration; (ii) prevent or treat macronutrient and micronutrient deficiencies; (iii) provide nutrition compatible with patients' metabolism; (iv) improve patient outcomes with regard to both morbidity and mortality (3).

Indications for Parenteral Nutrition

Parenteral nutrition is indicated in patients in whom the gut does not function, or in those who undergo any form of treatment which precludes the use of the gut for the foreseeable future. Parenteral nutrition improves the outcome in the short bowel syndrome, enterocutaneous fistulae with a large leak > 500 ml from the fistulae, major burns, and acute tubular necrosis. Nutritional support is also of value in necrotizing or suppurative pancreatitis (till such time as the gut can be used), sepsis, prolonged ileus from any cause, stomal dysfunction after surgery, and in large wounds causing loss of proteins from the wound surface. Nutritional support is often offered to selected patients with cancer, and to malnourished patients as a preparation for major surgery. Parenteral nutrition may be a supplement to enteral nutrition in many of these problems, so that caloric requirements and adequate protein intake are ensured. In many instances where the gut does not work or cannot be used, total parental nutrition (TPN) is employed.

Indications for Enteral Feeding

Patients with a functioning small bowel, who for any reason cannot take food orally, or who cannot meet their nutritional requirements, are given special supplements and/or tube feedings. The important indications, contraindications and further details of enteral nutrition, are discussed later in this chapter.

Nutritional Assessment

An assessment of the nutritional state of a critically ill patient is not always easy. The goal is to identify patients at risk for increased morbidity and mortality because of poor nutrition, thereby enabling the clinician to focus attention on nutritional support. There is no magic formula to determine the nutritional state of the patient. Clinical evaluation and laboratory findings should be combined to enable an overall assessment to be made (4).

Major parameters used in nutritional assessment are the patient's history, clinical examination, and the anthropometric measurements and laboratory data.

History and Clinical Examination

Important features in the history include the medical and surgical background of current and past illnesses with specific reference to conditions that could impair ingestion, digestion or absorption of nutrients. Physical examination should specifically seek clinical evidence of protein-calorie malnutrition, deficiency of essential fatty acids, anaemia, vitamin deficiencies, and deficiency of trace elements.

Anthropometric Measurements

A basic anthropometric measurement is that of height and body weight. This should be compared to the usual body weight rather than to the ideal body weight. Weight gain or loss may have important implications. However in the critically ill patient, fluctuations in body weight are often related to variations in hydration of the patient. Thus a critically ill patient who has lost a significant degree of lean muscle mass, may yet be normal in weight due to significant water retention. Other anthropometric measurements like the skin fold thickness and arm circumference, have proved to be of less value.

Biochemical Data

(i) Serum Proteins and Serum Albumin Levels

The serum albumin level in particular is a good marker or predictor of malnutrition, as it provides an index of the visceral and somatic protein stores in a critical illness. There are however a few important points to be remembered in interpreting low serum albumin levels. A fall in the serum albumin may be brought about by rapid intravenous hydration or an overhydrated state, rather than by a change in the nutritional status. Again, low albumin levels may occur with increased catabolism, decreased synthesis (as in liver disease), or in increased loss (as in burns, large wounds, in faeces or in urine), even when the patient has been adequately nourished. Finally even if a low serum albumin level in a critical illness serves as a marker for the initial nutritional state, it does not serve as a marker if the nutritional state has improved following nutritional support. This is because serum albumin has a half-life of 20 days and the plasma level does not rise significantly for 4–5 weeks following nutritional repletion.

(ii) Estimation of Levels of Serum Transferrin, Thyroxin-binding Prealbumin, Retinol-binding Protein and Fibronectin

Lowered levels of transferrin (half-life 8 days), thyroxin-binding prealbumin (half-life 2 days), retinol-binding protein (half-life 12 hours), and fibronectin (half-life 12 hours), have all been used in well-equipped laboratories as indices of malnutrition. A significant rise in these proteins following repletion, is observed fairly early and points to an improved nutritional state. We have never used these esoteric markers for reasons of cost. Though they may be of use, they cannot replace a holistic evaluation of the patient based on history, clinical examination, and on simple laboratory data.

(iii) Estimation of 24 hours Urinary Urea Nitrogen Excretion and Determination of Nitrogen Balance

This test evaluates somatic protein status. It provides a good index of protein breakdown, and if the protein intake is known, the nitrogen balance can easily be calculated.

$$\text{Nitrogen Balance} = \text{Nitrogen Intake} - \text{Nitrogen Excretion}$$

$$= \frac{\text{Protein Intake}}{6.25} - (24\text{ hrs Urinary Urea Nitrogen Excretion} + 4)$$

The 4 g are added to the urinary nitrogen loss to account for faecal and other losses in patients fed via the gut. Faecal loss of nitrogen is often much less. It is near zero to 1 g when patients receive total parenteral nutrition even when there is diarrhoea (5).

A urinary loss of less than 6 g is normal; loss of 6–12 g/day is mild; loss of 12–18 g is moderate and more than 18 g/day indicates severe catabolism. Since 1 g of urea nitrogen is equivalent to 6.25 g of nonhydrated protein, a total loss of 16 g nitrogen would mean that about 100 g protein needs to be given to maintain nitrogen balance.

The above concept holds as long as the urine is a major source of nitrogen loss. It does not hold in patients who lose large quantities of nitrogen through the gut as in diarrhoea, or through the surface of extensive weeping wounds. Nitrogen balance cannot be correctly evaluated by this equation in patients with nitrogen retention due to renal insufficiency.

Other Laboratory Data

Other laboratory data that need to be assessed include serum electrolytes, renal and hepatic function, pulmonary function, haematopoietic function, and basic parameters for evidence of osteoporosis or osteomalacia.

Nutritional Requirements

Caloric Requirements (6–9)

On an average most critically ill individuals expend and therefore need 25–35 kcal per kilogram ideal body weight per day. The resting metabolic expenditure can also be estimated by using the Harris-Benedict equation (10). This formula or equation is as follows.

In Males: $HB = 66.5 + 13.7\,W + 5\,H - 6.8\,A$
In Females: $HB = 66.5 + 9.6\,W + 1.7\,H - 4.7\,A$

where W = Weight (kg); H = Height (cm); A = Age.

The caloric requirement increases with the stress and catabolism of illness. Calvin Long's stress factors (8) take the catabolism of illness into consideration. Thus the caloric requirement is as follows:

$1.3 \times HB$ for sepsis or uncomplicated major surgery
$1.5 \times HB$ for complicated sepsis (with organ failure)
   and burns < 20 per cent
$2 \times HB$ for burns > 20 per cent

We are of the opinion that *it is quite unnecessary to use either the Harris-Benedict equation or the Calvin Long's 'stress factors'*. Predictive equations can be notoriously unreliable in critically ill individuals (11) and the use of 'corrective stress factors' invariably overestimates the caloric requirements of critically ill patients.

Measurement of Caloric Requirements by an Indirect Calorimeter

Indirect calorimetry computes the respiratory quotient (RQ) and the daily resting energy expenditure (REE), by measuring the respiratory gas exchange—oxygen consumption ($\dot{V}O_2$), the carbon dioxide production ($\dot{V}CO_2$) and the minute ventilation ($\dot{V}_E$). An apparatus called the 'metabolic cart' measures the oxygen concentration of inhaled oxygen, and the CO_2 concentration of exhaled gas. The metabolic cart can be wheeled to the patient's bedside, and devices to measure the $\dot{V}O_2$ and the $\dot{V}CO_2$ can be suitably connected to the ventilator tubings to measure gas exchange across the lungs. The REE is calculated thus:

$$\text{REE (kcal/min)} = 3.94\,(\dot{V}O_2) + 1.1\,(\dot{V}CO_2)$$
$$\text{REE (kcal/day)} = \text{REE} \times 1440$$

The gas exchange measurements are usually obtained over a 30 minute period, and the REE is extrapolated to 24 hours (12).

Indirect calorimetry provides an exact method of measuring caloric needs in a critically ill patient. However if the patient is at rest, this method usually underestimates the caloric needs by 10–15 per cent, as no allowance has been made for activity. The caloric requirement should therefore be stepped to 10–15 per cent more than the computed value. Indirect calorimetry is expensive, and time-consuming. At higher inspired fraction of oxygen (> 60 per cent) the values obtained are unreliable. Although theoretically, 'replacing energy expenditure' is reasonable, it is debatable whether such a balance is effective and improves outcome. We do not possess a 'metabolic cart' and employ a very simple approach to compute nutritional needs of critically ill patients in our unit.

We prefer to initially administer 25 kcal/kg per day in which total

Table 12.1.1. Caloric requirement in a critically ill adult

Nutrient	Quantity	Percentage of total calories	Initial requirement for 60 kg adult
Total calories	25 kcal/kg/day	100 per cent	1500 kcal/day
Protein, peptides and aminoacids	1–1.75 g/kg/day	15–25 per cent	60–70 g/day 240–280 kcal/day
Carbohydrates	3–3.5 g/kg/day	40–60 per cent	190 g/day 760 kcal/day
Fats	0.75–1 g/kg/day	20–30 per cent	50 g/day 450 kcal/day

Micronutritients in the form of vitamins, minerals and trace elements should also be adequately provided to meet the needs of the patient.

kilocalories in the day are split into 20 per cent protein, 30 per cent fats and 50 per cent carbohydrates. Current recommendations in ICU patients are to apportion 60 to 70 per cent of non protein calories as carbohydrates and 30–35 per cent as fat. Proteins and carbohydrates provide 4 kcal/g, and fats provide 9 kcal/g. (**Table 12.1.1**).

Carbohydrates

These are important and provide ready fuel for energy. Excessive glucose administration however has the following disadvantages:

(i) It increases norepinephrine secretion; this in turn increases energy expenditure, glucagon secretion and insulin resistance.

(ii) Glucose is poorly utilized in sepsis and other catabolic states. Excessive glucose and carbohydrate administration will thus lead to severe hyperglycaemia, particularly in diabetes (13).

(iii) Excessive glucose is converted to fat in the liver, and produces steatosis.

(iv) In critically ill patients, excessive use of glucose for non-protein calories nearly doubles the production of carbon dioxide. This increases pulmonary work load (14). Weaning therefore becomes difficult in patients on ventilator support.

Lipids

Lipids provide 30–50 per cent of ingested calories, and are as good as hypertonic glucose in improving protein synthesis in catabolic patients. Linoleic acid is the only essential fatty acid that must be provided for. It should constitute 4 per cent of the total caloric intake, else a fatty acid deficiency results (15). The latter is typically seen after a few weeks of fat-free intravenous alimentation. The clinical manifestations include an eczema-like rash with neutropaenia and thrombocytopaenia. The syndrome can be countered by the use of intravenous lipid emulsions or the oral intake of 10–15 ml/day of safflower oil.

Protein Requirements

The minimum protein intake is 0.5 g/kg/day. In most patients in the ICU, an intake of 0.75–1 g/kg/day suffices. In highly catabolic states the intake is between 1.5 to 2 g/kg/day. Perhaps severe burns and fulminant tetanus are the only catabolic states which might require an even higher intake of up to 2.5 g/kg/day.

Protein catabolism can be measured as stated earlier, by estimating the 24 hour loss of urea nitrogen in the urine. Nitrogen balance studies may help adjust protein intake. Nevertheless, it is generally impossible to prevent loss of lean muscle weight in critically ill catabolic patients. It is therefore unwise to use large quantities of proteins. This merely adds to the metabolic problems encountered during nutritional support. Attempts to provide adequate protein to patients in hepatic or renal failure may fail because of increasing azotaemia or worsening encephalopathy. Indications for a decrease in protein administration include a rising blood urea nitrogen that exceeds 100 mg/dl or an elevated serum ammonia level that is associated with encephalopathy.

Water and Electrolytes

Carbohydrates given to a malnourished patient reduce salt and water excretion. If sodium is also provided simultaneously, there is a significant expansion of the extracellular volume, resulting in weight gain. Many catabolic states may also be associated with diminished salt and water excretion. The possibility of a fluid overload must therefore be always kept in mind following the initiation of total parenteral nutrition.

Vitamins

Twelve essential vitamins need to be supplied. The daily requirements may be much higher in seriously ill or catabolic patients. Low serum values of vitamins were observed in 25 per cent of adult males in a surgical ICU (16). Intravenous replacement therapy even in large doses failed to correct these low values in as many as 40 per cent of these patients (16).

Thiamine deficiency, folate deficiency and deficiency of Vitamins A, C and E are fairly often observed (16, 17).

Trace Elements

The nine necessary trace elements that need to be included in nutritional support are iron, zinc, manganese, molybdenum, copper, chromium, selenium, iodine and cobalt. They are present in many enteral feed formulations, but some of these trace elements may need to be added to TPN solutions. Requirements of trace elements may increase in patients with diarrhoea or malabsorption. Supplements of manganese and copper are avoided or reduced in patients with liver cell dysfunction.

Total caloric requirement for either parenteral or enteral feeds and in particular the protein content supplied will depend both on the nature of the illness and the background nutritional state of the patient. The recommendations for nutritional requirement in different critical problems are discussed later in this chapter.

Methods of Nutritional Support

There are two methods of nutritional support—enteral and parenteral. When nutrition is provided totally by the parenteral (i.e. intravenous) route it is termed total parenteral nutrition (TPN). Parenteral nutrition is generally provided through a central vein; it could also be given via a peripheral vein. Both parenteral and enteral routes are often used in the same patient. Though both methods can provide equal nutritional support, the enteral mode or method is always to be preferred whenever this is possible. The following points need to be kept in mind:

(i) Parenteral nutrition alters the normal physiology of nutrition. Physiological changes during parenteral nutrition include an alteration in body composition, and an increased blood flow to the gut (18).

(ii) Hepatic dysfunction, in particular steatosis, is frequent with parenteral nutrition. There are also changes in the blood levels of pancreatic and gastrointestinal hormones.

(iii) The absence of direct enteral stimulation by nutrients during parenteral nutrition, can disturb the structural and functional integrity of the gut (19–23).

(iv) The absence of enteral nutrition reduces the immune function of the gut. The gut can be an important portal of entry for pathogens in critically ill patients. Translocation of bacteria from within the lumen to the mesenteric glands and then to the bloodstream is ordinarily prevented by gastric acid, intact peristalsis and normal bacterial gut flora. These factors are altered in an intensive care setting by antacids, H_2-antagonists, antibiotics, as also by disuse atrophy of the gut in patients on parenteral feeds. IgA normally present in the intestinal mucosa is also decreased in parenterally fed patients. This robs the gut of an important immune defence mechanism. It is likely that enteral feeds besides maintaining the absorptive function of the mucosa, also maintain the functional integrity of the mucosal barrier, and prevent translocation of bacteria outside the lumen of the gut. The latter aspect may be of great importance in critically ill patients in an ICU setting.

(v) Parenteral nutrition is far more expensive than enteral nutrition.

(vi) Both methods can be associated with complications—technical, infectious and metabolic. In our experience, parenteral nutrition has greater hazards when compared to enteral feeding.

(vii) Parenteral nutrition should be terminated once enteral feeds are tolerated.

Enteral Nutrition

Indications

Full enteral support is indicated in the following conditions (24):

(i) Malnourished patients whose oral intake is poor for 3–5 days.

(ii) Well nourished patients with poor oral intake for 7–10 days.

(iii) Inability for whatever reason to eat adequately: oropharyngeal lesions, oesophageal lesions, neurological disorders involving the upper GI tract.

(iv) Following massive small bowel resection (90 per cent)—enteral nutrition helps in the regeneration of small bowel mucosa.

(v) Enterocutaneous fistulae with an output of < 500 ml/day.

Enteral feeds allow absorption, and probably do not interfere with spontaneous closure of the fistulae.

(vi) Severe full thickness burns. There is some evidence that early enteral feeds limit sepsis and reduce protein loss from the bowel in these patients.

(vii) Following major upper GI surgery (total oesophagectomy or total gastrectomy), feeds administered through a tube catheter jejunostomy are necessary.

(viii) Following surgery for necrotizing, suppurative pancreatitis. Initial TPN in these patients is followed by jejunostomy feeds or feeds through a nasojejunal tube following recovery of small bowel function.

Although enteral feeds are generally well tolerated in critically ill individuals, there are case reports of bowel infarction during jejunal feeds in pressor-dependent patients (25). It was postulated that jejunal feeds increased oxygen demand in a segment of the bowel that was poorly perfused. It is therefore best to commence enteral feeds only after the patient is haemodynamically stable. Initial feeds should be small; they should be gradually increased if the patient tolerates them.

Contraindications

Enteral feeds are contraindicated in:

(i) Generalized suppurative peritonitis.

(ii) Complete intestinal obstruction.

(iii) Ileus from any cause.

(iv) Ischaemia to the bowel.

(v) Patients with severe shock.

(vi) Enterocutaneous fistulae with a large output.

(vii) Acute fulminant necrotizing pancreatitis (in the early phase).

In severe uncontrolled diarrhoea we give arrowroot, electral water (water + electrolytes), weak tea without milk orally, and give the main nutritional support through intravenous alimentation.

Access

Enteral feeds can be infused into the stomach, duodenum or jejunum. This can be achieved by a nasogastric tube, nasoduodenal or nasojejunal tube, a percutaneous feeding gastrostomy, or a jejunostomy. A feeding jejunostomy is fashioned through a tube or catheter (tube jejunostomy) at surgery.

Gastric Feeding. Enteral feeds infused into the stomach can have both advantages and disadvantages. The advantage is that the stomach initiates digestion though no nutrients are absorbed. Gastric acid secretion helps to sterilize gastric contents and the risk of bacterial contamination of the gut is reduced. The stomach can also protect the gut from an osmotic load. In the presence of hyperosmotic fluid, the motility of the stomach is reduced. Gastric secretions dilute the hyperosmolar load till it is iso-osmolar; the contents then pass through the pylorus into the duodenum and small gut.

The major disadvantage of enteral feeds infused into the stomach, is the development of gastric atony. Gastric atony is more frequent than atony of the small gut in critically ill patients. Feeds cannot be continued in the presence of severe atony, else there is the danger of aspiration pneumonia. When enteral feeds are infused into the stomach, gastric residual volume should be monitored frequently—every 2–4 hours. In spite of monitoring, acute gastric atony with dilatation can occur suddenly, and in critically ill patients can cause massive aspiration of gastric contents into the lungs. It is then mandatory to discontinue gastric feeds.

Duodenal Feeding is often preferred for the above reasons to gastric feeding. The feeding tube is inserted through the nostril or through a gastrostomy. At times in presence of gastric atony it is necessary to insert a separate nasogastric tube in order to aspirate gastric contents, or to administer sucralfate for treatment or prevention of bleeds caused by stress ulcers.

The earlier feeding tubes were large bore (14–16 French), rigid tubes placed in the stomach. For reasons of economy, we still have to make do with these tubes. The newer feeding tubes are narrow (8 French), flexible and are available in longer lengths for intubation of the small bowel (26). These tubes add to patient comfort and reduce the risk of reflux and aspiration pneumonia (27). Because of lack of easy availability and increased expense, we use the new narrow tubes only in rare instances. The finer tubes however have one disadvantage, and that is the risk of misplacement of the tube in the tracheobronchial tree, with disastrous consequences. The fine bore tubes require a stylet for insertion, and in ill patients with a blunted cough reflex, can quite easily go through the larynx and into the trachea. They can also pass by the side of the inflated cuff of an endotracheal or tracheostomy tube. If this goes unrecognized, a small bore feeding tube may find its way right into the pleural space. The tube position should therefore always be checked. The tip of the tube is radiopaque, and a chest X-ray should show the tube below the diaphragm. A lateral view of the chest should also be done if there is doubt about the tube placement. Aspiration of contents through the tube helps; if the aspirate has an acid pH (< 3), the tube lies within the stomach (28).

Jejunal Feeding is now being used frequently all over the world. It is used particularly in patients following major abdominal surgery, and severe trauma. The technique is either a needle jejunostomy or a tube (catheter) jejunostomy. A feeding jejunostomy allows full use of the gut despite ileus involving the stomach and the large bowel. When for any reason enteral feeds in the stomach are contraindicated, we prefer to infuse feeds through a jejunostomy. Technically, small bore tubes advanced through the pylorus into the small bowel, avoid quite a few problems associated with a direct feeding jejunostomy. It is often difficult to manoeuvre these newer fine bore tubes through the pylorus into the small bowel. The procedure is preferably done under fluoroscopic guidance.

Starting Tube Feeds

A test infusion is indicated to determine the safety of gastric feeds. A volume of N saline equivalent to the desired hourly feeding volume, is infused into the stomach (in patients with nasogastric tubes) over 1 hour. The feeding tube is clamped for 30 minutes, and the residual volume aspirated. If the volume is < 50 per cent of the infused quantity, gastric feeding can be started. If during feeds the aspirated residual volume increases, the feeds need to be given at a slower rate, or temporarily stopped. It is best to give the test volume as an infusion and not as a bolus. The latter causes gastric distension and can delay gastric emptying. The residual volume can then be greater than that observed if the volume load had been given by an infusion.

Feeding Patterns

Intermittent infusions are now frowned upon, though we admit to its use over years. The popular method of delivery is by a continuous infusion over 16 hours. This is believed to reduce the risk of aspiration and diarrhoea; it also produces more weight gain and a positive nitrogen balance (29).

Tube feedings are initiated by starter regimes that use less calories and a slower infusion rate. Both caloric intake and volume are then increased to desired levels over a few days. The rationale is to initially avoid the occurrence of diarrhoea by not overloading a gut which has had no nutrients to deal with for the preceding 4–7 days. Many units however forego starter regimes, and commence full enteral feeds from the outset, except in patients who have had no enteral feeds for several days. Starter regimes should always be used when enteral feeds are administered through a jejunostomy or through a nasojejunal tube. This is because the small bowel does not have the reservoir capacity of the stomach, and diarrhoea invariably results if feeds are not initiated through starter regimes. An isotonic feeding formula is diluted to a quarter of its strength, and started at 25 ml/hr (30). The infusion rate is increased by 25 ml every hour, till the target rate is achieved (31). The concentration of the feeding solution is now increased over the next few days, full nutrition being achieved within 4 days (30). Jejunal feeds are preferably given as an infusion over a 6 hour period.

Types of Enteral Feeds (Formulations) (32)

Unfortunately very few satisfactory special formulations for enteral feeds are available in our country. A frequently used formulation is *Ensure*, which is both lactose and gluten free. 1 ml of this formulation provides one calorie. The calories contained in one serving amount to 250 calories in 250 ml. Each serving of 250 calories contains 9 g of protein (14.2 per cent calories), 9 g of fat (31.8 per cent calories) and 34 g carbohydrates (54 per cent calories) + 200 g water + 24 key vitamins and minerals. 1500 ml of the formulation (i.e 6 servings) would thus give a caloric intake of 1500 calories with the distribution of protein, carbohydrate and fat as indicated above (i.e. 54 g protein, 54 g fat and 204 g carbohydrates). The formulation has an osmolarity of 379 mosm/l H_2O.

The formulation *Ensure Plus HN* provides a higher caloric and higher protein content. Each serving contains 355 calories in 237 ml, with 14.8 g protein, 11.8 g fat and 47.3 g carbohydrates together with vitamins and minerals. This formulation is hyperosmolar (1.5 kcal/ml), the osmolarity being 500 mosm/l H_2O.

When special formulations are available (as in Western countries), the following characteristics help in selecting the appropriate formula for the patient (33):

(a) Caloric Density and Osmolality: (i) The formulations that provide 1 kcal/ml are isotonic to plasma, and are preferred for small bowel feeds. They include preparations such as Osmolite or Isocal.

(ii) The formulations which provide 1.5–2 kcal/ml are hypertonic or high density formulas, and are preferred when fluid intake needs to be restricted. These feeds should be administered preferably into the stomach. Gastric secretions dilute the feeds and render them isotonic before they reach the small bowel. High caloric density formulations include Osmolite HN (2 kcal/ml) and Isocal HN (2 kcal/ml).

(b) *Protein Content.* Most enteral formulas provide up to 14–20 per cent of total calories as proteins. There is no evidence to suggest that a higher protein content improves morbidity or mortality. Intact protein is more difficult to absorb than hydrolysated protein. The latter is preferred in malabsorption and in the short bowel syndrome. Peptide based formulas can reduce diarrhoea from tube feedings (34).

(c) *Fat Complexity.* Median chain triglycerides are easier to absorb than long chain triglycerides, and are favoured in patients with malabsorption. Most enteral formulas have long chain triglycerides, but some have a combination of both (e.g. Isocal).

Classification of Enteral Feeds (32)

Enteral feeding formulas are classified according to the nature of nutrients, or the ease of absorption (33). The important enteral feeds and formulations available in the West are listed below.

(i) *Liquidized or Blenderized Food.* They are liquid forms of table food. We can use these enteral feeds for most patients (see below).

(ii) *Lactose-Free Formulas.* There are several standard feeding formulas available in the West. These standard formulations are indicated in patients with a normal GI tract who do not tolerate lactose. Examples: Isocal 1 kcal/ml; Sustacal HC 1.5 kcal/ml; Isocal HCN 2 kcal/ml.

(iii) *Chemically Defined Formulas.* These contain hydrolysated protein instead of intact protein, to facilitate absorption, and are indicated in patients with impaired ability to absorb nutrients. Examples: Criticare HN; Vital HN.

(iv) *Elemental Formulas.* The elemental formulas contain aminoacids. Most of the nutrients are well absorbed in the jejunum. These are indicated in patients with limited absorptive capacity and are often used for jejunal feeds. Example: Vivonex 1kcal/ml.

Liquefied or Blenderized Feeds

We have devised for our unit enteral feeds that contain naturally available nutrients. These nutrients include milk, whey, curds, fruit juice, protein powders, glucose, and liquidized potatoes, rice and vegetables. The protein content can be further increased in those intolerant to milk or milk products by liquidizing chicken or meat. Alternatively, high protein containing powders can be added. The commonly used protein preparations are listed in **Table 12.1.2.** Fat content is provided by measured quantity of butter. This cocktail is made up to a desired volume by the addition of water, and fed to the patient at the rate of 200 ml 2 hourly. It is easier to feed liquidized food in the above fashion through the old-fashioned nasogastric tube. The Buttermilk Diet (BMD) can be used for patients with increased caloric requirements (e.g. those with severe burns) (see **Table 18.2.4**); 1 l of BMD provides 1000 kcal, 60 g of

proteins and 340 g of carbohydrates. Jejunostomy feeds require more meticulous preparation before they can be given through the jejunostomy catheters. Nevertheless it is important to be aware of what is available in the outside world, even if these preparations remain at present of theoretical interest. It must needs be said that in our unit, the morbidity and mortality of critically ill patients given enteral nutritional support in the manner outlined above, is no higher than that observed in units in the West that use special feeding formulas. We do encounter diarrhoea with the liquidized food prepared as described above, but it is generally controllable.

A model nasogastric/jejunostomy blenderized tube feed administered in the ICU at the Breach Candy Hospital, Mumbai, is detailed in **Table 12.1.3.**

Table 12.1.2. Commonly used high protein preparations

* Simyl MCT Powder	– 14 g proteins/100 g powder
* GRD Biscuits	– 1.5 g protein/biscuit
* Threptin Biscuits	– 1.5 g protein/biscuit
* Trophox Powder	– 6 g protein/10 g powder
* Proteinex Powder	– 5.6 g protein/10 g powder
* Complan Powder	– 20 g protein/100 g powder
* Casein Powder	– 1.4 g protein/measure

Table 12.1.3. A model nasogastric/jejunostomy blenderized tube feed for a 70 kg adult administered in the ICU, Breach Candy Hospital, Mumbai

Time	Feed	Quantity
6 am	Milk + 1 Egg + 1 tbsp glucose	200 ml
8 am	Coccnut water + 1 tbsp glucose + 4 measures casein	200 ml
10 am	Fruit juice + 1 tbsp glucose	200 ml
12 noon	50 g pureed chicken + 15 g butter	200 ml
2 pm	Rice + Boiled mixed vegetables + 30 ml vegetable oil	200 ml
4 pm	Beaten curd + 1 tbsp glucose + 4 measures casein	200 ml
6 pm	Banana milk shake + 1 tbsp glucose + 4 measures casein	200 ml
8 pm	Pureed vegetable soup + 15 g butter	200 ml
10 pm	Rice + Boiled mixed vegetables + 30 ml vegetable oil	100 ml
11 pm	Stewed apple + 1 tbsp glucose + 4 measures casein	100 ml
4 am	Milk + 1 sachet of Ten-O-Lip + 2 tbsp glucose	200 ml

Total Quantity—2000 ml
Total Calories Supplied—1900 calories

Proteins —75 g	300 calories	
Carbohydrates—200 g	800 calories	
Fats—90 g	800 calories	

Complications of Enteral Feeding

(i) *Gastric Retention, Vomiting and Aspiration Pneumonia.* These are most often observed when feeds are infused into the stomach. The reported incidence of aspiration varies from 1 to 44 per cent (34). Aspiration is in our opinion, less likely when feeds are infused into the duodenum or jejunum. A trace of bright color may be added to feeds when aspiration is suspected. If respiratory secretions aspirated through a tracheostomy or endotracheal tube are similarly coloured, it is a pointer to definite aspiration.

(ii) Diarrhoea. This is the most frequent and most troublesome complication of enteral feeding.

The following steps should be taken to control the diarrhoea:

(a) Reduce the feeds by half. Avoid lactose in the feeds, and avoid bolus feeding. Use Pectokab (pectin and kaolin combination), and aluminum hydroxide; stop magnesium antacids if they are being administered. Examine stools for ova, parasites, and Cl. difficile toxin.

(b) Use isotonic and not hyperosmotic solutions.

(c) Check if antibiotics could possibly be causing diarrhoea.

(d) When available, special feeding formulas containing aminoacids alone, or in combination with small amounts of peptide, may be used. These may help in patients with poor digestion and absorption. In patients with pancreatitis, pancreatic enzymes need to be given with enteral feeds.

(e) If diarrhoea still persists, tincture opium 2–3 minims thrice daily, or 10 ml paregoric twice daily may be used for 2–3 days.

(f) If diarrhoea relents slowly, build feeds to the desired levels.

(g) If it continues for a week, it is best to shift to partial parenteral nutrition. As far as possible, it is wise to continue with small enteral feeds (arrowroot, whey, electral water). Total stoppage of enteral feeds often aggravates diarrhoea when enteral feeding is reattempted at a future date.

(iii) Mechanical Problems. Small bore feeding tubes become obstructed by plugs of nutrient material in 10 per cent of patients (**35**). The tube should therefore be flushed with water before and after infusion of nutrients (**36**). When the tubes are not being used for infusion, they are filled with water and plugged. If the tube is blocked and the block cannot be flushed out with warm water, a warm solution of 7.5 per cent sodium bicarbonate is used to flush the tube. If unsuccessful, the feeding tube needs to be replaced.

Parenteral Nutrition

The total caloric requirements, the protein content and the ratio of carbohydrates to fat in patients requiring TPN, have already been discussed. The indications for TPN have also been detailed earlier. The present section will briefly deal with access, type of solutions in use, methods of administration and complications.

Access

In an intensive care unit, TPN is generally given through a central vein. We prefer to secure the subclavian vein through the usual percutaneous technique. It is convenient for the patient who can move his head and neck freely, and allows better sterile dressings when compared to a catheter in the internal jugular vein. This central line once secured is reserved solely for infusing nutrients required for TPN. We never infuse drugs, antibiotics, crystalloids or colloid infusions through this line. All other infusions are given through a separate lumen if a triple lumen catheter is in place, or through a separate peripheral vein.

Parenteral nutrition may also be infused through peripheral veins. This is appropriate for short-term nutritional support or in patients in whom central veins are inaccessible. Thrombophlebitis is frequent when peripheral veins are used because of the high osmolality of the nutrient solutions. Nutrient solutions with an osmolality > 900 mosm/l invariably produce peripheral venous thrombophlebitis. Osmolality of nutrient solutions can be reduced by decreasing the glucose concentration and substituting lipid solutions to provide the necessary calories

Types of Solutions for Use

Dextrose. Dextrose solutions (10, 20, 50 per cent) supply 4 kcal/gram and constitute the carbohydrate content of parenteral therapy. Solutions with an osmolarity greater than 300 mosm/l are hyperosmolar. 500 ml of 20 per cent dextrose solution would provide 100 g of carbohydrate with a caloric value of 400 calories.

Lipid Solutions. Fat has a caloric equivalent of 9 kcal/g. Fat emulsions in use are rendered isotonic by addition of glycerol. The chief source of fatty acids in intravenous fatty emulsions is soya bean, with or without safflower. Linoleic acid constitutes 50–65 per cent and linolenic acid 4–9 per cent of the fatty acid content. Fatty emulsions marketed as Intralipid are available in India as either 10 per cent or 20 per cent fat emulsions.

Crystalline Aminoacids. The formulations available contain 40–50 per cent of essential aminoacids, and 50–60 per cent of non-essential aminoacids. Available concentrations of aminoacids vary from 3.5–10 per cent, with varying total nitrogenous content (5.4–16 g) of the solutions. The protein content is computed by multiplying the nitrogen content in g by 6.2, so that a nitrogen content of say 10 g would equal a protein content of about 60 g. The exact aminoacid and electrolyte profile may also vary in different formulations. From the clinical points of view all products are by and large similar. There are also solutions designed specifically for certain disorders. Solutions preferred for renal failure supply concentrated essential aminoacids and L-histidine. Those preferred for hepatic encephalopathy contain a high concentration of branched-chain aminoacids (valine, leucine, isoleucine). Vitamins, electrolytes, and trace elements should be provided as additives. Vitamins B and C are extremely important, as are B12, folate, vitamin A and vitamin D. Most vitamins are present in formulations of aminoacid mixtures. In large wounds and after major surgeries, extra vitamin C to the extent of 1 to 2 g/day should be given. Large doses of vitamin A and vitamin D can cause toxicity. 5000 units of vitamin A and 500 units of vitamin D on a weekly basis are generally adequate. Trace elements, in particular zinc, need to be given separately as deficiency in these elements may result. It is important that other than sodium, potassium and chloride, calcium, magnesium and phosphates also need to be replaced, and at times replenished in depleted body stores.

Administration

Dextrose, intralipid (lipid solution), aminoacid solutions can be given as separate solutions through a triple lumen catheter inserted into a central vein. The advantage of this method is that one can tailor the exact quantity of carbohydrate, fats, proteins and the total calories that need to be given to a critically ill patient. Currently, many manufacturers supply either all-in-one solutions or two-in-one solutions. All-in-one solutions contain dextrose, aminoacid

Table 12.1.4. Frequently used parenteral nutrition solutions

Product	Total Energy (kcal)	Non protein Energy (kcal)	Dextrose (g)	Nitrogen (g)	Lipids	Osmolality mOsm/l
All-in-one solutions						
Vitrimix (Central TPN—1000 ml)	1000	800	75	7	20% 250 ml	960
Celemix G* (Peripheral TPN—1000 ml)	1040	800	75	9.6	20% 250 ml	675
Kabiven (3-in-1 bag—100 ml)	900	800	100	5.4	Soyabean oil 40 g	1060
Two-in–one solutions						
Aminomix	1000	800	200	8.2	Nil	
PNA 10** (Central TPN solution 1000 ml)	1200	1000	250	8	Nil	1908
Nutriflex	790	600	150	6.8	Nil	1400
Lipid solutions						
Intralipid 10%*** (250 ml)	275					
Celepid 10%****	275					
Protein solutions						
Aminoven 10%				16		
Celemin 10%*****				16		

*Celemix containing sorbitol as carbohydrate is also available.
** PNA 7, PNA 8, PNA 12 and PNA 16 are also available.
*** Intralipid 20% and Intralipid 30% are also available. Also available as 500 ml.
****Celepid 20% is also available. Also available as 500 ml.
*****Celemin 5% is also available.

solution and lipid all in one pack so that all three are infused from one bag through a single lumen of a central vein catheter. An example of an all-in-one solution is Vitrimix. 1000 ml of Vitrimix provides for 1000 kcal; dextrose (75g) and lipids (20 per cent in 250 ml) supply non-protein energy, equivalent to about 800 kcal and the nitrogen content of the solution is 7 g (roughly equivalent to $7 \times 6.2 = 43$ g protein). The osmolarity of this all-in-one solution is 960 mOsm/l

A two-in-one solution has dextrose and an aminoacid solution in one pack; the fats would need to be infused (an intralipid infusion) separately through a separate lumen of a multilumen catheter.

Parenteral nutrition may also be infused through a peripheral vein. **Table 12.1.4** lists the frequently used 'all-in-one' and 'two-in-one' parenteral solutions, the kcal each supplies and the contents in relation to carbohydrate (dextrose), nitrogen and fat. It also lists intralipid solutions and aminoacid solutions available as separate infusions.

Monitoring the Patient

The frequency of monitoring depends on the stability of the patient's condition. Vital signs need the usual frequent monitoring. At the start of TPN a full biochemical profile, as also a full blood count, and platelet count should be done. A biochemical profile should include blood glucose, serum electrolytes, bicarbonate, blood NPN, creatinine, full liver function tests, and serum proteins, with special reference to serum albumin levels. Serum calcium, phosphorus, alkaline phosphatase, pH of arterial blood and arterial blood gases should also be done. When possible, a nutrition screen should include serum levels of transferrin, prealbumin, and retinol-binding protein. These tests may be repeated once or twice weekly. Serum electrolytes and tests for liver and renal function may need to be repeated more often, depending on the patient's clinical state. The adequacy of the nutritional regime should be assessed at weekly intervals. Nitrogen balance studies may be necessary in highly catabolic complicated cases.

Complications of Parenteral Nutrition (Table 12.1.5)

Complications fall into three groups—metabolic complications, catheter-related infections, and complications related to technical problems.

1. Metabolic Complications. These include disorders in glucose metabolism, chiefly hyperglycaemia, deficiency states and hepatic dysfunction. Deficiency states include in particular deficits of magnesium and phosphorus. Fluid and electrolyte disturbances are also observed, and are partly related to the background disease in the patient.

Hyperglycaemia. Hyperglycaemia constitutes the most frequent metabolic complication. It is often produced when 50 per cent dextrose infusions are used instead of 20 per cent dextrose infusions, so as to provide calories and reduce total fluid intake. Diabetics critically ill with catabolic problems, show hyperglycaemia in spite of large doses of insulin. Corticosteroids also enhance the hyperglycaemic state. Careful monitoring of blood glucose is mandatory and an insulin infusion is best started separately through a peripheral line, the dose being adjusted to keep the blood glucose levels between 150–200 mg/dl. Insulin, besides controlling the blood sugar, also has a beneficial effect on nitrogen balance. Large doses of insulin however may cause severe hypokalaemia. Potassium replacement is therefore important.

The appearance of hyperglycaemia in a previously stable patient often heralds the onset of sepsis. The latter may be clinically evident within 12 to 24 hours. The source of sepsis should be promptly identified and treated; the hyperglycaemic state is then easily controlled.

Uncontrolled increasing hyperglycaemia from one or more causes listed above, can lead to hyperosmolar non-ketotic coma. Fever, obtundation, focal neurological signs, seizures and death characterize the untreated syndrome. Mental obtundation without acidosis should always suggest the possibility of a hyperosmolar non-ketotic state. The blood sugar levels may vary from 450 to 1000 mg/dl.

Therapy consists of stopping dextrose infusions, administering large quantities of insulin intravenously in an infusion, and using half-strength saline infusions intravenously.

Hypoglycaemia invariably occurs if high concentrations of dextrose infusions are suddenly stopped. Parenteral infusions of dextrose should always be slowly tapered, and never suddenly stopped. Five per cent dextrose can be infused through a peripheral vein if necessary.

Hypomagnesaemia may clinically manifest with tingling in the limbs and around the mouth. Serum magnesium levels are often reduced to < 0.6 mg/dl. The average requirement of magnesium is 8–16 mEq/day. In patients whose stores need to be repleted, or in those with diarrhoea or hepatic dysfunction, the requirement of magnesium may be significantly increased.

Hypophosphataemia. Inadequate intravenous administration of phosphate may progress over a period of time to increasing phosphate deficiency. Severe deficiency leads to mental obtundation and coma. Lethargy and a slurred thick speech are early features. If unrecognized, the patient becomes increasingly obtunded and fully comatose. Haemolysis, rhabdomyolysis and heart failure may occur. The normal phosphate requirement is estimated to be 90 mEq/day. This level may be increased in hypercatabolic states, or when there is excessive loss of phosphates from body stores.

Hepatic Dysfunction. A rise in the serum transaminases and the alkaline phosphatase is often observed in patients on TPN. It is usually a self-limited, non-progressive complication. A progressive rise in the serum bilirubin is almost always not due to TPN. An ultrasound examination is necessary in such patients to exclude abdominal sepsis, biliary obstruction, acalculous cholecystitis or liver steatosis. The current use of glucose plus lipid solutions to share in the caloric requirement, has reduced the incidence of liver steatosis. Causes that could probably contribute to hepatic dysfunction during TPN include the effects produced by breakdown products of aminoacids and bacterial endotoxins, excessive carbohydrate administration, essential fatty acid deficiency, lack of enteral stimulation of the gut with altered levels of gut hormones (1), and the presence of complicating sepsis.

2. Catheter-related Infections

Catheter-related Sepsis. This is a dreaded complication of TPN. Infection can be bacterial, fungal or both. Aseptic care of the catheter, and restriction of use of the catheter solely for the purpose of TPN, has reduced the incidence of catheter-related sepsis from 6–27 per cent, to the current acceptable rate of 1–3 per cent (1). The subject is discussed at length in the Section on Fever and Acute Infections in a Critical Care Setting.

Thrombosis of the Subclavian Vein. The incidence of clinically apparent thrombosis is 2–5 per cent. Venographic studies have however shown an incidence as high as 20–50 per cent, the majority being asymptomatic (37). Catheter insertion may injure the intima of the vein and initiate thrombosis. A fibrin sleeve often forms around the tip of the catheter, extending for a centimetre or two proximally. This may constitute a nidus for a sleeve thrombus. Hypertonic infusions (particularly the use of 50 per cent dextrose) are irritant, and may also contribute to thrombus formation. The composition of the catheter has been incriminated in thrombosis of the subclavian vein. Polyvinyl catheters act as a strong irritant; silastic catheters have the least irritant effect. Finally, background diseases like sepsis or malignancy can lead to hypercoagulable states that promote thrombus formation.

Pain and swelling of the arm are clinical manifestations of subclavian vein thrombosis. The latter, as stated above, may however be asymptomatic. A subclavian vein thrombus may become infected, and cause a septic thrombophlebitis of the vein. Pulmonary embolization can also result.

Treatment involves prompt removal of the catheter, and anticoagulation with heparin. Treatment of septic thrombophlebitis involves in addition, the use of antibiotics.

3. Technical Complications. These have been discussed in the Section on Procedures and Monitoring in the Intensive Care Unit. They are related to the placement of the central venous catheter in the subclavian or jugular vein, by the percutaneous technique.

Table 12.1.5. Complications of parenteral nutrition

---

1. Metabolic Complications
   * Hyperglycaemia
   * Hypoglycaemia
   * Hypomagnesaemia
   * Hypophosphataemia
   * Hepatic dysfunction
2. Catheter-related Infections
   * Catheter-related sepsis
   * Thrombosis of the subclavian vein
3. Technical Complications
   * Related to placement of the central venous catheter (see Section on Procedures and Monitoring in the ICU)

Nutritional Support in Special Conditions (Table 12.1.6)

Renal Failure

Nutritional support in renal failure increases the risk of fluid overload, and uraemic symptoms. The following special points merit consideration:

(i) Nutritional support is absolutely necessary in hypercatabolic patients with renal failure. It should be begun early and should be combined with haemodialysis or haemofiltration. If the patient is haemodynamically unstable, continuous haemofiltration is used to control fluid overload and uraemia.

(ii) In patients who are not dialysed, and are in renal failure. The protein intake is restricted to 0.5 g/kg/day, and standard formulations are used. The fluid is restricted to 0.8–1 l/day if the urine output is low. In the absence of clinical improvement, haemodialysis or haemofiltration should be commenced. Once dialysis is begun, the protein intake is suitably increased to 1 g/kg/day, or even more in catabolic states.

(iii) If enteral feeding is used, the fluid intake and protein intake should be carefully calculated. A carbohydrate:fat ratio of 60:40 should be used to meet caloric needs. Insulin may be required to manage glucose intolerance in these patients.

(iv) During haemodialysis, there is a loss of 6–12 g of aminoacids per treatment, and a loss of 25–30 g of glucose during a 6 hour dialysis session. Haemofiltration results in the loss of 4 g aminoacids per day. When calculating nutritional requirements, these losses should be considered and made good. When dialysis is in the form of peritoneal dialysis, there is a net gain in glucose of 120–150 g/day from the dialysate fluid. This amount thus needs to be subtracted from the nutritional supplementation.

(v) The use of essential aminoacid formulas is controversial. The rationale for the use of essential aminoacids is that endogenous nitrogen can be used to synthesize non-essential aminoacids, thereby reducing the degree of rise in the blood urea nitrogen (BUN). Essential aminoacid formulations are probably only indicated when a patient in renal failure is a poor risk for dialysis, and when standard formulations produce a rapid rise in the BUN. Fluid overload remains a problem even with special aminoacid formulations. In less catabolic patients, the protein intake should be kept at 0.3 g/kg/day.

Hepatic Failure

If there is no encephalopathy, the protein intake is kept at 1 g/kg/day. In the presence of encephalopathy, the protein is restricted to 0.3 g/kg/day or even less of the standard formulations and solutions. It has been shown that the infusion of branched-chain enriched aminoacids improves encephalopathy in many patients. A meta-analysis of six large studies in patients with liver disease showed that the mortality in those receiving branched-chain enriched aminoacids was 24 per cent in contrast to 43 per cent in the control group (38). The intake of branched-chain aminoacids should start with 0.25–0.5 g/kg/day. In hypercatabolic states, this is gradually increased to 1 g/kg/day. The caloric requirement should be given by glucose and fat in the ratio of 60:40.

Respiratory Failure

Nutritional support is of importance in critically ill patients with respiratory failure. The aim is to improve respiratory muscle strength to help counter the impedance to ventilation produced by either severe restrictive disease as in ARDS, or by severe airways obstruction as in chronic bronchitis, emphysema. A poor nutritional state is an important cause of unsuccessful weaning from ventilator support.

Patients with chronic airways obstruction who are hypercapnic may experience a further rise in PCO_2 if carbohydrates are given in excess. This is because the metabolism of carbohydrates leads to CO_2 production. A significant increase in the volume of CO_2 produced can only be got rid off by an increase in alveolar ventilation. Patients with severe chronic airways obstruction may be unable to increase their alveolar ventilation to wash out the excess CO_2. The $PaCO_2$ therefore rises. Carbohydrates should be restricted in these patients, particularly when they are being weaned from ventilator support. The total caloric requirement and protein remains as described earlier but the carbohydrate:fat ratio should be 40:60.

Table 12.1.6. Recommendations for specific clinical conditions

Clinical Condition	Initial caloric requirement	Proteins	Comments
Multiple trauma	25–30 kcal/day	1.5 g/kg/day	Immune-modulating formula may be of benefit
Major cardiothoracic surgery	25 kcal/day	1.2–1.5 g/kg/day	Immune-modulating formula may be of benefit
Severe burns	30–35 kcal/day	1.5–2.5 g/kg/day	Higher protein intake improves outcome
Fulminant tetanus	30–35 kcal/day	1.5–2 g/kg/day	Higher calories and high protein intake helps blunt or reduce catabolism
Acute renal failure (not on dialysis)	25 kcal/day	0.5 g/kg/day	Restrict water, sodium and potassium
Acute renal failure (on dialysis)	25 kcal/day	1.5 g/kg/day	Protein needs higher because catabolic state and loss of protein in dialysis
Liver failure	25 kcal/day	0.5–1 g/kg/day	Use 0.5 g/kg/day in hepatic encephalopathy; branch chain aminoacid may improve CNS function
Acute hypercapnic respiratory failure	25 kcal/day	1.2 g/kg/day	Reduce carbohydrates to reduce VCO_2 in severe obstructive lung disease; reduce fats in TPN in ARDS
Pancreatitis	25 kcal/day	1–1.5 g/kg/day	Jejunal feeds (preferably with a peptide based formula) should be tried before initiating TPN
Inflammatory bowel disease	25 kcal/day	1–1.5 g/kg/day	Small bowel feeds (preferably with a peptide based formula) are well tolerated

On the other hand in patients with ARDS, lipid emulsions may interfere with gas exchange and it is preferable to restrict fats and keep the carbohydrate: fat ratio at 65:35 when the patient is on parental nutrition.

Cardiac Failure

The major feature in TPN is to restrict salt and water intake. Sodium, potassium and magnesium should be carefully monitored. TPN is started with half the caloric requirement over 3–4 days in order to avoid pulmonary oedema secondary to refeeding and increased metabolic rate. It is then gradually increased to the required level. The caloric and protein intake is as discussed in earlier sections, with a glucose: fat ratio of 60:40. Ischaemic myocardium derives its energy from anaerobic metabolism. The use of parental nutrition with adequate glucose, potassium and insulin may provide substrate delivery to such ischaemic areas.

Pancreatitis

Recent trials suggest that jejunal enteral feeds of a peptide-based diet are well tolerated in patients with severe pancreatitis. Enteral nutrition should be attempted before starting total parenteral nutrition in the majority of patients with acute pancreatits. In fact septic complications in necrotizing pancreatitis are reduced in those receiving enteral feeds when compared to those receiving total parenteral nutrition (**39**). However in fulminant pancreatitis with ileus and complicating sepsis, total parenteral nutrition is imperative. Jejunal enteral feeds should be started slowly when gut function returns.

Thermal Injury

Patients critically ill with severe burns need 30–35 kcal/kg daily and 2 to 2.5 g of protein per kg per day. Increased protein intake appears to reduce both morbidity and mortality in these patients. The gut should be used as far as possible; nutrition if need be can then be supplemented by parenteral therapy.

Metabolic Stress Syndrome and Diabetes

Metabolic stress syndrome is a condition of elevated blood glucose levels in non-diabetics in an ICU setting. It is not just due to caloric intake, but is related to increase in counter-regulatory hormones and insulin resistance. It should be countered by the use of a titrated dose of insulin, so as to keep blood glucose levels not > 110 mg/dl. In a prospective randomized study in 765 critically ill mechanically ventilated patients, a tight control over blood glucose with insulin, reduced mortality by 43 per cent and also resulted in a significant reduction in morbidity (**40**).

Diabetic patients receiving total parenteral nutrition frequently have serum glucose and electrolyte levels difficult to control. Insulin administration is vital for effective parenteral alimentation. TPN should be initiated in diabetics with just 150 g of glucose in 24 hours. A quarter to half of the patient's daily insulin requirement should be added to the TPN solution; further doses of subcutaneous insulin are given according to a sliding scale, the dose of insulin being based on bedside glucose estimations every 3 to 4 hours. It is always preferable to add insulin to the TPN solution to control elevated blood sugar levels. The use of separate intravenous infusions of insulin and TPN solution can cause severe hypoglycemia in these critically ill patients.

Immuno-nutrition or Immunity-enhancing Formulas

Combination of various nutrients which enhance immune activity and immune response have been in use over the last few years. These immuno-modulating nutrients include glutamine, arginine, omega-3 fatty acids, neucleotides and antioxidant vitamins. Glutamine which accounts for more than 60 per cent of the body's free aminoacid pool is markedly decreased in stress and starvation. Supplements of glutamine are believed to be of use in patients with multiple trauma, sepsis, severe burns, AIDS, inflammatory bowel disease. Glutamine supplements can be given by the enteral route or intravenously. Arginine plays a role in lymphocyte proliferation and wound healing. Omega-3 fatty acids may reduce production of inflammatory mediators by neutrophils, macrophages and endothelial cells. Neucleotides are believed to enhance immune function.

The use of immune-enhancing formulas is reported to be associated with lower rates of infection, decreased time on ventilator support and decreased length of stay in the ICU (**41**).

REFERENCES

1. Benson DW, Fischer JE. (1990). Nutritional Management. In: Handbook of Critical Care, 3rd edn (Eds Berk JL, Sampliner JE). pp. 573–617. Little, Brown and Company, Boston, Toronto, London.

2. Buzby GP. (1988). Case for preoperative nutritional support. Presented at the American College of Surgeons 1988 Clinical Congress Postgraduate Course 'Pre- and Postoperative Care: Metabolism and Nutrition,' Chicago, October 25–28.

3. Cerra FB, Benitez MR, Blackburn GL et al. (1997). Applied nutrition in the ICU: a consensus statement of the American College of Chest Physicians. Chest. 111, 769.

4. Detsky AS, McLaughlin JR, Baker JP et al. (1987). What is subjective global assessment of nutritional status? JPEN. 11, 8.

5. Allard JP, Jeejeebhoy KN. (1991). Nutrition in the Critically Ill. In: Current Therapy in Critical Care Medicine, 2nd edn (Ed. Parrillo JE). pp. 262–271. BC Decker Inc., Philadelphia, Hamilton.

6. Jequier E. (1987). Measurement of energy expenditure in clinical nutritional assessment. JPEN. 11(Suppl), 86S-89S.

7. Westenskow DR, Schipke CA, Raymond JL et al. (1988). Calculation of metabolic expenditure and substrate utilization from gas exchange measurements. JPEN. 12, 20–24.

8. Long CL, Schaffel N, Geiger JW et al. (1979). Metabolic response to injury and illness: Estimation of energy and protein needs from indirect calorimetry and nitrogen balance. JPEN. 3, 452–456.

9. Weissman C, Kemper M, Askanazi J et al. (1986). Resting metabolic rate of the critically ill patient: Measured versus predicted. Anesthesiology. 64, 673–679.

10. Harris JA, Benedict FG. (1919). Biometric studies of basal metabolism in man. Carnegie Institute of Washington. Publication # 279.

11. Christman JW, Mccain RW. (1993). Intensive Care Med. 129–136.

12. Marino PL. (1998). Nutrient and Energy Requirements. In: The ICU Book. pp. 721–736. Lippincott, Williams and Wilkins, USA.

13. Askanazi J, Carpentier YA, Elwyn DH et al. (1980). Influence of total parenteral nutrition on fuel utilization in injury and sepsis. Ann Surg. 191, 40–46.

14. Stein TP. (1985). Why measure the respiratory quotient of patients on total parenteral nutrition? J Am Coll Nutr. 4, 501–513.

15. Linscheer WG, Vergroesen AJ. (1988). Lipids. In: Modern Nutrition in Health and Disease (Eds Shils ME, Young VR). pp. 72–107. Lea and Febiger, Philadelphia.

16. Dempsey DT, Mullen JL, Rombeau JL et al. (1987). Treatment effects of parenteral vitamins in total parenteral nutrition patients. JPEN. 11, 229–237.

17. Campillo B, Zittoun J, de Gialluly E. (1988). Prophylaxis of folate deficiency in acutely ill patients: Results of a randomized clinical trial. Intensive Care Med. 14, 640–645.

18. Yeung CK, Smith RC, Hill GL. (1979). Effect of an elemental diet on body composition: A comparison with intravenous nutrition. Gastroenterology. 77, 652.

19. Bower RH. (1983). Hepatic complications of parenteral nutrition. Semin Liver Dis. 3, 216.

20. Dupre J, Curtis JD, Unger RH et al. (1969). Effects of secretin, pancreozymin, or gastrin on the response of the endocrine pancreas to administration of glucose or arginine in man. J Clin Invest. 48, 745.

21. Gimmon Z, Murphy RF, Chen M et al. (1982). The effect of parenteral and enteral nutrition on portal and systemic immunoreactivities of gastrin, glucagon and vasoactive intestinal polypeptide (VIP). Ann Surg. 196, 571.

22. Johnson LR, Copeland EM, Dudrick SJ et al. (1975). Structural and hormonal alterations in the gastrointestinal tract of parenterally fed rats. Gastroenterology. 68, 1177.

23. Levine GM, Deken JJ, Steiger E et al. (1974). Role of oral intake in maintenance of gut mass and disaccharide activity. Gastroenterology. 67, 979.

24. ASPEN Board of Directors. (1987). Guidelines for the use of enteral nutrition in the adult patient. JPEN. 11, 435–439.

25. Schunn CO, Daly JM. (1995). Small bowel necrosis associated with post-operative jejunal tube feeding. J Am Coll Surg. 180, 410.

26. Ramos SM, Lindine P. (1986). Inexpensive, safe and simple nasoenteral intubation—an alternative for the cost conscious. JPEN. 10, 78–81.

27. Metheny NA, Eisenberg P, Spies M. (1986). Aspiration pneumonia in patients fed through nasoenteral tubes. Heart Lung. 15, 256–261.

28. Raff MH, Cho S, Dale R. (1987). A technique for positioning nasoenteral feeding tubes. JPEN. 11, 210–213.

29. Jones BMJ. (1986). Enteral feeding: Techniques and administration. Gut. 27(Suppl), 47–50.

30. Sarr MG. (1988). Needle catheter jejunostomy: An unappreciated and misunderstood advance in the care of patients after major abdominal operations. Mayo Clin Proc. 63, 565–572.

31. Ryan JA, Page CP. (1984). Intrajejunal feeding: Development and current status. JPEN. 8, 187–198.

32. Marino PL. (1998). Enteral Nutrition. In: The ICU Book. pp. 737–53. Lippincott, Williams and Wilkins, USA.

33. Heimburger DC, Weinsier RL. (1985). Guidelines for evaluating and categorizing enteral feeding formulas according to therapeutic equivalence. JPEN. 9, 61–67.

34. Koruda M, Geunther P, Rombeau J. (1987). Enteral nutrition in the critically ill. Crit Care Clin. 3, 133–153.

35. Marcuard CP, Segall KL, Trogdon S. (1989). Clearing obstructed feeding tubes. JPEN. 13, 81–83.

36. Rombeau JL, Caldwell MD, Forlaw L, Geunter PA (Eds). (1989). Atlas of nutritional support techniques. pp. 77–106. Little, Brown and Company, Boston.

37. Bozzetti F, Scarpa D, Terno G et al. (1983). Subclavian venous thrombosis due to indwelling catheters: A prospective study on 52 patients. JPEN. 7, 560.

38. Marchesini G, Bianchi G, Rossi B. (2000). Nutritional treatment with branched-chain aminoacids in advanced liver cirrhosis. J Gastroenterol. 35 (Supplement 12), 7–12.

39. F Kalfarentzos, J Kehagias, N Mead. (1997). Enteral nutrition is superior to parenteral nutrition in severe acute pancreatitis: results of a randomized prospective trial. Br J Surg. 84(12), 1665–1669.

40. van den Berghe G, Wouters P, Weekers F et al. (2001). Intensive insulin therapy in critically ill patients. N Engl J Med. 345, 1359–1367.

41. Beale RJ, Bryg DJ, Bihari DJ. (1999). Immuno-nutrition in the critically ill: a systematic review of clinical outcome. Crit Care Med. 27, 2799–2805.

Fever and Acute Infections in a Critical Care Setting

13.1 General Considerations and Non-infective Causes of Fever in the ICU
13.2 Nosocomial Infections
13.3 Community-acquired Fulminant Infections Requiring Critical Care
13.4 Use of Antibiotics in the ICU
13.5 Treatment of Fungal infections in Critically Ill Patients

General Considerations and Non-infective Causes of Fever in the ICU

General Considerations

The incidence of acute infections requiring critical care is probably higher in the poor developing countries of the world than in developed regions. The nature of acute infections is also often different. In India, we see most of the infections that prevail in the West, as also other acute infections which the Western half of the world hardly ever encounters. This is related to differing geographical, environmental and socio-economic factors.

Patients with infection in intensive care units fall into three groups:

(a) *Patients with Severe Community-acquired Infections who need Critical Care.* These include in our part of the world, patients with severe tetanus, severe Pl. falciparum infections, severe community acquired pneumonia, disseminated haematogenous tuberculosis, violent Gram-negative infections chiefly originating in the gastrointestinal tract, fulminant amoebic infections, fulminant meningitis, haemorrhagic dengue fever, severe leptospiral disease and other miscellaneous acute infections.

(b) *Patients with Nosocomial (i.e. Hospital-acquired) Infections.* These can occur either in patients admitted to hospital wards, the infection being serious enough to merit critical care, or in patients already admitted to the ICU. In our ICU, the rate of nosocomial infection in patients requiring life support for more than 2 weeks, is 5-fold higher than in those admitted to the general wards, who do not require ICU care. However the proportion of nosocomial infection in the ICU vis-à-vis the general wards differs in different hospitals in Mumbai, and in different centres of this country.

(c) *The Immunocompromised, and in particular the Neutropaenic Patient in the ICU* falls in a separate category. Such patients are extremely vulnerable to nosocomial infections in the ICU, because of a 'hostile' environment where the risk of infection is high, and also because they lack appropriate defence mechanisms against infection.

Fever and infections in neutropaenic patients are dealt with in the Section on The Immunocompromised Patient. Important infections, and the background factors underlying these infections in the other 2 groups of patients are dealt with in subsequent chapters of this section. The present chapter deals with *nosocomial* *fever (i.e. fever that appears 24 to 48 hours after admission) in a critical care setting, unrelated to infection.*

The Febrile Response

The normal temperature ranges from 36°C (am) to 38°C (pm), with a mean temperature of 37°C (98.6°F). It is measured in the mouth as oral temperature and more reliably in the rectum as the rectal temperature. A febrile response is the hallmark of infection. It is however important to bear the following facts in mind when considering the febrile response.

(i) Fever and its attendant symptoms of malaise, together with leucocytosis can occur in the absence of infection. A careful consideration of the background clinical features of a patient with pyrexia in the ICU, and a search for non-specific causes of pyrexia is imperative, if unnecessary use of antibiotics (with all its attendant dangers) is to be avoided.

(ii) The height of the fever and the clinical appearance of the patient need not constitute a reliable guide either to the presence or severity of the infection. High fever with rigors could be due to a pyrogen reaction from an infusion, or to a drug reaction, while minimal temperature elevations and even normal or subnormal temperatures may be associated with life-threatening sepsis.

(iii) A normal oral and axillary temperature in a setting where fever is expected, should always prompt one to measure the rectal temperature. A very high rectal temperature with normal or only modest elevation of axillary temperature is a feature of fulminant tetanus, in many patients with Pl. falciparum infection, and in some patients with life-threatening sepsis. Rectal temperatures closely approximate the core temperature, and are standard measurements in most ICUs in Europe and the United States. Oral temperature is fairly reliable (1 degree < than rectal and 1 degree > axillary temperature), but in problem patients and in those with a marked discrepancy between the oral and the rectal temperatures, the latter should be monitored. Alternative methods for monitoring core temperatures are now available in the form of thermistors placed in bladder catheters, pulmonary artery catheters and ear probes. These however are expensive, and in a poor country like ours, unnecessary for patient care.

(iv) Infants and elderly patients may not respond with the expected temperature pattern even in serious infections.

Non-infective Causes of Fever in the ICU (Table 13.1.1)

In a pyrexial patient under critical care, the clinical background or setting should dictate the initial bedside evaluation of the fever. The following non-infective causes of pyrexia should come to mind, and should be carefully evaluated. Unnecessary, expensive investigations are avoided by a careful clinical examination.

Table 13.1.1. Non-infective causes of fever in the ICU

* Trauma (specially crush injuries)
* Post-operative
* Malignant hyperthermia
* Thromboembolism
* Blood in body cavities and large haematomas
* Post-cardiotomy syndrome / Dressler's syndrome
* Myocardial infarction
* Procedures or therapeutic measures e.g. blood transfusions, fluid infusions, haemodialysis, bronchoscopy
* Drug fever
* Pancreatitis
* Bowel infarction
* Other rare causes e.g. tumours, lymphomas, vasculitis, severe adrenal insufficiency or exacerbation of hyperthyroidism

Trauma

Trauma and in particular crush injuries, can induce a systemic febrile response even in the absence of infection.

Post-operative Fever

About 10 per cent of patients may develop an elevated temperature in the first week of surgery even in the absence of wound or other infection. Most such fevers are mild to moderate, occur as a single episode, and are short-lasting. Expensive investigations are best deferred if the wound is clean and clinical examination reveals no cause for the fever. A sterile serous collection beneath a portion of the wound may lead to a low grade fever mainly occurring in the afternoon or evenings for 8–12 days, till such time as the serous collection is absorbed or drained.

Malignant Hyperthermia

This is a very rare disorder caused by an abnormal release of calcium from skeletal muscles following the use of general anaesthetics and muscle relaxants (1). Initially it is characterized by muscle rigidity, tremulousness, tachycardia, labile blood pressure and ventricular arrhythmias. The striking muscle rigidity is due to the abnormal release of calcium from the sarcoplasmic reticulum of skeletal muscles (1). Cyanosis may be marked and pulmonary embolism may be wrongly diagnosed. Fever with shivering occurs in 30 per cent of patients; hyperpyrexia with temperatures ranging from 104–107°F may occur. If untreated, myoglobinuric renal failure may be observed. Immediate treatment with dantrolene reduces morbidity and mortality. An intravenous bolus of 1–2 mg/

kg of the drug is given and is repeated every 15 minutes if necessary to a maximum of 10 mg/kg. A maintenance dose of 1–2 mg/kg orally 4 times a day for 3 days is then administered.

Thromboembolism

A low-grade fever may be due to thromboembolism. This risk is highest in post-operative patients, patients immobilized for long periods of time, following cerebrovascular accidents, myocardial infarction and in patients with neoplastic disease. Careful examination for painful swelling of the calves and thighs, and for tenderness over the course of the large veins in the lower limbs is at times rewarding. Even so, pulmonary emboli may be shot out from thrombi in the deep veins of the leg, thigh or from thrombosed veins within the pelvis, without the presence of abnormal physical signs.

Blood in the Body Cavities and Large Haematomas

Accumulation of blood in the thorax, abdomen, and the presence of blood in the subarachnoid space produces fever. A large haematoma in any organ or tissue, occurring spontaneously as in certain diseases, or following trauma or rupture of a vessel, also produces pyrexia. A clot within a dissecting aneurysm of the aorta, is similarly associated with a low grade fever. An appropriate clinical background should suggest the correct aetiology for fever in these patients.

Post-cardiotomy Syndrome, Dressler's Syndrome

Following cardiac or open heart surgery, the persistence of a pericardial rub after 6–7 days, with fever, leucocytosis, and an ESR > 50 mm/hour, should suggest the diagnosis of a post-cardiotomy syndrome. A pleural rub with a pleural effusion in the left pleural space, or rarely bilaterally, may be present. The possibility that a pleuropulmonary shadow after cardiac surgery could be due to a post-cardiotomy syndrome should be kept in mind, else the diagnosis of a nosocomial pneumonia can be wrongly made.

Dressler's syndrome with fever, and precordial pain due to pericarditis can occur any time from 7 days to 6 weeks after a myocardial infarct. Pleurisy and pleuropulmonary shadows may also be observed, exactly as after cardiac surgery. The response to corticosteroids is dramatic both in the post-cardiotomy syndrome and in Dressler's syndrome. Response to nonsteroidal anti-inflammatory agents or to aspirin is also satisfactory in many patients.

Myocardial Infarction

A critically ill patient from any cause may develop a myocardial infarction. Pain in such individuals literally goes unnoticed, and a low-grade fever with leucocytosis may cause concern.

Procedures or Therapeutic Measures

The following procedures or therapeutic measures are associated with fever in the absence of infection:

(i) *Blood Transfusions or Intravenous Infusions of Fluids*. Fever is observed in about 5 per cent of patients receiving blood products. Febrile transfusion reactions are discussed in another chapter.

(ii) *Haemodialysis*. Temporary fever during dialysis is of uncertain aetiology. It could be due to non-infective causes, or to endotoxin contamination of the dialysis equipment, or due to bacteraemia by Gram-positive and/or Gram-negative organisms (2).

(iii) *Fever following bronchoscopy*. This occurs in 10 per cent of patients but should not last for more than one day.

Drug Fever

The diagnosis of drug fever is generally made after exclusion of other causes of fever—both non-infective and infective. The fever is usually low grade, but may be high, and may be associated with chills and rigors. A drug rash and/or peripheral eosinophilia, if present, allow for an easy diagnosis; however, Mackowiak and LeMaistre (3) noted a drug rash in only 18 per cent and peripheral eosinophilia in 22 per cent of patients with drug fever. Tachycardia is frequent and hypotension may also occur. Contrary to conventional teaching, a patient with drug fever can appear as ill as a patient with a serious infection (3). Any drug can theoretically speaking produce drug fever, but fever and drug reactions are most commonly observed with sulphas, quinine, quinidine, penicillin and its derivatives, other antibiotics, amphotericin B, furadantin, phenytoin and procainamide. If drug fever is suspected, the offending drug should be omitted; if the diagnosis is correct, the fever disappears in 2–3 days.

Pancreatitis

This can complicate the course of a critical illness in an ICU patient—particularly with multiple organ failure, or as a complication of viral hepatitis, or following the use of corticosteroid therapy, or in the presence of shock and hypoperfusion from any cause, or in burns with sepsis. The diagnosis may be missed in very ill patients and should be suspected if abnormal abdominal symptoms or signs, fever, or an unexplained worsening in the clinical picture is observed against a background where pancreatitis may be a possible complication. The serum amylase and lipase levels are both markedly elevated, and the diagnosis can be further confirmed by an ultrasound or CT of the abdomen which show an enlarged, often necrotic pancreas with pancreatic and peripancreatic inflammation [see Chapter on Acute (Fulminant) Necrotizing Pancreatitis].

Bowel Infarction

Ischaemia and/or infarction of the bowel due to occluded mesenteric vessels can produce fever which is accompanied by abdominal pain and tenderness, but these symptoms may be masked in patients who are critically ill or in those with an altered mental state. Fresh blood per rectum or maelena with normal upper GI scopy findings should suggest the diagnosis.

Other Rare Non-infective Causes

Other, less common, non-infective causes of fever encountered in an ICU setting include alcohol withdrawal, severe adrenal insufficiency precipitated by the stress of a critical illness, exacerbation of hyperthyroidism in a critically ill individual, and multiple organ failure due to a non-infective aetiology. Tumours and lymphomas can also produce fever, particularly during chemotherapy. Vasculitis of any aetiology, is another rare cause of fever in critically ill patients.

REFERENCES

1. Britt BA. (1983). Malignant hyperthermia. In: Complications in Anesthiology (Eds Orkin FK, Cooperman LH), pp. 291–307. J B Lippincott, Philadelphia.

2. Pollack VE. (1988). Adverse effects and pyrogenic reactions during hemodialysis. JAMA. 260, 2106–2107.

3. Mackowiak PA, LeMaistre CF. (1987). Drug fever: A critical appraisal of conventional concepts. Ann Intern Med. 106, 728–733.

Nosocomial Infections

General Considerations and Epidemiology

Nosocomial infections are those which manifest in patients 48 to 72 hours after admission to hospital. They are therefore hospital-acquired infections, in contrast to community-acquired infections. Nosocomial infections are directly related to diagnostic, interventional or therapeutic procedures a patient undergoes in hospital, and are also influenced by the bacteriological flora prevailing within a particular unit or hospital. Infections in patients occurring within 48 to 72 hours of discharge from hospital are also invariably nosocomial in origin. Nosocomial infections carry a significant morbidity and mortality, particularly when they affect patients in the ICU.

Critical care units increasingly use high technology medicine for patient care—haemodynamic monitoring, ventilator support, haemodialysis, parenteral nutrition, and a large battery of powerful drugs, particularly antibiotics to counter infection. It is indeed a paradox that the use of high-tech medicine has brought in its wake the dangerous and all too frequent complication of nosocomial infections.

By a strange quirk of circumstance, the better equipped an ICU for invasive procedures, the more frequently are these procedures performed for patient care, and the greater is the incidence of nosocomial infections. Prospective studies (1) have shown that various invasive devices play a far more important role in determining susceptibility to nosocomial infection than underlying disease. Again, though the concept of caring for critically ill patients in special units equipped to do so is sound, the disadvantages of such a milieu are also being increasingly realized.

The ICU milieu is uniquely conducive to nosocomial infections. It is a 'closed' milieu, constantly full of patients with life-threatening illnesses. It has a constant staff of nurses and doctors who over prolonged periods of time are exposed to and are in contact with an environment contaminated by antibiotic-resistant pathogens. In this 'closed milieu' the major reservoir of nosocomial organisms is the infected or colonized patient. Most bacteria, many viruses, and possibly even fungi are spread primarily via the hands of the medical, paramedical and nursing staff. Mycobacteria, Legionella, and in granulocytopaenic patients, Aspergillus are transmitted by the airborne droplets. Aspiration of infected pharyngeal and mouth secretions, exposure to invasive devices and procedures, surgery,

impairment of immune mechanisms or overwhelming illnesses amplify colonization and vulnerability to nosocomial infections, and promote their easy transmission. In most patients, antibiotic use promotes sooner or later antibiotic resistance to a number of organisms that prevail in a particular ICU. These resistant organisms contaminate the whole closed environment of the ICU; they can contaminate the curtains, the walls, floor and ceilings, the side tables, the wash basins and the soap dishes, the detergents used as antiseptics, and the clothing and hands of the ICU staff. Bacteria from colonized or infected patients can also be perpetuated in urine bottles, bedpans, commodes, respiratory therapy equipment, ventilators, chamber domes of transducers used in haemodynamic monitoring, and in bronchoscopes or other endoscopes.

In short, the closed milieu of the ICU provides an environment that is as conducive to the growth and preservation of resistant organisms as is a hothouse conducive to the growth and preservation of exotic flora. It is therefore not surprising that two-thirds of reported outbreaks of nosocomial infections have occurred in ICUs even though less than 10 per cent of all hospitalized patients require ICU care (2).

The epidemiology of nosocomial infection in illustrated in **Fig. 13.2.1**.

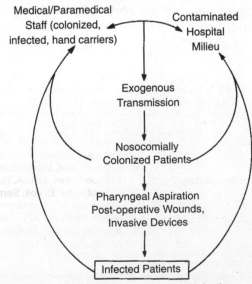

Fig. 13.2.1. Epidemiology of nosocomial infection.

Incidence

The more ill the patient, the greater the incidence of nosocomial infections. The rate of nosocomial infections is highest in burn units, surgical ICUs and ICUs for low birth weight neonates (15–30 per cent). The risk is intermediate in medical and paediatric ICUs (5–10 per cent), and lowest in coronary care units (1–2 per cent) (**2**).

The risk of nosocomial infections in the ICU is also markedly influenced by the length of stay; the latter varies in different institutions. The CDC has therefore advocated the use of nosocomial infection rates expressed per 1000 patient days, to enable comparison between different institutions. Again, increasing exposure to invasive devices increases the nosocomial infection rate. The CDC has therefore advocated that device-associated nosocomial infections should be expressed as infections per 1000 device days (**3–6**).

Profile of Nosocomial Infections

Urinary tract infections are the most frequent, accounting for more than 40 per cent of all nosocomial infection. Other nosocomial infections include nosocomial pneumonias, post-operative surgical wound infections, nosocomial bacteraemias, gastrointestinal infections, especially mucomembranous colitis due to clostridium difficile (**3**).

Different ICUs have different frequency profiles of nosocomial infections. Nosocomial infection and the frequency with which they are observed in the ICU at Breach Candy Hospital, over the last 3 years have been tabled in **Table 13.2.1**. Our overall incidence of nosocomial infections over the past 3 years (5905 patients) has been 2.1 per cent (124 patients). Septicaemia was found to be the most common form with an incidence of about 0.77 per cent (45 patients), followed by pneumonia with 0.65 per cent (38 patients) and wound infections with 0.43 per cent (25 patients). Till 1996, urinary tract infections headed our list of nosocomial infections, as in most ICUs all over the world. However, in the last 3 years, there has been a dramatic fall in UTIs, the incidence being 0.27 per cent (16 patients), accounting for only about 13 per cent of all nosocomial infections in our ICUs for the past 3 years. The fall in nosocomial UTI is probably related to great care of urinary catheters and possibly because most patients with an indwelling urinary catheter in the ICU receive antibiotics for one reason or another.

Table 13.2.1. Profile of organisms isolated from patients in the ICUs at the Breach Candy Hospital between 2000–2003

Site	Common Pathogens
Blood	Pseudomonas, MRSA, Acinetobacter, Klebsiella, MSSA, Enterobacter, Enterococcus, Diptheroids
Lower Respiratory Tract*	Pseudomonas, MRSA, Klebsiella, Enterobacter, E. coli, Serratia, Acinetobacter, S. pneumoniae
Surgical Wounds	MRSA, MSSA, E. coli, Pseudomonas, Acinetobacter, S. epidermidis
Urinary Tract	E. coli, Pseudomonas

*Tracheal secretions and sputum
Note: Candida has been isolated frequently, but true candidial infection is rare

Organisms Involved

More than 50 per cent of nosocomial ICU infections are caused by Gram-negative bacilli, chiefly the Pseudomonas aeruginosa and the Enterobacter species. Here again the nature and frequency of the Gram-negative organisms varies with different units. 10–20 per cent of nosocomial infections are caused by Gram-positive cocci. Most frequently the Staphylococcus aureus or coagulase-negative Staphylococci or Enterococci (**7**). Close to 5 per cent of infections are due to the Candida species. Aspergillus and Zygomycetes infection are occasionally reported from units caring for patients with haematological malignancies, or in organ transplant patients (**8, 9**).

The microbiology of nosocomial infections observed in our unit at the Breach Candy Hospital is given below. (**Fig. 13.2.2**)

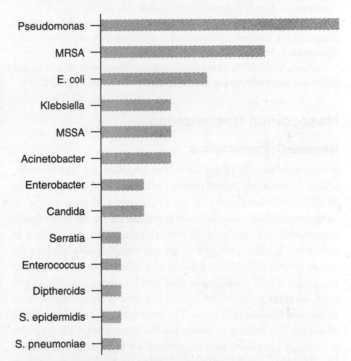

Fig. 13.2.2. Profile of organisms causing ICU nosocomial infections at the Breach Candy Hospital from 2001–2003.

Distinguishing between Colonization and Infection

It is extremely important that doctors in the ICU treat patients and not laboratory reports. Thus a urine culture, or a wound culture, or a sputum culture may show growth of pathogens which may merely represent colonization of the urinary tract or catheter, or of the wound or of the trachea respectively. A close liaison with the microbiology department is essential if correct interpretation of reports is to be made. Culture reports should always be correlated with clinical findings. At times however, it may be extremely difficult to determine whether a growth of pathogens in an individual patient represents true infection or not.

REFERENCES

1. Maki DG. (1989). Risk factors for nosocomial infections in intensive care. Arch Intern Med. 449, 30–35.

2. Maki DG, Weinstein RA. (2001). Nosocomial Infection in the Critical Care Unit. In: Critical Care Medicine (Eds Parrillo JE, Dellinger RP). pp. 981–1046. Mosby, USA.

3. Jarvis WR, Edwards JR, Culver DH et al. (1991). Nosocomial infection rates in adult and pediatric intensive care units in the United States. Am J med. 91 (suppl 3B), 185S.

4. Center for Disease Control. (1991). Nosocomial infection rates for interhospital comparison: limitations and possible solutions. Infect Control Hosp Epidemiol. 12, 609.

5. Maki DG. (1978). Control of colonization and transmission of pathogenic bacteria in the hospital. Ann Intern Med. 89, 777.

6. Wenzel RP, Osterman CA, Donowitz LG et al. (1981). Identification of procedure-related nosocomial infections in high-risk patients. Rev Infect Dis. 3, 701.

7. Horan T, Culver D, Jarvis W et al. (1989). Pathogens causing nosocomial infections. Antimicrobic newsletter. 23, 353.

8. Walsh TJ, Dixon DM. (1989). Nosocomial aspergillosis: environmental microbiology, hospital epidemiology, diagnosis and treatment. Eur J Epidemiol. 5, 131.

9. Castaldo P, Stratta RJ, Wood P et al. (1991). Clinical spectrum of fungal infections after orthotropic liver transplantation. Arch Surg. 126, 149.

Nosocomial Pneumonias

General Considerations

Nosocomial pneumonia is a dreaded complication which chiefly afflicts the most critically ill patients in a hospital (**1, 2**). Impairment of defence mechanisms of an ill patient and easy access of dangerous pathogens to the lower respiratory tract, are both equally responsible for nosocomial pneumonias. The ICU milieu is therefore the ideal setting for this major complication. Neiderman and co-workers (**3**) observed that in an intubated population treated in a surgical ICU, pneumonia developed in approximately 10 per cent, whereas in a medical ICU 20 per cent of intubated patients developed this complication. The true incidence of nosocomial pneumonias is difficult to determine chiefly because of the difficulty in reaching a precise diagnosis, particularly in patients who already have significant radiological shadowing within the lungs to start with—as in acute lung injury (ARDS).

The incidence of nosocomial pneumonias in various intensive care units in our country is undetermined, chiefly because few have bothered to answer this question, and little or no data is available. In our unit in Mumbai, nosocomial pneumonias are nowhere as frequent as reported from ICUs in the West, our incidence in the last 3 years being about 0.65 per cent. The incidence in our unit is about seven times greater in intubated patients compared to non-intubated patients and about 10 to 12 fold greater in patients on mechanical ventilation for more than 5 to 7 days. However in the ICUs of large municipal hospitals in the city, the incidence of nosocomial pneumonia in patients on mechanical ventilation for periods ranging over a week, is as high as 40 per cent. The reasons for this significant epidemiological difference need careful evaluation.

The risk of pneumonia as reported from Western countries is 7–20 fold greater in patients treated with endotracheal intubation (**4, 5**) than in other non-intubated patients in the hospital. As many as 66 per cent of patients with a tracheostomy and on mechanical ventilation were noted to develop pneumonia (**6**). Langer and colleagues (**7**) noted that the incidence of nosocomial pneumonias increased with the duration of mechanical ventilation. Thus fewer than 5 per cent developed pneumonia if they were treated for less than one day on a ventilator, and close to 70 per cent developed nosocomial pneumonias if mechanical ventilation extended for over 30 days. These figures seem shockingly high compared to those observed by us in our unit over the years. In patients who have normal lungs to start with (e.g. those with acute infective polyneuritis, poliomyelitis, head injury or poisonings), the incidence of nosocomial pneumonia is < 5 per cent, even with ventilatory support extending for over a month. In patients who have abnormal lungs to start with as in ARDS or fulminant infections like tetanus or falciparum malaria, the incidence though high, is still not > 10–15 per cent despite the patient being on prolonged ventilator support. In our study on 32 patients with severe fulminant tetanus, we found the incidence of nosocomial pneumonia to be 14 per cent. As explained later, the problems of reaching a correct diagnosis of nosocomial pneumonia in patients with ARDS, are often insurmountable. Even so, our incidence is remarkably low as compared to the incidence of 70 per cent reported by Seidenfeld and associates (**8**). The only possible explanations that can be offered for the differences in the incidence of nosocomial infections are: (i) the presence of a milieu which is probably less threatening from the point of view of prevailing organisms, to very sick patients; (ii) a quicker but judicious use of antibiotics in all patients in whom complications are anticipated, and in all those for whom prolonged mechanical ventilation seems virtually certain; (iii) the less frequent use of invasive monitoring procedures as compared to the practice prevailing in the West.

Pathogenesis (Fig. 13.2.3)

Aspiration Pneumonia

Almost always, nosocomial pneumonia is due to aspiration of infected secretions or particulate matter from the mouth and pharynx into the lower respiratory tract. Retained infected secretions within the large and small airways can also produce nosocomial pneumonias. In most sick patients in the ICU, the oropharynx is colonized by aerobic Gram-negative bacteria within 5 to 10 days, whereas in healthy adults the normal organisms are anaerobic bacteria, and harmless commensals like Neisseria pharyngitidis. The severity of the illness plays an important role in perpetuating this colonization. Invasive diagnostic and therapeutic procedures further promote the aspiration and transfer of infected, colonized oropharyngeal contents into the lower respiratory tract. The upper airway is usually colonized before the lower airway, but organisms such as Ps. aeruginosa can colonize the lower airway as a primary event (**9**). The reason for colonization of the mouth, oropharynx and airways by pathogenic bacteria and in particular by Gram-negative organisms, is the subject of research. In healthy individuals a film of fibronectin covers the epithelium lining the mucosa of the mouth and oropharynx, and prevents the Gram-negative bacteria from adhering to the epithelial cells. This protective coating

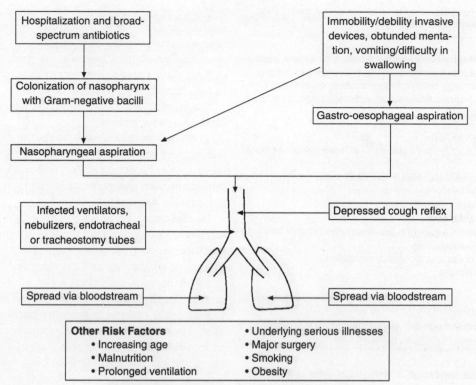

Fig. 13.2.3. Pathogenesis of nosocomial pneumonias.

is lost in very ill individuals, so that pathogenic Gram-negative organisms adhere to receptors present on epithelial cells of the mucosa and soon colonize it. The number of these bacterial receptors on both upper and lower airway epithelial cells is increased in many illnesses. This change is associated with increased colonization at these sites. Risk factors for increased colonization due to enhanced adherence of bacteria to mucosal cells in the airways include serious illnesses, smoking, azotaemia, surgery and malnutrition (**10**).

Gastric Colonization

The acid within the stomach serves as a major deterrent to bacteria swallowed in the saliva. If gastric acidity is suppressed by the use of antacids and H_2-antagonists, the bacteria within the stomach survive, multiply, and soon colonize the upper gastrointestinal tract. Gastric contents laden with Gram-negative bacteria could easily regurgitate and be aspirated into the lungs, causing aspiration pneumonia. This is particularly frequent in obtunded patients, sedated patients or following a large vomit. Prophylaxis and treatment of bleeding stress ulcers with sucralfate which does not significantly increase gastric pH in most patients, has resulted in a reduced incidence of nosocomial pneumonias (**11, 12**). Further research on the relationship between lowered gastric acidity and nosocomial pneumonias is necessary.

Haematogenous Pneumonia

Rarely infected emboli from a septic thrombophlebitis can lead to septic infarcts within the lung. Catheter related sepsis or any other source of sepsis can cause bacteraemia with haematogenous spread of infection into the lungs, causing pneumonia.

Inhalation Pneumonia

Contaminated respiratory equipment (nebulizers, humidifiers, ventilator tubing etc) is a source of infected aerosols. Infected particles 3–5 microns in size can be deposited into the terminal bronchioles and alveoli, thereby causing a lower respiratory tract infection.

Iatrogenic Causes

Lack of aseptic precaution during suction of tracheobronchial secretions, either through an endotracheal tube or tracheostomy is an important cause of lower respiratory tract infection.

Factors Predisposing to Nosocomial Pneumonias (Table 13.2.2) (13, 14)

These can be divided into:

(A) *Host Factors* in which defence mechanisms are suppressed by (i) overwhelming infections, serious illnesses e.g. severe sepsis, extra pulmonary infections, prolonged shock, burns or severe trauma, or following major surgery; (ii) background factors which are associated with a greater propensity to infection. These include underlying chronic lung disease (chronic bronchitis), diabetes mellitus, cardiac disease, renal failure, liver cell dysfunction, underlying malignancy, advanced age, malnutrition prior to the onset of a critical illness or occurring acutely during the course of an illness, and total parenteral nutrition.

(B) *Therapeutic Interventions.* The most important of these are endotracheal intubation, tracheostomy, and mechanical ventilation. Nasogastric tubes encourage gastric colonization with pathogens, and perhaps provide a scaffolding or conduit for these pathogens

Table 13.2.2. Factors predisposing to nosocomial pneumonia (also applicable to other nosocomial infections)

A. Host Factors
* Overwhelming infections/serious illnesses e.g. severe sepsis, prolonged shock, burns, severe trauma or following major surgery
* Background factors e.g. chronic lung diseases, diabetes mellitus, cardiac, renal or hepatic dysfunction, advanced age, underlying malignancy, malnutrition
* Total parenteral nutrition

B. Therapeutic Interventions
* Endotracheal intubation/tracheostomy with mechanical ventilator support
* Use of invasive procedures (including central lines)
* Nasogastric tube
* Use of corticosteroids/chemotherapy
* Prolonged use of antibiotics
* Colonization of upper GI tract with Gram-negative bacteria following use of antacids/H_2-antagonists
* Use of high FIO_2 whilst on mechanical ventilation

C. Environmental Factors
* Overcrowding
* Overall unclean environment (unfortunately so frequently seen in developing countries)
* Transmission chiefly through contaminated hands of ICU personnel
* Increased prevalence of multiple, resistant organisms

to reach the pharynx; aspiration of these pathogens or of infected particulate matter results in pneumonia. Corticosteroids/ antimitotic agents are immunosuppressants, and their use both encourages and masks infection. As mentioned earlier, there is evidence that excessive neutralization of acid to treat upper GI bleeds by antacids and H_2-antagonists also facilitates upper GI tract colonization with Gram-negative bacteria, and predisposes to pulmonary infection. The use of very high oxygen concentrations in mechanical ventilation over prolonged periods of time may also be detrimental to lung morphology and physiology, and may well predispose to infection. Prolonged antibiotic therapy can induce a superinfection by organisms resistant to conventional therapy, and lead to nosocomial pneumonia resistant to the usual antibiotics.

(C) *Environmental Factors* like overcrowding, an overall unclean environment (which unfortunately is frequently seen in developing countries), increased prevalence of multiple, resistant organisms, and transmission chiefly through the contaminated hands of ICU personnel, all predispose to the development of nosocomial infections.

Clinical Diagnosis (15)

The clinical diagnosis of nosocomial pneumonia, including Ventilator Associated Pneumonia (VAP), is difficult and often erroneous. This is proven by a post-mortem study showing that the clinical diagnosis of pneumonia was incorrect in 60 per cent of cases (16). The diagnosis of nosocomial pneumonia requires the presence of the following important features:

(i) Fever, leucocytosis, purulent sputum, or in the case of VAP, purulent tracheal secretions. At least two of these three clinical criteria should be present.

(ii) A chest X-ray which shows a new or progressive alveolar infiltrate (**Fig. 13.2.4**).

The presence of an abnormal radiographic infiltrate together with at least two of three clinical criteria stated above has a high degree of sensitivity but a low specificity. When all three clinical criteria are present in a patient with a fresh alveolar infiltrate on an X-ray chest, the specificity improves but the sensitivity falls to an unacceptable level (< 50 per cent) (**17**).

Diagnostic problems in an individual patient can be formidable for the following reasons:

(i) A systemic inflammatory response characterized by fever and leucocytosis may be present, but its absence does not exclude the diagnosis of pneumonia. Also, fever and leucocytosis can occur in infections other than pneumonia and in non-infective pathologies in a critically ill patient.

(ii) Absence of sputum or of significant lower respiratory tract secretions in patients with a tracheostomy (with or without ventilator support), does not exclude pneumonia in the presence of a recent infiltrate on an X-ray chest in a critically ill patient.

(iii) A 'shadow' on a chest X-ray is not necessarily inflammatory. Localized shadows in one or both lung fields can be due to pulmonary oedema, pulmonary haemorrhage, pulmonary infarction, ARDS, and other non-inflammatory causes. Atelectasis is often mistaken for pneumonia in a critically ill patient. A clearing of the shadow after vigorous physiotherapy differentiates infiltrates caused by atelectasis from those due to infection.

In a study of autopsy-proven VAP, no single radiographic sign had a diagnostic accuracy > 68 per cent (**18**). The presence of air bronchogram was the only sign that corresponded best with pneumonia, predicting 64 per cent of pneumonias in this study (**18**).

(iv) Nosocomial pneumonia in a patient with ARDS may be impossibly difficult to diagnose on a chest X-ray. A number of pathologies can cause asymmetric consolidation in patients with

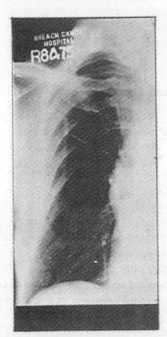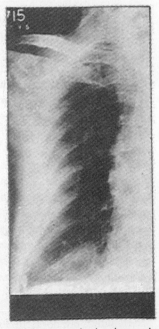

Fig. 13.2.4. X-ray of a patient with nosocomial pneumonia showing newly evolving infiltrates in right lower lobe. **(a)** X-ray on 21/3/95. **(b)** X-ray on 25/3/95.

ARDS. An air bronchogram on a chest X-ray in a patient with ARDS is not necessarily predictive of nosocomial pneumonia.

The above discussion suggests that clinical features combined with radiographic findings are of help, but lack sufficient specificity in the diagnosis of nosocomial pneumonia. Bacteriological evidence of pulmonary parenchymal infection is therefore also considered necessary to make a firm diagnosis. The cost-effectiveness of different methods used to obtain this bacteriological evidence and the relation of the evidence obtained to ultimate patient management and patient outcome are matters of continued discussion. These methods are briefly discussed below.

Bacteriological Examination of Respiratory Secretions

1. Sputum and Endotracheal Aspirate Examination

A. Microscopic Examination

This is useful in determining the presence and at times the site of infection (upper airways, lung parenchyma).

Leucocytes

More than 25 leucocytes per low power field denote infection, but not necessarily pneumonia. Marino (19) stresses the importance of using the presence of epithelial cells of the oral cavity in a sputum sample as markers of the mouth and upper airways, while alveolar macrophages and elastin fibres are used as markers of the distal airspaces and lung parenchyma respectively. The epithelial cells of the oral cavity are large flattened cells with abundant cytoplasm, and if a sputum sample contains many such epithelial cells, it is not suitable for further examination or culture. On the other hand, alveolar macrophages inhabit only distal airspaces so that their presence denotes that at least a part of the specimen being examined is from the lower respiratory tract. The presence of elastin fibres in the sputum sample is often used as evidence in favour of a necrotizing pneumonia (20). These fibres are filamentous structures visualized by placing a drop of KOH over the sputum sample. When present, the elastin fibres appear as clumps of interlocking filaments and denote a destructive parenchymal lesion within the lungs.

B. Significance of Sputum and Endotracheal Aspirate Cultures

It is always necessary to screen sputum samples before asking for cultures. Only samples that represent secretions from the lower respiratory tract (and are not from the oropharynx), are suitable for being cultured.

It is worth stressing that sputum cultures and cultures of aspirates through an endotracheal tube or tracheostomy tube which has been in situ for 5 to 7 days often grow Gram-negative organisms—in particular Pseudomonas aeurginosa, because of colonization of the trachea by these bacteria. A positive tracheal aspirate culture therefore does not necessarily indicate infection or pneumonia, nor does it necessarily indicate the organism responsible for the pneumonia, if a pneumonia is indeed present. The difficulties in interpreting sputum or tracheal aspirate cultures in relation to a possible nosocomial pneumonia, make one wonder as to how

cost-effective sputum and tracheal aspirate cultures are, and how frequently they should be ordered in poor developing countries.

We however, routinely perform qualitative cultures on tracheal aspirates when there is strong clinical suspicion of nosocomial pneumonia.

The reasons for doing so are listed below:

(i) The diagnostic test is non-invasive, cheap and requires no expertise, compared to invasive testing. Even a junior nurse can perform an aspiration procedure at the bedside (21).

(ii) Qualitative cultures of tracheal aspirates usually identify pathogenic organism found by invasive tests. They have therefore a high sensitivity. They however frequently identify non-pathogenic organisms, reducing the specificity and predictive value of the test (21).

(iii) If cultures are negative for pathogenic bacteria, VAP is unlikely, unless the patient has received antibiotics (22).

(iv) When quantitative cultures are performed in specimens, the sensitivity ranges from 38 to 100 per cent and specificity from 14–100 per cent (23).

The practical management of a patient with nosocomial VAP may be influenced by tracheal aspirate culture sensitivity tests under the following circumstances: (i) if there is an absence of response to empiric antibiotic therapy, a culture sensitivity test of the tracheal aspirate may help in the correct choice of antibiotics; (ii) if cultures of respiratory tract secretions grow Staphylococci an appropriate antibiotic against this organism should be used, rather than the usual antibiotic combination against Gram-negative organisms.

Even so, in vitro sensitivity of cultured organisms is not necessarily synonymous with in vivo sensitivity. If a patient with nosocomial pneumonia is doing well on antibiotics which on in vitro testing are shown to be ineffective against the organism grown on culture, it is wise to persist with the clinically effective antibiotics.

2. Invasive Diagnostic Tests (15, 21)

Role of PSB sampling

Samples of lower respiratory tract secretions can be collected by special protected brushes through a fibreoptic bronchoscope (PSB sampling). The brush is housed in a catheter that is plugged at the distal end. The protective housing allows the catheter to be advanced through a bronchoscope without coming into contact with the upper airways. Brushing should be obtained from the area of abnormal radiological shadows observed on the X-ray chest. The material should be stained by Gram's stain and cultured qualitatively and quantitatively. A culture yielding 10^3/ml or greater concentration of organisms supports the diagnosis of nosocomial pneumonia and identifies the pathogens (24, 25). The sensitivity for PSB tests ranges from 33–100 per cent, with a median of 67 per cent, and the specificity ranges from 50 to 100 per cent with a median of 95 per cent. PSB sampling therefore offers greater specificity and lesser sensitivity in the diagnosis of nosocomial pneumonia.

Bronchoscopic procedures even when performed expertly carry a risk to critically ill patients on ventilator support. The main complication is hypoxia during the procedure; this could lead to hypotension, arrhythmias and even death. Hypoxia may persist for several hours after the procedure, particularly in patients with ARDS.

Role of BAL

Brochoscopic alveolar lavage has also been used in the diagnosis of VAP. The sensitivity of quantitative BAL fluid cultures ranges from 42–93 per cent with a mean of 73 per cent. For quantitative cultures a CFU (colony forming units) count/ml of 10^3 to 10^5 is considered a positive result. The specificity ranges from 45–100 per cent with a mean of 82 per cent

Role of Blinded Invasive Procedures

The risk and expense entailed in bronchoscopic procedures has led to the development of other tests requiring less expense, expertise and risk. These tests include the following nonbroncho-scopic techniques: blinded bronchial sampling (BBS), mini-BAL, blinded sampling with PSB (BPSB). The sensitivity and specificity are reported to be similar to bronchoscopic techniques. We have no experience with blinded nonbronchoscopic invasive procedures.

3. Positive Blood Culture, Positive Culture of a Pleural Exudate

In a patient with clinical and radiological features compatible with nosocomial pneumonia, a positive blood culture is to be taken as a clear pointer to the nature of the organism causing the infection. Similarly cultures of an organism from a tapped pleural exudate is certain bacteriological evidence of nosocomial pneumonia. Unfortunately pleural effusions or empyemas are infrequent and blood cultures come positive only in a small minority of patients with nosocomial pneumonia.

In conclusion, the diagnosis of nosocomial pneumonia should be based on an overall perspective of clinical, radiological and bacteriological findings. There is no diagnostic criterion or proce-dure that serves as gold standard for the diagnosis of nosocomial (including VAP) pneumonia. There is no definite scientific evidence, or for that matter expert consensus, to show that antibiotic treat-ment based on bacteriological examination and cultures of lower respiratory secretions via special bronchoscopic procedures is superior to empiric treatment aided by culture sensitivity reports on sputum or on tracheal secretions aspirated through a trache-otomy or endotracheal tube (21). The only concession in favour of bronchoscopic diagnostic procedures is that specificity in diagno-sis is improved, and perhaps the unnecessary use of antibiotics is avoided for clinically insignificant organisms, or in situations where smears and cultures are negative. However patient outcome has not been altered for the better by the use of diagnostic invasive bronchoscopic procedures. In poor developing countries, it is therefore justifiable to treat nosocomial pneumonia (suspected on clinical and radiological evidence) empirically with a suitable planned antibiotic regime. Culture sensitivity of tracheal secretions in VAP may or may not be of help in empiric management.

Where expense is not in question and the expertise good and available, bronchoscopic bronchoalveolar lavage or protected bronchoalveolar lavage on protected brush specimens are stained and cultured to guide treatment. This second option in our opinion

is chiefly of use if done before starting antibiotics. Its efficacy is reduced, if the patient has already been receiving antibiotics. In any case, in critically ill patients, empiric therapy with antibiotics should commence promptly after the bronchoscopic procedure. Treatment should never await culture reports. A positive Gram's stain could however guide initial treatment. Treatment could be later modified, based on culture sensitivity reports.

In our unit we use empiric antibiotic therapy for nosocomial pneumonia. Bacteriologic examination of tracheal aspirates is done routinely but it is a moot point as to what extent this helps man-agement and patient outcome. We use PSB sampling for bacterio-logical evidence if a patient on empiric therapy fails to improve. The PSB sampling is done before changing antibiotic regime. Again, it is doubtful if this protocol influences patient outcome.

Antibiotic Therapy in Nosocomial Pneumonias

Though antibiotic therapy to start with is often empiric, the following factors need to be considered for optimal selection of antibiotics.

(i) *A knowledge and awareness of the prevalence of core organisms and their sensitivity to various antibiotics in a particular ICU set-up.* Core organisms responsible for nosocomial infection in units all over the world are predominantly Gram-negative bacteria. It is the exact prevalence of different Gram-negative organisms and their varying sensitivity to antibiotics that is important. This prevalence and sensitivity to antibiotics may vary from unit to unit. Also preva-lence and sensitivity patterns may vary in the same unit from time to time. A bacteriologic surveillance in every ICU is therefore of crucial importance. Also, the awareness of the nature of organisms generally responsible for VAP in a unit is of help in choosing ap-propriate antibiotic therapy.

(ii) *Clinical background* (15, 26). The following clinical features require special consideration.

(a) Presence or absence of *risk factors*. To give an example, nosocomial pneumonia is more likely to be caused by MRSA, if the patient has been receiving corticosteroids and antibiotics prior to the pneumonia, if he is on ventilator support for close to a week, or if there is an underlying COPD. On the other hand, nosocomial pneumonia occurring in patients with head injury is more often due to methicillin sensitive staphylococcus.

(b) The *severity* of pneumonia, whether mild to moderate or severe.

(c) In VAP, the *time of onset* of the nosocomial pneumonia— early onset or late onset.

(d) *Whether the patient has received antibiotics* prior to the onset of pneumonia.

In a recent study (27) in patients with early-onset VAP who had not received prior antibiotic therapy, the aetiological bacteria often found were Enterobacteriaceae, Haemophilus sp, MSSA or S. pneumonia. Monotherapy with a second generation cephalosporin (e.g. cefuroxime) or a third generation cephalosporin with no anti-pseudomonal activity (e.g cefotaxime or ceftriaxone), or the use of clavulinic acid with amoxycillin was appropriate in these patients.

In contrast, VAP occuring in patients after prolonged ventilator support (late onset) and after prolonged use of antibiotics is often caused by multiresistant pathogens such as P. aeruginosa, Acinetobacter, MRSA. A polymicrobial infection is often found in these patients. The appropriate antibiotic choice would be a broad-spectrum anti-Pseudomonas β-lactam, such as piperacillin-tazobactam or imipenem-cilastin or meropenem plus aminoglycoside plus vancomycin.

In patients with early onset VAP who have received antibiotics, Gram-negative organisms (Ps. aeruginosa and/or other Gram-negative core organisms), as also Streptococci and H. influenzae are often responsible for the infection.

Finally, in late onset pneumonia occurring without antibiotic use during 15 days prior to infection, Enterobacter, MSSA and occasionally Gram-negative bacteria are often causative agents.

In both the above groups i.e. early onset with previous antibiotic therapy and late onset without antibiotic therapy, an appropriate antiobiotic choice would be a combination of an aminoglycoside or ciprofloxacin with an anti-Pseudomonal β-lactam. Vancomycin need not be used. If nosocomial pneumonia is thought to result from aspiration of stomach contents, or if there is any other reason to suspect anaerobic infection, metronidazole or clindamycin should be added to the antibiotic regime.

(iii) *Information obtained from Gram's stain of respiratory secretions.* The presence of chiefly Gram-positive bacteria should direct treatment towards the staphylococcus, streptococcus, pneumococcus. The morphology of stained organisms is also of help in identification. Predominant Gram-negative bacilli direct an appropriate choice of antibiotics. Empiric therapy should start promptly without awaiting culture reports.

(iv) *Information obtained from culture sensitivity reports.* Though both sensitivity and specificity in identification of the aetiological agent in nosocomial pneumonia leave much to be desired, the culture report may be valuable in patient management, particularly if the empiric therapy decided upon does not prove beneficial.

Lack of Response to Antimicrobial Therapy (28)

There are several reasons for a lack of response to antibiotic therapy. These include a wrong diagnosis of pneumonia, or lack of antibiotic coverage against the causative organism. At times though the choice of antibiotic therapy is correct, *persistence of the aetiological agent* leads to a persistent or worsening pneumonia. Persistence of the offending micro-organism may be due to several factors; an important cause, is inappropriate dosing regime.

Superinfection pneumonia is a serious problem that often causes death. Superinfection follows prolonged broad-spectrum antibiotic therapy. Organisms causing superinfection are generally drug-resistant and therefore lethal. They include resistant strains of Pseudomonas and other Gram-negative bacteria, MRSA, Enterococci, fungi and multidrug-resistant Enterobacteriaceae.

Nosocomial pneumonia when severe can lead to *multiorgan dysfunction* and/or *septic shock*, situations where the mortality is high in spite of adequate antibiotic therapy

Prognosis

Nosocomial pneumonia is the leading cause of death due to hospital-acquired infections. Mortality rate ranges from 20 per cent to 70 per cent. High-risk organisms that lead to increased mortality include Pseudomonas aeruginosa, Acinetobacter, Enterobacter, other Gram-negative organisms, S. faecalis, S. aureus, Candida species, Aspergillus and polymicrobial infections. It must be however remembered that nosocomial pneumonia is more common in patients who are critically ill with multiple problems. To what extent death can be attributable to nosocomial pneumonia per se may be impossible to judge. It is likely that many critically ill patients die with pneumonia rather than die of pneumonia.

Death in nosocomial pneumonia can result from any one or more of the following—septic shock, multiple organ dysfunction, ARDS, cardiovascular instability, GI bleed. In VAP it could also be occasionally related to barotrauma pneumothorax.

Prevention

Prevention of nosocomial pneumonia is of great importance, both to reduce mortality and morbidity as also to reduce hospital cost. Prevention of aspiration, particularly in the aspiration-prone patient is crucial. Patients fed via nasogastric tube should have the head end of the bed elevated at 45°. Feeds should be withheld if the earlier feed is retained within the stomach.

Patients should be turned frequently; physiotherapy to the chest, deep breathing, increasing mobility in bed all help to prevent atelectasis and infection.

Meticulous asepsis should be observed during suction of tracheal secretions. As explained later, hand-washing before and after examining a patient is an important prophylaxis against transmitted infection. Humidifiers, nebulizers, and all other respiratory equipment should be disinfected or sterilized as necessary.

Oral hygiene is also of crucial importance and may reduce or perhaps prevent the growth of Gram-negative organisms within the oropharynx of critically ill patients.

REFERENCES

1. Rello J, Quintana E, Ausina V et al. (1991). Incidence, etiology and outcome of nosocomial pneumonia in mechanically ventilated patients. Chest. 100, 439–444.

2. Craven DE, Steger KA. (1989). Nosocomial pneumonia in the intubated patient: New concepts on pathogenesis and prevention. Infect Dis Clin North Am. 3, 843–866.

3. Niederman MS, Craven DE, Fein A et al. (1990). Pneumonia in the critically ill hospitalized patient. Chest. 97, 170–179.

4. Celis R, Torres A, Gatell JM et al. (1988). Nosocomial pneumonia: A multi-variate analysis of risk and prognosis. Chest. 93, 318–324.

5. Haley RW, Hooton TM, Culver DH et al. (1981). Nosocomial infections in US hospitals, 1975–1976: Estimated frequency by selected characteristics of patients. Am J Med. 70, 947–959.

6. Cross AS, Roup B. (1981). Role of respiratory assistance devices in endemic nosocomial pneumonia. Am J Med. 70, 681–685.

7. Langer M, Mosconi P, Cigada M et al. (1989). Long-term respiratory support and risk of pneumonia in critically ill patients. Am Rev Respir Dis. 140, 302–305.

8. Seidenfeld JJ, Mullins RC, Fowler SR et al. (1986). Bacterial infection and acute lung injury in hamsters. Am Rev Respir Dis. 134, 22–26.

9. Niederman MS, Mantovani R, Schoch P et al. (1989). Patterns and routes of tracheobronchial colonization in mechanically ventilated patients: The role of nutritional status in colonization of the lower airway by Pseudomonas species. Chest. 95, 155–161.

10. Niederman MS, Fein AM. (1990). Sepsis Syndrome, the Adult Respiratory Distress Syndrome, and Nosocomial Pneumonia: A Common Clinical Sequence. Clinics in Chest Medicine. 11(4), 633–656.

11. Driks MR, Craven DE, Celli BR et al. (1987). Nosocomial pneumonia in intubated patients given sucralfate as compared with antacids or histamine type-2 blockers. N Engl J Med. 317, 1376–1382.

12. Eddleston JM, Vohra A, Scott P et al. (1991). A comparison of the frequency of stress ulceration and secondary pneumonia in sucralfate- or ranitidine-treated intensive care unit patients. Crit Care Med. 19, 1491–1496.

13. Cook DJ, Kolef MH. (1998). Risk factors for ICU acquired pneumonia. JAMA. 279, 1605–1606.

14. Cook DJ, Walter SD, Cook RJ et al. (1998). Incidence and risk factors for ventilator associated pneumonia in critically ill patients. Ann Intern Med. 129, 433–440.

15. Chastre J, Fagon JY. (2002). Ventilator-associated pneumonia. Respir Crit Care Med. 165(7), 867–893.

16. Bryant LR, Mobin-Uddin K, Dillon ML et al. (1973). Missed diagnosis of pneumonia in patients needing mechanical respiration. Arch Surg. 106, 286–288.

17. Sutherland K, Steinberg K, Maunder R et al. (1995). Pulmonary Infection during the acute respiratory distress syndrome. Am J Respir Crit Care Med. 152, 550–556.

18. Wunderink RG, Woldenberg LS, Zeiss J et al. (1992). The radiographic diagnosis of autopsy-proven ventilator-associated pneumonia. Chest, 101(2), 458–463.

19. Marino PL. (1998). Nosocomial Pneumonia. In: The ICU Book. pp. 516–530. Williams and Wilkins, USA.

20. Salata RA, Lederman MM, Shlaes DM. (1987). Diagnosis of nosocomial pneumonia in intubated intensive care unit patients. Am Rev Respir Dis. 135, 426–432.

21. Grossman RF, Fein A. (2000). Evidence-based assessment of diagnostic tests for ventilator-associated pneumonia. Chest, 117(4) Suppl 2, 177–181.

22. El-Ebiary M, Torres A, Gonzalez J et al. (1993). Quantitative cultures of endotracheal aspirates for the diagnosis of ventilator-associated pneumonia. Am Rev Respir Dis. 148, 1552–1557.

23. Sauaia M, Moore F, Moore E et al. (1993). Diagnosing pneumonia in mechanically ventilated trauma patients: endotracheal aspirate versus bronchoalveolar lavage. J Trauma. 35, 512–517.

24. Fagon J-Y, Chastre J, Hance AJ et al. (1988). Detection of nosocomial lung infection in ventilated patients. Am Rev Respir Dis. 138, 110–116.

25. Richard C, Pezzang M, Bouhaja B et al. (1988). Comparison of non-protected lower respiratory tract secretions and protected specimen brush samples in the diagnosis of pneumonia. Intensive Care Med. 14, 30–33.

26. Lode HM, Schaberg T, Raffenberg M et al. (1998). Nosocomial pneumonia in the critical care unit. Crit Care Clin. 141, 119–133.

27. Trouillet JL, Chastre J et al. (1998). Ventilator-associated pneumonia caused by potentially drug-resistant bacteria. Am J Respir Crit Care Med. 157, 531–539.

28. Wunderink RG. (1995) Ventilator-associated pneumonia—Failure to respond to antibiotic therapy. Clin Chest Med. 16(1), 173–190.

Catheter-related Infections

Central venous lines, Swan-Ganz catheters and intra-arterial catheters are frequently used in the monitoring and management of patients in the ICU. These catheters provide for the infusion of fluids and electrolytes, for the infusion of antimicrobial agents, for short-term hyperalimentation and for haemodynamic monitoring in critically ill individuals.

Besides the use of central venous catheters which provide direct access to the large veins in the chest, metal needles and teflon or other synthetic short catheters are often inserted into peripheral veins for the infusion of fluids and the intravenous administration of drugs. The intravenous and intra-arterial access provided in ICU patients by catheters for purposes stated above is for a short-term period. They are ordinarily removed as soon as the critical phase of the patient's illness is over.

Central venous catheters used over a long period are of the Hickman type. These are used primarily for the administration of chemotherapy, and for total parenteral nutrition that needs to be continued for weeks or even months. Long-term catheters have a subcutaneous tunnel through which the catheter passes after entering the skin, before entering a large central vein. This subcutaneous tunnel reduces the risk of catheter-related infections considerably.

All catheters either entering central or peripheral veins or arteries, are foreign bodies and are prone to get infected; such infected vascular catheters constitute an important source of varying degrees of sepsis in all critical care units (1–3). In our unit, vascular catheters are responsible for 5–10 per cent of all hospital-acquired infections. Catheter-related sepsis is often difficult to diagnose with certainty. It involves the presence of clinical features of sepsis, for which no other cause is present; it also involves the profuse or dense growth of an organism from the tip of the catheter, the same organism being also grown on blood culture. Catheter-related sepsis needs to be distinguished from mere colonization of the catheter tip, in which there is a comparatively sparse growth of organisms on the catheter tip cultures. Blood cultures may or may not be positive. It is obvious that the distinguishing features are quantitative and perhaps arbitrary. Two facts are of crucial importance—the longer a catheter is used to provide vascular access, the greater the chances for infection. Suspicion of catheter related sepsis is often though not necessarily confirmed, when removal of the catheter results in a clearing of the features of sepsis or infection.

Risk Factors (Table 13.2.3)

A number of risk factors can be identified. A multilumen catheter offers more portals for the entry of infection than a single lumen catheter. Also, multilumen catheters are generally inserted in more severely ill patients who are subjected to more interventions, leading to an enhanced risk of infection.

Catheters introduced into the jugular vein are more frequently associated with infection compared to subclavian vein catheters. This could be related to increased motion at the jugular vein site and the difficulty in keeping this site clean due to soiling with oropharyngeal secretions.

The number of times a closed infusion system is opened, either to draw blood or to inject drugs, correlates with an increased risk of contamination and infection.

As mentioned earlier, the longer a catheter remains within a vein, the greater the risk. Repeated catheterization also increases

Table 13.2.3. Risk factors for catheter-related infections

* Prolonged use of catheters
* Multilumen catheters—provide more portals of entry for infection
* Frequent 'opening' of intravenous infusion sets
* Incorrect handling of intravenous infusions and catheters
* Frequent catheterizations
* Skin lesions/breach of skin in area of catheter
* Use of tightly occlusive dressings over the point of entry
* Sepsis at other sites (particularly intra-abdominal sepsis which causes 'seeding' of the catheter)

the risk. It is unwise to change the catheter every few days, yet in our opinion it is probably equally unwise to keep the catheter in for weeks with intent to change it only when infection occurs. Perhaps a via media would be to change the catheter over a guide wire every 8 to 10 days. Risk of catheter related infection increases in the presence of a suppurative focus in the body as it exposes the catheter to bactaermia. Occlusive dressing over the site of puncture can lead to a growth of micro-organisms and predispose to infection at the site of entry.

Physiopathology (4)

There are three possible mechanisms that can lead to infection of arterial or venous catheters:

(i) Contamination of the infused fluid. Micro-organisms can gain entry into the blood through breaks or contamination in bivalves or stopcocks. Rarely, the infusate is contaminated, particularly that used for hyperalimentation.

(ii) Organisms, and in particular those constituting normal skin flora can migrate from the entry site in the skin along the catheter tract, and colonize the intravascular portion and the tip of the catheter, which is often covered by a fibrin sheath. This fibrin sheath provides a protective environment for micro-organisms as it is not easily permeable to antibiotics or to drugs. Silicone catheters like the Hickman's and Broviac's catheters are less thrombogenic and less likely to have a fibrin coat on their intravascular portion. Though the above mechanism is considered the most frequent cause of catheter infection, it is difficult to comprehend how non-motile organisms e.g. Staphylococci, can migrate for long distances from the site of skin entry to the catheter tip.

(iii) Haematogenous seeding of the intravascular portion of the catheter by organisms already present in the blood stream. This seeding could either be a mere colonization of the catheter tip, or it could be the source of secondary sepsis and septicaemia. Haematogenous seeding of the catheter tip is common in patients with severe abdominal sepsis (e.g. septic peritonitis) even in the presence of negative blood cultures. More often than not, this merely represents colonization of the catheter tip rather than a catheter related sepsis. 'Seeding' of the catheter tip could also occur from organisms which gain entry into the bloodstream through the gastrointestinal tract. This translocation of bacteria from the gut into the blood stream occurs when there is an overgrowth of pathogenic bacteria in the gut. This is observed in critically ill individuals, particularly in patients whose gastric acidity is sharply reduced by H_2-antagonists and antacids. In many such very ill patients the mucosal barrier of the gut is devitalized or has small

breaks which allow the overgrowing bacterial flora to enter the bloodstream.

Microbiology

In our experience in our unit over the past 3 years, about 15 per cent of catheter related infections are due to the Staphylococcus—chiefly S. aureus. S. epidermidis and S. saprophyticus are coagulase-negative, are not usually pathogenic in normal subjects, but assume increasing pathogenicity in very sick individuals (5, 6). S. epidermidis produces a sticky substance which allows the organisms to adhere to foreign prosthetic materials like intravascular catheters. This could account for the prevalence of this organism on catheter tip cultures (5, 6). Unfortunately, a number of these Staphylococci are now found to be methicillin-resistant. In the West, the incidence of methicillin-resistant S. epidermidis can be as high as 80 per cent (5). S. aureus is not as frequent a source of catheter-related infection in our unit as compared to studies reported from the West (7). Gram-negative organisms constitute an even more frequent source of catheter-related infections—70–75 per cent. The most commonly seen organisms are the Pseudomonas followed by the Acinetobacter, Klebsiella, Enterobacter and Enterococcus.

Clinical Features

Catheter-related infections can produce three syndromes:

(i) *Infection at the Site of Entry* of the catheter through the skin. This is characterized by tenderness, erythema, induration, and at times exudation at the cutaneous entry site. If an exudate is present, its culture is often positive.

(ii) *Tunnel Infection* with long-term lines as in the Hickman's catheter. This is characterized by tenderness, induration, erythema, and warmth starting well beyond the cutaneous entry point of the catheter, without any discharge from the entry site. At times, tunnel infection may be associated with infection at the entry site.

(iii) *Catheter-related Sepsis* is characterized by fever, tachycardia, leucocytosis and occasional tachypnoea; if unrecognized and untreated, increasingly severe sepsis results, culminating at times in multiple organ failure. A positive blood culture is often but not always present. It is important to rule out any other cause of sepsis in the patient before diagnosing catheter-related sepsis. Frank pus at the entry site of the catheter in the presence of fever, chills and tachycardia, usually points to catheter-related sepsis.

Catheter-related infections in granulocytopaenic patients are even more difficult to diagnose. Systemic features are minimal, though some degree of fever is invariably present. These patients do

Table 13.2.4. Features suggesting catheter-related infection

* Local inflammation/phlebitis at catheter site
* Features suggestive of thrombosis of large veins (when vein is cannulated), or of distal embolic phenomenon (when artery is cannulated).
* Sepsis for which there is no other apparent cause
* Defervescence after catheter removal
* Microbiological evidence of a contaminated infusate
* 15 or more colonies on semiquantitative culture of catheter tips (Note: Catheter tip cultures are routinely done in all critically ill patients, or whenever there is suspicion of a catheter-related infection)
* Candidal retinitis in patients on total parenteral nutrition

not manifest the typical inflammatory features associated with entry site infection. Tenderness on palpation is however invariably present.

Features suggesting catheter-related infections are detailed in **Table 13.2.4**.

Laboratory Investigations

(a) *Blood Cultures*. Blood cultures should be done at least twice to detect bacteraemia in patients with catheter-related sepsis. At least 10 ml of blood is withdrawn each time for culture, so as to improve the yield for positive results (**8**). Blood cultures should not be taken from the suspected catheter because of the risk of false-positive cultures, but from other venepuncture sites (**5**).

(b) *Quantitative Blood Culture Techniques* (**9**). Catheter-related bacteraemia has been rather arbitrarily defined by using quantitative blood culture techniques: (i) More than a 10-fold increase in colony forming units (CFU) of bacteria per ml of blood obtained through the suspected catheter, as compared with blood samples drawn from distant peripheral veins is of clinical significance. (ii) In the absence of a positive peripheral blood culture, more than 1000 CFU/ml in blood obtained from the suspected catheter is also considered to be clinically significant.

(c) *Culture of the Catheter Tip*. When catheter-related sepsis is suspected, the catheter should be removed after cleansing the site of entry with alcohol, and the tip sent for culture. After withdrawal, the distal 2–3 cm of the catheter is cut with sterile scissors and the severed end placed in a sterile tube and promptly sent to the microbiology laboratory. Here, the severed end should be immediately plated directly on blood agar plates and the number of colonies of microbes on the plate quantified. This is a semiquantitative culture (**10**). Broth cultures are unreliable for distinguishing colonization of catheters from true catheter sepsis.

Maki et al. (**10**) have interpreted results of colony culture on agar plates as shown in **Fig. 13.2.5**. These workers maintain that when blood cultures are positive: (i) > 15 colonies of the same organism on the catheter tip suggest that the catheter is the source of infection—a true catheter related-sepsis; (ii) < 15 colonies on the catheter tip suggest that the source of septicaemia is elsewhere, and that the catheter tip is merely seeded, and then colonized by organisms from the blood stream.

When the blood cultures show no growth: (i) > 15 colonies on the catheter tip suggest a possible catheter-related sepsis. This can be confirmed if prompt removal of the catheter leads to a quick regression of sepsis; (ii) < 15 colonies on the catheter tip suggest that the tip is merely colonized and the cause of fever and sepsis if present, lies elsewhere.

As mentioned earlier, the above interpretation is arbitrary in a way, and abatement of sepsis following catheter removal is probably the closest one can get to relating sepsis to an indwelling catheter.

(d) *Gram's Staining of the Catheter*. Cooper and Hopkins (**11**) used Gram's stain on a removed catheter which had been longitudinally slit by sterile means. Both the internal and external surface of the catheter are stained. A positive stain for organisms gives a quick idea of the presence and nature of the infection. The surface of the catheter involved could provide information about the source of infection. Organisms on the inner surface suggest contamination of the infused fluids; organisms on the external surface suggest a cutaneous source or a bacteraemic seeding from a distant site. Though time consuming, this investigation may prove useful, and requires further evaluation.

Complications of Catheter-related Sepsis

Other than varying grades of bacterial sepsis, the two major complications are a septic thrombophlebitis (**12, 13**), and disseminated fungal infection.

Septic peripheral thrombophlebitis is obvious by the signs of inflammation and thrombosis of peripheral veins. Thrombophlebitis in central veins is often difficult to diagnose. Oedema proximal to the phlebitis is common and should promptly arouse suspicion. Localized pain, warmth and tenderness is an important feature, particularly when the internal jugular vein is involved. Blood cultures continue to be positive, and features of sepsis persist after removal of the catheter. Venography of a central vein may confirm the diagnosis. Small pulmonary emboli may complicate the picture, and in one of our patients sudden death occurred from pulmonary embolism, the source of embolism being an infected clot in the subclavian vein.

Disseminated fungal infection is often missed. It should always

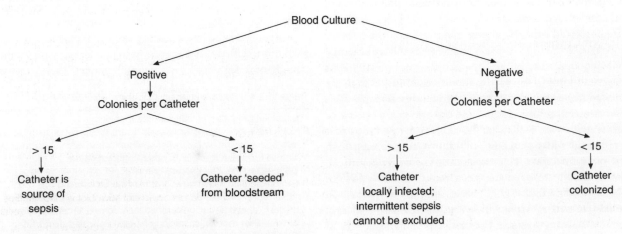

Fig. 13.2.5. Interpretation of semiquantitative cultures (reference **10**).

be suspected when fever and other features of sepsis continue in spite of removal of the catheter and the use of appropriate antibiotics (6). This is of particular importance in neutropaenic or immunocompromised patients. Fever persisting for more than 3–4 days in spite of the administration of broad-spectrum antibiotics and catheter removal in a critically ill neutropaenic patient, should prompt a trial with amphotericin B (14).

Treatment

Entry Site Infections. Short-term catheters suspected to be infected should be removed, but it would be unwise to remove a long-term Hickman's catheter as this catheter is often used as a lifeline for chemotherapeutic drugs and / or for hyperalimentation in very sick individuals. Entry site infection of long-term catheters should be treated with local bactericidal ointments and antibiotics given orally or intravenously. The choice of antibiotics depends on the organisms grown, aided by antibiotic sensitivity results.

Tunnel Infection. Patients with tunnel infection (e.g. with Hickman's catheter) require removal of the catheter (15). The tunnel needs to be surgically opened and the infection drained. One should not wait for culture reports before starting antibiotics. The antibiotic regime should preferably include vancomycin for a possible staphylococcal infection, and a third generation cephalosporin active against Ps. aeruginosa and other Gram-negative infections or an aminoglycoside.

Catheter-related Sepsis. Short-term catheters are promptly removed and antibiotics given. We prefer to give antibiotics for a period of 5–10 days depending on the clinical response. Empiric therapy generally includes a third generation cephalosporin (ceftazidime or cefoperazone) with an aminoglycoside. If features of sepsis persist, methicillin or vancomycin are added. The frequency of infection due to methicillin-resistant staphylococci is still low in our unit. In other units, particularly in oncology units, the incidence is high, necessitating the empiric use of vancomycin till blood and catheter tip culture sensitivity reports are available. If catheter sepsis is proven on culture reports, or is strongly suspected, and if the patient worsens in spite of using a broad-spectrum antibiotic cover, a decision to start amphotericin B should be taken.

Septic thrombophlebitis particularly of central veins, requires the use of intravenous heparin in addition to an appropriate combination of antibiotics as stated above.

Prevention of Catheter-related Infections (16) (Table 13.2.5)

(i) Percutaneous insertion of catheters into central and even into peripheral veins should be preceded by vigorous scrubbing of the skin around the insertion site with betadine or chlorhexidine. The solution should be allowed to 'stand' on the skin for 30 seconds before inserting the catheter. It has been shown that the risk of infection related to vascular catheters can be substantially lowered by disinfecting the skin before and after catheter insertion with 2 per cent chlorhexidine solution (17). Sterile gloves should always be used, and preferably a sterile mask and gown as well.

(ii) An inserted catheter should be cared for meticulously. We

Table 13.2.5. Prevention of catheter-related infections

* Thorough disinfection of skin around insertion site prior to inserting catheter. Allow the disinfectant to 'stand' on the skin for at least 30 seconds prior to inserting catheter
* Meticulous handwashing prior to touching infusion lines/catheter
* Sterile procedures for injecting drugs through bivalves
* Maintaining separate lines for intravenous hyperalimentation
* Early removal of central and peripheral lines

clip a sterile towel starting close to the entry point, and extending proximally for a distance of 1.5 feet.

(iii) Careful hand-washing or wearing sterile gloves before touching the catheter or the lines of infusion sets is mandatory (18). Sterile procedures should be followed for injecting drugs through bivalves. A central line used for intravenous alimentation should not as far as possible be used for injecting drugs or other fluids; drugs and other infusions should be administered through a separate line. Catheters used for hyperalimentation, in our experience, have a greater chance of being infected in spite of the strictest aseptic precautions. The site of skin puncture by a central line should be carefully treated with an antibacterial ointment or powder and suitably covered with a sterile gauze dressing anchored to the skin by a hypoallergenic tape. Occlusive skin dressings are popular, as they allow easy inspection of the puncture site. Their disadvantage is that they allow moisture to accumulate over the skin, promoting microbial colonization.

(iv) The duration for which the catheter is inserted in a central vein varies in different units. The current trend is not to recommend routine replacement of the catheter at regular intervals as this is believed to increase the risk of catheter-associated complications (19). Yet, there are patients who require a central line for several weeks. Would it be wise to keep a central line for a well-nigh indefinite period if the patient so requires it? In our set-up we opt for a via media and recommend that a central line catheter is not kept for a period longer than 10 days. A Swan-Ganz catheter is preferably removed within 3 to 4 days. If a central venous catheter is needed for a longer duration, a new catheter is inserted over a guide wire. It is not necessary to make a fresh percutaneous puncture for insertion of a new catheter, except when the same site has been used for over 2–3 weeks, or the earlier catheter has been removed because of the presence of a catheter-related infection, or when the previous catheter tip has shown a profuse bacterial growth on culture.

Catheters in peripheral veins are removed and changed if necessary after 5–7 days, or at the first sign of thrombophlebitis.

(v) The earlier central lines and even catheters in peripheral veins are removed, the lesser the chance of catheter-related infection.

REFERENCES

1. Maki DG. (1989). Pathogenesis, prevention and management of infections due to intravascular devices used for infusion therapy. In: Infections Associated with Indwelling Medical Devices (Eds Bisno A, Waldvogel F). pp. 161–177. American Society for Microbiology. Washington DC.

2. Eyers S, Brummit C, Crossley K et al. (1990). Catheter-related sepsis:

Prospective, randomized study of three methods of long-term catheter maintenance. Crit Care Med. 18, 1073–1079.

3. Norwood S, Ruby A, Civetta J et al. (1991). Catheter-related infections and associated septicaemia. Chest. 99, 968–975.

4. Henderson DK. (2000). Infection due to percutaneous intravascular devices. In: Principles and Practice of Infectious Diseases, 5th edn (Eds Mandell GL, Bennett JE, Dolin R). pp. 3005–3007. Churchill Livingstone.

5. Lowy F, Hammer Sm. (1983). Staphylococcus epidermidis infections. Ann Intern Med. 99, 834–839.

6. Marino PL. (1998). The Indwelling Vascular Catheter. In: The ICU Book. pp. 76–93. William and Wilkins, USA.

7. Hampton A, Sheretz RJ. (1988). Vascular-access infections in hospitalized patients. Surg Clin North Am. 68, 57–71.

8. Aronson MD, Bor DH. (1987). Blood cultures. Ann Intern Med. 106, 246–253.

9. Benezra D, Kiehn TE, Gold JW et al. (1988). Prospective study of infections in indwelling central venous catheters using quantitative blood cultures. Am J Med. 85, 495–498.

10. Maki DG, Weise CE, Sarafin HW. (1977). A semiquantitative culture method for identifying intravenous-catheter related infection. N Engl J Med. 296, 1305–1309.

11. Cooper GL, Hopkins CC. (1985). Rapid diagnosis of intravascular catheter-associated infection by direct gram staining of catheter segments. N Engl J Med. 312, 1142–1147.

12. Garrison RN, Richardson JD, Fry DE. (1982). Catheter associated septic thrombophlebitis. South Med J. 75, 917–919.

13. Verghese A, Widrich WC, Arbeit RD. (1985). Central venous septic thrombophlebitis—the role of medical therapy. Medicine. 64, 394–400.

14. Rubin M, Pizzo PA. (1989). Update on the management of the febrile neutropaenic patient. Resident & Staff Physician. 35, 25–43.

15. Olson ME, Lam K, Bodey GP et al. (1992). Evaluation of Strategies for Central Venous Catheter Replacement. Crit Care Med. 20, 797–804.

16. Pearson ML. (1996). Guideline for prevention of intravascular device related infections. Hospital Infection Control Practices Advisory Committee (HICPAC). Infect Control Hosp Epidemiol. 17, 438–473.

17. Maki DG, Ringer M, Alvarado CJ. (1991). Prospective, randomised trial of povidone-iodine, alcohol, and chlorhexidine for prevention of infection associated with central venous and arterial catheters. Lancet. 338, 339–343.

18. Garner JS, Farero MS. (1986). Guidelines for handwashing and hospital environment control. Infect Control. 7, 231–243.

19. Cobbs DK, High RP, Sawyer RP et al. (1992). A controlled trial of scheduled replacement of central venous and pulmonary artery catheters. N Eng J Med. 327, 1062–1068.

Urinary Catheter-associated Infections

The most important predisposing factor for such infections is the presence of an indwelling urinary catheter (1, 2). The longer a catheter remains in the bladder, the greater the risk of urinary infection. Unfortunately, the use of urinary catheters for long periods of time in very ill individuals is often necessary. The incidence of bacteriuria from urinary catheters varies from 5–10 per cent per day (1). In our experience, a significant growth of organisms in urine is present in almost every patient who has an indwelling catheter for more than 8 days. Many of these are asymptomatic, but a significant number are symptomatic. As with all nosocomial infections, it is difficult to distinguish between colonization by bacteria and actual infection. Urinary infection may take the form of a cystitis or urethretis or may involve the upper urinary tract and produce pyelonephritis.

Physiopathology (3)

The urinary catheter provides a ready passage for organisms present around the perineum and the urethral meatus to enter the bladder, colonize and infect it. Ascending infection from the bladder can result in a pyelonephritis. This theory is dubious as it assumes that bacteria with no means of locomotion can travel long distances on their own. Yet the fact is incontrovertible that not uncommonly the same organism found around the perineum or the urethral meatus, is also isolated from within the bladder (4, 5). Perhaps the presence of a catheter markedly depresses local tissue resistance, and this aids the passage and growth of organisms upwards into the bladder. Another likely factor in the pathogenesis of urinary tract infections is the ability of pathogenic bacteria to adhere to mucosal cells within the bladder. In healthy individuals, it is the harmless commensals which adhere to cells of the bladder mucosa; this prevents more dangerous pathogenic organisms from adhering to it (6). A catheter within the bladder is associated with reduced adherence of commensals to the bladder mucosa. There is therefore an increased propensity for pathogenic bacteria to adhere and multiply (1).

Microbiology

An analysis of urine cultures in individuals with catheters in our ICU showed that the commonest organism grown was E. coli followed by Enterococci, Klebsiella, Proteus mirabilis, Ps. aeruginosa and Enterobacteriaceae. A growth of Candida is not at all uncommon in very ill patients with indwelling catheters who have been deluged with powerful broad-spectrum antibiotics. Polymicrobial infections are also fairly frequent in catheterized patients. The presence of polymicrobial infections in the urine in non-catheterized patients, or in those who have not had any instrumentation done on their urinary tracts, is likely to be due to contamination.

Risk Factors

Risk factors for catheter induced bacteriuria (often accompanied or followed by infection) are prolonged duration of catheterization, a break in the closed system drainage with colonization of the urinary bag, poor catheter care, urethral trauma, a raised serum creatinine, diabetes, preuretheal colonization with potential pathogenic bacteria and immunocompromised states.

Clinical Features (7)

Catheter-related urinary tract infections may be asymptomatic, and may be detected only by a routine urine examination. A search for a possible urinary tract infection is however mandatory in a patient with clinical features of sepsis, or in one who has a pyrexia for which there is no other apparent cause. Burning in the urethra and pain in the suprapubic region are indications of urethritis and cystitis. Pain in the flanks with tenderness on palpation over the loins when associated with fever suggests a possible upper urinary tract infection.

Infection may be mild, moderate or fulminant in nature. Fulminant Gram-negative infections produced by catheter-related Ps. aeruginosa or Klebsiella, or any other Gram-negative infections may take the form of high fever with severe rigors, and may quickly progress to a state of mental obtundation, hypotension, septic shock and renal failure. *A rapidly progressive renal insufficiency may be the sole clinical manifestation of a severe catheter-related urinary tract infection both in very critically ill patients and in immunocompromised states.*

Complications

These include, as stated above, pyelonephritis, emphysematous pyelonephritis, renal abscess, perinephric abscess, Gram-negative bacteraemia with septic shock. Progressive renal failure may complicate urinary tract infections, and this is often compounded by the use of nephrotoxic drugs (e.g. aminoglycosides) used to treat such infections.

Urinary Findings

Microscopic Examination. Pyuria is an indicator of urinary infection. The presence of white blood cell casts indicate an infection of the upper urinary tract. The presence in unspun urine of more than 2 leucocytes per high power field and/or bacteria observed under oil immersion suggests infection, as these observations have a 95 per cent correlation with the presence of more than 100,000 CFU/ml of urine (8). The leucocytes in an unspun urine specimen can be quantified by using a haemocytometer counter grid. Stamm (9) suggests that the number of leucocytes counted helps to differentiate infection from colonization. According to him, a leucocyte count > 10 cells/mm^3 indicates infection, and < 10 cells/mm^3 indicates colonization. This can serve as a useful empiric guide regarding the decision to start therapy whilst awaiting culture reports. It is noteworthy that the absence of bacteria on microscopy (or < 5 bacteria/oil immersion field), does not exclude infection. The importance and relevance of the microscopic findings described above relate to unspun urine. The quantification of leucocytes in a spun sediment is not always reliable for differentiating between infection and colonization (10).

Urine Culture. The presence of bacteria in a concentration > 100,000 CFU/ml suggests infection. There are a few points however worth noting: (i) A *consistent* increase in the colony count to > 100,000 CFU/ml is important (11). (ii) In patients with indwelling catheters over a prolonged period, a colony count > 100,000 CFU/ml does not always signify infection (12). One should take the overall clinical picture into consideration, and pay particular attention to the results of microscopic examination of the urine. (iii) In some instances, urinary infection can exist with a colony count < 100,000 CFU/ml. (iv) Urine cultures for bacteria or fungi submitted to the microbiology laboratory should be processed promptly. Alternatively, the specimens should be stored at 4°C; at this temperature the organisms remain viable for about 24 hours. If urine sent to the laboratory is kept standing for over 2 hours before being cultured, the urinary bacterial count increases significantly, thus making the diagnosis of urinary infections increasingly difficult. Sensitivity tests to antibiotics are routinely performed whenever the colony count is > 100,000 CFU/ml. When a polymicrobial flora is grown, sensitivity tests for different organisms may need to be performed separately.

Other Laboratory Investigations

A blood count may show leucocytosis and blood cultures may detect bacteraemia, the source being an infected urinary tract.

Imaging Studies

Patients in the ICU with urosepsis, whether catheter related or not, often require evaluation for upper urinary tract disease. Ultrasonography is useful to establish the anatomy of the kidneys, and to exclude an obstructed ureter. Occasionally, an intravenous or retrograde pyelography may be necessary. A CT scan may establish the diagnosis of a suspected renal or perinephric abscess and may yield further evidence of any ureteric obstruction.

Differential Diagnosis

It is important as stated earlier to distinguish urinary tract colonization manifested by asymptomatic bacteriuria from a true urinary tract infection. Prostatitis, pelvic inflammatory disease and diverticulitis may mimic a catheter-related urinary tract infection in a very ill individual. Not uncommonly, a septic state in a moribund patient in the ICU is mistakenly attributed to the presence of a comparatively mild to moderate urinary infection, whereas the actual cause is more sinister e.g. an intra-abdominal abscess or a peritonitis resulting from a bowel perforation or infarction.

Treatment

Bacteriuria in Asymptomatic Patients

Antibiotic therapy is discouraged as bacteriuria will often recur after antibiotics are stopped, or superinfection with more virulent organisms may occur.

If however a profuse growth of urinary pathogens is observed in very ill but asymptomatic patients in the ICU, we prefer to remove the catheter and repeat the culture after a few days. If the culture is negative, the infection has cleared; if bacteriuria > 100,000 CFU/ml persists, a short course of antibiotic therapy is given. If it is not possible to remove the catheter, it is advisable to treat the patient if he already has a life-threatening illness.

It is debatable whether routine screening tests involving urine cultures are worth the while in asymptomatic patients with indwelling urinary catheters. We however do urine cultures at periodic intervals routinely in very sick patients admitted to our ICU.

Bacteriuria in Symptomatic Patients

In symptomatic patients the catheter is removed and suitable antibiotics commenced. If the patient needs an indwelling urinary catheter, a new one is inserted. In serious urinary tract infections it is important to commence therapy promptly after sending urine cultures, without waiting for the culture reports. Empiric therapy for urinary infection should also be given in those patients who are haemodynamically unstable, in the immunocompromised and neutropaenics, in poorly controlled diabetics, in patients with damaged or prosthetic valves, (for fear of complicating bacterial endocarditis), and in patients with deteriorating renal function.

Selection of Antibiotics

A Gram's stain of the urine may help decide the nature of the infection (whether Gram-negative as is common, or Gram-positive in occasional cases), well before culture reports are available.

The choice of antibiotics for Gram-negative infections is usually ceftazidime or cefoperazone, combined with an aminoglycoside. We prefer not to use the latter if renal function is impaired, more so as facilities for determining aminoglycoside levels are generally available in just a few medical centres. Ciprofloxacin is added to ceftazidime or cefoperazone in severe urinary tract infections with renal insufficiency. An alternative regime for severe Pseudomonas or other Gram-negative infections is the use of piperacillin-tazobactam combination or of merepenem

In Gram-positive infections, augmentin (amoxicillin-clavulanic acid) is generally used till such time as a culture report is available. Resistant staphylococcal infections are not common in our unit. If however infection with resistant staphylococci is suspected, the drug of choice is vancomycin, which covers both resistant Staphylococci as well as enterococci. Gentamicin may be added for mixed staphylococcal and Gram-negative infections.

Candiduria

The presence of candida in the urine requires careful interpretation.

Asymptomatic candiduria in an immunocompetent patient generally indicates mere colonization without infection. It clears when the catheter is removed and particularly when the antibiotics are stopped.

Symptomatic candiduria in immunocompetent patients or severe candiduria, even though asymptomatic in immunocompromised individuals, often spells danger. It could signify fungal infection of the bladder, an ascending fungal pyelonephritis, or disseminated candidiasis. The presence of disseminated candidiasis is difficult to diagnose as blood cultures are not necessarily positive. Fluffy white retinal exudates protruding from the retinal surface into the vitreous, and an endophthalmitis have been reported in 40–50 per cent of patients with disseminated candidiasis (13, 14), but we have never had the opportunity of observing these lesions. Clinical features that should make one suspect disseminated candidiasis are:

(i) A deterioration in the general condition with worsening renal function in a patient with persistent and profuse Candida in the urine.

(ii) Growth of Candida from two other sites (e.g. sputum, vascular catheter), besides the urine. In neutropaenic patients who are septic, growth of Candida from just two sites is sufficient evidence to start systemic amphotericin B therapy.

(iii) Profuse growth of Candida in the urine in a patient who has no indwelling catheter and who is deteriorating clinically at a very rapid rate.

Treatment

Suspected Candida infection of the upper urinary tract or suspected disseminated candidiasis requires the use of intravenous amphotericin B or intravenous fluconazole (see Chapter on Treatment of Fungal Infections in Critically Ill Patients). The indwelling catheter should be removed and a new one inserted, if a catheter is vital for patient management.

Candidiasis confined to the bladder should be treated with oral fluconazole and/or irrigation of the bladder with amphotericin B. Sobel (13) describes the following method for irrigation of the bladder with amphotericin B solution. 50 mg amphotericin B is mixed with 1 litre of sterile water and infused at a rate of 40 ml/hour, using a 3-way bladder catheter. The response is generally good and the irrigation can be stopped after 3–4 days. Systemic candidiasis or fungal involvement of the kidneys or the perinephric space requires the prompt use of amphotericin B.

Prevention of Urinary Catheter-related Infections (1, 15)

(i) Insert an indwelling catheter only if absolutely necessary. If condom drainage of the urine is satisfactory, and there is no urinary retention, it is wiser not to insert the catheter.

(ii) A urinary catheter must be inserted under complete aseptic conditions, and should be meticulously cared for once inserted. The catheter should not be pulled upon during nursing, and the sterile system should not be broken by obtaining samples of urine for examination from the urine collection bag. Urine samples should always be obtained from the proximal portion of the catheter or through the sample port of the catheter system. The urethral meatus should be coated with a bactericidal ointment—neosporin, soframycin or bacitracin. Care should be taken that the catheter is not contaminated by faecal matter or secretions on bedsheets or bedclothes.

(iii) We routinely change the Foley's catheter every 8–10 days. In suspected urinary infection, besides culturing the urine, we also send the tip of the removed urinary catheter for culture. The care and technique for tip culture is the same as that described for cultures of catheters inserted into vessels. Silicon catheters can be kept for much longer periods of time—as long as 6–8 weeks.

REFERENCES

1. Warren JW. (1987). Catheter associated urinary tract infections. Infect Dis Clin North Am. 1, 823–854.
2. Stamm WE. (1991). Catheter-associated urinary tract infections: Epidemiology, pathogenesis and prevention. Am J Med. 91, 65S-71S.
3. Wong ES. (1987). New aspects of urinary tract infections. Clin Crit Care Med. 12, 25–38.
4. Tambyah PA, Halvorson RT, Maki DG. (1999). A prospective study of pathogenesis of catheter-associated urinary tract infection. Mayo Clin Proc. 74, 131–136.
5. Sobel JD. (1987). Pathogenesis of urinary tract infections: host defences. Infect Dis Clin North Am. 1, 751–772.
6. Daifuku R, Stamm WE. (1986). Bacterial adherence to bladder uroepithelial cells in catheter-associated urinary tract infection. N Engl J Med. 314, 1208–1213.
7. Rosser CJ, Bare RL, Meredith JW. (1999). Urinary tract infection in

the critically ill patient with a urinary catheter. Am J Surg. 177, 287–290.

8. Witt MD, Anne Chu L. (2002). Infections in the Critically Ill: Urinary Catheter-Associated Infections. In: Current Critical Care Diagnosis and Treatment (Eds Bongard FS, Sue DY). pp. 417–419. McGraw-Hill, USA.

9. Stamm WE. (1983). Measurement of pyuria and its relation to bacteriuria. Am J Med. 75, 53–58.

10. Jenkins RD, Fenn JP, Matsen JM. (1986). Review of urine microscopy for bacteriuria. JAMA. 255, 3397–3403.

11. Stark RP, Maki DG. (1984). Bacteriuria in the catheterized patient. What quantitative level of bacteriuria is relevant? N Engl J Med. 311, 560–564.

12. Platt R. (1983). Quantitative definition of bacteriuria. Am J Med. 75, 44–52.

13. Sobel JD. (1988). Candida infections in the intensive care unit. Crit Care Clin. 4, 325–344.

14. Parke D, Jones D, Gentry L. (1982). Endogenous endophthalmitis among patients with candidaemia. Ophthalmology. 89, 789–792.

15. Cunin CM, McCormack RC. (1966). Prevention of catheter-induced urinary tract infections by sterile closed drainage. N Engl J Med. 274, 1155.

Antibiotic-associated Colitis

General Considerations

Diarrhoea in a patient under critical care, is most often due to antibiotics, to overzealous enteral feeding, or following chemotherapy for malignancy or myeloproliferative diseases. In hospitals and ICUs in poor countries, where kitchen hygiene leaves a lot to be desired, outbreaks or isolated instances of intestinal infection due to E. coli, Shigella, Salmonella, or trophozoites of E. histolytica may also be occasionally observed.

Antibiotic-associated diarrhoea is due to an overgrowth of various organisms in the gut. An overgrowth of clostridium difficile in the colon, leads to a potentially serious form of diarrhoea due to a pseudomembranous colitis. C. difficile acts by producing an enterotoxin (Toxin A) and a cytotoxin (Toxin B); the organism however is localized to the colon, and does not have any invasive properties (1, 2). Almost all antibiotics have been known to cause pseudomembranous colitis. Those most frequently incriminated are ampicillin, clindamycin and the cephalosporins. Pseudomembranous colitis due to C. difficile toxin also occurs after chemotherapy.

Clinical Features (3)

A low-grade fever and watery diarrhoea of varying severity are observed. This may occur during antibiotic therapy, or may occur some weeks after antibiotics have been stopped. The diarrhoea may be mild, or profuse causing both hypovolaemia, and fluid and electrolyte disturbances. Mucus, blood and shreds of colonic mucosa that have sloughed off from the colon, may be present in the stools. The clinical features may be indistinguishable from acute dysentery. In severe pseudomembranous colitis, all the features of a toxic megacolon may occur, culminating in perforation of the large bowel. This is more likely if the association of the above clinical features with the antibiotic used is not realized, and the drug is not immediately withdrawn.

Diagnosis

The diagnosis is made by detection of the toxin of C. difficile in the stools (4). Unfortunately very few laboratories, even in the large metropolitan cities of India, are equipped to do an assay of this toxin. A high index of suspicion is therefore necessary to make a clinical diagnosis. Yet, a life-saving antibiotic should not be needlessly omitted from a therapeutic regime. In suspected cases, a sigmoidoscopy is of help. It shows mucosal ulcerations covered by yellowish or whitish-yellow membrane-like plaques. Biopsy of the ulcers shows nonspecific inflammation. A careful search for trophozoites of E. histolytica should be made to exclude an amoebic infection.

Differential diagnosis includes infective diarrhoea or dysentery due to various organisms—E. coli, Shigella, Campylobacter jejuni, Salmonella and E. histolytica. These nosocomial infections of the gut may be rare in Western countries, but are not so uncommon in our part of the world. In the elderly, a differential diagnosis of ischaemic colitis must also be considered. Cytomegalovirus infections in immunocompromised patients may present with diarrhoea or with a haemorrhagic colitis. Noninfectious causes of nosocomial diarrhoea include enteral feeding, drugs increasing intestinal motility and alteration of the normal bowel flora following antibiotic use.

Management

Most patients improve quickly after withdrawing the antibiotic responsible for the diarrhoea. Specific therapy must be used in addition in patients with severe diarrhoea, or in those whose diarrhoea continues after stopping the antibiotic. Drugs useful in pseudomembranous colitis are metronidazole (5) 400 mg thrice daily for 14 days, erythromycin 500 mg four times a day for 10 days, or vancomycin (6) 250 mg thrice a day orally for 14 days. We generally obtain excellent results with metronidazole.

C. difficile, at least in Western countries, has been known to survive for prolonged periods on a variety of surfaces—walls, carpets, beds etc. It is also easily transmitted to patients by the hands of doctors, nurses and other paramedical personnel working in the ICU (7). Whether an outbreak of nosocomial diarrhoea in ICU patients could result from transmission of C difficile in this fashion is uncertain.

REFERENCES

1. Johnson S, Clabots CR, Linn FV et al. (1990). Nosocomial Clostridium difficile colonization and disease. Lancet. 336, 97–100.

2. Silva J, Iezzi C. (1988). Clostridium difficile as a nosocomial pathogen. J Hosp Infect. 11(Suppl A), 378–385.

3. Mylonaka E, Ryan ET, Calderwood SB. (2001). Clostridium difficile associated diarrhoea: a review. Arch Int Med. 161, 525–533.

4. Laughon BE, Viscidi RP, Gdovin SL et al. (1984). Enzyme immunoassay for detection of clostridium difficile toxins A and B in fecal specimens. J Infect Dis. 149, 781–788.

5. Pashby NL, Bolton RP, Sheriff RJ. (1979). Oral metronidazole in Clostridium difficile colitis. Br Med J. 1, 1605–1606.

6. Tedesco F, Markham R, Gurwith M et al. (1978). Oral vancomycin for antibiotic-associated pseudomembranous colitis. Lancet. 2, 226–228.

7. McFarland LV, Mulligan NE, Kurok RV et al. (1989). Nosocomial acquisition of Clostridium difficile infection. N Engl J Med. 320, 204–210.

Prevention and Control of Nosocomial Infections (1, 2)

Infection Control and Prevention Programmes

Ideally every hospital should have an Infection Control and Prevention Committee consisting of heads of major clinical services, pathologists, microbiologists, Hospital Matron, senior sisters of the ICU, registrars and physiotherapists. The basic function of such a committee is outlined in **Table 13.2.6** and comprises maintenance of surveillance of nosocomial infections, with special reference to the ICU, and formulation of policies and procedures for prevention and control of such infections. It is imperative to lay down a standard policy for sterilization of instruments and other invasive gadgetry used in the ICU. Frequent checks should be carried out to ensure that strict standards once formulated, are meticulously followed.

Table 13.2.6. The role of a nosocomial infection control committee

1. Surveillance of nosocomial infection, particularly in the ICU
2. Formulation of policies and procedures for prevention and control of such infections
3. Laying down of a standard, strictly followed policy for the effective sterilization of instruments and other gadgetry used in the ICU
4. Holding educational updates for nurses and house doctors on the correct use and management of invasive devices, or of other gadgetry contributing to nosocomial infection (see text)
5. Formulation of a broad policy on the use of antibiotics in the ICU
6. Investigation of a nosocomial epidemic
7. Implementation of immunization programmes (particularly against Hepatitis B virus), and protection against infection (all fulminant infections and HIV infection) of medical, nursing, paramedical and other hospital staff. Special emphasis should be laid on protection of those working in the ICU and other high-risk areas within the hospital

Frequent educational updates for nurses and house doctors on the correct use and management of invasive devices, or of other devices responsible for nosocomial infection, are of great help. These devices include urinary catheters, all varieties of intravascular catheters, equipment for haemodynamic monitoring and for haemofiltration, tracheostomy and endotracheal tubes, mechanical ventilators, nebulizers and other gadgets used for respiratory therapy. Instructions on the correct use and handling of gadgetry should be extended to the operating theatre staff, with special reference to the cardiopulmonary bypass machine, and the use of the intra-aortic balloon pump.

A policy should be formulated on the use of antibiotics in the ICU, though sufficient latitude needs to be given to the treating consultant within the framework of such a policy.

The Infection Control Committee should shoulder the responsibility of promptly investigating a nosocomial epidemic. Finally it should supervise and implement immunization programmes and protective measures against infection, for the medical, paramedical, nursing and other personnel working in the ICU and other high-risk areas of the hospital.

It is beyond the scope of this chapter to cover and discuss at length the various factors contributing to nosocomial infections in the ICU. Nevertheless, some basic practical points need to be emphasized (**Table 13.2.7**).

(i) Hand washing (3).

This is perhaps the most important measure for preventing nosocomial infection. Hands should be thoroughly washed with soap before touching or handling a very sick patient in the ICU. This is specially important before examining or dressing a wound, performing an invasive procedure, or touching invasive devices used in patient care. Hands should be washed again when one has finished with the patient, as contamination of the hands with pathogenic organisms will almost certainly have occurred. ICU personnel, in our experience, frequently carry Gram-negative bacilli and Staphylococci either on their skin or within their throats. Yet the habit of hand washing seems extremely difficult to inculcate in all workers (including doctors) in the ICU. Detergents or antiseptic solutions can be used instead of soap. In fact, three controlled trials have demonstrated that the use of a chlorhexidine-containing solution instead of soap, for routine hand washing in the ICU, significantly lowers the incidence of endemic nosocomial infections (3). In our country, thorough scrubbing of the hands with soap is cheaper, and suffices. Soap water must never be allowed to collect in the soap dish, as it easily becomes contaminated with pathogens.

(ii) The use of reliable chemical disinfectants and antiseptics

Perfect sterilization and disinfection encompass almost all measures aimed at preventing nosocomial infections. The failure of a disinfectant to sterilize or disinfect reusable respiratory apparatus, ventilator tubings, or a patient's skin prior to an invasive procedure, can be responsible for serious outbreaks of nosocomial infection. Like most units all over the world, we chiefly use povidone-iodine as a disinfectant, particularly for cleaning the patient's skin before an invasive procedure. Yet, contamination of povidone-iodine with Ps. aeruginosa has been responsible for four outbreaks of nosocomial infection in the USA in the past (4).

(iii) Careful use of invasive devices and other gadgetry known to cause nosocomial infections.

A few points need to be emphasized.

(a) It is tempting to use invasive gadgetry just because it is waiting to be used! Developing countries are fortunate in a way because not all ICUs are very well equipped, and invasive monitoring equipment like Swan-Ganz catheters are expensive. With greater experience, invasive monitoring is done only in selected problem patients, in whom diagnostic assessment is difficult, and whose management is therefore uncertain.

(b) Ventilator tubings should be changed and carefully sterilized every 48 hours. Bacterial filters in ventilators should also be changed every 48–72 hours. Every precaution should be taken to prevent nosocomial infections through nebulizers. Nebulizing solutions may sometimes be contaminated and cause nosocomial pneumonia. It is wrong to use nebulizers unless they are of clear benefit to the patient; routine use of nebulizers should be strongly discouraged.

Table 13.2.7. Prevention of nosocomial infections

---
* Thorough handwashing
* Use of reliable chemical disinfectants and antiseptics
* Care over central lines/urinary catheters
* Tracheostomy care and care of ventilator tubings, nebulizers, and all other respiratory equipment
* Judicious use of antibiotics
* Careful use of antacids and H_2-antagonists
* Isolation of patients with resistant bacteria or fulminant contagious infections
* Keep ICU environment as clean as possible
* Good nutritional support

(c) Central venous lines are removed as quickly as possible. It is best to remove a catheter in the radial artery (used for monitoring blood pressure) by the fifth day. When central lines are suspected to cause nosocomial infection, catheter tips should be cultured in a correct manner (see Subsection on Catheter-related Infections).

(d) Urinary catheters are the commonest cause of nosocomial infections. They should be meticulously cared for; we change a Foley's self-retaining catheter every 8–10 days.

(e) Tracheostomy tubes should be changed every 4 to 7 days. The no-touch technique for tracheal aspiration through a tracheostomy tube or through an endotracheal tube, is vital. Every single suction should be carried out like a surgical procedure. It is not necessary to wear gloves for suction, but the hands should be thoroughly scrubbed. Gloves however should be worn for changing a tracheostomy tube or for dressing a tracheostomy wound.

(iv) Carefully planned use of antibiotics

An indiscriminate use of antibiotics can cause an ecological disaster, characterized by the multiplication of resistant bacteria in the ICU. This has been observed all over the world. Resistant organisms include methicillin-resistant Staphylococci, Gram-negative bacilli including Proteus, Klebsiella, Enterococci and Ps. aeruginosa resistant to third generation cephalosporins and aminoglycosides, and fungi, in particular Candida. These resistant organisms cause great problems in management, and are the source of serious nosocomial infections that can wreak havoc in an ICU setting. The following principles are of help in formulating a policy for antibiotic use:

(a) Fever may occur without infection (as explained earlier), in an ICU patient. Antibiotics should not be used in such patients.

(b) There should be a logical reason for the use of antibiotics, and for the choice of one or more antibiotics in a patient. This should be freely discussed and noted.

(c) If the infecting organism is known, the most narrow-spectrum drug or combination of drugs, should be used against this organism.

(d) A protocol should outline the empiric use of one or more antibiotics in critically ill patients, depending on the nature of illness. This protocol varies in different ICUs, as it depends on the epidemiology of nosocomial organisms and infections seen in a particular unit.

(e) Antibiotics should not be continued indefinitely. An assessment of duration of therapy is important.

(f) Patients on broad-spectrum antibiotic combinations should be monitored for the possible occurrence of superinfection by resistant organisms—chiefly Gram-negative bacteria, staphylococci, and fungi.

(v) Circumspection and care in use of antacids and H_2-antagonists for upper GI bleeding

Since increasing the pH of gastric acid contents by antacids and H_2-antagonists promotes colonization of the stomach, it is wise not to use H_2-antagonists routinely in all critically ill patients as prophylaxis for GI bleeding. Severe GI bleeding due to acute or chronic gastric or duodenal ulcers can however pose a serious hazard to life, and H_2-antagonists with sucralfate are indicated. Some ICUs prefer to use sucralfate alone, as it prevents a significant change in the pH of gastric contents (5, 6).

(vi) Good nutritional support

This is vital if nosocomial infections are to be successfully treated. In our country, and in all other developing countries, critical illnesses manifest against a background of poor nutrition. Survival for example in severe tetanus or in nosocomial infections in severe tetanus, is absolutely impossible without adequate nutritional support.

(vii) Isolation of patients with fulminant infections and of patients infected by resistant bacteria.

This can help to prevent dangerous nosocomial epidemics. We do not have the facilities for complete isolation, but we have managed to contain and yet look after such infections through barrier nursing and by allocating special nurses and other special staff who only care for such patients when they are admitted to the unit.

(viii) Cleanliness of ICU environment.

It is vital to keep the ICU environment as physically clean as possible. The practice of changing shoes and wearing special slippers before entering the ICU is an eyewash, and perhaps contributes to additional nosocomial infections. It is more important to have the floor swabbed with a disinfectant every 3–4 hours through the day and night, to keep bedside tables clean and uncluttered, to keep ceilings, walls and curtains meticulously clean, and to have as little equipment as possible cluttering the unit.

The incidence of nosocomial infections in our intensive care unit is much lower compared to other units in Mumbai, and in this country. This could be partly due to the fact that in our unit, patient care in relation to washing and cleaning, is entrusted only to the nurses, who have been indoctrinated and trained to wash hands promptly after touching a patient. Intravenous lines or other invasive and non-invasive gadgets used for patient care are never touched without first scrubbing the hands. Bedpans and urinals are also solely handled by the nursing staff. In contrast, in all other units urinals and bedpans are handled by a special group of untrained men and women whose standards of hygiene, to say the least, are deplorable.

(ix) Selective decontamination of the GI tract

This was earlier reported to reduce the incidence of nosocomial pneumonias by preventing or reducing the colonization of the upper GI tract by Gram-negative organisms. The antibiotics commonly used orally are a combination of tobramycin, polymyxin and amphotericin B. Current work however suggests that selective decontamination does not influence the mortality in nosocomial infections (7, 8). The risk of breeding even more resistant organisms with this modality of treatment is significant. We have never used selective decontamination of the GI tract and will probably never do so.

REFERENCES

1. Centres for Disease Control. (1981). Guidelines for the Prevention and Control of Nosocomial Infections. US Department of Health and Human Services, Atlanta, GA.

2. Craven DE, Steger KA, Barber TW. (1991). Preventing nosocomial pneumonia: State of the art and perspectives for the 1990s. Am J Med. 91 Suppl 3B, 44S-53S.

3. Garner JS, Farero MS. (1986). Guidelines for handwashing and hospital environment control. Infect Control. 7, 231–243.

4. Maki DG. (1991). Nosocomial Infection. In: Current Therapy in Critical Care Medicine, 2nd edn (Ed. Parrillo JE). pp. 208–215. BC Decker Inc., Philadelphia, Hamilton.

5. Driks MR, Craven DE, Celli BR et al. (1987). Nosocomial pneumonia in intubated patients given sucralfate as compared with antacids or histamine type-2 blockers. N Engl J Med. 317, 1376–1382.

6. Eddleston JM, Vohra A, Scott P et al. (1991). A comparison of the frequency of stress ulceration and secondary pneumonia in sucralfate- or ranitidine-treated intensive care unit patients. Crit Care Med. 19, 1491–1496.

7. Gastinne H, Wolff M, Delatour F et al. (1992). A controlled trial in intensive care units of selective decontamination of the digestive tract with nonabsorbable antibiotics. N Engl J Med. 326, 594–599.

8. Vandenbroucke-Grauls CMJE, Vandenbroucke JP. (1991). Effect of selective decontamination of the digestive tract on respiratory tract infections and mortality in the intensive care unit. Lancet. 338, 859–862.

Community-acquired Fulminant Infections Requiring Critical Care

Important community-acquired fulminant infections requiring critical care in our unit include Pl. falciparum infections, tetanus, acute disseminated haematogenous tuberculosis, fulminant pneumonias, fulminant Gram-negative and amoebic infections, dengue haemorrhagic fever, fulminant leptospiral infections and acute infections involving the meninges and the neuraxis. Fulminant pneumonias requiring critical care are briefly discussed in the Section on Respiratory Problems Requiring Critical Care. Acute infections of the meninges and the neuraxis are dealt with in the Subsection on Neurologic Disorders Requiring Critical Care. Severe Pl. falciparum infections, tetanus and disseminated haematogenous tuberculosis are discussed in detail in this chapter. They are of immense importance in India and other poor countries of the world. This is followed by a brief description of fulminant Gram-negative food-borne infections, fulminant amoebic infection, dengue haemorrhagic fever and severe leptospiral infection.

Fulminant Plasmodium Falciparum Infection—Cerebral Malaria (1, 2)

General Considerations

Plasmodium falciparum malaria is now unfortunately endemic in many parts of India. It has even become endemic in the city of Mumbai and its suburbs, and in other major cities of Maharashtra and Gujarat. What is worse, strains resistant to chloroquine are frequently encountered. In certain cities of Gujarat like Navsari, Surat and Ahmedabad Pl. falciparum is more often than not resistant to chloroquine.

The global case fatality rate of falciparum infections is around 1 per cent or 2 million deaths per year (3). Pl. falciparum is the predominant malarial infection in highly endemic areas of Africa (4, 5), and has a high prevalence in South America and South Asia, including India and Thailand. Cerebral malaria is the most severe manifestation of Pl. falciparum infection, and is responsible for 80 per cent of 2 million global deaths. If unrecognized and not correctly treated, cerebral malaria is almost certainly fatal. It must however be realized that severe, Pl. falciparum infection can also cause death through a fatal involvement of other organ systems,

without necessarily producing a significant involvement of the central nervous system. An increasing number of patients with fulminant Pl. falciparum infection are now being treated in intensive care units all over Mumbai, as also in other metropolitan cities of the country.

Physiopathology

The pathological and clinical manifestations of severe Pl. falciparum infection are caused exclusively by the intraerythrocytic asexual form of the parasite. The parasite exerts a two-fold action:

(i) It induces the formation of protein-rich knobs on parasitized red blood cell surface membrane, causing these cells to adhere to the endothelial lining of the microvasculature, through proteins such as thrombospondin, intercellular adhesion molecules and CD36. This cytoadherence leads to a sequestration of the parasitized RBCs in the capillaries and post-capillary venules in the brain and other organs of the body. Obstruction to microcirculation in the brain and other organ systems leads to tissue hypoxia and lactic acid acidosis.

(ii) The interaction between the parasite and the host RBCs is believed to result in the liberation of tumour necrosis factor α, interleukins and other potentially toxic or pharmacologically active compounds such as reactive oxygen species and nitric oxide. These have deleterious local-cum-systemic effects.

It is a combination of the above two factors which is responsible for severe multiple organ dysfunction observed in fulminant falciparum infections. This obstruction to the microcirculation within the brain produces cerebral hypoxia and features of cerebral malaria. Cerebral oedema develops in some patients as a terminal event, and is not the chief cause of coma. Global cerebral blood flow is reduced in cerebral malaria, and there is increased cerebral anaerobic glycolysis with an increase in the cerebrospinal fluid lactate concentration.

Widespread damage to endothelial cells can perhaps trigger disseminated intravascular coagulopathy. Decreased antithrombin levels are noted in severe cases, and generally signify a poor prognosis.

Massive intravascular haemolysis with haemoglobinuria is due to heavy parasitaemia; haemolysis also occurs in patients with G6PD deficiency, particularly after the use of quinine.

Damage to the alveolar-capillary membrane due to parasitized red blood cells obstructing pulmonary capillaries and due to release of cytokines, leads to acute lung injury and non-cardiogenic pulmonary oedema.

Renal failure is an important feature of fulminant infection. Factors producing renal failure include sluggish circulation due to parasitized erythrocytes, renal vasoconstriction, haemoglobinuria and acute glomerulonephritis.

Hypoglycaemia is due to parasitaemia as also to quinine therapy. Children and pregnant women are particularly susceptible to hypoglycaemia which is often asymptomatic. The increased susceptibility in pregnancy is because of pancreatic islet cell hyperplasia, and other metabolic changes associated with the pregnant state.

Translocation of bacterial flora from the gut may be related to mesenteric ischaemia produced by parasitized erythrocytes. Gram-negative bacteraemia with secondary sepsis may occur. This is specially observed in the 'algid' form of Pl. falciparum malaria.

Clinical Features and Complications (6–9) (Table 13.3.1)

Severe falciparum infection is characterized by any one or more of the following features:

1. A parasite count > 5 per cent;
2. Cerebral malaria;
3. Haematocrit < 20 per cent;
4. Total serum bilirubin > 5 mg per cent;
5. Gross fluid and electrolyte abnormalities;
6. Other organ failure—e.g. cardiovascular, renal, respiratory, haematologic, metabolic;
7. Temperature > 39°C;
8. Complicating infection.

Cerebral malaria can strike with dramatic suddenness, or may be preceded by unremitting fever accompanied by chills. Usually 10 days after the fever, the patient has a generalized seizure followed by progressive coma. High fever alone can cause delerium and mental obtundation. The term cerebral malaria should be reserved for an encephalopathy due to Pl. falciparum infection, which leads to mental obtundation, often progressing to coma. Pl. falciparum infection can also induce coma which is post-ictal or is due to severe hypoglycaemia.

Hyperpyrexia, frequent or rarely continuous seizures, and in-

Table 13.3.1. Complications of fulminant falciparum malaria

---
* Cerebral malaria—pyrexia (at times > 105°F), mental obtundation, coma, seizures
* Renal failure
* Haemolytic anaemia
* Hypotension and shock
* Hypoglycaemia
* Hepatic dysfunction with jaundice
* Spontaneous bleeding from gums/GI tract; rarely DIC
* Pulmonary oedema/ARDS
* Metabolic acidosis
* Massive intravascular haemolysis with haemoglobinuria and renal shutdown (blackwater fever)
* Bacterial sepsis
---

creasing coma form a triad of symptoms observed in this dreadful disease. Mild neck stiffness is present at times, and Kernig's sign may be positive. There is generally no focal neurological deficit. Papilloedema is generally absent, but retinal haemorrhages may be seen. Dysconjugate gaze disturbances and in particular skew deviation of the eyes are common, but except in terminal cases the pupillary and corneal reflexes are preserved. Doll's eye movements and oculovestibular reflexes are also generally preserved. Muscle tone is increased, deep jerks are exaggerated, abdominal reflexes are absent, and the plantars are often bilaterally extensor. Extensor thrusts resembling decerebrate rigidity, associated oculugyric crisis, and stertorous breathing may occur in patients who are severely hypoglycaemic.

A rare presentation of falciparum malaria is cerebellar ataxia, without disturbance in consciousness.

Malaria psychosis is on rare occasions a presenting feature of the disease, though more often than not psychosis follows upon the use of mefloquine or chloroquine.

Fulminant Pl. falciparum infection often produces multiple organ dysfunction, and in our experience 80 per cent of patients with cerebral malaria have complications pointing to other organ system involvement. As has already been pointed out, some patients have severe multiple organ dysfunction without significant cerebral encephalopathy (9).

Hypoglycaemia is very frequent, and can occur spontaneously in severe infections with heavy parasitaemia, or can occur within a few hours to a few days of starting quinine. Pregnant women and children, as mentioned earlier, are very prone to this complication. Complicating bacteraemia also contributes to and worsens the condition.

Patients admitted to ICUs following Pl. falciparum infection occasionally present with hypotension and shock (algid malaria). Diarrhoea and severe gastrointestinal bleeds are often associated features. This state is believed to be due to Gram-negative endotoxaemia, probably due to translocation of bacteria from the gut.

The cardiovascular manifestations are often similar to those observed in endotoxin shock, and are typically characterized by hypotension, a lowered systemic vascular resistance (SVR) and an increased cardiac index (CI). A low CI with an increased SVR may be observed in terminally ill or in fulminant cases and is of ominous significance (**Fig. 13.3.1**).

The pulmonary manifestations (6) of the fulminant form of the disease are characterized by the evolution of acute lung injury, which may be mild, moderate or severe in intensity. The severe form of the disease is associated with a large right to left shunt in the lungs, and is generally fatal. Acute pulmonary oedema sometimes occurs suddenly (7, 8), and is observed with hyperpyrexia > 107°F; this is generally fatal within a few hours. Aspiration pneumonia is frequently seen in fulminant infections; nosocomial pneumonia may also occur particularly in patients on ventilator support. Other pulmonary complications include pulmonary oedema due to fluid overload and the occurrence of marked tachypnoea even in the absence of acute lung injury or ARDS. Tachypnoea in old, feeble, malnourished patients with hyperpyrexia invariably leads to respiratory muscle fatigue and respiratory

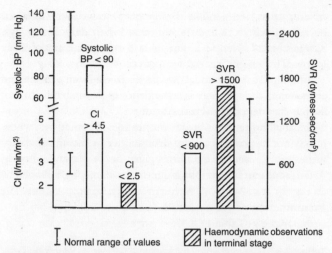

Fig. 13.3.1. Haemodynamic observations in fulminant falciparum infections

arrest. Elective intubation and respiratory support is life saving in these patients. Rarely death may occur from pulmonary embolism (**Table 13.3.2**).

The renal manifestations include oliguria, a rise in serum creatinine, and a mild to moderate renal insufficiency. Acute tubular necrosis with renal shutdown is occasionally observed, particularly in the presence of haemolysis.

Acute haemolysis can also occur in patients who do not have a G6PD deficiency, and who have not received quinine. It is probably due to heavy parasitaemia. Classical blackwater fever is the association of haemoglobinuria with severe manifestations of Pl. falciparum infection in a non-immune patient, who is not G6PD deficient.

Spontaneous bleeding from gums and the GI tract may be encountered. Fulminant malaria can also produce generalized bleeding due to a disseminated intravascular coagulopathy.

Jaundice is frequently present with the serum bilirubin being generally elevated to about 5 mg/dl, and this is accompanied by a modest rise in the serum transaminases. Deepening jaundice (serum bilirubin > 15 mg/dl), with a disseminated intravascular coagulopathy initially mistaken as viral hepatitis or obstructive jaundice, is an occasional presentation in intensive care units in Mumbai.

Hyponatraemia (due to inappropriate ADH secretion), and a lactic acid acidosis are seen quite frequently in severe infections.

Multiple organ systems are often involved, with increasing dysfunction, failure and ultimate death. In hyperfulminant cases, death may ensue within 24 hours.

Table 13.3.2. Pulmonary complications of fulminant falciparum infection

1. A fall in PaO_2–inappropriate to the X-ray changes observed
2. Acute lung injury of varying severity
   – chiefly a $\dot{V}/Q$ abnormality
   – a marked right to left shunt
3. Aspiration pneumonia
4. Fulminant pulmonary oedema due to hyperpyrexia
5. Pulmonary oedema due to fluid overload
6. Tachypnoea with respiratory muscle fatigue
7. Nosocomial pneumonia
8. Pulmonary embolism

Diagnosis

The clinical picture of an encephalopathy or of an encephalopathy with multiple organ dysfunction, should point to cerebral malaria particularly in an area endemic for Pl. falciparum infection. The spleen may or may not be palpable. In fulminant cases, there is probably no time for the spleen to enlarge. A palpable liver and spleen in the presence of the clinical features described above, are useful pointers however to the correct diagnosis. Repeated blood smears for malarial parasites should be done, and when a clinical diagnosis is highly suspect, specific treatment for falciparum infection should be promptly started. Diagnostic tests to confirm or establish any other diagnosis producing a similar clinical picture must be persisted with. It must be remembered that at times (on rare occasions), no parasites can be found in peripheral blood smears from patients suffering from fulminant falciparum infection. This may be related to partial antimalarial treatment, or due to sequestration of parasitized cells in vascular beds of different organ systems. The importance of starting empiric treatment in critically ill patients with an illness compatible with fulminant Pl. falciparum infection is obvious. Time is of essence in severe infections; a delay of 24 hours or even less, spells the difference between life and death.

Enzyme-linked immunosorbent assays (ELISA) and radioimmunoassays (RIA), can detect 0.0001 per cent of parasitaemia (**3**). Recently developed probes using genomic or synthetic P. falciparum DNA can detect as little as 0.01 mg of parasite DNA after just one week's exposure. These are basically for research and epidemiological surveys, and have no role in the management of acutely ill patients in intensive care units of poor developing countries.

Laboratory investigations should always include blood glucose levels; they should also include laboratory tests which monitor the function of different organ systems of the body. Fluid, electrolyte and acid-base studies are important, as derangement of these parameters can be easily rectified.

Though leucopaenia or a normal leucocyte count is the rule in fulminant falciparum infections, a mild neutrophilic leucocytosis does not exclude the diagnosis. Blood cultures for bacteraemia should always be done in the presence of a neutrophilic leucocytosis.

Differential Diagnosis. Mistakes in diagnosis are frequent, and would probably include consideration of a large cross-section of emergency medicine. Heat stroke in the hot summer months in North India bears a close resemblance to cerebral malaria. Acute pyogenic meningitis can be easily differentiated by a CSF examination. The algid form may be mistaken for heat exhaustion or food poisoning. Non-specific abdominal pain in fulminant infections has convincingly mimicked an acute abdomen. Icterus with fever may be mistaken for viral hepatitis. The presence of fever with multiple organ system dysfunction, may be mistaken for Gram-negative sepsis. Fulminant Pl. falciparum infection in fact constitutes protozoal sepsis.

Management (9)

Patients with fulminant Pl. falciparum infection, and in particular with cerebral malaria, require prompt admission to the ICU. A central venous line should be quickly secured, and all vital signs

Fever and Acute Infections in a Critical Care Setting

carefully monitored. If a clinical diagnosis is made, a careful search for malarial parasites by an experienced pathologist in thin and thick peripheral smears is almost always rewarding. Blood cultures, blood glucose, serum electrolytes and arterial pH and blood gas analysis are done. If rapid investigations reveal no clear cause for a clinical picture strongly suggestive of cerebral malaria, specific treatment should be promptly started.

Specific Therapy

Many cases of Pl. falciparum malaria in the city of Mumbai are chloroquine-resistant. It is therefore best to start with intravenous quinine in fulminant infections, and in cases of cerebral malaria. The recommended loading dose in a young adult is 20 mg salt/kg in 10 ml/kg of isotonic fluid infused intravenously over 4 hours, followed 8 hours after the start of the loading dose with 10 mg salt/kg infused intravenously over 4 hours, every 8 hours until the patient can swallow. The oral dose is 600 mg 8 hourly; the total duration of quinine therapy is 7 days. Many clinicians and intensivists in India prefer to use a lesser dose than that stated above—12 mg/kg being infused in 500 ml dextrose-saline over 6 hours followed by 8 mg/kg infused in dextrose-saline over 4 hours, 8 hourly, till the patient is conscious and can swallow. Since most deaths with falciparum infection occur within 4 days of starting therapy, it is important to quickly achieve paracidal levels of quinine in the serum. We have found that a loading dose of 12 mg/kg suffices to achieve this without undue side effects. The initial dose of quinine should not be reduced in patients with renal or hepatic insufficiency, but the maintenance therapy should be halved if parenteral therapy is needed for more than 48 hours.

If for any reason quinine cannot be given intravenously, the drug is given intramuscularly. 20 mg salt/kg is diluted to 60–100 mg/ml (loading dose) and is given intramuscularly into the lateral aspect of the thigh (half the dose in each leg). This is followed by 10 mg/kg every 8 hours till the patient can swallow and take the medication orally.

Hypoglycaemia is the most important complication of quinine therapy. Quinine also produces cinchonism, characterized by tinnitus, impaired hearing, blurred vision, tremors and giddiness. The most dangerous side effect of quinine, particularly when used intravenously is the occurrence of arrhythmias—in particular ventricular tachycardia. A prolonged QTc interval is a warning of the possible occurrence of such arrhythmias. ECG monitoring is therefore very necessary in critically ill patients. Rarely haemolysis, thrombocytopaenia and granulomatous hepatitis are observed. High blood concentrations can cause deafness, blindness and CNS depression, but these features are very rarely seen in patients treated for malaria. In patients who are G6PD deficient, quinine can cause severe haemolysis.

In patients who cannot tolerate quinine, particularly those with background cardiac disease or when it induces malignant arrhythmias or severe haemolysis, it is best to use artemisinin—either artesunate or artemether is used. This drug (an ancient Chinese drug extracted from the herb Artemesia annua) is very effective against chloroquine-resistant strains of Pl. falciparum.

Artesunate is given in a dose of 2–4 mg/kg intravenously, followed by 1.2 mg/kg at 12 and 24 hours and then daily for 5 days. Artemether is given in a dose of 3.2 mg/kg intramuscularly followed by 1.6 mg/kg/day for 5 days.

In critically ill individuals we prefer to use both quinine and artemisinin, though there is no evidence to prove that the use of both is superior to quinine used alone.

In small hospitals or health centres in poor countries, where it may not be possible to give drugs either by intramuscular or intravenous injection, quinine is given orally 600 mg 8 hourly. Artemisinin can be given by suppository 40 mg/kg followed by 20 mg/kg at 4, 24, 48, 72 hours or as an oral preparation. The chemotherapy of fulminant Pl. falciparum infection has been summarized in **Table 13.3.3**.

Table 13.3.3. Chemotherapy for fulminant falciparum infection

Drug	Dose
Quinine	20 mg/kg IV infusion over 4 hrs followed by 10 mg/kg over 4 hrs, 8 hourly for 7 days. If IV infusion not possible 10 mg/kg IM, 8 hourly. Later 600 mg tds orally
Artemisinin	
Artesunate	2.4 mg/kg IV or IM stat followed by 1.2 mg/kg at 12 and 24 hrs and then daily for 6 days
Artemether	3.2 mg/kg IM stat followed by 1.6 mg/kg/day for 6 days

Critical Care

Overall critical care is of vital importance. The central venous pressure is best maintained around 5–7 mm Hg, as overhydration carries the risk of inducing ARDS in these patients. Hyperpyrexia must be controlled with tepid sponging and paracetamol. Fluid, electrolyte and acid-base balance must be meticulously maintained. Intravenous dextrose is generally continued during quinine therapy to counter hypoglycaemia.

In patients with cerebral malaria, it is important to protect the airway by elective intubation; every effort must be made to prevent aspiration pneumonia. Intravenous mannitol is used if there is increase in intracranial pressure. Seizures are controlled by 20–40 mg diazepam given as a titrated infusion in 5 per cent dextrose. Dilantin sodium may be given intravenously in addition.

Ventilator support is always indicated in comatose patients particularly in the presence of seizures. It is also indicated in patients with ARDS or in severely tachypnoeic patients even when there is no evidence of acute lung injury.

Hypotension can be due to hypovolaemia, blood loss, haemolysis, septic shock, and hypoxia. Management consists of volume expansion with colloids, crystalloids and if necessary with packed cells. Inotropic support is invariably necessary. Suitable antibiotics are used against complicating bacterial sepsis. Proper arterial oxygenation and oxygen transport are important features of critical care.

Renal failure should be addressed by correcting pre-renal factors that can cause oliguria and azotaemia. Use of haemofiltration or dialysis may be necessary till kidney function has sufficiently recovered.

Disseminated intravascular coagulopathy is a dreaded complication. It should be treated with infusions of fresh frozen plasma, cryoprecipitate and platelet infusions.

Support to all organ systems is necessary for survival in critically ill patients.

When parasitaemia exceeds 20 per cent and the patient shows no improvement on conventional therapy, exchange transfusion has led to recovery.

Mortality (9)

In good, units, severe Pl. falciparum infections should not carry an overall mortality > 20–25 per cent. The mortality in our unit for just single organ failure is < 10 per cent. The mortality for two organ failure approximates 20 per cent; it increases to 50 per cent when three or more organs fail. Krishnan and Karnad (9) in an excellent study on 301 patients with severe Pl. falciparum infection observed a mortality of 48.8 per cent with two or more organ failure. Even so, this is one tropical condition where multiple organ dysfunction and failure is not necessarily associated with as forbidding a mortality as that reported in Western literature. We have observed that in patients seeking early admission, prompt treatment with quinine and good critical care can lead to survival even when SOFA scores are as high as 12–15 (see Chapter on Multiple Organ Dysfunction and Failure).

Mortality is not necessarily related to the degree of parasitaemia; yet, a parasite count > 500,000 ml carries a 50 per cent mortality. Severe ARDS carries a bad prognosis, as does complicating bacterial infection. Fulminant disseminated intravascular coagulopathy in association with severe ARDS is invariably fatal. Persistent lactic acid acidosis, profound persistent hypotension are associated with a high mortality.

REFERENCES

1. White NJ, Pukrittayakamee S. (1993). Clinical malaria in the tropics. Med J Aust. 159(3), 197–203.

2. Kampfl AW, Birbamer GG, Pfausler BE et al. (1993). Isolated pontine lesion in algid cerebral malaria: clinical features, management, and magnetic resonance imaging findings. Am J Trop Med Hyg. 48(6), 818–822.

3. Bradley DJ, Warrell DA. (2003). Malaria. In: Oxford Textbook of Medicine (Eds Warrell DA, Cox TM, Firth JD, Benz EJ Jr). pp. 545–551. Oxford University Press.

4. Soni PN, Sharp BL, Ngxongo S et al. (1993). Morbidity from falciparum malaria in Natal/KwaZulu. S Afr J Med. 83(2), 110–112.

5. Vitris M, Saissy JM, Demaziere J et al. (1991). Current aspects on cerebral malaria in the non-immune dysfunction in African endemic areas. Dakar Med. 36(1), 62–65.

6. Gozal D. (1992). The incidence of pulmonary manifestations during Plasmodium falciparum malaria in non-immune subjects. Trop Med Parasitol. 43(1), 6–8.

7. Salord F, Allaouchiche B, Gaussorgues P et al. (1991). Severe falciparum malaria. Intensive Care Med. 17(8), 449–454.

8. Charoenpan P, Indraprasit S, Kiatboonsri S et al. (1990). Pulmonary oedema in severe falciparum malaria. Haemodynamic study and clinicophysiologic correlation. Chest. 97, 1190.

9. Krishnan A, Karnand DR. (2003). Severe falciparum malaria: An important cause of multiple organ failure in Indian Intensive Care Unit Patients. Crit Care Med. 31, 2278–2284.

Tetanus

Tetanus is a killer disease afflicting the poor underprivileged people of developing third world countries. It is caused by contamination of a wound by Cl. tetani, which is a Gram-positive, anaerobic, spore-forming organism. The spores gain entry through any wound; only the wound may be so minor that it escapes notice. Patients with tetanus require critical care, and in the larger cities of India are admitted either to special tetanus wards (equipped as intensive care units), or to general medical intensive care units. The fulminant form of the disease is a challenge to all that critical care medicine stands for. Successful management necessitates the application of every basic tenet of critical medical and nursing care.

The mortality of neonatal tetanus worldwide, is close to 1,000,000 deaths each year. In our country, as also in other third world countries, the disease chiefly afflicts the younger age group between 17–30 years. In the West, the disease is extremely rare, and is nearly extinct in some countries. When it does occur, it is commoner in people older than 50 years, in whom the effects of immunization have worn off, in the non-immunized, in the impoverished and in drug addicts.

Tetanus is a disease of wounds; any wound however trivial can result in the disease. In fact 20 per cent of patients have no evidence of a wound, nor do they give a history of injury. Contamination of wounds by manure, garden soil, or rusty implements is particularly dangerous. In our part of the world, tetanus can complicate burns, middle ear infections, septic abortions, childbirth and surgery. Tetanus neonatorum is most often due to non-sterile obstetric techniques, and to the dreadful habit of application of infected material such as cowdung to the umbilical stump.

Physiopathology (1, 2)

Under anaerobic conditions, tetanus bacilli within a wound produce a neurotoxin called tetanospasmin. This toxin spreads to underlying muscles and is bound to receptors containing gangliosides on the neuronal membranes of the presynaptic nerve terminals. It is then internalized and transported intra-axonally and retrogradely within the peripheral nerves to the motor horn cells of the segment of the cord supplying the muscles. The toxin also invariably enters the blood stream. It does not cross the blood-brain barrier, but via the blood it reaches and is bound to numerous nerve terminals in muscles throughout the body. It is then transported intra-axonally and retrogradely along numerous peripheral nerves to reach the alpha motor neurones of the whole spinal cord and brain stem. It also reaches the sympathetic ganglia, the lateral horns of the spinal cord and the parasympathetic centres. After reaching the cell bodies in the spinal cord and the brain stem, the toxin crosses the presynaptic cleft, and is bound to receptors on presynaptic nerve terminals of inhibitory interneurones (**Fig. 13.3.2**). Tetanus toxin now blocks the release of inhibitory neurotransmitters (chiefly

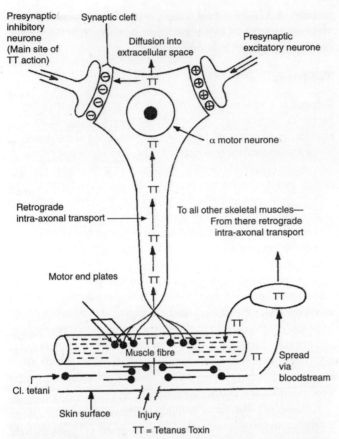

Fig. 13.3.2. Retrograde intra-axonal transport and main site of action of tetanus toxin (TT) in the central nervous system. The toxin ascends retrogradely along axons of the the peripheral nerves to reach the alpha motor neuron cell bodies. It then crosses the synaptic cleft to reach the terminals of the presynaptic inhibitory neurones where it exerts its main action by binding to receptors on the presynaptic membrane. Tetanus toxin also acts on the neuromuscular junctions of the peripheral nerves, as well as on the presynaptic excitatory neurons. The clinical picture of tetanus is however largely related to its main site of action.
(From Udwadia FE. 1994. Tetanus. Oxford University Press, Mumbai.)

glycine and gamma aminobutyric acid) from nerve terminals of inhibitory neurones.

The motor and autonomic neurones are now devoid of inhibitory control, which leads to an uncontrolled, disinhibited efferent discharge from motor neurones of the spinal cord and brainstem to both agonist and antagonist muscles, causing muscle rigidity and reflex muscle spasms that characterize the generalized forms of the disease. Disinhibited autonomic discharge leads to excessive sympathetic activity with increased catecholamine levels in the blood, as also to excessive parasympathetic activity. Medullary and other centres in the brainstem and the hypothalamus may also be affected by tetanus toxin. The direct action of tetanus toxin on organ systems has not been proven, but remains a distinct possibility.

Altered Haemodynamics (1–3)

Severe tetanus is characterized by a hypermetabolic, hyperdynamic, hyperkinetic circulatory state with tachycardia, and an increased

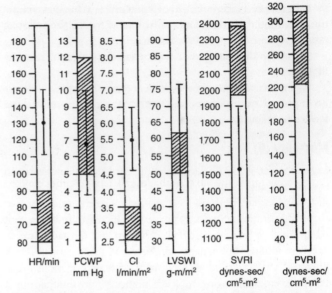

Fig. 13.3.3. Haemodynamic observations in 19 patients with **severe uncomplicated tetanus** (♦ = mean ± SD). Shaded areas show range of normal values. HR = heart rate; PCWP = pulmonary capillary wedge pressure; CI = cardiac index; LVSWI = left ventricular stroke work index; SVRI = systemic vascular resistance index; PVRI = pulmonary vascular resistance index.

cardiac output. The details of the haemodynamics in patients with severe uncomplicated tetanus are illustrated in **Fig. 13.3.3**.

Autonomic nervous system disturbances can profoundly affect the circulatory state. Autonomic 'storms' described under Complications, are characterized by a paroxysmal seizure-like discharge causing marked tachycardia and hypertension. A cessation of this discharge leads to bradycardia and hypotension. Increased parasympathetic activity is as integral a feature of tetanus as sympathetic overactivity. The imbalance between the sympathetic and parasympathetic systems, with fluctuations in tone and activity, leads to marked cardiovascular instability.

Our studies on tetanus suggest that though the myocardium responds well to volume load, the response is not as good as in control subjects (1–3). Myocardial function is thus suspect; whether this is related to tetanus toxin per se, or is related to factors common to any critical illness, is uncertain. Our experience also suggests that tetanus toxin may have a direct depressant effect on infranodal conduction causing infranodal block and arrest (1–3).

Clinical Features and Diagnosis

Generalized Tetanus

The two basic clinical features of tetanus are increased muscle tone and spasms. Fulminant tetanus is also invariably associated with autonomic disturbances.

Rigidity or increased muscle tone generally first involves the masseters, resulting in difficulty in opening the mouth—trismus or lockjaw. It soon involves the muscles of the face giving rise to the typical tetanus facies, with a 'risus sardonicus'. The muscles of the neck, trunk, back and extremities are all involved. The limbs are ramrod stiff, the abdomen may show board-like rigidity, and increased tone in the muscles of the neck and back can cause opisthotonos with retraction of the head, closely simulating meningitis.

Muscle spasms or seizures form the hallmark of severe tetanus. Seizures are easily induced by touch, noise or emotional stimuli. They often occur spontaneously, and vary in frequency and severity. Spontaneous seizures in the very severe forms of the disease occur at very brief intervals, so that the patient is often in a perpetually convulsed state. Protracted spasms often involve the pharynx, rendering swallowing impossible. Laryngeal spasms can lead to asphyxia. Powerful frequent spasms of the respiratory muscles render breathing impossible, so that the patient becomes hypoxic and even cyanosed.

Severe tetanus is a painful, febrile disease associated with tachycardia, sweating and an unstable cardiovascular system. Unless expertly managed, the patient succumbs to respiratory complications, circulatory failure, cardiac arrest, or to multiple organ failure.

Autonomic Nervous System Disturbances

These are intrinsic to severe tetanus. Tachycardia (ranging from 150–180/min) persisting for days on end, drenching sweats, frequent elevations in systolic and diastolic blood pressure, increased salivary and tracheobronchial secretions, and evidence of increased vagal tone and activity are the usual features pointing to autonomic disturbances in severe tetanus.

Grading the Severity of Tetanus

This is not just an academic exercise; it helps in both the prognosis and the management of the problem. The criteria described below are arbitrary, but have been used by us over many years, and have stood the test of time.

Grade I (Mild). Mild to moderate trismus; general spasticity; no respiratory embarrassment; no spasms; little or no dysphagia.

Grade II (Moderate). Moderate trismus; well marked rigidity; mild to moderate, but short-lasting spasms; moderate respiratory embarrassment with tachypnoea > 30–35/minute; mild dysphagia.

Grade III (Severe). Severe trismus; generalized spasticity; reflex and often spontaneous prolonged spasms; respiratory embarrassment with tachypnoea > 40/minute; apnoeic spells; severe dysphagia; tachycardia usually > 120/minute; a steady moderate increase in autonomic nervous system activity.

Grade IV (Very Severe). Features of Grade III plus violent autonomic disturbances often resulting in what may be aptly termed 'autonomic storms' involving the cardiovascular system. These include episodes of severe hypertension and tachycardia alternating with relative hypotension and bradycardia, or severe persistent hypertension (diastolic pressure > 110 mm Hg), or severe persistent hypotension (systolic pressure < 90 mm Hg).

Cephalic Tetanus (1)

This occurs after wounds to the face or head and is typified by unilateral facial paralysis, trismus, and facial stiffness of the unparalyzed side. Pharyngeal spasms causing dysphagia, and frequent laryngeal spasms are generally present. Rarely, facial palsy is bilateral. Occasionally there is also paresis of the glossopharyngeal, vagal, and rarely the oculomotor nerves. Cephalic tetanus often graduates to generalized tetanus.

Tetanus Neonatorum (1)

Even in the best of units this has a high mortality. The earliest symptom is a difficulty in suckling and swallowing due to stiffness of the masseters and the muscles of the pharynx. Stiffness extends to the face causing the classic tetanus facies. Skeletal muscle stiffness produces flexion at the elbows with the fists clenched and drawn to the thorax, extension of the knees with plantar flexion at the ankles and toes. There is retraction of the head with marked opisthotonos. Muscle spasms render breathing difficult. Autonomic disturbances occur, and death results from cardiorespiratory failure.

Local Tetanus

Rarely tetanus is confined to a group of muscles adjacent to a wound, or confined to one limb.

Natural History

The incubation period of tetanus averages 7–10 days, but may range from 2 days to 2 months. The shorter the incubation period, the more severe the disease.

The period of onset is the time interval between the first symptom and the occurrence of muscle spasms or seizures, and it ranges from 1–7 days. The shorter the period of onset, the more severe the disease. The period of onset is a more reliable prognostic guide than the incubation period. The disease increases to its maximum intensity over a period of 7–10 days, then plateaus over the next 1–2 weeks, and then gradually declines over the next 2 weeks. The natural history of the disease is punctuated by numerous complications which have been briefly outlined later. Tetanus is a severely catabolic disease, with the patient remaining in a hypermetabolic state for 3–4 weeks. Significant weight loss is observed even in those who recover, and even when every aspect of nutrition is assiduously cared for.

Complications (1)

The natural history and management of moderate, and in particular severe tetanus are bedevilled by numerous complications. As mentioned at the outset, any and every organ system can be involved. Respiratory and cardiovascular complications, and those involving the autonomic system are inherent to the disease. Others are related to the prolonged management of critically ill individuals who have been paralyzed by curare-like drugs, and maintained on ventilator support for periods extending from 4–6 weeks.

Respiratory Complications (1,4). These include atelectasis, aspiration pneumonia, and bronchopneumonia. Infection is generally due to Gram-negative organisms, chiefly Klebsiella and the Pseudomonas species. Prolonged laryngeal spasm can produce death from asphyxia. Episodes of acute respiratory distress with tachypnoea occur in both moderate and severe tetanus, and are probably related to release of inhibitory control over the respiratory centre, induced by the tetanus toxin. Unrelenting continuous spasms render breathing impossible, and unless correctly managed, produce death from acute hypoxia. The adult respiratory distress syndrome is now increasingly observed—it is chiefly due to iatrogenic sepsis, but can be due to tetanus per se. Complications related to tracheostomy and to prolonged ventilator support (chiefly pneumothorax and nosocomial pulmonary infections), are also observed.

Autonomic Cardiovascular Complications (**1, 3**). Marked tachycardia, as high as 180/min has already been commented upon. Severe hypotension, labile hypertension, or persistent severe hypertension are all observed. Hypertensive patients are almost always extremely sensitive to beta-blockers. Severe peripheral vasoconstriction with a shock-like state resulting in rapid death, is observed in a few fulminant cases. Autonomic 'storms' are characterized by episodes of sudden severe tachycardia with severe hypertension (BP =180–220/110–130 mm Hg), alternating within minutes with bradycardia (50–60/min) and a fall in systolic blood pressure to < 100 mm Hg. Marked cardiovascular instability results in, and is the forerunner of cardiac arrest and sudden death.

Increased vagal tone is invariably present and is manifested by increased tracheobronchial secretions, by sudden severe bradycardia and hypotension, and even arrest during suctioning of the trachea through the tracheostomy tube.

Cardiac arrhythmias are frequent and include supraventricular tachycardias, ventricular extrasystolies, junctional rhythms, and short spontaneously reverting bursts of ventricular tachycardia.

Sudden hyperthermia (rectal temperature > 41°C) can occur and result in cardiovascular collapse and death. Hypothermia may also be rarely observed. Sudden fluctuations in temperature are probably related to hypothalamic disturbance.

Sudden Death (**1, 4**). This remains the most dreaded complication of tetanus. In our experience, it constitutes the commonest cause of death in patients managed in well-equipped and well-staffed ICUs. Sudden death is related to the following factors:

(i) marked cardiovascular instability due to fluctuating sympathetic tone;

(ii) excessive vagal tone causing reflexly induced bradycardia, hypotension and cardiac arrest;

(iii) hypoxia due to unremitting seizures or to prolonged laryngeal spasms;

(iii) hyperpyrexia, often unsuspected and sudden, causing cardiovascular collapse and death;

(v) impaired infranodal conduction, probably related to the tetanus toxin per se;

(vi) massive pulmonary embolism;

(vii) an unrecognized iatrogenic complication, as for example, tension pneumothorax;

(viii) no obvious reason.

Multiple Organ Dysfunction. This is frequent in severe fulminant tetanus, multiple dysfunction was observed in 22 per cent of our cases. The system most frequently involved is of course the respiratory system, followed by the cardiovascular system, the gastrointestinal system, the liver and the kidneys. Changes can also occur in the haematopoietic system. Hypotension with systolic blood pressure < 70 mm Hg necessitating inotropic support, may persist for days. GI dysfunction is evinced by ileus and massive

bleeds. A rise in the liver enzymes to well above 100 IU, and of serum bilirubin up to 5 mg/dl is frequent. Mild elevations in the prothrombin time to one and half times the control value are also observed. Renal insufficiency is characterized by a rise in serum creatinine up to 3 mg/dl. Rarely acute renal failure requiring dialysis, is observed. It is indeed remarkable and noteworthy that multiple organ dysfunction, when not induced by obvious sepsis, does not carry the grim prognosis reported in Western literature, and recovery ensues provided excellent care is available.

Other Complications. These are chiefly iatrogenic and related to prolonged ventilator support in critically ill patients. These include sepsis, gastrointestinal complications (GI bleeds, diarrhoea, ileus), renal dysfunction, fluid and electrolyte disturbances, compression fractures of vertebrae, anaemia and hypoproteinaemia.

Miscellaneous complications include peripheral neuropathy,

Table 13.3.4. Respiratory complications in 265 patients with tetanus

	No. of patients
1. Bronchopulmonary infections	
Pneumonia and bronchopneumonia	36
Lung abscess	1
Pyopneumothorax with bronchopleural fistula	1
2. Significant pulmonary atelectasis*	26
3. Pneumothorax (iatrogenic)	5
4. Pneumomediastinum	5
5. Episodes of unexplained respiratory distress	29
6. Acute respiratory distress syndrome	9
7. Significant stridor	5
8. Accidental disconnection of ventilator	1

*Atelectasis (segmental or subsegmental) is an invariable feature of severe tetanus. 'Significant pulmonary atelectasis' includes only those patients where atelectasis persisted over a day in spite of repeated attempts to open up the involved segment or lobe.
From Udwdaia FE. (1994). Tetanus. Oxford University Press, Mumbai.

Table 13.3.5. Cardiovascular and autonomic complications in 233 patients at the JJ Hospital, and 32 patients at the Breach Candy Hospital

	JJH	BCH
1. Sustained tachycardia (> 150/min)	42	20
2. Hypotension (systolic BP < 90 mm Hg)	22	6
3. Hypertension (moderate and severe)	20	11
4. Episodic labile hypertension	12	8
5. Sudden cardiac arrest with death	13	1
6. Sudden cardiac arrest with successful resuscitation	6	3
7. Severe sweating	30	26
8. Severe vasoconstriction	15	1
9. Hyperpyrexia (> 42°C rectal)	12	11
10. Cardiac arrhythmias		
Paroxysmal SVT	6	7
Ventricular extrasystoles (frequent)	24	24
Nodal rhythm	–	3
Short runs of ventricular tachycardia	–	3
Idioventricular rhythm	–	1
11. Myocardial infarction	1	1
12. Severe hypothermia	–	1

Note: The lower incidence of arrhythmias in the 233 patients at the JJ Hospital was due to imperfect monitoring conditions as compared to the Breach Candy Hospital.
Source: as in Table 13.3.4.

Table 13.3.6. Other systemic complications in the 233 patients at the JJ Hospital, and 32 patients at the ICU, Breach Candy Hospital, Mumbai

	JJH	BCH
1. Septicaemia	5	7
2. Septic shock with DIC	4	2
3. Gastrointestinal		
GI bleed	56	4
Paralytic ileus	38	3
Diarrhoea	24	3
4. Renal failure	27	4
5. CNS complications		
Obtunded mentation	10	4
Peripheral neuropathy	4	2
6. Metabolic and electrolyte disturbances	23	10
7. Miscellaneous		
Keratitis	–	4
Corneal perforation	–	1
Fracture of vertebrae	2	2
Urinary tract infection	13	12

Source: as in Table 13.3.4.

infected bed sores, thrombophlebitis, corneal ulcers and deep vein thrombosis in the lower limbs; this can result in death due to pulmonary embolism.

A list of respiratory, cardiovascular autonomic, and other complications observed in 233 patients at the JJ Hospital, and in 32 patients with severe tetanus at the Breach Candy Hospital are given in **Tables 13.3.4–13.3.6**.

Diagnosis

The diagnosis is based on the clinical features; there is no laboratory test that can confirm tetanus. To the experienced eye, tetanus admits of no differential diagnosis. The tetanus facies is unmistakable. It occurs in no other disease, and it simply cannot be mimicked by even a trained malingerer for any length of time. Rarely, trismus may be an early feature of meningitis. A CSF examination clinches the diagnosis, as in tetanus the CSF is normal. Dystonic reactions produced by phenothiazines and metoclopramide bear no resemblance to tetanus, and can be easily distinguished from it. Cephalic tetanus may be mistaken for rabies because of dysphagia; however, hydrophobia is never present in tetanus.

Management (2)

Whenever possible, all patients with tetanus should be admitted to an ICU, or a specially equipped tetanus ward that functions as an ICU. Mild or Grade I tetanus poses no problems except when complicated by a serious or septic wound, which by itself can result in death. However mild (Grade I) tetanus can graduate over a few days to moderate (Grade II) or even severe (Grade III and IV) tetanus. Even mild cases therefore require close observation till the natural history of the disease is clearly established.

Use of Antiserum

Immediately on admission to our unit the patient is given antiserum. Human tetanus immunoglobulin (HTIG) is superior to the equine antiserum as it does not produce a hypersensitivity reaction, and should be given in the dose of 3000–5000 international units intravenously or intramuscularly. However in poor developing countries, equine antiserum is the only one generally available and 10,000 units are given intravenously after doing a skin sensitivity test. Fatal anaphylaxis can occur even in the absence of a positive skin test. Some workers infiltrate 3000 units of the antitoxin locally around the wound, but this is of doubtful efficacy.

Antibiotics

Two mega units of crystalline penicillin are given intravenously for 8 days. Metronidazole, 500 mg intravenously 8 hourly for 5–7 days has been currently recommended.

Management Strategies (Table 13.3.7)

Grade I or mild tetanus should be treated conservatively with the use of sedatives and muscle relaxants.

Grade II or moderate tetanus should have a tracheostomy done, in addition to the use of sedatives and muscle relaxants.

Grade III and Grade IV or severe tetanus require sedation, tracheostomy, neuromuscular paralysis with curare-like drugs, and ventilator support till such time as the disease resolves and recovery ensues.

Table 13.3.7. Management strategies according to severity of tetanus

* Mild or Grade I Tetanus	Sedatives + Muscle Relaxants
* Moderate or Grade II Tetanus	Sedatives + Muscle Relaxants + Tracheostomy
* Severe or Grades III and IV Tetanus	Sedatives + Tracheostomy + Induced Neuromuscular Paralysis + Ventilator Support

Use of Sedatives and Muscle Relaxants

This constitutes the traditional conservative management of tetanus. Even today, sedatives and muscle relaxants continue to be the only therapy available, even for severe cases, in many tetanus units in developing countries all over the world.

In good ICUs and in well-equipped tetanus wards, sedatives and muscle relaxants continue to form the basis of therapy for Grades I and II tetanus. We almost exclusively use diazepam as the drug of choice. The dosage in children and adults is 5–20 mg thrice daily, and in neonates 2 mg thrice daily. In moderate (Grade II) tetanus, the drug is used as an intravenous infusion over 24 hours. We prefer not to exceed a dose of 80–100 mg intravenously over 24 hours, even in the presence of marked rigidity. Many units both in India and in the West and South America, continue to use doses as high as 250–350 mg intravenously over 24 hours. In our wide experience with this disease over the years, we remain unconvinced that doses > 80–100 mg/day, given over many days, confer any further benefit, or reduce the mortality associated with this disease. In fact, we feel that very high dosage schedules, as explained later, may do more harm than good, and particularly in the absence of ventilator support, always seriously depress respiration.

Other muscle relaxants in use include chlorpromazine, phenobarbitone, paraldehyde, mephenesin and meprobamate. The last two drugs are hardly ever used. A few units use chlorpromazine, or a combination of diazepam with chlorpromazine or phenobarbitone, or prefer to use all three drugs to help achieve better control of severe rigidity. The dose of chlorpromazine is 50 mg intramuscularly, four times daily in adults, 25 mg in children and 12.5 mg in neonates. The dose of phenobarbitone is 200 mg in adults, 100 mg in children and 30 mg in neonates, given intramuscularly every 8–12 hours. Dantrolene is a relatively new muscle relaxant which has been used in tetanus; we however have no experience with this drug, but doubt that it has any significant additional advantage over diazepam.

Baclofen, a centrally acting muscle relaxant, has been used intrathecally by some workers, with satisfying results (5, 6). It has no special advantage (7) and in our opinion, its use is not practical for poor third world countries.

Sedatives and muscle relaxants are of symptomatic use. The ideal sedative and muscle relaxant schedule for each patient should be so tailored as to ensure sedation, muscle relaxation and sleep, yet allow the patient to be aroused to obey commands. A practical, objective guide to the degree of muscle relaxation desired in moderately severe tetanus, is the tone of the abdominal muscles, which should feel relaxed and much less stiff on palpation.

Laryngeal spasm should be countered by an intravenous injection of 10–20 mg of diazepam, or 50 mg chlorpromazine, or by intravenous succinylcholine.

Tracheostomy

We consider this necessary even for Grade II or moderate tetanus, and absolutely mandatory for Grades III and IV tetanus. In Grade II tetanus an important cause of death even in intensive care settings, is sudden, prolonged laryngeal spasm, which causes death by asphyxia. This is easily preventable by doing a tracheostomy. Inability of patients with moderately severe tetanus to swallow well, combined with the use of heavier sedation, are also indications for an elective tracheostomy.

Induced Paralysis with Ventilator Support

Severe tetanus should not be managed conservatively, solely with the use of sedatives and muscle relaxants. Conservative management in these patients carries an appallingly high mortality. These patients not only require an elective tracheostomy, but also need to be paralysed by neuroparalytic agents and kept on ventilator support. Pancuronium is the neuroparalytic agent generally available in poor countries. Pancuronium 2–4 mg is given intravenously, and the dose is so titrated for each patient, that the neuromuscular paralysis achieved allows for efficient ventilator support. This is checked by serial measurements of arterial pH and arterial blood gases. The PaO_2 should be maintained > 70 mm Hg, and the $PaCO_2$ between 35–40 mm Hg. The initial requirement of the neuroparalytic drug may be as frequent as $1/2$–1 hourly. With time the requirement falls to 2 hourly, and later still to even 6–8 hourly schedules. We prefer to use bolus injections in the manner stated above (as in our opinion these are better tolerated) rather than using a continuous intravenous infusion of the drug. Newer neuroparalytic drugs include vecuronium used in the dose of 6–8 mg/hr and atracurium (loading dose 0.23 mg/kg followed by an infusion of 5 µg/kg/min) (8). The high cost of these two drugs however precludes their use in poor developing countries where tetanus is still rampant.

The average period of ventilator support in severe tetanus in our experience varies from 10 days to 6 weeks. Once spasms abate, pancuronium is stopped; ventilator support is however continued till the patient is deemed fit to be weaned. Premature weaning in the presence of excessively stiff chest muscles is unwise, and leads to problems necessitating reintroduction of ventilator support. The tracheostomy tube is removed only when the patient can cough well, swallow satisfactorily, and can handle his upper respiratory secretions without difficulty.

Treatment of Autonomic Circulatory Disturbances

A number of drugs have been used to treat autonomic 'storms' producing severe cardiovascular instability in fulminant tetanus. These include beta-blockers (9), heavy sedation (10), intravenous morphine sulphate (11), intravenous clonidine (12), and intravenous infusions of magnesium sulphate (13). However these drugs do not alter the high mortality in fulminant disease. Our studies on the haemodynamics of severe tetanus have convinced us that it is best to rely on efficient cardiorespiratory support, and to avoid drugs that strongly depress the central or autonomic nervous systems. Hypotensive spells are treated with a volume load, and if this is inadvisable or ineffective, we use a titrated dose of dopamine sufficient to raise the systolic blood pressure just above 100 mm Hg. Hypertensive spells with systolic blood pressure > 200 mm Hg or a diastolic blood pressure > 110 mm Hg are best treated with 5–10 mg of oral propranolol, the dose being titrated to achieve an effective control over the heart rate and the blood pressure, or sublingual nifedipine (5 mg), or a combination of the above two. The use of intravenous beta-blockers is best avoided as these patients are extremely sensitive to these drugs, particularly when used intravenously. Bradyrhythms below 50/min are treated with intravenous atropine, and severe sinus tachyrhythms > 170–180/minute with verapamil 40 mg twice or thrice daily. In patients with a shock-like state with increased systemic vascular resistance and a reduced cardiac index, 2–5 mg morphine given intravenously helps sometimes in effectively reducing the systemic vascular resistance, and improving the cardiac output and tissue perfusion. The dose again needs to be titrated as per the patient's response, and the dose may be repeated if necessary. Patients with the above mentioned haemodynamic abnormality who do not respond to morphine, should be given a trial with a slow titrated infusion of sodium nitroprusside, so as to reduce the systemic vascular resistance. We invariably combine this with simultaneous dopamine inotropic support.

Severe tetanus is often associated with hypotension (systolic blood pressure < 70–80 mm Hg). Unless the intravascular volume is definitely depleted, it is unwise to use large fluid challenges to increase the arterial blood pressure. The compliance of both the systemic and pulmonary vasculature is markedly increased in these patients, and volume replacements are literally 'swallowed up' in the compliant vessels, or tend to produce non-cardiogenic pulmonary oeder... and the acute respiratory distress syndrome. The cardiac index may still be markedly raised in the presence of a low arterial blood pressure. Even so, the use of dopamine inotropic support is advocated so as to maintain the systolic blood pressure in young individuals between 90–100 mm Hg, and in older patients close to 120 mm Hg. This ensures adequate oxygen transport, and allows for an increased oxygen uptake by hypermetabolic tissues.

In our opinion, high doses of diazepam (150–300 mg/day intravenously) in severe tetanus are unwise, and may well contribute to a high mortality. Such high doses by strongly depressing the autonomic and central nervous systems, may predispose to cardiac arrest during episodes of bradycardia and hypotension, or could well prevent successful resuscitation following cardiac arrest. We advocate only 30–50 mg/day of intravenous diazepam in patients who are paralyzed and on ventilator support.

The management principles enunciated and discussed above have resulted in a mortality as low as 6 per cent in our ICU in patients with severe fulminant tetanus.

Treatment of Other Complications

Prevention, prompt recognition and treatment of the numerous complications that can involve almost each and every system, is vital if mortality is to be reduced.

Critical Care and Nursing

No other illness makes greater demands on a critical care unit than severe fulminant tetanus. Critical care of the patient as a whole, and expert nursing are of crucial importance. Special emphasis should be laid on meticulous care of the tracheostomy, and good physiotherapy. In addition to maintaining the arterial blood gases within the normal range, adequate oxygen transport must be ensured. Packed cells should be transfused to correct anaemia; cardiac output is enhanced by inotropic support, if necessary.

Nutrition

Tetanus is a severely catabolic disease, and generally occurs in patients with a poor nutritional state. Good nutrition is imperative for survival. A caloric intake between 2500–3000 calories/day,

with at least 75–100 g of protein is given in the form of liquid or semiliquid food through the nasogastric tube.

A summary of the management protocol in tetanus, has been tabulated below in **Table 13.3.8**.

Prevention

Tetanus is a dreadful disease which is almost totally preventable by proper active immunization and proper care of wounds. An attack of tetanus does not confer immunity from another attack. Immunization with tetanus toxoid should begin during convalescence. Some prefer to administer the first dose of toxoid soon after admission to the ICU.

Mortality

Mortality depends on the severity of tetanus. A short incubation period (< 4 days) and a short period of onset (< 2 days) signify severe disease and prognosticate a high mortality, often over 50 per cent. Tetanus neonatorum carries a mortality of 60–80 per cent. The overall mortality in tetanus, reported from different countries, ranges from 20–60 per cent. In Mumbai till 10 years back, overall mortality in a large teaching hospital was 30 per cent, and the mortality in fulminant tetanus was between 70–100 per cent. This high mortality was due to a failure to grasp the principles of critical care and ventilator support. With the management strategies outlined above, the overall mortality in the same teaching hospital fell to 12 per cent, and mortality in severe tetanus to 23 per cent (**4**). With better intensive care facilities the mortality of severe tetanus has been brought down to around 6 per cent (**3**). These results amply justify our management strategies discussed above.

REFERENCES

1. Udwadia FE. (1994). In: Tetanus. Oxford University Press. Bombay, Delhi, Calcutta.

2. Udwadia FE. (2003). Tetanus, In: Oxford Text Book of Medicine (Eds Warrell DA, Cox TM, Firth JD, Benz EJ Jr). pp. 545–551. Oxford University Press.

3. Udwadia FE, Sunavala JD, Jain MC et al. (1992). Hemodynamic studies

Table 13.3.8. Summary of the management protocol in tetanus

1. Antiserum—Equine antitoxin 10,000 units IV after test dose. If available, 3000–5000 IU of HTIG preferred
2. Antibiotics—Crystalline penicillin 2 mega units IV for 8 days + metronidazole 500 mg IV 8 hourly
3. Care of the wound according to general surgical principles
4. Sedatives and muscle relaxants—used for all grades of tetanus. The sedative most commonly used is diazepam, 20 mg 8 hourly IV, in adults. We do not exceed a dose of 100 mg/24 hrs
5. Tracheostomy—done in Grades II, III and IV tetanus
6. Induced paralysis + ventilator support—used in Grades III and IV tetanus. Pancuronium 2–4 mg IV as and when required (to start with, every half to one hour)
7. Treatment of autonomic circulatory disturbances
   - Hypotensive spells treated with volume load, or if this is ineffective or inadvisable, a titrated dose of dopamine is used for inotropic support. Maintain BP around 100–120/80 mm Hg
   - Hypertensive spells treated with 5–10 mg oral propranolol, or 5 mg sublingual nifedipine, or a combination of both drugs. Avoid IV propranolol. Morphine 2–5 mg IV, is used in patients with low CO and high SVR. Morphine in an IV infusion may also be used
   - Bradyrhythms < 50/min treated with IV atropine
   - Sinus tachycardia > 180/min treated with verapamil 40 mg thrice a day
8. Treatment of other complications
9. Overall critical care and nursing
10. Nutrition—Maintain a caloric intake of 2500–3000 cals/day, with 75–100 g of proteins/day

during the management of severe tetanus. Quart J Med. 83(302), 449–460.

4. Udwadia FE, Lall A, Udwadia ZF et al. (1987). Tetanus and its complications: Intensive care and management experience in 150 Indian patients. Epidem Inf. 99, 675–684.

5. Muller H, Zierski J, Borner U, Hempelmann G. (1988). Intrathecal baclofen in tetanus. Ann N Y Acad Sci. 531, 167–173.

6. Vitris M, Saissy JM, Demaziere J et al. (1991). Treatment of severe tetanus by repeated intrathecal injections of baclofen. Dakar Med. 36(1), 28–29.

7. Saissy JM, Demaziere J, Vitris et al. (1992). Treatment of severe tetanus by intrathecal injections of baclofen without artificial ventilation. Intensive Care Med. 18(4), 241–244.

8. Fassoulaki A, Eforakopoulou M. (1988). Vecuronium in the management of tetanus. Is it the muscle relaxant of choice? Acta Anaesthesiol Belg. 39(2), 75–78.

9. Prys-Roberts C, Corbett JL, Kerr JH et al. (1969). Treatment of sympathetic overactivity in tetanus. Lancet. 1, 542–546.

10. Cole LB, Youngman HR. (1969). Treatment of tetanus. Lancet. 1, 1017–1029.

11. Wright DK, Laloo UG, Nayiager S et al. (1989). Autonomic nervous system disturbances in severe tetanus: Current perspectives. Crit Care Med. 17(4), 371–375.

12. James MF, Manson ED. (1985). The use of magnesium sulphate infusions in the management of very severe tetanus. Intensive Care Med. 11, 5–12.

13. Sutton DM, Trenlitt MB, Woodcock TE et al. (1990). Management of autonomic dysfunction in severe tetanus: The use of magnesium sulphate and clonidine. Intensive Care Med. 16, 75–80.

Acute Disseminated Haematogenous Tuberculosis

General Considerations

The problem of acute disseminated haematogenous tuberculosis is of importance in critical care medicine in India, and in other developing countries. This is because of the wide prevalence of tuberculosis in poor countries, and the certain increase in incidence likely to occur with the spread of AIDS in these countries (1). According to the 2003 WHO report on tuberculosis, the incidence of tuberculosis in India is 38/1000 population (2). The diagnosis of acute disseminated haematogenous tuberculosis is easy in a patient with known tuberculosis in the recent past. When the problem presents de novo, or when it occurs in immunocompromised patients who are extremely prone to both community-acquired and opportunistic pathogens, the diagnosis can be extremely difficult.

Clinical Features and Diagnosis (Table 13.3.9)

Fever of unknown origin is the presenting feature. Clinical deterioration can occur over a period of months, but is observed in a matter of days in immunocompromised individuals (3). Pulmonary lesions are invariably present, but can be easily missed. Miliary shadows may be undetectable on a portable chest X-ray, and the sputum examination may not be possible, as the patient either has no expectoration, or is too ill to expectorate. At times,

the disease manifests with fever and bilateral diffuse shadows in both lungs on an X-ray of the chest. There may be little or no cough and there is generally no sputum. Tachypnoea is an important feature; the clinical picture is that of acute respiratory distress syndrome with well-marked hypoxaemic respiratory failure, necessitating intubation and mechanical ventilator support. The relation of these 'shadows' within the lung to tubercle can only be proven by examination of the BAL fluid obtained through fibreoptic bronchoscopy. The BAL fluid shows acid-fast bacilli and a transbronchial biopsy often shows caseating granulomas.

Over a varying period of time (15 days–1 month), patients who are critically ill invariably develop dysfunction of multiple organs. The liver and the spleen may both be palpable, and liver functions are frequently deranged with a rise in serum bilirubin to well beyond 5 mg/dl, a significant increase in the transaminases, and a prothrombin time more than one and a half times the control value. A liver biopsy may show caseating granulomas. Very ill individuals have a fall in systolic blood pressure below 90 mm Hg (often as low as 70 mm Hg), and require inotropic support. Gastrointestinal bleeds and ileus make maintenance of nutrition difficult. Anaemia and hypoproteinaemia are both invariably present; the former is due both to blood loss and to infection. The white blood cell count may not be of much help. Normal counts, leucopaenia, or a mild to moderate leucocytosis may be observed. The ESR however is invariably raised, and is in the region of 100 mm/hr by the Westergren method. There may however be exceptions to this rule, particularly in the early phase of the natural history of the disease.

The patient may be obtunded even when the CSF examination is normal, and even with no evidence of tuberculomas in the brain on a CT examination of the head. The clinical picture in the fully evolved disease is often indistinguishable from sepsis with multiple organ dysfunction.

The presentation with multiple shadows within the lung evolving into the acute respiratory distress syndrome with multiple organ dysfunction is generally observed in immunocompromised patients, including those on corticosteroids. Rarely it may occur in immunocompetent individuals as well.

Table 13.3.9. Features suggestive of disseminated haematogenous tuberculosis

* Fever of unknown origin lasting over a few weeks, with sudden deterioration specially in immunocompromised patients
* Tachypnoea
* Sputum scanty or absent
* Hypoxaemic respiratory failure—ARDS
* Initially a hyperdynamic circulation as in sepsis, soon followed by a fall in cardiac output and shock
* Miliary or scattered shadows within lung
* Diagnosis most often made by fibreoptic bronchoscopy
* AFB present in BAL fluid; caseating granulomas may be seen in transbronchial biopsies
* CT chest or abdomen may show evidence of lymphadenopathy
* CT head may show presence of tuberculomas in the brain
* Frequent evidence of liver cell dysfunction
* Multiple organ dysfunction indistinguishable from sepsis
* Recovery possible if diagnosed early and treated promptly

The *diagnosis* may be difficult and at times impossible to establish. Repeated blood cultures in the early phase of the illness for Gram-negative infections, and peripheral smears to exclude Pl. falciparum infection should be done. As has been already mentioned, a fibreoptic bronchoscopy with bronchoalveolar lavage and a transbronchial biopsy are in our experience, probably the most useful investigations (4). Acid-fast bacilli can be demonstrated in bronchial aspirates or grown on culture. Biopsies (including liver biopsy) may show caseating granulomas. CT examination of the chest and abdomen may provide tell-tale clues by demonstrating the presence of enlarged necrotic glands. A CT of the head may unexpectedly reveal tuberculomas in the brain (5). If the patient is not too ill and if the above investigations are negative, an open lung biopsy is of great help in the presence of pulmonary shadowing of undetermined aetiology. Tuberculosis may manifest in the most bizarre fashion, particularly in countries where the disease is common. It should never be forgotten as an important differential diagnosis in an acute, life-threatening obscure illness.

Management

The management is with all 5 antituberculosis drugs—streptomycin 0.75–1 g intramuscularly, rifampicin 450–600 mg, isoniazid 300 mg, pyrazinamide 1.5 g, and ethambutol 800–1200 mg per day. Unfortunately the presence of liver dysfunction complicates management. Very often it is impossible to use rifampicin, as liver function deteriorates further, and one may need to omit pyrazinamide as well. In general, isoniazid continues to be well tolerated in our country in spite of evidence of liver cell dysfunction. Unfortunately however, even this drug may need to be stopped at times if liver function deteriorates or is markedly poor to start with. One is then left with second line drugs like ethionamide or cycloserine. We always add ciprofloxacin to the drug regime in patients who cannot tolerate the first line drugs.

Critical care in these patients involves efficient ventilator support, inotropic support for the circulation, maintenance of pH and arterial blood gases, and maintenance of fluid and electrolyte balance. Repeated packed cell transfusions are necessary to keep the haemoglobin around 11 g/dl. Nutrition is of utmost importance, and patients with GI dysfunction may need intravenous alimentation till oral feeds can recommence.

It is remarkable that even with significant multiple organ dysfunction, the prognosis is not as bad as is observed with Gram-negative bacterial sepsis. If patients can tolerate the first line drugs, if liver function does not progressively deteriorate, and if expert critical care is available, the mortality is around 50 per cent. Mental obtundation, iatrogenic infection and persistent lactic acid acidosis are important features that point to a poor prognosis and a fatal outcome.

REFERENCES

1. Clark RA, Blakeley SL, Greer D et al. (1991). Hematogenous dissemination of Mycobacterium tuberculosis in patients with AIDS. Rev Infect Dis. 13(6), 1089–1092.

2. WHO World Report on Tuberculosis—Appendage 4 (2003).

3. Wirnsberger GH, Zitta F, Moore D et al. (1993). Tuberculosis of the small bowel with perforation and hematogenous spread in a renal transplant recipient. Z Gastroenterol. 31(6), 401–404.

4. Maartens G, Willcox PA, Benatar SR. (1990). Miliary tuberculosis: Rapid diagnosis, hematologic abnormalities, and outcome in 109 treated adults. Am J Med. 89(3), 291–296.

5. Arvind C, Korath MP, Raveendranadhan K et al. (1993). A retrospective study of 1247 cases of intracranial tuberculomata diagnosed by computerized tomography. J Assoc Physicians India. 41(9), 559–561.

Other Fulminant Infections

Other important fulminant infections in India requiring intensive care are fulminant salmonella infections, other Gram-negative infections, and fulminant infections due to Entamoeba histolytica, dengue haemorrhagic fever and severe leptospiral infections. A short but relevant description of these infections is given below with special reference to difficulties in diagnosis and management.

Gram-negative Fulminant Infections

Fulminant B typhosus and Salmonella Infections

Gram-negative infections occur all over the world. There are however some infections which are more common in tropical climes and in developing countries. An important Gram-negative infection in our part of the world is typhoid fever. This infection is generally treated in hospital wards except during a crisis produced because of a fulminant infection, or because of a delayed diagnosis.

Clinical Features. Patients with fulminant infection require intensive care as they may manifest with all the features of septic shock (see Chapter on Septic Shock). Unless promptly treated, severe peripheral vasoconstriction, hypotension, and lactic acid acidosis are observed. Rarely the patient is mentally obtunded or even unconscious, and may require ventilatory support. Acute respiratory distress syndrome is occasionally observed. Recovery is still possible, and the outlook is not hopeless in spite of severe multiple organ dysfunction. B. typhosus is the most frequent organism grown on culture. There are however a large number of pathogenic Salmonella strains. There is no epidemiological study regarding the frequency of life-threatening infections produced by these strains in developing countries.

Typhoid fever can lead to perforation of one or more typhoid ulcers within the ileum. The ensuing peritonitis causes sepsis and is fatal unless surgically treated. However fulminant typhoid infection can lead to a picture of severe sepsis and multiple organ dysfunction without any perforation of typhoid ulcers.

Management. Intensive care management consists of the treatment of shock and the use of specific antibiotics against the infection. A volume load should be given so that the filling pressures are maintained at optimal levels. Inotropic support is invariably needed. Over-vigorous infusions can precipitate ARDS. Acute renal failure, initially due to prerenal causes and subsequently to acute tubular necrosis, almost certainly spells a fatal outcome. Persistent lactic acid acidosis, in spite of adequate measures to improve circulation, also carries a grim prognosis. Acute respiratory distress syndrome needs efficient ventilator support.

In a patient with proven fulminant B. typhosus infection, the drug of choice is ciprofloxacin. It is given intravenously in a dose of 200 mg twice daily for 10–15 days. Ceftriaxone 2 g intravenously twice daily for 10 days should also be used in life-threatening infections. S. typhi and S. paratyphi, in our country, as also in most countries of South-East Asia, are resistant to both ampicillin and chloramphenicol. It is however remarkable that in our experience, drug sensitivity to chloramphenicol seems to be returning, probably because the drug has not been used in typhoid or Salmonella infections for the last 15 years or more. It is also a matter of concern that there is now a slowly increasing incidence of partial or complete resistance of B. typhosus to ciprofloxacin.

Food or Water-borne Gram-negative Infections

The other Gram-negative infection which is peculiar to our country, and which occasionally finds admission to a critical care unit, is food poisoning due to contamination by Gram-negative bacteria.

The usual clinical picture of fever, vomiting, and violent diarrhoea resulting in hypovolaemic shock, is easily diagnosed. Occasionally the natural history of these infections is different, though still recognizable.

Within a few hours of ingestion of the contaminated food, the patient has abdominal cramps, a few watery stools, fever, and becomes seriously ill over 24 hours. The picture is of Gram-negative sepsis. The noteworthy feature is that after the first 24 hours, abdominal symptoms are mild, or almost totally absent. Blood cultures are positive either for E. coli or Klebsiella. Tachypnoea, a moderately severe ARDS, raised serum bilirubin and transaminase levels in blood, and a moderate degree of renal dysfunction with serum creatinine levels elevated up to 3 mg/dl, are observed in these patients.

Management is with the use of a third generation cephalosporin 1–2 g intravenous 8 hourly + metronidazole 500 mg intravenous 8 hourly + ciprofloxacin 200 mg 12 hourly intravenously. Shock is treated on the usual lines. Ventilator support was necessary in all our patients. In spite of the presence of multiple organ dysfunction, we were fortunate that all our patients survived.

The epidemiology and frequency of Gram-negative infections producing the clinical picture described above, have not been studied. Considering the poverty, and lack of sanitation and hygiene in many third world countries, such infections may well be frequent and important.

Fulminant Amoebic Infections

Disease due to E. histolytica is rampant in India, Bangladesh, South-East Asia, Africa and other developing countries. Amoebic infections requiring critical care are acute necrotizing ulcerative amoebic colitis, and amoebic liver abscess or abscesses, which produce life-threatening complications.

Acute Necrotizing Ulcerative Amoebic Colitis

This carries a high mortality, particularly in poor, malnourished, middle-aged patients, admitted to intensive care units of large teaching hospitals in our country. Death in these patients is due to perforation of the large bowel; more than one perforation may be present.

Clinical Features. Watery diarrhoea and abdominal cramps with blood and mucus in the stools, are the prelude to colonic perforation. The clinical manifestations of sudden severe abdominal pain, tenderness, rigidity, with evidence of a painful inflammatory abdominal mass, or of spreading peritonitis with gas under the diaphragm, are easy to recognize. However, in a number of instances, the clinical signs of perforation are atypical. This is particularly observed in poorly nourished, immunocompromised, or old debilitated patients. Such a patient looks ill; his sensorium is often clouded; he is dehydrated and complains of vague abdominal discomfort. He usually gives a history of loose watery stools for some days, but poverty, ignorance and apathy may sometimes combine to make him deny a history of significant diarrhoea. Clinical examination reveals a distended abdomen with diffuse tenderness on palpation. Distension in acute amoebic colitis is always to be viewed with suspicion as it is often a sign of impending perforation. When perforation occurs, distension increases and bowel sounds become feeble or absent. Watery diarrhoea from a necrotic large bowel may however persist and fool the unwary into complacence. A toxic look, not unlike that observed with a toxic megacolon complicating non-specific ulcerative colitis, is observed terminally in some patients. Fluid and electrolyte disturbances are always present. Increasing tachycardia, hypotension, shock and death ensue. A leucocytosis may not be always present. One has often wondered why the clinical features of amoebic perforation of the large bowel are so atypical in some patients. The probable answer lies in the host-parasite relationship. A fulminant infection in dehydrated, malnourished, or immunocompromised patients literally swamps the body defence and does not allow any worthwhile defence reactions to manifest themselves. The presence of a mild icterus and a palpable tender liver further strengthen the diagnosis. An associated liver abscess is easily picked up by an ultrasound or CT of the abdomen. A sigmoidoscopy is invaluable as amoebic ulcers are always seen; amoebae can be demonstrated in scrapings of these ulcers.

Management. Treatment for amoebic perforations of the large bowel is surgery for the perforation, and specific antiamoebic treatment. The prognosis in perforation is indeed poor. The friability of the large bowel adds to the surgeon's difficulties, the sutures often cutting through when the perforation is sealed. The possibility of multiple perforations must always be brought to the surgeon's attention. Remarkably enough, amoebic liver abscess is uncommon in patients with necrotizing colitis. Post-operative complications are frequent and require overall critical care.

Specific Treatment. Emetine hydrochloride 60 mg intramuscularly is administered daily for a total of 10 injections. Dehydroemetine (DHE) in the same dose, is thought to be equally effective and less toxic. Hypotension, tachycardia, and myocarditis are reported complications of emetine. These are rare in the recommended doses; ECG monitoring is however advisable.

Metronidazole 500 mg intravenously 8 hourly, is also administered for 10 days. This drug is an extremely valuable amoebicidal drug, and is also effective against anaerobes.

Tetracycline 250 mg 6 hourly is a useful adjunct in the treatment. It acts by modifying the bacterial flora necessary for the survival of E. histolytica. Suitable broad-spectrum antibiotics need to be given to counter the peritonitis produced by a colonic leak.

Fluid and electrolyte imbalance must be promptly rectified.

Life-threatening Complications of Amoebic Liver Abscess

Amoebic liver abscess is an extremely common pathology in tropical countries. There are however 2 groups of patients with amoebic liver abscess who require critical care.

(a) Those with a large undiagnosed solitary abscess, or multiple liver abscesses causing a life-threatening illness. Fever may be high and spiking, or may be low grade. The diagnosis is promptly made in a good unit, both on clinical examination and on an ultrasound of the abdomen. A tender liver, intercostal tenderness, signs of a pleural rub or pleural effusion on the right side with a raised right dome of the diaphragm, are all pointers to the clinical diagnosis. A large centrally placed abscess or multiple small abscesses not approaching the diaphragm, may not produce signs in the chest. A left lobe abscess may cause involvement of the left pleural space. Multiple liver abscesses or a single huge abscess can produce increasing jaundice and progressively increasing liver cell dysfunction. This is particularly seen in the malnourished, in alcoholics, and always in the cirrhotic. The patient becomes increasingly dull, apathetic and finally moribund, from a combination of sepsis and liver cell failure (**1, 2**).

Management lies in the CT-guided aspiration of one or more abscesses and the use of specific antiamoebic treatment outlined earlier. General supportive care towards circulatory, respiratory and other organ systems is essential.

(b) Those with rupture of a liver abscess. This is a life-threatening emergency requiring critical care (**Fig. 13.3.4**).

Rupture may occur into the following sites—

(i) Into the peritoneal cavity, producing features of acute peritonitis. In some patients, the florid features observed with bacterial peritonitis may be absent, so that there is a moderate delay in diagnosis. A laparotomy is mandatory. Large drains are kept in the peritoneal cavity; the liver abscess must also be drained. If diagnosis and exploratory laparotomy are delayed, multiple organ system failure occurs and death ensues. If diagnosis is quick and treatment prompt, recovery is possible even if multiple organ dysfunction occurs in the post-operative phase.

(ii) Along the right paracolic gutter with tenderness in the right flank and over the right iliac fossa. A wrong diagnosis of an acute appendicitis is often made. Surgical opinion should always be sought; an exploratory laparotomy may be necessary.

(iii) Into the lesser sac and subphrenic spaces, causing a subphrenic abscess. A CT guided drainage or open surgical drainage is necessary.

(iv) Into the stomach, duodenum or colon; this is very rare, and surgical advice should be sought.

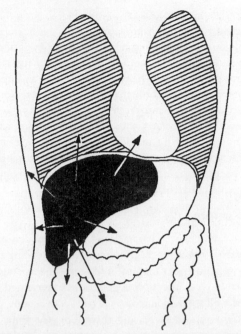

Fig. 13.3.4. Possible sites of rupture of an amoebic liver abscess (see text). From Vakil RJ and Udwadia FE. 1982. Diagnosis and Management of Medical Emergencies. OUP, Mumbai.

(v) Into the pleural space causing an empyema, or into the lung resulting in a lung abscess. The patient may cough up anchovy sauce pus. Management consists of repeated pleural taps to keep the pleura dry. The abscess within the liver should also be drained.

(vi) Into the pericardium—this is one of the most dreaded of medical emergencies, and is rapidly fatal. Heroic measures can however save the patient. The pus in the pericardial space must be promptly aspirated percutaneously and the liver abscess must also be quickly drained. The help of a thoracic surgeon must be sought so that open drainage of the pericardium can be performed, if percutaneous aspiration is inadequate.

REFERENCES

1. Vakil RJ, Udwadia FE. (1988). Amoebiasis. In: Diagnosis and Management of Medical Emergencies, 3rd edn. pp. 274–85. Oxford University Press, Delhi.
2. Kapoor, OP. (1979). Amoebic Liver Abscess. SS. Publishers, India.

Dengue Haemorrhagic Fever

Dengue haemorrhagic fever is a mosquito-borne (aedis aegypti is the carrier), flavivirus infection which afflicts 500,000 patients per year throughout the tropical regions of the world (**1**). Depending on epidemic activity, dengue and dengue haemorrhagic fever are observed with varying frequency in all parts of India. The average mortality is 5 per cent; the fulminant forms carry a much higher mortality. The disease can be caused by any one of four distinct dengue viruses—DEN1, DEN-2, DEN-3, DEN-4. Infection caused by one virus does not necessarily confer immunity to any one of the other viruses.

Pathogenesis

The pathogenesis underlying the features of dengue haemorrhagic fever is based in the presence of subneutralizing levels of dengue antibodies in the blood. This enhances the infectivity of a fresh dengue viral infection by increasing the binding and uptake of virus-antibody complexes through the Fc receptors on monocytes in the blood and on tissue macrophages. The immune response also involves cellular activation, with cytokine release and activation of complement. It is this primed immune response which is response for widespread capillary leakage, coagulopathy with extensive haemorrhagic manifestations and acute circulatory failure—the hallmarks of the illness.

Clinical Features (2)

The clinical features are characterized by the sudden onset of fever, bodyache and headache. It is impossible to distinguish this presentation from other tropical infections at this stage. The suspicion of a viral infection is generally entertained by the presence of well-marked leucopaenia (the WBC count may fall to < 2000/mm³) and increasing thrombocytopaenia. These early haematological features in a febrile patients should prompt the diagnosis of a possible dengue viral infection, more so in the presence of an outbreak of dengue in a particular area or district.

After two to seven days, there is a defervescence in the fever and at this crucial time the classic features of this infection are observed with varying degree and intensity. These are: (i) haemorrhagic manifestations due to thrombocytopaenia and coagulopathy; (ii) widespread capillary leak; (iii) acute circulatory failure—the dengue shock syndrome.

Haemorrhagic features are present in varying degree, the most common being purpuric lesions and ecchymosis. However, bleeding from thrombocytopaenia, coagulopathy and capillary damage often takes the form of severe epistaxis, haematemesis and haematuria. In fulminant cases we have observed bleeding into the pleural space, peritoneal cavity and into any organ system, including the brain.

The capillary leak is manifested by oedema of the feet and of the subcutaneous tissue, and at times by non-cardiogenic pulmonary oedema leading to acute lung injury and the acute respiratory distress syndrome (ARDS). Objective evidence of a capillary leak is provided by the presence of haemoconcentration (the haematocrit being elevated by 10–30 per cent).

Acute circulatory failure is characterized by the clinical features of shock. Tachycardia, tachypnoea, hypotension, oliguria, mental obtundation, lactic acid acidosis are all observed. Elevation of liver enzymes is invariably present; in fact liver enzymes are often raised well before the onset of haemorrhagic manifestations. Evidence of multiple organ dysfunction is frequent and progressive in fulminant fatal cases.

The duration of shock lasts for 2 to 4 days, culminating in recovery or death. Death can also occur from a severe bleed into an organ system (e.g. brain) or from multiple organ failure.

Diagnosis

The diagnosis depends on the demonstration of IgM antibodies (by the Elisa technique) to the dengue virus. Unfortunately not all patients develop IgM antibodies within the first week of the infection. In some patients a rise in IgM is observed after as long as 10 days.

Differential diagnosis of acute haemorrhagic fevers in the tropics may pose problems. Important infections other than dengue haemorrhagic fever that merit consideration are meningococal sepsis and meningitis, fulminant Gram-negative infections causing coagulopathy, fulminant falciparum infection, acute leptospiral infection, severe rickettsial infection, fulminant viral hepatitis, bacterial endocarditis and haemorrhagic exanthemas, as in haemorrhagic chicken pox and measles. Consideration of the clinical background, examination of peripheral blood smears, blood cultures, serological tests and other relevant laboratory investigations generally help in diagnosis.

Fortunately haemorrhagic fevers caused by the Ebola and Hanta viruses are restricted to well-defined areas of Africa. These highly infectious viral diseases cause fever with extensive haemorrhages, cellular death, multiple organ failure and have a mortality close to 80 per cent.

Thrombotic thrombocytopaenic purpura though rare, is often mistaken for a fulminant infection causing widespread purpura.

Management

Dengue haemorrhagic fever requires critical care; treatment is mainly supportive. No antimicrobial drug acts on the dengue virus. Haemorrhagic manifestations and coagulopathy are countered by replacement of deficient clotting factors and by platelet infusions. Anaemia is corrected by infusion of packed cells. Haemorrhage into the pleural space or peritoneal cavity may require drainage.

Signs of impending shock should be detected early and treated by prompt infusion of colloids, plasma and if necessary by inotropic support. Oxygenation should be well maintained and the delivery of oxygen to the tissues should be adequate. It is important to insert a central venous catheter early in the natural history of the disease, as puncture sites can bleed profusely. Volume replacement is guided by clinical examination and by measuring central venous pressure. Over-infusion of fluids can precipitate or worsen ARDS.

Patients with ARDS require intubation and ventilator support. Ventilator support is also necessary in patients who are in shock and acute circulatory failure.

Metabolic acidosis is frequent and should be corrected. All organ systems must be given adequate support.

Secondary bacterial nosocomial infection is observed in some patients, requiring suitable antibiotic treatment.

REFERENCES

1. Peterson LR, Gubler DJ. (2003). In: Oxford Textbook of Medicine (Eds Warrell DA, Cox TM, Firth JD, Benz EJ Jr). pp. 382–389. Oxford University Press.

2. Gubler DJ. (1998). Dengue and dengue haemorrhagic fever. Clin Microbiol Reviews. 11, 480–496.

Severe Leptospirosis

Leptospirosis is a worldwide zoonosis afflicting many mammals; rodents form the most important animal reservoir. The disease is common in the tropics and is frequently observed in India, South-East Asia, Africa, and South America. It is caused by a spirochaete, the pathogenic species being the Leptospira interrogans. There are several serotypes of this genus; some of these preferentially infect select mammalian hosts. Thus the serotype L. icterohaemorrhagica is associated with the rat, L. canicola with dogs and L. pomona with swine and cattle. Leptospira are excreted through the urine of the infected mammalian hosts. Transmission of infection from animal to man generally occurs through contaminated water or moist soil. Leptospira enter through abrasions in the skin (generally on the feet and legs), or rarely through the mucosa of the mouth, pharynx or oesophagus. The disease is therefore common in the monsoon particularly at the time of floods, in areas where there is a large population of rats.

In most cases, human infection is asymptomatic or mild and cures itself. However, 5 to 15 per cent of cases are severe or fatal (1).

Pathogenesis

The organisms after gaining entry, generally through abraded skin, enter the blood stream and are distributed to all organs of the body. The fulminant forms always severely affect liver function and often produce varying degrees of renal dysfunction. Leptospira can persist for months in the kidneys and ocular tissue.

The exact pathogenesis is unexplained as there are minor histopathological changes in the liver or kidney or other organ systems in the presence of severe functional derangement.

Clinical Features (2)

The severe and fulminant forms of the disease are observed in icteric leptospirosis (Weils disease). The illness is ushered by fever, headache, severe muscle pains and marked conjunctival injection. Jaundice with impaired liver cell function appears by the fifth to seventh day and may persist for a month. However death is very rarely related to liver cell failure.

All or many organ systems are affected. The most important organ involved is the kidney. Albuminuria, red blood cells are invariably present. Oliguria with acute renal failure occurs in severe cases.

The lungs frequently show haemorrhagic bronchopneumonia. We have seen a few patients presenting with acute intra-alveolar haemorrhage that can cause death from overwhelming hypoxia, unless the patient is promptly intubated and ventilated with a high FIO$_2$. Intra-alveolar haemorrhage may be the presenting feature of severe disease and is being increasingly recognized in Latin America (3).

Meningitis (the CSF showing pleocytosis with raised protein) is frequently observed. It is likely that meningeal involvement may be related to an immunological mechanism than to actual invasion of the leptospira in the meninges. Organisms may be found in the CSF without meningeal or CNS symptoms. An obtunded mental state is either due to aseptic meningoencephalitis or to uraemic encephalopathy.

Fulminant leptospirosis is characterized by a haemorrhagic diathesis. Petechiae, epistaxis, subconjunctival haemorrhage, haemoptysis are common manifestations. Death can occur from subarachnoid haemorrhage or from exsanguinating gastrointestinal bleeds. A coagulopathy with raised prothrombin time and thrombocytopaenia is frequent. Bleeding is related both to the coagulopathy and to capillary damage. The overall clinical picture in its fully evolved form often resembles Gram-negative bacterial sepsis.

There is marked leucocytosis in the peripheral blood; WBC counts as high as 30,000/mm^3 or more may be observed.

Diagnosis

The diagnosis should be suspected on clinical grounds in endemic areas. The triad of fever, conjunctival infection with subconjunctival haemorrhage and jaundice should arouse immediate suspicion. A further association of abnormal urinary findings with varying degrees of renal insufficiency renders the diagnosis even more likely. Muscle pains associated with muscle tenderness are observed in close to 80 per cent of patients. This is invariably associated with very high CPK levels in blood. Patients presenting with fever and intra-alveolar haemorrhage; invariably in our experience have very high CPK levels—a combination almost diagnostic of severe leptospiral disease. Leucocytosis is almost always present, but does not help in diagnosis.

The IgM for leptospiral infection (done by the Elisa technique) is generally positive by the fifth to seventh day. Immunfluorescent assays are also being used for diagnosis.

The main differential diagnosis is sepsis caused by other organisms, fulminant viral hepatitis, fulminant Pl. falciparum infection. The latter does not generally cause deep jaundice. When meningitis is a presenting feature the disease has to be distinguished from other forms of aseptic meningitis and from tuberculous meningitis. Patients presenting with acute intra-alveolar haemorrhage need to be distinguished from acute Wegners granulomatosis, systemic lupus erythematosus and other connective tissue disorders.

Treatment

Treatment in severe cases should be made on clinical suspicion. It should never await a laboratory diagnosis. Penicillin G is the drug of choice; 2 million units six hourly, are given intravenously for 8 to 10 days.

Intra-alveolar haemorrhage requires intubation and ventilator support. We have observed a dramatic improvement in the clinical state, chest X-ray and arterial oxygenation following pulsed therapy with 1 g methylprednisolone intravenously daily for 3 days, followed by oral prednisolone (40 mg/day), tapered and stopped after 10 days. Dramatic improvement occurs within a few hours of the administration of the drug and we strongly urge this therapy in patients presenting with severe life-threatening intra-alveolar haemorrhage. Acute renal failure may warrant dialysis till recovery ensues.

Critical care is vital, with support to all organ systems. Fresh frozen plasma and platelet infusions are necessary to treat coagulopathy.

If the patient recovers, kidney function and liver function return to normal. However anterior uveitus may occur days or weeks after recovery or may persist if present during the course of the acute illness.

REFERENCES

1. Watt G. (2003). Leptospirosis. In: Oxford Textbook of Medicine (Eds Warrell DA, Cox TM, Firth JD, Benz EJ Jr). pp. 600–604. Oxford University Press.

2. Ko Al et al. (1999). Urban epidemic of severe leptospirosis in Brazil. Lancet, 354, 820–825.

3. Zaki SR, Shiej WJ, The epidemic working group. (1996). Leptospirosis associated with outbreak of acute febrile illness and pulmonary haemorrhage, Nicargria. Lancet. 347, 535–536.

CHAPTER 13.4

Use of Antibiotics in the Intensive Care Unit

General Considerations

Patients are often admitted to the ICU for fulminant infections. Infection is also an important complication in patients admitted to the ICU for other life-threatening problems. In either situation, treatment of infection needs to be prompt, judicious and yet comprehensive.

There is today, an immense and ever-increasing array of antibiotics available to doctors caring for very ill patients. The belief that this ever-increasing array will reduce the incidence of infections in the critical care unit, is a mirage. There is an ecological balance between micro-organisms and man in a given environment. Eradication of one group of organisms often breeds resistant strains, or is associated with an increasing incidence of different unrelated infections. It is however necessary for the intensivist to be thoroughly familiar with the more important antibiotics in common use.

Choice of Antibiotics for Use in the ICU (1)

The antibiotic of choice is obviously the one that acts best against the infecting organism, or is the least toxic amongst several equally effective agents. At times, the choice of an antibiotic depends on its ability to penetrate better within an area or site of infection, when compared to other drugs. Thus infection within the CNS demands not only an antibiotic effective against the offending pathogen, but also one that has good penetration into the cerebrospinal fluid. Similarly fulminant biliary infections or urinary infections can only be controlled by drugs that can penetrate and achieve high concentrations in the biliary and urinary tracts respectively. In our country, as well as in other developing countries, cost is also an extremely important consideration. It is positively obscene in a poor country, to have a patient spend a fortune on very expensive, new, fancy drugs, when a simple cheaper drug has the same or even better effect.

There are a few other general considerations worthy of note in the treatment of infections in the ICU:

(i) Severe infections in the ICU are occasionally polymicrobial; these multiple pathogens may be difficult to identify even after investigations.

(ii) Patients are generally far more ill in the ICU; antibiotic therapy against infections should be started promptly, and is invariably administered by the parenteral route.

(iii) A combination of two or more antibiotics is often used. This is imperative in a virulent infection, if the identity of the offending pathogens is unknown. Empiric therapy in these circumstances is mandatory. Antibiotic coverage should be reasonably comprehensive in a given situation; yet drugs which are redundant or unnecesssary should be strictly avoided. It should be remembered that there are some inherent disadvantages in the use of multiple antibiotics. Each additional antibiotic added to a therapeutic regime can contribute to increasing toxicity, drug interactions, superinfection and cost. The number of drugs used in life-threatening infections should therefore be reduced as soon as it is felt safe to do so. This principle curtails the incidence of drug toxicity and drug interactions. Above all, this also reduces the incidence of colonization and overgrowth by drug-resistant bacteria and fungi. It is sad to see one life-threatening infection being eradicated and being replaced by an even more virulent superinfection by Pseudomonas, other multiple drug-resistant Gram-negative bacilli, or fungi. The overall increased prevalence in an ICU of such resistant microbiological flora spells danger to other critically ill patients in the unit (2).

(iv) The pharmacokinetics of an antibiotic used in a critically ill patient is likely to be distorted; drug interactions and toxicity are more frequently encountered.

The choice of antibiotics for empiric therapy in serious infections in the ICU is a matter of clinical judgement and experience. It depends on: (a) the site of infection; (b) whether the infection is community acquired or nosocomial; (c) if nosocomial, the epidemiology, prevalence and nature of microbiological flora in a given unit; (d) the presence or absence of hepatic and/or renal dysfunction; (e) a history of allergy to drugs—in particular to penicillins; (f) host factors—age, pregnancy, background disease, immunosuppression; g) the cost to the patient, all other factors being equal.

Table 13.4.1 details the empiric antibiotic regimens used for the initial treatment of life-threatening infections, while the causative organism is being sought.

Table 13.4.2 lists the antimicrobials of choice for commonly encountered organisms in the ICU.

Table 13.4.1. Empiric antibiotic regimes for common life-threatening infections in the ICU

Clinical Syndrome	Antibiotic Regime	IV Doses	Clinical Syndrome	Antibiotic Regime	IV Doses
1. Sepsis			**2. Intra-abdominal Sepsis**		
* Extra-Abdominal Source of Infection	(a) Ceftazidime or Ceftriaxone	1 g 6 hrly 1–2 g 12 hrly	* Community-acquired	(a) Amoxycillin-Clavulanic Acid	1.2 g 8 hrly
	+			+	
	Aminoglycoside† (Gentamicin or Amikacin)	60–80 mg 8 hrly 7.5 mg/kg 12 hrly		Aminoglycoside† (Gentamicin or Amikacin)	60–80 mg 8 hrly 7.5 mg/kg 12 hrly
				+	
– If there is strong suspicion of pseudo-monal infection, use (b)	(b) Piperacillin or Ticarcillin	3–4 g 4 hrly 1–3 g 4–6 hrly		Metronidazole (b) Ceftazidime	500 mg 8 hrly 1 g 6 hrly
	+			+	
	Aminoglycoside† (Gentamicin or Amikacin)	60–80 mg 8 hrly 7.5 mg/kg 12 hrly		Ciprofloxacin or Aminoglycoside† (Gentamicin or Amikacin)	200 mg 12 hrly 60–80 mg 8 hrly 7.5 mg/kg 12 hrly
				+	
* Intra-Abdominal Source of Infection	See under Point **2**			Metronidazole	500 mg 8 hrly
			* Hospital-acquired	(a) Piperacillin-Tazobactam or Cefpirome	3–4 g 4 hrly 2 g 12 hrly
* Infection of Unknown Aetiology	Ceftazidime or Ceftriaxone	1 g 6 hrly 1–2 g 12 hrly			
	+			Ciprofloxacin or Aminoglycoside† (Gentamicin or Amikacin)	200 mg 12 hrly 60–80 mg 8 hrly 7.5 mg/kg 12 hrly
	Ciprofloxacin or Aminoglycoside† (Gentamicin or Amikacin)	200 mg 12 hrly 60–80 mg 8 hrly 7.5 mg/kg 12 hrly		+	
	+			Metronidazole (b) Ticarcillin-Clavulanic Acid	500 mg 8 hrly 3.1 g 4 hrly
	Vancomycin	500 mg 6 hrly		+	
	+			Ciprofloxacin or Aminoglycoside† (Gentamicin or Amikacin)	200 mg 12 hrly 60–80 mg 8 hrly 7.5 mg/kg 12 hrly
	Metronidazole	500 mg 8 hrly		+	
				Metronidazole	500 mg 8 hrly
3. Pneumonias (also see Chapter 8.7 and 13.2)				+	
				Vancomycin (c) Imipenem-Cilastatin	500 mg 6 hrly 500 mg 6 hrly
* Community-acquired In young individuals— mainly pneumococcal, staphylococcal or H. influenza pneumonias	Penicillin G†† OR Ampicillin†† + Cloxacillin	1 MU 4 hrly 2 g 4 hrly 1 g 4 hrly		or Meropenem + Vancomycin	1 g 8 hrly 500 mg 8 hrly
If Legionella or atypical pneumonias suspected, add—	Erythromycin	1 g 6 hrly	**4. Catheter-related Sepsis**	Ceftazidime or Piperacillin-Tazobactam	1 g 6 hrly 3–4 g 4 hrly
In old, debilitated patients—mainly Gram-negative pneumonias	Ampicillin + Ceftazidime + Aminoglycoside† (Gentamicin or Amikacin)	2 g 4 hrly 1 g 6 hrly 60–80 mg 8 hrly 7.5 mg/kg 12 hrly		+ Aminoglycoside† (Gentamicin or Amikacin)	60–80 mg 8 hrly 7.5 mg/kg 12 hrly
If aspiration suspected, add—	Metronidazole	500 mg 8 hrly	If strong suspicion of MRSA present, add—	Vancomycin	500 mg 6 hrly
* Nosocomial	Ceftazidime + Aminoglycoside† (Gentamicin or Amikacin) + Metronidazole	1 g 6 hrly 60–80 mg 8 hrly 7.5 mg/kg 12 hrly 500 mg 8 hrly	**5. Urinary Tract Sepsis** * Suspected Gram-negative Infections	Ceftazidime + Aminoglycoside† (Gentamicin or Amikacin) OR Ciprofloxacin	1 g 6 hrly 60–80 mg 8 hrly 7.5 mg/kg 12 hrly 200 mg 12 hrly
If strong suspicion of MRSA present, add—	Vancomycin	500 mg 6 hrly	* Suspected Gram-positive Infections	Amoxicillin-Clavulanic acid	1.2 g 8 hrly

† A single daily dose is as effective as 8 hrly or 12 hrly doses and in the case of gentamicin leads to reduced renal toxicity;
†† Many units would prefer the use of amoxycillin & clavulanic acid 1.2 g 8 hrly to pencillin or ampicillin.

Table 13.4.2. Antibiotics of choice for commonly seen organisms in the ICU.

Organism	Drug of First Choice	Alternative Drugs
1. Gram-positive Cocci		
(a) *S. aureus or coagulase negative staphylococci*		
– Non-penicillinase forming	Penicillin G	First generation, cephalosporin, imipenem, vancomycin
– Penicillinase forming	Penicillinase-resistant e.g. cloxacillin	First generation cephalosporin, imipenem, vancomycin, ciprofloxacin, ampicillin-sulbactam, amoxicillin-clavulanic acid
– Methicillin-resistant	Vancomycin	Ciprofloxacin, linezolid, teicoplanin
(b) β-*haemolytic Streptococci* (Groups A,B,C,G)	Penicillin G, ampicillin	First generation cephalosporin, vancomycin
– *S. pneumoniae*	Penicillin G, ampicillin	Ceftriaxone, vancomycin
2. Gram-positive Bacilli		
(a) *Cl. difficile*	Vancomycin (oral)	Metronidazole (oral)
(b) *Cl. tetani*	Penicillin G	Metronidazole
3. Gram-negative Cocci		
(a) *N. meningitidis*	Penicillin G	Cefotaxime, cefoperazone, ceftriaxone, cefuroxime
4. Gram-negative Bacilli		
(a) *Bacteroids*		
– Oropharyngeal	Penicillin G	Metronidazole, clindamycin
– Gastrointestinal	Metronidazole	Imipenem, ampicillin-sulbactam, amoxicillin-clavulanic acid
(b) *Enterobacter sp*	Ceftriaxone, cefoperazone, ceftazidime	Ciprofloxacin, aminoglycosides, imipenem
(c) *E. coli*	Third generation cephalosporins, aminoglycosides	Piperacillin, ticarcillin, aminoglycosides
(d) *Ps. aeruginosa*	Antipseudomonal penicillins or ceftazidime + aminoglycosides	Ciprofloxacin or ceftazidime or imipenem + aminoglycosides
(e) *K. pneumoniae*	Ceftriaxone, cefoperazone, ceftazidime	Piperacillin, ampicillin-sulbactam, imipenem
(f) *H. influenzae*	Ceftriaxone, cefoperazone, ceftazidime	Piperacillin, ampicillin-sulbactam, imipenem
(g) *Proteus (indole +ve)*	Cefotaxime, ceftriaxone	Ticarcillin, piperacillin, aminoglycosides, ciprofloxacin, aztreonam

Mode of Action of Antimicrobial Agents

Microbacterial agents may be either bactericidal or bacteriostatic. Bactericidal agents kill micro-organisms, whereas bacteriostatic agents prevent multiplication of the micro-organisms, only while present within them. A critically ill patient in the ICU is often at a special disadvantage because of poor phagocytic function of the macrophages. There is also at times poor antibody function, as compared to less ill patients. Bactericidal agents should therefore be preferred; yet in many situations, bacteriostatic agents act just as well.

The mechanism of action of antimicrobial agents on micro-organisms varies, and may take the following forms:

(i) Interference with cell wall synthesis. This is the main mode of action of penicillins, cephalosporins, imipenem, monobactams and vancomycin.

(ii) Interference with cell membrane synthesis as with polymyxins and amphotericin B.

(iii) Prevention of DNA replication e.g. quinolones, rifampicin, metronidazole.

(iv) Interference with protein synthesis as seen with chloramphenicol, tetracyclines, erythromycin, clindamycin, aminoglycosides and fusidic acid.

(v) Folic acid antagonists e.g. sulphonamides, trimethoprim, co-trimoxazole.

The different modes of action of important antimicrobial agents have been illustrated in **Fig. 13.4.1.**

The remaining part of this chapter deals very briefly with the common antibiotics used for serious infections in the ICU. Treatment for fungal infections has been discussed separately.

I. The Penicillins

A. Penicillin G

In the ICU, this cheap and extremely effective antibiotic is used against acute pneumococcal infection, streptococcal infection, meningococcal infection, and infections by Gram-positive bacillary pathogens—chiefly the clostridia. It is no longer used for treating Staphylococcus infections, as these strains are generally resistant to the drug. In fulminanat infections in adults, the dose is 4,000,000 units intravenously 4 hourly.

B. Ampicillin

This is a broad-spectrum penicillin with a significant spectrum of activity against Gram-negative bacilli. It is also nearly as effective as penicillin G against Gram-positive and Gram-negative cocci, and Gram-positive bacilli. It can therefore be used in place of penicillin G to treat fulminant infections mentioned under penicillin G. It is the drug of choice for infections due to Enterococci. Ampicillin and aminoglycosides form an extremely effective combination against Enterococci, as these drugs are synergistic against these organisms. The chief drawbacks of ampicillin are: (i) susceptibility to beta-lactamase produced by Staphylococci and Gram-negative bacilli—most strains of S. aureus and more than 50 per cent of E. coli are ampicillin-resistant; (ii) the occurrence of hypersensitivity

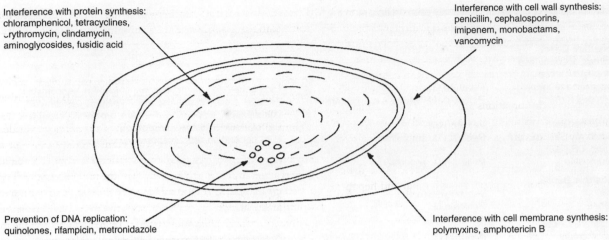

Fig. 13.4.1. Modes of action of important antimicrobials.

reactions. These are similar to those observed with penicillin G and are briefly described below.

In fulminant streptococcal or in other fulminant infections as in pneumococcal or meningococcal meningitis, the dose of ampicillin is 2 g intravenously 4 hourly—i.e. 12 g/day. In less fulminant cases, 1 g intravenously 4 hourly suffices.

C. Antistaphylococcal Penicillins—Cloxacillin, Flucloxacillin and Methicillin

These are not destroyed by penicillinases i.e. by beta-lactamase enzymes. They are therefore most useful against S. aureus, most of which produce penicillinase. They are however less effective against other Gram-positive organisms, and inconsistently effective against S. epidermidis. There is also an in vitro cross-resistance and cross-sensitivity between these three drugs, as also between these drugs and the cephalosporins.

Cloxacillin is only reserved for staphylococcal infections in our unit—the dose in serious infections being 1 g intravenously 4 hourly. The incidence of methicillin-resistant Staphylococci species (MRSA) is slowly increasing. In some other hospitals, notably those treating cancer patients, the incidence of MRSA is high. In all immunocompromised patients with staphylococcal infections, we prefer to use vancomycin instead of cloxacillin.

Side Effects of Penicillins

The penicillins described above occasionally produce reactions. Antibody-mediated hypersensitivity reactions in rare instances may cause fatal anaphylaxis. Though a skin sensitivity test is mandatory before starting penicillin therapy, a negative skin test does not exclude the possibility of anaphylaxis. Other antibody-mediated hypersensitivity reactions include fever, urticaria, serum sickness, and nephritis. Non-antibody-mediated reactions often occur in association with viral (notably Epstein-Barr) infections and take the form of fever with a measles-like rash.

Very large doses of penicillin, particularly in the presence of renal failure, may cause seizures, haemolytic anaemia, neutropaenia and thrombocytopaenia.

D. Antipseudomonal Penicillins—Piperacillin and Ticarcillin

These are the only two penicillins used against Ps. aeruginosa infection in our ICU.

Piperacillin has an extended spectrum of activity; its activity against Gram-positive cocci is similar to that of ampicillin. It is also active against a wide range of Gram-negative bacilli, Enterococci and anaerobes including certain strains of Bacteroides fragilis. It inhibits only 50 per cent of the strains of the Klebsiella species, but in vitro is the most active of all penicillins against Ps. aeruginosa. It is inactive against beta-lactamase producing staphylococci, and beta-lactamase positive Hemophilus influenzae.

In severe infections it is given intravenously in a dose of 3–4 g 6 hourly i.e. 12–16 g/day. We prefer to use the drug in combination with an aminoglycoside in a proven Pseudomonas infection, or in other life-threatening Gram-negative infections. Therapy in the latter situation is often empiric. It is often used to combat intra-abdominal and/or pelvic suppuration, and acute biliary infections—e.g. cholangitis or cholangitic abscesses. The only important side effect observed with piperacillin is thrombocytopenia.

Ticarcillin also has nearly the same activity against Ps. aeruginosa and other Gram-negative organisms. It is used in the dose of 1–3 g intravenously 4–6 hourly depending on the severity of the infection. It is generally used in combination with a beta-lactamase inhibitor—clavulanic acid.

E. Penicillins + Beta-lactamase Inhibitors

The major mechanism of beta-lactam resistance seen in both Gram-positive and Gram-negative infections is due to production of beta-lactamase (3). The three currently available betalactamase inhibitors are clavulanic acid, sulbactams and tazobactam (4, 5). The beta-lactamase inhibitor—beta-lactam antibiotic combinations available are ticarcillin-clavulanic acid, amoxicillin-clavulanic acid, and ampicillin-sulbactam. The last two combinations are effective against beta-lactamase producing strains of S. aureus, H. influenzae and B. fragilis (4, 5), as also against beta-lactamase producing Gram-negative bacilli. The important exceptions are Ps. aeruginosa and the Enterobacter species. We prefer to use any one of the above combinations in an identified Gram-negative infection sensitive to the drugs. Amoxicillin-clavulanic acid is given 1.2 g intravenously 8 hourly, and ampicillin-sulbactam is administered in a dose of 1.5 g intravenously 6 hourly. In mixed Gram-negative infections or in unidentified Gram-negative sepsis where empiric therapy is necessary, the above combinations are invariably inadequate.

The combination of ticarcillin-clavulanic acid (3.1 g intravenously 4–6 hourly), is useful against Ps. aeruginosa and other Gram-negative infections. It can be used in place of piperacillin, particularly when the sensitivity tests so indicate. The drug should be used with caution in patients with renal and hepatic dysfunction.

The combination of piperacillin with tazobactam has the advantage of being useful against beta-lactamase producing Gram-negative bacteria. It is used intraveneously in a dose of 2.25–4.5 g, 4–6 hourly. Both piperacillin and piperacillin with tazobactam should be used with caution in patients with renal and hepatic dysfunction.

II. Aminoglycosides

These are extremely useful against Gram-negative bacilli including Klebsiella and Pseudomonas aeruginosa. The aminoglycosides commonly used are gentamicin, tobramycin and amikacin. In severe fulminant Gram-negative infections, an aminoglycoside is always combined with another suitable antibiotic—either a third generation cephalosporin or ticarcillin or piperacillin. Gram-negative infections in neutropaenic patients should also preferably include an aminoglycoside in the therapeutic regime. The degree of resistance of Gram-negative organisms to aminoglycosides varies in different units. In our unit gentamicin-resistant organisms are frequently observed. We therefore prefer to use amikacin. Tobramycin offers no special advantage over gentamicin or amikacin.

In severe Gram-negative infections aminoglycosides should never be used alone; they should be combined with either a third generation cephalosporin like ceftazidime, or with piperacillin.

Dosage

The recommended dosage is given below in **Table 13.4.3**.

Aminoglycosides are excreted by the kidneys, and therefore dose adjustments are required when renal function is impaired. The easiest and most convenient method of adjusting the dose is by adjusting the dose interval thus:

Serum Creatinine × 8 = Dose Interval (in hours)

Table 13.4.3. Dose recommendations for aminoglycosides

	Loading Dose (mg/kg)	Daily Dose (mg/kg) (given in divided doses at 8 hourly intervals)	Serum Levels (µg/ml)	
			Peak	Trough
Gentamicin	1.5	3	4–6	1–2
Amikacin	5	15	20–30	5–10

Note: A single daily dose is as effective as 8 hrly or 12 hrly doses and in case of gentamicin leads to reduced renal toxicity.

Thus if the serum creatinine is 3 mg/dl, the interval for administration of each dose of the amninglycoside is 24 hours.

Toxic Effects

The major toxic effects of aminoglycosides are nephrotoxicity causing renal failure, and toxicity to the eighth cranial nerve causing deafness (**6–8**).

The nephrotoxicity is due to the action of the aminoglycosides on the renal tubules. It is a very important primary cause or a contributory cause of renal failure in patients in the ICU. Renal failure is generally (though not always) of the non-oliguric variety, the patient excreting > 1200 ml/day, yet showing a progressive rise in the serum creatinine. Both gentamicin and amikacin are equally nephrotoxic. Nephrotoxicity is related to drug levels in the blood. The likelihood of toxicity is thus related to the duration of time that the trough serum levels exceed 2 µg/ml for gentamicin, and 10 µg/ml for amikacin (**9**). The rise in serum creatinine occurs after 5–7 days, but can occur earlier in the presence of biliary obstruction (**8**), or if there is some degree of renal insufficiency to start with. The use of furosemide and the presence of hypovolaemia potentiate aminoglycoside nephrotoxicity (**10**). Aminoglycosides are best omitted if renal toxicity is apparent from a rising serum creatinine level. Acute renal failure generally resolves within a week; rarely it may take much longer to resolve, and the patient may then need to be supported by dialysis.

Early signs of renal toxicity include a fall in the urine output, proteinuria, and the presence of casts in the urine. These signs are however non-specific, and may be due to other causes operating in very ill patients in the ICU.

Ototoxicity from aminoglycosides results in nerve deafness, and is dose-related. The nerve deafness is enhanced by the use of furosemide (**9, 10**). Rarely aminoglycosides potentiate neuromuscular blockade. In clinical practice, this is only observed in patients with myasthenia gravis, or in those being given muscle relaxants.

Prevention of toxic effects of aminoglycosides is helped by maintaining a normal intravascular volume, and by the discriminate use of furosemide. Aminoglycosides should not generally be continued once the cultures are negative. In patients where renal failure is a likely hazard, one often prefers to use a safer antibiotic.

III. Glycopeptides

A. Vancomycin (11)

Vancomycin is the drug of choice for methicillin-resistant Staphylococcus aureus (MRSA), and methicillin-resistant Staphylococcus epidermidis (MRSE) infections and for serious infections in patients allergic to penicillin. The drug is also used for penicillin resistant pneumococcal meningitis and pneumonia. It also forms a second-line therapy for most Gram-positive infections. When used against Enterococci, the drug should be given together with an aminoglycoside.

There is a slow but definite emerging resistance of Enterococci to vancomycin in the USA; this has not been observed to a significant extent in India. An intermediate resistance of the S. aureus to vancomycin is also noted. Injudicious use of the drug could well lead to vancomycin-resistant Staphycoccal infections. This would be an unmitigated disaster. Monitoring of serum levels is advisable particularly in patients with renal insufficiency. The trough level should remain between 5–10 µg/ml if toxic effects are to be avoided.

Dosage

The dose is 500 mg 6 hourly, or 1 g 12 hourly intravenously. The drug is effective when used orally in a dose of 125–250 mg four times a day for Cl. difficile infections.

Side Effects

The major side effects are on the kidneys and on the eighth nerve. Renal insufficiency and ototoxicity are thus to be watched out for. The dose should be appropriately reduced on the basis of the creatinine clearance test. Drug levels should be monitored in the presence of impaired renal function. If the drug is given as a bolus, or even otherwise, it can cause a severe erythematous rash, flushing and transient hypotension (Red Man Syndrome).

B. Teicoplanin (11)

Teicoplanin is a new glycopeptide which has a similar spectrum to vancomycin. Its main use is again MRSA and MRSE infections. It is believed to be less toxic than vancomycin.

Dosage

An intravenous loading dose of 6 mg/kg is given slowly every 12 hours for 3 doses, followed by 400 mg intravenously daily.

Side Effects

It can cause both nephrotoxicity and ototoxicity (12). The dose should be suitably reduced in patients with renal insufficiency. Thrombocytopaenia can occur with higher doses.

IV. Newer Beta-Lactam Antibiotics

A number of new beta-lactam antibiotics have been developed against resistant facultative Gram-negative bacilli. Of these the commonly used ones are the third and fourth generation cephalosporins and the carbepenams.

A. Third Generation Cephalosporins (13)

Cefotaxime, ceftazidime, ceftriaxone and cefoperazone are the third generation cephalosporins which have been in frequent use against serious Gram-negative infections in the intensive care unit for the last several years. They penetrate well into the CSF, and are therefore the drugs of choice in Gram-negative bacterial meningitis. Ceftazidime provides a wider cover (which includes Pseudomonas), and is to be preferred particularly for empiric therapy against Gram-negative bacterial meningitis. Gram-negative nosocomial infections in the ICU, as also infection of unknown origin in neutropaenic patients, warrant the use of a third generation cephalosporin, together with an aminoglycoside or ciprofloxacin. Cefotaxime is useful against Gram-negative organisms particularly Klebsiella, but lacks activity against Pseudomonas. Ceftazidime on the other hand, has the greatest activity against Ps. aeruginosa, and some other Pseudomonas species. Cefoperazone also has anti-pseudomonas activity, and has significant activity against Gram-positive organisms including Staphylococci. Third generation cephalosporins are poorly active against B. fragilis, and display no activity against Enterococci, Listeria, and methicillin-resistant Staphylococci.

The third generation cephalosporins offer three other important advantages:

(i) A relatively slower emergence of bacterial resistance compared to the aminoglycosides or the newer quinolones.

(ii) Good tissue penetration. Penetration into the CSF has already been commented upon. Ceftriaxone and cefoperazone also reach high concentrations in the bile and may therefore be of special value in the treatment of severe cholangitis and cholangitic abscesses.

(iii) Reduced Nephrotoxicity. Cefotaxime, ceftriaxone and cefoperazone have little or no renal toxicity. Cefoperazone can thus be continued without any reduction in the dose in patients with renal failure. The dose of ceftazidime however needs to be reduced in patients with renal insufficiency; the degree of reduction is dependent on the serum creatinine levels and on creatinine clearance values.

Side Effects

The major side effect noticed in the ICU is the occurrence of reversible neutropaenia in 10 per cent of patients. This may cause confusion in the management of neutropaenic patients. A slight rise in the liver enzymes is occasionally encountered. Prolonged prothrombin time, and platelet dysfunction causing bleeding can sometimes occur, particularly with cefoperazone. Rarely, a positive Coomb's test is related to cephalosporin therapy.

Dosage

Cefotaxime is administered in a dose of 1–2 g 6 hourly. The dose of ceftazidime is 1–2 g 12 hourly. Ceftriaxone and cefoperazone have much longer half-lives, and have the added advantage of a once a day dosing of 2 g intravenously. In fulminant infections the dose can be increased to 4 g daily.

B. Fourth Generation Cephalosporins (14)

Cefepime and Cefpirome are the fourth generation cephalosporins. They have good activity (similar to that of ceftazidime), against Gram-negative pathogens, including Enterobacteriaceae and Pseudomonas aeruginosa. Some strains of Enterobacter, Citrobacter and Serratia resistant to ceftazidime, aztreonam are susceptible to cefepime and cefpirome. They are also active against Gram-positive organisms—Streptococcus pneumoniae, Streptococcus pyogens and methicillin sensitive Staph. aureus. This activity is similar to cefotaxime but better than ceftazidime. Like other cephalosporins they do not have activity against anaerobes. Compared to other second and third generation cephalosporins they have lower affinity for β-lactamases and are not inducers of chromosomal β-lactamases.

Indications

They are used in Gram-negative infections, as in nosocomial pneumonia, urinary tract infections, febrile neutropaenia, intra-abdominal infections (along with metronidazole).

Dosage

Cefepime 1–2 g 12 hourly, 2 g 8 hourly intravenously. Cefpirome 1–2 g 12 hourly intravenously. Both drugs require dosage adjustment in patients with renal dysfunction.

Side Effects

Side effects are similar to other cephalosporins. Cefpirome interferes with serum creatinine estimation by Jaffe's method. Hence falsely elevated serum creatinine levels will result, though BUN remains unaffected. Hence cefpirome should be administered after blood sample collection or the HPLC/enzymatic method should be used for estimating serum creatinine.

C. Imipenem

Imipenem is a carbapenem with the widest antibacterial spectrum of any available antibiotic (15, 16). The drug is inactivated by enzymes in the renal tubule so that the drug cannot achieve high concentration in the urine. This is overcome by combining imipenem with an enzyme inhibitor cilastatin. The combination of imipenem-cilastatin is commercially available as Primaxin. Imipenem is one of the most expensive antimicrobials in use today. It is active against most clinically important bacteria. It has no activity against Enterococcus faecium, Pseudomonas maltophilia, many strains of Ps. cepacia, and methicillin-resistant Staphylococci. It is therefore an extremely valuable drug to treat fulminant, unidentified infections in the ICU, or to treat fulminant infections due to multiple drug-resistant bacteria. It is particularly useful: (i) as empirical treatment of infection in severely immunocompromised patients; (ii) in intra-abdominal or pelvic sepsis involving mixed infections with aerobes, anaerobes, and Enterococci; (iii) infections with Enterobacter or Ps aeruginosa resistant to other antibiotics (17). It can probably be used as a single antibiotic in such patients. When the possibility of methicillin-resistant staphylococcal infection cannot be excluded, it should be combined with vancomycin.

The drug should be used with caution, restraint and circumspection as resistant bacteria are bound to emerge (15, 16).

Dosage

Imipenem is given intravenously in a dose of 500 mg 6 hourly. The dose should be reduced by 50–75 per cent in patients with renal failure (18).

Side Effects

The main side effects are skin rashes, phlebitis, gastrointestinal symptoms, and seizures, particularly in patients with renal insufficiency. Seizure disorders are reported in 1–3 per cent of patients (18). Patients with a previous history of seizure disorder are more prone to this complication.

D. Meropenem (19, 20)

Meropenem is a newer carbapenem similar to imipenem. It has the same range of activity against Gram-negative organisms and against anaerobes as imipenem.

Dose

The drug is given in a dose of 0.5–1 g 8 hourly in an intravenous infusion.

Side Effects

Incidence of seizures is reported to be less as compared to imipenem. The drug does not affect renal function.

V. Quinolones

A. Ciprofloxacin

The only quinolone we use for serious infections in the ICU is ciprofloxacin, which has the following advantages:

(i) An excellent activity against Gram-negative organisms, particularly against B. typhosus, Salmonella infections and Pseudomonas. It is therefore a useful alternative to aminoglycosides when combined with either piperacillin or ceftazidime or cefpirome in the treatment of Pseudomonas infections.

(ii) Activity against methicillin-resistant S. aureus and epidermidis. However strains of MRSA are now becoming increasingly resistant to ciprofloxacin.

(iii) Good tissue penetration, particularly in bones, lungs, bronchi, the hepatobiliary system, gut, prostate and the urinary tract. Penetration into the CSF is however poor. It is therefore useful against Gram-negative infections involving the above sites, particularly in severe osteomyelitis.

Ciprofloxacin lacks activity against B. fragilis and many non-aeruginosa species of Pseudomonas.

Dosage

In fulminant infections it is administered intravenously in a dose of 200 mg 12 hourly. Once the infection is under good control, it is given orally in a dose of 500–750 mg twice a day.

Side Effects

Gastrointestinal disturbances are frequent. Skin rashes, and transient gouty pains involving the fingers may be observed. A transient elevation in liver enzymes, and rarely in serum creatinine, may occur. The dose may need to be reduced in patients with renal insufficiency. CNS excitation may take the form of headache, confusion and seizures. Serious but very rare side effects include anaphylactoid reactions that may cause death, and possibly a hemorrhagic vasculitis (17).

The drug is best avoided (unless absolutely necessary) in children, and pregnant and lactating women.

Indiscriminate use of the drug is bound to breed resistance against Pseudomonas species, and other Gram-negative bacteria.

B. Newer Fluroquinolones (21)

The newer fluroquinolones include ofloxacin, levofloxacin (L-isomer of ofloxacin), gatifloxacin, moxifloxacin. These drugs are active against Gram-negative bacilli, including Salmonella, B. tyhosus, Shigella, H. influenzae and Pseudomonas strain. However among fluroquinolones, ciprofloxacin has the highest activity against Pseudomonas. While ciprofloxacin and ofloxacin are also active against Mycobacteria, the other fluroquinolones are active against Myoplasma, Chlamydia and Legionella. For serious Gram-negative infections in the ICU, we have restricted the use of quinolones to ciprofloxacin and ofloxacin. They are invariably used in combination with a third generation or fourth generation cephalosporin or with piperacillin. Ciprofloxacin or ofloxacin is the drug of choice in fulminant B. typhosus infection. However resistance of B. typhosus to these drugs is slowly on the rise.

Dosage

The intravenous dose of ofloxacin is 200–400 mg 12 hourly. Gatifloxacin is given intravenously—400 mg once daily. The intravenous dose of levofloxacin and moxifloxacin is 500–750 mg once daily and 400 mg once daily respectively.

Side Effects

The side effects of the newer quinolones are by and large similar to those of ciprofloxacin.

VI. Monobactams (19, 20)

Aztreonam

This is a narrow spectrum antibiotic to be used exclusively against Gram-negative aerobic organisms including β-lactamase producing strains and Pseudomonas aeruginosa. It does not have any activity against Gram-positive organisms and anaerobes. There is synergy reported between aztreonam and aminoglycosides against Ps. aeruginosa.

Indications

Intra-abdominal sepsis, urinary tract infections, nosocomial pneumonia.

Dosage

The dose is 1–2 g intravenously every 6–8 hours. The dosage needs to be suitably adjusted in patients with renal failure.

Side Effects

Side effects are minor. Rarely, a rise in serum liver enzymes and in serum bilirubin have been reported.

VII. Linezolid (11, 22, 23)

Linezolid is an oxazolidinone group antibiotic. It is bacteriostatic and acts by inhibiting the initiation of protein syntheses. It is predominantly effective against Gram-positive organisms like MRSA, vancomycin-resistant Enterococci, vancomycin intermediate resistance Staphylococcus aureus and penicillin-resistant pneumococci. It has 100 per cent bioavailability when administered orally.

Dosage

The dose is 600 mg intravenously or orally every 12 hours.

Side Effects

The drug can cause vomiting, diarrhoea and lead to candidal superinfection. Linezolid is a weak monoamine inhibitor and has a potential for interaction with adrenergic drugs. Resistance of organisms to the drug can occur on prolonged therapy; hence the routine use of this antibiotic should be discouraged.

VIII. Quinopristin/Dalfopristin (11)

This is a streptogramin antibiotic. The drugs are present in a fixed 30:70 ratio and are synergistic. It is active against Gram-positive bacteria including vancomycin-resistant Enterococcus faecium and MRSA. It is a bacteriostatic drug. It does not have activity against Enterococcus faecalis.

Dosage

The dose is 7.5 mg/kg intravenously 8 hourly for seriously ill patients, to be administered preferably through a central vein as local reactions may occur with use through peripheral veins.

Side Effects

The drug causes myalgias and arthralgias in up to 10 per cent of patients.

Drug Interactions

Most ICU patients receive multiple drugs. The possibility and the potential for drug interactions is therefore very significant, and should always be considered. **Table 13.4.4** provides information on important interactions involving antimicrobial drugs used frequently in very ill patients in the ICU.

Table 13.4.4. Important drug interactions in the ICU

Type of Interaction and Antibiotics	Affected/Displaced by	Effect
1. *Interaction at Tissue Site*		
* Aminoglycosides	Succinylcholine, Polymyxin, Ethacrynic acid, Furosemide	Nephrotoxicity Ototoxicity Ototoxicity
* Cephaloridine	Furosemide	Nephrotoxicity
2. *Competition for Binding Sites*		
* Isoniazid	Phenytoin, Rifampicin	Neurotoxicity Liver toxicity

Adjusting Dosage Schedules

Patients with hepatic or renal dysfunction often need modifications of drug dosage. **Table 13.4.5** gives details regarding the use of

Table 13.4.5. Modifications in dose and frequency of administration of important antimicrobial agents in patients with hepatic or renal dysfunction.

Antibiotic	Interval between doses with various Creatinine clearances (renal failure)			Dose altered by dialysis		Dose in hepatic failure
	Normal (100 ml)	Moderate (20–40 ml)	Severe (<10 ml)	Haemo-dialysis	Peritoneal Dialysis	
1. Penicillin	4 hr	NC	1 MU/6 hr	1 MU/ 6 hr	No	NC
2. Ampicillin	4 hr	NC	1 g/8 hr	0.5 g/6 hr	No	NC
3. Cefotaxime	6–8 hr	NC	1 g/12 hr	Yes	No	Reduce dose
4. Ceftazidime	8–12 hr	1g/12–24 hr	0.5 g/24–48 hr	Yes	No	NC
5. Imipenem	6–8 hr	6–12 hr	12–24 hr	Yes	Yes	NC
6. Gentamicin	8 hr	Use nomogram or serum levels		Yes	Yes	NC
7. Amikacin	8 hr	Use nomogram	Use nomogram	Check serum levels	—	NC
8. Ciprofloxacin	12 hr	Half dose/12 hr	Half dose/18–24 hr	No	Yes	NC
9. Vancomycin	6–12 hr	24 hr	4–6 days	No	No	NC
10. Isoniazid	24 hr	NC	Reduce dose	Yes	Yes	Reduce dose
11. Ethambutol	24 hr	Reduce dose	Stop drug	Yes	Yes	NC
12. Rifampicin	24 hr	NC	NC	No	—	Reduce dose
13. Amphotericin B	24 hr	3 days	5 days	No	No	NC
14. 5-Fluorocytosine	6 hr	12–24 hr	2 days	25 mg/kg	—	NC

NC = No change

antimicrobials against a background of renal or hepatic insufficiency in ICU patients.

Monitoring drug levels is particularly important in critically ill patients. Failure to attain therapeutic levels can have disastrous consequences, just as toxic levels add to the problems of a very ill patient. Monitoring drug levels so as to avoid toxicity, is specially necessary in a patient population in whom the pharmacokinetics of a drug is difficult to predict. This is particularly so in patients whose hepatic or renal function is suspect, or in those who have clear evidence of hepatic or renal dysfunction. Unfortunately in our set-up, monitoring drug levels is difficult, and till recently was non-existent. Fortunately laboratories have now started to estimate serum levels of important drugs used in the ICU. This is of great help in adjusting the appropriate dose of these drugs (including antimicrobials), in very ill ICU patients.

REFERENCES

1. Moellering RC. (2000). Principles of antiinfective therapy. In: Principles and Practice of Infectious Diseases (Eds Mandell GL, Bennett JE, Dolin R). pp. 223–235. Churchill Livingstone, USA.

2. Murray BE. (1991). New aspects of antimicrobial resistance and the resulting therapeutic dilemma. J Infect Dis. 163, 1184–1194.

3. Stone HH, Kolb LD, Currie CA et al. (1974). Candida sepsis: Pathogenesis and principles of treatment. Ann Surg. 179, 697.

4. Lode H, Kass EH. (Eds) (1986). Enzyme-mediated resistance to betalactam antibiotics: A symposium on sulbactam/ampicillin. Rev Infect Dis. 8(Suppl 5), S 465.

5. Neu HC. (Ed) (1985). Beta-lactamase inhibition: Therapeutic advances. Am J Med. 79(Suppl 5B), 1.

6. Sillix DH, McDonald FD. (1987). Acute renal failure. Crit Care Clin. 3, 909–925.

7. Kaloyanides GJ, Pastoriza-Munoz E. (1980). Aminoglycoside nephrotoxicity. Kidney Int. 18, 571–582.

8. Desai TK, Tsang TK. (1988). Aminoglycoside nephrotoxicity in obstructive jaundice. Am J Med. 85, 47–50.

9. Conte JE Jr, Barriere SL. (1988). Antibiotics and Infectious Diseases, 6th edn. Lea and Febiger, Philadelphia.

10. Pancoast SJ. (1988). Aminoglycoside antibiotics in clinical use. Med Clin North Am. 72, 581–612.

11. Lundstrom TS, Sobel JD. (2000). Antibiotics for Gram-positive bacterial infections. Vancomycin, Teicoplanin, Quinupristin/Dalfopristin and Linezolid. Infect Dis Clin North Am. 14(2), 463–74.

12. Chow AW, Azar RM. (1994). Glycopeptides and nephrotoxicity. Intensive Care Med. 20, S23–S29.

13. Donowitz GR. (1989). Third generation cephalosporins. Infect Dis Clin North Am. 3, 595–612.

14. Wilson WR. (1998). The role of fourth generation cephalosporins in the treatment of severe infectious diseases in hospitalized patients. Diagn Microbiol Infect Dis. 31(3), 473–477.

15. Geddes Am, Stille W (Eds). (1985). Imipenem: The first thienamycin antibiotic. Rev Infect Dis. 7(Suppl 3), S 353.

16. Remington JS (Ed) (1985). Carbapenems: A new class of antibiotics. Am J Med. 78(Suppl 6A), 1.

17. Kumana CR, Chau PY, French G (Eds). (1991). Antibiotic Guidelines. Adis International, Science Press, Hong Kong.

18. Hellinger WC, Brewer NS. (1991). Imipenem. Mayo Clin Proc. 66, 1074–1081.

19. Asbel LE, Levison ME. (2000). Cephalosporins, Carbapenems, and Monobactams. Infect Dis Clin North Am. 14(2), 435–447.

20. Hellinger WC. (1999). Carbapenems and monobactams: Imipenem, meropenem and aztreonam. Mayo Clin Proc. 74(4), 420–434.

21. Blondeau JM. (1999). Expanded activity and utility of the new fluroquinolones: A review. Clin Therapeutics. 21, 3.

22. Clemett D, Markham A. (2000). Linezolid. Drugs. 59, 815.

23. Diekema DJ, Jones RN. (2000). Oxazolidonones. Drugs. 59, 7.

CHAPTER 13.5

Treatment of Fungal Infections in Critically Ill Patients

Fungal infections occur not only in immunocompromised patients (see Chapter on The Immunocompromised Patient), but also in patients who are under critical care for various problems e.g. acute infections, trauma or major surgery, and who have a normal immune defence mechanism to start with. Perhaps the most important cause of fungal overgrowth, and any systemic or deep-seated fungal infection in these patients is the prolonged use of broad-spectrum antibiotics which alter the bacterial flora, and promote the growth of unusual resistant organisms and fungi. Acute or critical illnesses in the course of time, also temporarily depress the immune mechanisms within the body to some extent. Thus patients with unresolved or persistent septic infections, or long-standing untreated foci of infection e.g. undrained abscesses, show a decreased capacity to respond to immunological challenges. All major surgical procedures are also followed by a depressed immunological response; this is related to an increase in suppressor cells, a fall in T4 lymphocytes, and alterations in lymphokine production (1). These changes are however temporary, and are quickly reversed as recovery progresses. In the presence of complications, the post-operative changes noted above are protracted, and may well play a role in predisposing the patient to both bacterial and fungal infections. Finally, poor nutritional status further depresses the immune defence mechanisms. Thus a combination of various factors, varying in degree in each individual critically ill patient, form a background against which fungal infections can occasionally supervene. The environment too perhaps has some part to play—e.g. clear-cut nosocomial outbreaks of invasive aspergillosis have been described in critical care units, and these have been related to the marked increase in air-borne spores of Aspergillus fumigatus in these units (2–8).

The important fungal infections encountered in a critical care setting are candidal, cryptococcal and aspergillus infections. Occasionally, infections with the mucor species are observed, particularly in diabetics or other severely immunocompromised patients. Other fungal infections are being increasingly recognized in the West; in our country however, we are as yet blissfully unaware of their possible occurrence.

Antifungal Compounds

Amphotericin B is still the most important antifungal drug; it has a wide antifungal spectrum and remains the choice for life-threatening invasive fungal infection. The drug has however a number of adverse effects, particularly on the kidneys. Various lipid formulations have been therefore developed to reduce this toxicity and offer a better therapeutic index. All these lipid formulations seem to be as effective as amphotericin B, with the additional advantage of less adverse reactions and in particular less renal toxicity (9). Nevertheless these lipid formulations of amphotericin are dreadfully expensive, the cost being 10–13 times greater than amphotericin B.

Fluconazole belongs to the imidazole class of antifungal agents (together with itraconazole and ketoconazole). The drug has a wide-ranging antifungal activity and fewer toxic side-effects than amphotericin. It is therefore considered a safer alternative to amphotericin in the treatment of several fungal infections, particularly in high risk patients with renal insufficiency (10).

Flucytosine is a fluorinated antifungal agent which has helped in the management of disseminated cryptococcal infections and also perhaps in other infections.

Caspofungin is a recently introduced semisynthetic lipopeptide echinocandin compound effective in the treatment of invasive aspergillosis.

Research continues on newer antifungal agents; their impact on the treatment of critically ill patients remains poor. The chemical classes of antifungal agents have been given in **Table 13.5.1**.

Table 13.5.1. Chemical classes of antifungal compounds

I. Polyenes
  * Amphotericin B
  * Nystatin
  * Pimaricin
II. Fluorinated Pyramidines
  * Flucytosine
III. Imidazoles
  * Miconazole
  * Ketoconazole
  * Clotrimazole
IV. Triazoles
  * Fluconazole
  * Itraconazole
V. Echinocandins
  * Caspofungin

Treatment of Systemic Fungal Infections (11, 12)

If there is an obvious or even a suspected source from which the fungal infection can originate, it should be promptly eradicated. Two classical examples of this (as restressed later), are (i) the removal of a central venous line in a patient with candidaemia and (ii) the removal of a urinary catheter in a patient with a heavy monolilial growth in the urine. Antibiotics which promote fungal overgrowth (particularly the penicillin group of drugs) should as far as possible be omitted.

Most critical care units are of the opinion that the presence of fungus in any normally sterile body fluid or tissue in a critically ill individual, is an indication for starting amphotericin B therapy. *Amphotericin B* should be empirically added to the therapeutic regime in granulocytopaenic patients who are critically ill, and who remain febrile for over 48 hours in spite of a combination of broad-spectrum antibiotic therapy. Similarly in any severely immunocompromised patient, where the aetiology of infection is undetermined, amphotericin B should be added to the therapeutic regime if the patient does not respond within 48 hours to antibacterial therapy or if the patient deteriorates after an initial response.

In critically ill patients we start with a test dose of 1 mg in adults (0.5 mg in children < 30 kg), given over 1 hour. This is followed after 4 hours by a dose of 0.5 mg/kg administered over 3–4 hours. Even if the test dose does produce a reaction, we give 10 mg after 4 hours, and increase the dose by 10–15 mg daily, so that the dose of 0.5–1 mg/kg is reached within 3–7 days. This dose is then continued daily till a total dose of at least 1 g is administered. In granulocytopaenic patients empirically given amphotericin B should be continued till recovery from granulocytopaenia ensues. Deep visceral infections may require a total dose of 2–3 g.

Amphotericin B is given in a 5 per cent dextrose infusion. Electrolyte solutions should be avoided, as they cause precipitation of the amphotericin B suspension. Side effects are common; pyrexia with chills is the most frequent side effect observed. Intravenous hydrocortisone given at the time of infusion often controls a severe pyrexial reaction. Other important side effects include hypotension, nausea, thrombophlebitis, and renal dysfunction with a rise in the serum creatinine levels. A significant rise in the latter warrants a temporary stoppage of the drug; it is restarted when the creatinine levels fall. Permanent renal tubular damage may occur when large doses (3–4 g) of amphotericin B are used.

Amphotericin B does not achieve significant concentrations in the urine, CSF or peritoneal fluid. In cases of fungal meningitis, intrathecal administration of amphotericin B may be combined with intravenous therapy. The intrathecal dose is 0.5–1 mg dissolved in the CSF. The total dose should not exceed 15 mg. Arachnoiditis and motor or sensory disturbances may occur as complications. An Omaha reservoir is sometimes used for instillation of amphotericin B into the cerebral ventricles in patients with CNS fungal infection. The danger of introducing secondary bacterial infection is ever present with this mode of administration.

Fluconazole (13) is effective in candidal and cryptococcal infections, both in the immunocompromised patients, and in patients with an intact immune system. The drug is chiefly used in disseminated candidiasis. Many units prefer it as an alternative to amphotericin B particularly in the presence of renal insufficiency and in patients who do not tolerate amphotericin B. In immunocompromised individuals, systemic candidiasis and cryptococcal infections are preferably treated with a combination therapy of amphotericin B and fluconazole.

Fluconazole is frequently used in critical care units as a preventive agent against candidal and cryptococcal infections.

Dosage

The drug is given once daily in a dose of 200–400 mg/day. The dose should be halved in patients with renal failure. The drug interferes with the metabolism of phentoin and warfarin potentiating the action of both drugs.

Side Effects

The main side effect is on the liver; fatal drug-induced hepatitis can occur in very rare instances. More often a rise in liver enzymes is observed.

Flucytosine (5-fluorocytosine) is also effective against candida and cryptococcus. Though it is absorbed when given orally (150–200 mg/kg in 4 divided doses), in acute systemic fungal infections it is best given intravenously in a dose of 150 mg/kg/day. The main disadvantage of this drug is the development of either primary or secondary drug resistance in a significant number of fungal isolates from patients. It can cause bone marrow depression, and as it is excreted chiefly by the kidneys, the dosage should be suitably reduced in patients with renal dysfunction.

Though the drug can be used alone in urinary or peritoneal candidiasis, it is most useful in the treatment of acute fungal infections in combination with amphotericin B. The two drugs have a synergistic action, and this allows for a reduction in the dose of amphotericin B. This combination has been proven to be particularly useful in the treatment of cryptococcal meningitis (14). Amphotericin B in a dose of 0.3 mg/kg/day is combined with flucytosine in a dose of 150 mg/kg/day and is given over 6 weeks. This combination has been shown in a prospective randomized trial to result in a higher cure rate, a quicker disappearance of cryptococci from the CSF, and a lower incidence of nephrotoxicity, as compared to a regime where amphotericin B is given alone over a 10 week period (15).

Flucytosine in contrast to amphotericin B, penetrates well into the CSF. The above combination therapy has also been recommended for CNS candidiasis, disseminated candidiasis, renal or hepatosplenic candidiasis, invasive pulmonary aspergillosis, deep-seated fungal infections within the body and systemic fungal infections responding poorly to amphotericin B. The dose requirement of amphotericin B in these patients is high (total dose of 2–4 g); however, death from uncontrolled infection may still occur.

Other synthetic imidazole derivatives like miconazole, ketoconazole, fluconazole and itraconazole are also commonly used in the treatment of fungal infections. They have proved to be effective in coccidiomycosis, paracoccidiomycosis, candidiasis, histoplasmosis and cryptococcosis. Though these drugs may be used for localized fungal infections, their efficacy in critically ill individuals with fungal infections, has yet to be established.

Caspofungin (16, 17) as has already been mentioned, is the only new antifungal agent which shows promising activity against invasive aspergillosis. It is particularly indicated in patients with invasive aspergillosis who are refractory to or intolerant to other therapies (amphotericin B, lipid formulation of amphotericin B and/or itraconozole)

Dosage

A single 70 mg loading dose on the first day is followed by 50 mg daily thereafter. The drug is given in a slow intravenous infusion over one hour. Duration of treatment depends on the severity of the patient's illness and clinical response. No dosage adjustments are needed for patients with renal insufficiency.

Side Effects

Fever, nausea, vomiting, flushing are occasionally observed. A rise in the liver enzymes may also occur. The drug is remarkably well tolerated compared to amphotericin.

Table 13.5.2 given below provides a ready reference for drugs acting on common fungal infections.

Table 13.5.2. Treatment of common systemic fungal infections

Organism	Drug of choice	Dose (mg/kg/day)	Duration of therapy (weeks)
Candida sp	Amphotericin B	0.5–0.6	3–8
Aspergillus sp	Amphotericin B	1–1.5	8–12
Blastomyces dermatitidis	Amphotericin B	0.4–0.5	6–8
Coccidioides immitis	Amphotericin B	0.5–0.6	8–14
Cryptococcus neoformans	Amphotericin B + Flucytosine	0.3 + 3–5	6
Histoplasma capsulatum	Amphotericin B	0.4–0.5	8

Clinical Resistance to Amphotericin B

Clinical resistance to amphotericin B is observed in severely immunocompromised patients, in patients with infected prosthetic valves or other foreign bodies, and in advanced visceral fungal infections involving the liver, spleen or kidneys.

Hepatosplenic candidiasis is a clinically resistant infection which may prove resistant to even high doses of amphotericin B. The development of fever, abdominal pain, or liver cell dysfunction occurring in a patient recovering from granulocytopaenia should raise suspicion of candidal infection within the abdomen. Investigations should include ultrasound, CT and if necessary MRI imaging of the abdominal organs. A combination of amphotericin B and flucytosine or fluconazole should be promptly started.

Therapy may need to be continued for several months, and may still be unsuccessful.

Microbiological resistance to amphotericin B has been reported in Candida albicans, Candida tropicalis, other Candida species, as also against other fungi—Trichosporon beigelii, Fusarium species, and Pseudallescheria boydii species (15). Most polyene resistant strains of candida cause mucosal lesions, though some have been reported to cause life-threatening infections. In the West, Trichosporon beigelii, Fusarium species, and Pseudallescheria boydii species are increasingly recognized causes of systemic fungal infections (15). A combination therapy of high doses of amphotericin B with flucytosine or fluconazole is recommended as initial treatment. If unsuccessful, fluconazole plus flucytosine is advised for systemic fungal infections due to polyene resistant fungi (15).

Systemic fungal infections originating from an infected foreign body, viz. an infected prosthetic valve, can never be controlled unless the foreign body is first removed. Fungal valvular endocarditis invariably necessitates removal of the valve. Further examples where removal of infected foreign bodies is mandatory, include:

(i) Removal of central venous lines in patients with systemic fungal infection or candidaemia.

(ii) Removal of infected ventriculo-peritoneal shunts in patients with cryptococcal meningitis or infections of the CNS with other fungi.

(iii) Removal of urinary catheters in patients with systemic candidiasis or candidiasis involving the urinary tract.

(iv) Removal of a dialysis catheter in fungal peritonitis associated with peritoneal dialysis.

Parenteral lipid emulsions given through central lines have been reported to cause fungaemia and pulmonary vasculitis due to a lipophilic fungus Malassezia furfur (15). Discontinuation of the lipid emulsions with removal of the central venous line, is generally adequate for treatment.

It is not enough to use antifungal drugs in the treatment of systemic fungal infections in critically ill patients. As always, overall critical care is of vital importance. An assiduous search to determine why the systemic fungal infection occurred, and whether the source of infection can be controlled or eradicated is of great importance.

Systemic Fungal Infections in Patients with AIDS

Patients with AIDS are the most severely immunocompromised of all patients. They are prone to a number of fungal infections—particularly cryptococcal infections. Disseminated coccidioidomycosis and histoplasmosis are not observed in our country, but are increasingly prevalent in other parts of the world where these infections are endemic.

A combination of amphotericin B with flucytosine rarely results in a complete cure of cryptococcal infections in these patients. Outpatient administration of amphotericin B has however reduced the relapse rate of cryptococcal meningoencephalitis. Another alternative prophylactic regime, is the use of fluconazole 200–400 mg daily in adults; this may need to be continued indefinitely.

REFERENCES

1. Wilson RE. (1990). Management of the Critically Ill Immunodeficient Patient. In: Handbook of Critical Care, 3rd edn (Eds Berk JL, Sampliner JE). pp. 711–728. Little, Brown and Company, Boston, Toronto, London.

2. Rhame FS, Streifel AJ, Kersey JH et al. (1984). Extrinsic risk factors for pneumonia in the patient at high risk of infection. Am J Med. 76, 42–52.

3. Kyriakides GK, Zinneman HH, Hall WH et al. (1976). Immunologic monitoring and aspergillosis in renal transplant patients. Am J Surg. 131, 246.

4. Aisner J, Schimpff SC, Bennett JE et al. (1976). Aspergillus infections in cancer patients: Association with fireproofing materials in a new hospital. JAMA. 235, 411.

5. Arnow PM, Anderson RL, Mainous PD et al. (1978). Pulmonary aspergillosis during hospital renovation. Am Rev Respir Dis. 118, 49.

6. Mahoney DH Jr, Steuber CP, Starling KA et al. (1979). An outbreak of aspergillosis in children with acute leukemia. J Pediatr. 95, 70.

7. Lentino JR, Rosenkranz MA, Michaels JA et al. (1982). Nosocomial Aspergillosis; a retrospective review of airborne disease secondary to road construction and contaminated air conditioners. Am J Epidemiol. 116, 430.

8. Sarubbi FA Jr, Kopf HB, Wilson MB et al. (1982). Increased recovery of Aspergillus flavus from respiratory specimens during hospital construction. Am Rev Respir Dis. 125, 33.

9. Dupont B. (2002). Overview of lipid formulations of Amphotericin B. J Antimicrobiol Chemo. 49, Suppl 1, 31–36.

10. Terrell CL, Hughes CE. (1992). Antifungal agents used in deep-seated mycotic infections. Mayo Clin Proc. 67, 69–91.

11. Stevens DA, Bennett JE. (2000). Antifungal agents. In: Principles and Practice of Infectious Diseases (Eds Mandell GL, Bennett JE, Dolin R). Churchill Livingstone, USA.

12. Drutz D. (1988,1989). Systemic fungal infections: Diagnosis and treatment I and II. Infect Dis Clin North Am. 2, 779–969; and 3, 1–133

13. Bennett JE, Dismukes WE, Duma RJ et al. (1979). A comparison of amphotericin B alone and combined with flucytosine in the treatment of cryptococcal meningitis. N Engl J Med. 301, 126.

14. Rex JH, Bennet JE, Sugar AM et al. (1994). A randomised trial comparing fluconazole with amphotericin B for the treatment of candidemia in patients with neutropenia. Nosocomial infection Eng J Med, 331, 1325–1330.

15. Walsh TJ, Pizzo PA. (1991). Antifungal Therapy. In: Current Therapy in Critical Care Medicine, 2nd edn (Ed. Parrillo JE). pp. 224–232. BC Decker Inc., Philadelphia, Hamilton.

16. Hoang A. (2001). Capsofungin acetate: an antifungal agent. Am J Health Syst Pharm. 58 (13), 1206–1214.

17. Keating GM, Jarvis B. (2001). Capsofungin. Drugs. 61 (8), 1121–1131.

SECTION 14

Surgical Infections in the Intensive Care Unit

14.1 Post-operative Wound Infections

14.2 Nectrotizing Fasciitis and Clostridial Myonecrosis

14.3 Intra-abdominal Sepsis

Post-operative Wound Infections

Introduction

Surgical infections in the intensive care unit fall into 2 groups:

(i) Infections which Require Prompt Surgery

These include serious soft tissue infections like necrotizing fasciitis, acute inflammatory intra-abdominal disease, acute suppurative disease tucked away (and therefore not easily evident) in other parts of the human anatomy—e.g. the thorax, within the head and neck, or in the skeleton.

Acute inflammatory or acute suppurative disease within the abdomen accounts for most infections requiring definitive surgery. Important surgical problems within the abdomen include acute suppurative appendicitis, empyema of the gall bladder, pancreatic suppuration, and peritonitis following a leak from the bowel. Peritonitis may be generalized or may be localized, and may ultimately result in an intra-abdominal abscess. Such an abscess may be tucked away in any one of the nooks and corners within the abdomen. In a few critically ill patients it may go unrecognized, and is responsible for a hidden, or rather undiscovered source of systemic sepsis, septic shock and multiple organ failure. Pelvic suppuration is also an important and at times unrecognized source of systemic sepsis. Pelvic suppuration may present as a pelvic abscess or suppuration involving the organs within the pelvis—chiefly tubo-ovarian suppuration.

(ii) Wound Infections which Occur as a Complication of Surgery

Infected post-surgical wounds pose serious problems for critically ill patients in the ICU (1). Major surgery performed for problems totally unrelated to infection, can thus be complicated by wound infection. The rather hostile microbiological environment in the ICU, almost certainly encourages such wound infections. Besides nosocomial wound infections, the post-operative surgical patient is also exposed to other nosocomial infections prevalent in the ICU. These chiefly include nosocomial pneumonias, urinary infections, and catheter (central line) related sepsis. These nosocomial complications can drastically influence the morbidity and mortality of surgical patients in the ICU, and call for prompt diagnosis and treatment.

Post-operative Wound Infections

General Considerations

Wound infections account for about a quarter to a sixth of all nosocomial infections. Despite the most meticulous attention to surgical technique, a surgical incision exposes sterile tissue to some degree of contamination (2). The rate of infection of a surgical wound will in the main, depend on the nature of the wound. Operative wounds are classified as (i) clean; (ii) clean-contaminated; (iii) contaminated; (iv) dirty and infected, based on the degree of contamination at the time of surgery. The incidence of post-operative wound infections in clean wounds may be less than 2 per cent. On the other hand, in dirty and infected wounds, the incidence may be as high as 40 per cent (3). **Table 14.1.1** gives the classification of surgical wounds and the incidence of wound infection (3).

The propensity to infection in surgical wounds depends on a number of other factors:

(i) The degree of attention paid to pre-operative, intra-operative and post-operative asepsis; ensuring adequate tissue perfusion and eliminating tissue dead space, reduces the incidence of post-operative infections.

Table 14.1.1. Classification of surgical wounds and incidence of wound infection

Type of Wound	Characteristics	Incidence of Infection
1. Clean	Non-traumatic, inflammation absent, respiratory, genito-urinary or GI tracts not breached	< 2 %
2. Clean-Contaminated	GI, respiratory, biliary or genito-urinary tracts entered without significant spillage	2–8 %
3. Contaminated	Gross spillage from GI tract	8–15 %
4. Dirty and Infected	Acute bacterial inflammation present, traumatic wound with devitalized tissue, foreign body, faecal contamination, or delayed treatment	12–40 %

Adopted from Cruse PJ, 1988. Wound Infections: Epidemiology and Clinical Characteristics. In: Surgical Infectious Disease. (Eds Howard RJ, Simmons RL). p. 320. McGraw-Hill Companies, NY, with permission.

(ii) The stage of disease when surgery is performed. Surgery performed late in the natural history of a disease is often prolonged, complicated and more likely to result in post-operative infections.

(iii) The duration of pre-operative hospitalization influences the incidence of wound infections. The infection rate almost doubles with each week of hospitalization prior to surgery. Colonization with nosocomial and often resistant bacteria is common, particularly if the patient has been in the ICU prior to surgery.

(iv) The risk of wound infection increases with prolonged surgery, the liberal use of cautery, and the placement of drains.

(v) A concurrent but remote infection (e.g. pulmonary infection, urinary tract infection or skin infection) increases the likelihood of wound infection. It is always wise to postpone elective surgery till such infections are eradicated.

(vi) Infections are more likely in the old, feeble, diabetic, malnourished, anaemic patients, and those with chronic hepatitis or renal or cardiac dysfunction.

(vii) Immunosuppression because of disease or drugs (antimitotic drugs, corticosteroids) is associated with a far greater risk of wound infection.

(viii) A history of shock or prolonged hypotension during or soon after surgery is a risk factor—probably related to poor tissue perfusion.

(ix) An important factor which decides the nature and severity of wound infection, is the nature of organisms likely to contaminate the wound. Possible contamination with S. aureus, Gram-negative organisms, or anaerobes like clostridia, can give rise to violent tissue infections in spite of all the care in the world (1).

Factors predisposing to post-operative wound infections are listed in **Table 14.1.2.**

Table 14.1.2. Predisposing factors for post-operative wound infections

* Poor pre-operative, intra-operative or post-operative asepsis
* Prolonged or complicated surgery, or surgery performed late in the natural history of the disease
* Prolonged hypotension during or soon after surgery
* Prolonged period of hospitalization particularly in the ICU
* Presence of co-existing infection elsewhere in the body (lungs, skin, urinary tract)
* Adverse host factors e.g. old, feeble, malnourished, anaemic patients, and those with hepatic or renal dysfunction
* Immunocompromised patients
* Pathogenicity of infecting organism

Clinical Features

The diagnosis of wound infection is based on a history, physical examination and the results of Gram's stain and culture report of a discharge from the wound (1, 4–6). Wound pain due to infection may be difficult to distinguish from post-operative incisional discomfort. Most wound infections occur between the fourth to seventh day of surgery. Fever occurring two to four days after surgery should prompt examination of the wound, which may show erythema, oedema, tenderness, warmth, and often purulent discharge. Rarely a crepitus may be palpated. Deeper soft tissue infections may show no physical signs initially—particularly so in obese patients.

The microbiological spectrum responsible for wound infections is vast. Staphylococcal infections generally occur 4–6 days after surgery. The infection is well localized, painful and purulent (6).

Gram-negative wound infections usually present with fewer local inflammatory signs, but with systemic features of fever, tachycardia and leucocytosis. Systemic sepsis may follow depending on the virulence of the organisms, and the resistance of the host. Gram-negative infections are usually due to contamination by enteric bacilli as well as by anaerobic streptococci and by B. fragilis. The incubation period for most of these infections is 7–14 days (6). The potential gastrointestinal sources for such infections should be carefully looked for.

Fever, and severe pain in a surgical or traumatic wound accompanied by a progressively toxic state should lead to a suspicion of a wound infected by Group A streptococci or clostridia (5). Early diagnosis, use of appropriate antibiotics and prompt surgical treatment are life saving.

Treatment

(a) Surgical Drainage and Debridement

This should be left to the surgeon's expertise. The principle in management is drainage of infections and debridement of necrotic tissue. Drainage requires removal of skin sutures or staples, and laying the wound open. Dressings should be done daily or as often as instructed by the surgeon. The wound is allowed to granulate and heal by secondary intention. If the wound is clean and clear of infection, secondary suturing may be done.

(b) Antibiotics

Antibiotics are invariably used except for the very mild and superficial infections. The empiric choice of antibiotics in severe wound infections depends on the clinical picture and the nature of the surgery performed. Antibiotic therapy may be suitably modified after culture sensitivity reports of the discharge from an infected wound are available.

(c) Hyperbaric Oxygen

The use of hyperbaric oxygen in certain infections will be commented upon in the Section on Clostridial myonecrosis.

Antibiotic Prophylaxis (7, 8)

Prophylactic antibiotics decrease the incidence of wound infections. The selection of the antibiotic depends on the possible pathogens in a given situation, and should be left to the discretion of the surgeon. The commonly used antibiotics for prophylaxis include either a third generation cephalosporin like ceftazidime 1 g intravenously, or a second generation cephalosporin like cefazoline 1 g intravenously, or an aminoglycoside like gentamicin 60–80 mg intravenously. It is important to stress that the unnecessary, indiscriminate and prolonged use of powerful antibiotics for prophylaxis can cause untoward side effects. These include hypersensitivity reactions, possible toxic effects (as on the kidneys with the use of aminoglycosides), and above all the emergence of drug-resistant superinfections. A single agent generally suffices for prophylactic therapy. This should be given immediately prior to the skin incision and should be repeated during surgery if this exceeds 3 hours, or twice the half-life of the drug. Most surgeons in the West do not continue antibiotics beyond the first day, as they believe that continuing the drug does not confer any additional benefit. In our country many surgeons prefer to continue the antibiotic for 5–7 days. In contaminated wounds or dirty and infected wounds, the extended use of antibiotics for a number of days after surgery, as best judged by the surgeon, is accepted practice.

In clean surgical wounds involving open heart surgery or intracranial surgery, the use of antibiotics for more days, is also justified. It is however doubtful if extended use in these patients for more than 7 days confers any special benefit.

Mechanical cleansing of the bowel plus administration of a non-absorbable oral antibiotic, is generally done to reduce the bacterial load in the colon and the distal small bowel before colorectal surgery. Oral neomycin or amoxycillin is the antibiotic most often used. Metronidazole 400 mg thrice daily is also given for four days prior to surgery to reduce the load of anaerobic organisms within the large bowel. Most surgeons also use a systemic antibiotic for prophylactic purposes just before the skin incision. This combined approach of oral and systemic antibiotic prophylaxis reduces the bacterial flora within the gut, and helps to reduce the incidence of septic complications.

REFERENCES

1. Luke WP. (1986). Surgical infections—The general surgeon's perspective. Postgrad Med. 80, 74.

2. Nichols RL. (1991). Surgical wound infection. Am J Med. 91(Suppl 3B), 54S-64S.

3. Meakins JL.(1989). Elective Care, Infection, Guidelines for Prevention of Wound Infection. In: Care of the Surgical Patient (Ed. Wilmore DW). Scientific American.

4. Kunin CM. (1984). Genitourinary infection in the patient at risk: Extrinsic risk factors. Am J Med. 76, 131.

5. Norwood SH, Civetta JM. (1987). Evaluating sepsis in critically ill patients. Chest. 92, 137.

6. Simmons RL. (1982). Wound infection: A review of diagnosis and treatment. Infect Control. 3, 44.

7. Classen DC, Evans RS, Pestotnik SL et al. (1992). The timing of prophylactic administration of antibiotics and the risk of surgical wound infection. N Engl J Med. 326, 281–286.

8. Whittmann DH, Condon RE. (1991). Prophylaxis of post-operative infections. Infect. 19 (Suppl 6), 337–344.

Necrotizing Fasciitis and Clostridial Myonecrosis

Necrotizing Fasciitis (1–6)

This is a dreadful rapidly spreading infection involving the deep subcutaneous tissue, deep fascia and even the muscle (myonecrosis). It causes extensive necrosis and gangrene not only involving the skin but also extending into the fascia and muscle. Necrotizing fasciitis is classically due to Streptococcus pyogenes infection. However, infection can be polymicrobial. Polymicrobial infections are virulent and are caused by a synergism between facultative aerobes and anaerobic bacteria.

The disease is generally community-acquired, usually affects the upper or lower extremity, but occasionally involves the groin and the perineal area. The infection can however occur after surgery, presenting as a wound infection even after minor surgical procedures.

Risk factors are diabetes and the presence of a portal of entry. Portal of entry includes surgery, needle punctures as after injections (particularly with contaminated needles used by drug addicts), minor abrasions, childbirth and trauma. Blunt trauma or muscle strain with a haematoma formation is also implicated as a risk factor. Other risk factors postulated are advanced age, peripheral vascular disease, chronic alcoholism, cancer and patients on immunosuppressive drugs. It needs to be however stressed that the majority of patients afflicted with this disease have been previously healthy.

Clinical Features

The infection begins with fever and the appearance of a localized, red, indurated painful swelling at the site of minor trauma or at the site of a surgical wound. At times no evidence of even minor trauma is available both on history and physical examination. Pain is often a predominant feature and the significance of this is often ignored as the wound or infected area appears reasonably clean to start with. The infection spreads very rapidly with increasing pain, fever and toxaemia. Characteristic local features include oedema, violaceous discolouration, pain beyond the zone of the inflamed area, and the appearance of vesicles and haemorrhagic bullae. A palpable crepitus may be present and is a diagnostic feature. When the presence of crepitus is in doubt, an X-ray of the soft tissues, or better still an MRI, may demonstrate gas in tissue planes. Within a few days extensive necrosis and sloughing of skin, subcutaneous tissue, fascia and at times even muscle occur. Fever, tachycardia, tachypnoea and overwhelming sepsis are often present. The mortality is as high as 30–70 per cent; death being due to sepsis, septic shock and multiple organ failure.

Table 14.2.1 gives a classification of necrotizing soft tissue infections according to the anatomic depth and common organisms (7).

Investigations

Blood culture in severe cases reveals bacteraemia. There is marked leucocytosis. Severe anaemia is due to both haemolysis and infection. Sepsis can lead to disseminated intravascular coagulopathy with a deranged coagulation profile. With extensive involvement of muscle (myonecrosis), rhabdomyolysis occurs and contributes to renal failure. Investigations assessing function of different organ systems are necessary.

When the clinical diagnosis is in doubt a fine needle aspiration or an incisional biopsy should be performed. These procedures may demonstrate the organisms on Gram's stain. The material obtained should also be cultured on both aerobic and anaerobic media, and an antibiotic sensitivity of the organisms grown should be asked for.

Imaging Studies (8)

Soft tissue radiographs in particular may demonstrate subcutaneous emphysema. This finding is not necessary for diagnosis and in any case may occur late in the disease.

Treatment

1. Excision and Debridement

Necrotising fasciitis is a life-threatening infection in which extensive surgical excision, debridement, combined with appropriate antibiotic therapy and intensive critical care are necessary for survival (9). Delay in surgery significantly increases mortality. Debridement needs to be extensive, as infection is present well beyond the margins of involved skin area. Incomplete debridement leads to further spread of necrosis. The margins of the excised area must appear perfectly healthy. The wound should be lightly packed and dressed; planned surgery may be required every 24 to 48 hours to ensure that ongoing necrosis is not present. Further excision and debridement is performed if necessary.

Table 14.2.1. Classification of necrotizing soft tissue infections according to anatomic site and common pathogens

Organism	Anatomic Site	Soft Tissue Infection
1. Strep. pyogenes	– Dermis + Subdermis	Erysipelas
2. S. aureus	– Dermis + Subdermis	Folliculitis, abscess
	– Fascial planes	Carbuncle
	– Muscles	Abscess/pyomyositis
3. Staph. + Strep.	– Fascial planes	Necrotizing fasciitis
	– Muscles	Non-clostridial myonecrosis
4. Cl. perfringens	– Dermis + Subdermis	Clostridial cellulitis/abscess
	– Fascial planes	Clostridial cellulitis/abscess
	– Muscles	Clostridial myonecrosis
5. Mixed enteric bacteria	– Dermis + Subdermis	Tropical ulcer
	– Fascial planes	Necrotizing fasciitis
	– Muscles	Non-clostridial myonecrosis

Modified from Ahrenholz DH. 1988. Necrotizing Soft Tissue Infections, Surg Clin North Am. WB Saunders Co., PA.

2. Antibiotics

Streptococcus pyogenes infection causing necrolizing fasciitis responds best to penicillin G, 2 mega units intravenously every 4 hours. Clindamycin is a suitable alternative.

In fulminant cases or when a polymicrobial infection is suspected, it is best to cover for Gram-positive, Gram-negative and anaerobic infection to start with. Imipenem-cilastatin 500 mg 6 hourly intravenously is of value as it covers a wide range of Gram-positive, Gram-negative infections as well as anaerobes. It could be combined with an aminoglycoside and metronidazole. When staphylococcal infection is suspected vancomycin 500 mg intravenously 6 hourly, should be added to the therapeutic regime. Once culture reports are available, antibiotic therapy can be more precisely defined.

Critical Care

Critical care is vital for survival. These patients require fluid and electrolyte replacement and cardiovascular and renal support. Ventilator support is also often necessary. Critical care is as for severe sepsis and septic shock.

Table 14.2.1 gives a classification of necrotizing soft tissue infections according to the anatomic depth, and the common organisms.

REFERENCES

1. Hill MK, Sanders CV. (1998). Skin and soft tissue infections in critical care. Crit Care Clin. 14(2), 251–262.

2. Chapnik EK, Ater EI. (1996). Necrotizing soft tissue infections. Infectious Dis Clin North Am. 10(4), 835–855.

3. Green RJ. (1996). Necrotizing fasciitis. Chest. 110(1), 219–229.

4. Majeski JA. (1984). Necrotizing fasciitis of the extremities. Prob Gen Surg. 1, 500.

5. Stone HH, Martin JD. (1972). Synergistic necrotizing cellulitis. Ann Surg. 175, 702.

6. Asfar SK, Baraka A, Juma T et al. (1991). Necrotizing fasciitis. Br J Surg. 78, 838–840.

7. Arenholz DH. (1988). Necrotizing, soft-tissue infections. Surg Clin North Am. 68, 199–214.

8. Struk DW, Munk PL, Lee MJ et al. (2001). Imaging of soft tissue infections. Radiol Clin North Am. 39(2), 277–303.

9. Ajeski JA, Alexander JW. (1983). Early diagnosis, nutritional support, and immediate extensive debridement improve survival in necrotizing fasciitis. Am J Surg. 145, 784.

Clostridial Myonecrosis (1–6)

Clostridial myonecrosis is a quick spreading fulminant infection (7), also known as gas gangrene; it is fortunately rare. It follows gross contamination of traumatic wounds by manure and is more likely to occur in the presence of devitalized tissue and poor perfusion. It can also occur when surgery is performed in a non-sterile environment where there is little regard for asepsis. In poor developing countries, there are operation theatres in smaller towns where conditions for surgery leave a lot to be desired. Clostridial myonecrosis in our country, is a rare but important cause of wound infection in septic abortions. Operations on the gall bladder or large bowel can also rarely produce clostridial infection (1, 2). The wound in clostridial myonecrosis is pale, painful with a watery, serous, or a serosanguinous discharge; above all it has a putrid smell (3). Crepitus is frequent; however it may be absent in the early stages of infection. It is to be noted that crepitus in a wound infection can be produced by gas-forming organisms other than clostridia. Clostridial infection spreads rapidly and can lead to gangrene, overwhelming sepsis, shock and death. A Gram's stain of the discharge from the wound shows Gram-positive cocci and a few neutrophils. A quick diagnosis, the use of appropriate antibiotics, and rapid surgical excision and debridement are necessary as in necrotizing fasciitis.

Investigations

The WBC count is usually raised with an increase in the mature and immature neutrophils. Gram's stain and culture from the wound discharge help to identify the pathogens causing the wound infection. A sensitivity test to various drugs helps in the choice of an appropriate antibiotic. Most experienced surgeons can predict with a fair degree of accuracy, the nature of the infection from the history, the surgery performed, and the appearance of the wound.

Treatment

Crystalline penicillin alone in massive doses of 2–4 million units intravenously 4 hourly, can control clostridial myonecrosis and monomicrobial cellulitis. Critical care of the patient involves cardiorespiratory support and attention to the functions of other organ systems as outlined in the Chapter on Septic Shock. Critical care is vital for survival.

The Use of Hyperbaric Oxygen (8)

Hyperbaric oxygen as a mode of treatment has been recommended as an adjunct to surgery and to antibiotic therapy for clostridial myonecrosis and for other soft tissue necrotizing infections. Hyperbaric oxygen is bactericidal for Cl perfringens and bacteriostatic for other anaerobic bacteria. Hyperbaric oxygen has however no effect on the toxin already produced; it can only reduce further production of exotoxin. It leads to an arrest of further necrosis, and often produces a visible improvement in the wound. As many as 14–15 sessions in the hyperbaric chamber may be necessary. The difficulty often lies in transporting very ill patients to a distant centre.

REFERENCES

1. Hill MK, Sanders CV. (1998). Skin and soft tissue infections in critical care. Crit Care Clin. 14(2), 251–262.

2. Chapnik EK, Ater EI. (1996). Necrotizing soft tissue infections. Infectious Dis Clin North Am. 10(4), 835–855.

3. Green RJ. (1996). Necrotizing fasciitis. Chest. 110(1), 219–229.

4. Stone HH, Martin JD. (1972). Synergistic necrotizing cellulitis. Ann Surg. 175, 702.

5. Hart GB, Lam RC, Strauss MB. (1983). Gas gangrene. J Trauma. 23, 991.

6. Ajeski JA, Alexander JW. (1983). Early diagnosis, nutritional support, and immediate extensive debridement improve survival in necrotizing fasciitis. Am J Surg. 145, 784.

7. Simmons RL. (1982). Wound infection: A review of diagnosis and treatment. Infect Control. 3, 44.

8. Stephens MB. (1996). Gas gangrene: potential for hyperbaric oxygen therapy. Postgrad Med. 99, 217–220.

Intra-abdominal Sepsis

General Considerations

One of the most important surgical problems requiring intensive care is intra-abdominal sepsis. Patients with intra-abdominal sepsis requiring intensive care fall into 3 groups:

(i) Those with acute inflammatory pathologies within the abdomen, who are directly admitted to the ICU to start with. They require critical care before surgery, and if surgery is considered necessary, require intensive care and support in the post-operative period.

(ii) Those transferred to the ICU after surgery has been performed for acute abdominal inflammation or suppuration, because of an anticipated stormy post-operative course.

(iii) Those admitted to the ICU for an unrelated serious problem, but who develop intra-abdominal sepsis whilst in the unit. These patients are often difficult to diagnose and have an extremely high morbidity and mortality.

Intra-abdominal sepsis may occur in the peritoneal cavity, in the retroperitoneal space, or may be localized within the viscera, to form an abscess. The most frequent site of intra-abdominal sepsis is the peritoneal cavity. If generalized, it results in generalized peritonitis; if localized, it forms an intraperitoneal abscess. Perhaps the commonest site of an intraperitoneal abscess is in the right lower quadrant in association with acute appendicitis, or a perforated duodenal ulcer. Localized intraperitoneal abscesses also occur in the left lower quadrant, and the pelvic, subhepatic and subphrenic spaces. Less frequently they may be found in the lesser sac, or between the loops of the intestine.

Retroperitoneal abscesses occur in the space between the transversalis fascia and the retroperitoneum. They may occur posteriorly or anteriorly. Posterior retroperitoneal abscesses are usually related to suppuration within the kidneys, pancreas or the spine. Rarely they can be due to an infected blood clot. Anterior retroperitoneal abscesses occur following surgery performed for an intra-abdominal infection.

Visceral abscesses occur most often within the liver and the pancreas. An empyema of the gall bladder is also best considered an abscess. A tubo-ovarian abscess is an important focus of suppuration within the pelvis. Rarely visceral abscesses can form in other organs like the kidney or the spleen.

The grave danger of any form of intra-abdominal suppuration is progressive sepsis leading to septic shock and to multiple organ failure. Critically ill patients who develop intra-abdominal sepsis fall into 2 groups. The first consists of patients with less severe infections and good immune responses, so that the infection is contained and an intra-abdominal abscess results. These patients are less likely to progress to multiple organ failure (1). The second group comprises those whose defence mechanisms are either very poor, or suppressed, or those whose defences are overwhelmed by virulent pathogens. These patients often develop generalized peritonitis without the formation of a localized abscess, and progress rapidly to septic shock and multiple organ failure. Death often results in spite of good critical care, surgery, antibiotics and nutritional support (2).

Aetiology

The most common causes preceding intra-abdominal suppuration are perforated peptic ulcer, acute appendicitis, and acute diverticulitis. Perforation of any portion of the gut within the abdominal cavity, whatever the aetiology, leads to peritonitis and intra-abdominal sepsis. Besides a perforated peptic ulcer, other important perforations include appendicular perforation, diverticular perforation, perforation of the small bowel in enteric fever and perforation of a tuberculous ulcer. Corticosteroids can cause a peptic ulcer which may perforate, and non-steroidal anti-inflammatory drugs can induce perforation in any portion of the GI tract, including the large bowel. Occasionally, perforation with localized or generalized peritonitis can occur in inflammatory bowel disease.

Gangrene of the bowel from strangulation and obstruction, or from mesenteric vascular ischaemia or occlusion, are important causes of peritonitis.

Rupture of an empyema of the gall bladder or a gangrenous cholecystitis, also causes generalized peritonitis. Acute inflammatory disease within the pelvis initially causes pelvic peritonitis, which may progress to a generalized peritonitis. Acute salpingitis, tubo-ovarian abscess are the classic examples of inflammatory pelvic pathologies. Acalculous cholecystitis and acute pancreatitis can complicate the course of a critical illness and are believed to be related to poor perfusion states in critically ill patients. In our country, septic abortion and puerperal sepsis are important causes of peritonitis.

In a critical care setting, low perfusion states, as observed in cardiogenic shock, congestive heart failure or shock due to any cause, can cause ischaemia to the gut with a breach in its anatomic integrity.

Trauma to the abdomen, either blunt or penetrating, is also an important cause of intra-abdominal sepsis.

Post-operative peritonitis may be the direct result of abdominal surgery. It is more lethal than the other forms of peritonitis. Peritonitis following surgery is most commonly due to anastomotic dehiscence. Ischaemia, infection, haemorrhage can all singly or in combination, promote dehiscence. Excessive spillage and soiling of the peritoneum during handling of viscera during surgery, can also lead to post-operative intra-abdominal sepsis. In gynaecological operations on the pelvic viscera, an uncommon but important cause of post-operative peritonitis, is an ileal perforation a few inches above the ileocaecal junction. In my opinion, this is related to undue pressure on the ileocaecal area exerted by a retractor during surgery. A small area of the ileum is devitalized or suffers pressure necrosis, and this perforates on the third or fourth post-operative day. Diagnosis may be difficult and delayed, leading to disastrous consequences.

Primary peritonitis is due to a generalized peritoneal infection unrelated to any intra-abdominal perforation or septic pathology. The most important background against which primary bacterial peritonitis occurs is in patients with cirrhosis of the liver with ascites. Infection is generally due to Gram-negative organisms; it is probably haematogenous in origin. Primary bacterial peritonitis is also observed in patients with nephrotic syndrome, systemic lupus erythematosus and very rarely in immunocompromised individuals. A primary pneumococcal peritonitis is a dangerous entity in children, and is often mistaken for peritonitis following an appendicular perforation.

Table 14.3.1 lists the common causes of intra-abdominal sepsis.

Physiopathology (3)

The term peritonitis used without qualification, refers to acute bacterial suppurative peritonitis. Presence of sterile bile, blood, or gastric acid in the peritoneal cavity can also cause intense peritoneal irritation, and a chemical inflammation, which is clinically indistinguishable from surgical peritonitis. The notable difference in these situations is the absence of bacterial infection, which when present plays a crucial role in the evolution of the natural history and the fatal outcome.

Bacterial contamination of the peritoneum is countered by local peritoneal defences, and by a general immune response. The following physiopathological changes are observed in suppurative peritonitis:

1. Local inflammation of the peritoneum.
2. Adynamic ileus.
3. Hypovolaemia, chiefly related to (1) and (2) above.
4. Changes in other organ systems secondary to (1) and (2).

Table 14.3.1. Common causes of intra-abdominal sepsis

1. Gastrointestinal
   * Perforations
     – Perforated gastric or duodenal ulcer
     – Perforation of hollow viscus or any part of the gut
     – Enteric or tuberculous ulcer
     – Inflammatory bowel disease
     – Diverticulitis
     – Iatrogenic (corticosteroid and NSAID use)
   * Infection
     – Acute appendicitis
     – Diverticulitis
   * Impaired blood supply to the bowel
     – Gangrene from strangulation
     – Obstruction
     – Ischaemia to the bowel
2. Acute necrotizing pancreatitis
3. Cholecystitis (acute, acalculous, gangrenous)
4. Liver abscess (pyogenic, amoebic), splenic abscess
5. Pelvic pathologies
   * Acute salpingitis
   * Tubo-ovarian abscess
   * Septic abortions/Puerperal sepsis
6. Perinephric/Retroperitoneal abscesses
7. Trauma to the abdomen
8. Following abdominal surgery
9. Low-perfusion states (congestive cardiac failure, shock of any aetiology).
10. Primary bacterial peritonitis
    * Cirrhosis of liver with ascites
    * Nephrotic syndrome
    * SLE, other immunocompromised states
    * Pneumococcal peritonitis in children

5. Hormonal and metabolic changes related chiefly to the immediate and acute stress of infection.

6. The evolution of the sepsis syndrome.

This syndrome is a systemic response of the body to bacteria, their toxins and to other bacterial products. Sepsis and the semantics of clinical states closely associated with sepsis, have been discussed in the Chapter on Septic Shock. It is worth stressing that intra-abdominal sepsis can be fulminant, and can quickly graduate to septic shock, multiple organ dysfunction and death. In earlier years, before intensive care came into being, most patients with generalized suppurative peritonitis died before sepsis with multiple organ system failure could fully evolve. Sepsis is due to endotoxins and other toxins of bacteria and their products, having far reaching effects on all organ systems of the body. The syndrome however is not just the direct result of infection; it is also partly due to the unorchestrated response of the defence mechanisms of the body to infection.

This is dealt with at length in the Chapters on Septic Shock and Multiple Organ Dysfunction Syndrome. Localized undrained intra-abdominal abscesses (peritoneal, retroperitoneal or visceral), can also lead to the syndrome of sepsis and multiple organ failure. The tempo of the evolution of the syndrome with a localized abscess, is generally slower than with generalized suppurative peritonitis.

The section below briefly deals with the physiopathological changes listed under points (1) to (5). It then proceeds to mention the pathogenetic factors which determine the severity of intra-abdominal sepsis.

1. Local Peritoneal Inflammation

The local response to a peritoneal insult is characterized by hyperaemia of the peritoneum with vascular congestion, oedema and transudation of fluid from the extracellular interstitial compartment into the abdominal cavity. This transudation is accompanied by the diapedesis of polymorphonuclear leucocytes. It is followed by exudation of a protein-rich exudate containing large quantities of fibrin and other plasma proteins. Clotting of this protein-rich exudate results in sticking together of the bowel loops to other viscera and the parietes in the areas of inflammation. This helps to localize the area of peritoneal contamination, to some extent.

2. Adynamic Ileus

Initially there is a short period of bowel hypermotility; motility is then depressed, and is followed by a complete adynamic ileus. The gut distends and is filled with fluid and air, most of the latter being swallowed air. Fluid secretion into the gut is markedly enhanced, whilst absorption of fluid from the gut is markedly impaired. There is therefore sequestration of a large volume of fluid within the lumen of the gut.

3. Hypovolaemia

The loss and sequestration of fluid in the gut and in the peritoneal cavity, may be marked and results in a fall in the volume of the interstitial tissue compartment, and in the circulating volume within the vascular compartment. Fluid is also trapped as oedema beneath the mesothelium of visceral peritoneal linings, adding thereby to the volume of water, electrolytes and proteins translocated into the 'third space'. The degree of loss of extracellular fluid into this non-functional 'third space' is proportional to the surface area of the peritoneum involved. The volume of sequestrated fluid may be as large as 4–6 l in 24 hours.

4. Secondary Changes in Other Organ Systems

(a) Cardiac Response

Cardiac response is conditioned by hypovolaemia and progressive metabolic acidosis. Diminished venous return due to a fall in circulating volume leads to a fall in cardiac output, hypotension, a decrease in the oxygen transport, and to poor oxygenation of tissues. This promotes metabolic acidosis, which in turn further depresses cardiac function. The clinical importance of this should never be forgotten. Expanding the extracellular and intravascular compartments by intravenous infusions can reverse the above trends. In fact, if the patient is made normovolaemic and survives the initial crisis, the circulatory state often graduates to that typically seen in sepsis. The haemodynamic changes are then characterized by a high cardiac output, hypotension, and a low systemic peripheral vascular resistance (see Chapter on Septic Shock). Even so, the tissue demand for oxygen is often inadequately met, so that tissue hypoxia results.

(b) Renal Changes

These are secondary to hypovolaemia, fall in cardiac output, and the effects of increased secretion of the antidiuretic hormone and aldosterone (see below). Renal perfusion suffers and there is a fall in the glomerular filtration rate due to the prerenal factors stated above. Renal insufficiency develops to a varying extent, and enhances metabolic acidosis.

(c) Respiratory Changes

Abdominal distension due to ileus, together with restriction of diaphragmatic and intercostal movements due to pain, result in a fall in the tidal volume. This predisposes to atelectasis, which in turn results in a ventilation-perfusion mismatch, and a fall in the PaO_2.

5. Hormonal and Metabolic Changes

Peritonitis causes an almost immediate response from the adrenal medulla. There is an outpouring of epinephrine and norepinephrine into the blood, resulting in vasoconstriction, tachycardia and sweating. There is also an increased secretion of adrenocortical hormones for the first 2–3 days following a peritoneal insult. Secretion of antidiuretic hormone and aldosterone is also increased, causing a reduction in urine output with conservation of sodium and water. Water retention may exceed sodium retention, leading to hyponatraemia.

The metabolic rate is generally increased with a corresponding increase in oxygen demand by the tissues. For reasons stated above, the cardiopulmonary system is unable to achieve delivery of oxygen commensurate with the demand for oxygen by the tissues, resulting in tissue hypoxaemia and lactic acid acidosis.

Protein catabolism is also increased from the very start, and progressively becomes more severe. Weight loss of 25–30 per cent of lean body mass is observed if peritonitis persists. Though albumin synthesis is increased, serum albumin levels progressively fall, as albumin accumulates in the peritoneal cavity, and is lost to the general circulation.

If the above described general responses to suppurative peritonitis go unchecked, and if the hypovolaemic circulatory state is uncorrected, there is increasing tissue hypoxia, and increasing metabolic acidosis causing increasing dysfunction of all organ systems. Death results from irreversible hypovolaemic shock. The classical clinical description of peritonitis by Hippocrates corresponds to this terminal hopeless state.

The general and specific responses to peritonitis are illustrated in **Figs. 14.3.1** and **14.3.2**.

Factors Determining Severity of Intra-abdominal Sepsis (Table 14.3.2)

(i) Virulence and Microbiology of Pathogens

The larger the dose of pathogens, and greater their virulence, the more severe the infection. The microbiology of intra-abdominal sepsis is polymicrobial. This is always so when the peritoneal cavity is invaded from the gastrointestinal tract. The most common bacteria are coliform organisms (mainly E. coli), other enterococci,

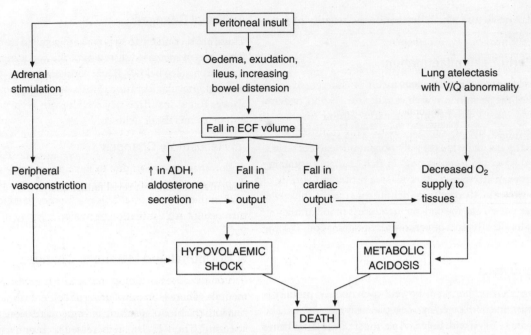

Fig. 14.3.1. General responses to peritonitis.

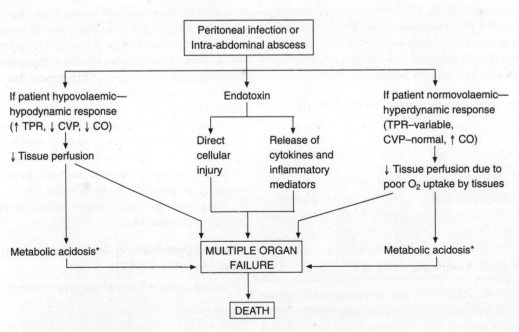

*If early treatment successful, recovery possible.

Fig. 14.3.2. Specific responses to peritonitis.

Table 14.3.2. Factors determining severity of intra-abdominal sepsis

* Virulence and microbiology of pathogens
* Extent of contamination
  – Maximal spillage in ileal and caecal perforation
* Presence of foreign bodies and blood
* Errors in management
  – Unrecognized, unsutured perforations and leaks
  – Inadequate surgical drainage and debridement
  – Administration of laxatives in abdominal sepsis
* An immunocompromised patient
* Co-morbid conditions—diabetes, chronic renal disease, cirrhosis of the liver, chronic alcoholism
* Elderly patients > 70–75 years

B. fragilis, anaerobic cocci and Clostridia. Other Gram-negative bacilli such as Klebsiella and Proteus species are often present, but form a small part of the total flora. There are an increasing number of fungal isolates in patients with prolonged sepsis and in immunocompromised hosts. Anaerobes always play an important role in contributing to the virulence of intra-abdominal and intra-peritoneal sepsis. It is important to note that a patient in whom peritonitis or an intra-abdominal abscess develops in the hospital whilst on antibiotics, may have a different aerobic flora. Klebsiella, Proteus and Pseudomonas often predominate, and may be resistant to antibiotics.

(ii) Extent of Contamination

The severity of peritonitis and intra-abdominal sepsis following spontaneous or traumatic perforation of the GI tract, depends on the size and location of the perforation. Ileal or caecal perforations with spillage, are associated with a greater contamination and greater morbidity than perforations of the very proximal or very distal parts of the GI tract. Proximally the gut has fewer bacteria, and distally the fecal contents are more solid, and the inflammation is more easily localized. On the other hand, ileal and caecal contents are liquid and have a high concentration of bacteria, and of residual enzymes, which prevent localization of the infection.

(iii) Presence of Foreign Bodies and Blood

The presence of a foreign body, or blood clots (which invariably get infected), increase the morbidity and mortality in peritoneal inflammation.

(iv) Errors in Management

The following errors need to be stressed, and should be avoided:

(a) Draining the peritoneal cavity at surgery, without also ensuring that all leaks from the GI tract or a ruptured viscus have been surgically sealed. A continuing source of peritoneal contamination always spells death.

(b) Attempting to control infection and sepsis by the use of antibiotics without adequate surgical drainage and debridement.

(c) An important error of commission is the administration of laxatives or enemas in abdominal sepsis. This increases the risk of rupture of an inflamed bowel segment.

(v) Immunosuppressed Patients

Cancer, the prior use of antimitotic drugs, radiation therapy, myeloproliferative disease, HIV infection lead to a poor immune response to acute infection. The extent, gravity and prognosis of intra-abdominal sepsis is worse compared to immunocompetent patients.

(vi) Co-morbid Conditions

The prognosis is comparatively poor when intra-abdominal sepsis occurs in uncontrolled diabetics, in cirrhotics, in alcoholics, in patients with chronic renal failure and in the elderly.

Clinical Features and Diagnosis

The clinical features of intra-abdominal sepsis depend on the age of the patient, the background disease against which intra-abdominal infection develops, and whether the patient is immuno-competent or immunosuppressed.

Peritonitis presents as an acute abdomen, but localized suppuration (intra-peritoneal abscess) may present with subtle manifestations.

Abdominal pain is the most important symptom of generalized peritonitis. It is severe and constant, the patient preferring to lie absolutely still in bed without any movement. Even turning in bed from one side to the other sharply increases the pain. To start with, the pain is maximal over the initial site of inflammation; it then spreads to involve the whole abdomen as generalized inflammation supervenes. Pain is often accompanied by nausea and vomiting.

The abdomen may show distension because of ileus. Abdominal movements on respiration are poor; the patient is tachypnoeic with shallow intercostal breathing. Tenderness on palpation, with guarding and rigidity are accompaniments of peritoneal irritation and inflammation. Rebound tenderness is present; percussion of the abdomen is painful, and is merely a gentler method of eliciting rebound tenderness. Free fluid in the abdomen is difficult to detect on clinical examination, but is often present. Auscultation typically reveals a silent abdomen; the heart sounds are clearly heard on abdominal auscultation. Rectal examination and pelvic examination may reveal tenderness or a painful inflammatory mass. The hernial orifices and the genitals must always be inspected and examined.

Systemic features include fever, tachycardia, tachypnoea and leucocytosis. None of these however may be present. Leucocytosis is generally observed but not always so. Leucopaenia if present, is of ominous significance.

Hypovolaemic Shock

Clinical features of hypovolaemia and hypovolaemic shock are often present in the first few days of acute generalized suppurative peritonitis. This is, as explained earlier, due to sequestration of fluid from the interstitial tissue compartment into the peritoneal cavity and the lumen of the gut. Hypotension, tachycardia, and oliguria with a rise in the non-protein nitrogen and creatinine levels are observed. If the circulatory state is uncorrected and if prompt surgery for the peritonitis is delayed, the patient rapidly deteriorates and dies. The Hippocratic facies—'hollow eyes, collapsed temples, the colour of the face brown, black, livid or lead coloured'—is the description of a patient about to die with generalized peritonitis.

If on the other hand, hypovolaemia is corrected, the circulatory haemodynamics restored, and critical care offered, the patient may proceed to develop all the features of prolonged sepsis. Sepsis may or may not respond to surgery and antibiotics. Sepsis will never respond if the cause or the source that seeds the peritoneum is undetected, or is not eradicated totally by surgical procedures. In patients with multiple bowel perforations, or in whom surgery has been delayed, or is inadequate, radical eradication of the sources of peritonitis are impossibly difficult. The very friable bowel loops with total obliteration of tissue planes, render the approach to the sites of perforation impossible. Death from multiple organ failure is inevitable in these patients. The better the critical care offered, the slower and more agonizing the death, particularly so in young patients. It is pathetic to helplessly watch the slow decline, and the final, inevitable disintegration of all organ system function in these patients.

Localized Peritoneal and Retroperitoneal Inflammation

In the form of an intra-abdominal abscess, localized peritoneal and retroperitoneal inflammation may show few or no clinical signs. A tender localized mass is not always palpable. A subphrenic abscess may present with dyspnoea, hiccups, referred shoulder pain, basal atelectasis or pleural effusion. A pelvic abscess may present with diarrhoea or urgency of micturition. A rectal and vaginal examination may elicit tenderness, by causing direct pressure over the inflamed mass or peritoneum. A psoas abscess may manifest as spasm and pain in the hip, when the psoas is stretched on extension of the hip (the psoas sign). Retroperitoneal perinephric abscesses are difficult to diagnose clinically till the abscess surfaces and produces warmth and tenderness over the loin posteriorly.

Systemic features include fever, often spiking in nature, and leucocytosis. If the abscess is undrained, sepsis is protracted, and leads to progressive multiple organ dysfunction, failure and death (see Chapters on Multiple Organ Dysfunction Syndrome and Septic Shock).

The diagnosis of intra-abdominal sepsis is particularly difficult in the following groups of patients:

(i) In the immunosuppressed patient inflammatory reactions and all immune responses are suppressed or muted. The usual abdominal signs may be barely elicitable. This is particularly so in severely neutropaenic patients. The presence of fever of undetermined origin in these patients should prompt a meticulous search for possible abdominal sepsis. Imaging studies are of great help in arriving at a correct diagnosis.

(ii) In patients who are critically ill in the ICU for unrelated problems, but who develop intra-abdominal sepsis as a complication, intra-abdominal sepsis may be fortuitous or iatrogenic (as peptic perforation in a patient on corticosteroids). It may also occur as a complication of a poor perfusion state or a low output syndrome. This can cause bowel ischaemia, a small leak from the bowel, and intra-abdominal suppuration. Acalculous cholecystitis or acute pancreatitis can also occur as a complication of a low output syndrome or due to poor perfusion of the abdominal viscera. Recognition of intra-abdominal suppuration is difficult because of the paucity of physical signs, the preoccupation with the primary critical illness for which the patient is admitted, and because of the frequent presence of a blunted sensorium in a very ill patient.

(iii) In the immediate post-operative patient. Intra-abdominal sepsis including peritonitis is difficult to diagnose if it occurs as a complication in a patient who has been operated upon very recently. This complication again may be fortuitous or iatrogenic (chiefly as a result of perforation of the bowel during surgery). The pain of the surgical wound is not immediately distinguishable from the pain of peritonitis. The persistence of paralytic ileus after surgery, should always suggest an underlying perforation with peritonitis, or a localized abscess within the abdominal cavity. Physical signs of tenderness, guarding and rigidity are often difficult to evaluate in these patients in the immediate post-operative period. When perforation of the gut with peritonitis occurs soon after a caesarean section for a full-term delivery, the diagnosis is doubly difficult. The stretched abdominal muscles (as a result of pregnancy) show minimal guarding, and little or no rigidity. A history of sudden pain in the abdomen a few days after surgery, the presence of ileus, rebound tenderness, and the demonstration of free fluid within the abdomen, should point to the correct diagnosis.

Differential Diagnosis (4, 5)

The differential diagnosis of intra-abdominal sepsis, is extensive and includes all other causes of acute abdomen—in particular acute bowel obstruction, acute bowel ischaemia, pancreatitis, and a ruptured ectopic pregnancy in a female patient. An intra-abdominal abscess may masquerade as systemic sepsis, the source of which is undetermined. In patients with cirrhosis of the liver, primary peritonitis (generally haematogenous in nature), needs to be distinguished from peritonitis secondary to perforation or inflammation of the abdominal viscera. Acute medical problems may present with acute abdominal pain and tenderness in the abdomen, and mimic intra-abdominal inflammation due to surgical pathologies. The most important of these problems are acute pneumonias which produce referred pain in the upper abdomen and at times even in the right iliac fossa, and acute viral hepatitis which can produce generalized abdominal pain, pain in the right iliac fossa and pain in the right upper abdomen. This is particularly observed in children and in young adults. Acute falciparum malaria can also present with abdominal pain. The latter is also a classic feature of severe diabetic ketoacidosis. The importance of a routine urine examination cannot be overemphasized. Acute glomerulonephritis in children often presents with abdominal pain or severe loin pain. Acute exanthemas in children often present with fever and generalized or even localized abdominal pain. The diagnosis is apparent with the appearance of a characteristic skin rash. Finally, other rare but important causes of severe abdominal pain (not generally associated with rigidity or rebound tenderness) are acute porphyria and acute adrenal crisis.

Laboratory Findings

Blood examination should include a complete blood count, platelet count, ESR, serum electrolytes, liver function tests, blood sugar, blood urea and serum creatinine. Systemic features of sepsis should warrant investigations on the clotting profile, arterial blood gas analysis and tests to evaluate functions of different organ systems. Cultures of blood, urine and peritoneal fluid are important investigations before starting empiric antibiotic therapy.

Imaging Studies

These are of crucial importance in the diagnosis of intra-abdominal inflammation, as also in the differential diagnosis of other causes of acute abdomen.

1. An X-ray of the Chest in the Upright Posture

This can exclude pneumonia as a cause of acute abdominal pain and fever. Gas under the diaphragm is indicative of a perforated viscus. Intra-abdominal suppuration often causes elevation of one or both domes of the diaphragm and basal atelectasis.

Pleural effusion is an important finding in a subphrenic abscess or in acute pancreatitis.

2. An X-ray of the Abdomen (AP) in the Erect Posture

Gas under the diaphragm is indicative of perforation of a hollow viscus. Fluid levels, often in a step-ladder fashion, point to an intestinal obstruction. Small bowel or large bowel obstructions can be diagnosed from the pattern of the bowel proximal to the obstruction. Three or more fluid levels in the abdomen should be considered significant, and point to some degree of obstruction within the gut. A follow-up X-ray needs to be done in such patients after some hours. Paralytic ileus, whether due to medical or surgical problems, is characterized by marked distension of the small gut. This may involve the colon as well. Acute dilatation of the stomach is demonstrated by the outline of a hugely distended stomach, with an air-fluid level.

If perforation of a viscus is suspected, and the patient is too ill for an X-ray in the erect posture, then a left lateral decubitus X-ray of the abdomen (with the left side down), is of help. It may show the presence of free air between the liver margin and the abdominal wall. An X-ray of the chest or abdomen with the patient in the supine posture, may not yield this crucial information, and may therefore be misleading.

Presence of free fluid and gas in the peritoneal cavity after perforation of the gut, is visible as a fluid collection (generally gravitating into the pelvis), with a clear horizontal air-fluid level.

Rarer findings in intra-abdominal suppuration on a plain X-ray include: (a) air in the wall of the gut—pneumatosis intestinalis is observed in some patients with gangrene of the gut; (b) air in the gall bladder lumen in patients with empyema caused by gas forming organisms; (c) thumb-printing of the colonic wall in ischaemic colitis; (d) marked distension of the colon in megacolon

and in Ogilvie's syndrome. The latter occurs after surgery, and is characterized by severe ileus involving the large bowel. Caecal distension may lead to perforation and peritonitis in some patients.

3. Ultrasonography of the Abdomen

This is a portable, non-invasive useful diagnostic tool. It is of special value in diagnosing acute cholecystitis, cholangitis, or stones in the gall bladder. Ultrasonography is useful in the diagnosis of acute pancreatitis, pancreatic fluid collections, intraperitoneal and retroperitoneal abscesses, pelvic abscesses, pelvic tumours and ruptured ectopic pregnancy. Unfortunately, the sensitivity of an ultrasound examination is lost or vitiated to an extent, by the presence of overlying gas in the bowel, by skin incisions and bulky dressings over surgical wounds. The presence of an ileostomy, colostomy or open wounds limits the use of this otherwise extremely valuable diagnostic investigation.

4. CT Scan

A CT scan is more sensitive and specific than an ultrasound for identification of abscesses within the abdomen (intraperitoneal, retroperitoneal or within a viscus). It is particularly useful for the correct diagnosis of pancreatic necrosis, or pancreatic and peripancreatic suppuration. The sensitivity of a good CT scan of the abdomen approaches 95–100 per cent.

5. Gastrograffin Studies

Oral gastrograffin is sometimes used in patients with intestinal obstruction, to determine the site of a small bowel obstruction just before surgery. If a patient operated upon for a perforation of the gut fails to improve, and shows continuing sepsis, it probably indicates the presence of one or more other perforations, or the formation of a new intra-abdominal abscess. Oral gastrograffin can demonstrate a perforation with a leak of the dye in the peritoneal cavity, or can outline the anatomic site of an enteric fistula.

Gastrograffin given rectally helps to distinguish between a terminal ileal obstruction and a proximal colonic obstruction.

6. Angiographic Studies

Acute intra-abdominal suppuration is sometimes associated or complicated by massive bleeds. This is particularly observed with suppurative pancreatitis which can cause bleeds within the gut, or outside it. Most patients are generally too ill for open exploratory surgery to stop such bleeds. The distortion of tissue planes also often makes this task impossibly difficult. Angiographic studies, with the catheter placed in the appropriate vessels can demonstrate the bleeding vessels, which can then be suitably embolized with gelfoam or other agents.

7. Radionuclide Scanning

This test holds no advantage over a good CT scan and ultrasound, for identifying occult intra-abdominal abscesses. Indium-III labelled autologous leucocyte scanning is reported to have a sensitivity of 80–93 per cent. However false positives and false negatives may result.

Management

Management consists of the following important features:

1. Quick restoration of the circulatory haemodynamics followed promptly by surgery for the intra-abdominal suppuration.
2. The use of appropriate antibiotics.
3. Critical care and support of different organ systems.
4. Maintenance of nutrition.

I. Management Prior to Surgery

1. Restoration of Circulatory Haemodynamics

Most patients are hypovolaemic from the massive sequestration of fluid into the peritoneum and into the lumen of the gut. Intravenous infusions of normal saline, dextrose saline, and Ringer lactate solutions should be given to raise the CVP, the filling pressures of the ventricles, and the cardiac output. Intake/output charts are carefully maintained. All vital signs, the arterial blood pressure in particular, are also carefully monitored. Abnormalities in electrolyte balance and acid-base equilibrium should be corrected. The haemoglobin should be raised by packed cell infusions and kept close to 11 g/dl. Deranged clotting mechanisms should be corrected by infusions of fresh frozen plasma.

Too rapid infusions in patients with overt cardiac dysfunction, can cause pulmonary oedema. Over-resuscitation of shock can cause hypervolaemia, and should be avoided as this can precipitate the subsequent development of ARDS.

2. Antibiotic Therapy (6, 7)

Empiric therapy should be started promptly after relevant cultures have been sent. One should never await culture results, as this would waste precious time. Different units have their own choice of empiric regimes for intra-abdominal sepsis. Any one of the following regimes can be used.

(a) Augmentin 1.2 g intravenously 8 hourly + aminoglycoside (gentamicin or amikacin) + metronidazole 500 mg intravenously 8 hourly.

(b) Ceftazidime 1 g intravenously 6 hourly + ciprofloxacin 200 mg intravenously 12 hourly or aminoglycoside (gentamicin or amikacin) + metronidazole 500 mg intravenously 8 hourly.

In patients who develop intra-abdominal infection while in hospital, or who develop intra-abdominal suppuration or infection whilst being treated in the ICU for some other unrelated serious illness, or who develop peritoneal sepsis following abdominal surgery, we prefer to use one of the following regimes: (i) a piperacillin derivative 3–4 g intravenously 6 hourly + aminoglycoside or ciprofloxacin + metronidazole; (ii) ticarcillin-clavulanic acid 3.1 g intravenously 4 hourly + aminoglycoside + metronidazole; (iii) imipenem-cilastatin or meropenem 500 mg intravenously 6 hourly + vancomycin 500 mg intravenously 6 hourly.

Each of these regimes provides a significant coverage against a wide range of pathogens. The choice of a particular regime depends on the aetiology of the intra-abdominal suppuration, the antibiotics used earlier, the microbiological flora of nosocomial infection in a particular unit, and the state of renal function in an individual patient.

II. Definitive Surgical Treatment

1. Surgery (8)

The definitive treatment of intra-abdominal sepsis lies in surgical eradication of the septic focus and debridement of necrotic tissues. Surgery should never be delayed unnecessarily. It is at times impossible to restore circulatory haemodynamics to even a semblance of normalcy, without first performing definitive surgery for intra-abdominal suppuration. Though the risk of surgery is high, it must be taken; the passage of time increases rather than decreases this risk. Surgery may necessitate removal or diversion of a part of the gut. The surgical procedure depends on the nature, extent and duration of the problem. At times multiple, planned laparotomies are necessary to identify and debride septic foci which are unrecognized at the start, or which develop during the post-operative period. In gross abdominal sepsis, where repeated surgeries appear inevitable from the outset, some surgeons prefer to leave the abdominal wound open (9). In this 'open wound' form of surgical procedure, the peritoneum is packed either with a special non-adhesive sheet or with paraffin gauze. The latter is cheap, available and better suited to developing countries. This technique favours easier watch over infection, and improves ventilation due to reduction in intra-abdominal pressure. The disadvantages are the need for excellent nursing, the occurrence of large fluid losses, and intestinal fistulae.

It is common practice to irrigate or to perform a lavage of the peritoneal cavity with antibiotic solutions at the time of surgery. This presumably helps to reduce the bacterial load within the abdominal cavity. Whether peritoneal lavage with antibiotics during or after surgery, plays a significant role in reducing the morbidity or mortality, has however not been definitely established.

2. Percutaneous Drainage of Abscesses (10)

Well-localized peritoneal or retroperitoneal abscesses that are easily accessible by percutaneous needle aspiration, can be drained in this fashion. Repeated aspirations can be done under ultrasound or CT guidance, or preferably, a large bore pigtail drain or a sump catheter is placed in the abscess cavity, again under ultrasound or CT guidance. The abscess cavity can then be intermittently irrigated with normal saline and appropriate antibiotics. The drain is removed when the drainage ceases and when the abscess cavity appears obliterated on a CT scan or a sinogram. Percutaneous drainage is obviously not to be used if the abscess cavity contains thick pus or a significant quantity of necrotic material. Drainage through a pigtail or sump catheter is likely to be unsuccessful if there are multiple pockets of pus. The drain is removed when the drainage has stopped or is less than 30 ml in the day. If the response to percutaneous drainage is inadequate, open surgical drainage with debridement of necrotic tissue should be performed.

III. Critical Care

This is vital both during the pre- and post-operative stages. Attention to *fluid, electrolyte and acid-base balance, and to nutrition* are vital. *Cardiorespiratory support,* and in particular *ventilator support,* are invariably necessary in critically ill patients. Haemodynamic monitoring which includes an arterial line and insertion of a Swan-Ganz catheter may be necessary. Antibiotics need to be continued for 2–4 weeks.

Persistent sepsis after abdominal surgery indicates one or more of the following:

1. An undetected perforation of the gut, or a new perforation.

2. A post-operative intra-abdominal abscess.

3. The presence of devitalized gut due to ischaemia involving a segment of the bowel.

A rising bilirubin with a rise in liver enzymes following abdominal surgery for a perforation, suggests that factors (1), (2), or both in combination, are present as post-operative complications. In my experience, this is invariably so if other organ systems show satisfactory function.

4. An ongoing peritoneal infection often due to resistant organisms.

5. *Fungal infection.* The occurrence of a superadded fungal infection should always be considered in unresolved intra-abdominal sepsis, particularly in immunocompromised patients or in those who have received prolonged broad-spectrum antibiotic therapy. The discharge from wounds, fistulae, should always be sent for fungal culture. Blood cultures for fungal infection may be positive even when discharge from the area of suppuration is negative. Appropriate antifungal treatment is life-saving in fungal infections.

6. *Nosocomial infection* (wound infection by resistant bacteria, pneumonia, catheter-related sepsis, urinary tract infections).

The role of monoclonal antibodies in the treatment of septic shock (**11, 12**) has been discussed briefly in the Chapter on Septic Shock.

REFERENCES

1. Fry DE. (1984). The diagnosis of intra-abdominal infection in the post-operative patient. Prob Gen Surg. 1, 558.

2. Norwood SH, Civetta JM. (1987). Evaluating sepsis in critically ill patients. Chest. 92, 137.

3. Walker AP, Condon RE. (1989). Peritonitis and Intra-abdominal Abscesses. In: Principles of Surgery, 5th edn (Eds Schwartz SI, Tom Shires G, Spencer FC). pp. 1459–1489. McGraw-Hill Book Company, New York, London, Toronto, Paris.

4. Liolios A, Oropello JM, Benjamin E. (1999). Gastrointestinal complications in the intensive care unit. Clin Chest Med. 20(2), 329–45, viii.

5. Podnos YD; Jimenez JC; Wilson SE. (2002). Intra-abdominal sepsis in elderly persons. Clin Infect Dis. 35 (1), 62–68.

6. Bohnen JMA et al. (1992). Guidelines for critical care: Anti-infective agents for intra-abdominal infection. Arch Surg. 127, 83–89.

7. Sawyer MD, Dunn DL. (1992). Antimicrobial therapy for intra-abdominal sepsis. Infect Dis Clin North Am. 6, 545–570.

8. Aprahamian C, Whittmann DH. (1991). Operative management of intra-abdominal infection. Infection. 19, 453–455.

9. Schein M, Saadia R, Decker GGA. (1986). The open management of the septic abdomen. Surg Gynecol Obstet. 163, 587–592.

10. vanSonnenberg E, Ferrucci JT Jr, Mueller PR et al. (1982). Percutaneous drainage of abscesses and fluid collections: Technique, results, and applications. Radiology. 142, 1–10.

11. Greenman RL, Schein RM, Martin MA et al. (1991). A controlled clinical trial of E5 murine monoclonal IgM antibody to endotoxin in the treatment of gram-negative sepsis. JAMA. 266, 1125–1126.

12. Ziegler EJ, Fisher CJ Jr, Sprung CL et al. (1991). Treatment of gram-negative bacteraemia and septic shock with HA-IA human monoclonal antibody against endotoxin. N Engl J Med. 324, 429–436.

SECTION 15

Organ System Dysfunction Requiring Critical Care

15.1   Multiple Organ Dysfunction Syndrome (MODS)

15.2   Renal Dysfunction in the Critically Ill

15.3   Critical Care in Fulminant Hepatitis

15.4   Acute (Fulminant) Necrotizing Pancreatitis

15.5   Acute Gastrointestinal Bleeds Requiring Critical Care

15.6   Haemorrhagic Disorders in the ICU

15.7   Transfusion (Blood Product) Therapy

15.8   Endocrine Dysfunction in the Critically Ill

15.9   Diabetes Mellitus in the Critically Ill Patient

15.10   Neurological Disorders Requiring Critical Care

      A. Increased Intracranial Pressure

      B. Cranial Trauma

      C. Acute Stroke

      D. Fulminant Neurological Infections

      E. Status Epilepticus

      F. Peri-operative Neurosurgical Care

CHAPTER 15.1

Multiple Organ Dysfunction Syndrome (MODS)

The syndrome of multiple organ dysfunction (also called multiple organ failure) has gained increasing importance over the last 20 years. It remains even today one of the major therapeutic challenges faced by physicians treating patients with critical illnesses due to widely differing aetiologies. Single organ failure was long recognized as an important cause of morbidity and mortality in surgical patients. In the late 1960s, extended organ failure sequentially involving the lungs, liver and kidneys, and finally resulting in death, was observed in patients suffering from severe trauma. In 1973, Tilney and colleagues reported on a case of failure of multiple organ systems causing death, following the repair of a ruptured aortic aneurysm (1). The syndrome of multiple organ failure as a distinct nosologic entity was increasingly recognized in the 80s (2–5), and today is rightly considered as an unsolved problem carrying a forbidding mortality in ICUs all over the world.

What is the reason for the increasing incidence of this frightening new entity over the last two decades? Ironically enough, the recognition and increasing incidence of this syndrome is to an extent related to better critical care in the early phase of a severe illness—critical care which enables the patient to weather the initial storm, and not succumb to it. It is only against such a background, where very ill patients are expertly cared for and supported over a period of time (this being virtually impossible 30 years ago), that the syndrome of multiple organ dysfunction or failure unfolds. In other words, this syndrome is a product of 'progress' in critical care, and 'progress' in life-saving technology. There are two other factors that are responsible for unmasking the increasing incidence and development of this syndrome. These are an increase in the high-risk patient population being cared for in intensive care units, and an activation of inflammatory and immune responses during the initial phase of an acute illness, through which the patient survives (6–9). These responses have far-reaching effects not only on the initial system involved, but also on multiple organ systems of the human body. They are poorly understood, and to date cannot be effectively countered, so that over a period of time they lead to progressively increasing dysfunction and failure of multiple organ systems, often culminating in a harrowing death (1, 10–13).

The syndrome of multiple organ failure illustrates perfectly the interdependence of different organs of the body—an idea that was intuitively grasped by ancient Ayurvedic physicians in India. The syndrome also illustrates the fact that no organ functions in isolation, that each organ influences the other, and that deranged function in one, has far-reaching effects on the other organs. It is this harmony of the whole, rather than the function of individual parts, which spells the difference between health and disease, as also between survival and death.

Definition and Concept

There is as yet no precise definition of multiple organ failure. Clinically it can be considered as the sequential or concomitant occurrence of severe derangement of function in multiple organ systems of the body, against a background of a critical illness. Various serious illnesses can induce multiple organ failure, the commonest and most frequent being sepsis, trauma, and shock from any cause. The syndrome semantically has been given various names—sequential organ failure (14), multiple organ failure (11), and multiple system organ failure (12). For reasons stated below, and in agreement with the recommendations of an ACCP/SCCM Consensus Conference on the subject (15), we prefer the term multiple organ dysfunction syndrome (MODS).

The difficulty in precise definition is directly related to defining what failure of function exactly means or signifies in various organ systems of the body. Parameters of one or more organ system failure vary with different investigators. The variability of indices constituting organ failure in different studies, prevents a correct interpretation and comparison between mortality figures and the effects of treatment. There is yet no universally acceptable classification system which defines parameters of organ specific failure. Knaus and colleagues (16–18) developed an Acute Physiologic and Chronic Health Evaluation Score II (APACHE II) system, which is considered by many to be a significant advance in this direction. The APACHE II scoring system gives precise measurements of organ specific failure in 5 systems, viz. the cardiovascular, pulmonary, renal, neurologic and the haematologic systems.

Since the initial description of the APACHE II system, there has been an increasing awareness of the role of the liver in multiple organ dysfunction and failure. Precise measurements defining severe liver cell dysfunction have therefore also been incorporated recently in the APACHE II score (**18**).

A modified APACHE II Criteria for organ system failure, which purports to define 'failure' of each specific organ system is given below in **Table 15.1.1**.

In our opinion the usefulness of the above system lies only in predicting ICU outcome. It merely forecasts well-nigh certain mortality when three or more organ systems have failed for more than three days. Even in this prognostication, there are, as will

Table 15.1.1. Modified APACHE II criteria for organ system failure*

Cardiovascular failure (presence of one or more of the following):
    Heart rate ≤ 54/min
    Mean arterial blood pressure ≤ 49 mm Hg (systolic blood pressure
      ≤ 60 mm Hg)
    Occurrence of ventricular tachycardia and/or ventricular fibrillation
    Serum pH ≤ 7.24 with a $PaCO_2$ of ≤ 40 mm Hg
Respiratory failure (presence of one or more of the following):
    Respiratory rate ≤ 5/min or > 49/min
    $PaCO_2$ ≥ 50 mm Hg
    (A-a) O_2 ≥ 350 mm Hg; (A-a) O_2 = 713 FIO_2 – $PaCO_2$ – PaO_2
    Dependent on ventilator or CPAP on the 2nd day of OSF (i.e., not
      applicable for the initial 24 h of OSF)
Renal failure (presence of one or more of the following)†:
    Urine output ≤ 479 ml/24 h or ≤ 159 ml/8 h
    Serum BUN ≥ 100 mg/100 ml
    Serum creatinine ≥ 3.5 mg/100 ml
Haematologic failure (presence of one or more of the following):
    WBC ≤ 1000/mm³
    Platelets ≤ 20,000/mm³
    Haematocrit ≤ 20 %
Neurologic failure
    Glasgow Coma Score ≤ 6 (in absence of sedation)
    Glasgow Coma Score: Sum of best eye opening, best verbal, and
      best motor responses

Eye	Open: spontaneously (4); to verbal command (3); to pain (2); no response (1)
Motor	Obeys verbal command (6); response to painful stimuli— localizes pain (5); flexion-withdrawal (4); decorticate rigidity (3); decerebrate rigidity (2); no response (1); movement without any control (4)
Verbal	Oriented and converses (5); disoriented and converses (4); inappropriate words (3); incomprehensible sounds (2); no response (1)
	If intubated, use clinical judgement for verbal responses as follows: patient generally unresponsive (1); patient's ability to converse in question (3); patient appears able to converse (5)

Hepatic failure (presence of both of the following):
    Serum bilirubin > 6 mg %
    Prothrombin time > 4 sec over control (in absence of systemic
    anticoagulation)

Abbreviations: WBC, white blood count; BUN, blood urea nitrogen; $PaCO_2$, partial arterial pressure of carbon dioxide; (A-a)O_2, arterial-alveolar difference in oxygen tension; FIO_2, fraction of inspired oxygen; PaO_2, partial arterial pressure of oxygen; CPAP, continuous positive pressure.
*If the patient had one or more of the following during a 24–hr period (regardless of other values), organ system failure(OSF) existed on that day.
†Excluding patients on chronic dialysis prior to hospital admission.
From: Matuschak GM. 1992. Multiple System Organ Failure. In: Principles of Critical Care (Eds Hall JB, Schmidt GA, Wood LDH). pp. 613–636. McGraw-Hill Inc., New York, with permission.

be discussed later, certain important exceptions that need to be carefully considered.

The APACHE III scoring system is a refinement of the APACHE II. Analysis of the APACHE III database of 17,440 patients indicates that a consideration of the features of the acute disease together with detailed physiological mapping perhaps provides better estimates of ICU mortality than the number of organs termed 'dysfunctional'. Also, different combinations of organ dysfunction could result in differing mortality. Thus mortality was 20 per cent in patients with cardiovascular and haematological dysfunction vis à vis 76 per cent in those with cardiovascular and neurological dysfunction.

There are important lacunae in our present day concept of the multiple organ dysfunction syndrome and these lacunae are briefly discussed below:

(**i**) The major criticism is that the parameters defined above take into consideration 'failure' of an organ system at only one point in time, when the disease process is perhaps too advanced to respond to treatment. The syndrome of multiple organ failure is in reality a dynamic ongoing process, so that consideration of disturbed function, without reference to the tempo and natural course of the disease, is unsatisfactory.

Each organ system in this syndrome has to tread a path of increasing dysfunction that can end in terminal failure, from which there is no return. Organ dysfunction may be mild, moderate or severe. Multiple organs may show varying dysfunction. The recognition and significance of early organ dysfunction is not just of academic interest; it may help to initiate treatment at an early stage in the natural history of the syndrome. It is important to test specific variables of function (both singly and in groups or combinations) of different organ systems against outcome. This concept should perhaps be mirrored semantically by using the term multiple organ dysfunction, rather than multiple organ failure. An ACCP/SCCM Consensus Conference which was held in 1991, *defined MODS as the 'presence of altered organ function in an acutely ill patient such that homeostasis cannot be maintained without intervention'* (**15**); we strongly concur with this definition.

(**ii**) A summative conceptual model of organ system dysfunction which merely stresses the number of organs that have critically 'failed' at one given point in time (as in the APACHE II system) is only of statistical prognostic value. It is relevant to consider varying degrees of dysfunction (from the mild to the hopelessly irreversible) in each organ system, at different points in time in the natural history of a critical illness, as also to consider, if possible, the interrelation between these failing organ systems. The Sequential Organ Failure Assessment system (SOFA score) offers to our mind, a clear insight and a more practical and realistic concept for predicting mortality in MODS (**19**) (**Table 15.1.2**).

(**iii**) The definition of organ failure is problematic in certain organ systems. Thus one could accept varying degrees of oliguria and azotaemia to reflect renal dysfunction and failure, just as one would accept a Glasgow coma score of < 6 to denote severe dysfunction involving the neurological system. But what constitutes dysfunction of the gastrointestinal system? How does one quantitate degree of dysfunction in this system? There is no measurement

Table 15.1.2. The Sequential Organ Failure Assessment (SOFA) score

	SOFA score				
	0	1	2	3	4
Respiration					
PaO$_2$/ FIO$_2$	> 400	≤ 400	≤ 300	≤ 200 with respiratory support	≤ 100 with respiratory support
Coagulation					
Platelets (× 10^3/mm^3)	> 150	≤ 150	≤ 100	≤ 50	≤ 20
Liver					
Bilirubin (mg/dl)	< 1.2	1.2–1.9	2.0–5.9	6.0–11.9	> 12.0
(μg/dl)	< 20	20–32	33–101	102–204	> 204
Cardiovascular					
Hypotension	No hypotension	MAP < 70 mm Hg	Dopamine ≤ 5 or dobutamine (any dose)	Dopamine > 5 or epi ≤ 0.1 or norepi ≤ 0.1	Dopamine > 15 or epi > 0.1 or norepi > 0.1
CNS					
GCS	15	13–14	10–12	6–9	< 6
Renal					
Creatinine					
(mg/dl)	< 1.2	1.2–1.9	2.0–3.4	3.5–4.9	> 5
(μmol/l)	< 110	110–170	171–299	330–440	> 440
or urine output				< 500 ml/day	< 200 ml/day

epi – epinephrine; norepi – norepinephrine.
*Adrenergic agents administered for at least 1 hour (doses given are in μg/kg/min).

today that reflects a breakdown of the mucosal barrier of the gut, permitting intraluminal bacteria and their products access to the portal and systemic circulations. Similarly hepatobiliary dysfunction and poor protein synthesis by the liver may not reflect and may well be dissociated from the phagocytic function of Kupffer cells, or production by the liver cells of inflammatory peptide and lipid mediators that produce far ranging effects in distant organ systems. We are thus abysmally ignorant of measurement of functions that may well play a crucial role in amplifying disturbed function in various organ systems.

(iv) Disturbed function in each organ system may not have equal pathogenetic significance in the evolution of the syndrome. If this be so, the view that the clinical expression of multiple organ dysfunction and its outcome merely depends on the numerical sum of specific organ failures, is simplistic and may not be true. The interdependency and interrelationship of organ systems, and the special importance of factors (related to organ dysfunction) which worsen host defence failure and further impair regulation of immune and inflammatory responses by the host, are crucial to the concept and evolution of the syndrome (**Fig. 15.1.1**).

Aetiology

Numerous reports and our own experience over many years, confirm that sepsis is the main predisposing cause of multiple organ dysfunction (**12, 13, 20–23**). However many causes other than sepsis and septic shock can also result in this syndrome. Trauma and shock from causes other than sepsis are classic examples in which the clinical features of multiple organ dysfunction may exist without any evidence of infection.

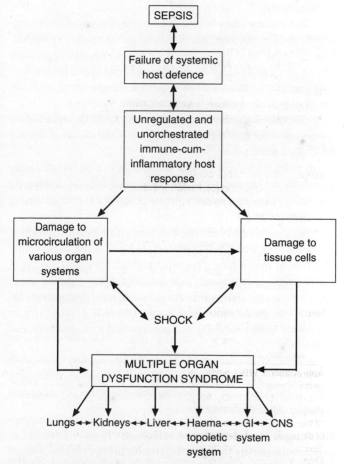

Fig. 15.1.1. Interrelationships between organ systems in the evolution of the multiple organ dysfunction syndrome (MODS).

The ACCP/SCCM consensus conference in our opinion, has given a valuable semantic classification of the terminology related to sepsis. The reader is referred to their description which is detailed in the Chapter on Severe Sepsis and Septic Shock.

In a tropical setting, the aetiology of multiple organ dysfunction is best classified thus:

I. Sepsis. Sepsis by definition is an expression of the systemic inflammatory response syndrome (see Chapter on Severe Sepsis and Septic Shock) due to infection. The commonest infection producing sepsis is a bacterial one, and the commonest sites of bacterial infection producing sepsis and related multiple organ dysfunction in our ICU are pulmonary infections, intra-abdominal sepsis and urosepsis. However, localized infection in the form of an abscess anywhere in the body, as also nosocomial infections, if undetected and untreated, result in sepsis which may evolve into multiple organ failure. Gram-positive and Gram-negative aerobic or anaerobic organisms can produce localized or generalized sepsis, and culminate in multiple organ dysfunction.

II. Tropical infections (24) (see Chapter on Community-acquired Fulminant Infections Requiring Critical Care). These are of special importance in our part of the world.

(a) The most important tropical problem responsible for multiple organ dysfunction and failure, is severe infection due to Pl. falciparum.

(b) Extensive miliary tuberculosis and disseminated haematogenous tuberculosis, particularly in immunocompromised individuals (as those on corticosteroids or other immunosuppressant drugs), can lead to a rapidly evolving multiple organ failure. The diagnosis may be missed if not suspected. The patient is generally too ill to provide sputum for examination.

(c) Tetanus is another important cause. Multiple organ failure is most often due to iatrogenic sepsis, but it could also result directly from the disease per se.

(d) Fulminant typhoid and salmonella infections can occur anywhere in the world, but are commoner in poor developing countries. They can result in a picture of sepsis and multiple organ dysfunction.

A peculiar though uncommon form of Gram-negative infection following the ingestion of contaminated food is also occasionally observed in the tropics. This results after a very brief period of gastrointestinal symptoms, in features of sepsis, culminating in acute lung injury. Liver cell dysfunction and renal dysfunction also often occur. Blood cultures if done early, may grow E. coli or Klebsiella. Early treatment and good critical care generally lead to recovery.

(e) Fulminant amoebic infections characterized by an amoebic abscess of the liver rupturing into the peritoneum and/or the lung or the pleural space, or necrotizing amoebic colitis can also cause multiple organ dysfunction.

III. Fungal, viral, leptospiral infections. These infections can produce the picture of sepsis with multiple organ failure. Fungal infections are assuming increasing importance. They should be particularly kept in mind in immunocompromised patients,

neutropaenic patients, in patients who have received antibiotic therapy and in those on intravenous hyperalimentation.

Fulminant dengue can lead to multiple organ dysfunction through haemorrhagic shock or through bleeding into various organ systems. Haemorrhagic viral fevers like the Ebola virus or the Hanta virus fevers are fortunately confined to specific areas in Africa. They are fulminant and frequently fatal; MODS and death resulting from bleeding and widespread cell necrosis in various organ systems of the body.

Multiple organ dysfunction syndrome in rabies is of academic interest, as patients die within 24 to 72 hours. One patient who was offered intensive care in our unit, survived for 26 days and then succumbed. MODS was observed in this patient (**25**).

Severe leptospiral infections can cause hepatic, renal and CNS dysfunction. ARDS may also occur and is at times due to severe intra-alveolar haemorrhage.

IV. Severe haemorrhage causing shock or shock from any cause can lead to multiple organ dysfunction.

V. Trauma. This is an extremely important cause of multiple organ dysfunction, perhaps second only to sepsis. In hospitals with trauma units, it constitutes the most important cause of MODS. Trauma can cause multiple organ dysfunction and failure, even in the absence of any evidence of infection. When infection does complicate trauma, it adds to the risk of multiple organ dysfunction.

VI. Other conditions not initiated by or due to infection
(a) Important conditions:
   (i) Burns
   (ii) Acute pancreatitis
   (iii) Multiple blood transfusions
   (iv) Poisonings, in particular organophosphorus poisoning
   (v) Following complications during cardiopulmonary bypass surgery
   (vi) Eclampsia
   (vii) Severe vasculitides
   (viii) Acute connective tissue disease
(b) Less common conditions:
   (i) Thrombotic thrombocytopaenic purpura
   (ii) Atrial myxoma
   (iii) Cholesterol emboli syndrome
   (iv) Steven-Johnson syndrome, toxic epidermal necrolysis

It is extremely important to rule out noninfectious causes of MODS, particularly in patients diagnosed as 'sepsis', whose blood cultures are negative and whose source of 'sepsis' is undetermined. In our experience, MODS caused by unusual poisonings, acute vasculitides (particularly acute Wegners granulomatosis), acute connective tissue disease, atrial myxoma, thrombotic thrombocytopaenic purpura, though rare, can be easily missed and wrongly diagnosed as sepsis with MODS.

VII. Severe derangement in the function of any one major organ system can lead in time to dysfunction of multiple organ systems. A classic example is acute liver cell failure, irrespective of its aetiology (e.g. drugs, poisons, viral causes). In a short span of time, multiple organ dysfunction is observed. Similarly, persistent

Table 15.1.3. Incidence and Mortality of Multiple Systems Organ Failure

Study	Patients	ICU population[2]	Incidence n (%)	Mortality Rate per No. of Organ Systems Failed		
				1	2	≥3
Knaus et al. (18)	5815	M, S[2]	819 (15)	40	60	100
ECMO[a]	490	M, S[3]	74 (15.1)	40[1]	55	80–100
Fry et al. (12)	553	S[4]	38 (6.9)	30[1]	60	85–100
Montgomery et al.[b]	207	M, S[3]	22 (10.6)	NE	NE	NE
Pine et al.[c]	106	S[5]	21 (19.8)	10	50	100
Bell et al.[d]	84	M, S[3]	40 (47.6)	40	54	80–100

[1]Multiple systems organ failure (MSOF) defined as severe acquired dysfunction in ≥ 2 organ systems during critical illness or after trauma/major operation.
[2]Random ICU admissions prospectively followed.
[3]Patients at risk for ARDS or with established ARDS prospectively identified.
[4]Emergency surgical patients retrospectively reviewed.
[5]Patients with trauma or intra-abdominal sepsis retrospectively reviewed.
[6]Patients with pre-existing intra-abdominal sepsis prospectively followed.
Abbreviations: M, medical patients; S, surgical patients; NE, not evaluable.
Source as in Table 15.1.1.
[a]National Heart, Lung and Blood Institute, Division of Lung Diseases (1979), Extracorporeal support for respiratory insufficiency: a collaborative study. NIH, Bethesda, MD.
[b]Montgomery AB, Stager MA, Carrico CJ, Hudson LD (1985). Causes of mortality in patients with adult respiratory distress syndrome. Am Rev Respir Dis. 132, 485.
[c]Pine RW, Wertz MJ, Lennard ES et al. (1983). Determinants of organ malfunction or death in patients with intra-abdominal sepsis. Arch Surg. 118, 242.
[d]Bell RC, Coalson JL, Smith JD, Johansson WG Jr (1983). Multiple organ system failure and infection in adult respiratory distress syndrome. Ann Intern Med. 99, 293.

or prolonged severe cardiac dysfunction, or acute renal failure can result in MODS. Again, trauma to the lungs with massive contusions produces a primary respiratory failure. Over a period of time, other organ systems can be secondarily involved.

Epidemiology

As mentioned earlier, the incidence of multiple organ dysfunction syndrome continues to show a steady rise. A busy, efficient ICU which is equipped with good life-support systems and is engaged in looking after critically ill patients, will have a high incidence of MODS. The incidence and mortality rate in the West is illustrated in **Table 15.1.3**. If multiple system organ failure (MSOF) is defined as severe acquired dysfunction in at least two organ systems lasting for at least 24 to 48 hours during the course of a critical illness, infection or injury, then MSOF complicates 7 per cent—15 per cent of all ICU admissions in the West (**12, 18**). We have noted that approximately 10 per cent of all the admissions in our ICU develop MSOF.

Natural History and Clinical Features

Sepsis, severe trauma or ischaemia to tissues, shock from any cause and severe inflammation as in acute pancreatitis, are important causes of multiple organ dysfunction and failure. In these conditions, the natural history of multiple organ dysfunction syndrome (MODS) in an ICU setting, may evolve through the following 4 phases—shock, resuscitation, a hypermetabolic phase, and finally the clinical evolution of multiple organ dysfunction, which culminates either in death or recovery. This need not however always be so. Polytrauma, sepsis, ischaemia to a limb and even pancreatitis can result from the very start in the systemic inflammatory response syndrome, progressing to a slow or quickly evolving

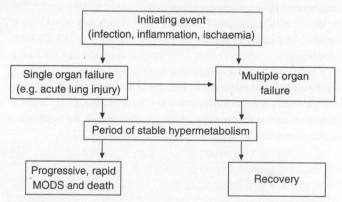

Fig. 15.1.2. Natural history of multiple organ dysfunction syndrome (MODS).

multiple organ dysfunction without causing shock to start with. If shock does however occur as the first phase, resuscitation is generally achieved in a number of patients, provided that infection or any other aetiological factor is controlled and the patients are adequately supported during this phase. In a small group of resuscitated patients the illness next enters a hypermetabolic phase. The natural history of MODS is illustrated in **Fig. 15.1.2**.

The clinical features of the hypermetabolic phase include all the features of the systemic inflammatory response syndrome (SIRS)—fever, leucocytosis, tachycardia and tachypnoea (**15**). In fact, the seeds of multiple organ dysfunction are sown during this stage, or probably even earlier. The hypermetabolic state that characterizes the systemic inflammatory response syndrome may be associated with obvious evidence of a single organ dysfunction (typically the lung or kidney) or very subtle clinical or laboratory findings of early dysfunction of more than one organ system. Recovery can still ensue though the mortality with well-marked single organ dysfunction is between 10 to 30 per cent.

The final stage of multiple organ dysfunction is characterized by sequential or at times, well-nigh concomitant failure of other organ systems. It is almost certain that at least in acute infections and sepsis there is global cellular injury; however different organ systems manifest overt or clinical features of dysfunction at differing times. More often than not, the lung shows the first manifestation of dysfunction. Whether this is due to a special vulnerability of this organ system, or whether this early involvement is more apparent than real, is undecided. Lung dysfunction related to disturbed gas exchange is easily detected both on clinical grounds, and on standard laboratory measurements.

The tempo of the natural history is dependent both on the aetiology and the host response to 'insult' or 'injury'. Multiple organ system dysfunction in our experience, can evolve quickly, and kill the patient within a week despite the best of care and support. At other times, sequential organ failure is observed, and the natural history may extend from 2 to 6 weeks before death or recovery ensue.

The ACCP/SCCM Consensus Conference (15) suggested that MODS 'develops by 2 relatively distinct, but not mutually exclusive pathways'. Primary MODS is due to direct injury or insult to an organ system. Organ dysfunction occurs early, and is directly due to this insult. Examples of primary MODS due to a direct injury or insult to one organ system include pulmonary injury following inhalation of noxious fumes, or following contusion of the lungs as a result of trauma, coagulopathy induced by multiple blood transfusions, and acute renal shutdown due to drugs. In primary MODS the role of an abnormal and excessive host inflammatory response, both at the onset and during progression of the syndrome, is not so evident as in secondary MODS (**Fig. 15.1.3**).

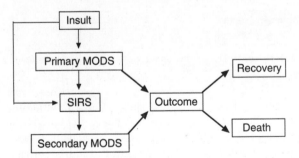

Fig. 15.1.3. Outcome of primary and secondary multiple organ dysfunction syndrome (MODS).

Secondary MODS is due to an indirect injury to one or more organ systems. It is in fact a consequence of the host response, which results in an immunoinflammatory response in organs distant from the site of the initial insult. Secondary MODS is observed in acute infections, sepsis, shock, and trauma or ischaemia to tissues.

Risk factors in the development of the MODS have been arrived at from a study of 5815 randomly selected ICU admissions from 13 United States medical centres, using the APACHE II scoring system (17, 18). The major risk factors for the development of this syndrome are: (i) severity of disease; (ii) presence of sepsis or infection at time of ICU admission; (iii) age > 65 years.

Table 15.1.4. Clinical risk factors for the development of MODS

* Severity of disease (grading according to APACHE II score)
* Presence of sepsis or infection at time of admission
* Age > 65 years
* Severe, persistent shock of any aetiology
* Major, prolonged surgery, trauma, presence of devitalized tissue
* Severe burns
* Persistent hypotension (>24 hours) after admission
* Persistent liver or renal dysfunction
* Uncontrolled diabetes
* Immunocompromised patients
* Malnutrition

Other major risk factors observed in our unit include severe, persistent shock from any cause, persistent hypotension, prolonged major surgery, trauma, burns, pre-existing chronic disease of a major organ system, in particular liver cell dysfunction, immuno-compromised patients, and a background of poor nutrition. These factors are tabulated in **Table 15.1.4**.

The clinical recognition of multiple organ dysfunction is easy to the trained eye. An important feature in the diagnosis of early dysfunction is the recognition of background factors known to cause the development and evolution of this syndrome.

Carrico and colleagues (26) have tabled a brief clinical description of increasing severity of multiple organ dysfunction (**Tables 15.1.5–15.1.8**). The greatest flaw in this tabulated description of Stages I, II, and even III of MODS, is the assumption that each organ system fails at the same pace, and at the same time. This presumption is an exception rather than the rule. In clinical practice just 2 organ systems may show severe or Stage III changes, with barely any involvement of other organ systems for many days—at times right up to the time of death. Yet in some instances, concomitant or a quickly sequential failure of one organ system after another may be observed.

Table 15.1.5. Stage 1 of MODS

General appearance	Normal or mildly restless
Cardiovascular function	Increased volume requirements
Respiratory function	Mild respiratory alkalosis
Renal function	Oliguria, limited diuretic responsiveness
GI function	Distension
Hepatic function	Normal or mild cholestasis
Metabolism	Hyperglycaemia, insulin requirement
CNS	Confusion
Haematology	Variable

Source as in Table 15.1.1 (reference **26**).

Table 15.1.6. Stage 2 of MODS

General appearance	Ill-appearing, restless
Cardiovascular function	Hyperdynamic, volume-dependent
Respiratory function	Tachypnoea, hypocapnia, hypoxaemia
Renal function	Fixed output, minimal azotaemia
GI function	Intolerence to enteral feeding
Hepatic function	Hyperbilirubinaemia, prolonged PT
Metabolism	Severe catabolism
CNS	Lethargy
Haematology	Thrombocytopaenia, leukopaenia, leukocytosis

Source as in Table 15.1.1 (reference **26**).

Table 15.1.7. Stage 3 of MODS

General appearance	Obviously unstable
Cardiovascular function	Shock, decreased cardiac output, oedema
Respiratory function	Severe hypoxaemia, ARDS
Renal function	Azotaemia, indication for dialysis
GI function	Ileus, stress ulceration
Hepatic function	Clinical jaundice
Metabolism	Metabolic acidosis, hyperglycaemia
CNS	Stuporous
Haematology	Coagulopathy

Source as in Table 15.1.1 (reference **26**).

Table 15.1.8. Stage 4 of MODS

General appearance	Moribund
Cardiovascular function	Vasopressor dependent, oedema, rising SvO$_2$
Respiratory function	Hypercapnia, barotrauma
Renal function	Oligo-anuria, instability on dialysis
GI function	Diarrhoea, ischaemic colitis
Hepatic function	Transaminase elevations, deepening jaundice
Metabolism	Muscular wasting, lactic acidosis
CNS	Coma
Haematology	Uncorrectable coagulopathy

Source as in Table 15.1.1 (reference **26**).

Physiopathology (see Chapter on Severe Sepsis and Septic Shock)

Multiple organ dysfunction syndrome (MODS), can be considered to result from a combination of impaired host defences, and inappropriate, uncontrolled host regulation of immunoinflammatory, vascular, neural, metabolic, endocrine responses, which have far-reaching deleterious effects on the organ systems of the body. The body response to 'injury' whether related to sepsis or non-infectious causes, is remarkably similar (**27**). Also the type of organisms causing infection (e.g. Gram-negative bacilli, Gram-positive cocci, viruses, protozoa or fungi), does not make any difference to the final expression of the syndrome. Unfortunately the vicious downward spiral of worsening organ function culminating in death, is not necessarily arrested by identifying and successfully treating the aetiological factor responsible for the syndrome.

The initiating cause of SIRS and MODS can induce:

(a) Direct injury to cells.

(b) Indirect injury through activation of serum factors.

(c) Indirect injury due to cellular activation.

(d) Endothelial injury and dysfunction which worsens inflammation and induces coagulation.

(a) Direct injury to cells

This is illustrated in sepsis when the lipopolysaccharide fraction of the endotoxin of Gram-negative organisms during the period of endotoxaemia, can directly damage endothelial capillary cells in different organs, and perhaps even directly impair tissue cell function.

(b) Activation of serum factors

Activation of complement can result not only from the effects of endotoxin in sepsis, but also from other diverse initiating factors, viz. trauma, ischaemia, or poor generalized tissue perfusion as in shock. Complement kinin-kallikrein coagulation and fibrinolysis cascades can lead to widespread tissue injury (**28, 29**). Complement activated neutrophil mediated injury is also important in the genesis of organ dysfunction.

(c) Cellular activation

Platelets, polymorphonuclear leucocytes, and macrophages when activated can produce and release different mediators, which if uncontrolled can induce and amplify damage to cells in various organ systems of the body. Great attention has been focused on the role of activated mononuclear cells and on the activated macrophage system, both in the systemic inflammatory response syndrome (SIRS), and in the MODS. More than 30 different mediators, produced and released endogenously, have been identified (**30–33**). These can have local and systemic actions. The role of cytokines in the regulation of the inflammatory response of the body to 'injury' is of proven importance. The term 'cytokine' refers to cell derived peptide molecules which cause a target cell to alter its functional activities. The tumour necrosis factor (TNF), interleukin-1, and interleukin-6 are cytokines credited with an important pro-inflammatory role in SIRS and MODS (**34–36**). Platelet activating factor, products of arachidonate metabolism, and in particular metabolites produced through the cyclo-oxygenase pathway, have important effects on the vasculature, and on other mediators (**37–39**). It is just not the effect of individual mediators that matters, but the interaction and inter-relation between them that is important. The polymorphonuclear cell, though a crucial factor in the defence against bacterial invasion, can also play an important role in mediating cell injury. Neutrophils can cause injury to other cells by the release of reactive metabolites to oxygen (superoxides, oxidants), and the release of proteolytic enzymes during degranulation.

(d) Endothelial injury

The role and metabolic activity of the endothelium is also of great importance in the development of SIRS and MODS. Injury to the endothelium can be direct as in endotoxaemia or indirect as in shock. Endothelial injury promotes coagulation and reduces fibrinolysis that ordinarily counters the tendency to coagulation. Previously, 'inflammation' caused by release of cytokines and pro-inflammatory mediators was considered the dominant feature in the cascade of events that led to MODS. The current concept is that inflammation, coagulation and fibrinolysis act together in the disease process. Investigations into the time course and extent of coagulation and fibrinolytic abnormalities in severe sepsis and their relation to endothelial dysfunction have pointed to the crucial role of an imbalance in haemostatic mechanisms. This imbalance results in a coagulopathy and microvascular thrombosis, which may well be a vital driving force in the evolution of progressive multiple organ dysfunction and death (**Fig. 15.1.4**).

In conclusion, the pathogenetic mechanisms responsible for diffuse cellular injury and MODS are as yet poorly understood. The host responses to infection or 'injury' that lead to MODS are dynamic, variable, interconnected and according to a current

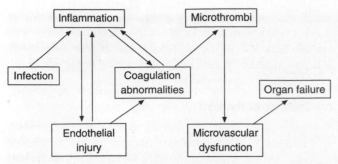

Fig. 15.1.4. Physiopathology of sepsis.

concept, perhaps non-linear in nature (**40**). If this be so, an analytical approach may fail to evaluate the emergent properties of this network or system. This may well explain the lack of response to various anti-mediator therapies observed in numerous clinical trials. It appears that organs 'talk' to each other and that cells within them do likewise at the molecular level. It is this 'communication system' which probably adjusts the balance between health and disease. We need to decipher this 'communication system' if we are to find means to arrest the downward spiral frequently observed in severe multiple organ dysfunction syndrome.

The Role of the Gut and Liver in MODS

What causes an ongoing stimulation of mediator response? This continues to exercise the minds of many researchers in this field. Attention is being increasingly focused on the gastrointestinal tract

as a source that fuels the inflammatory response (**26**). The gut is an effective barrier which prevents bacillary organisms and their products from entering the systemic circulation and injuring the host. It is suggested that in shock, trauma, burns or sepsis, changes occur in this protective barrier, resulting in a bacterial translocation. This allows a continuous uncontrolled release of bacteria, antigens and endotoxin into the lymphatics and the circulation, to which the body responds by the stimulation and release of inflammatory mediators (**41**). The liver may ordinarily 'detoxify' or destroy these products if the Kupffer cell function is adequate. These Kupffer cells represent 70 per cent of the fixed macrophage population of the body, and in addition influence hepatocyte functions such as protein synthesis (**42, 43**). Ischaemia to the gut from any cause also depresses the immunological function of the gut, further enhancing the activity of the bacterial flora within it. Factors predisposing to bacterial translocation are given in **Table 15.1.9.** The sequence of events in the gut-liver axis leading to septicaemia is illustrated in **Fig. 15.1.5.**

Table 15.1.9. Factors predisposing to bacterial translocation

* Change in normal flora
* Impaired cell-mediated immunity
* Severe malnutrition
* Severe shock
* Total parenteral nutrition
* Sepsis—mainly intra-abdominal sepsis
* Severe burns
* Intestinal obstruction

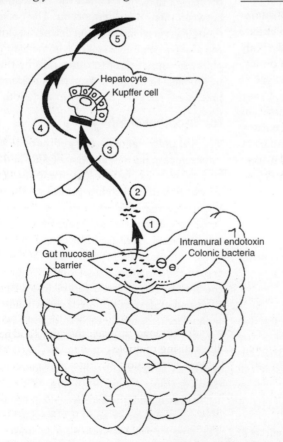

1. Mesenteric ischaemia
2. ↑ Portal venous endotoxaemia
3. Kupffer cell uptake blockade
4. ↓ Endotoxin clearance with spillover
5. Endogenous endotoxaemia

Fig. 15.1.5. Sequence of events in gut-liver axis leading to septicaemia (Source as in Table 15.1.1).

The crucial role of the liver in the pathogenesis of MODS is evident in the above situation. A poorly functioning liver due to current or pre-existing liver disease, or a liver whose Kupffer cells are unable to cope with the load of bacteria or their products caused by translocation, can lead to an overwhelming invasion of the systemic circulation, by the bacteria and their products. These wreak havoc by their direct effect on endothelial cells and tissue cells, or act indirectly through stimulation of inflammatory mediators. Mechanisms that impair hepatocellular function in MODS are detailed in **Table 15.1.10**.

Table 15.1.10. Factors which impair hepatocellular function in MODS

* Significant pre-existing liver cell disease
* Bacterial translocation
* Mesenteric/hepatic ischaemia

Metabolic dysregulation in the SIRS (42)

Metabolism is controlled to a significant extent by inflammatory mediators, and is less responsive to the normal regulatory mechanisms within the body. As a consequence there is:

(i) a rise in energy demands manifested by increase in oxygen consumption, and an increased production of carbon dioxide with metabolic acidosis;

(ii) increase in gluconeogenesis and lipolysis;

(iii) energy production by the process of aerobic glycolysis;

(iv) a severe catabolic state characterized by a loss in lean body mass, that does not respond to exogenous aminoacid or protein administration. There is also a redistribution of the body nitrogen to the areas of active protein synthesis e.g. viscera or wounds (44).

SIRS and MODS are in continuum, and the transition from SIRS to MODS is often characterized by the following features:

(i) Worsening liver function, possibly affected by activated Kupffer cells (42, 43).

(ii) Impairment of extraction and utilization of oxygen at the microcirculatory level, which could be related to capillary damage or to disturbed cellular function at the tissue level. Hypoxia to tissue cells leads to progressive worsening of organ function.

(iii) The clinical expression of the above feature is an increase in the mixed venous oxygen saturation ($S\bar{v}O_2$).

Prognosis

Most investigators show that the greater the number of organ failure, and the longer the duration, the greater is the mortality (**Table 15.1.3**) (12, 18). Knaus and colleagues (17, 18) from a study of their large database, and using the APACHE II scoring system, noted that any single organ system failure lasting for more than one day, resulted in an in-hospital mortality of approximately 40 per cent; persistent failure in two organs over the same period led to a 60 per cent mortality; failure of any three systems led to a mortality approaching 100 per cent. This study also supported the view that a predisposition to MODS, and mortality due to MODS, increased with age (> 65 years). The APACHE III system is an even more recently designed scoring system to objectively assess risk for mortality in critically ill hospitalized patients (45) (see Section

1). It is a complicated system using seventeen physiological variables, and its utility vis-à-vis clinical judgment based on experience, needs to be proved.

There are some important reservations that need to be discussed in relation to the above stated mortality figures.

(a) The outcome of the scoring system in predicting mortality in individual patients admitted to the ICU, can be misleading. The scoring system may be wrongly computed and marked, leading to a nihilistic approach to potentially salvageable patients. Both the APACHE II and the Mortality Prediction Models (MPM) developed by Teres et al. (46) have a misclassification rate as high as 15 per cent.

(b) The dismal outcome predicted holds true for the advanced stage of MODS—i.e. when organ dysfunction and the natural history of the disease are very severe or well beyond the point of return.

(c) Mortality figures with lesser degrees of multiple organ dysfunction, as judged for example by the use of SOFA scores, are not as dismal as those quoted above.

(d) Most patients in the large database studied by Knaus and colleagues (17, 18), had sepsis, shock, trauma, and gross disturbances in tissue perfusion. Most of their experience with sepsis was related to bacterial infections, particularly Gram-negative bacterial infections. A closer study of other aetiological factors in relation to the ultimate prognosis in MODS, is urgently required.

(e) The mortality figures reported in severe multiple organ dysfunction occurring in the West, do not necessarily apply to multiple organ dysfunction and failure occurring in tropical problems (17, 18). A severe degree of multiple organ dysfunction often involving three or more organ systems, is thus often present in Pl. falciparum infections. The organ systems frequently involved are the CNS, the CVS, the kidneys, the haematopoietic system, the lungs and the liver. The mortality with severe dysfunction, in our experience, is about 33 per cent even when more than 3 organs are involved for over a week. In a similar fashion, in our experience, mortality in severe tetanus with multiple organ failure, does not exceed 29 per cent. Mortality in multiple organ failure in disseminated haematogenous tuberculosis lasting for many days, is about 50 per cent. Our last 4 patients with disseminated haematogenous tuberculosis and multiple organ failure, all survived; one patient had evidence of more than four organ system dysfunction for over 3 weeks, and yet recovered. All our patients with severe typhoid infection causing sepsis and multiple organ failure recovered; all our patients with severe Gram-negative infection and multiple organ failure following ingestion of contaminated food, also recovered. Fulminant amoebic infections and necrotizing amoebic colitis causing multiple organ failure, have a comparatively bad prognosis with a mortality rate of 50 per cent.

In our rather small series of 50 patients with different fulminant tropical problems causing MODS, a SOFA score of 16 was associated with a 50 per cent mortality. In contrast, a study by Vincent and colleagues, in which 74 per cent of the patients with four organ failure had bacterial infection, a SOFA score of 16 was associated with greater than 80 per cent mortality (19). The improved mortality in MODS due to tropical problems in our unit could be related to prompt good critical care soon after the onset of symptoms, and the availability of specific therapy for many tropical problems—quinine for malaria, a proven effective management protocol for severe tetanus, anti-TB drugs for disseminated haematogenous tuberculosis, ceftriaxone and quinolones for typhoid, and specific drugs for amoebic and leptospiral infections. However, the present impression that MODS due to tropical infections causes a lesser mortality compared to bacterial infections needs to be confirmed by a larger prospective study.

(f) Any scoring system used for predicting prognosis is arbitary. A scoring system must be stringent, but must also take into consideration milder or more moderate forms of MODS. A larger base of exact variables, and of various combinations of variables of organ dysfunction, in relation to outcome, merits further study to predict a more realistic prognosis of MODS.

(g) A nihilistic approach to severe MODS is against the basic tenet of critical care medicine. Many an individual patient has defied perfectly derived statistical figures, so that he or she survives when clearly expected to die.

Management

The treatment of MODS is unsatisfactory. There are three reasons for this:

(i) The cause or underlying aetiology responsible for initiating MODS, very frequently cannot be eradicated. This is particularly so in patients with abdominal sepsis related to multiple perforations, which cannot be permanently tackled due to technical reasons. Unless the peritoneal leak from a diseased section of the bowel is permanently sealed, no treatment is of avail. The better the support and care offered to such unfortunate patients, the more protracted the agony prior to death. Another example is abdominal sepsis related to acute suppurative pancreatitis. Despite the best surgical techniques available, it may be impossible to totally eradicate all sources of infection in a critically ill individual.

(ii) When the cause of SIRS and MODS can be eradicated, the chances of recovery improve. Even so, a number of patients progress to worsening multiple organ dysfunction, and ultimately die.

(iii) Beyond a certain stage in the natural history of MODS, there is a point of no return, perhaps because the underlying mechanisms responsible for organ injury, are self-perpetuating. Currently, we have no means to arrest this downward trend leading to death. This perhaps explains why eradication of the cause responsible for initiating the pathophysiological cascade, does not necessarily lead to recovery.

The importance of possible prevention of this syndrome is thus self-evident.

Prevention

Only a few basic principles are outlined in this chapter. Perhaps the most important preventive measure, is the rapid, appropriate resuscitation of shock, whatever its aetiology. Since MODS is common in surgical patients, it is wise to optimize organ function before major surgical procedures, as this decreases the incidence of both peri-operative and post-operative complications (47). Accurate monitoring and maintenance of organ function during surgery, and above all good surgical techniques in poor risk patients, go a long way in prevention of disastrous post-operative sequelae. The importance of appropriate management of early pulmonary dysfunction, so that ventilation-perfusion inequalities stand corrected, and adequate arterial oxygen saturation is maintained or restored, is being increasingly realized. One should never hesitate to offer ventilator support to achieve this objective.

Management protocols designed to support or treat one organ system, should not result in possible dysfunction of some other organ system.

Selective gut decontamination using a combination of oral antibiotics (e.g. tobramycin, polymyxin, nystatin, or amphotericin) continue to be used in many critical care units as a means of sterilizing the bowel and reducing the risk of nosocomial pneumonias, and translocation of bacteria from the gut. Though a few prospective studies have shown a decreased risk for nosocomial infections, there has been no improvement in either the incidence or overall mortality of MODS (48–50). Though Rocha and colleagues (51) showed fewer nosocomial infections, there was an increase in resistant bacterial isolates from the treated group, and there was no improvement in the cost-benefit ratio. We have never used selective decontamination of the gut in the treatment of these patients, and are perhaps happier for it.

Treatment

The treatment of an evolved MODS is basically supportive and the following five features need to be emphasized.

   I. Eradication, or at least control of the aetiology responsible for the syndrome.

   II. Maintenance of maximal oxygen transport to the tissues.

   III. Use of activated Protein C in severe sepsis.

   IV. Use of corticosteroids in severe sepsis.

   V. Metabolic support.

   VI. Support to organ systems viewed from an overall perspective.

   VII. Notwithstanding the grim prognosis forecast for patients with three or more organ failure lasting for three days or more, according to the APACHE II scores (17, 18), a nihilistic attitude to these patients is unjustified and ethically wrong.

I. Eradication or control of underlying aetiology. Recovery is impossible if the source or origin of this syndrome remains uncontrolled in a patient. An abscess must thus be drained however ill the patient, or the source of acute peritonitis must be removed in so far as this is possible, or a full thickness burn excision with skin grafting must be undertaken in spite of the patient being critically ill.

II. Maintenance of oxygen transport (see Chapter on Severe Sepsis and Septic Shock and Chapter on ARDS). Though controversial, in patients with sepsis and MODS, oxygen consumption is not always related to tissue needs (as should normally be the case), but is dependent on oxygen delivery. Also, in severe sepsis and MODS, oxygen consumption is reduced in spite of adequate oxygen delivery, suggesting an inability of the tissues to utilize oxygen. The resuscitation of shock should therefore take into paramount consideration the maintenance of maximal oxygen transport. As mentioned in earlier chapters, increase in oxygen transport involves maximizing oxygen content and cardiac output. Oxygen content is increased by (a) maintaining a high arterial PaO_2 (preferably ≥ 70 mm Hg), and an oxygen saturation of over 90 per cent; (b) maintaining the haemoglobin at 11 g/dl. Cardiac output is maximized by taking into consideration the preload, contractility, and afterload, and by treating disturbances in rate and rhythm which may adversely affect the cardiac output. It is advocated that oxygen consumption should be measured, and even if this appears adequate, oxygen delivery (transport) should be further increased till a plateau in oxygen consumption is reached. In other words, the objective is to achieve a supramaximal oxygen delivery so as to ensure that tissues have enough oxygen for their metabolic demands. A good pointer to the need for supramaximal oxygen transport or delivery is the presence of increased lactic acid levels in these patients (see Section on Clinical Shock Syndromes). Pre-and post-operative results in some studies continue to indicate a decrease in mortality, infections, complications, and incidence of MODS when the above principles are put into practice (52–54). There are however limitations to the concept of maximizing oxygen transport, and a recent study does not prove that increasing oxygen transport to supramaximal levels is associated with a reduced morbidity and mortality. This has been discussed in the Chapters on Septic Shock and Acute Lung Injury (ARDS).

III. Use of Human Recombinant Activated Protein C. The use of drotrecogen alpha (activated) has been discussed at length in the Chapter on Severe Sepsis and Septic Shock. The PROWESS study showed that use of activated Protein C resulted in a 6.1 per cent absolute reduction and a 19.4 per cent relative risk reduction in 28 day all cause mortality (55).

IV. Use of Corticosteroids in MODS due to Severe Sepsis. This aspect has been dealt with in the Chapter on Severe Sepsis and Septic Shock. The present consensus is to use hydrocortisone in a dose of 50 mg intravenously 8 hourly, preferably in the early stage of severe sepsis and septic shock for 5 to 10 days.

V. Metabolic Support. Patients with MODS suffer tremendous weight loss and lose a great deal of lean muscle mass during the course of their illness. This problem is indeed more acute when the syndrome evolves against a background of poor nutrition or malnutrition, as is often the case in third world countries. It is however suggested that nutritional support does not alter the course of the underlying disease. Nevertheless our experience with MODS in tropical countries has convinced us that nutritional support reduces both morbidity and mortality. This is perfectly illustrated in the management of fulminant tetanus in patients from a poor strata of society with poor nutritional status (56).

Reduction in morbidity and mortality following good nutritional support has also been reported by other workers (2, 3, 57).

The principles of nutritional support in patients with SIRS and MODS are to some extent being revised. Current concepts are briefly enunciated below:

(a) The objective in these hypermetabolic, hypercatabolic patients is to attain nitrogen equilibrium using nutritional formulae that offer the maximum benefit with the least morbidity (58). It is now believed that too many calories and the wrong combination of caloric substrates can do more harm than good (58).

(b) It is not necessary to use excessive daily total caloric intakes—the recommendations vary greatly. We use 30 to 50 calories/kg body weight with not more than 5 g/kg/day as glucose or carbohydrates. Excessive carbohydrate intake should be avoided because of the higher risks of hepatic lipogenesis and excessive carbon dioxide production.

(c) Fat emulsions (n-6 polyunsaturated fatty acids) are restricted to 0.5–1 g/kg/day. The use of larger quantities of fat emulsions chiefly consisting of n-6 long-chain polyunsaturated fatty acid triglycerides can lead to hypoxaemia, bacteraemia and immune suppression (59–61).

Arachidonic acid is an omega-6 polyunsaturated fatty acid which is produced from linoleic acid and is commonly found in soybean oil and safflower oil emulsions. Products of arachidonic acid metabolism include prostaglandins and leucotrienes. A few leucotrienes produce platelet aggregation and adherence of polymorphs to endothelial cells; excess prostaglandin-E_2 can reduce lymphocyte antigen responsiveness. These factors thus promote further immunosuppression commonly found in SIRS and MODS (58). The use of lipids high in fish oil that contain omega-3 polyunsaturated fatty acids may reduce leucotrines and prostaglandin-E_2 production, as also perhaps reduce the release of interleukin-1 and TNF (38, 62, 63). These should theoretically benefit patients with an evolving MODS.

(d) Administration of proteins should not exceed 1.5–2 g/kg/day (64). The use of preparations with an increased content of branched-chain amino acids has allowed increased nitrogen retention with quick and smooth achievement of nitrogen equilibrium (65–67). This is particularly useful in excessively hypercatabolic states during which the patients may lose more than 10 g nitrogen in the urine.

(e) Good nutritional support should ensure a rising or normal range of hepatic protein synthesis as judged by plasma albumin and transferrin levels.

(f) Administration of vitamins, minerals and trace elements is an integral feature of nutritional support.

Omega-3 fatty acids (found in fish oil), arginine, and dietary nucleotides have been combined into special formulated enteral feeds. A recent multicentric trial has shown significantly fewer acquired infections, a shorter hospital stay, improvement in protein metabolism and in immune responsiveness in patients receiving these specially formulated feeds (68).

The above principles of nutritional support are applicable to both enteral and parenteral feeds. Enteral feeds are unquestionably superior, should be started as early as possible, and are always to be preferred.

VI. Support of organ systems viewed in an overall perspective. It is important to treat the patient as a whole and not to confine treatment to a specific organ system. This is often lost sight of even in very good ICUs, where superspecialists are very common and where each one thinks exclusively of the organ under his charge. Not uncommonly the organ survives, but the patient dies. The relative importance of different problems in a patient, should never be lost sight of; the one posing the maximum danger needs to be considered as a priority bearing in mind the patient as a whole.

VII. A nihilistic approach to MODS when three or more organs are involved, is unjustified and wrong. We predict that the future will show that the prognosis of MODS, to an extent will depend on the predisposing factors in a given patient, the nature and magnitude of the 'insult' or aetiological agent, the nature and magnitude of the host response (about which we are in almost abysmal ignorance), the number and degree of organ involvement and perhaps even the combination of organ systems that are 'dysfunctional'. Our experience in this syndrome with infections peculiar or commoner to our part of the world, justifies this prediction. We also predict that newer scoring systems will be devised to include the less severe forms of MODS. The SOFA scoring system is a step in the right direction.

Future Prospects

It was stated at the outset of this chapter that this syndrome is the end-result of impaired host defences, and the uncontrolled, inappropriate regulation of immune and inflammatory responses by the host. Research continues to be directed at solving the puzzle of the poorly orchestrated inflammatory mediators, that perpetuate the process of increasing organ dysfunction and failure. It is not simply the individual actions of these mediators of destruction, but their interaction and inter-relation which pose problems for research.

Antagonists to important pathogenetic mediators have been tried without significant success. Attempts to control production and release of these mediators are also being made, again without much success.

Monoclonal antibodies have been developed against a number of mediators. Initial studies using human IgM antibodies to endotoxin (derived from the J5 strain of E. coli) showed promising results in Gram-negative bacteraemia and sepsis (**69**). Murine IgM monoclonal antibodies were also shown to be useful in a subset of patients with sepsis—those with septic shock (**70**). However the use of monoclonal antibodies in sepsis or septic shock has not yet gained universal approval, and is not sanctioned for use by the health authorities in the United States. Monoclonal antibodies have also been developed and tried against interleukin-1 and the tumour necrosis factor, again without overall encouraging results (**71–73**). Competitive inhibition of the platelet-activating factor has also been attempted (**32**). Methods and agents to prevent adherence of polymorphs to endothelial cells is also being researched

upon. Tissue injury is often related to oxidants produced by polymorphonuclear leucocytes. Antioxidants used to counter toxic oxygen radicals include allopurinol, iron chelation, ibuprofen, vitamin E and catalase. Their use is limited and of unproven value (**30, 74**).

Modulation of immune function of the host through the use of proper nutrients and nutritional support has already been commented upon.

So far, the only intervention that has been shown to clearly reduce mortality in severe sepsis and MODS is the use of human activated Protein C. This is indeed encouraging; perhaps the use of more than one agent (besides activated Protein C) to counter either mediator or cytokine effects, or to counter the effects of endothelial dysfunction may further improve prognosis. Research continues and there appears perhaps a little more light at the end of the tunnel. For the present, we must rest content by attempting to prevent the syndrome, by promptly treating aetiological factors whenever possible and by offering maximal support to all organ systems as the syndrome evolves.

REFERENCES

1. Tilney NL, Batley GL, Morgan AP. (1973). Sequential organ system failure after rupture of abdominal aortic aneurysms: An unsolved problem in post-operative care. Ann Surg. 178, 117–122.

2. Cerra FB. (1987). Hypermetabolism, organ failure, and metabolic support. Surgery. 101(1), 1.

3. Cerra FB. (1988). The syndrome of multiple organ failure. In: New Horizon III: Cell Injury and Organ Failure (Eds Cerra FB, Bihari D). pp. 1–14. Society of Critical Care Medicine, Fullerton, CA.

4. McMenany RC, Birkhahn R, Oswald G et al. (1981). Multiple systems organ failure I: The basal state. J Trauma. 21(2), 99.

5. Moyer AD, Border JR, Cerra FB et al. (1981). Multiple systems organ failure V: Alterations in the plasma proteins as a function of amino acid infusion in the trauma septic patient: Contrasts between survival and death. J Trauma. 21, 645.

6. Tracey KJ, Fong Y, Hesse DG et al. (1987). Anticachetin/TNF monoclonal antibodies prevent septic shock during lethal bacteraemia. Nature. 330, 662–664.

7. Okusawa S, Gelfand JA, Ikejima T et al. (1988). Interleukin-1 induces a shock-like state in rabbits: Synergism with tumor necrosis factor and the effect of cyclooxygenase inhibition. J Clin Invest. 81, 1162–1172.

8. Wallace JI, Steel G, Whittle BJR et al. (1987). Evidence for platelet-activating factor as a mediator of endotoxin-induced gastrointestinal damage in the rat: Effects of three platelet activating factor agonists. Gastroenterology. 93, 765–773.

9. Sculier JP, Bron D, Verboven N et al. (1988). Multiple organ failure during interleukin-2 and LAK cell infusion. Intensive Care Med. 14, 666–667.

10. Skillman JJ, Bushnell LS, Goldman II et al. (1969). Respiratory failure, hypotension, sepsis and jaundice: A clinical syndrome associated with lethal hemorrhage from acute stress ulceration of the stomach. Am J Surg. 117, 523–530.

11. Eiseman B, Beart R, Norton L. (1977). Multiple organ failure. Surg Gynecol Obstet. 144, 323–326.

12. Fry DE, Pearlstein L, Fulton RL et al. (1980). Multiple system organ failure: The role of uncontrolled infection. Arch Surg. 115, 136–140.

13. Bell RC, Coalson JJ, Smith JD et al. (1983). Multiple organ system failure and infection in the adult respiratory distress syndrome. Ann Intern Med. 99, 293–298.

14. Baue AE. (1975). Multiple, progressive, or sequential systems failure: A syndrome of the 1970's. Arch Surg. 110, 779–781.

15. The ACCP/SCCM Consensus Conference. (1992). Definitions for Sepsis and Organ Failure and Guidelines for the Use of Innovative Therapies in Sepsis. Chest. 101(6), 1644–1655.

16. Knaus WA, Draper EA, Wagner DP et al. (1985). APACHE II: A severity of disease classification system. Crit Care Med. 13, 818.

17. Knaus WA, Draper EA, Wagner DP et al. (1985). Prognosis in acute organ-system failure. Ann Surg. 202, 685.

18. Knaus WA, Wagner DP. (1989). Multiple organ system failure: Epidemiology and prognosis. Crit Care Clin. 5, 221.

19. Vincent JL, de Mendonca A, Cantraine F et al. (1998). Use of the SOFA score to assess the incidence of organ dysfunction/failure in intensive care units: results of a multicenter, prospective study. Crit Care Med. 26 (11), 1793–1800.

20. Montgomery AB, Stager MA, Carrico CJ et al. (1985). Causes of mortality in patients with the adult respiratory distress syndrome. Am Rev Respir Dis. 132, 485.

21. Meakins JL, Wicklund B, Forse RA et al. (1980). The surgical intensive care unit: Current concepts in infection. Surg Clin North Am. 60, 117.

22. Wiles JB, Cerra JB, Siegal JH et al. (1980). The systemic septic response: Does the organism matter? Crit Care Med. 8, 55.

23. Marshall J, Sweeney D. (1990). Microbial infection and the septic response in critical surgical illness: Sepsis, not infection, determines outcome. Arch Surg. 125, 17.

24. Udwadia FE. (1993). Acute lung injury—experience in the tropics. Paper read at the XVIIth World Congress of Chest Diseases, Amsterdam.

25. Udwadia ZF, Udwadia FE, Katrak SM et al. (1989). Human rabies—clinical features, diagnosis, complications and management. Crit Care Med. 17, 834–836.

26. Carrico CJ, Meakins JL, Marshall JC et al. (1986). Multiple organ failure syndrome. Arch Surg. 121, 196–208.

27. Goris RJA, te Boekhorst TPA, Nuytinck JKS, Gimbrere JSF. (1985). Multiple organ failure: Generalized autodestructive inflammation? Arch Surg. 120, 1109–1115.

28. Nuytinck JKS, Goris JA, Real H et al. (1986). Post-traumatic complications and inflammatory mediators. Arch Surg. 121, 886–890.

29. Zimmerman T, Laszik Z, Nagy S. (1989). The role of the complement system in the pathogenesis of multiple organ failure in shock. Prog Clin Biol Res. 308, 291–297.

30. Cipolle MD, Pasquale MD, Cerra FB. (1993). Secondary organ dysfunction: From clinical perspectives to molecular mediators. Crit Care Clin. 9, 261–298.

31. Dinarello CA, Mier JW. (1987). Lymphokines. N Engl J Med. 317, 940–945.

32. Anderson BO, Bensard DD, Harken AH. (1991). The role of platelet-activating factor and its antagonist in shock, sepsis and multiple organ failure. Surg Gynecol Obstet. 172, 415–424.

33. Bone RC. (1991). The pathogenesis of sepsis. Ann Intern Med. 115, 457–469.

34. Dinarello CA. (1984). Interleukin-1 and the pathogenesis of the acute-phase response. N Engl J Med. 311, 1413–1418.

35. Heinrich PC, Castell JV, Andus T. (1990). Interleukin-6 and the active-phase response. Biochem J. 265, 621–636.

36. Beutler B, Cerami A. (1987). Cachectin: more than a tumor necrosis factor. N Engl J Med. 316, 379–385.

37. Cook JA. (1989). Arachidonic acid metabolism in septic shock. In: New Horizon III: Cell Injury and Organ Failure (Eds Cerra FB, Bihari D). pp. 101–124. Society of Critical Care Medicine, Fullerton, CA.

38. Alexander JW, Saito H, Trocki O, et al. (1986). The importance of lipid type in the diet after burn injury. Ann Surg. 204, 1–8.

39. Endres S, Reza G, Kelley VE et al. (1989). The effect of dietary supplementation with omega-3 polyunsaturated fatty acids on the synthesis of interleukin-1 and tumor necrosis factor by mononuclear cell. N Engl J Med. 320, 265–271.

40. Seely AJE, Christou NV. (2000). Multiple organ dysfunction syndrome: Exploring the paradigm of complex nonlinear systems. Crit Care Med. 28(7), 2193–2200.

41. Border JR, Hassett J, LaDuca J et al. (1987). The gut of origin septic states in blunt multiple trauma in the ICU. Ann Surg. 206, 427–448.

42. Keller GA, West MA, Cerra FB et al. (1985). Multiple system organ failure: modulation of hepatocyte protein synthesis by endotoxin-activated Kupffer cells. Ann Surg. 201, 87–95.

43. Cerra FB, West MA, Billiar TR et al. (1989). Hepatic dysfunction in multiple systems organ failure as a manifestation of altered cell-cell interaction. Prog Clin Biol Res. 308, 563–573.

44. Cerra FB. (1992). The Syndrome of Hypermetabolism and Multiple System Organ Failure. In: Principles of Critical Care (Eds Hall JB, Schmidt GA, Wood LDH). pp. 656–665. McGraw-Hill, New York.

45. Knaus WA, Wagner DP, Draper EA et al. (1991). The APACHE III Prognostic System. Risk prediction of hospital mortality for critically ill hospitalized adults. Chest. 100, 1619–1636.

46. Teres D, Lemeshow S, Harris D, Klar J. (1989). Mortality prediction models (MPM) for ICU patients. In: Prognostic scoring systems in the ICU. Problems in critical care (Ed. Farmer JC). p. 585. Lippincott, Philadelphia.

47. Berlauk JF, Abrams JH, Gilmour IJ et al. (1991). Preoperative optimization of cardiovascular hemodynamics improves outcome in peripheral vascular surgery. Ann Surg. 214, 289–299.

48. Kerves AJH, Rommes JH, Mevissen-Verhage EAE et al. (1988). Prevention of colonization and infection in critically ill patients: a prospective, randomized study. Crit Care Med. 16, 1087–1093.

49. Gastinne H, Wolff M, Delatour F et al. (1992). A controlled trial in intensive care units of selective decontamination of the digestive tract with nonabsorbable antibiotics. N Engl J Med. 326, 594–599.

50. Cerra FB, Moddaus MA, Dunn L et al. (1992). Selective gut decontamination reduces nosocomial infection and length of stay but not mortality or organ failure in surgical ICU patients. Arch Surg. 127, 163–169.

51. Rocha LA, Martin MJ, Pita S et al. (1992). Prevention of nosocomial infection in critically ill patients by selective decontamination of the digestive tract: a randomized, double-blind, placebo-controlled study. Intensive Care Med. 18, 398–404.

52. Shoemaker WC. (1985). Hemodynamic and oxygen transport patterns in septic shock: Physiologic mechanisms and therapeutic implications. In: New Horizons: Perspectives in Sepsis and Septic Shock (Eds Sibald W, Sprung C). pp. 203–234. Society of Critical Care Medicine, Fullerton, CA.

53. Shoemaker WC, Appel PL, Kram HB. (1989). Tissue oxygen debt as a determinant of lethal and non-lethal post-operative organ failure. J Crit Care Med. 16, 1117.

54. Eyer SD, Cerra FB. (1987). Cost-effective use of the surgical intensive care unit. World J Surg. 11, 241.

55. Bernard GR, Vincent JL, Laterre PF et al. (2001). Efficacy and safety of recombinant human activated protein C for severe sepsis. N Engl J Med. 344 (10), 699–709.

56. Udwadia FE, Lall A, Udwadia ZF et al. (1987). Tetanus and its complications: intensive care and management in 150 Indian patients. J Epidemiol Infections. 99, 675–684.

57. Cerra FB, Siegal JH, Border JR. (1979). The hepatic failure of sepsis: Cellular vs. substrate. Surgery. 86, 409.

58. Beal AL, Cerra FB. (1994). Multiple Organ Failure Syndrome in the 1990s. Systemic Inflammatory Response and Organ Dysfunction. JAMA. 271(3), 226–233.

59. Hunt CE, Gora P, Inwood RJ. (1981). Pulmonary effects of intralipid: the role of intralipid as a prostaglandin precursor. Prog Lipid Res. 20, 199–204.

60. Fraser I, Neoptolemos J, Darby H et al. (1984). Effects of intralipid and heparin on human monocyte and lymphocyte function. JPEN J Parenter Enteral Nutr. 8, 381–384.

61. Hamawy KJ, Moldawer LL, Georgieff M et al. (1985). Effect of lipid emulsions in reticuloendothelial system function in the injured animal. JPEN J Parenter Enteral Nutr. 9, 559–565.

62. Billiar TR, Bankey PE, Svingen BA. (1988). Fatty acid intake and Kupffer cell function: fish oil alters eicosanoid and monokine production to endotoxin stimulation. Surgery. 104, 343–349.

63. Kinsella JE, Lokesh B. (1990). Dietary lipids, eicasanoids and the immune system. Crit Care Med. 18, S94–S113.

64. Ronco JJ, Fenwick JC, Wiggs BR et al. (1993). Oxygen consumption is independent of oxygen delivery by dobutamine in septic patients who have normal or increased plasma lactate. Am Rev Respir Dis. 147, 25–31.

65. Cerra FB, Mazuski JE, Teasley K et al. (1983). Nitrogen retention in critically ill patients is proportional to the BCAA load. Crit Care Med. 11, 775–778.

66. Cerra FB, Mazuski JE, Chute E et al. (1984). Branched chain metabolic support: a prospective randomized double-blind trial in surgical stress. Ann Surg. 199, 286–291.

67. Cerra FB, Blackburn G, Hirsch J et al. (1987). The effect of stress level, amino acid formula and nitrogen dose on nitrogen retention in traumatic and septic stress. Ann Surg. 205, 282–287.

68. Cerra FB, Lehman S, Konstantinides N et al. (1991). Improvement in immune function in ICU patients by enteral nutrition supplemented by arginine, RNA and Menhaden oil is independent of nitrogen balance. Nutrition. 7, 193–199.

69. Ziegler EJ, Fisher CJ, Sprung L et al. (1991). Treatment of gram-negative bacteraemia and septic shock with HA-IA human monoclonal antibodies against endotoxin: a randomized, double-blind placebo-controlled trial. N Engl J Med. 324, 429–436.

70. Greenman RL, Schein RMN, Martin MA et al. (1991). Controlled clinical trial of E-5 murine monoclonal IgM antibody to endotoxin in the treatment gram-negative sepsis. JAMA. 266, 1097–1102.

71. Dinarello CA. (1991). Interleukin-1 and Interleukin-1 antagonism. Blood. 77, 1627–1652.

72. Exley AR, Cohen J, Buurman W et al. (1990). Monoclonal antibody to TNF in severe septic shock. Lancet. 335, 1275–1277.

73. Fisher CJ, Opal SM, Dhaimaut JF et al. (1993). Influence of an anti-tumor necrosis factor monoclonal antibody on cytokine levels in patients with sepsis. Crit Care Med. 21, 318–327.

74. Revhaug A, Hamish RM, Manson JM et al. (1988). Inhibition of cyclo-oxygenase attentuates the metabolic respose to endotoxin in humans. Arch Surg. 123, 162–170.

Renal Dysfunction in the Critically Ill

Acute Renal Failure

General Considerations (1)

The kidneys play a major role in fluid and electrolyte balance, and help to keep the H^+ ion concentration of arterial blood within physiological limits. Renal dysfunction is common in the critically ill, and when present the morbidity and mortality are both significantly increased. Early detection of renal dysfunction, measures to correct the early dysfunction if this is at all possible, and/or measures to prevent further deterioration in renal function, are of great importance in ultimate prognosis. Delay in recognition and management often results in increasing renal failure requiring dialysis till such time as kidney function improves.

An absolute requisite for the diagnosis of renal dysfunction or failure is an elevated plasma creatinine concentration. An early sign of renal dysfunction and impending failure is a fall in the urine output. Oliguria is defined as a fall in urine output to < 400 ml/ 24 hours, or a fall in urine output to < 20 ml/hr. *Though oliguria is a frequent accompaniment of renal failure, the latter can also occur and progress (with increasing plasma creatinine levels), in the presence of a normal urine output.*

This chapter is not a treatise on acute renal failure. It basically stresses the approach to diagnosis and management of oliguria with impending or progressive renal dysfunction in ill individuals in an ICU setting. It deals briefly with the principles in the medical management and in the management by dialysis, of established severe acute renal failure. It touches upon important clinical syndromes characterized by acute progressive renal failure; these are invariably critical illnesses demanding intensive care. Finally, the chapter concludes with a brief section on critical illnesses requiring intensive care in patients with underlying chronic renal failure.

Causes of Oliguria (2, 3)

Oliguria with a rise in serum creatinine, and non-protein nitrogenous (NPN) products can be due to prerenal causes, intrinsic renal disorders, and postrenal conditions characterized by obstruction to the renal outflow system (**Table 15.2.1**).

Table 15.2.1. Causes of acute renal failure

1. Prerenal Causes
   * Hypovolaemia – fluid or blood loss
                    – sequestration of fluid into third space
   * Loss of effective circulating volume in distributive shock (sepsis, anaphylaxis)
   * Low-output syndromes with poor pump function and low cardiac output
2. Intrinsic Renal Diseases
   * Acute tubular necrosis (after shock, sepsis, severe haemolysis, or surgery)
   * Toxic factors (drugs, haeme pigment, contrast media)
   * Acute interstitial nephritis
   * Acute glomerulonephritis; acute pyelonephritis
   * Vascular causes (vasculitis, obstruction to large vessels, TTP, DIC, HUS, malignant hypertension)
   * Crystal precipitation (acute uric acid nephropathy)
   * Plasma cell dyscrasias (e.g. tubules obstructed by myeloma protein)
3. Postrenal Causes
   * Ureteral or bladder outlet obstruction
   * Traumatic rupture of the bladder with extravasation of urine

Prerenal Causes

Prerenal causes act by inducing a fall in perfusion pressure within the vessels perfusing the kidneys. Important prerenal causes are hypovolaemia, low-output syndromes related to acute heart failure and severe vasodilatation with a reduction in the arterial blood pressure and perfusion pressure within the kidneys.

Hypovolaemia has been discussed in an earlier chapter (see Chapter on Fluid and Electrolyte Disturbances in the Critically Ill). It can be due to loss of extracellular fluid as in vomiting, diarrhoea, burns, blood loss. Hypovolaemia can also result from sequestration of fluid in the 'third compartment' as in intestinal obstruction, pancreatitis, peritonitis, post intra-abdominal surgery, crush injuries to muscles. A fall in effective circulating volume also occurs in distributive shock (sepsis, anaphylaxis), characterized by peripheral vasodilatation, hypotension and a fall in renal perfusion.

Poor pump function of the heart, due to any aetiology, is also an important cause of pre-renal azotaemia.

Intrinsic Renal Disorders

The *three important renal disorders* causing acute oliguric renal failure (AORF) in an ICU setting are—acute tubular necrosis (ATN), drug toxicity particularly related to the use of aminoglycosides, and acute interstitial nephritis, either allergic or infectious in aetiology. The important causes of ATN observed in our unit are shock, severe sepsis, major surgery and acute haemolysis. Acute severe haemolysis results in ATN because of the toxic effect of haeme pigments on renal tubular cells, blockage of renal tubules by pigment casts, and impaired perfusion of kidneys. Acute glomerulonephritis is also an important cause of AORF, but is rare in an intensive care setting. Acute fulminant pyelonephritis is at times a feature of urosepsis and 'results in acute renal failure. Renal vascular disorders causing acute renal failure, though uncommon in the ICU, are easily missed. They include obstruction to large renal vessels (embolism or thrombosis) or to small vessels as in vasculitis of any aetiology, thrombotic thrombocytopaenic purpura (TTP), DIC, haemolytic uraemic syndrome (HUS), malignant hypertension. In oncology units, acute oliguric renal failure is observed following precipitation of uric acid within urinary tubules causing an acute uric acid nephropathy. Plasma cell dyscrasias (in particular myeloma) may present with quickly evolving renal failure due to obstruction of renal tubules by protein deposits.

Drug toxicity is an important cause of acute renal failure (ARF) in the ICU. Important drugs that can do so are listed in **Table 15.2.4**. The need for taking a proper history of drugs the patient has received cannot be over-stressed. Radiocontrast agents, aminoglycosides, amphotericin, nonsteroidal anti-inflammatory agents (NSAIDS), and ACE inhibitors are the drugs most frequently observed to precipitate ARF in our unit. NSAIDs and ACE inhibitors induce a form of prerenal azotaemia. NSAIDs inhibit cyclooxygenase, leading to a depletion of eicosanoids which normally counteract the constrictive effect on afferent arteriolar tone due to increased renal adrenergic drive and lipid derived constrictors. Severe afferent arteriolar vasoconstriction in ARF can occur particularly in the presence of hypotension, volume depletion, sepsis or heart failure. ACE inhibitors reduce angiotensin II levels, leading to a lowering of renal perfusion pressure and a dilatation of efferent arterioles. This lowers glomerular filtration pressure and causes ARF, particularly in patients with bilateral renal artery stenosis or in unilateral renal artery stenosis with a contralateral diseased kidney. Generally, the prerenal azotaemia induced by NSAIDs and ACE inhibitors is reversible if the drug is promptly stopped.

Postrenal Conditions

Postrenal disorders include obstructive lesions within the renal outflow system. They include papillary necrosis, ureteric obstruction by calculi or retroperitoneal fibrosis or tumours, and bladder outlet obstruction. Extravasation of urine as after rupture of the bladder, is another postrenal disorder presenting with acute oliguric renal failure. Obstruction is an uncommon but important cause of acute oliguric renal failure, and should be considered in all patients who are known to have a solitary functioning kidney.

Bedside Approach to the Evaluation of Acute Renal Failure in the ICU (Table 15.2.2)

Acute renal failure generally comes to the attention of the physician either because of the finding of a raised serum creatinine or blood urea nitrogen (BUN) level or because of oliguria. It needs to be however re-stressed that all forms of ARF—prerenal, renal, postrenal can be non-oliguric in nature. A normal urine output is therefore not a reliable indicator of adequate renal function. Non-oliguric renal failure is particularly observed in ARF precipitated by the use of aminoglycosides. The approach to diagnosis and management in both oliguric and non-oliguric renal failure is similar. A patient with ARF who is non-oliguric is at an advantage compared to the oliguric patient, because fluid and electrolyte management is easier. There is a greater leeway for fluid administration and lesser danger of fluid overload.

Table 15.2.2. Evaluation of a patient with acute renal failure

1. Thorough clinical examination with maintenance of input/output charts
2. History of administration of nephrotoxic drugs or nephrotoxic insult in recent past
3. Urine analysis
4. Serum creatinine and BUN levels; creatinine clearance test
5. Other urinary and blood indices of renal function—urine osmolality, urinary sodium (mEq/l), urine/plasma creatinine, BUN/serum creatinine, fractional excretion of sodium
6. Evaluation of circulatory haemodynamics
7. Imaging studies—particularly for kidney size, urinary stones, obstructive uropathy, perinephric/intrarenal abscesses
8. Renal biopsy (in rare selected problems)

I. Clinical Evaluation

A clinical evaluation is always of utmost importance.

(a) The background factors and the aetiology of oliguria with azotaemia should be ascertained through a careful history, a thorough clinical examination and other relevant investigations. Intake/output charts should be evaluated. The role of nephrotoxic drugs should be kept in mind. The history of a recent hypotensive episode, or a recent nephrotoxic insult, e.g. the use of a contrast dye in radiological investigations, are important pointers to the cause and nature of acute renal failure.

(b) In a patient admitted to the ICU with a rise in serum creatinine, it is important to determine whether the renal failure is acute or chronic, or acute on chronic. A sudden oliguria always points to an acute disturbance in renal function.

(c) It is vital to determine whether oliguria with azotaemia is due to prerenal factors, due to intrinsic renal disease or due to postrenal causes. All prerenal causes of oliguria, if left uncorrected, have the potential to cause intrinsic renal damage (ATN). Hence the presence of prerenal aetiological factors, by no means excludes intrinsic renal damage. For this a careful evaluation of the urine should be performed as outlined below.

Urine Evaluation

When diminished renal perfusion is the cause of oliguria with azotaemia, there is an increase in sodium reabsorption by the renal tubules with a marked decrease in urinary sodium excretion to usually below 20 mEq/l (4). An examination of urinary sodium concentration of a random urine sample is therefore of great help.

Conversely, intrinsic renal disease causing acute oliguric renal failure is associated with impaired sodium absorption by the renal tubules, with an increase in the urinary excretion of sodium. A random urine sample in these patients generally shows a urine sodium concentration of above 40 mEq/l.

There are however certain important provisos to the above statements. A urinary sodium of 40 mEq/l or more can occur in prerenal oliguria and azotaemia, if the effect of a recently administered diuretic persists, or in patients who have prior renal dysfunction. Elderly patients can also sometimes show a high urine sodium (40 mEq/l) in the presence of diminished renal blood flow.

The urinary sodium concentration therefore is an important pointer, but should not be considered in isolation in the diagnosis of oliguric acute renal failure due to intrinsic renal disease (4).

Fractional Excretion of Sodium (FENa)

The fractional excretion of sodium represents the fraction of sodium filtered at the glomerulus that is excreted in the urine (5). It is determined by comparing the urinary sodium clearance to the urine creatinine clearance.

$$FENa = \frac{U/P\,Na}{U/P\,Cr} \times 100$$

where U is the urinary concentration and P the plasma concentration. In prerenal azotaemia, the FENa is < 1 per cent; in acute renal failure it is > 2 per cent.

The FENa is the best and most reliable single urinary test for acute renal failure (5, 6), but again should not be considered in isolation. AORF following the use of contrast agents and myoglobinuria can occur with the FENa < 1 per cent (5).

Microscopic Examination of the Urine

Microscopic examination of the sediment of a freshly voided urine sample, is elementary but of great value.

(i) The presence of epithelial cells and of epithelial cell casts (in particular muddy brown casts), suggests acute tubular necrosis.

(ii) In prerenal azotaemia the urinary sediment shows non-specific hyaline casts or finely granular casts.

(iii) In acute interstitial nephritis the urine shows many white blood cells and white blood cell casts.

(iv) In acute glomerulonephritis the urine contains albumin, plenty of red blood cells, white blood cells, and above all red blood cell casts.

(v) The presence of bacteria with a positive culture showing a high colony count, points to infection in the urinary tract.

(vi) Modest proteinuria (up to 1 g/dl) is common in many forms of acute renal failure, but proteinuria in the nephrotic range (> 3.5 g/dl) is most often due to glomerular disease, except when associated with Bence-Jones proteinuria in multiple myeloma. Urine protein electrophoresis will distinguish between Bence-Jones protein and albumin, in a suspected case of multiple myeloma.

II. Determining Degree of Renal Dysfunction

In patients with acute renal failure it is important to determine the degree of renal dysfunction and also to determine the changes in the internal milieu brought about by renal dysfunction.

(a) *Blood Creatinine Levels.* This is the simplest and most valuable guide to renal dysfunction. In critical care medicine, a rise in creatinine levels (> 1.6 mg/dl) signifies renal dysfunction. Even so, the normal glomerular filtration rate must be reduced by about half before there is a significant rise in the serum creatinine levels. Modest degrees of renal dysfunction may thus go undetected if a creatinine clearance test is not done. During the acutely evolving phase of renal failure, serum creatinine levels may rise by 2 mg/dl every 24 hours. More rapid increases can occur in rhabdomyolysis. A misleading increase in serum creatinine without a fall in the glomerular filtration rate may occur when cephalosporin or certain ketones (acetoacetate), interfere with the calorimetric method used for its measurement (7). Cimetidine and trimethoprim-sulfamethoxazole compete with tubular secretion of creatinine and result in increased creatinine values without a fall in the glomerular filtration rate (7).

(b) *Blood Urea.* Urea is the major nitrogen containing metabolite of protein metabolism and is excreted chiefly by the kidneys. 35–50 per cent of filtered urea is reabsorbed by the tubules. In the presence of hypovolaemia or decreased renal perfusion from any prerenal cause, the reabsorption of urea can increase to as high as 90 per cent. In contrast, creatinine is not reabsorbed by the renal tubular cells. When measured as blood urea nitrogen (BUN) in mg/dl, the normal ratio of BUN to creatinine in serum is 10:1. An increase in this ratio to 20:1 or more, points to prerenal azotaemia. Blood urea levels are also related to the amount of protein intake and degree of protein catabolism. Inadequate caloric intake, corticosteroid administration, and the stress of a hypermetabolic critical illness can result in endogenous protein catabolism, and increase in blood urea levels even with normal renal function. Gastrointestinal haemorrhage with resulting absorption of blood protein is another important cause of elevated blood urea levels.

(c) *Creatinine Clearance Test.* Creatinine clearance test using a 24 hour urine collection is a reliable index of renal function.

Creatinine Clearance (ml/min) =

$$\frac{Urine\ Creatinine\ (mg/dl) \times Urine\ vol\ (ml/min)}{Serum\ Creatinine\ (mg/dl)}$$

(d) *Other Urinary and Blood Indices.* Other urinary and blood indices are often used to distinguish between prerenal azotaemia and acute oliguric renal failure. The urine osmolality, the urine/plasma urea nitrogen ratio, and the urine/plasma creatinine ratio increase in prerenal azotaemia, whereas urine sodium and the fractional excretion of filtered sodium remain low. The indices which help to distinguish between prerenal azotaemia and acute oliguric renal failure are listed in **Table 15.2.3**.

(e) *Serum Electrolytes.* Estimation of serum sodium, potassium,

Table 15.2.3. Urinary indices which differentiate prerenal azotaemia from oliguric acute renal failure

Urinary Indices	Prerenal Azotaemia	Oliguric Acute Renal Failure
* Urine Osmolality (mOsm/kg H_2O)	> 500	< 350
* Urine Sodium (mEq/l)	< 20	> 40
* Urine/plasma urea nitrogen	> 8	< 3
* Urine/plasma creatinine	> 40	< 20
* Fractional excretion of Na	< 1	> 1

chloride, bicarbonate, calcium, magnesium, phosphate, should be done. Their monitoring forms an important feature in the management of acute renal failure.

(f) *Arterial pH and Blood Gas Analysis* should always be done to determine the presence and degree of acidosis, as also to determine any abnormality in blood gas exchange within the lungs.

III. Evaluating Circulatory Haemodynamics

The haemodynamics of the circulation should be carefully evaluated. A central venous line is invariably inserted in these patients and provides a guide to the central venous pressure. In oliguric patients, it is important that the filling pressures are maintained at an optimal level. When there is doubt about hypovolaemia with low left-sided filling pressures contributing to azotaemia, a Swan-Ganz catheter may need to be inserted to determine the pulmonary capillary wedge pressure. A volume load can then be so adjusted as to keep this wedge pressure around 12–15 mm Hg.

IV. Imaging Studies

(a) An ultrasound imaging is invaluable for two reasons: (i) It gives the size of the kidneys—small kidneys suggest underlying chronic renal disease; (ii) it can pick up ureteric obstruction and hydronephrosis, and is invaluable in the diagnosis of oliguria due to postrenal causes; (iii) in fulminant urinary infections, an ultrasound examination helps in the detection of a renal or perinephric abscess.

(b) An abdominal X-ray demonstrates the presence of radioopaque kidney stones and may pick up other associated diseases within the abdomen.

(c) Imaging studies involving the use of contrast dyes are contraindicated in acute renal failure, because of the toxicity of the contrast dye to the kidneys. A retrograde pyelography may however be necessary in patients with obstruction to the ureters, resulting in postrenal oliguria and renal failure. A CT study may help to localize a perinephric abscess, or diagnose a fulminating pyelonephritis.

V. Renal Biopsy

We never do a renal biopsy in critically ill patients with acute renal failure except (a) when there is strong suspicion of acute vasculitis, or a rapidly evolving autoimmune disorder; (b) in patients with acute tubular necrosis in whom renal failure fails to resolve within 6–8 weeks.

Management Protocol For Acute Oliguria in Critically Ill Patients

(a) It is important to ensure that urinary catheters in critically ill patients do not get blocked, thereby giving a false impression of oliguria.

(b) It is vital to ensure that the haemodynamic status of the patient is satisfactory. He should have a normal circulating volume, normal filling pressures in the right and left heart chambers, and an adequate cardiac output. In critically ill patients, we at times need to ascertain this with a Swan-Ganz catheter and give enough volume infusion to maintain the pulmonary capillary wedge pressure around 15 mm Hg. The 'pump' in other words must be optimally primed.

If oliguria persists despite the pump being fully primed, and if facilities so exist, the cardiac output should be measured. If this is found to be low, the cause of this should be ascertained. Cardiac output can be increased by using inotropic support with dopamine (5–10 µg/kg/min) or dobutamine (10–20 µg/kg/min); at times both can be used together.

If the cardiac output is normal or high, but the patient is hypotensive as with sepsis or other forms of distributive shock, the vascular resistance is increased with dopamine at 10–15 µg/kg/min or the use of noradrenaline.

(c) Whilst the patient's haemodynamic state is brought to as optimal a level as possible, a clinical assessment and the urinary evaluation described earlier, is simultaneously carried out to determine if there is any intrinsic renal damage causing acute renal failure. The importance of estimating urinary sodium concentrations and FENa values has already been emphasized.

The persistence of oliguria after normal filling pressures and normal haemodynamics have been restored, suggests acute renal failure. An attempt is often made in many units to increase the urine flow by trying the following measures:

(i) Use of low-dose intravenous dopamine at 2–3 µg/kg/min to stimulate dopaminergic receptors and thereby increase urine flow (**8**). It used to be believed that low-dose dopamine could also increase renal blood flow, but the evidence for this in critically ill patients is lacking (**9**).

(ii) Furosemide 100–200 mg is either given intravenously or as a continuous infusion of 10–40 mg/hour over 24 hours. At times the combination of furosemide and low-dose dopamine may initiate a satisfactory diuresis (**10, 11**).

(iii) Mannitol infusions act through an osmotic diuresis and have also been tried to promote increased urine flow.

Saline infusions designed to maintain a urine output > 150 ml/hour have been found to be useful in acute rhabdomyolysis. Mannitol (together with intravenous sodium bicarbonate) is often used to add to this diuretic effect, in the hope of preventing blockage and damage to renal tubules.

There is however no evidence to show that either low-dose dopamine or intravenous furosemide or mannitol infusions can prevent, or influence for the better the natural course of acute renal failure (**12–14**). In fact it has been suggested that the incidence of acute renal failure is increased in some patients at risk (**15**).

The only preventive measures for acute tubular necrosis in a critical care setting, are the prompt correction of pre-renal factors before ischaemic damage to the kidney occurs, the avoidance of nephrotoxic drugs and of radiocontrast dyes for imaging purposes.

Even so, both low-dose dopamine infusion and intravenous furosemide can in some patients promote a satisfactory diuresis in oliguric patients converting an oliguric ARF to a non-oliguric one. This is a decided advantage as it allows easier management of fluids, electrolytes and nutrition in these patients. If this diuretic effect is not observed the drugs should be withdrawn.

Further management now lies in offering circulatory support and maintaining the haemodynamic state and internal milieu as close to normal as possible, till such time as renal function improves and diuresis starts. If renal function continues to worsen and if dangerous changes are observed in fluid, electrolyte or acid-base balance, dialysis becomes necessary.

Drugs in Patients with Persistent Oliguria

All nephrotoxic drugs should be withheld. Aminoglycosides in particular should always be stopped right at the start when oliguria and azotaemia first appear. Imipenem and aztreonam are equally effective in countering Gram-negative sepsis including that due to Ps. pyocyaneus. In systemic fungal infections there is no substitute for amphotericin B, but the drug can be stopped temporarily, and then restarted at half or quarter of the usual dose. A list of drugs which are preferably stopped or not administered in acute renal failure is given below in **Table 15.2.4.**

Table 15.2.4. Drugs which should be discontinued in acute renal failure (alternative drugs in parenthesis)

A. Nephrotoxic drugs
 * Aminoglycosides (Imipenem/Aztreonam)
 * Amphotericin B (Fluconazole)
 * Pentamidine (Trimethoprim-Sulphamethoxazole)
B. Drugs that can cause allergic interstitial nephritis
 * Penicillin and allied drugs (Erythrocin/Vancomycin)
 * Cephalothin (Vancomycin)
 * Trimethoprim-Sulphamethoxazole (Pentamidine)
 * Cimetidine (Sucralfate, other antacids)
 * Avoid radiocontrast dyes for imaging
C. Drugs impairing intrarenal flow (afferent arteriolar constriction)
 * Non-steroidal Anti-inflammatory Drugs (Paracetamol)
 * ACE inhibitors (Calcium channel blockers)

If nephrotoxic drugs must need be administered, their dosage is modified as per the creatinine clearance. A list of common ICU drugs excreted by the kidneys, with modifications in their dose, is detailed in **Table 13.4.5.**

Management of Persistent Oliguric Acute Renal Failure

The principles of management are:
 (i) To maintain body homeostasis with particular reference to fluid, electrolyte and acid-base balance.
 (ii) To maintain nutrition.

(iii) To recognize and treat complications occurring in the course of acute renal failure.
(iv) To use specific treatment for some forms of acute glomerulonephritis.
(v) To use dialysis when indicated, and to decide on the type of dialysis best suited to the patient.

(i) Maintaining Homeostasis

Acute tubular necrosis (ATN) is the commonest form of oliguric acute renal failure observed in critical care units. The oliguric phase may last for a period ranging from a few days to as long as 4 to 6 weeks. This is followed by a period or phase of relative diuresis.

Fluid Balance

The greatest danger is fluid overload. The fluid intake should not exceed the urine output plus the fluid output from other sources (e.g. nasogastric suction, fluid loss from diarrhoea, sweating, surgical drains), plus the insensible water loss. In a well-nigh anuric patient who has no fluid loss from other sources, the fluid intake should not exceed 500–700 ml.

In a patient who already has been in oliguric renal failure some days prior to admission to the ICU, it is often impossible to determine the degree of fluid imbalance present prior to hospitalization. In these patients, as also in critically ill patients in whom acute renal failure is a complication of severe underlying disease (e.g. acute lung injury or sepsis), it is often necessary to measure the filling pressures of the right and left heart through a Swan-Ganz catheter. Fluid intake should then be adjusted to ensure that the left-sided filling pressure (as measured by the pulmonary capillary wedge pressure) does not exceed 15 mm Hg.

Critically ill patients may require large quantities of intravenous fluids—for hyperalimentation, administration of vasopressors and antibiotics. Fluid overload is certain in these patients and methods involving dialysis are then necessary to ensure that fluid overload does not occur.

Sodium Balance

Sodium balance is maintained by replacing the sodium that is lost. Urinary losses of sodium can be exactly measured by 24 hour collection of urine. An approximate method of estimating urinary sodium loss is by determining the sodium concentration in a random sample and multiplying this by the urine volume over 24 hours. Gastrointestinal losses are difficult to measure but can be roughly estimated. The approximate sodium content of body fluids is given below in **Table 15.2.5.**

In oliguric renal failure, hyponatraemia is the most frequent electrolyte abnormality; this is invariably a dilutional hyponatraemia due to a water overload.

Table 15.2.5. Sodium content of important body fluids

 * Sweat: Na$^+$ 20–100 mEq/l
 * Gastric Fluid: Na$^+$ 30–90 mEq/l
 * Diarrhoea: Na$^+$ 50–110 mEq/l
 * Small Bowel Ostomy: Na$^+$ 70–150 mEq/l
 * Biliary Drainage: Na$^+$ 120–170 mEq/l

Potassium

Except in individuals who lose a large quantity of fluid through nasogastric suction or diarrhoea, hyperkalaemia is always to be anticipated and promptly corrected. Potassium should be invariably restricted in these patients except in those who have potassium losses from the above-mentioned sources (see Section on Fluid and Electrolyte Abnormalities in the Critically Ill).

Acid-Base Balance

Uraemic acidosis is an expected feature of oliguric renal failure, and is related to protein catabolism. 1 mEq of H^+ ion is retained for every gram of protein catabolism, and on a normal diet, 70 mEq of H^+ ion are produced in the body. With poor renal function H^+ ions accumulate and cause acidosis. Patients may develop a substantial base deficit > 15 mEq/l, and the pH may drop to below 7.15 in spite of a compensatory fall in the $PaCO_2$ produced by hyperventilation. It is prudent to correct significant acidosis with 50–100 mEq of intravenous sodium bicarbonate (see Chapter on Acid-Base Disturbances in the Critically Ill). If serum calcium levels are low, 10 ml of calcium gluconate is given intravenously before administering sodium bicarbonate.

Lactic acid acidosis often occurs in critically ill patients with acute renal failure, particularly in those with sepsis. Lactic acid production in very ill patients maybe as high as 50 mEq/hr, and can reduce plasma bicarbonate at the rate of 1–2 mEq/l/hr. In the presence of marked oliguria, replacement of large quantities of bicarbonate almost always results in fluid overload and in hypernatraemia, requiring dialysis. All efforts should be made to maximize oxygen transport and tissue perfusion in these patients.

Calcium, Magnesium, Phosphates

It is important to maintain these electrolytes within normal limits. Hypocalcaemia may occur following the use of intravenous bicarbonate, but otherwise tetany is rare. Hypercalcaemia is observed in oliguric renal failure associated with multiple myeloma.

Magnesium excretion is reduced during renal failure, and magnesium containing antacids should be avoided.

Phosphate levels increase with increasing duration of oliguric renal failure. When serum phosphate levels exceed 6 mg/dl, aluminum hydroxide 30 ml 8 hourly is effective in binding phosphates within the gut. Once phosphate levels are < 6 mg/dl, calcium carbonate can be given in a dose of 500 mg 8 hourly, after meals.

If intravenous alimentation is used for purposes of nutrition, it is best to avoid phosphates in the intravenous fluids till such time as the high phosphate levels have returned to normal.

(ii) Maintain Nutrition (16)

In an intensive care setting, patients with oliguric acute renal failure are invariably catabolic. Nutritional therapy should include adequate calorie and nitrogen (protein) administration so as to minimize negative nitrogen balance. The calorie requirement varies from 35–50 kcal/kg/day. The protein requirement can be given orally as 0.75 to 1.2 g/kg/day of high biologic value protein or intravenously as 10–20 g/day of essential aminoacids. Patients with

severe burns or severe tetanus require a higher protein intake. The non-protein calories should be divided equally between carbohydrates and fats. The enteral route of nutrition is always to be preferred. If for any reason enteral feeds are not possible, parenteral administration should be started early. This is of essence in the management of severely catabolic patients in acute renal failure. All such patients require dialysis or haemofiltration to allow the necessary administration of a large fluid intake associated with parenteral nutrition, and to allow a larger protein intake without precipitating uraemic symptoms. Appropriate nutritional support is vital as it helps in renal recovery and improves overall survival in acute renal failure. However, nutrition should be administered in a form and volume so that it does not lead to complications that may well outweigh its benefits. Excessive protein intake > 2 g/kg/day is unnecessary and may do more harm than good. In non-catabolic patients with ARF the nutritional requirement is 30–35 kcal/kg/day with 0.5 g/kg/day of high biologic value protein.

(iii) Recognize and Treat Complications

Complications may arise as a result of the primary disease causing acute renal failure, or may be directly related to acute renal failure. Rapidly progressive acute renal failure has a high morbidity even when it occurs as a primary event. It can ultimately so derange homeostatic mechanisms, as to lead to multiple organ failure and death.

Important complications associated with acute oliguric renal failure are listed in **Table 15.2.6**. They should be anticipated, if possible prevented, and when they do occur, should be promptly treated.

Dose adjustments of all drugs during acute oliguric renal failure are of great importance, else drug toxicity is inevitable. Uraemic patients bleed easily. GI bleeding is common; bleeding from other sites due to platelet dysfunction also occurs. If this is observed, or if more effective haemostasis is required for any operative or invasive procedure, the prophylactic use of desmopressin acetate 0.3 µg/kg intravenously or the use of sufficient quantity of cryoprecipitate, and platelet concentrates shortens the bleeding time appreciably (17). Prophylaxis against GI bleeding due to acute erosive gastritis is generally recommended. Sucralfate is preferable to the use of other antacids. In the presence of active bleeding, an H_2-antagonist or omeprazole should be used.

Kidney recovery in ATN is heralded by the onset of the diuretic phase. In some patients diuresis may be as high as 5–6 l/day. Blood creatinine and urea may remain high for some days in spite of the diuresis. Fluid and electrolyte balance should be maintained as per the principles outlined above. With progressive recovery, homeostasis is finally achieved.

(iv) Specific Treatment for Certain Specific Forms of Glomerulonephritis

Specific treatment for some forms of autoimmune glomerulonephritis, immune-complex disease, and acute renal disease due to various forms of vasculitides includes the use of cytotoxic agents, corticosteroids, antiplatelet drugs, and plasma exchange (18).

Table 15.2.6. Complications associated with acute renal failure

1. Metabolic
   * Hyperkalaemia
   * Hyponatraemia
   * Hypocalcaemia
   * Hyperphosphataemia
   * Hypermagnesaemia
   * Acidosis/Alkalosis
   * Hypoglycaemia
2. Gastrointestinal
   * Nausea, vomiting, diarrhoea
   * GI haemorrhage, paralytic ileus
3. Cardiovascular
   * Fluid overload with water retention
   * Hypertension
   * Congestive cardiac failure
   * Pulmonary oedema
   * Cardiac arrhythmias
   * Myocardial infarction
   * Pericarditis
4. Haematologic
   * Anaemia
   * Platelet dysfunction
   * Bleeding from various sites
5. Neurologic
   * Neuromuscular irritability
   * Mental obtundation and coma
   * Seizures
6. Multiple Organ Dysfunction
7. Infections
   * Sepsis
   * Pneumonia
   * Catheter-related infections
   * Urinary tract infections
   * Wound infections

(v) The Use of Dialysis (19)

Dialysis enables homeostasis of fluid, electrolytes, acid-base and nitrogen balance, when this is difficult or impossible with the medical measures outlined above. Certain principles of management need to be stressed.

(i) The cause of acute renal failure should as far as possible be determined and postrenal causes should be excluded before commencing dialysis.

(ii) Attention should be given to preserving and maintaining a satisfactory haemodynamic state, so that renal perfusion is adequate.

(iii) Sepsis should be vigorously treated.

(iv) The dosage of all drugs administered to the patient are modified according to the degree of renal failure and the type of dialysis in use.

Three types of dialysis (renal replacement therapy) are available—intermittent haemodialysis, continuous haemofiltration/haemodiafiltration, peritoneal dialysis (intermittent or continuous). They work on the principle of enabling water and solute clearance through a semipermeable membrane and discarding the waste products so produced. The mode of replacement therapy chosen for a particular patient depends on the nature and degree of homeostatic imbalance, the haemodynamic status and the background disease or complications present.

Indications for Dialysis

(a) Fluid Overload. This is the most important indication for dialysis. When fluid overload produces increasing pulmonary congestion and oedema, dialysis needs to be performed urgently.

In haemodynamically stable patients, intermittent haemodialysis provides the quickest method of removing fluid—1–2 l/hr by ultrafiltration. In haemodynamically unstable patients peritoneal dialysis or continuous haemofiltration is safer and therefore preferable. Peritoneal dialysis can remove 2–3 l/day, and this allows for intravenous alimentation or the intravenous administration of drugs. Fluid removal in excess of 5 l/day may cause hypernatraemia, as the fluid removed by peritoneal dialysis is hyponatraemic as compared to plasma. In patients presenting with massive fluid overload, continuous haemofiltration is probably the best as it allows a large quantity of fluid to be removed, and the ultrafiltrate is iso-osmotic with plasma.

(b) Electrolyte Abnormalities. Hyperkalaemia is an important indication for dialysis, if it is marked, persistent or rapidly progressive. Rapid potassium removal is only possible by machine haemodialysis, the clearance rate of potassium being 100–200 ml/min. Peritoneal dialysis or continuous haemofiltration does not allow a clearance rate of potassium > 20 ml/min, and these forms of dialysis should be used to counter modest hyperkalaemia, or for maintaining potassium balance.

Toxic serum levels of calcium, magnesium and phosphates are also rapidly corrected by haemodialysis. Severe hypophosphataemia may complicate all forms of dialysis, if phosphates are absent in the diet or in the intravenous alimentation fluids.

(c) Acid-Base Abnormalities. Uraemic acidosis and lactic acid acidosis can both be temporarily corrected by haemodialysis. Acidosis recurs quickly (particularly in patients with lactic acid acidosis) in the interdialysis period. Continuous arteriovenous haemofiltration provides continuous correction of acidosis, and is the treatment of choice in septic patients in acute renal failure, who have both fluid overload and a lactic acid acidosis.

(d) Uraemic Symptoms. Dialysis is indicated with BUN levels > 100 mg/dl, particularly in the presence of uraemic symptoms—pericarditis, encephalopathy, bleeding tendency, neuromuscular irritability, and seizures.

The current practice is to initiate dialysis early rather than late in acute renal failure. It is bad medicine to await serious complications of uraemia before starting dialysis. Most ICUs would consider dialysis when any one of the following is present: severe oliguria (<5 ml/kg/day), anuria for over 12 hours, pulmonary oedema not responding to diuretics, metabolic acidosis < 7.2, uraemic symptoms, such as increasing obtundation, or encephalopathy, or pericarditis, or severe GI symptoms. The presence of any two of the above would be considered by most as a clear indication for dialysis.

It must be however remembered that an over-aggressive approach to the very early commencement of dialysis in ARF does not necessarily equate with a reduction in mortality. In fact an over-aggressive approach in units that lack either experience or expertise can do more harm than good.

Intermittent haemodialysis may be necessary every other day or even daily, in hypercatabolic patients. Dialysis needs to be continued till recovery ensues. This usually takes place within 2–8 weeks. Dialysis should be withheld if there is evidence of irreversible vital organ failure, or severe cerebral damage.

Modes of Dialysis

The mode of renal replacement therapy in an ICU for a given patient, depends not only on the underlying medical problem but on local resources, expertise and experience. We increasingly tend to use continuous haemofiltration/haemodiafiltration in preference to intermittent haemodialysis or peritoneal dialysis. Continuous haemofiltration/haemodiafiltration offers the following advantages:

(a) use of biocompatible membrane;

(b) greater haemodynamic stability;

(c) ability to control the quantum of removal of water over prolonged time;

(d) a leeway for increased fluid intake necessary both for hyperalimentation and for administering drugs intravenously;

(e) prevention of cerebral oedema and increase in intracranial pressure (20, 21).

A brief description of intermittent haemodialysis, peritoneal dialysis and continuous haemofiltration is given below. The techniques and the details regarding vascular access and performance of different forms of dialysis are best left to the nephrologist and trained nursing staff. The physician in the ICU must however be aware of the principles underlying the effectiveness, advantages and disadvantages of each form of dialysis and the complications that can be encountered during dialysis in the ICU.

Haemodialysis
Advantages and Effectiveness

The major advantage of haemodialysis is its highly efficient solute removal, and its ability to remove fluid overload within a short period of time. Most modern dialyzers allow 150–200 ml/min of urea clearance with blood flows between 200–300 ml/min. More rapid solute clearance can be obtained with newer filters when operated at a higher flow of 400 ml/min. As much as 1–3 l of fluid can be removed per hour—fluid withdrawal is however limited by the patient's haemodynamic state. A very rapid fluid withdrawal can produce disastrous consequences in critically ill patients. Ordinarily a 4 hour haemodialysis should reduce pretreatment urea levels by about 50 per cent.

Disadvantages

The major disadvantage is the rapidity of fluid withdrawal which is unsuitable in a haemodynamically unstable patient. The need for a large-bore vascular access, and the need for anticoagulation, are other disadvantages. The latter specially poses problems in patients who are actively bleeding.

Complications (22)

The following complications are often met with during, or immediately after haemodialysis.

(i) **Hypotension.** This is related to poor tolerance of fluid removal. Poor tolerance to the acetate used in the dialysate fluid can potentiate hypotension. Bicarbonate based dialysates are always preferred in haemodynamically unstable patients.

Hypotension resistant to volume replacement, together with respiratory distress, can in rare instances be due to relative bio-incompatibility between cuprophane and cellulose-based membranes. This has been dubbed the 'first use syndrome', and is treated with subcutaneous epinephrine and intravenous aminophylline. Definitive management consists in using more biocompatible materials.

Hypotension during dialysis should be treated by decreasing the blood flow, and administering a volume load with either colloids like albumin, or crystalloids like dextrose or normal saline.

(ii) **Arrhythmias.** Cardiac arrhythmias are particularly prone to occur in haemodynamically unstable patients. Digitalis toxicity is another cause, and is precipitated by the rapid lowering of serum potassium levels. Abnormalities in serum levels of magnesium and calcium, hypoxia, myocardial ischaemia, and acetate toxicity are other causes of cardiac arrhythmias. Cardiac arrest is a dreaded complication in critically ill patients. Arrhythmias should be promptly recognized and treated.

(iii) **Hypoxaemia.** Arterial hypoxaemia can be due to 2 causes—

(a) The loss of CO_2 through the dialyzer with subsequent diminishing of the respiratory drive. Oxygen administered through nasal prongs corrects the hypoxia.

(b) The occurrence of the 'first-use syndrome' caused by activation of complement and of leukoagglutination within the lungs, can cause severe bronchospasm with hypoxia. Dialysis needs to be promptly discontinued, and the bronchospasm should be countered by adrenaline or a beta-2 adrenergic agonist and intravenous aminophylline.

(iv) **Haemorrhage.** If serious haemorrhage occurs, previously administered heparin should be neutralized by protamine. 1 mg of protamine ordinarily neutralizes 100 International Units of heparin. Protamine infusions should preferably be limited to a maximum of 15 mg over 5 minutes, to minimize the risk of anaphylactic reactions.

(v) **Dialysis Disequilibrium Syndrome.** This syndrome is characterized by headache, nausea, twitchings, mental obtundation, delerium and seizures, following rapid correction of severe uraemia. Shorter duration of treatment to start with, using slower blood flow rates of < 200 ml/min, helps to minimize or prevent this syndrome.

Peritoneal Dialysis
Advantages and Effectiveness

In patients in whom vascular access is difficult or impossible, peritoneal dialysis is a possible alternative. Haemodynamically unstable patients can withstand peritoneal dialysis without further compromise of their circulatory system, as the rate of fluid removal is much slower than with haemodialysis.

The effectiveness of peritoneal dialysis is not as good as intermittent haemodialysis. Solute removal depends on the volume of the dialysate, and dwell time within the peritoneal cavity. An aggressive schedule incorporates 2 l exchange every hour, providing 24 l of urea clearance per day. Less aggressive schedules involving 2 l exchanges every 4 hours, result in 8–10 l of urea clearance per day. Fluid removal depends on the concentration of glucose in the dialysate, and the dwell time allowed. Higher concentrations of glucose (4.25 per cent solutions), can provide a fluid removal of 500 ml/hour. A major advantage of this technique is that no anticoagulation is required. The method therefore is safer than haemodialysis in bleeding patients.

Severe fluid overload producing pulmonary oedema is however best managed by intermittent dialysis or continuous arteriovenous haemofiltration.

Disadvantages and Complications (23)

(i) An important disadvantage and complication is impaired drainage. Problems can be particularly serious when the catheter allows unimpeded inflow, but the outflow is markedly reduced. This may be due to malpositioning of the catheter, or a ball-valve obstruction produced by omentum wrapped round the perforations in the catheter.

(ii) Infection with resulting peritonitis is a serious complication. As opposed to peritonitis resulting from intrinsic disease, dialysis-induced peritonitis can be successfully managed by intraperitoneal antibiotics. When suspected, the WBCs in the effluent should be estimated. A WBC count > 100 granulocytes/μl points to infection. Gram's stain of the effluent for organisms is also of help. A suitable antibiotic is added to the dialysate depending on the nature of infection present. The choice and dosage of antibiotics in the dialysate should be decided upon by the nephrologist. Gentamicin is preferred for Gram-negative infections, and vancomycin or cefazole for staphylococcal infections.

(iii) Protein loss can be considerable in peritoneal dialysis.

(iv) Compromised pulmonary function due to elevation of the diaphragm and hydrothorax, is frequently observed. Peritoneal dialysis cannot be effectively used in breathless patients with pulmonary disease.

(v) Abnormal blood sugar levels and electrolyte disturbances may be induced during peritoneal dialysis.

(vi) Peritoneal dialysis is very slow and ineffective in patients who are severely hypercatabolic, and who are in acute renal failure, or when dangerous abnormalities in fluid and electrolyte balance need very prompt correction.

Continuous Haemofiltration (CHF)

CHF is being increasingly used as the mode of dialysis in critically ill patients who have a large fluid overload, and in those who are haemodynamically unstable. It is also indicated when the use of intravenous alimentation necessitates the administration of large volumes of fluid.

In CHF a highly permeable membrane acts as an artificial glomerulus by permitting hydrostatically driven ultrafiltration. The ultrafiltration leads to loss of water, solutes, urea, and waste products in the ultrafiltrate. This method of solute clearance is termed convective clearance.

A large volume of fluid can be removed in a fluid-overloaded critically ill patient, without inducing hypotension or other circulatory disturbances because treatment lasts continuously throughout the day. The procedure can be carried out at the bedside and this is an added advantage. The need for an access to large vessels, for excellent nursing and for continuous anticoagulation with heparin are the main drawbacks.

Continuous Arteriovenous Haemofiltration (CAVH)

This is perhaps the most commonly used mode of haemofiltration. In CAVH blood is driven through the filter by the patient's own blood pressure, either via a large bore femoral artery cannula or via the arterial limb of an arteriovenous Scribner shunt. The blood traverses the biocompatible permeable filter, undergoes ultrafiltration and is returned to the circulation via a cannula in the femoral vein or via the venous limb of the Scribner shunt. Solute clearance and removal of nitrogenous waste products is not as efficient as in haemodialysis. Even so, significant and often adequate clearance of nitrogenous waste products is achieved because treatment is continuous throughout the day.

Continuous Arteriovenous Haemodiafiltration (CAVHD)

Numerous modifications have been incorporated to improve solute clearance in the CAVHD circuit. The most effective way of increasing solute clearance is to add dialysate flow countercurrent to the haemofiltration current. This can double solute clearance through diffusion of solutes. This technique is termed continuous arteriovenous haemodiafiltration (CAVHD).

Continuous Venovenous Haemofiltration (CVVH) and Haemodiafiltration (CVVHD)

In CVVH access to the circulation is obtained via a double lumen catheter inserted into the femoral, or subclavian or internal jugular vein. Blood is pumped by a roller pump from the arterial limb of the double lumen catheter into the filter and after ultrafiltration and purification returns to the circulation via the venous limb of the double-lumen catheter.

If a counter-current dialysate flow is added to the CVVH current, solute clearance is further increased. This technique is termed continuous venovenous haemofiltration (CVVHD).

Large amount of fluid can be removed by the various techniques of continuous haemodiafiltration. A careful hourly measurement of fluid removed in relation to fluid replaced is mandatory and a frequent estimation of serum electrolytes is also necessary. Good nursing, and constant attention are required for good results.

Clinical Syndromes Associated With Acute Renal Failure

1. Pigment Nephropathy due to Rhabdomyolysis or to Acute Haemolysis (24)

Rhabdomyolysis is observed most frequently after severe traumatic crush injuries. In an intensive care setting it also occurs in patients with fulminant tetanus, acute polymyositis, and rarely in severe leptospiral infections. Myoglobinuria with precipitation of myoglobin casts in renal tubules is the cause of acute renal failure. Volume depletion from any cause (e.g. crush injuries) promotes precipitation of myoglobin within the tubules. Rhabdomyolysis is associated with painful muscles, and elevated creatinine kinase and aldolase levels in the blood.

Acute severe haemolysis in our part of the world, is most frequently due to three causes—the inadvertent administration of incompatible blood transfusion, the use of certain drugs in patients who are G6PD deficient, and acute haemolysis in falciparum malaria and blackwater fever. Acute viral and salmonella infections can also induce severe haemolysis in G6PD deficient patients with resulting acute renal shutdown. The presence of severe anaemia, a high reticulocyte count, rise in serum bilirubin and haptoglobin, are features of acute haemolysis. In the absence of detectable red blood cells on urinanalysis, a dipstick test positive for haeme is diagnostic of myoglobinuria or haemoglobinuria. Patients with myoglobinuria and haemoglobinuria have dark brown and at times almost black urine. The serum in patients with myoglobinuria is clear, whilst in severe haemoglobinuria the spun serum sample is pink, free haemoglobin is detected in the serum, and the serum enzymes particularly the LDH, are raised.

Treatment

The most important step is to restore circulating volume quickly, and to attempt a forced diuresis with mannitol 250 ml intravenously, or furosemide 250–500 mg intravenously. Hydration with forced diuresis should aim for a urine output over 100 ml/hr. Alkalinization of the urine with intravenous sodium bicarbonate in patients with acute haemolysis may prevent precipitation of the haeme pigment within the renal tubules.

Once oliguric renal failure has set in, it is unwise to persist with repeated use of mannitol or furosemide. Treatment is then continued on the lines mentioned earlier.

Hypocalcaemia and severe hyperkalaemia are frequent features of rhabdomyolysis and acute haemolysis.

2. Hepatorenal Syndrome (25, 26)

This syndrome is characterized by renal failure with normal tubular function in a patient with chronic liver disease. It usually afflicts patients with alcoholic cirrhosis. Renal failure is related to increased preglomerular vascular resistance which leads to a reduced glomerular filtration rate (GFR), with diversion of blood flow away from the renal cortex. This occurs even in the presence of a normal or increased cardiac output. Oliguria, a low urine sodium concentration, a highly concentrated urine, a progressively increasing azotaemia, and the frequent presence of hyponatraemia are characteristically observed. Renal failure in cirrhotic patients is precipitated by haemorrhage, or paracentesis, or diuretic therapy, or following a slight fall in the intravascular volume as produced by diarrhoea. It can occur without any fall in arterial blood pressure.

Prevention is of crucial importance, as treatment of the fully evolved hepatorenal syndrome is of no avail. Hypovolaemia should be prevented in cirrhotic patients, and if it does occur, should be promptly treated. Treatment of hepatic failure is on the usual lines. Infection should be recognized and treated; nephrotoxic drugs such as aminoglycosides and non-steroidal anti-inflammatory drugs, should be stopped. Mannitol has been tried to expand intravascular volume, but is of little use and may result in intracellular acidosis. High doses of furosemide fail to act. Dialysis does not help and may in fact precipitate hypotension, shock and gastrointestinal bleeding. In a fully evolved hepatorenal syndrome death is inevitable, and is preceded by hypotension, hyponatraemia and mounting azotaemia.

3. Syndromes with Pulmonary and Renal Involvement

A quickly evolving renal failure requiring intensive care, occasionally occurs in association with a pulmonary pathology. Thus pulmonary vasculitides are often associated with progressive renal failure. A classic example is Wegener's granulomatosis (27) associated with an arteriolitis within the kidneys, or associated with a rapidly progressive glomerulonephritis. Other pulmonary vasculitides with renal involvement include the Churg-Strauss syndrome, polyarteritis nodosa, and small vessel vasculitis. Autoimmune disorders which involve the lung and produce renal failure include systemic lupus erythematosus, and the Goodpasture's syndrome. Sepsis from any cause can result in acute lung injury and produce progressive renal dysfunction and failure. In the tropics, fulminant falciparum infection is an important cause of multiple organ dysfunction, with the CNS, the lungs and the kidneys bearing the brunt of the infection. A few poisons including the herbicide Paraquat can produce pulmonary oedema and anuria due to acute tubular necrosis (28).

Diagnosis is dependent on a careful consideration of the clinical features, radiological studies of the lungs, special diagnostic tests, a lung biopsy, and in some instances a kidney biopsy. The antineutrophilic cytoplasmic antibody (ANCA) test is positive in Wegener's disease and in small vessel vasculitis. The ANF and anti-DNA tests are positive in systemic lupus erythematosus. Immunofluorescent studies of material from kidney biopsy show IgG immune complex deposits in SLE. The diagnosis of Goodpasture's syndrome can be made by detection of anti-glomerular basement membrane antibodies in the serum. A kidney biopsy shows the presence of linear immunofluorescence in the glomerular basement membrane in Goodpasture's syndrome.

Treatment in acutely ill patients is difficult if a diagnosis is not established. Acute renal failure should be treated on lines mentioned earlier. Severe haemoptysis and progressive renal failure in Goodpasture's syndrome are treated with corticosteroids (pulsed doses of methylprednisolone, 15–20 mg/kg/day for 3 days, are used initially in critically ill patients), cyclophosphamide (1.5 mg/kg body weight), and plasmapheresis.

Acute renal failure occurring in severe forms of Wegener's disease and other forms of severe vasculitides, is treated with corticosteroids and cyclophosphamide, as in the Goodpasture's syndrome.

Pulsed doses of methylprednisolone are used for rapidly evolving renal failure in systemic lupus erythematosus.

In poisonings involving the lungs and the kidneys, gastric lavage with the use of charcoal adsorbents is of use. Charcoal haemoperfusion and continuous arteriovenous haemofiltration may be tried in suitable cases.

Acute Renal Failure in the Transplant Patient (29)

Renal failure may occur early in a transplant recipient—sometimes within 10 days of the transplant, or late (after 10 days of the transplant). Acute renal failure occurring early can be due to (i) hyperacute immune rejection of the graft; (ii) acute tubular necrosis of the transplant; (iii) problems related to surgery e.g. obstruction, leak or infection. Cyclosporine toxicity particularly in those receiving high intravenous doses of the drug, presents with hypertension and prerenal azotaemia; this should be differentiated from the other causes of acute renal failure listed above.

Acute renal failure occurring in the late period after transplant, may be due to acute immune rejection, renal artery stenosis, ureteric obstruction, cyclosporine toxicity, or to recurrence of the original renal disease.

Acute rejection of the transplant is diagnosed by the presence of tenderness and swelling over the transplanted kidney, fever, a fall in the urine output and increasing azotaemia. Imaging studies and nuclear scans help in distinguishing between the different causes of acute renal failure in a transplant patient. At times, a kidney biopsy may be necessary to reach a definitive diagnosis.

Management is specialized, and should be in consultation with a nephrologist, and the transplant surgeon.

Critical Illnesses in Patients on Chronic Dialysis

Patients on maintenance dialysis, are often admitted to a critical care unit for an acute illness. The following problems are frequently encountered:

(i) *Acute Hypertension.* This is often caused by an increased ingestion of salt and water by the patient, in the interdialysis period. Acute left ventricular failure, and hypertensive encephalopathy may occur. These complications mandate admission to an ICU and appropriate treatment. Pulmonary oedema is generally unresponsive to diuretic therapy, and requires removal of the extra fluid by dialysis.

(ii) *Acute Hypotension and Arrhythmias.* Acute hypotension, arrhythmias and even cardiac arrest may occur at times during, or immediately after haemodialysis, necessitating emergency transfer to the ICU. If the patient is hypotensive, he should be given a volume load. A bradyrhythm is countered by intravenous atropine

0.5–1 mg. Sudden atrial fibrillation with a very rapid ventricular rate needs intravenous digoxin (see Chapter on Tachyarrhythmias in the ICU).

(iii) *Upper GI Bleeds* are extremely common; antacids containing magnesium are best avoided, and the dose of H_2 blockers may need to be adjusted.

(iv) *Electrolyte Disturbances.* Occasionally a patient is admitted for acute hyperkalaemia or acute acidosis (see Sections on Fluid and Electrolyte Disturbances and Acid-Base Disturbances in the Critically Ill). Hyperkalaemia can pose a serious life-threatening emergency, requiring prompt recognition and treatment.

(v) *Acute Hypoglycaemia.* This is observed at times in patients with chronic renal failure. Sudden drowsiness, mental obtundation, abnormal behaviour, unconsciousness, generalized seizures or even focal neurological signs, should alert the clinician to this possibility. We have observed recurrence of hypoglycaemia after the discontinuation of intravenous dextrose. An increased incidence of hypoglycaemia observed in our patients, may perhaps be related to the fact that glucose is not used in the dialysate fluid, and that glucose may be lost from the blood during dialysis, with resultant hypoglycaemia. This is more frequently observed in diabetics on insulin.

(vi) *The Use of Acetate in the Dialysis Fluid* sometimes produces life-threatening clinical features during or immediately after haemodialysis. The patient becomes increasingly breathless due to severe acidosis; hypotension, arrhythmias, and cardiac instability may be observed. The problem is generally solved by replacing the acetate by bicarbonate in the dialysate fluid.

(vii) *Acute Infections.* Patients in chronic renal failure on maintenance dialysis are immunosuppressed, and are prone to infections (see Section on The Immunocompromised Patient). Antibiotics have more prolonged therapeutic levels in these patients and nephrotoxicity of antibiotics and other drugs, is not of major importance in these patients.

Infection of the vascular access is common in patients on haemodialysis. Though pain, local erythema and tenderness are common over the access site, physical signs may be minimal. Systemic sepsis and septicaemia may originate from an apparently non-infected site of vascular access. This should always be kept in mind in patients with systemic infection. Successful treatment of infection of the access site is generally possible with prolonged administration of antibiotics. Antibiotic regimes for such infections generally include vancomycin, since this drug is poorly dialysable, and a single dose results in adequate serum levels for 7 days.

(viii) *Thrombosis of a Vascular Access Site.* This is another complication observed in critically ill patients who are on chronic dialysis. At times a prolonged period of hypotension results in thrombosis. At other times, infection at the site, or venepunctures at or near the site, lead to thrombosis. Venepunctures should always be done on the contralateral arm, and avoided on the arm which has a graft or a surgically fashioned fistula. If an access site is found to be thrombosed (absent thrill or bruit), immediate surgical consultation is necessary. Thrombolytic therapy with intravenous urokinase may at times obviate the need for surgical treatment.

Fluid and Electrolyte Restriction in Patients on Chronic Haemodialysis

Fluids should be restricted between 700 ml, to a maximum of 1 l. The degree of fluid restriction is dictated by the tendency of the patient to develop hypertension, or pulmonary oedema during the interdialysis period.

Nutritional Requirements

Once on dialysis, the patient is encouraged to eat well. Protein requirements are about 1 g/kg/day. In an average adult, total caloric requirement is about 2000 calories per day, or 35 kcal/kg/day.

REFERENCES

1. Siegel NJ, Shah SV. (2003). Acute Renal Failure: Directions for the next decade. J Am Soc Nephrol. 9(2), 1293–1294.

2. Ellison DH, Bia MJ. (1987). Acute renal failure in critically ill patients. J Intens Care Med. 2, 8–24.

3. Brezis M, Rosen S, Epstein FH. (1991). Acute Renal Failure. In: The Kidney, 4th edn (Eds Brenner B, Rector FC). Saunders, Philadelphia.

4. Sillix DH, McDonald FD. (1987). Acute renal failure. Crit Care Clin. 5, 909–925.

5. Linton AL, Clark WF, Driedger AA et al. (1980). Acute interstitial nephritis due to drugs. Ann Intern Med. 93, 735–741.

6. Steiner RW. (1984). Interpreting the fractional excretion of sodium. Am J Med. 77, 699–702.

7. Kaplan AA. (2002). Renal Failure. In: Current Critical Care Diagnosis and Treatment (Eds Bongard FS, Sue DY). pp. 342–75. McGraw-Hill, USA.

8. Schwartz LB, Gewertz B. (1988). The renal response to low dose dopamine. J Surg Res. 45, 574–588.

9. Mykes PS, Buckland MR, Schenk NJ et al. (1993). Effect of renal dose dopamine on renal function following cardiac surgery. Anaes Int Care. 21, 56–61.

10. Corwin HL, Bonventre JV. (1988). Acute renal failure in the intensive care unit. Parts 1 and 2. Intensive Care Med. 14, 10–16; 86–96.

11. Lindner A. (1983). Synergism of dopamine and furosemide in diuretic-resistant oliguric renal failure. Nephron. 33, 121–126.

12. Kellum JA, Decker JM. (2001). Use of dopamine in ARF: A meta-analysis. Critical Care Medicine 29(8), 1526–1531.

13. Conger JD. (1995). Interventions in clinical acute renal failure: what are the data? Am J Kidney Dis. 26, 565–576.

14. Rudes ML, Zarovitz BJ. (1997). Low dose dopamine in acute oliguric renal failure. Am J Med. 102, 320–322.

15. Solomon R, Werner C, Mann D et al. (1994). Effects of saline, mannitol and furosemide to prevent acute decreases in renal function induced by radiocontrast agents. New Engl J Med. 331, 1416–1420.

16. Mizock BA. (2001). Nutritional Support. In: Critical Care Medicine (Eds Parrillo JE, Dellinger RP). pp. 1458–1472 Mosby, USA.

17. Nowbar S, Anderson AJ. (2001). Acute Renal Failure. In: Critical Care Medicine (Eds Parrillo JE, Dellinger RP). pp. 1133–1156. Mosby, USA.

18. Jennette JC, Falk RJ. (1990). Diagnosis and management of glomerulonephritis and vasculitis presenting as acute renal failure. Med Clin North Am. 74, 893–908.

19. Maher JF. (1989). Pharmacologic considerations for renal failure and dialysis. In: Replacement of Renal Function by Dialysis, 3rd edn (Ed. Maher JF). Kluwer Academic Publishers.

20. Arief AI. (1994). Dialysis dysequilibrium syndrome: current concepts on pathogenesis and prevention. Kidney Int. 45, 629–635.

21. Davenport A, Will EJ, Davidson AM. (1993). Improved cardiovascular stability during continuous modes of renal replacement therapy in critically ill patients with acute hepatic and renal failure. Crit Care Med. 21, 328–338.

22. Blagg CR. (1989). Acute complications associated with hemodialysis. In: Replacement of Renal Function by Dialysis, 3rd edn (Ed. Maher JF). Kluwer Academic Publishers.

23. Holley JL, Piraino BM. (1990). Complications of peritoneal dialysis. Diagnosis and management. Semin Dialysis. 3, 245–248.

24. Knochel JP. (1992). Rhabdomyolysis and acute renal failure. In: Current Therapy in Nephrology and Hypertension (Ed. Glassock RJ). BC Decker, Mosby YearBook.

25. Sherlock S. (1997). Ascites. In: Diseases of the Liver and Biliary System (Eds Sherlock S, Dooley J). pp. 119–34. Blackwell Scientific Publications, Oxford, London, Edinburgh, Boston, Melbourne.

26. Epstein M. (1989). Hepatorenal Syndrome. In: The Kidney in Liver Disease (Ed. Epstein M). Williams and Wilkins.

27. Hoffman GS, Kerr GS, Leavitt RY et al. (1992). Wegener's granulomatosis: An analysis of 158 patients. Ann Intern Med. 116, 488–498.

28. Winchester JF. (1990). Paraquat and the bipyridyl herbicides. In: Clinical Management of Poisoning and Drug Overdose (Eds Haddad LM, Winchester JF). Saunders, Philadelphia.

29. Yoshimura N, Oka T. (1990). Medical and surgical complications of renal transplantation: Diagnosis and management. Med Clin North Am. 74, 1025–1037.

CHAPTER 15.3
Critical Care in Fulminant Hepatitis

Fulminant hepatic failure is the clinical syndrome produced by sudden and severe liver cell dysfunction in a previously healthy individual. It is characterized by hepatic encephalopathy and coagulopathy. Multiple organ dysfunction involving the kidneys, heart, lungs, and metabolic abnormalities are also observed. Admission or transfer to an ICU is mandatory in patients with sudden severe liver cell dysfunction. Critical care is also often necessary in patients with chronic liver cell dysfunction (as in cirrhosis), who develop acute encephalopathy, a severe gastrointestinal bleed, a complicating infection or who become oliguric or azotaemic.

Definitions

The original and a generally accepted definition of fulminant hepatic failure is the occurrence of encephalopathy and other features of severe liver cell failure (notably coagulopathy) within 8 weeks of the first symptoms or jaundice.

Currently, acute liver failure (ALF) is defined as a rapid deterioration in liver cell function manifested by an increase in prothrombin time and a decrease in Factor V without evidence of hepatic encephalopathy. In fulminant hepatic failure, the time interval between the onset of liver cell failure as manifested by jaundice and the development of encephalopathy is less than 2 weeks (1). Rarely though importantly, encephalopathy may herald the onset of fulminant hepatic failure and may precede jaundice.

Subfulminant hepatic failure is severe hepatic failure in which the time interval between jaundice and encephalopathy is between 3 and 12 weeks.

In 1993, O'Grady (2) suggested a slight change in the definition of liver cell failure.

Hyperacute liver cell failure—if the interval between the appearance of jaundice and the development of encephalopathy is 0 to7 days.

Acute liver cell failure—if the interval between jaundice and encephalopathy is 8 to 28 days.

Subacute liver cell failure—if the interval between jaundice and encephalopathy is between 29 days to 12 weeks.

The time frame in the evolution of severe liver cell dysfunction is not just of semantic importance. The prognosis of patients with hyperacute liver cell failure is better than that of patients with acute or subacute failure.

Aetiology

In our country fulminant hepatic failure is most commonly due to an acute viral infection. Virus A, B, C, E can each produce fulminant hepatitis. The proportion of fulminant cases due to each of the viruses varies with geographical area under study. Virus A and virus B are responsible for roughly an equal number of patients with fulminant hepatitis. Fulminant hepatitis caused by virus C is rare in the West but accounts for 40–60 per cent of patients in the far East (3). Recent studies in India have found hepatitis C to be present in about 7–14 per cent of cases of fulminant hepatitis (4, 5). In a number of patients with hepatitis B infection, a fulminant course is precipitated by an acute infection or superinfection with the delta virus. Hepatitis E is particularly prone to cause fulminant hepatitis in pregnant women. Though very rare in the West, this does occur in Asia and Africa.

Other viruses can cause fatal hepatic necrosis in immunocompromised patients. These include the cytomegalovirus, the herpes simplex virus, varicella, and the Epstein-Barr virus (6, 7). Rarely, fulminant hepatitis can be due to leptospiral infection and P falciparum infection. An important cause of acute fulminant liver cell failure, particularly in the large teaching hospitals of Mumbai, is acute alcoholic hepatitis.

After viral infections, idiosyncratic drug reactions are the next most important cause of fulminant hepatitis. The most frequent drugs incriminated are isoniazid given with rifampicin, anaesthetic agents, non-steroidal anti-inflammatory drugs and anti-depressants.

In an intensive care setting progressive liver cell failure is also seen in patients with cardiac disease with a very low cardiac output. The longer the duration of cardiovascular support given to these patients, the more frequently is the picture of liver cell failure observed. Low output states due to shock from any cause also produce progressive severe liver cell dysfunction; this is always worsened by associated sepsis.

Poisonings causing acute or fulminant hepatic failure are rare in our country. In contrast, paracetamol poisoning (with suicidal intent) is an important cause of fulminant hepatic failure in the West, particularly in the United Kingdom. In India, phosphorus poisoning in children due to ingestion of fire crackers containing phosphorus, and a combination of phosphorus and arsenic poisoning due to ingestion of rat poisons (in an attempt at suicide), are rare but important causes. They should always be suspected in children and young adults where the viral markers are persistently negative. Industrial poisons and solvents can cause fulminant hepatic failure, but these are rarely encountered.

Acute fatty infiltration of the liver in full-term pregnant women and eclampsia may also present with fulminant hepatic failure. Acute Wilsons disease should always be excluded in a patient less than 40 years old, particularly in the presence of haemolysis and when all viral markers are negative. Acute autoimmune hepatitis can also cause fulminant hepatic failure. Rarely, fulminant hepatic failure is noted with extensive haematogenous tuberculosis massively involving the liver and in severe metastatic disease or lymphoma involving the liver. In about 10–12 per cent of cases of fulminant hepatitis, no cause can be found even after investigations. Such cases are classified as cryptogenic fulminant hepatitis.

The important causes of acute or fulminant hepatitis have been listed in **Table 15.3.1.**

Table 15.3.1. Causes of acute (fulminant) liver cell failure

1. Infections
   * Viral hepatitis (A, B, non-A, non-B)
   * Other viral infections (e.g. CMV, herpes simplex, EB virus)
   * Leptospiral and Pl. falciparum infections
2. Poisons, Chemicals and Drugs
   * Acetaminophen, tetracycline, paracetamol, phosphorus, halothane, isoniazid, rifampicin, methyldopa, non-steroidal anti-inflammatory drugs
   * Alcoholic hepatitis
   * Rat poisons (containing phosphorus, anticoagulants, arsenic); accidental ingestion in children of fire crackers containing phosphorus; mushroom poisoning
3. Ischaemia and Hypoxia
   * Pump failure, acute circulatory failure (shock of any aetiology)
4. Miscellaneous
   * Acute fatty liver of pregnancy; eclampsia
   * Reye's syndrome
   * Acute Wilsons disease; acute autoimmune hepatitis
   * Rarely extensive haematogenous tuberculosis involving the liver
   * Rarely extensive metastatic disease or lymphoma involving the liver

Clinical Features and Diagnosis

Neuropsychiatric features, progressively deepening jaundice with a shrinkage in liver size, cerebral oedema with symptoms of brain stem dysfunction, and bleeding due to disturbances in the normal coagulation mechanisms, dominate the clinical picture. Worsening liver cell function ultimately leads to multiple organ dysfunction—respiratory failure, renal failure and cardiovascular instability with hypotension and death ultimately ensue.

Neuropsychiatric features predominate in the early evolving phase of fulminant liver cell failure. They are due to stimulation of the reticular system of the brain, followed by depression of brainstem function. Neuropsychiatric features may be rarely present even in the absence of jaundice. A change in the personality, nightmares, excitability, drowsiness, and unruly behaviour are all common. Mental obtundation is punctuated by periods of extreme irritability, dementia or even mania. Spontaneous seizures may occur. The slightest stimulation (as an attempt to examine the patient), may provoke shouting, and violent behaviour. Flapping

tremors may be very transient, and generally disappear with increasing mental obtundation. Fetor hepaticus however is always present.

Disturbances in the conscious state should be charted and graded as follows (8):
Grade 1—Confused, altered mood or behaviour with psychometric deficit.
Grade 2—Drowsy, increasing behavioural changes.
Grade 3—Stuporose, confused, incoherent, but still obeying simple commands.
Grade 4—Coma cannot be aroused.

Cerebral oedema with increase in intracranial pressure is invariably present in patients with Grade III and IV encephalopathy. Increased intracranial pressure can lead to brainstem herniation, and this is the commonest immediate cause of death in fulminant hepatitis. Cerebral oedema results from interruption of the blood brain barrier with leakage of plasma into the CSF, and cytotoxic cellular changes that increase by osmosis the water uptake by brain cells.

Cerebral oedema and brainstem dysfunction can produce sustained or intermittent systolic hypertension, myoclonic jerks, convulsions, dysconjugate eye movements, skew deviation of the eyes, decerebrate posturing with extension of the legs, and extension and hyperpronation of the upper limbs. Decerebrate posturing can occur spontaneously, or on painful stimulation. Plantars are generally flexor, but an extensor response may occur. Depressed brainstem function ultimately leads to absent doll's eye movements, and absent vestibulo-ocular reflexes. Pupillary reaction is sluggish but present. A loss of pupillary reaction to light is generally terminal.

Jaundice in the early days may be mild and even undetectable. Fulminant hepatic failure can occasionally result in death with very minimal elevation in the serum bilirubin. If the patient survives for some days, the jaundice increases in intensity. Jaundice is extremely marked in patients with G6PD deficiency, where severe haemolysis contributes to the sharp rise in serum bilirubin. We have seen recovery in patients with bilirubin levels > 60 mg/dl.

Nausea and vomiting are very common. Abdominal pain can occur, particularly in children; it may be acute and may be first felt in the right iliac fossa. Occasionally an appendectomy is done with disastrous post-operative sequelae. Enlargement of the liver in the first few days can result in acute tenderness in the epigastrium and the right hypochondrium. As hepatic necrosis progresses, the liver shrinks and is then not palpable. The liver dullness in the midclavicular line, which is normally present in the fifth intercostal space, is percussed in the sixth or seventh intercostal spaces. Ultimately, in patients with severe liver necrosis, the liver dullness cannot be percussed.

Hypoglycaemia is common with worsening liver function. Drowsiness and other features of hypoglycaemia, if unrecognized, are mistaken for increasing severity of hepatic encephalopathy.

Acute haemorrhagic necrotizing pancreatitis can complicate fulminant hepatic failure and may cause death.

Severe bleeding from the GI tract, body orifices, injection sites, and internal bleeding into tissues and organ systems occur with severe hepatic necrosis. The coagulopathy of liver cell failure is due not only to a deficiency of clotting factors (the liver synthesizes all factors except factor VIII), but to enhanced fibrinolytic activity due to intravascular coagulation. A picture indistinguishable from severe DIC can result. Thrombocytopaenia may be due to reduced production in the marrow or to coagulopathy. Platelet function may also be impaired.

The development of tachypnoea in a patient with hepatitis is an ominous sign, pointing to impending severity of hepatic necrosis and failure. Increasing tachypnoea with a fall in PaO_2 points to respiratory failure. ARDS is an ominous complication. Atelectasis, infection, aspiration pneumonia may occur.

Infection is invariably present in patients with Grade III or more encephalopathy and contributes to increasing mortality. Renal dysfunction (oliguria with mounting azotaemia), cardiac dysfunction characterized by hypotension and arrhythmias, severe metabolic disturbances, are all features of multiple organ failure and are generally a prelude to death.

The major clinical features of fulminant hepatitis are listed in **Table 15.3.2**.

Table 15.3.2. Major clinical features of fulminant hepatitis

1. Neuropsychiatric features
2. Features of cerebral oedema and brainstem dysfunction
3. Progressively deepening jaundice
4. Bleeding disorders
5. Deteriorating liver function with multiple organ dysfunction

Investigations

The grading of the comatose state, and the intake/output charts should be carefully maintained.

Biochemical investigations should include serum bilirubin, serum transaminases (AST, ALT), serum alkaline phosphatase, and serum proteins with the albumin:globulin ratio. The serum transaminases though high to start with, fall with worsening liver function, as there is less viable liver tissue left. The prothrombin time is extremely useful for gauging the degree of liver cell dysfunction, and as a prognostic guide. A prothrombin time more than double the control carries a bad prognosis. The blood ammonia level is frequently raised in hepatic encephalopathy and coma. Serum electrolytes, Ca, P, Mg, urea, creatinine, glucose and serum amylase should also be done; biochemical tests should be repeated as and when necessary. Arterial pH and blood gas estimation are important.

Haematological investigations include haemoglobin estimation, blood and platelet count, and blood group. When bleeding tendencies are manifest, relevant tests for clotting factor disturbances and disseminated intravascular coagulopathy are also done.

Microbiological tests include viral markers for hepatitis A, B, C and E. These include tests for hepatitis B surface antigen, IgM anticore antibody, serum antidelta, hepatitis A IgM antibody, hepatitis C IgM antibody and hepatitis E IgM antibody. Hepatitis C antibodies may be absent as they may take some weeks to be detected. Hepatitis C RNA by the polymerase chain reaction should therefore be done. It is to be noted that in fulminant hepatitis due to virus B infection the hepatitis B surface antigen may be cleared and therefore negative. The IgM antibody to the core antigen should always be done to prove the diagnosis. Serum HBV DNA is usually negative. Rapid viral clearance indicates a good immune response and perhaps a better prognosis.

Blood cultures are necessary, particularly if secondary infection is suspected. Similarly, cultures of urine, sputum or other body secretions should be done and repeated as and when necessary. ECG, X-ray chest, ultrasonography of the abdomen to monitor liver size, are necessary.

Other relevant blood tests may be necessary to establish the aetiology in obscure cases.

If available, a portable EEG is useful to gauge the degree of hepatic encephalopathy. Increasing unconsciousness is characterized by increasing amplitude and decreasing frequency of the EEG tracings. Triphasic waves are observed in deep coma; these waves are only observed in patients over 20 years of age, and are of ominous significance. Decreasing amplitude of the EEG tracing is observed in terminal cases; finally there is a total absence of rhythmic activity.

Diagnosis

The diagnosis is generally easy. An early mistake is to suspect an acute abdomen, particularly in the presence of severe abdominal pain. Even when icterus is absent, these patients invariably demonstrate a rise in the serum transaminases. This finding should immediately alert the surgeon.

In areas endemic for P falciparum infection, particularly when the patient has high fever, a blood smear examination for malarial parasites should be done.

In patients with severe muscle pains, conjunctival injection, and with urinary findings suggestive of glomerulonephritis, leptospiral infections should be kept in mind.

Immunocompromised patients are susceptible to uncommon viral infections (cytomegalovirus in particular), that may rarely cause fulminant hepatitis.

The diagnostic evaluation of fulminant hepatitis is given in **Table 15.3.3**.

Table 15.3.3. Diagnostic evaluation of fulminant hepatitis

* History, including history of drugs and possible poisons ingested; clinical examination
* Haematological—Hb, platelet count, CBC, blood group, bleeding time, clotting time, prothrombin time, quantitative estimation of clotting factors
* Biochemical—Blood glucose, serum bilirubin, AST, ALT, serum proteins, blood urea, serum phosphates, serum electrolytes, serum calcium, serum phosphorus, serum amylase
* Microbiology—Hepatitis B antigen and IgM anticore antibody, antiserum delta, hepatitis A (IgM) antibody, Hepatitis C (IgM) antibody, Hepatitis C DNA, blood, sputum, urine cultures; smear for malarial parasites, IgM for leptospiral antigen
* Arterial Blood Gas Analysis—Arterial pH and arterial blood gas measurements
* Others—ECG, X-ray of chest and abdomen, ultrasound of the abdomen, EEG
* Special tests for obscure causes

Management

Intensive care is mandatory in fulminant hepatic failure. It is best to admit the patient to a good ICU as soon as definitive neuropsychiatric features become evident. It is wrong to avail of intensive care facilities only when the patient is comatose, as critical care in the early phases may prevent the evolution into deep coma in some patients with severe hepatic necrosis. Even though the survival rates in a good ICU setting have improved, the mortality is still forbiddingly high.

A short summary of the management protocol is given **Table 15.3.4**.

Table 15.3.4. Management of fulminant hepatic failure

1. Overall critical care
   * Nasogastric tube
   * Central venous line for administration of IV fluids and monitoring of CVP
   * Self-retaining catheter for monitoring of urine output
   * Monitoring of temperature, pulse, BP, CVP, ECG, input/output charts
2. Maintain fluid, electrolyte and acid-base balance
3. Management of hepatic encephalopathy
   * Avoid sedation/diuretics
   * Stop protein feeds
   * Amoxycillin 500 mg qds + metronidazole 400 mg thrice daily, given through nasogastric tube
   * Lactulose 10–30 ml 8 hourly orally
   * Daily large bowel wash/enema
4. Reduce cerebral oedema with IV mannitol
5. Treat hypoglycaemia using continuous IV infusion of 10–20% dextrose
6. Management of bleeding tendencies
   * Transfusion of fresh blood, packed RBCs, fresh frozen plasma, cryoprecipitate, Vitamin K, specific deficient clotting factors
7. Maintenance of nutrition—stop all proteins.
   * Give carbohydrates, strained vegetable soup, IV 20% dextrose, Vitamins B and C and multivitamins
   * Correct hypoalbuminaemia with IV salt-free albumin infusions
8. Support other organ systems
9. Control of infection
10. Diagnose and treat complications
11. Consider (when facilities available) a liver transplant in selected cases

General Measures

The patient is barrier-nursed in the ICU; special care, with nurses and attendants using masks and gowns, is necessary. Patients with fulminant virus B hepatitis should be nursed by staff vaccinated against the hepatitis B virus.

In a drowsy patient, or in a patient with a disturbed sensorium, the following general measures are promptly implemented: (i) A nasogastric tube is passed and the stomach deflated. Vigorous suction of the nasogastric tube is avoided; the stomach is best kept empty by gravity drainage. (ii) A self-retaining catheter is introduced into the bladder to allow an accurate intake/output chart to be maintained. (iii) A central venous line is introduced for administration of intravenous fluids, and for monitoring central venous pressure. The earlier this line is inserted, the safer it is. Even in comatose bleeding patients, a central line is mandatory, despite the risk of bleeding that the procedure may entail.

Monitoring of the Patient

Clinical monitoring should include a chart of the grade of the disturbed consciousness, the presence and degree of flapping tremors, the presence of foetor hepaticus, the liver size as obtained by palpation and percussion of the lower edge, as also by percussion of liver dullness in the thorax, the presence of free fluid within the abdomen, the degree of icterus, the urine output in relation to the intake, and the physical examination of the various organ systems of the body. Special emphasis should be laid on close monitoring of the respiratory rate, heart rate and rhythm, blood pressure, central venous pressure, ECG, temperature and the intake-output chart.

Hepatic Encephalopathy

Sedation is avoided at all costs, however violent the patient, as even the mildest sedation appreciably increases the depth of coma. The patient however should be nursed in very quiet surroundings. Protein feeds are totally stopped. Metronidazole 400 mg 8 hourly is given orally through the nasogastric tube; amoxycillin 500 mg qds may also be given. Neomycin is best avoided because of possible nephrotoxic and ototoxic effects.

Lactulose 10–30 ml 8 hourly is administered orally, and the dose so adjusted as to allow 2–4 semisolid stools/day. Lactulose reaches the caecum unchanged, where it is broken down by bacteria to fatty acids. The drop in fecal pH promotes the growth of lactose fermenting organisms, but suppresses the growth of ammonia-forming bacteria. Lactulose may also detoxify short-chain fatty acids produced in the presence of blood and proteins within the gut. It significantly increases the colonic output of bacterial mass and soluble nitrogen (9); the latter thus becomes unavailable for absorption as ammonia.

Lactulose may cause significant diarrhoea leading to hypernatraemia and to volume depletion. The latter is to be avoided at all costs, as it compromises circulation and adversely affects renal function. Lactitol is similar to lactulose, and is often more palatable and acceptable to the patient.

A large bowel (colonic) wash or enema is given daily to evacuate the large bowel of nitrogenous products. Phosphate enemas are advised but we have no experience with their use.

In patients who have a GI bleed, lost blood should be promptly replaced.

Lactulose and/or a mild purgative helps to 'hurry' intestinal contents, and a bowel wash removes nitrogenous products released from the blood within the colon.

Furosemide should be avoided as far as possible, and fluid and electrolyte balance should be well maintained; if disturbed, it should be quickly restored to normal.

Cerebral Oedema

Cerebral oedema with brainstem or cerebellar coning is present at autopsy in 80 per cent of patients with hepatic coma (10). Decerebrate posturing, disturbances in ocular gaze or pupillary size, and sudden deepening of the unconscious state, should be countered by 150 ml of intravenous mannitol given over 1 hour. 100 ml mannitol may be repeated intravenously once or twice in the day; it is best not to exceed 400 ml in 24 hours. Intracranial pressure monitoring is used in some units to help control cerebral oedema.

Focal persistent neurological signs with evidence of raised intracranial tension, should raise the suspicion of intracranial haemorrhage; prognosis in these patients is hopeless.

Maintenance of Fluid and Electrolyte Balance

Fluid and electrolyte balance should be assiduously maintained. Serum sodium levels tend to be low in fulminant hepatic failure. Severe persistent hyponatraemia is a pointer to impending cell death. Hyponatraemia due to obvious salt loss from the body (as with the use of diuretics), is corrected by the use of normal saline; hypertonic saline should be avoided as far as possible.

Hypokalaemia and metabolic alkalosis are frequently observed. The latter potentiates ammonia toxicity. Hypokalaemia is due to nasogastric suction, loss of K^+ from the urine and stools, to the use of intravenous dextrose-insulin, and to a poor intake of potassium. In the presence of a good urine output, 80–120 mEq of potassium may need to be given in an infusion daily. In the terminal stages, or in the presence of renal failure, hyperkalaemia is observed.

Serum calcium levels may be low; 10 ml of 10 per cent calcium gluconate may need to be given intravenously once or twice daily.

Total fluid intake should balance urine output and the loss of other secretions. The central venous pressure should be maintained around 7–8 mm Hg, and should as far as possible not exceed 12 mm Hg. Salt-free albumin is often given intravenously to counter hypoalbuminaemia, and to maintain an effective circulating volume.

Nutrition

All dietary protein should be stopped till recovery ensues. A few days to a few weeks of protein deprivation is well tolerated by these patients. 1500–2000 calories are supplied daily as 20 per cent dextrose through a gastric drip. Strained vegetable soup, also given through the nasogastric tube, provides the necessary minerals and some additional carbohydrates. 20 per cent dextrose is given intravenously through a central line; potassium may be added to the dextrose drip. If blood sugar levels are high, an appropriate dose of insulin may be added to the dextrose infusion. Vitamins B, C and K, together with a multivitamin preparation are also given intravenously daily.

Vegetable proteins are started only when recovery is evident. 10 g are given orally to start with; this is gradually increased as recovery progresses.

In massive hepatic necrosis, there is an increase in the plasma levels of the aromatic aminoacids methionine, tyrosine, and phenylalanine, and a decrease in the branched chain aminoacids leucine, isoleucine and valine. Infusion of branched chain aminoacids has been recommended in the management of hepatic coma, but is not of proven value. Branched chain aminoacids contained in specially made formulations, can also be used orally.

Hypoglycaemia

Persistent intractable hypoglycaemia is of ominous significance (11), and can cause sudden death in these patients. It is countered by a continuous infusion of 20 per cent dextrose. 100 ml of 50 per cent dextrose may need to be given in addition, and should be repeated when blood glucose levels are below 70 mg/dl.

Acid-Base Disturbances

Lactic Acid Acidosis is frequent in patients who are deeply comatose. It may occur even with a normal arterial blood pressure, and is due perhaps to arteriovenous shunting, to capillary endothelial damage, and to poor uptake and utilization of oxygen by tissue cells. This is also of ominous significance, and is countered by improving oxygen delivery or transport to the optimal level. The use of sodium bicarbonate grants only a temporary reprieve.

In the early phases of fulminant hepatic failure, respiratory alkalosis is common. In the presence of hypokalaemia, a mixture of respiratory and metabolic alkalosis may produce a significant increase in the pH. Potassium should be replaced by a slow intravenous infusion. Metabolic acidosis ultimately occurs either due to lactic acid acidosis, or to uraemic acidosis, or to both factors. Mixed acid-base disorders may be frequently observed.

Bleeding

Bleeding is a certain complication of fulminant hepatitis. Spontaneous bruising, bleeding from puncture sites, the mucosa, and into various organ systems, including the brain, is common.

Prevention is possible to a degree by (i) avoiding local trauma, including avoidable needle punctures; (ii) avoiding a tracheostomy; (iii) draining stomach contents by gravity rather than by suction; (iv) avoiding corticosteroids; (v) administering 10 mg Vitamin K intravenously once or twice daily; (vi) using 100 mg ranitidine intravenously 8 hourly, prophylactically.

Treatment consists of infusing fresh blood to replace the lost blood, and by countering defects in clotting factors by infusing fresh frozen plasma. 4–10 packs of fresh frozen plasma or even more may need to be given daily to replenish clotting factors. Severe thrombocytopaenia is treated by platelet infusions. Disseminated intravascular coagulopathy is characterized by an increase in the fibrin degradation products, and by thrombocytopaenia. It should be treated by transfusion of packed cells, and infusion of fresh frozen plasma, cryoprecipitate and platelet concentrates.

Respiratory Failure

Respiratory failure requires expert management. Lung function is impaired for various reasons. Infection, aspiration of gastric contents, atelectasis, and non-cardiogenic pulmonary oedema, all play a part and contribute to a low PaO_2. Patchy shadows develop within the lung and continue to increase. Acute lung injury (ARDS) is the most dreaded of all complications, as it is always fatal when it occurs secondary to fulminant hepatic disease.

It is vital to secure the airway by endotracheal intubation, as soon as the gag reflex is impaired and the patient is slightly obtunded. We prefer the early use of mechanical ventilation to ensure full oxygen saturation of arterial blood.

Circulatory Failure

Volume depletion should be guarded against and promptly corrected. Large quantities of volume infusion to maintain blood pressure, often precipitates acute lung injury (ARDS). If filling pressures are adequate and arterial blood pressure is still below 100 mm Hg, inotropic support with dopamine should be commenced. We always use a low dose dopamine support (for its diuretic effect), in all patients with hepatic coma.

Arrhythmias are frequent in the terminal phase. Hypo- and hyperkalaemia are easily correctible causes of dangerous arrhythmias.

Renal Failure

Fifty-five per cent of patients develop prerenal azotaemia that may ultimately cause acute tubular necrosis (10, 12). Hypovolaemia, blood loss, sepsis and deep jaundice all contribute to renal failure. Treatment is on lines outlined in the Chapter on Acute Renal Failure. Continuous arteriovenous haemofiltration (CAVH) may be necessary in patients with marked oliguria, to allow an adequate fluid intake and to provide nutritional support. Hyperkalaemia or fluid overload in the presence of severe oliguria, also necessitates the use of CAVH.

Infection

Urinary infection, respiratory infection and sepsis iatrogenically introduced through central lines and catheters, are frequent in spite of the best intensive care offered to these patients. Patients with fulminant hepatic failure are immunocompromised to some extent, and acute Gram-negative bacterial sepsis is often observed. Appropriate antibiotics are invariably necessary. Aminoglycosides should not be used as far as possible in the presence of renal dysfunction. Blood cultures, cultures of catheter tips, bacteriological examination of urine and sputum, are always performed. Fungal infections may be overlooked as blood cultures are not always positive. They should be suspected when the patient deteriorates after an initial improvement, and in the presence of leucocytosis, renal dysfunction and pyrexia not responding to antibiotics. Antifungal agents should be used with care because of potential hepatic and renal toxicity. Scrupulous attention to aseptic suction through the endotracheal tube, and to careful handling and protection of central venous lines must be given to prevent iatrogenic infection.

Acute Pancreatitis

This is a dreaded complication of fulminant hepatitis. It should be suspected in the presence of (i) severe upper abdominal pain; (ii) a sudden deterioration in the clinical state; (iii) a marked tenderness in the abdomen; (iv) rapid development of free fluid within the abdomen. A marked rise in serum amylase is observed in most, but not all patients. Pancreatitis in fulminant hepatic failure can be due to the hepatitis virus, to shock, sepsis, corticosteroid therapy, or bleeding within the pancreas. It carries virtually a hopeless prognosis.

Corticosteroids are not found to be of any use in fulminant hepatic failure; in fact, they may well produce further complications (13)—gastric erosions, infection, pancreatitis. Interferon is not indicated in fulminant hepatitis B or delta virus, as the virus has already been eliminated, and hepatic necrosis is immunologically mediated (10).

Exchange blood or plasma transfusions, or charcoal haemoperfusion, do not improve overall mortality in patients with fulminant hepatic failure.

Hepatic Transplantation (14, 15)

Hepatic transplant needs to be considered in all patients with Grade III and IV encephalopathy. The survival rate of these patients on conservative management is 20 per cent even in good centres offering excellent critical care. Currently, the survival rate is about 60 per cent after a hepatic transplant. Results in hepatitis B infection are better because the disease does not recur in the transplanted liver. Recurrence in the transplant has been noted in non-A, non-B hepatitis. Transplants have also been successfully performed in hepatic failure due to drugs, poisons, and in the acute form of Wilson's disease. In practice, it is difficult at times to gauge not only the need for a transplant, but the correct time for surgical intervention. In India, hepatic transplants have just begun to be performed. The poor availability of donor organs, the lack of infrastructure which hinders the prompt use of donor organs for transplant purposes, are some of the hurdles that afflict transplant surgery in this country.

The King's College modified criteria for transplantation in acute liver cell failure are given below. (**Table 15.3.5**)

Table 15.3.5. King's College Modified Indications for Liver Transplantation in Acute Liver Failure

---

Aetiology: Liver Failure Unrelated to Acetaminophen
Indicators
1. PT INR > 6.5 with any degree of encephalopathy or
2. Three of the following variables with any degree of encephalopathy:
   Age < 10 or > 40 years of age
   Etiology: Idiopathic nonviral hepatitis; idiosyncratic drug reactions
   Serum bilirubin > 17.5 mg/dl (> 300 µmol/l)
   PT INR > 3.5

Aetiology: Acetaminophen
Indicators
1. PT INR > 6.5
2. Serum creatinine > 3.4 mg/dl (> 300 µmol/l) in patients with grade III or IV encephalopathy or
3. pH < 7.3, with any degree of encephalopathy

From: Shakil AO, Kramer D, Mazariegos GV et al. (2000).
Liver Transpl. 6(2): 163–169, with permission of Wiley-Liss, Inc., a subsidiary of John Wiley & Sons, Inc.

In transplant centres, the chief contraindications to hepatic transplant include a cerebral perfusion pressure less than 50 mm Hg for > 2 hours despite therapy, ongoing sepsis, ARDS, an FIO_2 ≥ 60 per cent, uncal herniation with dilated pupils, and brain damage caused by an intracranial bleed (16).

Patients desperately needing a transplant may need to wait for lack of a donor organ, and may die before this is available. The current strategies in transplant centres that help to tide over this possible waiting period are the use of artificial or bioartificial livers, hepatocyte transplantation and extracorporeal perfusion.

Critical Care of Complications in Chronic Liver Cell Failure

Patients with chronic liver cell dysfunction need intensive care when they develop an acute hepatic encephalopathy (i.e. acute on chronic liver failure), a severe gastrointestinal bleed, an acute infection, or develop oliguric renal failure. More than one of these complications often co-exist in the same patient.

Acute Hepatic Encephalopathy

Acute hepatic encephalopathy in a cirrhotic patient may occur spontaneously in the natural course of events, usually as a terminal feature in a patient who has ascites and is deeply jaundiced. More often than not, acute encephalopathy in cirrhotics is precipitated by factors which further depress liver cell function, and increase nitrogenous material within the gut. These precipitating factors should be sought for, recognized and rectified as a matter of immediate priority after admission to the ICU.

The precipitating factors are:

(i) *Use of furosemide or other diuretics, volume loss, and subtle electrolyte disturbances* even in the absence of significant hypovolaemia, trigger acute neuropsychiatric features in these patients.

(ii) *Paracentesis* involving removal of a large quantity of ascitic fluid is an important precipitating cause of coma. Again electrolyte imbalance following removal of large quantities of electrolytes and water, hypotension and changes in the hepatic circulation may be contributory factors. These changes are not necessarily reflected by disturbances in serum electrolytes.

(iii) *Fluid and electrolyte loss* from vomiting, diarrhoea or from inadequate fluid intake.

The above precipitating factors can be corrected by intravenous infusions of fluid and electrolytes, and restoring electrolyte balance. Correction of hyponatraemia and hypokalaemia are of prime importance. Hypovolaemia can be quickly corrected by the intravenous infusion of salt free albumin. Hypotension, which persists after volume replacement should be treated by inotropic (dopamine) support.

Therapeutic paracentesis for ascites should not be performed in patients who are severely ill with chronic liver cell dysfunction, as this can precipitate both hepatic encephalopathy and acute oliguric renal failure.

The indications and precautions for therapeutic paracentesis (17) are tabled below (**Table 15.3.6**).

(iv) *Gastrointestinal bleeds* or blood loss from any other source

Table 15.3.6. Selection of patients for therapeutic paracentesis

* Tense ascites
* Preferably with oedema
* Child's Grade B
* Prothrombin > 40%
* Serum bilirubin < 10 mg/dl
* Platelets > 40,000/mm^3
* Serum creatinine < 3 mg/dl
* Urinary sodium > 10 mEq/24 hours

From: Sherlock S, 1989. Diseases of the Liver and Biliary System. Blackwell Scientific Publications, London, Oxford.

is one of the most important precipitating factors. It may be occult and may not manifest immediately. A rectal examination may reveal the presence of melaena and should always be performed as part of a routine examination. Coma in these patients may be due to hypovolaemia, hypotension, presence and absorption of increased proteins and their breakdown products from blood within the gut, and also to anaemia if there is a significant drop in the haemoglobin. We are of the opinion, that even a mild gastrointestinal bleed in decompensated cirrhotics needs to be replaced by a blood transfusion. A laxative to evacuate the intestinal contents of blood, and a bowel wash, should also be promptly given.

(v) *Infection.* This is an important precipitant; its source and nature should be sought for, identified and treated. Commonly, infection involves the lungs and urinary tract. Spontaneous bacterial peritonitis is characterized by the presence of infected ascitic fluid in the absence of a recognizable cause of secondary peritonitis (**18**). It can result in a rapidly evolving acute encephalopathy in cirrhotics, and should always be suspected when a patient with cirrhosis deteriorates suddenly without any apparent cause. The clinical features include pyrexia, diffuse or localized abdominal pain on palpation. These features may however be absent, and the diagnosis is made only when a high index of suspicion results in the examination of ascitic fluid which shows > 250 polymorphs/mm^3. The association of a pH < 7.3 and polymorphs > 500/mm^3 in the ascitic fluid, is diagnostic of bacterial peritonitis (**19, 20**). The infection is generally blood borne and usually monomicrobial (**17**). Patients with cirrhosis are immunocompromised and prone to bacteraemia. Ascitic fluid is a good culture medium for bacterial growth. If the opsonic activity of ascitic fluid is very low, there is poor opsonic coating of bacteria within the fluid; bacteria are therefore not destroyed by polymorphs, and produce a peritonitis. Culture of ascitic fluid in our limited experience, is rarely positive. At times infection of the peritoneum is not blood borne, but occurs through the gut wall, pointing to poor immune defences that allow a breach or perforation of the gut wall by intestinal flora. Infecting organisms are Gram-negative E. coli or streptococci.

Broad-spectrum antibiotics (we prefer the third generation cephalosporin, cefotaxime) should be used under the following conditions: (a) when clinical features are typical of spontaneous bacterial peritonitis; (b) when the ascitic fluid shows polymorphs > 250/mm^3 and the clinical picture is compatible with a bacterial peritonitis; (c) when the ascitic fluid shows a polymorph count > 500/mm^3 even in the absence of symptoms or signs of peritonitis (**21**). Therapeutic paracentesis should be done.

Prognosis is grave; it depends on the severity of bacterial infection of the peritoneum, the degree of underlying liver cell dysfunction, and the degree of clinical deterioration precipitated by the infection. The survival rate over a year in those patients who are discharged from the hospital, is dismal, being less than 21–38 per cent (**18**).

(vi) *Stress* in the form of surgery, trauma, fracture, shock or anaesthesia can further depress hepatic function.

(vii) *Acute alcoholic bouts.* Ingestion of alcohol precipitates drowsiness and coma both by producing an associated acute alcoholic hepatitis, and by depressing cerebral function. Sudden alconol withdrawal can also precipitate neuropsychiatric disturbances which may be difficult to distinguish from hepatic encephalopathy.

(viii) *Sedatives,* even if mild or in small doses, are an important cause of neuropsychiatric symptoms and acute encephalopathy. They should be strictly avoided in all cirrhotics.

(ix) *Constipation,* in our experience, sometimes triggers encephalopathy probably by increasing the nitrogenous content within the bowel and providing for a larger source of ammonia products.

(x) *A large protein meal* acts in a similar fashion, and its effect is accentuated by the presence of constipation.

Hepatic encephalopathy is treated on the lines already elaborated upon in acute fulminant hepatitis. It is obvious that the prognosis is better if a precipitating factor is identified and quickly corrected.

In the absence of a past history it is often difficult to determine whether acute encephalopathy, jaundice and deranged liver cell functions are due to acute hepatocellular dysfunction in a patient with a previously normal liver, or are due to acute on chronic liver cell failure. A poor nutritional state, a firm enlarged spleen, a firm and at times irregular liver with presence of spider nevi, point to acute on chronic liver cell dysfunction.

Neuropsychiatric features in acute on chronic liver cell failure are commonly misdiagnosed as acute alcoholic intoxication or alcohol withdrawal syndrome. A wrong diagnosis of a manic/depressive psychosis may also be made. Symptoms are at times bizarre, and may be transient lasting for only 8–12 hours. We have seen such abnormal neuropsychiatric behaviour necessitating admission, after ingestion of a large meal or following constipation, in patients with cirrhosis. A good clinical examination for gynaecomastia, liver palms, spider nevi, and for other clinical and biochemical evidence of liver cell dysfunction will always clarify the diagnosis.

Severe Gastrointestinal Bleeding

Acute gastrointestinal bleeding in a cirrhotic patient is a dreaded emergency requiring critical care. GI bleeds are most commonly due to bleeding oesophageal or gastric varices. They could also result from acute gastroduodenal erosions, a Mallory-Weiss syndrome, or a chronic peptic ulcer. The present discussion is related to the diagnosis and management of variceal bleeding in cirrhotics in an intensive care setting.

Diagnosis

The diagnosis is made by the presence of:

(i) Features of blood loss causing hypovolaemia and a lowered haemoglobin concentration.

(ii) The presence of a deteriorating liver cell function—encephalopathy, increasing jaundice and increasing ascites. Deteriorating liver cell function is due to hypovoiaemia, diminished hepatic arterial flow, increased nitrogen content in the gut due to the presence of blood within, and lowered haemoglobin content, which further accentuate hypoxic damage to the regenerating liver nodules in these patients.

(iii) Presence of blood in the nasogastric tube aspirate or the presence of melaena. These need not always be present. A slow ooze may fill the gut with blood before the bleed can be recognized. A rectal examination may demonstrate melaena, and may allow an earlier diagnosis to be made in a cirrhotic who has suddenly deteriorated.

Endoscopy is vital to determine the source of bleeding. Routine ultrasound examination of the abdomen is also done to determine the patency of the portal and hepatic veins, and to exclude a hepatocellular malignancy.

Routine biochemical tests to evaluate liver cell function should always include prothrombin time, and serum proteins with albumin and globumin levels. Baseline values of CBC, PCV, Hb, serum electrolytes, urea and creatinine are also mandatory.

Prognosis

The prognosis of a severe bleed from oesophageal varices is grim. The association of jaundice, ascites and encephalopathy in a variceal bleed carries an 80 per cent mortality. Prognosis can be classified according to Child into three risk grades (22). The one year survival in good risk patients (Child A and B) is about 70 per cent and in bad risk patients (Child C) about 30 per cent (**Table 15.3.7**).

Management (Fig. 15.3.1)

The patient with a GI bleed is promptly graded according to Child's classification. Blood transfusions should be promptly given to correct hypovolaemia; 4–10 units of blood may be necessary. Clotting factors are deficient in many of these patients; if possible, transfusion of fresh blood or fresh packed cells is preferred. Fresh frozen plasma may also be necessary. Over-expansion of the blood volume is avoided for fear of rebleeding (due to raised portal vein pressure) or pulmonary oedema. The central venous pressure must be maintained around +7 to + 10 mm Hg. In patients with pulmonary congestion, or in those in whom left ventricular dysfunction is suspected, it is preferable to monitor the left

Table 15.3.7. Child's classification of hepatocellular function in cirrhosis

	Se Bilirubin (mg%)	Se Albumin (g%)	Ascites	Neurological Disorder	Nutrition
Group A	< 2	> 3.5	Absent	Absent	Excellent
Group B	2–3	3–3.5	Well controlled	Minimal	Good
Group C	> 3	< 3	Poorly controlled	Advanced coma	Poor (wasting)

From: Sherlock S, 1989. Diseases of the Liver and Biliary System, Blackwell Scientific Publications, London, Oxford.

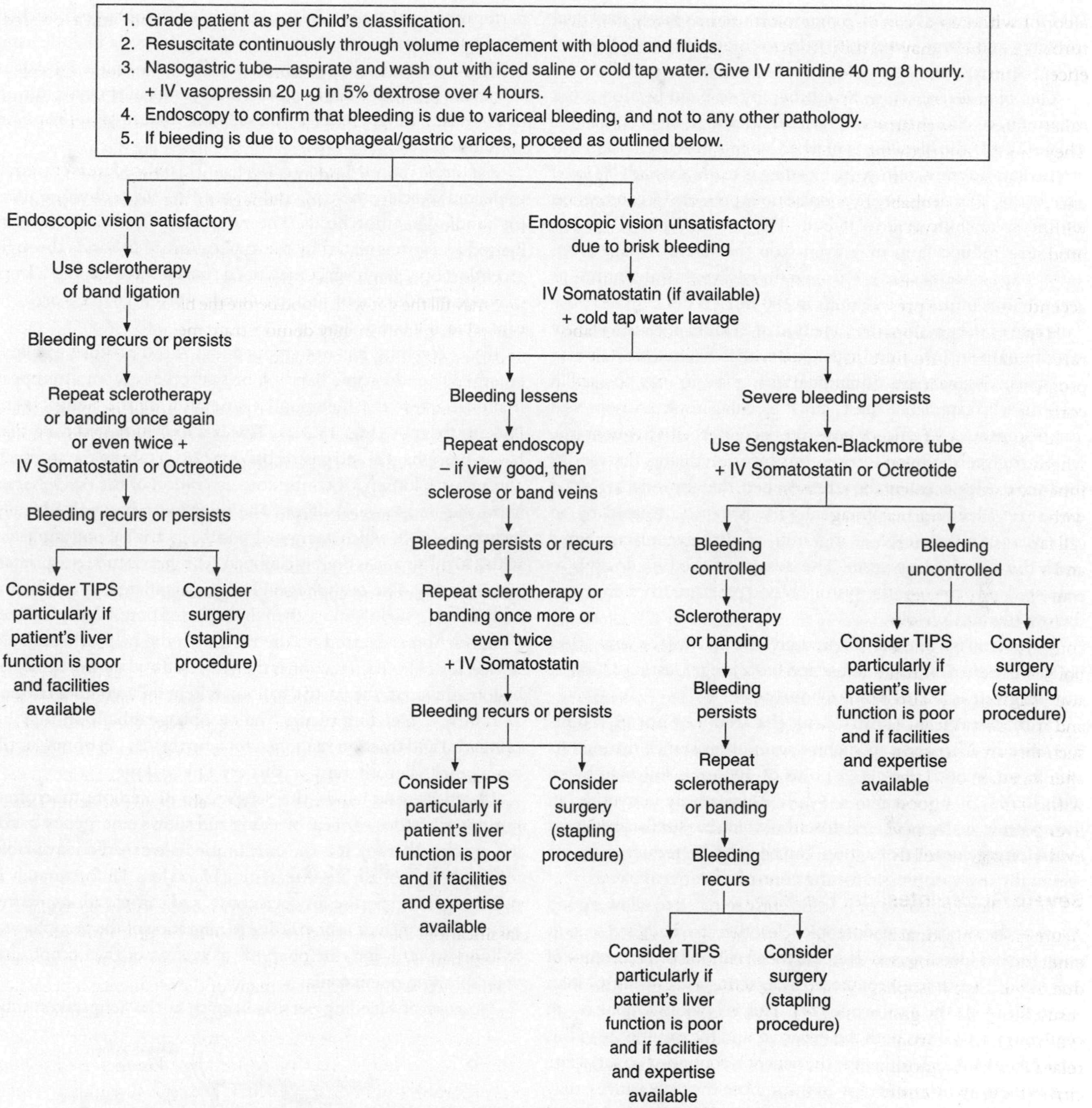

1. Grade patient as per Child's classification.
2. Resuscitate continuously through volume replacement with blood and fluids.
3. Nasogastric tube—aspirate and wash out with iced saline or cold tap water. Give IV ranitidine 40 mg 8 hourly.
   + IV vasopressin 20 µg in 5% dextrose over 4 hours.
4. Endoscopy to confirm that bleeding is due to variceal bleeding, and not to any other pathology.
5. If bleeding is due to oesophageal/gastric varices, proceed as outlined below.

Endoscopic vision satisfactory

Use sclerotherapy of band ligation

Bleeding recurs or persists

Repeat sclerotherapy or banding once again or even twice + IV Somatostatin or Octreotide

Bleeding recurs or persists

Consider TIPS particularly if patient's liver function is poor and facilities available

Consider surgery (stapling procedure)

Endoscopic vision unsatisfactory due to brisk bleeding

IV Somatostatin (if available) + cold tap water lavage

Bleeding lessens

Repeat endoscopy – if view good, then sclerose or band veins

Bleeding persists or recurs

Repeat sclerotherapy or banding once more or even twice + IV Somatostatin

Bleeding recurs or persists

Consider TIPS particularly if patient's liver function is poor and if facilities and expertise available

Consider surgery (stapling procedure)

Severe bleeding persists

Use Sengstaken-Blackmore tube + IV Somatostatin or Octreotide

Bleeding controlled

Sclerotherapy or banding

Bleeding persists

Repeat sclerotherapy or banding

Bleeding recurs

Consider TIPS particularly if patient's liver function is poor and if facilities and expertise available

Consider surgery (stapling procedure)

Bleeding uncontrolled

Consider TIPS particularly if patient's liver function is poor and if facilities and expertise available

Consider surgery (stapling procedure)

Fig. 15.3.1. Flow chart summarizing the management of variceal bleeding.

ventricular filling pressures through a Swan-Ganz catheter. The pulmonary capillary wedge pressure should be around 12 mm Hg and should not exceed 15 mm Hg.

Intravenous ranitidine 50 mg 8 hourly is started in the hope that it will prevent bleeding from stress-induced gastroduodenal mucosal erosions (**22**).

Sedatives are avoided as far as possible. If the patient is an alcoholic, alcohol withdrawal may precipitate neuropsychiatric disturbances. Distinguishing alcohol withdrawal from hepatic encephalopathy due to a severe GI bleed, may be difficult and at

times impossible. Flapping tremors and fetor hepaticus, if present, point to hepatic encephalopathy. A markedly raised prothrombin time (close to twice the control value) always points to severely impaired liver cell function.

Measures to prevent or treat an encephalopathy have been already detailed. Dietary proteins are stopped. A nasogastric tube should be promptly passed and the stomach kept empty. Ice cold lavage of the stomach, with 1–2 ml of adrenaline added to the wash, are given in the hope of arresting bleeding. This can be performed as frequently as necessary. Lactulose is given orally

10–30 ml 8 hourly. Milk of magnesia is used to hurry intestinal contents, and a large bowel wash helps to empty the colon of altered blood. Amoxycillin 500 mg four times a day is given orally.

Control of Haemorrhage. Sclerotherapy or band ligation is the treatment of choice for acute variceal bleeding, but is impossible to perform if the bleeding is marked, as this obscures vision. An immediate attempt to stop the bleeding is made through *the use of vasopressin.* This drug lowers portal venous pressure by constriction of the splanchnic arteriolar bed. The lowered portal venous pressure reduces and may even stop the haemorrhage from oesophageal varices (**23**). Vasopressin is given as a continuous intravenous infusion of 20 units in 100 ml of 5 per cent dextrose (at a rate of 0.4 µg/min) over a period of 2 hours. It causes colicky abdominal pain, pallor, and in patients with ischaemic heart disease can cause anginal pain. Sublingual nitroglycerin may be used in patients who experience chest pain. If bleeding restarts, vasopressin can be repeated; its efficacy however decreases with frequent use.

Nitroglycerine in an intravenous infusion dilates the venous bed and to a lesser extent the arteriolar bed, thereby reducing blood pressure. Bleeding oesophageal varices can be treated by an intravenous infusion (20–40 mg/min) of nitroglycerin combined with the use of vasopressin. The dosage of the two drugs is so adjusted as to prevent the systolic blood pressure from dropping below 100 mm systolic.

Glypressin is a costly synthetic derivative that has the same effect as vasopressin. It is more stable and has a longer lasting action. It can be given as a 2 mg bolus 6 hourly.

Somatostatin is a costly drug that reduces portal venous pressure by increasing splanchnic arterial resistance through its action on smooth muscle. A bolus of 500 µg is followed by an infusion of 250 µg/hour for 4–5 days. Alternatively, octreotide (an octapeptide analogue of somatostatin) which has similar properties but a longer duration of action, can be used. To reduce costs, we generally use vasopressin for the control of variceal bleeds.

If the bleeding stops, or is sufficiently reduced to allow a good view of the varices, an endoscopic sclerotherapy is advised so as to stop further bleeding and decrease the likelihood of recurrence of the bleed. The varix is thrombosed by injecting a sclerosing solution introduced via the endoscope (**24**). This is obviously done by an endoscopist who has both the expertise and the experience in this procedure. After sclerotherapy the patient is continued on sucralfate 1 g twice daily. Sclerotherapy to thrombose multiple varices, may need to be done over 2–3 sessions. Control of bleeding is observed in 71–88 per cent of patients (**25**). Sclerotherapy is felt to be superior to tamponade and the use of vasopressin and nitroglycerin, though rebleeding and survival are no different (**25**). In patients classed as Grade C of Child's classification, there was no difference in survival after sclerotherapy as compared to controls (**26**).

Complications following sclerotherapy include mucosal ulcers that have opened in a submucosal venous channel. Rebleeding is seen in 30 per cent of cases, either from the remaining varices or from ulcers. The former requires further sclerotherapy; omeprazole helps to arrest bleeding from ulcers. Oesophageal stricture may result from chemical oesophagitis, and acid reflux. Rarely

perforation of the oesophagus, or even an oesophago-bronchial fistula may result (**27**). Pulmonary complications include aspiration pneumonia, pleural effusion and mediastinitis. Pyrexia is frequent after sclerotherapy, and bacteraemia may occur during or following the procedure, necessitating the use of appropriate antibiotics.

Endoscopic Variceal Banding or Ligation. This procedure is currently preferred to sclerotherapy, and is based on the technique used for banding haemorrhoids. The varices are identified and then ligated and strangulated by the application of O bands through an endoscope. Each varix may need two to three bands. Ulcers may occur at the site of previous bands. Torrential haemorrhage can occur if a band 'slips'.

If the bleeding has not stopped and is too profuse to allow emergency endoscopic banding or sclerotherapy, an attempt is made to arrest the bleeding by insertion of the Sengstaken-Blakemore tube (**Fig. 15.3.2**). This is a four-lumened tube that has an oesophageal and gastric balloon (**28**), a tube in the stomach and a fourth lumen for continuous aspiration of the oesophagus above the oesophageal balloon. The lubricated tube is passed orally into the stomach which is emptied, and the gastric balloon is inflated with 250 ml air and is doubly clamped. The gastric tube is aspirated continuously. The oesophageal balloon is inflated to a pressure of 40 mm Hg slightly more than the expected portal vein pressure. Firm traction is exerted on the tube with the help of a suitable device, for 24 hours. Traction is then released and the oesophageal balloon deflated; the gastric balloon is kept inflated for a further 24 hours. If bleeding recurs, the oesophageal balloon may be reinflated and traction reapplied for a further 24–48 hours, or till emergency sclerotherapy or surgery can be done.

In experienced hands, the Sengstaken-Blakemore tube often temporarily stops variceal bleeding and allows emergency banding or sclerotherapy. It is the only immediate expedient available for stopping profuse life-threatening blood loss. Unfortunately it requires great expertise for correct use, and complications are frequent. These include asphyxia due to migration of the oesophageal balloon upwards into the pharynx, ulceration of the oesophagus and aspiration pneumonia.

However if bleeding persists in spite of the Sengstaken tube

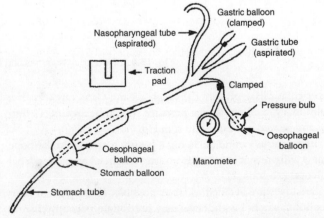

Fig. 15.3.2. Sengstaken-Blakemore oesophageal compression tube.

so that banding or sclerotherapy is not possible, or if the bleeding continues following sclerotherapy, TIPS or emergency surgery is warranted.

TIPS (**29**). The transjugular intrahepatic portosystemic shunt (TIPS) is a new non-operative therapeutic option for the management of variceal bleeding in patients with poor liver function (Grade C of Child's classification), particularly those awaiting a liver transplant. It is important to attempt TIPS to arrest variceal bleeding only if full medical treatment (use of vasoactive drugs, sclerotherapy or banding) has failed. The procedure is performed under sedation and local anaesthesia using ultrasound control. The middle hepatic vein is catheterized through the transjugular route and a needle is inserted through the catheter (under ultrasound guidance) and through the liver parenchyma, into a main portal vein branch. A guide wire is introduced through the needle and the catheter advanced into the portal vein. The needle is removed and the portal vein gradient measured. The needle tract is dilated by a balloon, and a self-expanding metal stent is inserted and expanded to 8–12 mm. A porto-systemic shunt is thus established; reduction in portal vein pressure should arrest variceal bleeding. TIPS seems more effective in controlling and preventing variceal bleeding than sclerotherapy (**30**).

The mortality during or soon after the procedure is less than 1 per cent in experienced hands. Complications chiefly include haemorrhage (intra-abdominal, biliary, or through the liver capsule), infection, and stent stenosis or occlusion. Early occlusion is seen in 12 per cent and is usually due to thrombosis within the shunt. Shunt occlusion results in recurrence of variceal bleeding. Late occlusion is due to intimal proliferation at the hepatic venous end of the stent. Other complications are—TIPS encephalopathy (due to porto-systemic shunt), renal failure (due to excessive intravenous contrast used). Hepatic infarction can occur from misplacement of the stent into the right hepatic artery. In conclusion, TIPS is a relatively new method to control bleeding in gastrooesophageal varices when conventional methods using vasopressors and banding or sclerotherapy have failed. TIPS in experienced hands, controls bleeding, reduces the rate of rebleeding but has little effect on survival (**31**). We are on a learning curve with regard to the TIPS procedure, and so far our results have been unsatisfactory.

Emergency Surgery. Emergency surgery for bleeding oesophageal varices has been considerably reduced following the use of vasoactive drugs, sclerotherapy, balloon tamponade and TIPS. When these fail or if the expertise for performing TIPS is unavailable in patients who rebleed after banding or sclerotherapy, emergency surgery is warranted. Oesophageal transection using the stapling procedure is the surgery of choice. Stapling arrests haemorrhage, but death occurs in 30–40 per cent of patients from hepatocellular failure. Alternative emergency surgical procedures are performing a mesocaval or portocaval shunt. Both are associated with a high mortality and a high incidence of hepatic encephalopathy in Grade C patients. In our set-up we rarely advocate emergency surgery in patients categorized as under Grade C of Child's classification.

Prevention of Bleeding. Propranolol decreases the risk of recurrent variceal bleeding but has little effect on survival. It is of value in gastropathy. Nadolol and isosorbide mononitrate have shown better results than sclerotherapy in reducing the risk of rebleeding (**32**).

Various portal systemic shunt procedures are used to prevent recurrent gastro-oesophageal variceal bleeding. These include portocaval, mesocaval or splenorenal shunts. For poor risk patients the mortality is 50 per cent; in good risk patients it is about 5 per cent. Hepatic encephalopathy is an important complication of portocaval shunts. Myelopathy with paraplegia and a Parkinsonian picture are other complications.

Hepatic transplant is perhaps the optimal solution to recurrent bleeding varices in cirrhotic patients. Previous sclerotherapy or porto-systemic shunts do not affect post-transplant survival (**33**).

Acute Infections

Patients with chronic liver cell dysfunction need intensive care if there is a serious, often life-threatening infection. Bacteraemia with sepsis is an important, life-threatening complication in these patients. The source of bacteraemia is generally undetermined. The role of translocation of bacteria from the gut in patients with impaired liver cell function, may have a significant role both in initiating and perpetuating sepsis. As mentioned earlier, acute infections involving any organ system, invariably worsen liver cell function and may well precipitate hepatic encephalopathy. In cirrhotics, body responses to infection may not be as vigorous as in patients who are normal to start with. Fever may be low grade, physical findings may be meagre, and leucocytosis may be absent. In the absence of a definite source of infection, the possibility of a specific bacterial peritonitis should always be excluded by examination of the ascitic fluid (see previous section of this chapter). Patient care demands the prompt use of empiric therapy with antibiotics after blood cultures and other relevant cultures and microbiological tests have been sent for examination. The antibiotics frequently used are a third generation cephalosporin plus ciprofloxacin. If there is a possibility of a staphylococcal infection, vancomycin needs to be added (see Chapter on the Immunocompromised Patient).

Acute Oliguric Renal Failure

Acute renal failure could be due to prerenal causes or to acute tubular necrosis. Prerenal causes include hypovolaemia, blood loss, hypotension from any cause, or fluid and electrolyte disturbances. Paracentesis of a large volume of ascitic fluid or over-vigorous diuretic therapy often precipitates oliguric renal failure. Acute tubular necrosis may occur in some of these patients. The hepatorenal syndrome as mentioned earlier, is characterized by progressive acute oliguric renal failure in the presence of normal tubular function.

Volume replacement, replacement of blood loss and the use of low dose dopamine infusions to improve the urine output, should be prompt. The prognosis of a fully evolved hepatorenal syndrome is well-nigh hopeless.

Iatrogenic and other potentially correctible problems causing

Table 15.3.8. Iatrogenic causes of oliguric renal failure (and their treatment) in chronic liver cell failure

Causes	Treatment
1. Drugs	
* Diuretics/Lactulose	Volume expansion
* Non-steroidal anti-inflammatory drugs	Stop drugs
* Aminoglycosides	Stop drug
* Cyclosporine	Haemodialysis
2. Paracentesis of large volume of ascitic fluid	Volume expansion
3. Volume depletion (blood loss/ vomiting/diarrhoea)	Volume replacement

oliguric renal failure are listed in **Table 15.3.8**. They should be carefully assessed and as far as possible corrected. Even so the prognosis in the presence of azotaemia is grim.

REFERENCES

1. Bernuau J, Reuff B, Benhamou JP. (1986). Fulminant and subfulminant liver failure: definitions and causes. Semin Liver Dis. 6, 97.

2. O'Grady JG, Schalm SW, Williams R. (1993). Acute liver failure: redefining the syndromes. Lancet. 342, 273.

3. Chu CM, Sheen IS, Liard YF. (1994). The role of hepatitis C virus in fulminant viral hepatitis in an area with endemic hepatitis A or B. Gastroenterology. 107, 189.

4. Khuroo MS. (2003). Aetiology and Prognostic factors in acute liver failure in India. J Viral Hepat. 10(3), 224–231.

5. Jain A, Kar P, Madan K. (1999). Hepatitis C virus in sporadic fulminant viral hepatitis in North India: cause or co-factor? Eur J Gastroenterol Hepatol. 11(11), 1231–1237.

6. Purtilo DT, White R, Filipovich A et al. (1985). Fulminant liver failure induced by adenovirus after bone marrow transplantation. N Engl J Med. 312, 1707.

7. Taylor RJ, Saul SH, Dowling JN et al. (1981). Primary disseminated herpes simplex infection with fulminant hepatitis following renal transplantation. Arch Intern Med. 141, 1519.

8. Sherlock S, Dooley J. (1997). Hepatic Encephalopathy. In: Diseases of the Liver and Biliary System (Eds Sherlock S, Dooley J). pp. 95–115. Blackwell Scientific Publications, Oxford, London, Edinburgh, Boston, Melbourne.

9. Weber FL, Banwell JG, Fresard KM et al. (1987). Nitrogen in fecal bacterial fiber, and soluble fractions of patients with cirrhosis: effects of lactulose and lactulose plus neomycin. J Lab Clin Med. 110, 259.

10. Sherlock S, Dooley J. (1997). Fulminant Hepatic Failure. In: Diseases of the Liver and Biliary System (Eds Sherlock S, Dooley J). pp. 103–117. Blackwell Scientific Publications, Oxford, London, Edinburgh, Boston, Melbourne.

11. Samson RI, Trey C, Timme AH et al. (1967). Fulminanting hepatitis with recurrent hypoglycemia and hemorrhage. Gastroenterology. 53, 291.

12. Ring-Larsen H, Palazzo U. (1981). Renal failure in fulminant hepatic failure and terminal cirrhosis: a comparison between incidence, types and prognosis. Gut. 22, 585.

13. EASL Study Group (1979). Randomised trial of steroid therapy in acute liver failure. Gut. 20, 620.

14. Van Thiel DH. (1993). When should a decision to procede with transplantation actually be made in cases of fulminant or subfulminant hepatic failure: at admission to hospital or when a donor organ is made available? J Hepatol. 17, 1.

15. Williams R, O'Grady JG. (1990). Liver transplantation: results, advances and problems. J Gastroenterol Hepatol. Suppl 1, 110.

16. Shakil AO, Mazariegos GV, Kramer DJ. (1999). Fulminant hepatic failure. Surg Clin North Am. 79, 77.

17. Sherlock S, Dooley J. (1997). Ascites. In: Diseases of the Liver and Biliary System (Eds Sherlock S, Dooley J). pp. 119–134. Blackwell Scientific Publications, Oxford, London, Edinburgh, Boston, Melbourne.

18. Hoefs JC, Canawati HN, Sapico FL et al. (1982). Spontaneous bacterial peritonitis. Hepatology. 2, 399.

19. Gitlin N, Stauffer JL, Silvestri RC. (1982). The pH of ascitic fluid in the diagnosis of spontaneous bacterial peritonitis in alcoholic cirrhosis. Hepatology. 2, 408.

20. Strassen WN, McCullough AJ, Bacon BR et al. (1986). Immediate diagnostic criteria for bacterial infection of ascitic fluid. Evaluation of ascitic fluid polymorphonuclear leukocyte count, pH and lactate concentration, alone and in combination. Gastroenterology. 90, 1247.

21. Conn HO. (1982). Acidic ascitic fluid: a leap forward (or a step?) Hepatology. 2, 507.

22. Sherlock S. (1989). The portal venous system and portal hypertension. In: Diseases of the Liver and Biliary System (Ed. Sherlock S). pp. 151–207. Blackwell Scientific Publications, Oxford, London, Edinburgh, Boston, Melbourne.

23. Shaldon S, Sherlock S. (1960). The use of vasopressin ('pitpressin') in the control of bleeding from esophageal varices. Lancet. ii, 222.

24. Snady H. (1987). The role of sclerotherapy in the treatment of esophageal varices: personal experience and a review of randomized trials. Am J Gastro. 82, 813.

25. Westaby D, Hayes PC, Gimson AES et al. (1989). Controlled clinical trial of injection sclerotherapy for active variceal bleeding. Hepatology. 9, 274.

26. Larson AW, Cohen H, Zweiban B et al. (1986). Acute esophageal variceal sclerotherapy. Results of a prospective randomized controlled trial. J Am Med Assoc. 255, 497.

27. Tabibian N, Schwartz JT, Lacey Smith J et al. (1987). Cardiac tamponade as a result of endoscopic sclerotherapy: report of a case. Surgery. 102, 546.

28. Pitcher JL. (1971). Safety and effectiveness of the modified Sengstaken-Blakemore tube: a prospective study. Gastroenterology. 61, 291.

29. La Berge JM, Somberg KA, Lake JR et al. (1995). Two-year outcome following transjugular intra-hepatic portosystemic shunt for variceal bleeding: results in 90 patients. Gastroenterology. 108, 529.

30. Merli M, Riggio O, Capocaccia L et al. (1994). Transjugular intrahepatic portosystemic shunt versus endoscopic sclerotherapy in preventing variceal rebleeding: preliminary results of a randomized controlled trial. Hepatology. 20, 107A.

31. Rossle M, Deibert P, Haag K et al. (1994). TIPS versus sclerotherapy and β-blockade: preliminary results of a randomized study in patients with recurrent variceal haemorrhage. Hepatology. 1994. 20, 107A.

32. Villanueva C, Balanzo J, Novella MT et al. (1996). Nadolzol plus isosorbide mononitrate compared with sclerotherapy for the prevention of variceal rebleeding. N Engl J Med. 334, 1624.

33. Ho K-S, Lashner BA, Emond JC et al. (1993). Prior oesophageal variceal bleeding does not adversely affect survival after orthotopic liver transplantation. Hepatology. 18, 66.

Acute (Fulminant) Necrotizing Pancreatitis

Acute inflammation of the pancreas can be of varying severity. Mild or acute oedematous pancreatitis has a good prognosis and recovery almost always ensues. These patients can be managed in the general wards of a hospital. However in about 30 per cent of patients the inflammation is severe and necrotizing, and often complicated by retroperitoneal sepsis. The mortality in fulminant necrotizing pancreatitis approaches 50 per cent. Critical care is mandatory in these patients. It ensures early aggressive resuscitation, close monitoring of the patient, and prompt diagnosis and management of complications frequently observed in the fulminant forms of the disease.

Aetiology

The two important causes of acute pancreatitis are gallstone disease and excessive alcohol consumption. Pathogenesis in gallstone disease may be related to obstruction of the pancreatic duct during passage of a gallstone. This obstruction results in ductal hypertension which through rather obscure mechanisms leads to zymogen activation. Activated pancreatic enzymes cause pancreatic inflammation, tissue destruction and various complications observed in the disease.

The pathogenesis of pancreatic inflammation in alcohol abuse, is obscure. Alcohol may have a direct action on acinar cells or may produce spasm of the sphincter of Oddi, with ductal hypertension. Alcohol-induced pancreatitis is directly related to the quantity and duration of alcohol consumption.

Pancreatitis may occasionally follow abdominal surgery, particularly surgery on the biliary tree. Early detection may be difficult, as the clinical features in these patients are often atypical. Persistent pain or unexpected prolonged ileus following abdominal surgery should raise the possibility of pancreatitis.

Endoscopic retrograde cholangiopancreaticography (ERCP) results in acute pancreatitis in 2 per cent of cases.

There are numerous other causes of pancreatitis listed in **Table 15.4.1.** These include drugs, viral and other infections, trauma, pancreatic tumours, autoimmune disease and metabolic causes (hypercalcaemia, hyperlipidaemia). Pancreatitis is also associated with Type I and Type V hyperlipoproteinaemias. Hypertriglyceridaemia may be the underlying mechanism in these patients.

Table 15.4.1. Aetiology of acute pancreatitis

* Alcohol
* Gallstones
* Following surgery, specially after biliary tract surgery
* Trauma
* Post-ERCP
* Drugs—corticosteroids
* Hypercalcaemia
* Hyperlipidaemia
* Infections e.g. mumps, coxsackie virus
* Polyarteritis nodosa and other collagen disorders
* Low flow states/embolic
* Idiopathic

Rarely, autoimmune disease can cause or be associated with pancreatitis. In spite of an elaborate work-up, 7 to 10 per cent of patients have idiopathic pancreatitis, where the cause is undetermined.

Patients in the ICU with acute pancreatitis, fall into two groups:

1. Those who were in reasonably good health, and who are now stricken with the disease and require intensive care. These patients are admitted primarily for acute severe pancreatitis.

2. Those who are already seriously ill in the ICU with a critical illness, and in whom pancreatitis develops as a further complication. The list of critical illnesses in the ICU that form a background to a complicating pancreatitis continues to grow, and is shown in **Table 15.4.2.**

Table 15.4.2. Important critical illnesses and problems in the ICU that predispose to acute pancreatitis

* Major upper abdominal surgery
* Shock of any aetiology
* Cardiopulmonary bypass
* Repair of abdominal aortic aneurysm
* Kidney/liver transplantation

The reason why seriously ill patients with diverse critical illnesses should develop the unrelated and potentially lethal complication of acute pancreatitis, is poorly understood. Multifactorial causes are probably responsible (1–10). Review of possible mechanisms of acute pancreatitis in critically ill patients suggests that hypoperfusion injury plays an important pathogenic role. Warshaw and O'Hara (11) go so far as to suggest that shock from any cause is a risk factor for the development of acute pancreatitis. The mechanisms that relate hypoperfusion states to release of activated pancreatic enzymes, and to pancreatic inflammation, are not known.

Physiopathology

The pancreas secretes a number of digestive enzymes, which are secreted as inactive proenzymes or zymogens. When activated enzymes come in contact with tissues outside their usual milieu, they have the potential to produce inflammation, necrosis and cellular death. This is normally prevented by the storage of inactive pancreatic zymogens and enzyme activators in separate cytosol granules. Once the integrity of this protective compartmentalization is lost, autodigestion due to enzymatic activation occurs, initiating a self-perpetuating inflammatory reaction. Activated enzymes, which include proteases such as trypsin, chymotrypsin and elastase, can in turn activate proenzymes in the inflammatory and complement cascades. Lipase produces fat necrosis and liberates phospholipid remnants. Inflammation and necrosis is not confined to the pancreatic and peripancreatic area, but can occur in various organ systems, leading to multiple organ dysfunction and death.

Sepsis frequently complicates necrotizing pancreatitis. Systemic toxicity is related to the release of several mediators, including arachidonic acid metabolites, interleukin-1 and other cytokines.

Clinical Features and Diagnostic Evaluation

Clinical assessment is initially directed towards establishing a diagnosis and determining the severity and prognosis of acute pancreatitis. Further diagnostic evaluation is then necessary to identify the presence of pancreatic necrosis and pancreatic and peripancreatic suppuration. The timing and nature of surgical intervention in some of these patients is indeed a matter of fine judgement based on clinical features, results of diagnostic tests, and experience.

Abdominal pain and vomiting are invariably present. Unlike the pain of a perforated peptic ulcer, the severity of which is maximal almost from the start, the pain of acute pancreatitis often builds up to a crescendo over a matter of hours. The pain is classically initially felt in the upper abdomen. It is however often poorly localized, and may be felt all over the abdomen, as also in the back. Rarely it is experienced more in the back than the abdomen. Low grade fever is often present. Abdominal distension and tenderness on palpation are present, but guarding and rigidity denoting peritonitis, are late in developing and may be absent to start with. Abdominal findings in any case, do not necessarily indicate the severity of the retroperitoneal inflammatory process. Localized 'ileus' may cause gastric dilatation which worsens vomiting. Localized effect of inflammation on the distal transverse colon leads to distension of the loop of the transverse colon with the 'colon cut off' sign on X-ray of the abdomen. In fulminant cases when retroperitoneal inflammation extends beyond the pancreas, erythema around the flanks may occur. Ecchymosis of the flanks (Grey-Turner's sign), and of the umbilicus (Cullen's sign), has been described, but is rarely observed. It is due to bleeding into the pancreatic bed or retroperitoneal space.

All patients with severe pancreatitis show circulatory changes of hypovolaemia, characterized by tachycardia, hypotension, cold peripheries and a falling urine output. Hypovolaemia is due to transudation of fluid into the retroperitoneal space, peripancreatic and extrapancreatic tissues, to sequestration of fluid in the ileum and to ascites. In fact, the diagnosis of acute pancreatitis should be always considered in any patient with abdominal pain and a compromised circulation.

Peripancreatic fluid collections occur in up to 50 per cent of patients. Pseudocysts are better defined collections of fluid within the lesser sac, and occur in 10 to 15 per cent of patients. Pseudocysts can compress the stomach, duodenum and rarely the bile duct. Pseudocysts can leak into the peritoneal cavity, or track into the retroperitoneal space, pleural cavity or even rarely into the pericardial space.

Necrosis of a part of the inflamed pancreas is termed acute necrotizing pancreatitis. If volume replacement has been adequate, necrotizing pancreatitis is characterized by clinical features of the systemic inflammatory response syndrome and is associated with a hyperdynamic circulation, tachycardia, tachypnoea, hypotension and fever.

Pulmonary complications are an intrinsic feature of almost every patient with severe necrotizing pancreatitis. Tachypnoea is invariably present. Hypoxia may occur without significant changes in an X-ray of the chest. Raised diaphragms, basal atelectasis are commonly observed. Pleural effusions (usually left sided) are frequent; the pleural fluid is an exudate with a high amylase content.

Complications

Complications may be local (within the abdomen), or systemic (taking the form of the multiple organ dysfunction syndrome—MODS). We would consider 'complications' to be really a progressive evolution of the pathology and natural history of fulminating pancreatitis.

Local Complications

(i) Local fluid collections have been already commented upon.

(ii) Erosion of mesenteric vessels can lead to massive colonic bleed, to haematemesis, or to severe melaena. Haemorrhage into the pancreas, pancreatic duct or pancreatic bed can also occur.

(iii) Pancreatico-enteric or pancreatico-colonic fistulas may occur.

(iv) Necrotizing pancreatitis is often associated with infection in the necrotic area, leading to increasing sepsis. Suppuration within the pancreas leads to a localized abscess. Suppuration can also involve the peripancreatic area. Local fluid collections can also suppurate.

Multiple Organ Dysfunction Syndrome

This is the most dreaded and frequent complication of severe necrotizing pancreatitis, particularly if the necrotic areas are infected. All organs can be involved. ARDS occurs in more than 20 per cent of patients and is associated with a mortality of over

60 per cent. Oliguric renal failure is associated with a mortality greater than 50 per cent. Liver cell dysfunction is often observed. Disseminated intravascular coagulopathy has a grim prognosis. Metabolic complications include hyperlipidaemia, hyperglycaemia, hypocalcaemia and metabolic acidosis. Rarely coma results from a pancreatic encephalopathy.

In critically ill patients already under intensive care, the sudden added complication of acute pancreatitis may go unrecognized for a length of time. Abdominal pain and vomiting may not be severe enough to draw attention to the nature of the problem. The patient may develop non-specific features of fever, leucocytosis, haemodynamic instability, and hypotension necessitating increased fluid requirements. Yet the classic major abdominal signs may be still absent. A quick deterioration in an already ill individual is observed. Diagnosis is possible only if there is a high index of suspicion.

Severe pancreatitis may be clinically difficult to distinguish from perforation, bowel obstruction, bowel infarction, and a leaking abdominal aortic aneurysm. Each one of these pathologies, except acute pancreatitis, requires immediate surgical intervention. The importance of a correct diagnosis can therefore never be overstressed.

Laboratory Investigations

Elevated serum amylase and lipase levels are found in a number of patients, but these tests lack both good sensitivity and specificity. A normal serum amylase does not exclude acute pancreatitis, and enzyme elevation is often also observed in a perforated ulcer, postoperative states, bowel obstruction and infarction, renal insufficiency and ruptured ectopic pregnancy. Serum amylase levels > 1000 Somogyi units are however most frequently observed only in acute pancreatitis. The measurements of isoenzymes of amylase lend some further specificity to elevated amylase levels, but the sensitivity is not what it should be. Amylase levels in blood may fall to normal within a few days after pancreatitis. Serum lipase levels remain elevated for 7 to 10 days; lipase activity is perhaps more sensitive and specific compared to amylase activity. Elevated lipase levels have been reported in bowel obstruction and cholecystitis.

Patients with gallstone pancreatitis have generally much higher AST, ALT and alkaline phosphatase levels, compared to pancreatitis due to other aetiologies.

Other routine blood and biochemical tests are done as for any patient with a serious illness; none of these are diagnostic. A low serum calcium level is often observed. Arterial pH for determining metabolic acidosis and arterial blood gases should always be estimated.

Patients presenting with suspected acute pancreatitis should undergo routine abdominal and chest X-rays, which help in differentiating pancreatitis from intestinal obstruction and perforation. Pleural effusions in a patient with severe abdominal pain should suggest pancreatitis. Pancreatitis may also be suggested by localized jejunal or colonic ileus, a widened duodenal C loop, associated radio-opaque gallstones, free fluid within the abdomen, and gas in the pancreatic bed, suggestive of a pancreatic or peripancreatic abscess.

Imaging Studies

Imaging the pancreas by ultrasound and CT scan studies are far more sensitive diagnostic tests than the serial estimation of enzyme levels in blood. Demonstration of an enlarged pancreas by imaging techniques confirms a diagnosis. Imaging abnormalities, even in mild cases, often persist for one week so that this modality is useful for the retrospective diagnosis of acute pancreatitis. Both ultrasound and CT imaging should be used, as they are complimentary to each other. The presence of bowel gas or obesity interferes with the examination of the retroperitoneum by ultrasonography. Subtle changes in tissue density denoting necrosis, haemorrhage and suppuration are not easily defined by this imaging technique (12). However valuable information about the biliary tree can be obtained, and ultrasonography has more sensitivity than the CT scan in picking up stones obstructing the biliary tree. CT scanning is invaluable for a study of the retroperitoneal space. Its crucial value lies in the recognition and follow-up of local complications of acute pancreatitis. It thus identifies pancreatic necrosis, haemorrhage and pancreatic and peripancreatic suppuration with precision. It is also superior to ultrasonography in identifying high density fluid collections in the transverse mesocolon, small bowel mesentery, pararenal, perirenal, renal and paracolic spaces (13) (see Section on Imaging in the Critical Care Unit).

Severity of Disease

It is important for the critical care physician not only to establish a diagnosis of acute pancreatitis but also to assess its severity. Ranson's criteria (14) have been used since 1976 to assess the severity and prognosis of a patient who presents with, and is admitted for acute pancreatitis. These criteria are difficult to evaluate in a patient who is already critically ill and who then develops pancreatitis as an added complication. Many of Ranson's criteria are directed towards the systemic effects of the disease. In patients who are critically ill to start with, many of these criteria may already be present prior to the onset of pancreatitis. They are therefore of little value in assessing the prognosis and severity of the disease under the circumstances stated above. **Table 15.4.3** lists Ranson's diagnostic criteria.

The APACHE II scoring system has also been used to assess the severity and prognosis of acute pancreatitis. Increased APACHE II scores correlate with increased risk of in-hospital mortality, but lack sensitivity in determining acute severe pancreatitis.

Table 15.4.3. Ranson's early objective prognostic signs used for estimating risk of death or major complications in acute pancreatitis

On Admission	During First 48 Hours
* Age > 55	* Haematocrit fall > 10 percentage points
* WBC > 16,000/mm^3	* BUN rise > 5 mg/100 ml
* Blood sugar > 200 mg/100 ml	* Serum calcium < 8 mg/100 ml
* Serum LDH > 350 IU/l	* PaO$_2$ < 60 mm Hg
* SGOT > 250 U/dl	* Base Deficit > 4 mEq/l
	* Estimated fluid sequestration > 6 l

From: Ransom JHC et al. 1976. Prognostic signs and non-operative peritoneal lavage in acute pancreatitis. Surg Gynecol Obstet (now called J of Am College of Surgeons). 143, 209.

The difficulties with scoring systems led to a new classification system adopted at the Atlanta International Symposium **Table 15.4.4**. This classification system focuses heavily on organ system failure, but takes into consideration other scoring systems, as also local complications of pancreatitis (**15**).

Table 15.4.4. Clinically based classification defining severe acute pancreatitis

Systemic Complications	Values Defining Complications
Cardiovascular	Systolic blood pressure < 90 mm Hg
Respiratory	PaO$_2$ < 60 mm Hg
Renal	Creatinine > 177 μmol/l (2 mg/dl) after hydration
Gastrointestinal haemorrhage	> 500 ml/24 hours
Coagulation	Platelets < 100,000/mm^3 or fibrinogen < 1 g/l or fibrin split products > 80 μg/ml.
Metabolic	Calcium < 1.87 mmol/l (7.5 mg/dl)

Multiple Organ System Dysfunction Defined by	
Ranson criteria	≥ 3
APACHE II score	≥ 8

Clinical Signs or Pancreatic Collections	
Pancreatic collections	Pancreatic necrosis, abscess, or acute pseudocyst
Clinical signs	Epigastric mass, Grey Turner's sign, Cullen's sign

From: Bradley EL. (1993). A clinically based classification system for acute pancreatitis. Arch Surg. 128, 586–590. American Medical Association.

Numerous blood tests have been suggested as indicators of severity of the disease and of pancreatic necrosis. These include plasma levels of cyclic adenosine monophosphate, albumin, methaemalbumin (**16**), C reactive protein, and fibrinogen (**17, 18**). The volume and colour of a peritoneal diagnostic aspirate has also been found to be useful (**19**). Currently, scoring systems based on CT appearances of the diseased pancreas and its surroundings have been developed. Clinical assessment of the patient together with serial CT scan studies, probably remain the best predictors of severity and outcome, particularly in an ICU setting (**20, 21**).

Identification of Local Pancreatic Complications

In a patient who progressively deteriorates, or who after a phase of significant improvement lasting for 8–10 days, again starts to deteriorate, pancreatic complications should always be suspected. These fortunately can be proven by the CT appearance of increasing pancreatic necrosis and suppuration. CT guided percutaneous needle aspiration of areas of pancreatic necrosis, or of pancreatic and peripancreatic fluid collections is now the recommended approach for exact diagnosis and further management. Microscopic examination with Gram's stain and culture of aspirated material for aerobic and anaerobic organisms should be done (**22, 23**). At least 40 per cent of necrotic collections are found to be infected at the time of initial intervention. Gram-negative infections particularly due to E. coli, Klebsiella and Ps. aeruginosa are most frequent. However a wide variety of Gram-positive and Gram-negative organisms, both aerobic and anaerobic, and occasionally fungi have

been isolated on culture. Sensitivity tests to different antibiotics guide medical management.

Evaluation of Other Organ Systems

Acute necrotizing pancreatitis is an important cause of multiple organ dysfunction syndrome. Each organ system therefore needs careful evaluation and daily follow-up both through clinical examination and relevant laboratory tests. Involvement of the respiratory system is part and parcel of the features of severe pancreatitis. Hypoxic respiratory failure may occur without ARDS (**24**). A CT scan of the lower chest often shows presence of pulmonary involvement which has been undetected on a chest X-ray.

The evolution of ARDS is characterized by an increasing alveolar-arterial gradient, bilateral pulmonary shadows and an increasing right to left shunt within the lungs.

Renal function, liver function, metabolic abnormalities, arterial pH and blood gas changes, CNS function and alteration in the coagulation profile need careful evaluation.

The numerous possible complications of fulminant pancreatitis are given below in **Table 15.4.5**.

Table 15.4.5. Complications of acute (fulminant) pancreatitis

A. Local
  * Pancreatic/peripancreatic suppuration and necrosis
  * Pancreatic abscess
  * Pseudocyst formation
  * Enteric fistulae
  * Catastrophic GI bleeds or bleeding into retroperitoneal tissues due to pancreatic/peripancreatic inflammation destroying vessel walls, or causing erosion of splenic or other large vessels

B. Systemic
  * Respiratory—Pleural effusion, V̇/Q̇ abnormalities, acute lung injury
  * Renal dysfunction, multiple organ dysfunction syndrome
  * CNS—Pancreatic encephalopathy

Management

Management includes:
(a) Careful monitoring of the patient.
(b) Relief of pain.
(c) Correction of haemodynamic defects—chiefly correction of volume depletion and electrolyte abnormalities. It is essential to maintain adequate oxygen transport and tissue perfusion to important organ systems during the period of acute illness, and during resolution of the inflammatory process within the pancreas.
(d) Correction of metabolic abnormalities.
(e) Control of pancreatic enzyme secretion as far as possible.
(f) Support to all other organ systems, particularly the respiratory and renal systems.
(g) Nutritional support.
(h) Use of antibiotics.
(i) Treatment of local complications arising from acute pancreatitis.

Ongoing evaluation of the patient requires close cooperation between the physician and an experienced surgeon in the surgical management of abdominal complications. The decision regarding the timing and nature of the surgical intervention is based not only on the clinical features, biochemical investigations, and CT appearances, but also on clinical experience and judgement.

(a) Careful Monitoring of the Patient

In critically ill patients, full haemodynamic monitoring is of great value, and should include heart rate, arterial blood pressure, ECG, central venous pressure, and hourly urine output. In patients with large volume deficits, or in those who are haemodynamically unstable, or have sepsis or pulmonary complications, a Swan-Ganz catheter may be necessary to measure and monitor pulmonary capillary wedge pressure, cardiac index, vascular resistances and oxygen derived variables.

Frequent examination of the CBC, blood chemistry, serum electrolytes and arterial blood gases are necessary to detect complications, to evaluate the function of various organ systems, and to judge the adequacy of treatment.

Serial ultrasounds and CT scans are of great importance in evaluating retroperitoneal complications.

(b) Relief of Pain

Pain can be excruciating in the early phase. Pethidine 25 mg intravenously or 100 mg intramuscularly is preferred to morphine, as the latter can contract the sphincter of Oddi, and can theoretically worsen the pancreatitis. Buprenorphine 150 µg diluted in 10–20 ml of N saline and given slowly 8 hourly via an epidural catheter, is also effective in relieving pancreatic pain.

(c) Fluid and Electrolyte Restitution and Correction of Haemodynamic Defects

Volume replacement is of crucial importance. Acute fulminant pancreatitis is in effect a massive retroperitoneal burn with an ongoing loss of fluid into the retroperitoneum, peritoneal cavity, and into the gut. Volume requirements vary. In severe cases it may be > 8–10 l within a period of 24 hours. The adequacy of fluid replacement in severe cases should be judged clinically, and by monitoring the central venous pressure and the pulmonary capillary wedge pressure. The latter should be kept between 12–15 mm Hg. Fluids used for volume replacement include both colloids and isotonic crystalloids.

Potassium replacement is also invariably necessary. Blood transfusions may be necessary to counter retroperitoneal haemorrhage produced by proteolytic enzyme extravasation. Hypoalbuminaemia when present, should be treated by intravenous infusions of albumin. Successful fluid resuscitation should result in warm peripheries, a good pulse volume, a normal arterial blood pressure, a good urine output and an improved mixed venous oxygen tension ($P\bar{v}O_2$).

If the patient is still hypotensive in spite of adequate fluid replacement (as judged by the CVP and PCWP), inotropic support is mandatory. Dopamine 10–15 µg/kg/min in a slow intravenous infusion, offers good cardiovascular support. Dobutamine may be preferred to dopamine in patients who are already vasoconstricted. Both these drugs can be used for inotropic support. It is important to maximize oxygen delivery or transport, in the hope that perfusion improves, and oxygen uptake and oxygen utilization by tissues are increased. Evaluation of organ perfusion is difficult. Perfusion of tissues may be inadequate even in the presence of a normal arterial blood pressure. A low $P\bar{v}O_2$ (< 35 mm Hg), and/or the presence of lactic acid acidosis, are additional pointers to hypoperfusion.

(d) Correction of Metabolic Abnormalities

Metabolic acidosis, hyperglycaemia, hypocalcaemia and hypomagnesaemia must be recognized and treated. Restoration of fluid volume, arterial blood pressure and perfusion, generally suffice to correct the metabolic acidosis.

(e) Control of Pancreatic Enzyme Secretion

There is no definite way of reducing pancreatic enzyme secretion in acute pancreatitis. Nasogastric suction is advisable in severe cases; it is absolutely indicated in the presence of ileus and continuous vomiting. It decreases the risk of aspiration, and may perhaps help in reducing pancreatic secretions. We also routinely use a H_2-antagonist intravenously to help reduce gastric acid secretion. This decreases the chances of bleeding from acute erosions, and may perhaps also help to reduce pancreatic secretions. Somatostatin in an intravenous bolus dose of 500 µg, followed by an infusion of 250 µg over 4 hours, has also been shown to suppress pancreatic secretion. However its high cost precludes its use for many patients in our part of the world.

(f) Support to Other Organ systems

Respiratory Support

Patients who are severely tachypnoeic with a respiratory rate > 30/min, or who have a PaO_2 < 60 mm Hg in spite of getting oxygen at 6–8 l/min through nasal prongs or a face mask, need to be intubated and kept on ventilator support. Mechanical ventilation ensures a high PaO_2 and maximum oxygen saturation of arterial blood. The evolution of acute lung injury and ARDS requires expert care till such time as the complication resolves. Increased alveolar-arterial oxygen gradients may occur in pancreatitis, without necessarily progressing to ARDS.

Renal Support

Renal function may deteriorate despite adequate haemodynamic resuscitation. A low-dose dopamine infusion to enhance urine output is recommended in those with a low urine output. In patients with increasing azotaemia, temporary haemodialysis or haemofiltration should be carried out till renal function returns. Recovery following a complicating acute tubular necrosis is possible with good critical care.

(g) Nutritional Support

All oral feeds or nutrients are stopped in severe pancreatitis as pancreatic exocrine secretion is stimulated by intragastric and intraduodenal stimuli. The first priority is the restitution of fluid and electrolyte loss and restoration of haemodynamic stability.

Once this is achieved patients are started on nutritional support. The recent trend is to use total enteral nutrition (TEN) through a naso-jejunal tube. It is suggested that early use of the gut maintains mucosal integrity and prevents translocation of intestinal bacteria into the pancreatic bed, thereby reducing the incidence of pancreatic infection, an important cause of morbidity and mortality in this disease.

Ideally the patient should be maintained in a positive nitrogen balance, though this may at times prove impossibly difficult. A total caloric intake of 25 to 30 kcal/kg should suffice. Proteins should supply 1 to 1.5 g/kg and 50–60 per cent of the nutrient mixture should consist of carbohydrate. Hyperglycaemia should be controlled by insulin so that blood sugar levels are < 150 mg/dl. In patients fed enterally, a low fat diet, with fats constituting less than 20 per cent of total calories is preferable as this minimizes pancreatic stimulation. Elemental diets that contain fat in the form of medium chain triglycerides should be used to minimize pancreatic stimulation (25).

Enteral nutrition may be impossible in the presence of fulminating disease associated with vomiting, distension, ileus, peritonitis and severe sepsis. In these patients nutritional support with caloric intake outlined above should be given by total parenteral nutrition. Intravenous lipid emulsions are not harmful in patients with severe pancreatitis. Nosocomial sepsis through central catheter related infections are a grave potential danger in patients on parenteral nutrition.

Vitamins, minerals, calcium, magnesium, antioxidants also need to be given for nutritional support.

Criteria for starting oral feeds are: (i) absence of abdominal pain; (ii) reduction of amylase and lipase to normal levels; (iii) absence of complications like pancreatic fistulas; (iv) resolution of ileus with return of bowel sounds.

(h) Antibiotics

A Gram-negative infection in and around the retroperitoneal necrotic pancreatic area, invariably supervenes in patients with fulminant pancreatitis. In our protocol, we use a third generation cephalosporin, metronidazole and either ciprofloxacin or an aminoglycoside from the very start of the illness. Imepenem or meropenem are antibiotics with a good penetration within pancreatic tissue and are often used in combination with metronidazole.

(i) Critical Care Management of Complications of Pancreatitis

The complications that should be anticipated are (i) pancreatic necrosis; (ii) infected necrosis, pancreatic abscess and peripancreatic suppuration; (iii) pseudocyst formation; rarer complications include (iv) enteric fistulae and (v) castastrophic bleeds.

(i) Pancreatic Necrosis

Patchy devitalization with necrosis of the pancreatic gland occurs from within a few days to a few weeks of the onset of acute inflammation. The clinical picture is one of persistent low grade fever, abdominal pain and leucocytosis. The diagnosis is made on a CT scan which shows local areas of nonenhancement. It may be impossible to determine whether the necrotic area is infected or not. Therefore a CT guided needle aspiration with microbiological examination of the aspirate is mandatory. The growth of aerobic and/or anaerobic organisms signifies infection. A negative culture however, does not always exclude the presence of infection in a necrotic area. Only 40 per cent of patients with pancreatic necrosis get infected (26). Surgery should not be done if the patient has only a low grade fever, the CT findings are not suggestive of an infected necrosis or abscess, and if a CT guided aspiration of the necrotic area is sterile.

(ii) Infected Pancreatic and Peripancreatic Necrosis, Pancreatic Abscess

Contamination of the necrotic pancreas by bacteria (presumably from the transverse colon) leads to infected pancreatic necrosis. Liquefaction of the necrotic areas produces an abscess which can be generally made out on a CT scan. CT guided needle aspiration is positive for bacteria on Gram's stain and/or a culture. The clinical course in patients with retroperitoneal sepsis can be rapidly downhill, with spiking fever, leucocytosis, tachycardia and tachypnoea.

Surgical Debridement of Infected Pancreatic Necrosis. The mortality in patients from infected pancreatic necrosis is 15–40 per cent (27, 28). Death in the majority of these patients is due to fulminant sepsis with progressive multiple organ dysfunction syndrome. Surgery in fulminant necrotizing pancreatitis should be reserved only for pancreatic sepsis. Persistent gallstone pancreatitis can be effectively dealt with by endoscopic sphincterotomy and is no longer an indication for surgery.

Currently, experience of several surgeons in the field of pancreatic surgery has led to the following guidelines for surgical debridement in pancreatic sepsis.

(i) Surgery should not be done within the first seven days of the onset of fulminating pancreatitis—death is almost inevitable.

(ii) The longer the surgery is delayed the less the surgical mortality. Those operated upon within 15 days of the onset of pancreatitis suffer over twice the mortality as compared to those operated on later (28, 29). Of late, placement of wide-bore percutaneous drainage for pancreatic suppuration thereby delaying surgery to around 28 days is being advocated. Antibiotics, nutritional support and support to all organ systems is mandatory during this period.

(iii) A rapidly progressive MODS with features of severe sepsis may however force the surgeon to an earlier intervention. The details of surgical procedures are beyond the scope of this book.

(iii) Pancreatic Pseudocyst

Fluid collections within and around the lesser sac are easily picked up by ultrasound and CT examinations of the abdomen. When sufficiently large, these collections can be palpated per abdomen. Diagnosis of a pancreatic pseudocyst does not necessitate treatment unless the cyst is infected, bleeds or ruptures into the peritoneal cavity or bowel. Repeated percutaneous aspirations of the pseudocyst may however be necessary. Definitive surgery, even for a large pseudocyst, should be delayed preferably for at least six weeks, by which time the patient is stable, and the cyst wall thick enough to allow anastomosis between the cyst and the gut.

(iv) Enteric Fistulae

These occur during the phase of severe retroperitoneal inflammation associated with fulminant pancreatitis. The retroperitoneal inflammation can cause thrombosis of vessels supplying the gut; the middle colic vessels supplying the transverse colon are particularly vulnerable. Necrosis of the colonic wall leads to colonic fistula. Gastric, duodenal and small bowel perforation and fistulae can also occur. Awareness of a possibility of enteric fistulae as a major hazard of acute pancreatitis allows a quicker diagnosis and planned surgical treatment.

(v) Catastrophic Bleeding

Severe bleeding occurs when pancreatic and peripancreatic inflammation destroys vessel walls within the retroperitoneal space or causes erosion of the splenic or other large vessels. Surgical control of bleeding may be virtually impossible in the midst of inflamed distorted tissue planes. Embolization of the vessels employing angiographic techniques to identify the bleeding vessels, is the treatment of choice. Ischaemic necrosis of the transverse colon can also cause bleeds into the large bowel.

REFERENCES

1. Colon R, Frazier OH, Kahan BD. (1988). Complications in cardiac transplant patients requiring general surgery. Surgery. 103, 32.

2. Feiner H. (1976). Pancreatitis after cardiac surgery: A morphologic study. Am J Surg. 131, 684.

3. Moneta GL, Misbach GA, Ivey TD. (1985). Hypoperfusion as a possible factor for the development of gastrointestinal complications after cardiac surgery. Am J Surg. 149(5), 648.

4. Mikhailidis DP, Hutton RA, Jeremy JY et al. (1983). Hypothermia and pancreatitis. J Clin Pathol. 36, 483.

5. Rose DM, Ranson JHC, Cunningham JN, Spencer FC. (1984). Patterns of severe pancreatic injury following cardiopulmonary bypass. Ann Surg. 199, 168.

6. Greenbaum RA, Barradas MA, Mikhailidis DP et al. (1987). Effect of heparin and contrast medium on platelet function during routine cardiac catheterization. Cardiovasc Res. 21, 878.

7. Grace AA, Barradas MA, Mikhailidis DP et al. (1987). Cyclosporine A enhances platelet aggregation. Kidney Int. 32, 889.

8. Dandona P, Junglee D, Katrak A et al. (1985). Increased serum pancreatic enzymes after treatment with methylprednisolone: Possible evidence of subclinical pancreatitis. Br Med J. 291, 24.

9. Victor DW, Rayburn JL, McCready RA et al. (1988). Pancreatitis following aneurysmectomy. J Ky Med Assoc. 86(6), 285.

10. Frick TW, Fryd DS, Sutherland DER et al. (1987). Hypercalcemia associated with pancreatitis and hyperamylasemia in renal transplant recipients. Am J Surg. 154, 487.

11. Warshaw AL, O'Hara PJ. (1978). Susceptibility of the pancreas to ischemic injury in shock. Ann Surg. 188, 197.

12. Jeffrey RB. (1989). Sonography in acute pancreatitis. Radiol Clin North Am. 27(1), 5.

13. Balthazar EJ. (1989). CT diagnosis and staging of acute pancreatitis. Radiol Clin North Am. 27(1), 19.

14. Ranson JHC, Rifkind KM, Turner JW. (1976). Prognostic signs and nonoperative peritoneal lavage in acute pancreatitis. Surg Gynecol Obstet. 143, 209.

15. Bradley EL III. (1993). A clinically based classification system for acute pancreatitis. Summary of the International Symposium on Acute Pancreatitis, Atlanta, Sept. 11–13, 1992. Arch Surg. 128, 586.

16. Kelly TR, Klein RL, Porquez JM et al. (1972). Methemalbumin in acute pancreatitis: An experimental and clinical appraisal. Ann Surg. 175, 15.

17. Bery AR, Taylor TV, Davies GC. (1982). Diagnostic tests and prognostic indicators in acute pancreatitis. J R Coll Surg Edinb. 27, 345.

18. Buchler M, Malfertheimer P, Schoetensack C. (1986). Sensitivity of antiproteases, complement factors and C-reactive protein in detecting pancreatic necrosis. Int J Pancreatol. 1, 227.

19. McMahon MJ, Pickford IR, Playforth MJ. (1980). Early prediction of severity of acute pancreatitis using peritoneal lavage. Acta Chir Scand. 146, 171.

20. Balthazar EJ, Ranson JHC, Naidich DP. (1985). Acute pancreatitis: prognostic value of CT. Radiology. 156, 767.

21. Kivisarri L, Somer K, Standertskjold-Nord-Enstam CG. (1980). Early detection of acute fulminant pancreatitis by contrast enhanced computed tomography. Scand J Gastroenterol. 15, 633.

22. Gerzof S, Banks P, Spechler S. (1984). Role of percutaneous aspiration in early diagnosis of pancreatic sepsis. Dig Dis Sci. 29, 950.

23. Karlson KB, Martin EC, Fanuchen EI. (1982). Percutaneous drainage of pancreatic pseudocysts and abscesses. Radiology. 142, 619.

24. De Coninck B et al. (1991). Scintigraphy with Indium-labelled leukocytes in acute pancreatitis. Acta Gastroenterol Belg. 54, 176–183.

25. Keith RG. (1980). Effect of a low fat elemental diet on pancreatic secretion during pancreatitis. Surg Gynecol Obstet. 151, 337–343.

26. Berger HG, Krauzberger W, Bittner R. (1985). Results of surgical treatment of necrotizing pancreatitis. World J Surg. 9, 972.

27. Beger HG, Rau B, Mayer J et al. (1997). Natural course of acute pancreatitis. World J Surg. 21, 130–135.

28. Bhansali SK, Shah SC, Desai SB et al. (2003). Infected necrosis complicating acute pancreatitis: experience with 131 cases. Indian J Gastroenterol. 22, 7–10.

29. Bradley EL III. (1994). Surgical indications and techniques in necrotizing pancreatitis. In: Acute Pancreatitis: Diagnosis and Therapy (Ed. Bradley EL III). pp. 105–117. Raven Press, New York.

Acute Gastrointestinal Bleeds Requiring Critical Care

Upper Gastrointestinal Bleeding

General Considerations

Upper gastrointestinal (GI) bleeds are a frequent cause of emergency admission to hospitals. By upper gastrointestinal bleeing is meant bleeding from the oesophagus, stomach or duodenum, arising from above the ligament of Treitz. Occassionally blood arising from the nose, oropharynx, larynx or lungs is swallowed and either vomited as 'haematemesis' or passed through the rectum as 'melaena'. A careful examination and relevant investigations should distinguish such spurious 'GI bleeds'.

Not all patients with GI bleeds require critical care. In at least 75–80 per cent of patients bleeding stops spontaneously and does not recur. However about 20 per cent of patients do not stop bleeding, or have a recurrent bleed. It is indeed difficult to predict which patient will continue to bleed or will have a recurrent haemorrhage. Intensive care is indicated in all severe bleeds, bleeds that continue or recur, bleeds in patients with cirrhosis of the liver, in elderly patients, in patients with serious background diseases, for example ischaemic heart disease, or renal failure.

Major Causes of Upper GI Bleed (1–3)

More than 70 per cent of upper GI bleeds are due to acid-peptic disease—duodenal or gastric ulcer, gastric or duodenal erosions, stress ulcers or reflux oesophagitis. About 15 per cent of upper GI bleeds are due to oesophageal or gastric varices or a gastropathy caused by portal hypertension. The remaining 10–15 per cent of bleeds are due to various aetiologies. These include the Mallory-Weiss syndrome, cancer of the oesophagus or stomach, vascular anomalies of the upper GI tract (e.g. Rendu Osler Weber disease). Acute pancreatitis may occasionally present as an acute severe GI bleed. Rarely a blood dyscrasia or a coagulation defect may present as a GI bleed.

The important causes of an upper GI bleed are listed in **Table 15.5.1**.

Clinical Manifestations

Bleeding from the upper GI tract, from a lesion at or above the ligament of Treitz manifests in one or more of the following ways.

(i) Haematemesis, which is the vomiting of fresh blood or of altered coffee ground blood.

Table 15.5.1. Important causes of upper GI bleeds commonly encountered in the ICU

* Acid-peptic disease—duodenal and gastric ulcers and erosions, stress ulcers, reflux oesophagitis
* Portal hypertension—oesophageal or gastric varices, gastropathy
* Mallory-Weiss tear
* Vascular abnormalities in the upper GI tract—e.g. Rendu Osler Weber disease
* Carcinoma of stomach/oesophagus
* Rarely acute pancreatitis, blood dyscrasias, or coagulation defects

(ii) Melaena, which is the passage of altered blood in the form of tarry black stools. It must however be stressed that in massive upper GI bleeds, maroon or bright right blood may be passed from the rectum mimicking a bleed from the small bowel (usually ileum) or colon. Fresh blood from the rectum due to an upper GI bleed, is however always associated with shock and haemodynamic instability.

(iii) The presence of fresh blood or altered blood in the nasogastric aspirate. This may be observed (a) when an upper GI bleed complicates a separate critical illness for which the patient is under intensive care; (b) when a patient is admitted for shock related to a GI bleed which till the time of admission has not resulted in haematemesis or melaena.

(iv) Major bleeding in rare instances may not be easily evident, particularly in older patients. Syncope, dizzy spells, unstable angina, undue breathlessness on exertion, increasing pallor, may be the initial outward manifestations of a bleed. Confusion and focal neurological signs suggesting transient ischaemic attacks may occur in those with cerebrovascular disease. Rectal examination in these old patients may reveal the presence of melaena.

The manifestations of blood loss in upper GI bleeds depend on the degree and rapidity of blood loss. Hypovolaemic and haemorrhagic shock have been discussed at length in the Section on Clinical Shock Syndromes.

The Clinical Approach to an Upper GI Bleed

The fundamental clinical approach should consider the following features.

(i) Determine the severity of the bleed and assess its effect on the haemodynamics of the circulation, and immediately initiate resuscitation by fluid replacement and transfusions in patients with moderate to severe blood loss.

(ii) Identify high risk patients.

(iii) Determine the cause of the bleed by appropriate investigations and diagnostic steps. It is of interest that diagnostic procedures and therapeutic strategies are often simultaneously performed in the management of GI bleeds.

(i) Assessment of Severity of Bleed

This has been discussed in the Section on Clinical Shock Syndromes. As has been emphasized earlier, changes in pulse rate, blood pressure, skin temperature, urine output, arterial pH are all of help in estimating the degree of blood loss. Some assessment of the severity of the haemorrhage can also be made by examination of the vomitus, nasogastric aspirate and the degree of melaena. Passage of fresh blood from the rectum in an upper GI bleed always signals a massive bleed. Continuous aspiration of bright red blood through the nasogastric tube is ominous, as it signifies fresh brisk arterial bleeding.

Laboratory investigations in an acute bleed do not help, as the haematocrit and the haemoglobin may not show a significant change for many hours.

(ii) Identification of High Risk Patients

It is important to identify high risk patients as soon as possible. Management in these patients should be as per a planned protocol if morbidity and mortality are to be reduced. The following factors are indicators of poor prognosis in upper GI bleeds.

(a) Increased Age—patients over 60 years of age are at greater risk, particularly in severe bleeds or recurrent bleeds.

(b) The presence of shock (in particular a systolic BP < 90 mm Hg) and the necessity for multiple transfusions.

(c) Variceal bleeding in a cirrhotic patient—the poorer the liver function, the worse the prognosis (See Chapter on Critical Care of Complications in Chronic Liver Failure).

(d) The presence of a continuing bright red nasogastric aspirate, or the passage of fresh blood via the rectum.

(e) Bleeding from a large (> 2.5 cm) gastric or duodenal ulcer.

(f) Haematocrit < 30 per cent.

(g) Recurrent bleeding during the same admission.

(h) The presence of a coagulopathy.

(i) The need for emergency surgery.

The factors indicating poor prognosis are listed in **Table 15.5.2**.

Table 15.5.2. Factors indicating poor prognosis in upper GI bleeding

* Increased age (> 60)
* Presence of shock (systolic BP < 90 mm Hg) and necessity for multiple transfusions
* Severe variceal bleeding in a cirrhotic patient
* Recurrent bleeding in presence of continuing bright red nasogastric aspirate, or passage of fresh blood via rectum
* Bleeding from a large (2.5 cm) gastric or duodenal ulcer
* Haematocrit < 30 per cent
* Recurrent bleeding during the same admission
* Presence of a coagulopathy
* Need for emergency surgery

(iii) Determining the Cause of the Bleed

Haematemesis always indicates an upper GI bleed. So does the presence of fresh or altered blood in the nasogastric aspirate in a patient who only has melaena. Melaena in the absence of haematemesis or blood in the nasogastric aspirate may also occur in a bleed from a lesion in the small bowel, caecum or ascending colon. Though fresh blood is most often seen in a lower GI bleed, (particularly in a bleed from the large bowel) it can also occur with a massive upper GI bleed. In the latter instance, haemodynamic instability is always present. The presence of hyperactive bowel sounds and a disproportionate rise in blood urea, suggests an upper GI lesion. In any case, an upper GI endoscopy should prove or disprove the presence of a lesion in the oesophagus, stomach or duodenum responsible for a bleed.

History and physical examination may occasionally suggest the specific disease. Stigmata of liver cell dysfunction should be carefully searched for. The abdomen should be carefully palpated for tenderness, guarding and rigidity, and percussed for the presence or absence of free fluid; auscultation for bowel sounds should never be omitted. It is important to do a complete physical examination to determine the circulatory state, and to look out for chronic background disease involving major organ systems of the body. Relevant blood and other investigations should be promptly sent for. These have been listed in the Subsection on Management.

Once adequate restitution of volume and of blood has been instituted and the patient is haemodynamically stable, an *upper GI endoscopy* should be performed. Oesophagogastroduodenoscopy provides a diagnosis in more than 90 per cent of patients scoped within 24 hours of a bleed. If the procedure is delayed for more than 48 hours the diagnostic sensitivity drops to 33 per cent. Endoscopy is not completely without risk. The complication rate is about 0.9 per cent with an incidence of 1 death per 700 examinations in the acutely bleeding patient (4). When aspiration of stomach contents is a major risk the procedure should be done under anaesthesia, after electively intubating the patient with an endotracheal tube. Continuous ECG monitoring and oxygen saturation monitoring though oxymetry is imperative during the procedure.

Selective angiography is infrequently used in the diagnosis of upper GI bleeds because patients with torrential bleeding should be promptly considered for surgery. However, in very poor risk patients, selective angiography is an alternative to surgery to help diagnose the source of bleeding, with a view to therapeutic selective arterial embolization.

Management (Fig. 15.5.1)

Major upper GI bleeds are best managed jointly by experienced physicians (the team should include a GI specialist), an endoscopist, and a surgical team. Obviously such bleeds require intensive care. Indications for transfer to critical care in a patient admitted to the wards for a GI bleed have been mentioned earlier.

On admission, blood is withdrawn for grouping and cross-matching, as also for routine baseline haematological and biochemical parameters. A large bore venous cannula is inserted into a peripheral vein, and volume replacement by infusion of colloids or crystalloids started (see Chapter on Hypovolaemic and Haemorrhagic Shock). Investigations should include a blood count, haematocrit, platelet count, and a basic coagulation profile—clotting time, prothrombin time, partial thromboplastin time. It should always include full liver function tests including serum proteins and serum albumin concentration; serum electrolytes, blood urea, and creatinine should also be estimated. Arterial blood gas analysis is done as a baseline study and an ECG tracing obtained. A serum amylase should always be done, as in rare instances acute pancreatitis may present with a severe upper GI bleed. An X-ray of the abdomen in the standing posture (if this is possible) is a routine investigation. Continuous ECG monitoring is advised, particularly in older patients, in those with a history of cardiac disease, and in those whose ECG tracing is abnormal. A Foley's catheter is inserted so that an hourly urine output chart is maintained. Intake/output charts are mandatory.

A central venous line is also promptly secured and connected to a pressure monitor. We generally do not monitor the left ventricular filling pressures except in those receiving massive transfusions, in older patients, and in those with known left ventricular disease or dysfunction. In the above high risk group of patients, a Swan-Ganz Catheter is inserted so that infusions of fluids and blood are carefully monitored to prevent pulmonary oedema.

A nasogastric tube should be passed expeditiously, immediately after a peripheral vein has been secured and volume replacement started. The stomach is aspirated, the contents with regard to their nature and quantity are noted. A half hourly or one hourly chart of aspirated contents is maintained. Gastric lavage is performed through the wide bore nasogastric tube. We prefer to use iced saline to which adrenaline or noradrenaline has been added. Cold tap water probably does just as well; in fact the current trend is to use cold tap water for lavage instead of ice cold saline. Frequent aspiration following lavage is important not only to note the degree of continuing bleed, but also to prevent aspiration into the lungs, and to allow a good view for endoscopy. At times blood gets clotted within the stomach, and cannot be aspirated even through a very wide bore tube. This is a grave obstacle both in endoscopic diagnosis and management.

After a good lavage, an upper GI endoscopy is done to determine the site and exact nature of the bleed.

Meanwhile, volume replacement should be rapid and its effects should be apparent by a stable blood pressure, improved urine output and improved tissue perfusion. To replace the loss of Hb, or in a massive bleed, urgent blood transfusions are indicated. In cases where there is no time for grouping and cross-matching, O Rh-negative blood is transfused. It is preferable to give packed cell infusions instead of whole blood whenever these are available. Over-transfusions carry the immediate risk of pulmonary oedema. One unit of fresh frozen plasma should be preferably administered for every 3 units of packed red cells. The details of volume replacement have been dealt with in the Chapter on Hypovolaemic and Haemorrhagic Shock.

The following therapeutic modalities are advocated to arrest haemorrhage in those who continue to bleed, or in those who rebleed. It will be noted that diagnostic procedures and therapeutic strategies are often performed at the same time.

Use of Drugs (5, 6)

Antacids and H₂-Antagonists. In gastroduodenal bleeds caused by the peptic ulcer group of diseases (chiefly acute gastroduodenal erosions, duodenal ulcer, gastric ulcer, oesophagitis and hiatal hernia), antacids and H_2-antagonists should be used. Aluminum hydroxide or magnesium hydroxide is given 4 hourly. Ranitidine, 50 mg, is given intravenously 8 hourly, or in a continuous infusion. Famotidine may be used in place of ranitidine; it reliably maintains pH above 4.0 in critically ill patients (7). A randomized, controlled trial of 220 patients in our country showed that early therapy with omeprazole, a proton-pump inhibitor, 40 mg orally every 12 hours, significantly reduces the frequency of rebleeding and of surgery in patients with bleeding ulcers (8).

Sucralfate (9). Sucralfate is preferred in many units to antacids. Sucrafate is an aluminum hydroxide salt of sucrose octasulfate. It forms a polymer which binds to positively charged proteins at pH less than 4.0. This action prevents gastric acid from gaining access to the base of ulcers in the gastroduodenal mucosa. Sucralfate acts best at acidic pH, so that concomitant use of antacids and H_2-antagonists is best avoided. Sucralfate is probably as effective as antacids and H_2-antagonists. The incidence of nosocomial infections is probably reduced with sucralfate, as it does not increase the pH of gastric contents and therefore prevents an overgrowth of bacterial organisms within the upper GI tract.

In our experience *it is doubtful if any of the drugs mentioned above significantly affect a severe upper GI bleed. They are probably useful in the prevention of a rebleed in the peptic ulcer group of diseases.*

Other Drugs. Other drugs that have been used in severe exsanguinating bleeds include the antifibrinolytic agent tranexamic acid, and somatostatin (4). Consistent benefit has not been demonstrated by their use. Vasopressin is of no benefit in nonvariceal haemorrhage. Studies have shown that the eradication of H pylori infection reduces the risk of rebleeding (10).

Endoscopic Methods to Arrest Bleeding (11–15)

Therapeutic procedures are performed at the same time as the diagnostic endoscopy. Endoscopic management of upper GI bleeding is successful in 80–90 per cent of patients with bleeding peptic ulcers. It is also often successful in the management of bleeding gastric or duodenal erosions in bleeding oesophageal ulcers and in patients with GI bleeds due to the Mallory-Weiss syndrome, Dieulafoy's erosions, and Rendu Osler Weber disease. Therapeutic options through an endoscope include application of haemostatic agents to bleeding points, injection with vasoconstricting and sclerosing agents, the use of thermal probe, bipolar coagulation, and of argon and laser coagulation. Therapeutic endoscopy in a bleeding acid-peptic disease is most effective when an actively bleeding vessel is visible. An injection of epinephrine or epinephrine + human thrombin around the base of an ulcer may arrest a severe bleed long enough to allow resuscitation, and reduce the risk of a more definitive surgical approach. Sclerotherapy or banding has

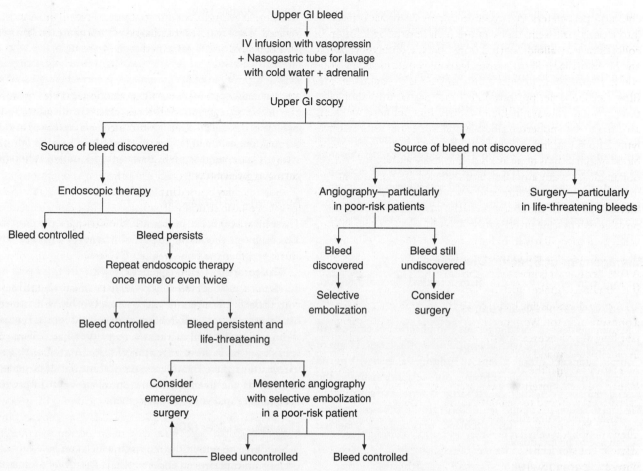

Fig. 15.5.1. Algorithm for the management of upper GI bleeds.

already been commented upon in an earlier chapter. 10 to 20 per cent of endoscopically treated patients will rebleed, generally within 72 hours. A repeat therapeutic endoscopy is effective in 50 per cent of patients. There is a significant reduction in morbidity and mortality in patients treated successfully endoscopically (including those requiring a repeat endoscopy) when compared to those treated surgically.

Clinical trials do not prove a significant difference in results with the different modalities of therapeutic endoscopy. Most endoscopists in our country have either little experience with argon and neodymium—YAG lasers. It is doubtful whether these are more effective than electrocoagulation, or the use of a heater probe. Lasers are expensive gadgets and their expense precludes their widespread use. The application of any of these expensive techniques requires both experience and expertise.

Selective Angiography and Transcatheter Arterial Embolization

Ordinarily, surgery is advised in a torrential upper GI bleed where endoscopic diagnosis has not been possible or where therapeutic endoscopy has failed. Diagnostic mesenteric angiography, followed by selective arterial embolization can control bleeding in 80 per cent of these patients (16). Arterial embolization is however associated with high rebleeding rates and other long-term com-

plications. It should therefore be reserved only for patients unfit for surgery, provided there is good local expertise in this interventional procedure.

Surgery

Surgery is most often needed for gastric or duodenal ulcers which continue to bleed. The mortality of emergency surgery is high (between 10 to 30 per cent), regardless of whether surgery is done promptly after admission to hospital, or is done following a recurrent bleed. By contrast, elective surgery for a peptic ulcer has a mortality of less than 2–3 per cent. Indications for emergency surgery are:

(i) Severe persistent bleed causing hypotension and shock. Endoscopic techniques to arrest bleeding should be inappropriate, unsuccessful or not available.

(ii) Age over 60 years, with a bleeding peptic ulcer, if the bleed is not promptly arrested by endoscopic measures.

(iii) Recurrence of a bleed at the same admission, uncontrolled by therapeutic endoscopy.

(iv) Age under 60 years, with a persistent and very brisk bleed from an active peptic ulcer, if the bleed is not arrested by endoscopic techniques.

(v) Loss of over 25–30 per cent of estimated blood volume and/or the requirement of > 6 units of blood in the first 24 hours.

(vi) When oesophageal or gastric varices continue to bleed in spite of banding or sclerotherapy and the intravenous use of vasopressin and somatostatin (see Chapter on Critical Care of Liver Cell Dysfunction).

(vii) In exsanguinating massive upper GI bleeds, emergency surgery may be the only option. Whenever possible an endoscopy should be performed before laparotomy. The basic aim of an emergency laparotomy is to stop the bleeding by ligating or undersewing bleeding vessels. The decision of whether to proceed with more definitive surgery for a bleeding peptic ulcer, depends on the clinical state of the patient and is left to the surgeon's judgement. If the bleeding is arrested and the patient is haemodynamically stable, a vagotomy with a drainage procedure carries the lowest post-operative mortality, and reduces the risk of a rebleed.

Management of Specific Disorders

Management of a few specific disorders needs special mention.

Bleeding Oesophageal Varices

The management of this dangerous complication of cirrhosis of the liver has been dealt with in another chapter (Critical Care of Complications in Chronic Liver Cell Failure). Patients with portal hypertension may also bleed from a diffuse abnormality of the gastric mucosa, a condition called portal hypertensive gastropathy. Medical measures to counter acute bleeds are the same as in variceal bleeding. Prevention of future rebleeds may perhaps be helped by the use of propranolol.

Stress Ulcers (17–19)

Single or multiple superficial gastric, duodenal, or gastroduodenal ulcers often occur in critically ill patients. They can on occasions bleed profusely, and carry a significant mortality. It is important to prevent these ulcers from bleeding and if possible from forming. Patients at risk from these lesions include those with burns, head injury, multiple trauma, acute liver cell failure, acute renal failure, Gram-negative sepsis and disseminated intravascular coagulopathy. Patients on prolonged mechanical ventilation, and those suffering from acute or fulminant illnesses (tetanus, Pl falciparum infections), are also prone to acute mucosal erosions.

We use either oral antacids and intravenous H_2-antagonists, or oral sucralfate for prevention of bleeds from stress ulcers. The reported advantage of using sucralfate has already been mentioned. In our unit, bleeding acute erosive gastroduodenitis from any cause is treated by a continuous infusion of cold milk containing magnesium hydroxide and norepinephrine, given through the nasogastric tube. This generally stops bleeding. In critically ill patients in whom oral feeds are contraindicated, endoscopic methods to stop bleeding may prove effective. Failing this, angiographic therapy, either in the form of a vasopressin infusion into the left gastric artery, or embolization of the left gastric artery should be tried. Every effort should be made to avoid surgery in these patients, as surgery carries a forbidding mortality.

Mallory-Weiss Tear

Mallory-Weiss tear is most often observed along the oesophagogastric junction. It is most common in young males who most often give a history of severe vomiting or retching, coughing or straining, prior to the haematemesis. A correct diagnosis is easily made at endoscopy. Most tears stop bleeding spontaneously. Some may however continue to bleed massively. Bleeding in these patients is controlled by balloon tamponade, endoscopic electrocoagulation, or the injection of vasopressin into the left gastric artery. If these methods fail, arteriographic embolization or surgery may be necessary.

Aorto-enteric Fistula (4)

These invariably occur in patients who have an aortic graft in situ. The diagnosis should be suspected whenever a patient with an aortic prosthesis suffers an upper GI bleed.

The communication is generally with the third part of the duodenum and the patient has both haematemesis and melaena, with all the haemodynamic effects of a severe bleed. Aorto-enteric fistula usually occurs following graft-related sepsis. Endoscopy should be performed to exclude more proximal lesions. A CT scan shows gas in the retroperitoneal space. Aortography may fail to reveal the fistula. Treatment is surgical and should be performed as soon as the haemodynamic state has been improved by immediate rapid volume replacement.

Dieulafoy's Ulcer (20)

A bleeding site within the stomach which can be easily missed even by an experienced endoscopist, is Dieulafoy's lesion in the fundus of the stomach. This lesion bleeds intermittently (one reason why it can be missed on endoscopy), and is characterized by the presence of a small arteriole (1 to 3 mm in size) protruding above the mucosa. It is dealt with endoscopically by electrocoagulation or heat coagulation.

Massive upper GI bleeds besides producing haemorrhagic shock, can (because of severe volume depletion) precipitate myocardial infarction, acute renal shut down or a stroke, particularly in older patients.

Even a moderate sized bleed complicating a critical illness can markedly enhance its gravity, and ultimately be responsible for the patient's death. Finally, patients with upper GI bleeds who have large clots in their stomach are at considerable risk for sepsis. Most of these patients have received large doses of antacids, and the additional presence of blood clots forms an excellent medium for the overgrowth of dangerous Gram-negative organisms. We have seen Gram-negative sepsis kill these patients, even after definitive surgery has been successfully performed.

Lower Gastrointestinal Haemorrhage

General Considerations

Lower GI bleeding occurs from a source below the ligament of Treitz. The source of haemorrhage could therefore be the small bowel, caecum, large bowel, rectum, or the anal canal. Only about 10–20 per cent of GI bleeds severe enough to merit critical care are lower GI bleeds, the rest being upper GI bleeds. However, most patients with severe lower GI bleeds are much older, often past 60 years and cannot tolerate severe blood loss.

Before the advent of endoscopy and interventional radiography, severe lower GI bleeds were invariably diagnosed as bleeds from diverticular disease. Investigations were few, treatment conservative, chiefly consisting of replacement of blood loss, and if massive bleeding continued, a hemicolectomy or total colectomy was performed. The mortality was high and recurrence of bleeding fairly common. The advent of colonoscopy and diagnostic angiography has changed our concepts and our approach to lower GI bleeds. It was observed that lower GI bleeds could result from a number of pathologies besides diverticular disease. It was also observed that even if diverticular disease was present, bleeding could occur from diverticuli in the right colon, and not necessarily from diverticuli in the left colon. Finally, as in upper GI bleeds, diagnostic procedures in lower GI bleeds (colonoscopy and selective arteriography) could be combined simultaneously with therapeutic strategies. If these strategies were successful, radical or definitive surgery on the large bowel could be avoided, or at least conveniently delayed to a time when the patient was more fit for major surgery.

Major Causes of Lower GI Bleeds

In our experience diverticular disease is still the most common single pathology accounting for more than 30 per cent of massive lower GI bleeds. Bleeding from colonic diverticuli ceases in 75 per cent but recurs in 38 per cent (21). Other important causes include angiodysplasia, inflammatory bowel disease, severe amoebic or other infective colitis, pseudomembranous colitis, ischaemic colitis, polyps, neoplasma, postpolypectomy bleeding, NSAID-induced colonic ulceration, radiation colitis, solitary rectal ulcer. Angiodyaplasia accounts for 3–12 per cent of lower GI bleeds (22). Bleeding can also occur after the use of anticoagulants like warfarin, heparin, streptokinase, urokinase.

Bleeding from the small bowel severe enough to merit critical care is much less common than bleeding from the large bowel and its source is more difficult to diagnose. Aetiological factors in a small bowel bleed include, Meckel's diverticulum, angiodysplasia,

Table 15.5.3. Important causes of lower GI bleeds commonly encountered in the ICU

* Diverticular disease
* Angiodysplasia
* Inflammatory bowel disease
* Severe amoebic or other infective colitis
* Pseudomembranous colitis
* Ischaemic colitis
* Polyps, neoplasms
* Post-polypectomy bleeding
* NSAID-induced colonic ulceration
* Radiation colitis
* Solitary rectal ulcer
* Use of anticoagulants

diverticuli, ischaemic bowel, ulcers (typhoid ulcer, tuberculous ulcer, Crohn's disease, solitary jejunal ulcer (of unknown aetiology)), tumours, non-Hodgkins lymphoma (23).

Clinical Manifestations

Bleeding from the lower GI tract manifests as follows:

(i) Massive bleeding, with the passage of fresh bright red blood or deep maroon stools from the rectum (haematochaezia).

(ii) Intermittent bouts of bleeding—bleeding may be in the form of fresh blood per rectum or melaena. Melaena in a large bowel bleed invariably signifies that the site of bleeding is the caecum or the ascending colon.

Chronic or occult blood loss from the large bowel can over a period of time, lead to significant blood loss and severe anaemia. This manifestation of a lower GI bleed is not considered in this chapter.

It is important to restress that both melaena and/or fresh blood per rectum may also be manifestations of bleeds from either the stomach or duodenum. A definite diagnosis as to the site of the GI bleed, may in many instances only be arrived at after full investigations. However, clinical considerations at the bedside are often of immediate help.

(i) When a continuing bleed from the stomach or duodenum or from the portion of the jejunum adjoining the duodenum, is severe enough to cause fresh blood to flow out of the rectum, the patient invariably has an unstable circulation, is haemodynamically compromised, and is in shock or soon goes into shock. Therefore fresh blood from the rectum with a stable circulation, invariably points to a lower GI bleed.

(ii) Fresh persistent bleeding from the rectum in the presence of a gastric aspirate (obtained through a nasogastric tube) which *persistently shows normal gastric contents also containing bile*, is against the diagnosis of a bleed proximal to the ligament of Treitz. Rarely a large bleeding duodenal ulcer may be associated with an absence of blood in the gastric aspirate.

An oesophagogastroscopy should invariably either prove or exclude an upper GI bleed.

Clinical Approach and Management (24–26)

The clinical approach is very similar to that observed in upper GI bleeds. It consists of:

(i) Assessing the severity of the bleed, with prompt replacement of volume loss by appropriate infusions and transfusions.

(ii) Determining the cause and site of bleed with management strategies to arrest the bleed. Diagnostic and therapeutic procedures are often performed more or less simultaneously in many patients with lower GI bleeds.

(i) Assessment of the Severity of the Bleed

The details have been discussed in the Chapter on Hypovolaemic and Haemorrhagic Shock. Assessment should be clinical as outlined earlier for upper GI bleeds, and in the Chapter on Hypovolaemic and Haemorrhagic Shock; it should also be based on the volume of blood loss, as judged from the degree of melaena or rectal bleed.

Most patients with lower GI bleeds are old and therefore poor risk patients. The additional presence of ischaemic heart disease, cerebrovascular disease, pre-existing anaemia, chronic respiratory disease, renal failure, liver cell dysfunction markedly worsen prognosis. Resuscitation through volume replacement is a matter of urgent priority. It should therefore be urgently undertaken as even mild to moderate blood loss in these patients can aggravate underlying illnesses.

(ii) Determining the Cause and Site of the Bleed

Management strategies to arrest this bleed. The site and cause of bleeding are determined by proceeding systematically with evaluation of the history, physical examination, and by proceeding with a series of investigations according to a strict protocol. Resuscitation measures should never be interrupted during the diagnostic work-up of the patient.

History. More often than not the history is non-contributory, though occasionally it may throw light on the nature of the disease. A past history suggestive of inflammatory bowel disease or a history suggestive of diverticulitis is important. Evidence of diffuse atherosclerotic disease, in association with episodes of abdominal pain may suggest ischaemia to the small or large bowel. Painless severe bleeding is commonly observed in diverticulosis, angiodysplasia, Meckel's diverticulum or a colonic polyp. Recurrent fresh bleeding per rectum extending over many years, may suggest common anorectal lesions or a colonic polyp. In patients with severe portal hypertension, massive haematochaezia can be due to haemorrhoids. Fresh bleeding associated with a change in bowel habits in an elderly patient suggests a mitotic lesion in the bowel.

Physical Examination. This should be done with the following objectives:

(a) Determining the haemodynamic and circulatory state.

(b) Careful examination of the abdomen for any palpable lumps, tenderness on palpation, and for evidence of local or generalized peritonitis. Inspection of the anorectal area and a rectal examination should be done; the presence of fresh blood or melaena staining the examining finger should be noted.

(c) Examination of all major organ systems to determine the presence of associated disease involving one or more of these organ systems.

Preliminary Investigations. Routine blood examination and biochemical tests, and a basic coagulation profile should be sent for, exactly as listed for a GI bleed.

X-ray Investigation. X-ray of the abdomen should be done with special reference to (a) a study of the colonic gas outline; this may provide information in patients with ischaemic colitis, or toxic megacolon, (b) radiological evidence of colonic perforation.

Further Investigations. These include a direct visualization of the GI tract, and should be planned and carried out as follows:

(a) If there is fresh blood per rectum which is mild to moderate, the patient is haemodynamically stable, and the gastric aspirate obtained through a nasogastric tube is normal, a sigmoidoscopy is performed. Anorectal lesions if present, should be obvious on a sigmoidoscopy. The presence of haemorrhoids does not exclude a more proximal lesion. At the same time in a patient with bleeding haemorrhoids, the presence of blood above the anorectal region does not necessarily imply that a more proximal lesion has to be present. There are instances where blood from bleeding haemorrhoids can track up the colon, as far proximal as the caecum.

(b) Anorectal lesions are common and though they bleed frequently, they are rare causes of severe GI bleeds. If sigmoidoscopy is negative as is generally the case, then in the presence of brisk fresh blood from the rectum or the presence of melaena, it is best to proceed with an upper GI scopy and exclude an upper GI bleed. This should be done even if the nasogastric aspirate does not show fresh or altered blood.

(c) If the upper GI scopy is negative, one should proceed to examine the lower GI tract with colonoscopy, angiography or radionucleide scan.

Colonoscopy. Colonsocopy allows a good view of the large bowel if bleeding has stopped at the time of examination, or even in the presence of mild to moderate haematochaezia. Colonoscopy is difficult, unrewarding and carries a risk of perforation in the presence of a brisk bleed or when the large bowel is tightly filled with blood. Preparation of the bowel with a bowel wash, oral lavage preparations allows a clearer view of the colon. In expert hands, colonoscopy provides a diagnosis in 70–85 per cent of patients with massive haematochaezia (**27, 28**).

Angiography. Selective angiography is indicated when endoscopy fails to reveal the cause of a lower GI bleed, the endoscopic view being obscured by active bleeding or by plenty of blood in the colon. An extravasation of the contrast medium during angiography points to the site of bleed. Angiography particularly picks up areas of abnormal vasculature as in angiodysplasia, Rendu-Osler-Weber syndrome, pseudoxanthoma elasticum, Ehler Danlos syndrome.

The success rate of angiography in localizing difficult lower GI bleeds varies in different units. Detection is only possible in the presence of active bleeding at the rate of at least 0.5–1 ml/minute. The test has been reported positive in 12–72 per cent; the success rate depends on patient selection and timing of the procedure (**29, 30**). The order of cannulation in selective angiography is generally the superior mesenteric, the inferior mesenteric and the coeliac artery. In an analysis of pooled data from 14 studies, complications were observed in 10 per cent of patients and included renal failure and transient ischaemic attacks (**20**).

Angiography is particularly useful in the diagnosis of lesions causing a severe bleed from the small bowel, which is inaccessible to the colonoscope. These lesions, as stated earlier, include carcinomas, arteriovenous malformations, ulcers, bleeding from Meckel's diverticulum and lymphomas.

Radionuclide Scan. Labelling of the patient's red blood cells with 99 m Tc for a tagged red blood cell scan can identify the location of extravasated blood in the GI tract. Positive findings include a 'blush' and extravasation of contrast into gut lumen. The technique is believed to identify bleeding at rates < 0.5 ml/min. Though nuclear scans are reported to be positive in 50 per cent of lower GI bleeds, our experience is unsatisfactory. Also, because of lack of in-house facilities, we prefer to opt straight for arteriography when colonoscopy fails to offer a diagnosis of the site and cause of a lower GI bleed.

Further Investigations for Small Bowel Bleeds. Angiography and tagged red blood cells scans often do not identify the source of bleeding in small bowel lesions. If bleeding is intermittent or has stopped, a carefully performed small bowel contrast study (small bowel enema), double contrast evaluation using enteroclysis, CT scanning, enteroclysis coupled with CT scanning are investigational modes which may help identify the site and nature of the lesion. The overall yield by these methods is less than 10 per cent.

Endoscopic evaluation of the small bowel is achieved through push enteroscopy, sonde enteroscopy or intraoperative enteroscopy. Push enteroscopy involves using of a longer endoscope that allows visualization beyond the ligament of Treitz up to the distal jejunum (31). It cannot therefore evaluate ileal lesions.

Sonde endoscopy uses a small calibre enteroscope passed through the nose into the small bowel. Insufflation of a balloon at the tip allows for intestinal peristalsis to push the scope passively to the distal small bowel. The procedure may improve yield, but is difficult, may take 6 to 8 hours, is extremely inconvenient and lacks therapeutic ability.

We have no experience with enteroscopies. When confronted with a severe life-threatening GI bleed not identified by an upper GI scopy, colonoscopy and a selective mesenteric or celiac artery angiography, we opt without hesitation for an operative enteroscopy (performed through a colonoscope), as the best means for evaluating the small bowel.

Wireless Capsule Endoscopy (32, 33). This new technique to identify the site of a 'hidden' GI bleed has been used when radiography, endoscopy, colonoscopy, push enteroscopy have been futile. The procedure will not yield reliable results during a massive bleed, with the bowel choked with blood.

The procedure has 3 components—a capsule endoscope, an external receiving antenna with attached portable hard-drive, and a personal computer work station with software for review and interpretation of images. The capsule is swallowed on a fasting stomach and images are reviewed as the capsule makes its way down the GI tract.

Adverse effects include failure of the capsule to progress through the bowel; gastrointestinal obstruction or pseudo-obstruction are contraindications to capsule endoscopy. Capsule endoscopy is reported to have a success rate of about 67 per cent in identifying the source of obscure GI bleeds (34, 35). We have very little experience with its use. More work needs to be done to determine its role and efficacy in the diagnosis of severe GI bleeds.

Management (Fig. 15.5.2)

Therapeutic procedures are planned with the diagnostic procedures of colonoscopy and arteriography.

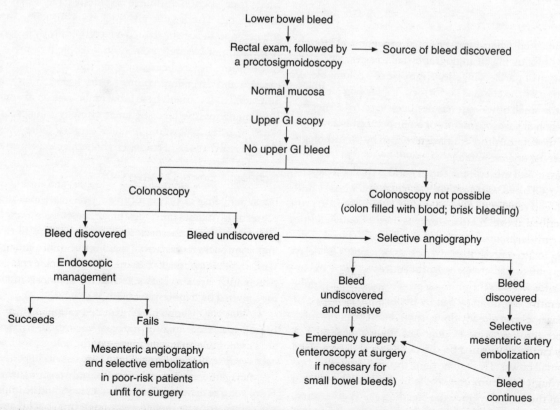

Note: If after colonoscopy or mesenteric arteriography the bleed is undiscovered, a push enteroscopy or wireless capsule enteroscopy may be tried to determine the source of the bleed provided the bleed is not massive and life-threatening and the necessary expertise is available. Push enteroscopy can be combined with therapeutic endoscopy (see text).

Fig. 15.5.2. Algorithm for the management of lower GI bleeds.

Medical Measures

Severe bleed from inflammatory bowel disease is treated with intravenous corticosteroids, rest to the bowel by using a liquid diet. Appropriate antibiotics may be necessary in some patients.

Endoscopic Management

Bleeding from vascular anomalies such as angiodysplasia are treated by electrocoagulation, heater probe, or laser therapy. Bleeding polyps are treated by polypectomy. The major complication is perforation, particularly when thermal, coagulation techniques are used for angiodysplasia involving the caecum. Culprit lesions within the small bowel identified either by 'push enteroscopy' or by enteroscopy at surgery, can be dealt with by standard endoscopic methods.

Angiography

Once the bleeding site is determined by selective angiography, infusion of vasopressin will stop bleeding in over 70 per cent of lower GI bleeds due to angiodysplasia or diverticulosis. Occlusion of a bleeding vessel through selective embolization with gelfoam can also arrest bleeding. Recurrence of bleeding is particularly common with diverticular disease.

Successful interventional procedures make the difference between survival and death in poor-risk, old enfeebled patients who are critically ill.

Surgery

Surgery is indicated when interventional procedures through colonoscopy or following an angiography fail to arrest bleeding. After localization of the bleeding site, in the case of a colonic bleed, partial resection of the colon is performed. If bleeding has been localized to the small bowel but has not been arrested either by selective infusion of vasoconstrictors or attempts at embolization, the nature of the surgical procedure is determined by the pathology discovered on the operation table.

The ultimate and most desperate scenario is that of a patient with a massive GI bleed who continues to bleed, and whose cause and site of bleed remain undetermined by the diagnostic procedures described above. A laparotomy is then essential. Some advocate an *early laparotomy* in a continuing massive bleed without resorting to attempts at mesenteric angiography. The delay caused in organizing such special procedures in such exsanguinating bleeds worsens the ultimate prognosis. At laparotomy, an intra-operative colonoscopy can be performed; an upper GI scopy if it has not been already done, should also be performed. If these procedures show no evidence of the site of bleed, an enteroscopy can be performed on the table in search of a bleed within the small bowel. This can be done through a colonoscope inserted through the ileum; the whole of the small bowel can be viewed in this manner. Once the bleeding site is discovered, appropriate surgery to stop the bleed is performed. Empiric resection of a part or whole of the colon in lower GI bleeds is bad surgery. It carries a high mortality and a high rate of recurrent bleeding.

Specific Lesions

Diverticular Disease (36)

Diverticulosis is common so that bleeding from diverticular disease should be diagnosed only if active bleeding is observed to originate from diverticuli at colonoscopy. Bleeding from diverticuli in the right colon is also fairly frequent. Hence the futility of doing a left hemicolectomy in the hope of stopping bleeding in a patient with diverticular disease. Bleeding in some of these patients can be massive so that colonscopy is non-informative. Arteriography may demonstrate the bleed in these instances. Temporary control of bleeding may be obtained by local infusion of vasopressin at angiography. Embolization yields more long term satisfactory results. In poor risk patients, control of bleeding by the interventional radiologist has obvious advantages. If the patient is haemodynamically stable and a fairly good operative risk, surgical excision of the bleeding site is recommended.

Angiodysplasia (37–39)

Arteriovenous malformations become increasingly common with age. The lesions are focal, submucosal and most often present in the caecum. Multiple lesions occur in less than 25 per cent of patients. Lesions are also often found in the ascending colon and may occur in other parts of the gut, including the small bowel as well. Angiodysplasia can cause a steady constant ooze of blood, which over a period of time in an elderly patient may prove life-threatening. The lesions are frequently visualized through a colonoscope and can be treated endoscopically by heat or electro-coagulation of bleeding points. Endoscopic treatment however carries some hazard because of the thinness of the wall of the caecum and ascending colon. As the lesion is focal, it is also amenable to treatment by arterial embolization at angiography. Continuing massive bleeding, unarrested by colonoscopic procedures or by embolization, requires surgery. Since these lesions chiefly involve the right colon, a right hemicolectomy is indicated.

Ischaemic Bowel Disease (40)

Ischaemic colitis can cause recurrent pain, diarrhoea and bleeding per rectum. At times the clinical picture resembles ulcerative colitis. Old age, diffuse atherosclerotic disease, atrial fibrillation are important background factors in ischaemic colitis. Younger patients with diabetes, connective tissues disease, sickle cell disease and pancreatitis, are also at risk. Ischaemia in older patients is often precipitated by hypotension from any cause.

Colonoscopy shows purplish discoloration of segments of the bowel, with focal areas of mucosal ulceration. Barium contrast studies may reveal thumb-printing of the colonic wall. Mesenteric angiography may show arterial or venous occlusion.

Management is conservative. It should ensure that the patient is not volume depleted. The cardiac state should be improved, and the ventricular rate slowed appropriately if there is atrial fibrillation. Fulminant disease leads to necrosis of the colonic wall, and will require surgical resection. These patients invariably have serious background disease; multiple organ failure is a common complication. The mortality in severe ischaemic colitis necessitating surgery is often close to 50 per cent.

REFERENCES

1. Kupfer Y, Cappell MS, Tessler S. (2000). Acute gastrointestinal bleeding in the Intensive Care Unit: The Intensivist's perspective.

2. Laine L. (1991). Upper gastrointestinal hemorrhage. West J Med. 155, 274–279.

3. Quigley EMM. (1989). Acute upper gastrointestinal hemorrhage. In: Clinical Gastroenterology (Ed. Turnberg LA). pp. 54. Blackwell Scientific, Oxford.

4. Schaffner JA. (2001). Gastrointestinal Bleeding. In: Critical Care Medicine (Eds Parillo JE, Dellinger RP). pp. 1370–1386. Mosby, USA.

5. McQuaid KR, Isenberg JI. (1992). Medical therapy of peptic ulcer disease. Surg Clin North Am. 72, 285–316.

6. Yacyshyn BR, Thomson AB. (2000). Critical review of acid suppression in non-variceal, acute, upper gastrointestinal bleeding. Dig Dis. 18, 117–128.

7. Aoki T. (1987). Clinical benefits of intravenously administered famotidine in the treatment of upper gastrointestinal hemorrhage caused by peptic ulcer and stress ulcer disease. Scand J Gastroenterol. 22(Suppl. 134), 41–45.

8. Khuroo MS, Yattoo GN, Javid G et al. (1997). A comparison of omeprazole and placebo for bleeding peptic ulcer. N Engl J Med. 336, 1054–1058.

9. Shea-Donohue T, Steel L, Montcalm E et al. (1986). Gastric protection by sucralfate: Role of mucus and prostaglandins. Gastroenterology. 91, 660–666.

10. Graham DY, Hepps KS, Ramirez FC et al. (1993). Treatment of Helicobacter pylori reduces the rate of rebleeding in peptic ulcer disease. Scand J Gastroenterol. 28, 939–942.

11. NIH Consensus Conference. (1989). Therapeutic endoscopy and bleeding ulcers. JAMA. 262, 1369–1372.

12. Fleischer D. (1986). Endoscopic therapy of upper gastrointestinal bleeding in humans. Gastroenterology. 90, 217–234.

13. Sugawa C. (1989). Endoscopic diagnosis and treatment of upper gastrointestinal bleeding. Surg Clin North Am. 69, 1167–1183.

14. Editorial. (1988). The role of endoscopy in the management of upper gastrointestinal hemorrhage. Guidelines for clinical application. Gastrointest Endosc. 34 (Suppl), 44–55.

15. Fromm D. (1987). Endoscopic coagulation for gastrointestinal bleeding. N Engl J Med. 316, 1652–1654.

16. Toyoda H, Nakano S, Suga T et al. (1995). Transcatheter arterial embolization for massive bleeding from duodenal ulcers not controlled by endoscopic haemostasis. Endoscopy. 27, 304–307.

17. Cook DJ, Witt LG, Cook RJ et al. (1991). Stress ulcer prophylaxis in the critically ill: A meta-analysis. Am J Med. 91, 519–527.

18. Durham RM, Shapiro MJ. (1991). Stress gastritis revisited. Surg Clin North Am. 71, 791–810.

19. Peura DA, Koretz RL. (1990). Prophylactic therapy of stress-related mucosal damage: Why, which, who and so what? Am J Gastroenterol. 85, 935–937.

20. Arnell TD. (2002). Gastrointestinal Bleeding. In: Current Critical Care Diagnosis and Treatment (Eds Bongard FS, Sue DY). pp. 756–767. McGraw-Hill, USA.

21. McGuire HH. (1994). Bleeding colonic diverticula: A reappraisal of natural history and management. Ann Surg. 220, 653–656.

22. Zuckerman GR, Prakash C. (1999). Acute lower intestinal bleeding: Part 2. Etiology, therapy and outcomes. Gastrointest Endosc. 49, 228–238.

23. Feldman M, Scharschmidt BF. (1998). Sleisenger and Fordtran's Gastrointestinal and Liver Disease (Eds Feldman M, Scharschmidt BF). pp. 214–5. WB Saunders, Philadelphia, USA.

24. Potter GD, Sellin JH. (1988). Lower gastrointestinal bleeding. Gastroentero! Clin North Am. 17, 341–355.

25. Leitman IM, Paull DE, Shires GT. (1989). Evaluation and management of massive lower gastrointestinal hemorrhage. Ann Surg. 209, 175–180.

26. Peterson WL. (1989). Gastrointestinal bleeding. In: Gastrointestinal Disease: Pathophysiology, Diagnosis and Management (Eds Sleisenger MH, Fordtran JS). pp. 397. WB Saunders, New York.

27. Schrock TR. (1989). Colonoscopic diagnosis and treatment of lower gastrointestinal bleeding. Surg Clin North Am. 69, 1309.

28. Rossini FP, Ferrari A, Spandre M et al. (1989). Emergency colonoscopy. World J Surg. 13, 190.

29. Leitman IM, Paull DE, Shires GT. (1989). Evaluation and Management of massive lower gastrointestinal haemorrhage. Ann Surg. 209, 175.

30. Browder W, Cerise EJ, Litwin MS. (1986). Impact of emergency angiography in massive lower gastrointestinal bleeding. Ann Surg. 204, 530.

31. Waye JD. (1997). Enteroscopy. Gastrointest Endosc. 46, 247–256.

32. Iddan G, Meron G, Glukhovsky A, Swain P. (2000). Wireless capsule endoscopy. Nature. 405; 725–729.

33. Gong F, Swain P, Mills T. (2000). Wireless endoscopy. Gastrointest Endosc. 51, 725–729.

34. Jensen DM, Dulai G, Lousuebsakul V et al. (2002). Diagnostic yield of capsule endoscopy in patients with severe GI bleeding of obscure origin, subsequent recommendations, and outcomes. Gastrointest Endosc. 55, AB127.

35. Delvaux MM, Saurin JC, Gaudin JL et al. (2002). Comparison of wireless endoscopic capsule and push enteroscopy in patients with obscure occult/overt digestive bleeding: results of a prospective, blinded, multicenter trial. Gastrointest Endosc. 55, AB88.

36. McQuire HH, Haynes BW. (1972). Massive hemorrhage from diverticulosis of the colon. Ann Surg. 175, 847.

37. Lanthier PH et al. (1989). Colonic angiodysplasia: Follow-up of patients after endoscopic treatment of bleeding lesions. Dis Colon Rectum. 32, 296–298.

38. Roberts PL, Schoetz DJ Jr, Coller JA. (1988). Vascular ectasia: Diagnosis and treatment by colonoscopy. Am Surg. 54, 56–59.

39. Steger AC, Galland RB, Hemingway A et al. (1987). Gastrointestinal hemorrhage from a second source in patients with colonic angiodysplasia. Br J Surg. 74, 726–727.

40. Guttormson NL, Burbick MP. (1989). Mortality from ischemic colitis. Dis Colon Rectum. 32, 469–472.

CHAPTER 15.6

Haemorrhagic Disorders in the ICU

General Considerations

Bleeding and haemorrhagic disorders are frequently observed in an intensive care unit. They are almost invariably acquired and are due to underlying disease, or are iatrogenically induced, most frequently by drugs. Rarely a congenital defect in the bleeding or clotting mechanism is uncovered for the first time in a patient admitted for an acute problem unrelated to this defect. Equally rarely, a patient with a congenital disturbance in his clotting mechanism may be admitted for the critical care of an acute severe bleed. A past history of bleeding, and relevant investigations are necessary to determine the exact nature of the congenital defect. This chapter briefly outlines the inherited defects in platelet function and in coagulation that can cause severe bleeding. It also discusses at greater length the acquired disorders of platelets and acquired coagulation disorders which are far more frequently encountered in critical care units when compared to inherited disorders.

Haemorrhagic disorders in the ICU are due to one or more of the following: (i) thrombocytopaenia; (ii) a qualitative defect in the platelets; (iii) damage to capillary endothelial cells; (iv) coagulation defects.

There are some diseases, particularly renal failure, sepsis, and multiple organ failure, which cause or are associated with two or more of the above defects. An awareness of the nature of acquired disorders in bleeding and clotting mechanisms peculiar to important common critical illnesses, is of great importance in management. This is because in poor developing countries, very few centres have facilities for doing detailed coagulation profiles, or studies on platelet function. Even when these facilities are available, there is a lag of precious time between the sampling of the blood, and the actual results of the analysis. Treatment in severely bleeding patients is therefore empiric. It is however always wise to collect blood for a proper analysis of haemorrhagic disorders, before starting such empiric treatment. Results of such analysis may then help to suitably modify treatment.

Clinical Approach

History

A good history is all-important, particularly with reference to spontaneous bleeding in the past, or to excessive bleeding following an injury or surgery. Rarely a background suggesting a possible congenital defect in bleeding/clotting, or an acquired one as in immune thrombocytopaenic purpura, will be uncovered. Previous coagulation profiles and platelet counts done in the course of an acute illness are also of help in comparing values. A meticulous history regarding intake of drugs is invaluable, as drug-induced disturbances are an extremely important cause of thrombocytopaenia in an intensive care setting. Aspirin, non-steroidal anti-inflammatory drugs, the newer synthetic penicillins, ticlopidine, clopidogrel, platelet glycoprotein IIb-IIIa inhibitors, and antihistaminics are amongst the more frequently used drugs responsible for either thrombocytopaenia or a qualitative defect in platelet function.

Coagulation defects may be congenital or acquired. Congenital defects when marked are generally evident from the history of frequent bleeds since childhood. Acquired coagulation defects are far more frequently encountered in an intensive care unit than congenital defects. As detailed later, acquired coagulation defects occur against a background of severe liver or renal dysfunction, or following consumption of coagulation factors, or in Vitamin K deficiency, or rarely due to circulating inhibitors of coagulation. A detailed history coupled with a careful physical examination should help uncover most of the background diseases known to produce acquired coagulation defects that result in a bleeding disorder.

Though drugs frequently affect platelets, they very rarely alter coagulation factors qualitatively or quantitatively. There are however several cephalosporins which diminish the production of Vitamin K dependent coagulation factors. These include cefaperazone, cefamandole and the monolactams. Patients on oral anticoagulants (e.g. warfarin) or on heparin have as expected, an altered coagulation profile. It is worth remembering that in rare instances, catastrophic bleeding can occur in a patient on warfarin, even when the alteration in the coagulation profile (i.e. the prothrombin time [PT]), is within the therapeutic range.10 per cent of these patients may bleed, and in 1–2 per cent of these cases, the bleeding may be intracranial with catastrophic results.

Physical Examination

Physical examination should have four important objectives:

(i) To determine clinically or on relevant tests, the nature of the background disease or critical illness. This suggests the cause and nature of the associated haemorrhagic disorder which results from the disease.

(ii) To carefully inspect the site of bleeding or haemorrhage. Petechiae, bleeding from catheters or drains, and bleeding from the GI tract, urinary tract and mucous membranes is more commonly observed with thrombocytopaenia or a qualitative defect in platelet function. Defects in coagulation factors can also cause bleeding from these sites, but are also associated with deep soft tissue bleeds, retroperitoneal haemorrhage, haemarthrosis, or bleeds into internal organs.

(iii) When bleeding occurs from one local site, e.g. the GI or the urinary tract, it is important to clearly exclude an anatomic cause for the bleed, even in patients with thrombocytopaenia or a clotting defect. Not uncommonly, a local pathology and a haemostatic disorder may both be contributory to such a bleed.

(iv) Inherited disorders of platelets or of coagulation are comparatively rare in the ICU. A good family history, absence of background disease known to cause platelet and coagulation abnormalities and detailed laboratory haematological investigations generally provide an accurate diagnosis.

Laboratory Investigations

Basic screening tests include a CBC, template bleeding time (BT), prothrombin time (PT), activated partial thromboplastin time (PTT), platelet count, thrombin time (TT), and serum fibrinogen levels. More elaborate tests which take time are performed in special laboratories. These include estimation of qualitative defects in platelets and a quantitative estimation of all coagulation factors.

Basic screening tests and even the more elaborate tests on the coagulation profile are now routinely done in the major cities of our country. However meagre facilities permit merely an estimation of the BT, CT, and PT in many of the smaller cities and district hospitals in poor countries all over the world.

Principles in Management (1, 2)

The intensivist must determine whether the haemorrhagic disorder is related to a qualitative or quantitative defect in platelets or to a coagulation disorder. The former is associated with a prolonged bleeding time, the latter with an abnormal coagulation profile. Not uncommonly thrombocytopaenia and/or platelet dysfunction coexist with a coagulopathy. Bleeding due to thrombocytopaenia or platelet dysfunction should be treated with platelet infusions. Bleeding due to a coagulopathy by transfusion of coagulation factors through fresh frozen plasma and/or cryoprecipitate. The nature of the coagulation defect is invariably suggested by the background disease responsible for the overall clinical problem in a given individual. Besides the routine laboratory tests stated above, a blood sample should be collected and sent to a reference laboratory for a study on qualitative platelet functions and for coagulation factor assays if there is a detectable abnormality in the screening tests. *Treatment of the underlying disease responsible for the haemorrhagic disorder is imperative.*

Patients with bleeding or clotting disorders should not be given intramuscular injections. Blood loss should be roughly estimated

and replaced. CBC and PCV should be done at necessary intervals to estimate the degree of blood loss. It may take 12–24 hours or even more, for the full effect of blood loss to manifest by a fall in the Hb or PCV, in a critically ill patient. Clinical evaluation of blood loss is therefore of prime importance.

The subsequent sections of this chapter now deal with platelet dysfunction (inherited and acquired), thrombocytopaenia, and with inherited and acquired coagulation disorders.

Inherited Platelet Dysfunction

Platelets are essential for normal haemostasis. Defects in platelet adhesion, aggregation, secretion or procoagulant activity can lead to impaired haemostasis that results in bleeding. Inherited platelet dysfunction is extremely rare, follows autosomal recessive inheritance patterns, and results in varying degrees of bleeding in neonates or in childhood. These defects are associated with a prolonged bleeding time or absent platelet aggregation in response to platelet agonists like ristocytin, ADP, adrenaline, collagen. The coagulation profile is normal.

Bleeding associated with prolonged bleeding time can occur with von Willebrand's disease. Inherited platelet dysfunction needs to be distinguished from acquired dysfunction. Platelet aggregation studies help distinguish these two conditions. Bleeding occurring for the first time in an adult is extremely unlikely to be related to inherited platelet dysfunction.

Treatment for bleeding is the infusion of normal platelets.

Acquired Platelet Dysfunction

Various conditions can lead to defects in platelet adhesion, aggregation, secretion or procoagulant function without causing a significant fall in the platelet count. The most important of these are drugs. Aspirin inactivates cyclooxygenase and thereby prevents the production of Thromboxane A_2 which mediates both platelet secretion and aggregation. Most individuals on aspirin will have a slightly prolonged bleeding time but serious clinical bleeding is rare unless there are other haemostatic defects. However it is always wise to stop aspirin for 5 to 7 days before major surgery and also before cataract surgery. Ticlopidine and clopidogrel selectively affect platelet aggregation, increase bleeding time and may induce significant mucosal bleeds. Platelet glycoprotein IIb/IIIa inhibitors are increasingly used particularly at and after angioplasty in the management of ischaemic heart disease. The use of these inhibitors is often combined with the use of anticoagulants and can at times cause catastrophic bleeding. We have seen two deaths from intracranial haemorrhage following the combined use of platelet glycoprotein inhibitors and heparin.

Acquired platelet dysfunction is common in renal failure as judged by prolonged bleeding time and by defects in platelet aggregation. Remarkably enough the risk of bleeding does not necessarily correlate with the degree of disturbance in platelet function. The exact biochemical nature of platelet dysfunction in renal failure or hepatic disease remains unknown.

Cardiopulmonary bypass induces both platelet dysfunction and thrombocytopaenia. These disturbances rectify themselves within a few hours after surgery. Transient coagulation disorders also occur in the immediate post-operative period. Bleeding therefore is accentuated not only by platelet dysfunction and thrombocytopaenia, but by coagulation defects and perhaps by incomplete haemostasis.

Myeloproliferative disorders, myelodysplastic syndromes, acute leukaemias may result in the production of intrinsically defective platelets. Multiple myeloma, Waldenstrom's macroglobinaemia are associated with the production of abnormal immunoglobulins which can also interfere with platelet function. Important causes of acquired qualitative platelet dysfunction are listed in **Table 15.6.1**.

Table 15.6.1. Important causes of qualitative platelet defects

---

1. Associated background disease
   - Uraemia, liver cell failure
   - Myeloproliferative disorders, acute leukaemia
   - Dysproteinaemias
2. Cardiopulmonary bypass
3. Drugs
   - Aspirin, non-steroidal anti-inflammatory drugs
   - Dipyridamole
   - Ticlopidine, clopidogrel
   - Platelet glycoprotein IIb/IIIa inhibitors
   - Dextrans
   - Antihistaminics, furosemide, propranolol
   - Ethanol

Clinical Features

The clinical features are characterized chiefly by mucosal bleeding or post-traumatic or surgical bleeding. The total platelet count is within normal limits and the coagulation profile is normal. The bleeding time is raised. In vitro platelet aggregation studies require both experience and expertise for reliable results. They should be resorted to only in special cases with unexplained increase in bleeding time or in patients with obscure bleeding with a normal bleeding time and a normal coagulation profile.

Treatment

Drug-induced platelet dysfunction is treated by withdrawal of the offending drug. Desmopressin (0.3 μg/kg intravenously) is useful in the management of bleeding due to platelet dysfunction observed in uraemia, liver disease and following cardiopulmonary bypass. Aprotinin, a plasmin inhibitor is also often used to combat post-operative bleeding after cardiopulmonary bypass surgery.

Renal failure is one of the commonest causes of platelet dysfunction, and is an important cause of active serious bleeding in an ICU setting. Uraemia produces a qualitative defect in platelet function, and also affects platelet adhesiveness to the capillary endothelium, by causing a defect in von Willebrand's factor. Transfused platelets may be life-saving in severe bleeds (particularly when the bleed occurs into organ systems), in uraemic patients. Cryoprecipitate (10 U) (**3**) and desmopressin (DDAVP) (0.3 μg/kg) (**4**) can both cause release of von Willebrand's factor into the circulation, and are also used to arrest the bleeding in uraemia.

The bleeding time (BT) generally decreases within 1–2 hours after infusion of cryoprecipitate, and within 1–4 hours after desmopressin use. Estrogens in high doses (0.6 mg/kg/day for 5–7 days), also reduce the BT in uraemic patients (**5**). Bleeding in renal failure, is often due both to platelet dysfunction and to defects in clotting factors. The latter need to be replaced by the infusion of fresh frozen plasma or of appropriate coagulation factors. The bleeding tendency in patients with renal failure is decreased and more easily controlled in patients on regular dialysis and with the use of erythropoeitin.

Platelet infusions should be used to counter severe bleeding due to platelet dysfunction, whatever the aetiology, or for planned surgery. Drugs (in particular aspirin) known to cause platelet dysfunction should be scrupulously avoided and the underlying disease known to cause defects in platelet function should be treated as best as possible.

Thrombocytopaenia

Thrombocytopaenia i.e. a fall in the platelet count, results from decreased production of platelets in the marrow, destruction or utilization of circulating platelets, or sequestration of platelets within the spleen. Important causes of thrombocytopaenia are listed in **Table 15.6.2**. Decreased production by the marrow invariably affects all haemopoeitic cells so that anaemia and leucopaenia are associated with thrombocytopaenia. Decreased production is classically observed in extensive metastatic disease involving the marrow, lymphoproliferative diseases, myelofibrosis, myelodysplastic syndromes, aplastic anaemia and B_{12} or folic acid deficiency. Chemotherapy, exposure to radiation, drugs, fungal,

Table 15.6.2. Causes of thrombocytopaenia

A. Decreased Production
1. Marrow infiltration or replacement
   - Metastatic ca, myelofibrosis, lymphoma, leukaemia, aplasia
2. Toxic exposure
   - Chemotherapy, radiation, alcohol, chemicals
3. Drugs
   - Thiazide diuretics
4. B_{12}, folate deficiency
   Myelodysplasia
5. Infections
   - Bacterial, fungal, viral, protozoal sepsis
B. Increased Destruction or Utilization
1. Mechanical
   - Disseminated intravascular coagulopathy (DIC)
   - Abnormal heart valves
   - Cardiopulmonary bypass
   - Thrombotic thrombocytopaenic purpura
   - Haemolytic uraemic syndrome
   - Vasculitis
2. Immunological
   - Autoimmune thrombocytopaenia
   - SLE, antiphospholipid syndrome
   - Drug-induced e.g. quinine, quinidine
   - Chronic lymphatic leukaemia, Hodgkins
   - HELLP syndrome
3. Bacterial, viral, fungal, protozoal sepsis
4. Massive transfusions
5. Sequestration—hypersplenism

---

protozoal and viral sepsis can also suppress platelet production.

Increased destruction or utilization can either be mechanical or immunological. Important mechanical causes include cardiopulmonary bypass, disseminated intravascular coagulopathy, abnormal heart valves and vasculitis. Immunological destruction may result from drugs, multiple transfusions, autoimmune disease (e.g. systemic lupus erythematosus). Immune thrombocytopaenic purpura is characterized by an immunological destruction of platelets occurring as an isolated disorder. Mechanical destruction of platelets is often associated with haemolytic anaemia and with red blood cell fragmentation in the peripheral smear.

Sequestration of platelets can occur in many conditions causing splenomegaly and hypersplenism. The classical example of thrombocytopaenia due to hypersplenism is seen in cirrhosis of the liver with portal hypertension and splenomegaly. Anaemia and leucopaenia may be associated with thrombocytopaenia in many patients with hypersplenism.

Clinical Features

Thrombocytopaenia can cause bleeding, and the bleeding is generally from mucocutaneous surfaces. Epistaxis, bleeding gums, haematuria may occur. Petechia are generally observed only when thrombocytopaenia is marked. Spontaneous bruising is seen but soft-tissue haematomas (common in coagulation disorders) are rare in thrombocytopaenia. Haemarthrosis does not occur. Severe thrombocytopaenia can cause bleeding within organ systems, the most dreaded being an intracerebral bleed. Bleeding from surgical wounds or during or immediately after surgery is an important feature of thrombocytopaenic purpura.

The risk of bleeding is to an extent unpredictable and depends (a) on the degree of thrombocytopaenia, (b) the presence or absence of any qualitative defects in platelets, (c) the presence or absence of an associated coagulation disorder, (d) the presence or absence of associated mucosal lesions, vascular injury or trauma.

Platelet counts > 100,000/mm^3 do not cause bleeding. In fact surgery is safe with thrombocytopaenia of this degree provided the platelets are qualitatively normal and there is no coagulation defect.

Platelet counts over 50,000/mm^3 do not cause bleeding problems, though it would be wise to avoid major surgery till the count is close to 100,000/mm^3.

Platelet counts between 30,000 to 50,000/mm^3 generally do not cause increase in bleeding except after trauma or surgery.

When the count ranges between 20,000/mm^3 to 30,000/mm^3, the risk of spontaneous mucocutaneous bleeding increases—epistaxis, menorrhagia, haematuria, bleeding from the mouth and gums can occur.

Platelet counts below 20,000/mm^3 and particularly below 10,000/mm^3 are dangerous, can lead to severe life-threatening GI bleeds and spontaneous bleeds into viscera (e.g. intracranial haemorrhage).

Diagnosis depends on the presence of a prolonged bleeding time, thrombocytopaenia of a sufficient degree, mucocutaneous bleeding and/or petechiae, absence of other haemostatic defects and the presence of a background or associated disease known to cause thrombocytopaenia.

A careful complete blood count and examination of the peripheral smear are important. Isolated thrombocytopaenia is mostly due to an immunological cause but may occur in acute alcoholic intoxication and in hypersplenism. The presence of both nucleated red blood cells and immature white blood cells in association with thrombocytopaenia suggests bone marrow infiltration. Fragmented red blood cells in the peripheral blood point to intravascular trauma to cells as seen with mechanical prosthetic valves, thrombotic thrombocytopaenic purpura, HELLP syndrome. Palpable purpuric lesions are often observed in vasculitis. Macrocytosis and pancytopaenia are observed in B$_{12}$ deficiency, particulary in strict vegetarians whose B$_{12}$ intake is very poor. Bone marrow aspiration and biopsy will help uncover important diseases that reduce production of platelets.

A coagulation disorder should be excluded by doing basic tests such as prothrombin time (PT) and the partial thromboplastin time (PTT). Disseminated intravascular coagulopathy is asscociated with an increase in both PT and PTT as also a thrombocytopaenia. Other severe coagulation disorders are associated with an abnormal coagulation profile and a normal platelet count.

Von Willebrand's disease or a qualitative defect in platelet function should be considered when mucosal bleeding is associated with a prolonged bleeding time but with no thrombocytopaenia.

Treatment

The principles of treatment are as follows:

(i) To diagnose and treat the critical illness responsible for the platelet disorder. Thus steroids are used in idiopathic thrombocytopaenic purpura or for SLE; myeloproliferative diseases responsible for thrombocytopaenia, merit specific treatment.

(ii) To omit drugs which may be primarily responsible for, or which could accentuate an existing qualitative or quantitative defect in platelets.

(iii) To replace platelets with platelet infusions.

The mere occurrence of thrombocytopaenia does not merit platelet infusions. Patients do not usually bleed unless platelet counts are less than 20,000–30,000/mm^3. Platelet counts between 50,000–80,000/mm^3 are generally safe for minor invasive ICU procedures e.g. inserting or changing central lines. If surgery is necessary for a critically ill patient in the ICU, platelet levels between 80,000–100,000/mm^3 are considered safe. These levels should be maintained during the surgical procedure and for 48 hours after surgery; the same levels should also be maintained during episodes of active bleeding (6).

Platelet infusions can increase the platelet count in thrombocytopaenia. Ordinarily the infusion of one unit of platelets in an adult, should produce a rise in the platelet count by 5000–10,000/mm^3. If this increase is not observed, single-donor pharesis platelets or group-specific platelets may be given. Intravenous IgG (1 g/kg for 3–5 days), may also be given (7), though it is effective in < 50 per cent of cases. Platelet infusions should preferably be given only when thrombocytopaenia causes bleeding, or when surgery is planned in a thrombocytopaenic patient. Platelet transfusions should also be given prophylactically, particularly in critically ill individuals, whose platelet counts are < 20,000/mm³.

Platelet transfusions are not generally indicated in idiopathic thrombocytopaenic purpura, which is treated with corticosteroids (60–80 mg prednisolone daily) and intravenous IgG. However platelet infusions may need to be given initially, to counter a life-threatening bleed in these patients. Platelet transfusions should as far as possible be avoided and may in fact be harmful in thrombotic thrombocytopaenic purpura, haemolytic uraemic syndrome and heparin-induced thrombocytopaenia.

Very occasionally heparin, which is used very frequently as an anticoagulant in the ICU, can cause thrombocytopaenia (8), and can result in venous and even arterial thrombi. This is due to heparin-induced platelet aggregation. Thrombocytopaenia (< 50,000/mm³), necessitates withdrawal of the drug, and oral anticoagulation should be substituted for heparin.

Platelet replacement by infusions, has one major drawback. The half-life of platelets is short, so that within a day or two, fresh replacements are necessary. Antibodies to transfused platelets soon develop, and besides causing untoward reactions, further reduce the life-span of the transfused platelets.

Inherited Coagulation Disorders

Inherited coagulation disorders are uncommon and rarely met with in a critical care unit. The pattern of inheritance is either dominant or recessive, autosomal or X-linked; rarely it results from a new mutation of a gene. In the latter instance the family history is non-contributory to the diagnosis. A personal history often reveals previous episodes of bleeding except when the inherited defect is mild or there has been no previous challenge to haemostasis (e.g. trauma or surgery). Inherited coagulation disorders can involve any one of the several coagulation factors responsible for blood clotting. The three commonest and most important of these disorders are von Willebrand's disease, haemophilia A and haemophilia B.

Von Willebrand's disease results from the deficiency of von Willebrand's factor due to an inherited autosomal dominant defect in its production. This factor is essential for platelet aggregation and also serves as a carrier for procoagulant factor VIII. The disease therefore affects both platelet function and coagulation. Severe defects can cause serious bleeding similar to that observed in patients with haemophilia A.

Haemophilia A is the commonest of inherited coagulation defects and is believed to occur in 1 in 5000 men. It is due to inheritance of an X-linked autosomal recessive mutation in the factor VIII gene that results in a mild (> 5 per cent activity), moderate (1–5 per cent activity) or severe (< 1 per cent activity) deficiency in the production of this factor. Haemophilia is a disease of males; the female serving as the carrier. Very rarely it may occur in females from the inheritance of two abnormal X chromosomes—one from the affected father and one from a carrier mother.

Haemophilia B results from the inheritance of an X-linked autosomal recessive mutation in the factor IX gene which results in a diminished production of factor IX. It exactly resembles haemophilia A; however a severe deficiency of factor IX occurs only in 50 per cent of cases. Haemophilia B is ten times less common than haemophilia A, occurring in about 1 in 50,000 men.

Inherited deficiencies of other coagulation factors are autosomal and generally recessive in nature. They are extremely rare and are observed in consanguineous marriages. Bleeding disturbances are usually not as severe as in haemophilia A and B, and as mentioned earlier are very rarely met with in critical care units.

Clinical features

A careful personal history and a family history will suggest the nature of the coagulation disorder as also its pattern of inheritance.

Bleeding can occur spontaneously but it often occurs or is reported after dental extraction, trauma or surgery. In von Willebrand's disease platelet function is also affected, so that easy bruising often occurs. In haemophilia spontaneous bleeding from the nose, the GI tract, the urinary tract and most importantly into joints (haemarthrosis) is common. In patients in whom factor VIII is grossly deficient exsanguinating haemorrhages can occur spontaneously into soft-tissues, retroperitoneally, and into various organ systems. Intracranial haemorrhage is catastrophic and generally fatal.

Laboratory Tests

Deficiency of factors II, V, VII, VIII, IX, X, XI, XII, XIII can be determined by special techniques. The diagnosis of von Willebrand's disease is made on the basis of a low von Willebrand factor antigen, an abnormal ristocetin co-factor activity and a factor VIII activity which is generally reduced. Quantitative defects in von Willebrand's factor can be distinguished from qualitative defects by special techniques.

Differential Diagnosis

Bleeding from inherited coagulation disorders must be distinguished from bleeding caused by acquired coagulation disorders. The differentiation is evident from the history and the presence of background disease in patients with acquired coagulation defects.

It is to be remembered that abnormal coagulation tests are not always associated with bleeding. Thus lupus anticoagulant deficiencies or contact deficiency can lead to abnormal coagulation tests but are associated with thrombotic rather than bleeding phenomena.

Mild coagulation defects may be associated with minimally prolonged or normal coagulation tests and may result in bleeding only in the event of vascular injury.

Bleeding in the presence of normal coagulation times suggests thrombocytopaenia, or a qualitative defect in platelets, an underlying vascular defect (if there is bleeding from a single source), excessive fibrinolysis or factor XIII deficiency.

In patients with inherited coagulation defects, the frequent infusions of a deficient factor may induce antibodies to this factor so that subsequent infusion of this factor may not be as effective as before. Antibodies or inhibitors to factor VIII in haemophilia A can cause problems in the management of this serious disorder.

Management

Factor Replacement. Patients with inherited coagulation disorders need replacement of the appropriate deficient factor either when they bleed or in preparation for surgery as also in the post-surgical period (**Table 15.6.3**).

Surgical procedures in these patients should be performed only in centres with good laboratory facilities and good blood banks. Intramuscular injections and aspirin are avoided in patients with coagulation defects. Patients who develop inhibitors to the deficient factor can cause problems in management. The problem is usually circumvented by using larger volumes of the deficient factor as replacement therapy or by using products that bypass the factor inhibitor—e.g. activated prothrombin complex concentrate with factor VIII inhibitor bypassing activity, recombinant factor VII a or porcine factor VIII in patients who develop inhibitors to factor VIII in haemophilia A. Plasmapheresis is at times resorted to in order to reduce the circulating inhibitory factor.

Adjuvant Factors. Adjuvant factors of help are desmopressin, antifibrinolytic agents (aminocaproic acid) and topical agents such as fibrin glue, and collagen preparations applied to local sites of bleeding.

Desmopressin (0.3 µg/kg intravenously over 15–30 minutes) raises both von Willebrand's factor and factor VIII to 2–5 times the prevailing level within 30 minutes. It is useful to arrest bleeding in von Willebrand's disease and in patients with mild factor VIII deficiency. The use of desmopressin may obviate the need for factor replacement in mild bleeding episodes and may reduce the quantity of factor replacement in patients with moderate and severe bleeding episodes. It is to be noted that severe haemophilics or patients with a qualitative defect in von Willebrand's factor will not respond to desmopressin and will need factor replacement therapy.

Some units use antifibrinolytic agents as adjuncts to factor replacement therapy to control severe bleeding in inherited coagulation disorders. Contraindications to their use are the occurrence of intravascular coagulopathy or the use of prothrombin activated complex. The dose of aminocaproic acid for the control of active bleeding is 1 g/hour till bleeding is controlled (maximum 24 g), followed by a maintenance dose of 6 g intravenously or orally every 6 hours for 7 to 10 days. Tranexamic acid is an antifibrinolytic agent given in a dose of 10 mg/kg intravenously or 25 mg/kg orally three to four times a day one day before surgery or during bleeding. It should be continued for 2 to 7 days.

Acquired Coagulation Defects

Coagulation defects in critically ill patients in the ICU are most frequently observed in liver disease, renal disease, sepsis, disseminated intravascular coagulopathy, and following massive transfusions. They may also be observed with Vitamin K deficiency. Oral anticoagulants like uniwarfarin are given in a dose sufficient to produce a controlled coagulation defect. As mentioned earlier, severe and even catastrophic bleeding can occur even when the altered clotting mechanism is within the therapeutic range. Very rarely inhibitors against various coagulation factors may develop, and lead to a serious bleeding diathesis.

From the overall clinical point of view, acquired coagulation disorders or defects are invariably characterized by deficiency of multiple factors, and are also frequently associated with thrombocytopaenia and/or a qualitative defect in platelet dysfunction. The clinical features are varied and often dominated by the background disease—an abnormal coagulopathy is just one manifestation of this underlying disease process.

Table 15.6.3. Principles for factor replacement in inherited coagulation disorders

Factor deficiency	Haemostatic requirement	Source	Dose	Interval between doses
Factor VIII	25–30%	Purified factor VIII	10–15 units/kg—minor bleeds 30–40 units/kg—major bleeds	12 hours
		Recombinant factor VIII	10–15 units/kg—minor bleeds 40–50 units/kg—major bleeds	
Factor IX	20–30%	Purified factor IX Recombinant factor IX	10–20 units/kg 100 units/kg, then 7.5 units/kg/hour	24 hours
Factor II	20–40 %	FFP Purified PCC	15 ml/kg; then 5–10 ml/kg 20 units/kg, then 10 units/kg	24 hours
Factor V	15–25 %	FFP	20 ml/kg, then 10 ml/kg	12–24 hours
Factor VII	10–20%	FFP Recombinant Factor VII Purified PCC	20 ml/kg, then 10 ml/kg 60–100 µg/kg 30 units/kg, then 10 units/kg	4–6 hours
Factor X	10–20%	FFP Purified PCC	15–20 ml/kg 10 units/kg	24 hours
Factor XI	10–20%	FFP	15–20 ml/kg	12–24 hours
Factor XIII Fibrinogen	3–5 %	FFP Cryoprecipitate	5 ml/kg 1–2 bags/10 kg	1–2 weeks 48 hours
Von Willebrand's factor	25–50 %	Desmopressin Cryoprecipitate	0.3 µg/kg/30 minutes 30 units/kg	24–48 hours 12 hourly for a day, then every 24 hours

Clinical Diagnosis

A good clinical history, physical examination and basic laboratory screening tests to determine the coagulation profile generally suffice to help diagnose the nature of the coagulation defect.

The clinical features are characterized by bleeding, the presence of background disease known to cause an acquired coagulation defect, and the laboratory evidence of a coagulation disorder.

Bleeding can be spontaneous, or excessive bleeding may result from surgical procedures. A disruption of vascular or mucosal integrity can lead to profuse bleeding. This is particularly observed in cirrhotics with varices due to portal hypertension or those with one or more mucosal ulcers in the GI tract. These patients bleed profusely into the gut and present with exsanguinating haematemesis or melaena.

Spontaneous bleeding may occur from the mucosa at various sites, can result in bruising of the skin, soft-tissue haematomas, retroperitoneal haematomas, and haematomas or bleeds into organ systems. However, petechiae so often seen in severe thrombocytopaenia or platelet dysfunction do not generally occur in patients with acquired coagulation defects.

Disseminated intravascular coagulopathy (DIC) is one condition in which bleeding may be associated clinically with intravascular thrombosis in various organ systems.

A brief resume of the nature of clotting defects found in the clinical conditions mentioned earlier is given below.

Liver Disease (9, 10)

Multiple coagulation abnormalities are invariably present in patients with advanced liver cell dysfunction. The liver synthesizes all coagulation factors except factor VIII and von Willebrand factor. It also synthesizes other regulatory proteins including α_1 antiplasmin, protein C, protein S, antithrombin III. The liver is responsible for the clearance of activated clotting factors and the degradation products of fibrin and fibrinogen. Liver dysfunction prevents Vitamin K from being effective in the synthesis of Vitamin K dependent clotting factors resulting in a functional Vitamin K deficiency. There is also impaired fibrin polymerization due to increased fibrin degradation products and accelerated fibrinolysis. Finally, thrombocytopaenia or a qualitative defect in platelet function may be associated with the coagulation abnormalities described above.

Bleeding in severe liver disease is therefore multifactorial and is invariably due to a deficiency of several coagulation factors. The prothrombin time is elevated; it is a sensitive index of liver cell function. Later the activated partial thromboplastin time is also prolonged due to low levels of factors IX and X. Patients with severe liver disease cannot utilize Vitamin K; the prothrombin time therefore remains high and unchanged after Vitamin K therapy. The decreased levels of protein C and a decreased clearance of activated clotting factors predispose to the development of disseminated intravascular coagulopathy. The accelerated fibrinolysis and the associated thrombocytopaenia and platelet dysfunction can contribute strongly to bleeding in some patients.

Treatment of severe bleeding in liver disease may be individu-alized according to the deficiency of one or more factors, as evinced from a study of the coagulation profile. This may not be possible if an elegant sophisticated laboratory back-up is unavailable. In any case, acute bleeding necessitates urgent replacement of clotting factors. This is best achieved by infusion of fresh frozen plasma. 6–10 units of fresh frozen plasma may have to be infused to raise the clotting factors to a level that arrests the haemorrhage. The short half-life of clotting factors necessitates frequent use of fresh frozen plasma, which may easily precipitate a fluid overload in critically ill patients. When patients cannot tolerate the large volume of fresh frozen plasma necessary to stop the bleed, exchange transfusions with replacement by fresh frozen plasma may be life-saving. Continuous arteriovenous haemofiltration is an alternative method of reducing fluid overload in such patients. An infusion of cryoprecipitate (8 to 10 units) becomes necessary when the fibrinogen level falls close to or below 100 mg/dl.

Platelet transfusions may also be necessary because of quantitative or possible severe qualitative defects observed in liver cell dysfunction. Thrombocytopaenia in chronic liver cell disease is however often due to hypersplenism. In these patients platelet infusions do not produce the expected increase in the platelet count.

Factor IX concentrates (activated prothrombin complex concentrates) which are rich in Vitamin K dependent factors, can be selectively used to counter haemorrhage in acute hepatocellular failure. The main advantage is a reduced volume load. The disadvantages are the risk of blood borne viral infections, and of thrombotic complications, including disseminated intravascular coagulopathy.

Prophylactic infusions of fresh frozen plasma or of selective clotting factors found to be deficient in patients with liver disease, need to be given before any emergency or elective major surgery.

Renal Disease (3)

Uraemia in renal failure very frequently produces platelet dysfunction and a deficiency of clotting factors. Management of platelet dysfunction has been outlined earlier. Clotting factors are replaced by fresh frozen plasma, or by selective replacement of one or more deficient factors. Haemodialysis improves bleeding tendencies in renal failure. In the presence of acute bleeding requiring emergency infusions of large volumes of fresh frozen plasma and of packed red blood cells, a continuous arteriovenous haemofiltration is necessary to avoid fluid overload. Recent evidence suggests that haemostasis may be improved in uraemia after treatment with recombinant human erythropoietin (11).

Disseminated Intravascular Coagulopathy (12–14)

Disseminated intravascular coagulopathy (DIC) occurs as a result of abnormal activation of coagulation and clotting factors because of vascular injury, release of precoagulant factors into the blood, or both. This leads to consumption of coagulation factors (consumption coagulopathy), and of platelets, and is accompanied secondarily by increased fibrinolysis. A generalized bleeding tendency results, with bleeding from the mucosa, puncture sites and surgical wounds. The clinical spectrum ranges from small thrombi in multiple organ systems that can result in organ dysfunction on the one hand, to profuse bleeding on the other. Evidence of both thrombi and active bleeding may be present. The presence of small thrombi in the microcirculation leads to tissue hypoxia. Widespread thrombi together with bleeding, produce the features of purpura fulminans, with skin necrosis and gangrene of fingers and toes, or even of distal portions of the extremities. Multiple organ dysfunction chiefly involves the kidneys, liver, lungs, skin and the central nervous system.

There are numerous causes of disseminated intravascular coagulopathy. The most important cause is bacterial sepsis, and in tropical countries, fulminant Pl. falciparum infections. Other fulminant infections can also produce a DIC. The next most common cause observed by us in our setting, is the presence of obstetric complications—in particular eclampsia, retained dead foetus, and abruptio placenta. In southern India, and in other snake-infested regions of the world, viper bites are an important cause of DIC. Severe burns, crush injuries, trauma, malignancies and acute leukaemias are other conditions causing DIC. A consumption coagulopathy should always be suspected whenever there is bleeding, or evidence of thrombotic episodes, or both, in the clinical conditions tabled below (**Table 15.6.4**).

Table 15.6.4. Important background diseases causing disseminated intravascular coagulopathy in the ICU

1. Infections—bacterial, fungal, viral, protozoal e.g. Pl. falciparum infection
2. Obstetric complications—ectopic pregnancy, abruptio placenta, retained dead fetus, septic abortion, amniotic fluid embolism
3. Massive trauma, crush injuries
4. Burns
5. Snake bite
6. Neoplasms, acute leukaemias
7. Vascular disorders, presence of prosthetic devices, giant haemangiomas, aortic aneurysm
8. Miscellaneous causes e.g. acute lung injury, acute pancreatitis, blood transfusions, hyperthermia, hypothermia, severe hypotension, hypoxia.

The laboratory diagnosis of DIC is not always easy. In low grade DIC the synthesis of coagulation factors and platelet production keep pace with the increased consumption. Screening coagulation studies may be normal in these patients. The only laboratory abnormality may be a rise in the fibrin degradation products.

In the more severe form of DIC that is generally observed in an ICU setting, bleeding is invariably present. The patients show a prolonged PT and PTT, thrombocytopaenia, hypofibrinogenaemia and increased fibrin degradation products. None of these tests are sensitive or specific enough to conclusively establish a diagnosis of DIC. Coagulation defects in severe liver disease may at times be impossibly difficult to differentiate from those in DIC. The factor VIII levels are generally not significantly diminished in liver cell failure, but are severely decreased in DIC. Also, the presence of circulating fibrin monomers as judged by a positive protamine sulphate test or the presence of cross-linked fibrin as judged from a positive D-dimer test generally points to DIC.

Schistocytes (fragmented RBCs) may be found in patients with DIC. When present, DIC should be distinguished from microangiopathic haemolytic anaemia. The latter condition is observed in thrombotic thrombocytopaenic purpura, haemolytic uraemic syndrome and the HELLP syndrome (haemolytic anaemia, elevated liver enzymes, lowered platelet count). Microangiopathic haemolytic anaemia is however characterized by haemolytic anaemia, fragmented red blood cells in the blood smear, thrombocytopaenia, without alteration of the coagulation profile. It can therefore be distinguished from DIC.

In the final analysis, it is the clinical background which prompts the diagnosis of DIC in a critically ill, bleeding patient, who has an elevated PT, a reduced platelet count and an increase in the serum levels of fibrin degradation products.

Management

DIC is a manifestation of a serious underlying disorder, and management should always be primarily directed towards the disease. Sepsis needs to be countered by appropriate antibiotics, and surgical drainage or intervention should be promptly instituted whenever indicated.

Serious bleeding is countered by fresh blood transfusions and by transfusions of fresh frozen plasma, in sufficient quantity so as to decrease the PT to within 2–3 seconds of normal. Cryoprecipitate may be infused to maintain fibrinogen levels above 100mg/dl, and platelet concentrates given to raise the platelet count to > 50,000/mm³. Unfortunately, as stated earlier, both platelets and clotting factors have a short half-life, so that the effects of these infusions are very transient. We have never used heparin in DIC. Its use in lower doses, has been advocated in purpura fulminans, in DIC complicating acute leukaemia, and in patients with low grade DIC due to solid tumours manifesting as small widespread thrombi in various organs of the body. Secondary fibrinolysis invariably accompanies DIC. Antifibrinolytic agents are generally contraindicated because of the risk of inducing widespread thrombosis. Some units however persist with the use of epsilonaminocaproic acid in patients with severe fibrinolysis and with no evidence of thrombotic complications.

It should be noted that massive external or internal bleeding can cause a consumption of clotting factors and mimic DIC. In this situation, though the consumption and depletion of clotting factors and platelets may result in a serious increase in bleeding tendency and a rise in the fibrin degradation products, formation of thrombi in the microvasculature of various organ systems does not occur.

Primary fibrinolysis is a very rare bleeding disorder and results in a rapid dissolution of fibrin clots, destruction of fibrinogen and consumption of plasminogen and its inactivators. It has to be distinguished from DIC. Primary fibrinolysis is not associated with intravascular thrombi nor with thrombocytopaenia.

Massive Transfusions

Patients receiving large volumes of blood in the form of packed RBCs or stored whole blood, will develop thrombocytopaenia, and a deficiency of labile clotting factors (**15**). Platelet infusions must be given to these patients to maintain a platelet count close to 100,000/mm³, and fresh frozen plasma infused to counter Factor V, VIII, and other clotting factor deficiencies. If necessary, cryoprecipitate should also be infused to maintain fibrinogen levels above 100 mg/dl. Usually one unit of fresh frozen plasma is given after every 5 units of packed red blood cells, and 4–6 units of platelets after every 10 units of packed red blood cells. If the patient continues to bleed in spite of adequate replacement, other causes for bleeding should be sought. Local pathologies in the gut, notably stress ulcers, are often responsible for severe GI bleeding. Bleeding in patients who have sustained severe traumatic injuries, or who have been in shock due to poor tissue perfusion, could be due to a DIC.

Vitamin K Deficiency

Vitamin K is necessary for the synthesis of a number of clotting factors—Factors II (prothrombin), VII, IX, X and Proteins C and S. This vitamin is present in green vegetables, and is also synthesized by bacteria in the intestinal lumen. Vitamin K deficiency occurs in seriously ill patients, particularly when they are on broad-spectrum antibiotics. Obstructive jaundice can also lead to Vitamin K deficiency. Malabsorption from any cause does the same. Patients on oral anticoagulants (like warfarin) have an induced Vitamin K deficiency, as these anticoagulants inhibit its metabolism in the liver. Aspirin in high doses, as well as certain cephalosporins are known to induce a deficiency of Vitamin K dependent coagulation factors; this can be reversed by administration of Vitamin K.

Vitamin K deficiency results in a deficiency of all Vitamin K dependent clotting factors. Factor VII is depleted first because it

has the shortest half-life. This leads to an increase in the PT. Factors IX and X are depleted next, causing an increase in the activated PTT. If the patient's liver function is normal, Vitamin K$_1$ given as an intravenous infusion over 10–15 minutes, will normalize the PT in 6–24 hours, and the PTT in 24–48 hours. Parenteral Vitamin K$_1$ reverses the effects of oral anticoagulants like warfarin, in the same period of time. If correction of prothrombin time does not occur within 24–48 hours, liver functions are invariably deranged. In severe bleeding resulting from Vitamin K deficiency, fresh frozen plasma should be administered in addition to Vitamin K to help increase the levels of depleted clotting factors.

Circulating Inhibitors to Coagulation Factors

Circulating inhibitors pose significant problems in the management of bleeding disorders. As with the treatment of haemophilia A, management consists of using high doses of the particular deficient coagulant factor or using factors that bypass the factor that is being inhibited (use of activated prothrombin complex or recombinant factor VII a). The titre of the inhibitor factor can be reduced by plasmapheresis or by immunosuppression. In patients with multiple myeloma, the abnormal myeloma protein prevents fibrin polymerization. Chemotherapy against myeloma can rectify this abnormality; plasmapheresis is useful as a temporary measure.

Table 15.6.5 gives important laboratory findings in acquired coagulation disorders.

Table 15.6.5. Laboratory findings in acquired coagulation disorders

	DIC	Liver Disease	Kidney Disease	Vitamin K Deficiency	Inhibitors	Primary Fibrinolysis
PT prolonged	+	+	+	+	+	
PTT prolonged	+	+	+	+	+	
TT prolonged	+	+				+
FDP elevated	+	+			+	+
D-dimer present	+	+				
Protein C/S diminished	+	+		+		
Antithrombin III diminished	+	+				
Fibrinogen diminished	+	+				+
Associated thrombocytopaenia	+	+				
Red blood cells	schistocytes present	target cells, macrocytes present	schistocytes present			

Inhibitor screen: Mix with normal plasma. If no correction—inhibitor present
If correction—factor deficient
The coagulation profile in severe liver disease is very similar to that in DIC; however, in liver disease the factor VIII levels are not significantly reduced, while in DIC, they are severely reduced.

REFERENCES

1. Ratnoff OD, Forbes CD. (1990). Disorders of Haemostasis. Grune and Stratton, New York.
2. Williams WJ, Beutler E, Erslev AJ et al. (1989). Hematology, 4th edn. McGraw-Hill, New York.
3. Janson PA, Jubelier SJ, Weinstein MJ et al. (1980). Treatment of the bleeding tendency in uremia with cryoprecipitate. N Engl J Med. 303, 1318.
4. Mannucci PM, Remuzzi G, Pusineri F et al. (1983). Deamino-8-D arginine vasopressin shortens the bleeding time in uremia. N Engl J Med. 308, 8.
5. Liu YK, Kosfeld RE, Marcum SG. (1984). Treatment of uremic bleeding with conjugated estrogen. Lancet. ii, 887.
6. Baron JM, Baron BW. (1998). Bleeding Disorders. In: Principles of Critical Care (Eds Hall JB, Schmidt GA, Wood LH). pp. 1043–1056. McGraw-Hill, USA.
7. Bussel JB, Kimberly RP, Inman RD et al. (1983). Intravenous gamma-globulin treatment of chronic idiopathic thrombocytopenic purpura. Blood. 62, 480.
8. Kelton JG, Warkantin TE. (1989). Heparin-induced thrombocytopenia. Annu Rev Med. 40, 31.
9. Horne MK, Fu CL. (2001). Hemorrhagic and thrombotic disorders. In:

Critical Care Medicine (Eds Parrillo JE, Dellinger RP) pp. 1402–1415. Mosby, USA.

10. Joist JH. (1987). Hemostatic abnormalities in liver disease. In: Hemostasis and Thrombosis, 2nd edn (Eds Colman RW, Hirsh J, Marder VJ, Salzman EW). pp. 861. Lippincott, Philadelphia.

11. Moia M, Mannucci PM, Vizzotto L et al. (1987). Improvement in the hemostatic defect of uremia after treatment with recombinant human erythropoietin. Lancet. 2, 1227.

12. Marder VJ, Martin SE, Francis CW et al. (1987). Consumptive thrombohemorrhagic disorders. In: Hemostasis and Thrombosis, 2nd edn (Eds Colman RW, Hirsh J, Marder VJ, Salzman EW). p. 975. Lippincott, Philadelphia.

13. Bick RL. (1988). Disseminated intravascular coagulation and related syndromes: A clinical review. Semin Thromb Hemost. 14, 299–338.

14. Levi M, ten Cate H. (1999). Disseminated intravascular coagulation. N Engl J Med. 341, 586–592.

15. Harrigan C, Lucas CE, Ledgerwood AM et al. (1982). Primary hemostasis after massive transfusion for surgery. Am Surg. 48, 393.

Transfusion (Blood Product) Therapy

Whole blood or blood products are of extreme therapeutic value in critical care units. However despite all care and attention in the collection, preparation and storage of blood products, there is an inherent risk in the administration of these products. The benefits in appropriate clinical settings invariably outweigh the risks. Even so, the hazards of transfusions should always be borne in mind, so that blood products are only transfused when absolutely indicated.

The greatest hazard of transfusions is the transmission of viral infections, notably the AIDS virus, and the Hepatitis B and C viruses. Cytomegalovirus, the Epstein-Barr virus and other viruses can also be transmitted through transfusions, though not with the same disastrous effects as transmission of HIV I or Hepatitis B and C viruses. Blood is now screened for antibodies to the human immunodeficiency virus (HIV I) as also for HIV II. It is also screened for Hepatitis B surface antigen, syphilis and for malarial parasites. Unfortunately, few blood banks and laboratories in our country screen blood donors for Hepatitis C virus. This is unfortunate because of the significant risk of hepatocellular dysfunction and hepatocellular carcinoma in patients infected with Hepatitis C virus, through transfusion of Hepatitis C positive blood. Liver functions are also routinely tested in our laboratory on all donor samples, and donors showing a rise in the liver enzymes are rejected for blood donations. Donor screening coupled with tests on donor blood, ensure maximal possible safety with regard to transfused blood. However there can never be a guarantee of 100 per cent safety. A small but definite risk for the transmission of viral diseases (in particular the AIDS virus) (1), as also the potential hazards of transfusion reactions, still remain.

Blood Products

The text below outlines the blood products available, and indications for their use (Table 15.7.1) (2).

Red Blood Cells (3, 4)

Red blood cell concentrates are prepared by removing most of the plasma from a unit of whole blood. This is the blood product of choice when increase in the oxygen carrying capacity of blood is desired, as in an anaemic patient. Each unit contains 200–225 ml of red cells, and should raise the haematocrit by 3 per cent. In a bleeding patient, who is given packed red blood cells, volume

Table 15.7.1. Commonly available blood products and main indications for their use

Blood Product	Main Indications
1. Red Blood Cells	Restoration of oxygen carrying capacity
2. Whole Blood	Restoration of oxygen carrying capacity + restoration of blood volume
3. Leukocyte-poor Red Cells	Restoration of oxygen carrying capacity, prevention of febrile transfusion reactions
4. Frozen/Deglycerolyzed Red Cells	Used in patients who are extremely sensitive to plasma, e.g. those with congenital absence or marked deficiency of IgA
5. Platelets	Actively bleeding patient with thrombocytopaenia, thrombocytopaenic patient undergoing surgery, prophylactically in patient with platelet count < 20,000/mm^3
6. Leucocytes	In patients having neutropaenia with sepsis (hardly ever used; the granulocyte-stimulating factor is more effective)
7. Fresh Frozen Plasma	Replacement of multiple coagulation factor deficiencies e.g.in patients with uraemia, liver disorders, DIC, and following multiple blood transfusions
8. Cryoprecipitate	Haemophilia A, von Willebrand's disease, hypofibrinogenaemia
9. Specific Clotting Factors	
– Factor VIII Concentrate	Haemophilia A
– Prothrombin Complex Concentrate	Deficiency of Factors II, VII, IX, or X
10. Other Blood Products	
– Human Albumin	Expansion of plasma volume as in burns, to increase serum albumin levels in patients with hypoalbuminaemia
– IV Immunoglobulin	In patients with ITP, or congenital deficiency of immunoglobulin

replacement should be supplemented by infusion of colloids or crystalloids. Besides acute blood loss, RBC transfusions are indicated in severe anaemia with a Hb of < 5 g/dl. The decision to transfuse cells is based not only on the haematocrit or Hb value, but also on the clinical state of the patient.

The volume of blood loss, the rate of blood loss, and the presence or absence of ongoing blood loss, are of crucial importance in determining the need for transfusions and estimating the number of units that require to be transfused. The patient's age, and cardiopulmonary status also need to be carefully considered. Young patients tolerate blood loss far better than the aged and debilitated. Any condition that impairs the ability of the patient to increase stroke volume, cardiac output and intravascular volume, will result in poor tolerance of acute blood loss or severe anaemia. Patients with ischaemic heart disease or poor pump function may be unable to maintain satisfactory tissue perfusion to the myocardium and to other vital organs after blood loss, and need more urgent blood transfusions. Patients with respiratory disease causing a low PaO_2 require urgent replacement of blood loss, as the latter produces a sharp fall in the oxygen content of blood. Patients with chronic liver disease are tipped into liver cell failure with even a minor blood loss in the GI tract, and need prompt transfusions to replace even minor losses. In the acutely bleeding patient, who runs a risk of dying due to exsanguination within a short time, uncrossmatched O negative red cells may be transfused till properly typed and crossmatched blood is available.

Whole Blood

Whole blood contains both red blood cells and plasma. Transfusion of whole blood increases both the oxygen carrying capacity of blood, as also the volume. Whole blood is to be preferred in the severely bleeding patient, and when transfused it should be ABO identical with that of the patient. The use of whole blood in a patient who is not bleeding profusely, exposes the patient unnecessarily to plasma, and prevents donor blood from being processed into other blood components. Platelets and clotting factors, particularly Factors V and VII are not adequate in whole blood.

Leucocyte-poor Red Cells

This product is prepared in a manner that eliminates most leucocytes and platelets, but retains at least 80 per cent of the RBCs. The leucocyte count is $< 5 \times 10^8$ per unit. The method of preparation of leucocyte-poor red cells is by centrifugation and washing, or by more elaborate filtration methods. Filters and filtration methods if available, are now more frequently used in well-equipped blood banks. Leucocyte-poor red cells are valuable in patients who have recurrent febrile reactions after transfusion of the usual packed RBCs. Such reactions are believed to be caused by sensitization to human leucocyte antigen (HLA) present in donor leucocytes, as also to other surface antigens on leucocytes and platelets in donor blood. Such sensitization is common in patients receiving multiple blood transfusions. The advantage of leucocyte and platelet free red blood cells is two-fold: (i) it reduces the incidence of HLA alloimmunization caused by blood products (5); (ii) it reduces (but does not completely eliminate) the risk of transmission of CMV from the donor to the recipient.

Frozen/Deglycerolyzed Red Cells (6)

Red cells can be frozen and stored if glycerol is used as an intracellular cryoprecipitant. When they need to be used, the red cells are thawed, and the glycerol removed by extensive washing, a process that removes all plasma, leucocytes, and platelets. This prod-

uct is used for patients who are known to be extremely sensitive to plasma, as in those who have a congenital absence or marked deficiency of IgA. Ordinary packed cell or whole blood transfusions can cause almost life-threatening reactions in IgA deficient patients. Frozen/deglycerolyzed red blood cells are difficult to obtain, extremely expensive to prepare and store, and have no additional advantage for routine use.

Platelet Transfusions (7, 8)

Platelet transfusions can control bleeding in patients with severe thrombocytopenia or in those with qualitative defects in platelet function. One unit of blood ordinarily yields platelets sufficient to raise the platelet count by about $10,000/mm^3$ per square metre of body surface area. This amounts to a rise of 5000–7000 platelets/mm^3 in a 70 kg adult. Ordinarily 6–8 units of platelets are administered to produce a significant rise in the platelet count. It is necessary to do a platelet count 1 hour and 24 hours after transfusion, so that the effectiveness of the transfusion in raising the platelet count can be estimated. Antibodies to platelets from alloimmunization can lead to rapid destruction of transfused platelets. Fever, sepsis, drugs, liver cell dysfunction, uraemia and hypersplenism probably shorten even further the life-span of transfused platelets.

The indications for platelet transfusions which have been briefly touched upon earlier, are recapitulated below:

(i) The actively bleeding patient with thrombocytopaenia. A platelet count of $50,000/mm^3$ in these patients generally ensures haemostasis unless there is a co-existing qualitative defect in platelet function.

(ii) For elective or emergency surgery in patients with thrombocytopaenia, platelet infusions are necessary to raise the platelet count to $80,000–100,000/mm^3$. This level should be maintained for at least 48 hours after surgery.

(iii) Platelet transfusions are often used prophylactically when the platelet count falls to $< 20,000/mm^3$. Infusions may be given even when platelet counts are higher than $20,000/mm^3$, if there is a past history of serious bleeding. It is however quite remarkable how patients can tolerate counts as low as $10,000–15,000/mm^3$ without actively bleeding.

(iv) Alloimmunization to platelet antigens often results in poor survival of transfused platelets, and a poor response is inevitable. HLA matching can improve platelet survival in 70 per cent of alloimmunized patients. Obtaining HLA matched platelets is difficult because of the heterogenicity of HLA antigens, and requires technicians and doctors with experience and expertise.

(v) Platelets are of no use in the treatment of bleeding due to idiopathic thrombocytopaenic purpura, a condition in which there is autoimmunization to platelet antigens. These patients need specific treatment with corticosteroids. It is remarkable how counts as low as $5000–10,000/mm^3$ are tolerated without active bleeding in these patients. This is perhaps related to the production of young 'extra sticky' platelets by the bone marrow. These platelets are very effective in securing haemostasis during their short period of survival.

(vi) Desmopressin administered intravenously increases the

level of von Willebrand's factor; this improves platelet function in uraemia and following cardiopulmonary bypass.

Fresh Frozen Plasma (2, 9)

Fresh frozen plasma (FFP) is prepared from whole blood, and is frozen within 6 hours of collection of the donated unit. Each unit of FFP contains 250 ml plasma, all the clotting factors, and 400 mg of fibrinogen. FFP infusions are indicated to replenish deficiency of multiple clotting factors as observed in uraemia, liver disease, DIC and coagulopathy following multiple blood transfusions. FFP (together with intravenous Vitamin K) is also useful in reversing the coagulopathy produced by warfarin, and may be beneficial in treating thrombotic thrombocytopaenic purpura, and antithrombin III deficiency.

One unit of FFP increases the level of clotting factors by 3 per cent in an adult. Excessive bleeding is controlled and generally stops when clotting factor levels are over 30 per cent and the PT and PTT are reduced to about 1.5 times normal. It is therefore not necessary to aim at restoring clotting factors to absolute normal levels. The efficacy of FFP infusions should be monitored by coagulation assays—at least for the PT and the PTT. Specific factor deficiencies may be treated by infusion of specific factors. The short half-life of clotting factors and the dangers of fluid overload have been commented on earlier.

Cryoprecipitate (6)

When FFP is thawed at 4°C, a precipitate is formed. This cryoprecipitate is separated from the supernatant plasma, resuspended in a small volume of plasma, and then refrozen at –18°C. The cryoprecipitate can be stored for a year. Each bag or unit of cryoprecipitate (about 50 ml), contains 100–250 mg fibrinogen, 80–100 units of Factor VIII, 40–70 per cent of von Willebrand's Factor concentrate, and Factor XIII in a concentration 2–4 times that present in FFP.

Cryoprecipitate transfusions are indicated in bleeding due to severe hypofibrinogenaemia (< 100 mg/dl), in patients with deficiency of von Willebrand's Factor, in haemophilia and in Factor XIII deficiency. It is particularly useful in achieving haemostasis in patients with uraemia or chronic liver disease with low serum fibrinogen levels, and in patients with DIC.

Fibrinogen levels should be kept > 100 mg/dl to counter bleeding due to fibrinogen deficiency. 2–3 bags of cryoprecipitate per 10 kg will raise fibrinogen concentration by about 100 mg/dl. Maintenance doses of 1 bag/15 kg body weight can be given daily till the bleeding is controlled. Bleeding due to deficiency of von Willebrand's Factor stops if this factor level is increased to 50 per cent, and the prolonged BT is corrected. Factor XIII replacement requires transfusion of 4–6 bags of cryoprecipitate every 3 weeks.

Specific Clotting Factors

Factor VIII concentrate and Factor IX (prothrombin complex) concentrate are prepared by fractionation and lyophilization of pooled plasma. Factor VIII is used in the treatment of haemophilia A. It is not used in an intensive care setting except for bleeding haemophilics requiring critical care. All current methods of pre-

paring Factor VIII, inactivate the human immunodeficiency virus (HIV I), and decrease the incidence of transmission of Non-A, Non-B hepatitis. Bleeding haemophilics who have antibodies to Factor VIII can be given porcine Factor VIII concentrate, or activated prothrombin complex concentrates that bypass Factor VIII in the coagulation cascade.

Factor IX concentrates contain Factors II, VII, IX and X, and can be used in patients with selective deficiency of these factors.

Other Blood Products

These are prepared by fractionation of large pools of plasma. They include intravenous immunoglobulin used to treat congenital immunoglobulin deficiency, and idiopathic thrombocytopaenic purpura.

Intravenous human albumin preparations are chiefly indicated in hypovolaemic states (e.g. burns) to expand the volume of the vascular compartment, and thereby support circulation. They are also used to increase serum albumin levels in patients with hypoalbuminaemia.

Transfusion Reactions (10)

Transfusion reactions occur in about 5 per cent of patients. They may be very mild and permit continuation and completion of the transfusion; occasionally they may be severe and life-threatening, necessitating immediate stoppage of the transfusion and institution of emergency measures to counter these reactions.

The important immune-mediated transfusion reactions are summarized in **Table 15.7.2**.

Table 15.7.2. Important immune-mediated acute transfusion reactions

Reaction	Symptoms	Aetiology
1. Anaphylactic	Choking in throat, bronchial spasm, constricting chest pain, anxiety, shock	Antibodies to donor plasma proteins (severe); often anti-IgA
2. Febrile Non-haemolytic	High fever, chills	Antibodies to donor leukocytes or plasma proteins
3. Acute haemolytic	Fever, flank pain, chest tightness, shock, hypotension, oliguria, renal shut-down	Antibodies to donor red cell antigens

(i) Anaphylactic Reactions

These are frightening. A choking feeling in the throat, constricting chest pain, and a state of shock quickly supervene. Overwhelming bronchial spasm may choke the patient to death within a few minutes. The transfusion should be stopped immediately. Adrenaline 1 mg is administered subcutaneously or slowly intravenously, and is followed by 300 mg of intravenous efcorlin. The airway should be secured, and oxygen administered at a high flow rate. Circulatory support with volume infusions and inotropes is necessary. The blood bank should be immediately informed about the untoward reaction.

(ii) Febrile Non-haemolytic Reactions

High fever with chills is an extremely distressing transfusion reaction even in the absence of haemolysis. Temperatures as high as 105°F may occur, and the patient has tachycardia, tachypnoea, and in severe cases may show some degree of cyanosis. These reactions are related to antibodies to donor leucocytes, or to plasma proteins. Leukoagglutinin reactions may occasionally produce pulmonary infiltrates, which may be mistaken for pulmonary oedema on chest X-ray, particularly in the presence of tachypnoea and auscultatory crackles. Some degree of bronchospasm may add to the difficulty in differentiating these reactions from acute left ventricular failure. A normal ejection fraction on 2-D echocardiography under the above circumstances, is suggestive of leukoagglutinin reactions, rather than left heart failure.

The transfusion should be promptly stopped. Antipyretics are given. The efficacy of antihistaminics is doubtful, but it is better to administer them intramuscularly or intravenously. Leukoagglutinin reactions are more frequent in patients who have received multiple blood transfusions. If these reactions occur, leucocyte-poor blood cells should be transfused.

(iii) Acute Haemolytic Reactions (11)

Acute haemolytic reactions are almost always due to human error due to transfusion of incompatible blood. ABO incompatibilty is the most common, as anti-A, anti-B antibodies occur naturally. However other antibodies due to prior sensitization can also cause acute haemolysis. Incompatible blood transfusions can be prevented by adhering to a strict protocol for blood collection, labeling, storage, release and the final checking of the correctness of the unit, prior to administration to the patient.

Haemolytic transfusion reactions may vary from the mild to the fulminant and fatal. Back pain, fever, and chest tightness, are the warning complaints in conscious patients. If the patient is undergoing surgery under general anaesthesia, unexplained hypotension, tachycardia, fever, and red scanty urine are observed. Recovery from anaesthesia may be slow. High fever with chills, sometimes accompanied by seizures may occur in this stage. There may also be generalized oozing from venepuncture sites due to an evolving DIC.

Acute haemolytic transfusion reactions often produce acute oliguric renal failure. Haemoglobinuria is present, and there is an increase of free haemoglobin in the blood. Cardiovascular collapse and DIC are important complications, which are due to immune complex deposition and stimulation of the coagulation cascade, resulting in a consumption coagulopathy. In severe cases, the perfusion to vital organ systems is grossly impaired leading to tissue hypoxia and damage. The degree of damage is dose-related. For this reason, even mild febrile reactions occurring in a patient receiving a transfusion, should prompt a stopping of the transfusion, checking the label and group of the blood product being used, and checking with the blood bank regarding the possibility of incompatibility. This is particularly important if the patient is being transfused for the first time, or has never exhibited transfusion reactions in the past.

Management of an acute severe haemolytic reaction requires critical care. Vital signs are monitored, and a volume load infused to maintain adequate blood pressure and renal perfusion. Furosemide 40–100 mg intravenously together with intravenous fluids and mannitol should be used to help maintain a urine output of 100 ml/hr or more. Furosemide should be given in a continuous intravenous infusion at the rate of 20–40 mg/hour if the urine output falls. Renal function should be monitored, and baseline coagulation studies should be done and repeated at periodic intervals. If acute renal shutdown due to acute tubular necrosis occurs in spite of the above measures, treatment is as for acute renal failure. DIC may need to be treated by replacement of clotting factors and/or by infusion of cryoprecipitate. Haemodialysis may be necessary for renal support till such time as renal function returns to normal.

(iv) Delayed Haemolytic Reactions

These are mild and generally occur one week after transfusion. Initial crossmatching fails to detect antibodies to donor red cell antigens. Prior sensitization by transfusion of red blood cell antigens not belonging to the ABO group results in a transient rise in antibodies. The titer of these antibodies wanes within a few weeks, and may not be detectable. A second transfusion with a repeat exposure to the red cell antigen provokes an anamnestic rise of the antibody to a degree sufficient to cause haemolysis.

(v) Transmission of Infection (12, 13)

The risk of transmitting infections through blood transfusions can never be entirely eliminated. Possible transmissions of HIV I, HTLV I and Virus B and C Hepatitis, as has already been mentioned, can occur despite tests on donor blood to check for these infectious complications. The risk of transmission of HIV is between 1 in 40,000 to 1 in 200,000, with maximum preventive control (14). It is far greater in poor developing countries where safeguards and protocols for checking on donor blood, are substandard in many hospitals. The risk of transmitting hepatitis is much higher—around 2–3 per cent. Tests for hepatitis C on donor blood should reduce the incidence further (15). The risk of transmission of CMV is also present, though its effects except in immunocompromised patients are not as disastrous. In tropical countries, additional risks include transmission of malaria, salmonella and other infectious diseases.

REFERENCES

1. Pisciotto PT. (1989). Blood Transfusion Therapy: A Physician's Handbook, 3rd edn. American Association of Blood Banks. Arlington, VA.

2. Cummings PD, Wallace EL, Schorr JB et al. (1989). Exposure of patients to human immunodeficiency virus through the transmission of blood components that test antibody-negative. N Engl J Med. 321, 941–946.

3. The National Blood Resource Education Program's Transfusion Alert. (1991). Indications for the use of red blood cells, platelets and fresh frozen plasma. US Department of Health and Human Services. NIH Publication No. 91–2974a.

4. Audet AM, Goodnough LT. (1992). Practice strategies for elective red blood cell transfusion: Clinical guideline. Ann Intern Med. 116, 403–406.

5. Welch HG, Meehan KR, Goodnough LT et al. (1992). Prudent strategies for elective red blood cell transfusion. Ann Intern Med. 116, 393–402.

6. Murphy MF, Metcalfe P, Thomas H et al. (1986). Use of leucocyte-poor blood components and HLA-matched-platelet donors to prevent HLA alloimmunization. Br J Hematol. 62, 529.

7. Baron BW, Baron JM. (1998). Blood products and plasmapheresis. In: Principles of Critical Care (Eds Hall JB, Schmidt GA, Wood Lawrence DH). pp. 1021–1031. McGraw-Hill, USA

8. Tomasulo PA, Petz LD. (1989). Platelet transfusions. In: Clinical Practice of Transfusion Medicine, 2nd edn (Eds Petz LD, Swisher SN). pp. 432. Churchill Livingstone, New York.

9. National Institutes of Health. (1987). Platelet transfusion therapy: Consensus Conference. JAMA. 257, 1777–1780.

10. National Institutes of Health. (1985). Fresh-frozen plasma: Consensus Conference. JAMA. 253, 551–553.

11. Holland PV. (1989). The diagnosis and management of transfusion reactions and other adverse effects of transfusion. In: Clinical Practice of Transfusion Medicine, 2nd edn (Eds Petz LD, Swisher SN). pp. 728. Churchill Livingstone, New York.

12. Greenwalt TJ. (1981). Pathogenesis and management of hemolytic transfusion reactions. Semin Hematol. 18, 84–94.

13. Barbara JAJ, Contreras M. (1990). Infectious complications of blood transfusion: Bacteria and parasites. Br Med J. 300, 386–389.

14. Barbara JAJ, Contreras M. (1990). Infectious complications of blood transfusion: Viruses. Br Med J. 300, 450–453.

15. Klein HG, Higgins MJ. (2001). Use of Blood Components in the Intensive Care Unit. In: Critical Care Medicine (Eds Parrillo JE, Dellinger RP) pp. 1416–1438. Mosby, USA.

Endocrine Dysfunction in the Critically Ill

Acute Adrenal Crisis

General Considerations

Acute adrenal crisis or adrenocortical insufficiency is due to a severe lack or deficiency of adrenocortical hormones. It is a critical illness requiring intensive care, and is quickly fatal unless promptly recognized and treated (1). Early diagnosis is essential, but so protean are the manifestations, that delay in diagnosis is common. An awareness of the background factors against which acute adrenal crisis suddenly unfolds, should make one suspect the diagnosis. Suspecting adrenal crisis, is in fact, a major step towards arriving at the correct diagnosis.

Acute adrenal insufficiency is rather infrequently encountered in patients under critical care. It does however occur under the following situations:

(i) Following sudden withdrawal of corticosteroids in a patient whose own adrenal glands have been suppressed by prolonged administration of corticosteroids. If these patients undergo 'stress' in the form of surgery or an acute infection, they require a larger dose of corticosteroids. Sudden withdrawal of the drug can precipitate an acute crisis, which if not promptly recognized, can prove fatal. More often than not, the drug is not administered in the ICU simply because the physician is unaware that the patient was on a maintenance dose of corticosteroids.

(ii) Acute stress in a patient with latent adrenocortical insufficiency. The stress may be in the form of prolonged anaesthesia and major surgery, acute infection, trauma, and occasionally following a difficult, protracted delivery in females. Relative adrenocortical insufficiency has been shown to exist in critically ill patients with severe sepsis; cortisol levels may be normal, but do not rise appropriately after ACTH stimulation (2).

(iii) As a complication in a patient with overt chronic adrenocortical failure. This is not as uncommon as is believed to be, in India. A frequent cause of chronic adrenocortical insufficiency, in our part of the world, is tuberculous destruction of both the adrenal glands. In the West, autoimmune disease destroying the adrenals, is far more frequent.

(iv) Acute bilateral destruction of the adrenal glands by haemorrhage (3). This occurs after trauma, and in fulminant infections (Waterhouse-Friderichsen syndrome). Meningococcal septicaemia is an important cause of the Waterhouse-Friderichsen syndrome. Adrenal haemorrhage has also been reported in pneumococcal, staphylococcal and H influenzae infections. Ps aeruginosa infection in children is also an important cause of sepsis producing adrenal haemorrhage. Other causes of bilateral adrenal haemorrhage include anticoagulant therapy, and disseminated intravascular coagulopathy.

(v) Acute adrenal insufficiency following bilateral adrenalectomy, or following removal of an unilateral adrenocortical tumour which has suppressed the opposite gland does not pose problems in diagnosis.

(vi) Very rarely we have observed shock, peripheral failure and a collapsed state following haemorrhage into the pituitary (pituitary apoplexy), which causes acute adrenocortical failure.

Clinical Features

The clinical features are protean, and at times bizarre, so that diagnosis depends on a high index of suspicion.

The onset may be explosive, and at times is characterized by fever, confusion, and drowsiness graduating to severe mental obtundation and even coma. In some patients the temperature is subnormal, and severe asthenia predominates, so that the patient is unable to even turn on his own in bed. Abdominal symptoms are very frequently present. Abdominal pain may be severe, and may mimic an acute abdomen. Nausea, vomiting and diarrhoea are often observed, and confuse the clinical picture. However the most striking feature in all patients, is the rapid development of peripheral failure and shock, characterized by a rapid thready pulse, and progressive hypotension. The shock resembles hypovolaemic shock, but is not corrected by volume replacement, or the use of inotropic support; quick improvement only follows after the use of adrenocortical steroids.

In the Waterhouse-Friderichsen syndrome, the explosive onset with high fever, headache, vomiting and prostration, is accompanied by purpuric skin rashes. These rashes may be confluent producing large areas of haemorrhage. Respiratory distress, cyanosis and a quickly evolving irreversible state of shock are observed, with death occurring within 24–48 hours.

Laboratory Investigations

(i) A moderate degree of hyponatraemia may be present; it may be associated with hyperkalaemia. Hyponatraemia is most often related to an associated mineralocorticoid deficiency. These patients however become hyponatraemic even in the presence of a positive sodium balance. This indicates inability to excrete free water due to glucocorticoid insufficiency.

(ii) Urea, creatinine and non-protein nitrogen levels in the blood are raised due to prerenal factors.

(iii) Hypoglycaemia is often observed. Glucocorticoids play an important role in gluconeogenesis, and counter the action of insulin.

(iv) Blood cortisol levels are very low, and do not show an adequate response to the ACTH stimulation test. Recent data suggest that any cortisol value equal to or greater than 20 µg/dl, during or before the ACTH test, is compatible with normal adrenal function (4, 5).

Primary adrenocortical insufficiency should be distinguished from secondary adrenal insufficiency. The aldosterone response to ACTH stimulation is impaired in primary adrenocortical insufficiency, but preserved in secondary adrenocortical insufficiency. Also, ACTH levels in blood are raised in primary adrenocortical insufficiency and below normal in secondary adrenocortical insufficiency. The clinical features of hyperpigmentation of the mucosa and skin and the presence of hyperkalaemia are characteristics of primary adrenocortical insufficiency. They do not occur in secondary adrenocortical insufficiency.

(v) Adrenocortical insufficiency may be associated with hypothyroidism and other hormonal deficiencies. If clinical suspicion exists; relevant tests for other hormonal deficiencies should be done.

(vi) In the Waterhouse-Friderichsen syndrome, blood cultures are generally positive. Organisms may be seen in petechial scrapings.

Diagnosis (6)

The possibility of acute adrenocortical insufficiency should always be considered when faced with any acute illness in the ICU, which is characterized by protean mainfestations and peripheral circulatory failure. The background against which acute adrenal insufficiency occurs, should always be kept in mind as it affords an invaluable clue to the diagnosis. Inexplicable shock occurring after a straightforward operation (e.g. appendicectomy or herniorrhaphy), or in a patient with an ordinary infection, should always suggest the possibility of acute adrenal crisis.

An important cause of hyperpyrexia with prostration and collapse, is acute adrenocortical failure. In such cases, the diagnosis is often confused with an acute infection like malaria, pneumonia, sepsis or even meningitis. Quite often an acute infection precipitates adrenocortical failure, so that the confirmed presence of the former, in no way excludes the latter.

In patients who are drowsy or mentally obtunded, the differential diagnosis of poisoning, cerebrovascular accidents, or other causes of a semiconscious state should be considered.

The occurrence of acute abdominal pain and vomiting contin-

ues to fox the most experienced of clinicians. An earlier history of asthenia, hypotension, mucosal pigmentation, and pigmentation of the exposed parts, particularly the creases of the palms, and of the skin over the knuckles, should suggest the diagnosis.

The diagnosis of an acute adrenal crisis requires a high index of suspicion, and is necessarily clinical. In most ICUs in our country, the diagnosis cannot be immediately confirmed by objective laboratory tests. Treatment should be immediate and vigorous. If possible, a blood sample should be collected for cortisol assay, and this can be repeated after 2 hours of ACTH stimulation. The patient however needs to be given a glucocorticoid without awaiting results. Dexamethasone 4 mg intravenously given as a bolus dose, does not interfere with cortisol assays. Recovery of the patient following correct treatment is probably the sole and most reliable objective pointer to a correct diagnosis.

Treatment

Treatment should be prompt. If the ACTH stimulation test has been done, dexamethasone 4 mg intravenously is administered, without awaiting the results of the test.

(i) Use of Glucocorticoids

Hydrocortisone hemisuccinate in a dose of 100 mg, is given intravenously 6 hourly over the first 24 hours. The drug may be given either as a continuous intravenous infusion, or as a bolus intravenous injection. The dose of intravenously administered hydrocortisone over the next 24 hours, should also be 300 mg. By this time recovery is apparent, so that from the third day onwards, the dose is reduced by 25–50 mg/day, and within the next 8–10 days, the patient is on a maintenance dose of 100 mg hydrocortisone daily. Once the crisis is over, the patient is put on oral prednisolone + mineralocorticoid therapy (fludrocortisone 0.05 to 0.1 mg/day), and intravenous hydrocortisone is omitted. The above is a general outline of dosage requirements in patients in an acute crisis. The dosage may need to be modified according to the patient's response. As a general rule, adrenal insufficiency is one of those rare situations where it is safer to overtreat than to undertreat. A careful watch on the side effects of corticosteroid therapy must be maintained.

An acute crisis can be prevented, if patients with underlying adrenocortical insufficiency (on a maintenance dose of corticosteroids) are given larger doses during the stress of surgery or acute infection (7). Emperic recommendations are 25 mg/day of hydrocortisone for mild stress, 50–75 mg/day for 2 to 3 days for moderate stress and 100–150 mg/day for 2 to 3 days for severe stress. After recovery from 'stress', patients are placed on a maintenance dose of 15–30 mg/day (7), tapered further to 7.5–10 mg/day.

(ii) Restoration of Fluid and Electrolyte Balance

Dehydration and salt depletion characterize an adrenal crisis, and it is important to quickly correct these abnormalities. During the first 24 hours, the usual requirement is at least 2 litres of normal saline. The administration of fluid and electrolytes should be monitored by clinical examination, by central venous pressure measurements, and by estimation of serum electrolytes. Many patients who have not been correctly diagnosed, or diagnosed late, are often already excessively volume loaded, in an attempt to correct the shock and hypotension. Further volume loading in these patients is unnecessary, and may precipitate acute pulmonary oedema.

Serum potassium may fall during recovery from a crisis. This is particularly likely if large doses of glucocorticoids continue to be used; potassium replacement is necessary in these patients.

Vomiting is often present and precludes oral feeds in the first 24–48 hours. Nutrition is poor in many of these patients, and this should be carefully supplemented once oral feeds are tolerated.

(iii) Dextrose Infusion

Hypoglycaemia, though generally not marked, needs to be countered by an intravenous infusion of dextrose. We generally use 1 litre of 10 per cent dextrose in the first 24 hours, and 500 ml of the same solution in the next 24 hours. By this time the patient is generally out of the crisis, and can take glucose orally in fruit juice or other liquids.

(iv) Treatment of Precipitating Factors

It is important to identify and treat these factors. Infection in particular, is the most important precipitating cause, and needs the use of appropriate antibiotics. Fulminant infections causing bilateral adrenal haemorrhage are often fatal. They require the use of antibiotics in massive doses, chosen according to the nature of the infection, and expert overall critical care. A few patients with adrenocortical insufficiency also have other endocrinopathies, which should be identified and treated.

The treatment of an acute adrenal crisis is summarized in **Table 15.8.1.**

Table 15.8.1. Treatment of acute adrenal crisis

1. Intravenous hydrocortisone 100 mg 6 hourly in the first 24–48 hours; this is gradually reduced over the next 5 days. Use oral prednisolone + a mineralocorticoid subsequently
2. Restore fluid and electrolyte balance
   (a) 2 l of N saline in the first 24 hours—monitor volume infusions clinically and with CVP, particularly in patients who have received large volume loads prior to arriving at the correct diagnosis
   (b) Correct hypokalaemia during recovery
3. IV dextrose infusions to counter hypoglycaemia. 1 l of 5% dextrose is generally necessary over 24 hours
4. Diagnose and treat precipitating factors—chiefly infection

Complications during Treatment of an Adrenal Crisis

(i) Overhydration occurs when a massive volume load has been administered prior to establishing a correct diagnosis. This is generally done as a measure of desperation to reverse shock. Once a diagnosis is made in these patients, the combination of further infusions of N saline with large doses of intravenous hydrocortisone, can produce cerebral oedema or pulmonary oedema. Cerebral oedema may result in seizures and unconsciousness; pulmonary oedema may be fatal.

(ii) Severe hypokalaemia with increasing asthenia, flaccid muscle weakness of the limbs, abdominal distension and arrhythmias may complicate recovery from a crisis. Serum potassium levels, as explained earlier, should be carefully monitored, and if present, hypokalaemia should be corrected by administration of potassium.

(iii) Hyperpyrexia may occur as part of an acute adrenal crisis. Rarely it is observed during recovery following the use of intravenous corticosteroids and saline infusions.

(iv) Important and frequently encountered side effects of corticosteroid therapy include acute gastrointestinal bleeding, and acute psychotic reactions.

REFERENCES

1. Knowlton AI. (1989). Adrenal insufficiency in the intensive care setting. J Intensive Care Med. 4, 35.
2. Shenkar Y, Skatrud JB. (2001). Adrenal insufficiency in critically ill patients. Am J Res Crit Care Med. 29, 310–316.
3. Rao RH, Vagnucci AH, Amico JA. (1989). Bilateral massive adrenal hemorrhage: Early recognition and treatment. Ann Intern Med. 110, 227.
4. Bhasin S, Tom L, Mac P. (2002). Endocrine Problems in the Critically Ill Patient. In: Current Critical Care Diagnosis and Treatment (Eds Bongard FS, Sue DY). pp. 607–21. McGraw-Hill, USA.
5. May ME, Carey RM. (1985). Rapid adrenocorticotropic hormone test in practice: Retrospective review. Am J Med. 79, 679–684.
6. Mattingly D, Sheridan P. (1976). Simultaneous diagnosis and treatment of acute adrenal insufficiency. Lancet. 1, 432–433.
7. Salem M, Tanish RE Jr, Bromberg J et al. (1994). Peri-operative glucocorticoid coverage: Reassessment 42 years after emergence of problem. Ann Surg. 219, 416–425.

Thyroid Dysfunction and Emergencies Meriting Critical Care

Life threatening problems in thyroid disease requiring critical care include the following:

(i) Thyroid storm or 'crisis' occurring in a patient with a hyperfunctioning thyroid gland.

(ii) Sudden atrial fibrillation with a very fast uncontrollable ventricular rate leading to acute congestive failure, occurring as a complication of hyperthyroidism.

(iii) Myxoedema coma due to a markedly poor function of the thyroid gland.

(iv) Haemorrhage into one or more nodules of a nodular goitre can lead to acute compression of the trachea in the neck, and haemorrhage into a substernal goitre can lead to acute mediastinal compression, necessitating urgent surgical intervention.

The first three conditions requiring critical care are discussed in this chapter. This is followed by a brief description of the Euthyroid Sick Syndrome, a commonly encountered abnormality in a critical care setting.

Thyroid Crisis (Thyroid Storm)

A thyroid crisis or storm is a life-threatening metabolic storm resulting from a marked increase in free thyroxine circulating in the blood (**1, 2**). The thyroid gland runs amuck, berserk with marked increase in its activity and its hormonal output, producing thereby an excessive metabolic rate, which the body cells cannot withstand.

The fulminant forms of thyroid crisis which can kill a patient within 24–48 hours, usually occur following surgery on an uncontrolled hyperfunctioning thyroid gland. These are now fortunately rare since surgery on a hyperfunctioning thyroid gland is never done without prior control of thyroid activity by proper medical treatment. In present days a 'crisis' is most often precipitated in a patient with hyperthyroidism by an acute infection or by the stress of major surgery. Other precipitating causes include trauma, severe psychological stress, diabetic ketoacidosis, treatment of uncontrolled hyperthyroidism with radioactive iodine, or withdrawal of drugs given to control hyperthyroidism. The patient may be admitted to the ICU for a thyroid crisis. At times a patient with underlying undetected hyperthyroidism is admitted for another life-threatening problem. A 'crisis' in this situation is precipitated by some of the factors outlined above, following admission to the unit. In these critically ill patients even if the degree of hyperthyroidism does not amount to an acute crisis, it is sufficient to add significantly to the gravity of the clinical situation. Thyrotoxicosis can also be induced in critically ill patients following the use of iodine rich drugs—amiodarone, povidone-iodine, and radiographic contrast agents (**3, 4**).

Table 15.8.2 lists the important precipitating factors of an acute thyroid crisis.

Table 15.8.2. Important precipitating factors of acute thyroid crisis

* Acute infection
* Stress of trauma/major surgery
* Severe psychological stress
* Diabetic ketoacidosis
* Sudden withdrawal of drugs used to control hyperthyroidism
* Treatment of uncontrolled hyperthyroidism with radioactive iodine
* Following surgery on uncontrolled hyperfunctioning thyroid gland

Clinical Features

The clinical picture is characterized by a marked increase in all the symptoms and signs encountered in thyrotoxicosis. Fever, marked restlessness, irritability and tachycardia that may be as high as 160–200/min, dominate the picture. In hot climes, hyperpyrexia with temperature of 108°F may be noted. Atrial fibrillation with a fast ventricular rate, as also other forms of supraventricular tachycardia are common. The circulation is hyperdynamic with tachycardia, warm peripheries, bounding high volume pulse, and a high pulse pressure due to elevation in the systolic reading and lowering of the diastolic pressure reading.

Abdominal pain and vomiting may occasionally usher a crisis. In these patients or even otherwise, diarrhoea may be a presenting feature. Patients in a crisis do not eat well and may have anorexia. This should never negate the diagnosis of severe hyperthyroidism.

In elderly patients a thyroid crisis may just present with marked apathy, extreme weakness and unexplained fever. Diarrhoea is frequent and paroxysmal disturbances in cardiac rhythm are common. Death in a thyroid crisis may be due to hyperpyrexia or cardiac failure.

Diagnosis

A thyroid crisis precipitated by surgery is often missed for an acute post-operative infection or a transfusion reaction. With a known background history of hyperthyroidism, the diagnosis of a sudden spurt in hyperthyroid activity should always be given prior consideration in a patient who develops a febrile illness, or does poorly following surgery.

Patients first seen in a crisis, who are unaware of a hyperthyroid background may pose difficulties in diagnosis. Common errors are to mistake thyroid crisis for sepsis, heat stroke, an acute gastrointestinal infection or ischaemic heart disease.

A careful clinical examination for tell-tale features of hyperthyroidism is invariably rewarding. Atrial fibrillation with an uncontrolled fast ventricular rate which is not slowed with digitalis, should always arouse suspicion. An extremely valuable sign that helps in the diagnosis of a thyroid crisis is the presence of an enlarged thyroid gland, or the presence of one or more palpable nodules in the thyroid gland. This enlargement is often not obvious and requires careful clinical palpation. Clinical examination should also be directed towards determining the precipitating cause of thyroid crisis.

Laboratory Investigations

The T_3, T_4 concentrations are high, but these are not necessarily greater in a thyroid storm than in the usual thyrotoxic state (**5**). There is however a marked increase in the free thyroxine levels, perhaps related to a defect in binding to thyroxine binding globulin (**6**). There are no other laboratory abnormalities characteristic of a thyroid storm. Hypercalcaemia, hyperglycaemia, and a rise in alkaline phosphatase may be noted. Hyperglycaemia is due to gluconeogenesis. There is decreased glucagon suppression and impaired insulin response to hyperglycaemia (**7**). The ECG may show atrial fibrillation or atrial flutter with a fast ventricular rate.

Management: Prevention

Surgery on a hyperthyroid gland should never be performed until the thyrotoxic state is controlled with neomercazole or by the thiouracil group of drugs. Neomercazole (carbimazole) is stopped 8 days before planned surgery, and Lugol's iodine substituted during these 8 days in a dose of 0.1–0.3 ml thrice daily. Following the above precautions, thyroid crisis following surgery on a hyperthyroid gland is extremely rare. The awareness of the fact that all stressful situations (physical or mental), in hyperthyroid patients are potential triggering factors for a thyroid crisis, goes a long way in the prevention of this serious problem.

Treatment of Thyroid Crisis

(i) Control of the Hyperthyroid State

Use of Thiouracils, Carbimazole, Methimazole. Propylthiouracil is the drug of choice. It is given in a loading dose of 600 mg, followed by 250 mg six hourly. Carbimazole or methimazole if used, are given in a dose of 20 mg three to four times a day. All three drugs have a rapid onset of action and act by inhibiting iodide oxidation and organification by thyroid peroxidase. Propylthiouracil has the additional advantage of being able to an extent, to inhibit the peripheral conversion of T_4 into T_3. Common side effects of antithyroid drugs are rash, urticaria, arthralgia, fever. Rarely agranulocytosis and hepatic toxicity may be observed.

Use of Iodine. Intravenous sodium iodide is the quickest method to control thyroid activity in a thyroid storm. Iodine acts by blocking the synthesis and release of thyroid hormones, but is safe to administer only after organification of iodine is arrested by propylthiouracil. It should therefore be given one to two hours after the first dose of propylthiouracil or carbimazole or methimazole.

Sodium iodide is given in a dose of 1 g in 500 ml dextrose over 8–12 hours. A total dose as high as 3 g may be given over the first 24 hours.

A maintenance dose of 0.5 g may then be given daily for the next 2 days. Lugol's iodine may be given orally if sodium iodide is not available for intravenous use. The dose is 3–5 drops (6 mg/drop) thrice daily. Potassium iodide can substitute for Lugol's iodine, and is given in a dose of 200 mg twelve hourly. We prefer to stop iodine after 5–7 days.

Recent studies have shown that ipodate sodium (an iodine-containing radiocontrast agent) when given orally, has an extremely rapid onset of action, resulting in a lowering of T_3 levels within 6 hours with normal T_3 levels within 24–48 hours. The dosage is 500 mg four times a day. We have no experience with its use, but this drug when available has replaced Lugol's iodine and potassium iodide in the treatment of severe hyperthyroidism. Ipodate sodium should be given one to two hours after the first dose of propylthiouracil or carbimazole or methimazole.

Use of Beta-blockers. Beta-blockers play a vital role in treatment. They particularly control the psychomotor and cardiovascular manifestations of a thyroid storm. Propranolol is given in a dose of 1 mg intravenously very slowly, with a careful watch on the blood pressure. If well tolerated, the dose is repeated not exceeding a total dose of 5 mg. Propranolol can also be given orally 20–80 mg 6 hourly, to control symptoms. In addition to the benefits produced by beta-blockade, propranolol prevents conversion of T_4 to T_3, improves glucose tolerance and reduces negative nitrogen balance.

Reserpine 1–2 mg 8 hourly was found to be of use in a thyroid crisis. The drug has now been replaced by beta-blockers.

Use of Adrenocortical Hormones. Glucocorticoids are useful to prevent adrenocortical insufficiency. The rate of utilization of adrenocortical hormones is excessive in a thyroid crisis, and it is possible that some patients may have a relative conditioned deficiency of these hormones. Hydrocortisone is given routinely in a dose of 100 mg intravenously 8 hourly till the crisis is controlled. Besides offering adrenocortical support, glucocorticosteroids are of benefit because they inhibit peripheral conversion of T_4 to T_3.

(ii) Control of Atrial Fibrillation

Atrial fibrillation with a fast ventricular rate generally does not respond satisfactorily to digitalis. Propranolol given in the manner described above is the drug of choice. Metoprolol is longer acting and may also be given intravenously in an initial dose of 5 mg given at a rate of 1–2 mg/min, to a total dose of 10–15 mg.

In an acute haemodynamic crisis with a barely recordable blood pressure and the presence of features of cardiogenic shock, a synchronized DC shock should be promptly administered. It generally restores sinus rhythm. Once this is achieved, a beta-blocker is used as mentioned earlier.

Digoxin (even though the response is generally unsatisfactory), and diuretics may also be used in atrial fibrillation with congestive cardiac failure. If atrial fibrillation persists anticoagulants should be given to prevent embolic epoisodes.

(iii) Treatment of Hyperpyrexia

Symptomatic treatment of hyperpyrexia is necessary in a few patients, else death can result before more definitive therapy can take effect.

(iv) Control of Restlessness, Excitability, Irritability

Restlessness is controlled by the use of phenobarbitone sodium 60 mg intramuscularly or chlorpromazine hydrochloride 25–50 mg intramuscularly. This dose is repeated as and when necessary.

(v) Maintenance of Fluid and Electrolyte Balance

Patients suffering a thyroid storm sweat profusely. This is even more marked in hot tropical climes. A tremendous loss of water, sodium and chloride occurs. Potassium loss is also marked because of diarrhoea and a poor intake. A fluid intake well over 3 l and at times exceeding 4 l is necessary. It is however worth recording that pulmonary oedema is an important complication of thyroid crisis. A close monitoring of the cardiovascular status, renal function and urine output is necessary. Fluid and electrolyte replacement should be based on clinical considerations and on serum electrolyte estimations.

Since hepatic glycogen is used up quickly in a thyroid crisis, fluid replacement should include at least 1 l of 10 per cent dextrose. The hypermetabolic state in a thyroid crisis places an excessive demand on nutrients and vitamins necessary for proper functioning of different tissues in the body. The demand particularly for thiamine may be great. In poorly nourished individuals so commonly encountered in the tropics, an acute thiamine deficiency may arise, particularly if large quantities of dextrose are given intravenously and an adequate dose of thiamine (200–500 mg) is not supplied.

(vi) Use of Oxygen

The demand and consumption of oxygen are excessively increased in the hypermetabolic state that characterizes a crisis. The patient is given oxygen at a flow rate of 6–8 l/minute.

The management of an acute thyroid crisis is summarized in **Table 15.8.3**.

Hyperthyroidism Contributing to the Morbidity of Other Critical Illnesses in the ICU

Undetected hyperthyrodism in patients admitted to the ICU for other critical illnesses can pose diagnostic problems, and can add to the morbidity of the critical illness. The stress of a critical illness often increases the degree of hyperthyroidism in a patient, so that mild or latent hyperthyroidism now becomes clearly manifest. The features of such co-existing hyperthyroidism often merge, and may well be indistinguishable from the features of the critical illness for which the patient is admitted.

Hyperthyroid activity in these patients generally takes the following forms:

Table 15.8.3. Management of acute thyroid crisis

1. Control of hyperthyroid state
   (a) 1 g sodium iodide in 500 ml dextrose, given as an IV infusion, followed by a maintenance dose of 0.5 g daily for next 2 days. Alternatively, 3–5 drops (6 mg/drop) of Lugol's iodine are given orally thrice daily. Start iodine 1–2 hours after first dose of propylthiouracil or carbimazole
   (b) Propylthiouracil 250 mg 6 hourly, or carbimazole 30 mg 6 hourly
   (c) Propranolol 1 mg given slowly IV; the dose may repeated to a maximum of 5 mg. Alternatively, oral propranolol 20–80 mg 6 hourly may be used
   (d) Hydrocortisone 100 mg is given IV 8 hourly
2. Control of atrial fibrillation
   (a) Propranolol (as above), or metoprolol 5 mg IV (at rate of 1–2 mg/min) up to a total dose of 10–15 mg
   (b) Synchronized DC shock given in acute haemodynamic crisis
3. Symptomatic treatment of hyperpyrexia
4. Control of restlessness and irritability with phenobarbitone sodium 60 mg IM, or chlorpromazine 25–50 mg IM, repeated as and when required
5. Maintenance of fluid and electrolyte balance
   (a) 3–4 l of fluid infused over 24 hours after monitoring the patient's cardiovascular status and urine output
   (b) Correct hyponatraemia, hypokalaemia
   (c) IV dextrose—at least 1 l of 10% dextrose required in 24 hours
   (d) Administer 200–500 mg thiamine, particularly in poorly nourished patients
6. Administer oxygen at flow rate of 6–8 l/minute

(i) Pyrexia of unknown origin, which fails to respond to antibiotics given because of a mistaken diagnosis of infection.

(ii) An unstable hyperdynamic circulation which is generally attributed to the critical illness for which the patient was admitted, or to complicating sepsis.

(iii) Rhythm disturbances with or without congestive cardiac failure, or the evolution and persistence of congestive cardiac failure with a fast ventricular rate. The following points help in correct diagnosis:

(a) The possibility of hyperthyroidism should always be considered at any age when a patient develops atrial fibrillation, a fast ventricular rate and congestive cardiac failure, which does not promptly respond to digitalis. Most such patients are past 40 years in age and may complain of cardiac pain due to relative coronary insufficiency produced by a very rapid ventricular rate. This often makes the unwary fall into the trap of diagnosing ischaemic heart disease causing atrial fibrillation and congestive heart failure. Even if the patient has proven ischaemic heart disease, as viewed from the past history and ECG recordings, this does not always exclude a co-existent hyperthyroid state.

(b) Paroxysmal atrial fibrillation, or any form of paroxysmal supraventricular tachycardia in a patient admitted to the intensive care unit for a serious illness, should suggest the possibility of a co-existing hyperthyroid state.

(c) Hyperthyroidism should always enter into the differential diagnosis of congestive heart failure of undetermined aetiology. A careful examination may reward the clinician with a few tell-tale signs, as for example the presence of a slight stare, a lid leg, a warm moist skin and a palpably enlarged thyroid gland.

Raised T_3, T_4 levels prove the diagnosis of a hyperthyroid state in these patients.

The importance of a correct diagnosis is obvious. Manifestations of excessive thyroid activity can only be controlled by the specific measures stated earlier. They remain uncontrolled with conventional therapy used for atrial fibrillation or for congestive heart failure. It is important to control co-existing hyperthyroidism in critically ill patients. Control reduces the metabolic demands of the critical illness and should improve the chances of recovery.

Myxoedema Coma

Myxoedema coma is invariably the culmination of long standing hypothyroidism. It may occur as the terminal event in the natural history of severe myxoedema. It may however also be precipitated by exposure to cold, by infection and by the unwise use of sedatives to which patients with myxoedema are extremely susceptible. Other precipitating factors include trauma, surgery, stroke, hypovolaemia from any cause, and congestive heart failure. **Table 15.8.4** lists the important precipitating factors of myxoedema coma.

Table 15.8.4. Important precipitating factors of myxoedema coma

* Infection
* Exposure to cold
* Injudicious use of sedatives
* Surgery/Trauma
* Cerebrovascular accident
* Hypovolaemia due to any cause
* Congestive heart failure

Diagnostic Clinical Features

The onset is gradual particularly when myxoedema coma is the terminal event of long standing progressive hypothyroidism. It may be fairly abrupt if the problem is triggered by the precipitating factors listed above. The hallmark of myxoedema coma is hypothermia—the rectal temperature being often < 80°F. This is missed as it will not be recorded by a clinical thermometer; the degree of hypothermia can be ascertained with a chemical thermometer.

The cardiovascular system on examination shows marked bradycardia. The stroke volume and cardiac output are decreased; there is an increased peripheral vascular resistance with decreased blood volume and diminished flow to vital organs. The heart size is often enlarged; pericardial effusion is frequently observed. The blood pressure to start with, may be non-contributory in the diagnosis. Terminally hypotension is invariably observed. There may be a rise in the creatinine kinase (CK) and lactic acid dehydrogenase enzymes (LDH), so that a diagnosis of myocardial infarction can be wrongly made.

The respiratory system shows important changes. Hypoventilation with resulting hypoxia and hypercapnia are invariably present. There appears to be a decreased response to hypercapnia (8), so that uncontrolled oxygen therapy can complicate the picture by inducing hypercapnic narcosis and worsening the obtunded state. There are probably a number of causes for hypoventilation in myxoedema coma. The most important reason is in all probability, a diminished central respiratory drive (9), followed by poor muscle power, poor tone and poor contraction of the respiratory muscles (10). Contributory causes may be extreme obesity and obstruction to the upper airways due to macroglossia and to oedema of the oropharynx. Marked sensitivity to the effects of sedatives and tranquilizers, narcotics and anaesthetic agents can trigger both coma and hypoventilation in patients with myxoedema.

The other tell-tale features are all there for those who have eyes to see; it is astonishing how these features are explained away! The dry, cool, puffy skin, the myxoedematous facies, the constant drowsiness and confusion that precede coma, the loss of scalp and body hair (which includes the axillary hair), the macroglossia, and delayed relaxation of the ankle reflex, are all present.

Constipation is a non-specific symptom but is almost always present. Ascites is uncommon, but if present may lead the unwary to a wrong diagnosis.

A normocytic, normochromic anaemia is present and the white blood cell count may be decreased. Inability to raise the core temperature or to generate a leucocytosis in response to infection, renders the diagnosis of a complicating infection doubly difficult.

The clinical diagnosis of myxoedema coma should be proved by low T_3, low T_4, and high TSH values. These values however need be no different from those observed in a patient with obvious myxoedema.

The basic features necessary for a clinical diagnosis and a summary of laboratory changes in patients with myxoedema coma are summarized in **Table 15.8.5**.

Table 15.8.5. Clinical features and laboratory abnormalities in patients with myxoedema coma

1. Hypothermia (except in presence of infection)
2. Clinical features of myxoedema
   * Dry, cool, puffy skin
   * Typical myxoedematous facies
   * Loss of scalp and body hair
   * Drowsiness/mental obtundation preceding coma
   * Macroglossia
   * Delayed ankle reflexes
   * Marked bradycardia
3. Hypoventilation
4. Hypotension in terminal stages
5. Laboratory abnormalities
   * Normocytic, normochromic anaemia, decreased WBC count
   * Hyponatraemia, hypoglycaemia, elevated levels of CK, LDH
   * T_3, T_4 levels decreased; TSH increased
   * ABG—PaO_2 decreased; $PaCO_2$ increased
6. Radiological abnormalities
   * Chest X-ray—cardiomegaly, pericardial effusion
   * Ultrasound of the abdomen—ascites may be present
7. Haemodynamic parameters
   * Decreased stroke volume and cardiac output
   * Increased peripheral vascular resistance
   * Decreased blood flow to vital organs

The principles of treatment of myxoedema coma are:
  (i) Quick replacement of thyroid hormone
 (ii) Use of adrenocortical steroids
(iii) Respiratory and cardiovascular support
 (iv) Treatment of infection, a common precipitating factor
  (v) Countering hypothermia
 (vi) Overall critical care

(i) Rapid Replacement of Thyroid Hormone. Use of L triiodothyronine sodium (T_3). This is a rapid acting hormone whose main use is in severe myxoedema or myxoedema coma (11). Thyroxine (T_4) given orally acts far too slowly and by the time the drug takes effect, the patient may succumb. The recommended dose of triiodothyronine is 10 μg every 4 to 6 hours; this can be given intravenously or by nasogastric tube till clear improvement is observed. The intravenous preparation is not easy to come by, but if available, is to be preferred as absorption of both triiodothyronine (T_3) and thyroxine (T_4) from the gut is erratic and unpredictable. If the intravenous preparation is not available, oral triiodothyronine (T_3) is preferred to oral thyroxine (T_4), as the former is quicker acting. If oral triiodothyronine is also unavailable, then one has to rest satisfied with the oral use of thyroxine. In Western countries, an intravenous thyroxine preparation is available. The dose for myxoedema coma is 500 μg as an intravenous bolus dose, followed by 50–100 μg daily. The dosage of the replacement hormones may need modification if anginal pains are frequent. We use isosorbide dinitrate 10 mg thrice daily, with triiodothyronine. After recovery the patient is kept on a maintenance dose of either triiodothyronine or thyroxine.

(ii) Use of Adrenocortical Steroids. There is a possibility that patients with severe myxoedema have a poor adrenocortical reserve. What is more, it is difficult in an emergency situation to distinguish hypopituitary coma from a myxoedema coma. To use thyroid hormones as the sole replacement hormones in a pituitary coma would provoke disaster, as the thyroid hormones would increase the metabolic rate and precipitate a severe adrenal crisis in such a patient. Hydrocortisone in a dose of 100 mg is therefore given intravenously every 8 hours.

(iii) Respiratory and Cardiovascular Support. Hypoventilation with hypercapnic respiratory failure needs to be treated by endotracheal intubation and mechanical ventilator support. This may need to be continued for 10–15 days. The airway must be kept patent, particularly if the patient lacks the strength to cough, or is mentally obtunded with a poor cough reflex.

Hypotension needs to be countered by a volume load provided there is no pulmonary oedema. Inotropic support with dobutamine should preferably not exceed 5–7 μg/kg/min, as these patients are invariably severely vasoconstricted. Further vasoconstriction can jeopardize tissue perfusion.

(iv) Treatment of Infection. Infection is a common precipitating cause, and may not be clinically evident because of hypothermia, and the frequent absence of leucocytosis. Infection should be countered by the use of appropriate antibiotics. Terminal bronchopneumonia is common in such patients.

(v) Raising the Body Temperature. Marked hypothermia may have to be corrected as an emergency measure. The body temperature should be raised very gradually; whenever possible, electric blankets or a heat cradle should be used. Sudden rewarming can cause peripheral vasodilatation and a crash in the already low arterial blood pressure. Ultimately, only a rise in the metabolic rate produced by the thyroid hormones can result in a sustained elevation of body temperature.

(vi) Overall Critical Care. This is of great importance. Hyponatraemia is often present and needs to be corrected. Hypertonic saline is avoided except under exceptional circumstances. Support to various other organ systems is often necessary.

Euthyroid-sick Syndrome (Sick Thyroid Syndrome)

Thyroid function changes rapidly in critically ill patients (12). A number of these patients have the euthyroid-sick syndrome. This syndrome is characterized by a low serum T_3 and T_4, and an increase in the L-reverse tri-iodothyroxine (rT_3) (13). The free fractions of T_3 and T_4 remain normal. This biochemical abnormality is due to inhibition of thyroid hormone binding to protein, and to diminished 5'-deiodinase activity. In healthy individuals, this enzyme catalyzes T_4 into the usual active T_3 in organs and tissues. On the other hand, the enzyme 5-deiodinase acts on T_4 and converts it to rT_3. 5-deiodinase, unlike 5'-deiodinase, is not affected by a critical illness. Therefore T_3 levels are low, and rT_3 levels are increased in a critical illness. These patients are clinically euthyroid, and have normal TSH levels.

The euthyroid-sick syndrome is an adaptive phenomenon to a serious illness. The low T_3 levels limit oxygen utilization and reduce tissue breakdown. Administration of thyroid hormone is not indicated in these patients, and may do harm as it promotes a negative nitrogen balance (14, 15). In an ICU setting, it becomes important to distinguish the euthyroid-sick syndrome which does not require thyroid replacement therapy, from true hypothyroidism which does. The serum TSH is usually normal in the euthyroid-sick syndrome patients, and high in true hypothyroidism. In critical illnesses in which hypothyroidism is co-existent, TSH values are however not always reliable, as these values are not consistently elevated. A reliable method of estimating thyroid function in a critical illness is to estimate the free thyroxine levels (normal in the euthyroid-sick syndrome, and low in true hypothyroidism), or to perform the thyrotropin-releasing hormone (TRH) test. The free thyroxine index can be estimated directly by the equilibrium dialysis method, or is computed approximately by multiplying the T_4 concentration by the T_3 resin uptake. The TRH test is performed at the bedside by administering 250–500 µg of TRH intravenously. TSH levels are measured after 30 minutes. The patient with a euthyroid-sick syndrome has a 2–3 times increase in the TSH after a TRH test. A hypothyroid patient has a rise of 6–8 times in the TSH concentration after a TRH test.

REFERENCES

1. Roth RN, McAuliffe MJ. (1989). Hyperthyroidism and thyroid storm. Emerg Med Clin North Am. 7, 873–883.

2. Bhasin S, Tom L, Mac P. (2002). Endocrine Problems in the Critically Ill Patient. In: Current Critical Care Diagnosis and Treatment (Eds Bongard FS, Sue DY). pp. 607–621. McGraw-Hill, USA.

3. Leger AF, Massin JP, Laurent MF et al. (1984). Iodine-induced thyrotoxicosis: Analysis of eighty-five consecutive cases. Eur J Clin Invest. 14, 449.

4. Martino E, Aghini-Lombardi F, Mariotti S et al. (1987). Amiodarone: A common source of iodine-induced thyrotoxicosis. Horm Res. 26, 158.

5. Brooks M, Waldstein S, Bronsky D, Sterling K. (1975). Serum triiodothyronine concentration in thyroid storm. J Clin Endocrinol Metab. 40, 339.

6. Brooks M, Waldstein S. (1980). Free thyroxine concentrations in thyroid storm. Ann Intern Med. 93, 694.

7. Lam KSL, Yeung RTT, Ho PWM, Lam SK. (1987). Glucose intolerance in thyrotoxicosis: Roles of insulin, glucagon and somatostatin. Acta Endocrinol. 114, 228.

8. Wilson W, Bedell G. (1960). The pulmonary abnormalities in myxedema. J Clin Invest. 39, 42.

9. Massumi R, Winnacker J. (1964). Severe depression of the respiratory centre in myxedema. Am J Med. 36, 876.

10. Blum M. (1972). Myxedema coma. Am J Med Sci. 264, 432.

11. Chernow B, Burman KD, Johnson D et al. (1983). T_3 may be a better agent than T_4 in the critically ill hypothyroid patient: Evaluation of transport across the blood-brain barrier in a primate model. Crit Care Med. 11, 99.

12. Chernow B, Alexander HR, Thompson WR et al. (1987). Hormonal responses to graded surgical stress. Arch Intern Med. 147, 1273.

13. Woeber KA, Maddux BA. (1981). Thyroid hormone binding in nonthyroidal illness. Metabolism. 30, 412.

14. Burman KD, Wartofsky L, Dinterman RF et al. (1979). The effect of T_3 and reverse T_3 administration on muscle protein catabolism during fasting as measured by 3-methyl-histidine excretion. Metabolism. 28, 805.

15. Gardner DF, Kaplan MM, Stanley CS et al. (1979). The effect of triiodothyronine replacement on the metabolic and pituitary responses to starvation. N Engl J Med. 300, 579.

Diabetes Mellitus and the Critically Ill Patient

General Considerations

Patients with diabetes mellitus in the intensive care unit generally present with the following problems:

(i) Complications of poorly controlled disease—particularly diabetic ketoacidosis and coma, and hyperosmolar non-ketotic diabetic coma.

(ii) Hypoglycaemia induced by insulin or by an overdose of antidiabetic oral medications.

(iii) One or more organ dysfunction associated with, or directly related to poor control of diabetes.

(iv) An unstable blood sugar with swings between hypoglycaemia and hyperglycaemia, induced by the stress of an unrelated critical illness.

The present section deals with diabetic ketoacidosis and coma, and with hyperosmolar non-ketotic diabetic coma.

Diabetic Ketoacidosis and Coma (1, 2)

Diabetic ketoacidosis is due to a lack or deficiency of insulin. Failure to take insulin, or to meet the increased need for insulin during the acute stress of infection or surgery, is the commonest cause of diabetic ketoacidosis. It is a common fallacy amongst insulin dependent diabetics, that if they do not eat they should not take insulin. This only serves to worsen the diabetic state, and increase the ketosis which in turn causes more nausea and vomiting.

Severe diabetic ketoacidosis is the forerunner to diabetic coma. A conscious diabetic with severe ketoacidosis should therefore be regarded and treated with the same urgency as one with diabetic coma. The dividing line between precoma and coma is thin and tenuous. Thus a few patients remain conscious in spite of severe ketoacidosis till just some hours before death, whilst others with the same degree of ketoacidosis lapse quickly into coma which may be prolonged for 24 to 72 hours.

Present day management has reduced the mortality of severe diabetic ketoacidosis and coma to 5 per cent. Remarkably enough there has been no further reduction in mortality. Further reduction is only possible if ketoacidosis is recognized early and treated promptly.

Physiopathology

The physiopathology of diabetic ketoacidosis is due to severe insulin deficiency combined with an excess of hormones that increase the blood glucose levels. Thus insulin deficiency is associated with an increase in glucagon. This change in the insulin-glucagon ratio alters carbohydrate, fat and protein metabolism. In addition to the marked increase in glucagon levels there is also a significant increase in the level of stress hormones including cortisol, growth hormones and catecholamines.

Insulin lack is furthermore associated with a varying degree of resistance to the action of insulin in diabetic ketoacidosis. The net result is an enhancement of the hyperglycaemic state. Glucagon acts predominantly in the liver. It increases the activity of carnitine acyltransferase I, and enhances transport of long chain fatty acids into the mitochondria. Cortisol increases gluconeogenesis and promotes insulin resistance. Catecholamines enhance lipolysis and ketogenesis, and also accelerate gluconeogenesis. Growth hormone also increases lipolysis and contributes to insulin resistance.

Hyperglycaemia

This as already explained is chiefly due to a marked increase in glucose production in the liver (gluconeogenesis). It is also in part due to poor utilization of glucose by the tissues. A factor that determines the degree of hyperglycaemia in diabetic ketoacidosis is the extent of glucose loss through the kidneys. As long as the circulatory state is satisfactory and the kidneys remain well perfused, there is a ready leak of glucose from the blood and the extracellular space via the urine. This helps to limit hyperglycaemia. Volume depletion could however lead to impaired renal perfusion, a lowered urine output and consequently a diminished leak of glucose in the urine. This could result in a sharp increase of glucose in the extracellular space, even though the hepatic glucose production remains unchanged.

Ketosis and Metabolic Acidosis

Ketosis is chiefly due to increased lipolysis in fat depots providing a source of free fatty acids as fuel. These free fatty acids are converted to ketones under the influence of glucagon. The predominant ketoacids are betahydroxybutyrate and acetoacetic acid, the ratio of these two ketoacids being 3:1.

Metabolic acidosis in uncontrolled diabetes is due to

(i) *Uncontrolled Ketosis with Ketonaemia.* This results in an increase in the anion gap because of the buffering by bicarbonate of the hydrogen ion.

(ii) *Hyperchloraemic Acidosis.* Many patients have a reduction in bicarbonate which is in excess of the increase in the anion gap. This indicates the association of a non-anion gap hyperchloraemic acidosis. The latter has been recognized for quite some time as a complication occurring in the later treatment stages of diabetic ketoacidosis. It may however also occur early, particularly in patients who are not so severely volume depleted. It is important to recognize hyperchloraemic acidosis as it takes longer to resolve because ketoacids are metabolized to generate equimolar quantities of bicarbonate. Hyperchloraemic acidosis stands corrected only through increased generation of bicarbonate by the kidneys.

(iii) *Lactic Acid Acidosis.* Increased lactic acid production contributes to the metabolic acidosis of severe diabetic ketoacidosis, when tissue perfusion is impaired because of a poor circulatory state.

Fluid and Electrolyte Abnormalities

Fluid and electrolyte loss form an important feature of diabetic ketoacidosis. This loss is consequent to the osmotic diuresis produced by glycosuria that follows from severe hyperglycaemia. Fluid loss may amount to 4–8 l in an average patient. There is also a marked depletion of sodium, potassium and chloride that may amount to 300–600 mEq or more. Phosphates and magnesium are also lost but in smaller quantities. The degree of electrolyte loss may not be manifested in the serum electrolyte levels, which may be only slightly reduced in concentration. Hyponatraemia may however be observed. Hypernatraemia pointing to excessive water loss in comparison with sodium loss, is rare. This is because of the shift of water from the intracellular compartment to the hyperosmolar extracellular and vascular compartments. The hyperosmolarity of the extracellular space which induces this shift, is due to hyperglycaemia. Shift of water from the intracellular compartment is accompanied by a shift of potassium from the cells into the interstitial and vascular compartments. Metabolic acidosis accentuates the shift of potassium from the intracellular to the extracellular compartment. Serum potassium levels may thus be normal or high, in spite of a gross overall deficit of potassium in the body. Chloride loss in the urine is less than the sodium loss, because sodium is additionally lost as an accompanying cation when ketones are excreted in the urine. Serum chloride concentration may thus not be significantly reduced.

Altered Mental State

This has not been well explained in patients with diabetic ketoacidosis. In all probability altered mentation, obtundation, drowsiness, and coma are at least partly related to serum osmolality. Patients with an altered mental state have an osmolality > 350 mosm/l. Ketonaemia with metabolic acidosis also probably contributes to the altered mentation.

Clinical Features (3)

Nausea and vomiting are frequent presenting manifestations, and may precede drowsiness and coma by a few days. Abdominal pain may also occur and in some patients is severe enough to mimic an acute abdomen. Respiration is of Kussmaul's type—deep and laboured, and there is a fruity smell of acetone in the breath. A history of polyuria, polydipsia, polyphagia, and muscle cramps in the immediate past, may be given by the patient or his relatives. The mental state is often confused and obtunded. Drowsiness progressing to coma can occur over a few hours to a few days.

Clinical examination reveals evidence of dehydration. The skin is dry, inelastic, and the tongue dry and furred. The eyeballs are soft; there is tachycardia, hypotension and oliguria. The untreated patient often progresses to drowsiness and coma from which he cannot be aroused by even the most painful stimuli. The corneal reflexes may then be lost, and the plantars become extensor. The blood pressure continues to drop, so that terminally it is unrecordable. Death results from peripheral circulatory failure or cardiac arrest.

Severe diabetic ketoacidosis is often triggered by precipitating factors, the main ones being acute infection, omission of insulin due to vomiting or diarrhoea, or to poor food intake, and poor compliance. Important precipitating factors are listed in **Table 15.9.1.**

Table 15.9.1. Important precipitating factors for diabetic ketoacidosis

1. Recent onset of insulin-dependent diabetes mellitus
2. Reduction or omission of insulin dose due to
   * Vomiting/diarrhoea
   * Poor food intake
   * Poor compliance
3. Infections e.g. pneumonia, carbuncle, urinary tract infection
4. Acute critical illnesses
   * Trauma
   * Acute pancreatitis
   * Acute myocardial infarction
   * Cerebrovascular accident
   * Sepsis from any cause
5. Oral or parenteral use of corticosteroids
6. Hyperthyroidism
7. Sudden severe stress

Laboratory Investigations

The urine shows glycosuria and ketonuria. The blood shows hyperglycaemia, the blood sugar usually being > 450 mg/dl. It is however important to stress that severe hyperglycaemia is not always present. In the presence of acidosis, the diagnosis should be suspected even if the blood sugar levels are not very high. This is particularly observed in patients who eat poorly and imbibe a large quantity of alcohol, and in pregnant females. In the latter, blood sugar levels may occasionally be modestly elevated even in the presence of severe ketoacidosis.

Ketonaemia is present, and the presence of metabolic acidosis is mirrored by a sharp fall in arterial pH (to as low as 7.0), a fall in the bicarbonate content (often < 10 mEq/l), and to a marked increase in the base deficit as computed by the Astrup technique.

There are some points to be noted in relation to acidaemia and ketonaemia in diabetic ketoacidosis.

(i) A deceptively mild acidaemia may be observed in diabetic ketoacidosis if there has been sufficiently severe vomiting to produce a metabolic alkalosis. The latter neutralizes the effect of metabolic acidosis. Mixed acid-base disturbances should therefore be correctly interpreted with reference to the clinical findings.

(ii) Absence of ketones in a patient with acidosis, hyperglycaemia and volume depletion, should suggest predominance of betahydroxybutyric acid as the predominant ketone in the plasma. In the presence of lactic acid acidosis (due to hypoperfusion), the acetoacetate is largely converted to betahydroxybutyrate. The nitroprusside test (a semiquantitative test), only recognizes acetone and acetoacetate, so that ketonaemia due to betahydroxybutyrate may go undetected. In these patients treatment with insulin and fluid replacement, reduces the ketonaemia. Betahydroxybutyrate is first converted to acetoacetic acid before being metabolized. Paradoxically thus, though the patient is improving, the nitroprusside test will now show a stronger positivity to plasma ketones. A clinical assessment, and monitoring of the pH of arterial blood, gives the correct perspective in these patients.

The blood urea, creatinine, and NPN are generally elevated; the azotaemia is prerenal due to dehydration and to endogenous tissue breakdown. Serum sodium and chloride are generally modestly reduced. Hyponatraemia is occasionally more marked, in which case the serum sodium is < 125 mEq/l. Very rarely one encounters hypernatraemia when water loss significantly exceeds sodium deficit. The serum potassium in majority of untreated cases is normal or slightly elevated, even though there is an overall deficit in body potassium. Some patients may however, present with hypokalaemia right from the start. Hypokalaemia is often present *during* treatment with insulin. Less than 10 per cent of patients have hypophosphataemia to start with; 10 per cent of patients may also present with hypomagnesaemia. Hypocalcaemia is frequent and the serum invariably shows hyperosmolality.

Well marked leucocytosis is often present (15,000–30,000/mm³) even in the absence of infection.

Diagnosis

The most important clinical differential diagnosis is a hypoglycaemic coma due to insulin reaction or an overdosage with oral antidiabetic drugs. Severe sweating is the hallmark of hypoglycaemic coma. Twitchings, seizures, the presence of a decerebrate state and even neurological focal signs are observed with hypoglycaemic coma, but not in diabetic coma. Deep laboured breathing with a fruity odour of ketones in the breath, should further help distinguish diabetic ketoacidosis from hypoglycaemic coma. When doubt exists, blood should first be withdrawn for estimating the blood glucose level, and 50 ml of 50 per cent dextrose is then injected intravenously. The patient becomes alert quickly in hypoglycaemic coma, but remains unchanged in diabetic coma.

Ketonuria and ketonaemia can also occur in starvation and following alcohol ingestion (4). There is no glycosuria in starvation ketosis, the blood sugar is normal or low, and the ketonaemia is very mild.

Alcoholic ketoacidosis may occasionally bear a strong resemblance to diabetic ketoacidosis. There is well marked ketonaemia and ketonuria, but blood sugar levels are normal or low. Severe diabetics who eat poorly and continue to ingest alcohol may have severe diabetic ketoacidosis with only modest elevations in blood sugar levels.

Coma due to metabolic acidosis with a large anion gap may also occur in uraemia and in some poisonings (notably methylsalicylate poisoning). The absence of ketonaemia and ketonuria in these conditions, and a careful clinical and laboratory assessment clarify the diagnosis.

A diabetic patient may become comatose following a head injury or a cerebrovascular accident. A subarachnoid haemorrhage in a diabetic is often missed, and the patient is treated for diabetic coma. This is because of the increase in hyperglycaemia triggered by the bleed. Neck stiffness, a positive Kernig's sign, and continuing drowsiness after correction of metabolic abnormalities, point to the correct clinical diagnosis.

Finally ketoacidosis with coma in a diabetic should be distinguished from the rare hyperglycaemic hyperosmolar non-ketotic coma.

Principles of Management

The principles of management are:

(i) To administer sufficient insulin, so that acidosis is quickly corrected and the blood sugar is brought down to near normal levels. Insulin corrects hyperglycaemia and ketosis by correcting the basic abnormalities in metabolism—it stops ketogenesis and lipolysis, reduces neoglucogenesis, and increases the peripheral utilization of glucose.

(ii) To replace the loss of water and electrolytes which characterize the severe diabetic state. Dehydration is corrected by rapid intravenous infusions of normal saline, and hypokalaemia which is often encountered during recovery from diabetic coma, by a monitored infusion of potassium chloride.

(iii) To correct severe metabolic acidosis. Insulin is mandatory for this purpose; however intravenous sodium bicarbonate may need to be used as an emergency measure in patients who are deeply unconscious and severely acidotic.

(iv) To correct shock if present, by the emergency infusion of plasma or colloids. The circulatory haemodynamics will ultimately stand corrected only if adequate replacement of fluid and electrolytes is quickly achieved.

(v) To determine the precipitating factor causing severe diabetic ketoacidosis with coma, and to treat this factor. It is extremely important to search for infection, a common and important precipitating factor.

(vi) To monitor patients carefully and meticulously through all phases of management.

Details of Management

(a) Monitoring the Patient

Close monitoring is important for easy and successful management. Once the diagnosis of diabetic coma is established, blood is withdrawn from a peripheral vein through a large needle, and sent for estimation of glucose, ketones, electrolytes, urea, creatinine, blood counts and other relevant biochemical tests. 25 units of actrapid insulin are injected through the same needle; this is followed by the starting of an intravenous infusion of normal saline. Arterial blood is also promptly collected and sent for measurement of arterial pH, blood gases and bicarbonate content. It is important to secure a good peripheral vein immediately after admission. In addition, we always have a central venous line with the venous catheter in the superior vena cava. This allows infusion of fluids, as well as measurement of the central venous pressure. In patients who are markedly hypotensive from fluid and electrolyte loss, we generally secure one more peripheral vein to aid in the rapid replacement of fluids.

A nasogastric tube is passed into the stomach, which is washed out by sodium bicarbonate. A Foley's catheter in the bladder allows the maintenance of an hourly urine output chart, as also examination of the urine for sugar and ketones.

The patient should be monitored as for any critical illness with special emphasis on intake-output charts, vital signs, evidence of pulmonary congestion, serum electrolytes, arterial pH and blood gases, renal function, and above all, blood glucose and plasma ketones.

Blood glucose should be monitored hourly at the bedside, and 2–3 hourly in the laboratory. This initially provides information as to whether the insulin administered is adequate to cause a fall in the high blood glucose levels at the rate of 75–100 mg/dl/hour. Later, estimating the blood glucose enables the physician to adjust insulin administration so that blood glucose levels are maintained between 150–250 mg/dl, and both hypoglycaemia or a return to hyperglycaemia, are avoided. Arterial pH, blood gases and serum electrolytes are monitored as often as necessary. The latter should preferably be monitored every 4–6 hours till the patient is well on the way to recovery. All data should be charted on a flow sheet for easy evaluation.

(b) Insulin Therapy for Correction of Hyperglycaemia and Ketosis

After the initial intravenous bolus of 25 units of actrapid insulin, this drug is promptly started at a rate of 6–8 units/hr (0.1–0.15 units/kg), in a continuous infusion of normal saline. The blood glucose levels should be monitored as stated above. In most patients the recommended dose is adequate to control hyperglycaemia and ketosis. If the blood glucose and ketone levels do not start to fall in the first 2 hours, the infusion rate should be doubled. This may rarely need to be doubled once again every 1–2 hours, if an adequate fall in blood glucose is not achieved. In very rare cases of insulin resistance we have needed to progressively double or even quadruple the rate of infusion per hour, so that insulin requirements over 24 hours are astronomical. Frequent blood sugar and ketone estimations are mandatory under such circumstances. We aim at a fall of at least 50–75 mg/dl/hr. When the blood sugar levels are between 180–230 mg/dl, a 5 per cent dextrose infusion is started, but the insulin infusion is continued till ketosis clears. This is important, as decreasing the insulin infusion at this

juncture may result in a persistence of ketosis for a much longer period of time. A situation may well arise during the treatment of diabetic ketoacidosis, when the blood glucose level is normal or less than normal, and yet ketonaemia and ketonuria are very evident. This is countered by an intravenous infusion of 5 per cent or even 10 per cent dextrose, and simultaneous continuation of the insulin infusion. It should never be forgotten that the main battle is to be waged against ketosis and resulting acidosis, which strongly disturb the homeostasis of the mileu interieur. Hyperglycaemia is generally controlled within 12 hours; ketosis may take longer to be controlled—18–24 hours, or even more.

It is often difficult to determine when ketosis is controlled. Serum ketone measurements are useful, but positive tests for plasma ketones may persist well after acidosis is resolved. Perhaps this is because acetone is cleared more slowly than acetoacetic acid and betahydroxybutyric acid. The sodium nitroprusside test is a measure of the acetone in the plasma, and can give persistently positive readings for ketones, even though acetone does not alter acid-base balance. Therefore to determine whether the ketosis has cleared, it is important to monitor the anion gap, and the arterial pH. An abolition of the anion gap and a normal arterial pH, signifies the clearance or control of ketosis.

Once ketosis is controlled and the patient is conscious and able to take oral feeds, a switch over to subcutaneous insulin is made. The patient is given a suitable dose (depending on the dose of insulin required during an intravenous infusion) subcutaneously, 30 minutes before a meal, and the insulin infusion is stopped once the meal is begun. Stopping the infusion before giving the subcutaneous insulin, can lead to low plasma insulin levels, and can result in rebound hyperglycaemia and ketosis. Initially actrapid insulin is used subcutaneously before each meal. Subsequently it may be combined with a slower acting insulin, and administered either once in the morning before breakfast, or twice a day, before breakfast and dinner.

(c) Fluid and Electrolyte Replacement

Severe diabetic ketoacidosis is always associated with fluid losses that may be as high as 4 to 8 l. It is vital to start fluid therapy immediately with N saline. 2 l are given over 2 hours in severely volume depleted patients. This is followed by another 2 l over the next 4–8 hours. Further infusions of 2–4 l may be necessary over the next 24 hours.

Volume replacement needs to be individually assessed and often modified or adjusted in each patient on clinical grounds, and on central venous pressure readings (5). One has to be extra careful in older patients or in those with cardiac dysfunction for fear of inducing acute pulmonary oedema. In some instances, a Swan-Ganz catheter is used to monitor pulmonary capillary wedge pressures to adjust the volume load.

Very rarely the serum sodium at admission is >150 mEq/l. This only means that the water loss is far greater than the sodium loss in these patients, with resulting hypernatraemia. We prefer to replace fluid losses in these patients as well, with N saline as outlined above, because restoration of blood volume and of circulatory haemodynamics is always of immediate and prime importance. Once this is achieved and if hypernatraemia is still present, half-strength saline or 5 per cent dextrose covered by an insulin infusion is used to counter the hypernatraemic state (see Chapter on Fluid and Electrolyte Disturbances in the Critically Ill).

Potassium Replacement. In the early stages of untreated diabetic coma, the serum potassium may be high in spite of a total body deficit of potassium. Once the diabetic ketoacidosis comes under control, hypokalaemia may develop. This is due to passage of glucose (and with it of potassium), from plasma to cells during conversion of glucose to glycogen under the influence of insulin, and also to a loss of potassium in urine following an improvement in urine output. Hypokalaemia during recovery from coma should be corrected by a slow intravenous infusion of potassium chloride in dextrose. Generally not more than 40–60 mEq of potassium are needed over 24 hours. Potassium administration must be monitored by an ECG and by checking the serum potassium levels periodically.

Phosphate Administration. Though phosphate levels in serum are known to fall during treatment of diabetic ketoacidosis, in our experience, replacement of phosphates is rarely necessary. There is however one group of patients in whom phosphate replacement is considered to be essential. This is a small group of probably < 5–10 per cent who have hypophosphataemia (< 1.5 mg/dl) at the time of admission. A further fall during treatment with insulin could lead to manifestations of hypophosphataemia. These include muscle weakness, respiratory failure due to respiratory muscle weakness, decreased myocardial contractility, haemolysis and rhabdomyolysis. Phosphate replacement during therapy is achieved by adding 5–10 ml of potassium phosphate solution (3 mmol/ml) to the replacement fluids used for replenishing the hypovolaemic state. 1–4 ml of potasium phosphate are added to one litre of N saline. Phosphate administration may occasionally produce a fall in serum calcium with resulting tetany. Serum calcium levels are monitored,and a drop in the serum calcium is treated by intravenous administration of 10–20 ml of 10 per cent calcium gluconate.

(d) Use of Sodium Bicarbonate

Metabolic acidosis is invariably corrected with insulin therapy. Sodium bicarbonate should therefore not be used routinely to combat acidosis. In fact, bicarbonate therapy often can do more harm than good. The complication of cerebral oedema is more likely in diabetic ketoacidotic children treated with intravenous sodium bicarbonate. Bicarbonate therapy can also result in sodium overload, hypocalcaemic tetany, a fall in pH in the cerebrospinal fluid and a rebound metabolic acidosis.

The only indication for intravenous bicarbonate is a pH < 7, as this poses an immediate threat to life. A pH < 7 can cause myocardial dysfunction, cerebral depression, intractable hypotension, resistance to insulin and tissue cell injury. 100 mmol of sodium bicarbonate in 400 ml distilled water is given at the rate of 200 ml/hour to counter a pH < 7. The routine use of bicarbonate in diabetic ketoacidosis is unnecessary and perhaps harmful.

(e) Treatment of Circulatory Collapse

In addition to the rapid infusion of normal saline it may be necessary to use colloids—plasma, albumin, and other plasma expanders, to counteract severe shock and urgently increase the volume within the vascular compartment. Vasopressors should be avoided as far as possible, as increasing the degree of peripheral vasoconstriction worsens tissue hypoxia.

(f) Detection and Treatment of the Precipitating Factor

It is important to determine the precipitating factor causing diabetic ketoacidosis and coma. An acute infection like pneumonia, a lung abscess, a carbuncle or acute dysentery, should be recognized and treated. It is to be noted that though well marked diabetic ketoacidosis can by itself cause a significant leucocytosis (up to 20,000/mm³), fever does not occur in these patients in the absence of infection. The presence of fever is an indication for the use of empiric antibiotic therapy if the source of infection is unidentified.

(g) Meticulous Nursing and Critical Care

This is vital for survival. Frequent changes in posture are imperative, and a clear airway should be maintained at all cost, as hypoxia due to ventilation-perfusion mismatch worsens the prognosis.

Complications during Treatment of Diabetic Coma

Important complications of diabetic ketoacidosis and coma are listed in **Table 15.9.2**.

(i) An overdose of insulin can result in *hypoglycaemic coma*. A frequent periodic check of blood glucose should prevent this problem. Severe sweating in a patient being treated with insulin for diabetic ketoacidosis, should always suggest the possibility of insulin-induced hypoglycaemia.

(ii) *Irreversible shock and circulatory failure* may complicate the course of diabetic coma. This is observed when patients are brought in very late, and when severe tissue hypoxia has been present for a prolonged period.

(iii) *Sudden death due to cardiac arrest or ventricular fibrillation* during recovery from diabetic coma is generally due to hypokalaemia. Frequent ventricular ectopics during recovery should suggest hypokalaemia. Severe hypophosphataemia may potentiate the effects of hypokalaemia.

Table 15.9.2. Important complications of diabetic ketoacidosis and coma

* Hypoglycaemic coma (overuse of insulin)
* Irreversible shock and circulatory failure
* Sudden death due to cardiac arrest or ventricular fibrillation, generally due to hypokalaemia
* Acute myocardial infarction, or cerebrovascular accident
* Cerebral oedema
* Acute lung injury and ARDS
* Acute vascular insufficiency in one or both lower limbs, particularly in older patients with atherosclerotic disease
* Acute renal shutdown
* Aspiration pneumonia
* Thromboembolism, particularly in older patients
* Infections

(iv) *Acute myocardial infarction or a cerebrovascular accident* may occasionally complicate the course of diabetic coma. Failure to recover consciousness after ketosis has been controlled, should suggest the possibility of a stroke. The persistence of shock after rapid correction of fluid, electrolyte and metabolic abnormalities should make one suspect a myocardial infarction or pulmonary embolism.

(v) *Cerebral oedema* is a dreaded complication (**6**). It is manifested by a deteriorating level of consciousness at a point in time when the metabolic abnormalities (including ketosis) show clear evidence of improvement. It is more often observed in children and young adults, and carries a mortality of nearly 90 per cent. Experimental studies have suggested that cerebral oedema is associated with greater reduction in blood sugar levels during treatment. Hence the wisdom of starting a 5 per cent dextrose infusion when the blood glucose level approaches 200 mg/dl during treatment with insulin.

(vi) A rare complication of ketoacidosis is *acute lung injury (ARDS)* (**7**). This is generally observed in older patients and in our opinion, is invariably triggered by excessive volume replacement. Other unknown factors are also probably responsible for contributing to increased pulmonary capillary permeability. Acute lung injury manifests with non-cardiogenic pulmonary oedema and refractory hypoxia that needs ventilatory support. Under the above circumstances it has a forbidding mortality.

(vii) Recovery from coma can be complicated by *acute vascular insufficiency in one or both lower limbs*. This is particularly likely to occur in old patients with atherosclerotic disease, following prolonged hypotension.

(viii) *Acute renal shutdown* may complicate recovery from diabetic ketoacidosis and coma.

(ix) *Aspiration pneumonia* particularly in obtunded and comatose patients is a common complication of diabetic ketoacidosis.

(x) *Thromboembolism* may be a complication particularly in older patients. Arterial thrombosis if it occurs, chiefly involves the lower limb vessels. Femoral vein thrombosis is an important cause of sudden death from massive pulmonary embolism.

(xi) *Infections*. Diabetic patients are prone to infection. Urinary tract infections, respiratory tract infections are common. Nosocomial sepsis with positive blood culture is occasionally encountered. A rare but frequently fatal infection in severe diabetes and diabetic ketoacidosis is mucormycosis, caused by the fungus rhizopus. The presence of a black necrotic area around the eye, nasal cavity, nose, or the presence of conjunctival injection with circumocular oedema and sinusitis are strongly suggestive of mucormycosis. Proptosis of the eye with restricted ocular movements are late features. This fungus has a tendency to invade vessels causing thrombosis and infarction. Unless recognized very early and promptly treated, death generally ensues.

Hyperglycaemic Hyperosmolar Nonketotic Diabetic Coma

This is a rare cause of coma in diabetes. It is characterized by marked hyperglycaemia (often > 700 mg/dl), with little or no reduction in the plasma bicarbonate (**8–10**). There is also marked hypernatraemia with serum sodium levels over 150–155 mEq/l. The plasma shows little or no ketonaemia and ketone bodies in urine are absent, or at most present in traces (**11**). A large overlap exists in the clinical presentation of diabetic ketoacidosis and hyperosmolar non-ketotic coma. Thus there are patients with hyperosmolar coma who have a fair degree of ketoacidosis, just as there are patients with typical ketoacidosis with significant hypernatraemia and hyperosmolarity.

The patient with typical hyperglycaemic hyperosmolar nonketotic coma is generally beyond 50 years of age, and often presents with neurological manifestations (**11**). These may include seizures, haemiparesis, and drowsiness progressing to coma. Dehydration is invariably present, and tachycardia with hypotension is common. Since renal perfusion is diminished, there is a fall in urine output with a resultant decreased escape of glucose via the kidney. However, the rate of production of glucose in the liver is high, and this can lead to increasingly high blood glucose levels. Severe hyperglycaemia and hyperosmolarity result.

Management

Insulin is given in an infusion exactly in the same manner as in diabetic ketoacidosis. Plasma glucose concentrations should decrease at the rate of 75–100 mg/dl per hour, and the dose and rate of insulin is adjusted so as to ensure this decrease. Fluid replacement should preferably be with normal saline rather than with hypotonic saline. Quick volume replacement is important to correct hypotension that may result from shifts of water from the extracellular to the intracellular compartment. These shifts of water often accompany the transport of glucose into the cells under the influence of insulin. Once dehydration is corrected by an adequate volume load, and hyperglycaemia is well controlled, hypernatraemia may be countered by using infusions of half-strength saline or half-strength dextrose, given under cover of insulin. In patients presenting with severe hypotension, infusions of plasma or of colloids (like dextran) may be necessary. Many of these patients are old and feeble and may well have cardiac dysfunction. Volume replacement should be monitored by central venous pressure readings and if necessary by pulmonary capillary wedge pressure measurements made through a Swan-Ganz catheter.

Most of these patients have a large potassium deficit. Serum potassium levels should be carefully monitored before and during therapy, and potassium replacement should be provided if necessary.

The mortality in hyperglycaemic, hyperosmolar non-ketotic diabetic coma is high. Death often results from infection or from thrombotic complications.

REFERENCES

1. Alberti KG. (1989). Diabetic Emergencies. Br Med Bull. 45, 242–263.
2. Foster DW, McGarry JD. (1983). The metabolic derangements and treatment of diabetic ketoacidosis. N Engl J Med. 309, 159.
3. Walker M, Marshall SM, Alberti KG. (1989). Clinical aspects of diabetic ketoacidosis. Diabetes Metab Rev. 5, 651–663.

4. Fulop M. (1989). Alcoholism, ketoacidosis, and lactic acidosis. Diabetes Metab Rev. 5, 365.

5. Adrogue HJ, Barrero J, Eknoyan G. (1989). Salutary effects of modest fluid replacement in the treatment of adults with diabetic ketoacidosis. JAMA. 262, 2108–2113.

6. Rosenbloom AL. (1990). Intracerebral crises during treatment of diabetic ketoacidosis. Diabetes Care.13, 22–33.

7. Hansen LA, Prakash UBS, Colby TV. (1989). Pulmonary complications in diabetes mellitus. Mayo Clin Proc. 64, 791.

8. Marshall SM, Alberti KGMM. (1988). Hyperosmolar non-ketotic diabetic coma. In: The Diabetes Annual, 4th edn (Eds Alberti KGMM, Krall LP). p. 235. Elsevier.

9. Pope DW, Dansky D. (1989). Hyperosmolar hyperglycaemic nonketotic coma. Emerg Med Clin North Am. 7, 849.

10. Wachtel TJ, Silliman RA, Lamberton P. (1987). Predisposing factors for the diabetic hyperosmolar state. Arch Intern Med. 147, 499.

11. Udwadia FE. (1972). Hyperosmolar non-ketotic diabetic coma. J of Assoc Phys India. 10(12), 937–942.

Neurological Problems Requiring Critical Care

Contributed by

Dr S.M. Katrak, MD, DM, Hon. Professor and Head of Department of Neurology, Grant Medical College and JJ Group of Hospitals, Consultant Neurologist, Jaslok Hospital and Research Centre, and Breach Candy Hospital & Research Centre, Mumbai,

Dr Sohrab K. Bhabha, MD, DM, Retired Consultant Neurologist, P. D. Hinduja Hospital and Research Centre, Mumbai.
and

Dr Noshir H. Wadia, MD, FRCP (London), FAMS (India), FNA, FASc, Retired Professor of Neurology, Grant Medical College, and JJ Group of Hospitals, Mumbai. Consultant Neurologist for Life, Grant Medical College, and JJ Group of Hospitals, Mumbai. Director of Neurology, Jaslok Hospital and Research Centre, Mumbai. Consultant Neurologist, Breach Candy Hospital and Research Centre, Mumbai.

A. INCREASED INTRACRANIAL PRESSURE

Dr Sarosh M. Katrak & Dr Noshir H. Wadia

Introduction

Raised intracranial pressure (ICP) is an important common feature in many untreated intracranial problems (**Table 15.10.1**). This constitutes a sizeable number of patients presenting with neurological emergencies. Clinical assessment is more often than not unreliable in judging the intracranial pressure. In the non-traumatic brain damaged patient, there may or may not be a history of *de novo* headaches, vomiting, visual disturbance, sixth cranial nerve palsy or papilloedema. The absence of papilloedema does not exclude raised ICP in patients with acute problems. In one series only 4 per cent had disc swelling suggestive of raised ICP, whereas 50 per cent had raised ICP on monitoring (**1**). Papillary dilatation, bradycardia, hypertension, alteration in the level of consciousness and decerebrate posturing are unfortunately late signs of the raised ICP and occur either with central or uncal herniation. In fact, the classic Cushing triad—hypertension, bradycardia and irregular respiration—is usually a later phenomenon associated with raised ICP particularly if the intracranial pressure is transmitted to the posterior fossa with distortion of the lower brainstem. Hence, clinical examination for raised ICP, though important, is unreliable, and may only be evident in the late stages by which time cerebral perfusion pressure (CPP) is affected leading to focal ischaemia and permanent brain damage. Thus the gold standard is to measure the intracranial pressure.

An understanding of the pathophysiology of the intracranial (IC) vault is necessary for proper management of the patient with raised ICP. The simplest approach would be to consider the clinical features caused by a rise in pressure within the intracranial vault as a variety of compartment syndrome. Under normal conditions the IC volume includes the brain and interstitial fluid—

Table 15.10.1. Common causes of raised intracranial pressure

1. Head Injury	Intracranial haematoma
	Diffuse brain swelling
	Cerebral contusion
2. Cerebrovascular disease	Subarachnoid haemorrhage
	Intracerebral haematoma
	Major cerebral / cerebellar infarct
	Cerebral venous thrombosis
3. Hydrocephalus	Congenital
	Obstructive due to tumour
	Communicating following tuberculous meningitis
4. Tumour	Late stages with central or uncal herniation
5. Metabolic encephalopathy	Hypoxic-ischaemic following cardiac arrest
	Reye's syndrome
	Hepatic or renal encephalopathy
	Severe hyponatraemia—SIADH
6. Status epilepticus	

80 per cent, the CSF—10 per cent, and blood—10 per cent. In pathological states, primary injury produces swelling of the brain compartment. Hence, approximate equal decrease in volume of other compartments occurs to maintain normal ICP. Secondly, primary injury tends to be self-limiting and it is the role of the specialist to prevent secondary injury produced by increased compartment pressure and organ ischaemia.

Pathophysiological Principles

In order to understand this approach, it is important to understand the relationship between the IC volume and the ICP (**Fig. 15.10.1**).

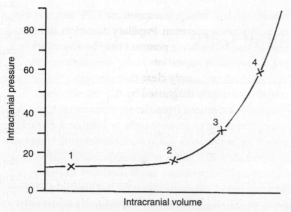

Fig. 15.10.1. Illustration of the relationship between intracranial volume and intracranial pressure. Note that beyond point 3, even a small increase in the intracranial volume produces a marked elevation of intracranial presssure.

At normal IC volume, the ICP is low (point 1 on **Fig. 15.10.1**), and remains so for an increment in volume. Thus compensatory mechanisms are adequate and hence 'compliance' (ratio of change in volume to resultant change in ICP) is high. With further addition of volume, compensatory mechanisms are exceeded. The ICP is still within normal limits, but compliance is low (point 2). From this point onwards, further addition of small volumes to the IC vault will produce elevation of ICP (point 3), which can go to dangerous limits (point 4).

The importance of any increase in ICP becomes evident when it is realized that it affects cerebral blood flow, which in turn is dependent on cerebral perfusion pressure (CPP). Conventionally, CPP is defined as mean arterial blood pressure (aBP) minus the mean ICP. Thus CPP = aBP–ICP. Because cerebral blood flow (CBF) is autoregulated, it remains constant over a fairly wide range of blood pressure, presuming that the ICP remains within normal limits. However, any increase in ICP has the potential of reducing CBF by reducing the CPP, and this indeed happens when CPP is reduced below the level of autoregulation, or when autoregulation fails and CBF is determined by the actual perfusion pressure. Thus an abnormal increase of ICP can result in a reduction of CBF to the point of producing ischaemic organ injury (**2**).

Based on this, three strategies can deal with increased ICP: (i) decrease brain oedema; (ii) decrease CSF volume; and (iii) decrease cerebral blood volume (**Table 15.10.2**). Administration of mannitol, steroids and diuretics have all been shown to decrease cerebral oedema, and thus lower ICP and improve CPP. Likewise, removal of even small amounts of CSF have helped in decreasing ICP. Nevertheless, the most important advance has been the understanding of how controlled ventilation helps in altering cerebral blood volume (CBV) and ICP, by modulating cerebral blood flow. Cerebral blood flow in normal humans is autoregulated (no influence of the autonomic nervous system) and is determined by an interaction between CPP (aBP–ICP) with the partial pressure in the arterial blood of both oxygen (PaO_2) and carbon dioxide ($PaCO_2$). Hence CBF remains constant with the range of CPP of approximately 60–160 mm Hg. Below this level, CBF will decrease

Table 15.10.2. Medical therapies for increased intracranial pressure

1. Decrease Cerebral Oedema
   (a) Mannitol
   (b) Non-osmotic diuretic
   (c) Steroids
2. Decrease CSF volume
   (a) CSF drainage via a ventricular catheter
   (b) Decrease CSF production—acetazolamide
3. Decrease Cerebral Blood Volume
   (a) Hyperventialtion
   (b) Head elevation
   (c) High dose barbiturates

and that is why so much attention is given to increased ICP as a cause of decreased CPP. Injury to the brain—trauma, hypoxia, drugs—all have the ability to abolish autoregulation. Hence in the injured brain, CBF is directly proportional to CPP, which in turn depends on the ICP and its relationship to PaO_2 and $PaCO_2$ (**Fig. 15.10.2**).

With regard to PaO_2, the brain is no different from other tissues. As PaO_2 falls and approaches 60 mm Hg, cerebral vasodilatation takes place with increased cerebral blood flow and volume with a consequent rise in ICP. Hence the importance of maintaining a normal PaO_2 in the setting of neuro-intensive care.

The most clinically useful tool for manipulation of CBF is control of $PaCO_2$. As can be seen, there is practically a linear relationship between CBF and $PaCO_2$. Hence with elective intubation, followed by hyperventilation, the $PaCO_2$ can be reduced to the low 20s, thereby reducing the CBF and hence the ICP. Perhaps there is some question about the extent of hyperventilation and the ability of hyperventilation to continue to control CBF over days or weeks. Nonetheless, there is no doubt about its usefulness in lowering ICP in the acute phase of neurological injury associated with increased ICP (**2**).

The concept of the simple volume-pressure (V-P) curve (**Fig. 15.10.1**) can be misleading, as the factor of rate of volume change

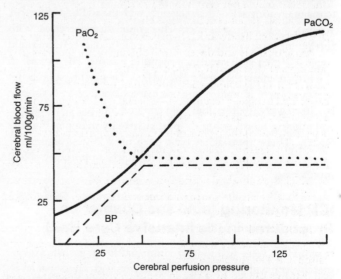

Fig. 15.10.2. In the injured brain, cerebral blood flow is directly proportional to the cerebral perfusion pressure, which in turn depends on intracranial pressure and its relationship to PaO_2 and $PaCO_2$.

is not given. Once this rate is taken into account, the simple V-P curve becomes a series of curves (**Fig. 15.10.3**). These curves help to explain why a suddenly appearing blood clot increases the ICP (curve t) much more rapidly than the same volume of a slowly growing brain tumour (curve 4t). Lastly the type of added volume also has a differing influence on the ICP. For example, addition of equal volume of CSF and tumor mass do not result in the same increase of ICP (**3**). CSF may be quickly moved down the spinal theca, out of the IC vault, or absorbed via the blood, whereas a tumour is not so easily displaced and may obstruct CSF pathways, further raising the ICP.

In summary, the pathophysiology of the increased pressure

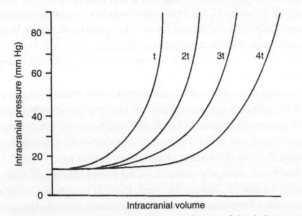

Fig. 15.10.3. This figure illustrates that the degree of rise in intracranial pressure depends on the rate at which intracranial volume increases. A sudden rise in intracranial volume increases the intracranial pressure (curve t) much more rapidly and to a greater extent, than a similar or even greater increase in intracranial volume occurring over a more prolonged period of time (curve 4t).

in the IC vault is that it is a variety of compartment syndrome in which the addition of volume in one compartment (brain) induces displacement from the others (CSF and/or cerebral blood volume) to maintain normal ICP. Subsequently, with the addition of further volume, the ICP remains normal but compliance decreases. With further increase in volume, compliance fails and there is a rapid rise in ICP even with small increments in volume. The increase in ICP, in turn, affects the cerebral blood flow. Therapeutic approaches to regulation of IC volume include manipulation of brain volume by altering brain interstitial fluid content, altering CSF volume, and altering blood volume—particularly by manipulating the $PaCO_2$. These approaches have been used in neuro-intensive care with significant success, and underlie the importance of ICP monitoring.

ICP Monitoring (also see Chapter on Procedures in the Intensive Care Unit)

It would be ideal to monitor abnormal focal/global cerebral metabolism and blood flow in all patients with abnormal levels of consciousness. Until this is possible it is important to maintain adequate CPP (> 50 mm Hg); to estimate CPP, it is mandatory to monitor ICP.

Elevations of ICP which compromise CPP are not always apparent on clinical examination. Pupillary dilatation, bradycardia, hypertension and decerebrate postures may be absent while ICP is rising (**4, 5**), or usually appear late in the clinical picture (**6**). Since 1960 (**7**), it has become amply clear that elevation in ICP can be accurately and promptly diagnosed by ICP monitoring.

ICP is usually measured from the supratentorial space. It can be measured from the cisterna magna or lumbar subarachnoid space, only if an intracranial lesion or noncommunicating hydrocephalus is excluded. ICP varies with position, and fluctuates with systolic arterial blood pressure, respiration and straining. ICP is normally < 10 mm Hg when measured at the level of the foramen magnum in the supine position; and sustained elevation of the ICP baseline above 15 mm Hg is abnormal.

Characteristic variations in ICP have been observed over a period of time, the most significant of which are a subclass of plateau waves called 'A waves'. These are due to a sustained elevation of ICP of 60 mm Hg or more. These waves are now shown to be an autoregulatory response to insufficient CPP (**8**) which in turn produces cerebral vasodilatation in an attempt to increase the cerebral blood flow. The resultant increase in cerebral blood volume produces a sustained rise of ICP. These A waves are of ominous significance, and precede loss of control over elevated ICP with subsequent circulatory arrest and brain death.

General Principles of ICP Monitoring

The modified compartmental model of ICP described earlier, presumes that the craniospinal compartments are watertight. If the system is *not* watertight, increase in ICP to abnormal levels may not occur till a substantial volume is added to the IC vault, or not at all in spite of brain herniation. This disparity between measured ICP and clinical signs occurs when a 'leak' allows bulk flow movement of the brain along a pressure gradient e.g. rostral to caudal brain herniation after lumbar puncture with CSF leak, in the presence of a supratentorial lesion. It may also occur when a strategically located mass (temporal lobe tumour) physically distorts neighbouring brain tissue (3rd nerve palsy), before raising the ICP. Thirdly, pressure throughout the craniospinal axis is normally coupled by free flow of CSF. At times the location of a mass may obstruct the flow of CSF. In this event, measurement of ICP from another compartment (uninvolved site), may not reflect the pressure in the compartment of interest (site of mass lesion). Therefore ICP monitoring should be performed within the compartment of interest, i.e. on the side of a lesion whenever possible, in the setting of a unilateral supratentorial mass lesion.

Devices for ICP Monitoring

Invasive ICP monitoring can be classified by the site where ICP is monitored—extradural, subdural, intraparenchymal and intraventricular, or by the means by which ICP is delivered to the measurement device—fluid coupled and non-fluid coupled systems.

The advantages of a fluid coupled system (ventricular catheter) are that it is simple, accurate, inexpensive and compatible with the existing equipment. Disadvantages include occasional infection (more so with long-term monitoring), epidural and subdural haematomas, and occlusion of the catheter. Non-fluid coupled systems are many, but are expensive and require a greater degree of expertise. However they are accurate, with facility of handling. Further details of ICP monitoring are given in an excellent review (9).

Management of Raised Intracranial Pressure

As mentioned earlier, the insult to the brain is usually self-limiting, and it is the duty of the specialist to attempt to maintain the ICP within a reasonable range, so as to maintain the CPP and avoid secondary ischaemic damage to the brain. Measures for controlling ICP can be divided into those which rapidly reverse acute rise of ICP, and those which maintain ICP within a reasonable range. The rapidly acting measures include hyperventilation, osmotic diuresis with mannitol, CSF drainage, and high dose barbiturates. Maintenance therapy includes fluid restriction, sedation and paralysis, control of blood pressure, seizure prophylaxis, prevention of fever, and head positioning.

Hyperventilation

Hyperventilation is one of the most effective and rapid methods of reducing ICP; it can do so in a matter of minutes. However many patients with head injury or meningitis hyperventilate on their own, and induced hyperventilation may be avoided.

Hyperventilation results in hypocarbia which in turn induces vasoconstriction through serum and CSF alkalosis (10). This results in a reduction of CBF and hence CBV, and a rapid reduction in ICP. An initial reduction in $PaCO_2$ by 5–10 mm Hg, produces a 25–30 per cent reduction in the ICP, but this rate of reduction cannot be maintained for long as systemic acid-base buffering mechanism produces compensation. Hyperventilation is produced by increasing the ventilator rate and keeping the tidal volume at 12–14 ml/kg. Only normal areas with intact blood-brain barrier respond well, as injured areas have diminished vascular reactivity to hypocarbia. The inability of hyperventilation to reduce ICP is suggestive of a grave prognosis, as other methods to reduce ICP also fail, and death rapidly follows from uncontrolled ICP. Once the ICP is rapidly reduced, the $PaCO_2$ must be maintained at the same low level till the original problem is resolved. Fever, not only increases CBF and CBV, but also increases CO_2 production. Hence it must be controlled with judicious use of antibiotics and antipyretics.

A safe initial range of $PaCO_2$ is 28–35 mm Hg. The ventilator rate may then be increased to bring the $PaCO_2$ to 22–25 mm Hg, till the ICP is reduced. Hyperventilation should not be stopped suddenly as a rapid increase in $PaCO_2$ will increase the ICP as rapidly, as reduction lowers it. Hyperventilation should be gradually reduced over 24–48 hours. If the ICP suddenly rises for any reason, hyperventilation may be used again once the $PaCO_2$ is around 35 mm Hg.

An occasional patient with positive end-expiratory pressure (PEEP) may show an increase in ICP because of the transmission of the positive pressure through the thoracic veins. This potential adverse effect of PEEP can be minimized by raising the head of the patient by 20–30 degrees. In this position the thoracic pressure

must exceed the ICP to have a deleterious effect (refer to Head Position later). Secondly, PEEP reduces cardiac filling, and consequently the cardiac output and blood pressure fall. To avoid this adequate hydration and intravascular volume should be maintained.

The beneficial effects of chronic hyperventilation are less clear (11). The compensatory mechanisms for CSF alkalosis begin in a few hours and are completed by 24 hours. For this reason, hyperventilation becomes ineffective after more than six hours. The addition of weak bases and buffers such as tromethamine, may sustain CSF alkalosis and cerebral vasoconstriction, but its use in prolonged hyperventilation is controversial.

In conclusion, hyperventilation remains the mainstay for rapid and effective control of ICP in an ICU setting. It is maximally effective in traumatic brain injury.

Osmotic Agents and Diuretics (12)

In some patients restriction of fluids to half of maintenance requirements is enough to control ICP. If osmotic agents are required, avoid dehydration by using iso-osmotic fluids to maintain adequate intake. Normal saline (310 mOsm/l) is the ideal fluid. Other fluids such as 5 per cent dextrose (250 mOsm/l) and Ringer's Lactate (275 mOsm/l) are hypo-osmolar as compared to serum, and should be avoided. Besides with acute ischaemic brain damage dextrose produces hyperglycaemia, and the anerobic oxidation of glucose produces more lactic acid and free radicles, which further damage the brain (13).

Mannitol with hyperventilation is the mainstay of therapy for ICP, particularly in the acute phase. It is impermeable to the blood-brain barrier and therefore draws water out of oedematous brain into the plasma. It is most effective in oedematous brain tissue with a defective blood-brain barrier. With reduction in the ICP, the CPP improves with a consequent increase in the CBF, but not to dangerous levels so as to increase the ICP. Osmotic infusions also reduce the CSF production, but this effect is clinically insignificant.

Although effective in the acute phase, prolonged administration of mannitol should be avoided as equilibrium is rapidly reached in the brain, and it becomes less effective. The maximum action in reducing ICP occurs between 20 and 60 minutes after infusion. Smaller doses (0.25 g/kg/dose) reduce ICP as effectively as large doses (1 g/kg/dose), but the effect is less prolonged (4 hours instead of 6 hours). Therefore smaller and more frequent doses of mannitol are to be encouraged (14). Initially 0.75 g/kg should be given followed by 0.25 g/kg every 3–5 hours depending on the ICP, CPP, serum osmolality and the clinical condition. If the ICP is markedly raised, restrict fluids with mannitol, but avoid dehydration, electrolyte imbalance, renal dysfunction, and hypotension. Central venous pressure (CVP) should if necessary be increased by an infusion of normal saline rather than dextrose or Ringer Lactate; pressor agents should as far as possible be avoided.

Corticosteroids (15)

Intravenous dexamethasone 4–6 mg 6 hourly, reduces cerebral oedema caused by intracranial tumours and mass lesions. The drug is also used to reduce raised intracranial pressure in cerebral haemorrhage or infarction, but is of unproven value in these situations.

Removal of CSF

Removal of CSF through an intra-ventricular catheter is a rapid method of reducing ICP, particularly when there is a hydrocephalus. Once hyperventilation and mannitol have stabilized a patient, a CT scan should be done to visualize the ventricular system, and then an intraventricular catheter is inserted. This is done because the ventricular system may be distorted by an intracranial mass, or cerebral oedema may compress the ventricular system. CSF drainage is most useful for brief periods to reduce the ICP during plateau waves. The main drawback of this method is the risk of intracranial infection, and this method is less frequently used than a decade ago.

High Dose Barbiturate Therapy

Of all the intravenous agents, barbiturates induce the most significant decrease in cerebral blood flow and metabolism, thereby reducing ICP (16). Their action is prompt when given intravenously. This therapy has been tried in patients who are comatose and have failed to respond to all conventional therapy to reduce ICP. High dose barbiturates require monitoring of blood pressure and ICP. The complications of such high doses of barbiturates include hypotension from decrease in venous tone, and decreased sympathetic baroreflex responsiveness. In an ICU setting, hypotension may be exaggerated by mannitol-induced dehydration, and decrease in cardiac filling secondary to mechanical ventilation.

The assessment of a comatose patient becomes difficult as the reflex activity of the brain is abolished by high doses of barbiturates. After stopping high dose barbiturate therapy, the reflex activity reappears in the following order—pupillary reaction to light, deep tendon reflexes, breathing, corneal reflex, oculocephalic reflexes, and lastly motor movements.

Failure of raised ICP to respond to increased doses of barbiturates, is a sign of poor outcome. But this therapy is usually used in comatose patients who have not responded to the conventional methods, i.e. in a small number of patients with features of a poor outcome. Hence high dose barbiturates used intelligently may prevent death from raised ICP in a few of these patients with a poor prognosis to start with (17).

During the care of comatose patients, frequent noxious stimuli increase the ICP in patients with poor intracranial compliance. These noxious stimuli include endotracheal intubation, coughing, endotracheal suction and chest physiotherapy. In this situation, thiopental (1–5 mg/kg) reduces the ICP within seconds, and the effect lasts for a few minutes after a single dose. Repeated large doses or continuous infusion should be avoided as the effect is less and drug accumulation with prolonged untoward effects occurs. Hence repeated small doses of thiopental may be used effectively to avoid these frequent bursts of rise in ICP in comatose patients.

Maintenance Therapy

Maintenance therapy for raised ICP includes fluid restriction and diuretics, sedation and paralysis, blood pressure control, seizure

prophylaxis, prevention of fever. The head is kept in a neutral position, and any constriction of the neck is avoided.

Fluid Restriction and Diuretics

Fluid restriction and diuretics are the mainstay of maintenance therapy for ICP. Furosemide and acetazolamide can be used to improve water clearance. The initial aim is to produce isovolaemic hyperosmolarity i.e. to elevate serum osmolarity without reducing the intravascular volume. Hence free water loss is replaced with isotonic solutions. The best fluid for this purpose is normal saline with added KCl. Whole blood or albumin solutions could also be used to advantage, if required. Potassium, magnesium and phosphate may need to be replaced. The effect of diuretic therapy can last up to two weeks while brain compliance returns to normal, as there is no tolerance to the diuretic effect of furosemide and acetazolamide. They also help in reducing the risk of rebound cerebral oedema after stopping mannitol. Another method of restricting fluids and maintaining serum osmolality is to use high caloric oral feeds (2 kcal/ml) through a nasogastric tube.

Sedation and Muscle Relaxants

Agitation, coughing, straining and fighting the ventilator raises the ICP significantly, at times to dangerous levels. In such patients sedation and the use of non-depolarizing muscle relaxants are indicated. Narcotics may produce miosis and suppress ventilation but these disadvantages are outweighed by the reduction in ICP. Besides, mechanical ventilation obviates the adverse effect of respiratory depression. Most intravenous sedatives, benzodiazepines, barbiturates and butyrophenones reduce ICP. Ketamine is a notable exception as it raises the ICP because of vasodilatation and increased CBF and should be avoided in such patients.

Pancuronium (0.1 mg/kg) is perhaps the drug of choice for muscle relaxation/paralysis, because of its shorter duration of action and lack of side effects. It may be used prior to endotracheal intubation, provided the procedure is rapidly and smoothly performed. Paralysis may also facilitate nursing care and may permit a movement artefact-free EEG. Muscle relaxants do not alter the pupillary reflex but the other brainstem reflexes are affected. Hence the clinician must weigh the advantages before paralysing the patient. However their effects can be neutralized in a matter of minutes if neurological evaluation is mandatory, and their use is more often beneficial than detrimental.

Control of Blood Pressure

The blood pressure should be appropriately controlled in brain damaged patients. If one recalls that CPP is the difference between the mean arterial blood pressure and ICP, then with a raised ICP, hypotension can result in cerebral ischaemia, and moderate hypertension may increase CPP in damaged areas and exaggerate oedema. To what extent should one treat the blood pressure? After brain damage, there is reactive hypertension, but the hypertension tends to subside over the first few days and often does not require aggressive therapy (18, 19). It is hazardous to produce a precipitate drop in the blood pressure in the acute phase, as in the presence of raised ICP, this will further reduce CPP and produce ischaemic brain damage. If a patient remains hypertensive for several days, an attempt should be made to lower the blood pressure *slowly*.

Many drugs are used to control blood pressure. In the agitated, restless patient, sedatives and analgesics may suffice. Small doses of intravenous thiopentone or pentobarbital would reduce not only the blood pressure, but also ICP—an ideal situation. However this should only be done in the comatose, intubated patient (20). Vasodilators (nitroprusside, hydralazine) and some calcium-channel blockers (verapamil, nifedipine) also cause cerebral vasodilatation and may increase ICP (21, 22). Beta-blockers (propranolol, atenolol, labetalol) and ACE-inhibitors (enalapril) are effective and do not increase ICP.

Seizure Prophylaxis (23)

Seizures cause an increase in metabolic requirements of the brain, and hence increase CBF and therefore CBV and ICP (24). Therefore seizures should be treated even in a paralyzed patient. Tonic/clonic seizures may be obvious but subtle myoclonic jerks may be missed. The EEG may help in detecting this subtle seizure activity.

The first step in seizure control is to remove the cause, if that is obvious, e.g. fever, hypoglycaemia, or metabolic derangement. While the cause is being investigated, intravenous phenytoin is given slowly (25 mg/min) up to 200–400 mg bolus depending on the severity and frequency of the convulsions. Intravenous diazepam is an excellent short-term anticonvulsant, but respiratory depression must be prevented, specially in the elderly. Intravenous lorazepam 4 mg 12 hourly, may be more suitable, if the seizures are more protracted. If necessary, phenobarbitone may be given in small doses. Thiopental may be necessary for patients in protracted status epilepticus. Multifocal myoclonic jerks after an ischaemic arrest have a poor prognosis, and are difficult to control. High doses of barbiturates or clonazepam are occasionally effective (see under Status Epilepticus).

Prevention of Fever

The cerebral metabolic rate increases by 5–7 per cent per degree celsius rise in body temperature (25). Hence hyperthermia must be vigorously treated in patients with increased ICP. Antipyretics and cooling methods must be used appropriately and infection should be treated vigorously with antibiotics.

On the other hand, hypothermia reduces cerebral metabolism. In fact at 30°C, cerebral metabolism is reduced to 50 per cent. The beneficial effect of hypothermia before a cerebral insult is borne out by the many reports of survivors of near drowning in cold water without any neurological deficit. However induction of hypothermia *after* a brain injury, has not been shown to improve the outcome. Secondly prolonged hypothermia has its own set of complications viz. hypovolaemia, metabolic acidosis and cerebral oedema during rewarming (26). Besides infection would be more difficult to detect.

Head Position

The brain damaged patient is best nursed in the supine position. However, if a patient has ventilatory support with high airway pressure, e.g. PEEP, elevating the head by 30 degrees may have the benefit of reducing the ICP. Care must however be taken to prevent a drop in arterial blood pressure.

REFERENCES

1. Miller JD. (1987). Normal and increased intracranial pressure. In: Northfield's Surgery of the Central Nervous System, 2nd edn (Ed. Miller JD). pp. 7–57. Blackwell, London.
2. Rogers MC. (1978). Management of intracranial pressure. John Hopkins Med J. 142, 99.
3. Sullivan HG, Miller JD, Griffith RL III et al. (1978). CSF pressure transients in response to epidural and ventricular volume loading. Am J Physiol. 234(5), R167–R170.
4. Bruce DA, Berman WA, Schut L. (1977). Cerebrospinal fluid pressure monitoring in children: physiology, pathology and clinical usefulness. Adv Pediatr. 24, 233–290.
5. Marshall LF, Smith RW, Shapiro HM. (1978). The influence of diurnal rhythms in patients with intracranial hypertension: implications for management. Neurosurgery. 2, 100–102.
6. McDowall DG.(1976). Monitoring the brain. Anesthesiology. 45, 117–134.
7. Lundberg N. (1960). Continuous recording and control of ventricular fluid pressure in neurosurgical practice. Acta Psychiatr Scand. 36(suppl 149), 1–193.
8. Rosner MJ, Becker DP. (1984). Origin and evolution of plateau waves. J Neurosurg. 60, 312–324.
9. Barnett GH. (1993). Intracranial pressure monitoring devices: principles, insertion, and care. In: Neurological and Neurosurgical Intensive Care, 3rd edn (Ed. Ropper AH). Raven Press, New York.
10. Shapiro HM. (1975). Intracranial hypertension: therapeutic and anesthetic considerations. Anesthesia. 43, 445–471.
11. Muizelaar JP, Marmarou A, Ward JD et al. (1991). Adverse effects of prolonged hyperventilation in patients with severe head injury: a randomized clinical trial. J Neurosurg. 75, 731–739.
12. Procaccio F, Stochetti N, Citerio G et al. (2000). Guidelines for the treatment of adults with severe head trauma (part I). Initial assessment: evaluation and pre-hospital treatment: current criteria for hospital admission: systemic and cerebral monitoring. J Neurosurg Sci. 44, 1.
13. Longstreth WT Jr, Diehr P, Cobb LA et al. (1986). Neurologic outcome and blood glucose levels during out-of-hospital cardiopulmonary resuscitation. Neurology. 36, 1186–1191.
14. Marshall LF, Smith RW, Rauscher LA et al. (1978). Mannitol dose requirements in brain-injured patients. J Neurosurg. 48, 169–172.
15. Bullock R, Chestnut R, Clifton G et al. (1996). Brain Trauma Foundation Guidelines for the management of severe head injury. New York.
16. Lafferty JJ, Keykhah MM, Shapiro HM. (1978). Cerebral hypometabolism with deep pentobarbital anesthesia and hypothermia (30 degree C). Anesthesia. 49, 3–8.
17. Eisenberg HM, Frankowski RF, Conant LP, et al. (1988). High dose barbiturate control of elevated intracranial pressure in patients with severe head injury. J Neurosurg. 69, 15–23.
18. Clifton GL, Ziegler MG, Grossman RG. (1981).Circulating catecholamines and sympathetic activity after head injury. Neurosurgery. 8, 10–14.
19. Robertson CS, Clifton GL, Taylor AA, Grossman RG. (1983). Treatment of hypertension associated with head injury. J Neurosurg. 59, 455–460.
20. Hayashi M, Kobayashi H, Kawano H et al. (1988). Treatment of systemic hypertension and intracranial hypertension in cases of brain haemorrhage. Stroke. 19, 314–321.

21. Tinker JH, Michenfelder JD. (1976). Sodium nitroprusside: pharmacology, toxicology and therapeutics. Anesthesia. 45, 340–354.

22. Bedford RF, Dacey R, Winn HR et al. (1983). Adverse effect of a calcium entry blocker (verapamil) on intracranial pressure in patients with brain tumours. J Neurosurg. 59, 800–802.

23. Scheirhout G, Roberts I. (1998). Prophylactic antiepileptic agents after head injury: A systematic review. J Neurol Neurosurg Psychiatry. 64, 108.

24. Seisjo BK, Carlsson C, Hagerdal M et al. (1976). Brain metabolism in the critically ill. Crit Care Med. 4, 283–294.

25. Vandam LD, Burnap TK. (1959). Hypothermia. N Engl J Med. 261, 546–553.

26. Bloch M. (1967). Cerebral effects of rewarming following prolonged hypothermia: Significance for the management of severe cranio-cerebral injury and acute pyrexia. Brain. 90, 769–784.

B. CRANIAL TRAUMA

Dr Sohrab K. Bhabha

Introduction and Definition

Critical care of severe craniospinal trauma is both mandatory and rewarding, for several reasons. First, the predisposed populations are the young and middle-aged; no effort can or must be spared to salvage this productive segment of the population. Second, such trauma *must* be viewed and managed in the setting of polytrauma and *never* viewed in isolation. Third, the results of timely and appropriate management more than justify the resource outlay and are invariably gratifying. It is estimated that, by 2020, road traffic accidents will have moved from its present position of ninth to *third* in the world disease burden ranking, as measured in disability adjusted life years, and will be ranked second in developing countries (1). UK figures indicate a fairly steady hospital admission rate of 100 severely head injured persons per million population per year. This is the group which requires skilled critical care management. Similar figures show that 63 per cent of such persons harbour evidence of polytrauma. The recognition and management of polytrauma has a positive effect on the outcome of head injury.

Severe head-injury is *operationally defined* when a person with trauma is found to have a Glasgow Coma Scale Sum score of 8 or less, *postresuscitatively* at admission or during the ensuing 48 hours. An important current issue is the appropriate application of the Glasgow Coma Scale to *intubated* patients. The timing of *initial* scoring is another area of discussion. Despite its drawbacks, the Glasgow Coma Scale remains the most universally utilized level of consciousness scale worldwide (2).

Pathophysiology

Traditionally, the applied pathophysiology of brain injury is viewed from primary and secondary angles. Brain insult which is more or less complete *at impact*, is termed primary. The *ensuing* insult is termed secondary. Primary insults may be *focal* or *diffuse*. Focal (frontal, temporal, cortical-impact lesional) contusions or lacerations invariably progress to brain necrosis and gliosis. *Diffuse* axonal injury, triggered by brain shearing stress associated with acceleration forces, results over time in axolemmal disruption, altered axoplasmic flow, axonal retraction and notable disruption in neuroaxonal function. This latter process may finally lead to Wallerian degeneration.

Secondary insult is extremely common during the early post injury period, especially if this is associated with polytrauma. Hypotension, alterations in blood gases, pH, fever, anaemia, hyponatraemia and infection-related coagulopathies are among the systemic causes of secondary brain insult. Intracranial causes include brain oedema, intracranial hypertension, haematomas, dysautoregulation and vasospasm, infection and seizures. Secondary insults largely culminate in ischaemic-hypoxic pathological changes.

A growing and impressive body of evidence suggests that the brain, though not irrevocably damaged on initial impact, is subject to a series of cytotoxic processes, which portend gravely for outcome. Such processes include the release of free-radicals, lipid peroxidation of cell membranes, calcium-mediated cytosolic damage, cytokine release and the metabolism of free fatty acids to vasoactive substances, which lead to ischaemia. A state of *metabolic-perfusion mismatch* may thus exist, leading to generalized or focal neuropathologic alterations.

Free radicals are highly reactive molecules implicated in the pathology of traumatic brain injury, through a mechanism known as oxidative stress. After brain injury, reactive oxygen and reactive nitrogen species may be generated through several different cellular pathways. Increased production of free radicals will lead to oxidation of lipids, proteins, and nucleic acids, which may alter cellular function in a critical way. Substantial experimental data link oxidative stress with other pathogenic mechanisms such as excitotoxicity, calcium overload, mitochondrial cytochrome release, caspase activation, and apoptosis in central nervous system trauma (3). Antioxidant anaesthetics, such as thiopental and propofol, directly scavenge reactive oxygen species and inhibit lipid peroxidation, which has prompted re-evaluation of their utility in this setting (4).

We now have evidence of fairly close correlation between an initial Glasgow Coma Scale score of 8 or less and (18) F-FDG Positron Emission Tomography, performed within 5 days of injury, demonstrating a significant decrease in glucose metabolism in the thalamus, brain stem, and cerebellum. Further, the metabolic rate of glucose in these regions significantly correlated with the level of consciousness at the time of PET (5).

It appears prudent at this stage to accept that regeneration *does* occur, particularly in patients with diffuse axonal injury in whom there has been little disruption of the cellular skeleton of brain tissue. This may account for the late improvements observed in some patients with cranial trauma.

Assessment and Investigations

The goal of assessment is to define head and allied trauma as well as to determine the risk of ensuing deterioration in brain function. At the earliest opportunity, resuscitation and stabilization of vital parameters are undertaken. This is essential for *risk-free further evaluation*. Neurological assessment is made by using the Glasgow Coma Scale for best eye opening response, verbal and best motor responses, noting asymmetric responses in the latter (see Section on An Introduction to Critical Care). Painful stimuli must be applied both above the neck and on the limbs, preferably supraorbital, mastoid and nail beds of fingers and toes. The pupillary response to light is important to note; bilateral impairment may indicate a brain stem lesion. Unilateral impairment indicates optic or oculomotor nerve lesion, which must be further differentiated with the comparison of consensual and direct responses. Papilloedema is rare though intracranial hypertension is truly common. Clinical evidence of a focal neurological deficit must be carefully sought. The neck must be most gently handled, if at all, for fear of worsening associated cervical cord trauma (the best practice calls for using a collar routinely). The conclusions drawn from neurological examination are only valid if blood pressure and oxygenation are normalized. There has been some concern expressed over the validity of the Glasgow Coma Scale sum-score in *intubated* persons, since a verbal score is difficult to assign. This has led to greater weightage being given to motor responses in particular (**2, 6**). The early assessment of polytrauma is essential and must include thoracoabdominal assessment; this is an often neglected factor, which can have an adverse effect on neurological outcome. Routine haematological and biochemical investigations are always in order and must always include arterial blood gas estimation as well as serum osmolality.

The CT scan has added much logic to the management of head injury and should be requested in every severe case. The wider indications of CT scanning are any person with Glasgow Coma Score of 14 or less at 24 hours post-injury or with seizures or focal neurodeficit. Plain radiology of the cervical spine is also mandatory (if cervical CT is not obtained at the outset), as are chest films and clinically-indicated skeletal radiology.

A careful analysis of the brain CT scan in severe head injury yields valuable information. *Compression* or *obliteration* of the basal cisterns is associated with a sustained rise in intracranial pressure greater than 30 mm Hg early in their hospital course, in *55 per cent* and *75 per cent* of persons, respectively. The traditional classification of CT findings differentiates patients with intracranial haematomas or large contusions from patients with little or no obvious intracranial pathology. Haematomas are further classified into extradural, subdural or intracerebral. Contemporary experience suggests that severely head injured persons without intracerebral mass lesions with *major diffuse injury* form a non-homogenous group, whose CT findings may be further classified on the basis of cisternal morphology and midline shift, to yield useful early information on outcome (**7**). Those with no visible injury on CT have a fair-to-good outcome in 60 per cent of cases and mortality of less than 10 per cent. Those whose cisterns are preserved, who may have < 5 mm of midline shift and an estimated volume of < 25 ml of high or mixed density parenchymal lesions, have a fair-to-good outcome in up to 35 per cent of cases and about 14 per cent mortality. Those whose cisterns are compressed or obliterated, though midline shift may be < 5 mm and the volume of high or mixed density parenchymal lesions are < 25 ml, have a fair-to-good outcome in only 16 per cent of cases and a mortality of 34 per cent. When persons with cisternal changes have in addition a midline shift exceeding 5 mm in the absence of an evacuable mass lesions, a fair-to-good outcome is attained in but 6 per cent and mortality is around 55 per cent. Similarly, the reliability of the Traumatic Coma Data Bank CT scan classification (which grades the severity of injury as follows: I = normal, II = diffuse injury,

III = diffuse injury with swelling, IV = diffuse injury with shift, V = mass lesion surgically evacuated, or VI = mass lesion not operated) in predicting the outcome of severe head injury has been established (**8**). The most valid predictor of outcome in diffuse brain swelling is *intracranial pressure* (ICP) and its efficient treatment when elevated. This emphasizes the need for ICP monitoring, since prompt treatment of small rises in pressure may prevent the subsequent development of uncontrolled *intracranial hypertension* (ICH).

The other aspect of CT scanning is to confirm skull integrity. The discovery of fluid in the sphenoid sinus, intracranial air, penetrating head wound or depressed fracture all have implications on management and impending complications e.g. spinal fluid leak. MR imaging provides infinitely superior structural assessment of parenchymal brain insult (particularly of the brain stem, the craniovertebral region and to a variable extent, the cervical spinal cord) and is exquisitely sensitive in detecting blood and blood products. Emerging literature indicates statistically significant correlations between patterns of MR-identified brain injury and outcome (**9**). MR angiography of neck and brain vessels, an essentially non-invasive technique, is another powerful tool. The utility and scope of functional MR imaging still remain to be fully explored in traumatic brain injury. The drawbacks of MR imaging are its availability, inferior visualization of bony structures, time and patient co-operation required and problems associated with the use of exclusively nonferromagnetic resuscitative apparatus in the MR suite. Invasive angiography may have a limited role in assessment.

Critical Care

In the light of contemporary understanding of the pathophysiology of traumatic brain insult, treatment must be directed at early limitation of the cascade of brain events which invariably follow *primary* brain damage, prevention, early detection and control of *secondary* factors and the maintenance of optimal brain perfusion and metabolic milieu, in line with general systemic homeostasis.

To ensure that the *airway* is patent and tissue oxygenation adequate, early endotracheal intubation and ventilatory support are being increasingly employed. This implies that the *pre-intubation* clinical assessment (the initial Glasgow Coma Scale score) be carefully recorded before the administration of sedative or relaxant drugs. Vital parameters *must* be normalized, as far as is possible. The impact of suboptimal blood pressure on neurological outcome cannot be overemphasized. It is a safe rule to presume that hypotension (systolic blood pressure < 90 mm Hg) indicates injuries other than brain injury.

Monitoring Considerations

Traumatic brain injury impairs several brain and systemic regulatory mechanisms. In addition, the injured brain is extremely vulnerable to transient dysequilibrium in vital functions. For example, a single episode of raised ICP or systemic hypotension lasting a few minutes may be sufficient to jeopardize brain circulation critically. Subsequent restoration of these factors may be unable to arrest the inexorable progress to brain death. Thus, a *pre-emptive* approach is essential to the management of traumatic brain injury.

Current methods used to assess brain physiology and its derangements include the continuous monitoring of mean systemic arterial pressure, ICP, *cerebral perfusion pressure* (CPP) and cerebral metabolism and oxygenation. Further, the effect of systemic events on brain function must be assessed as they are detected. Arterial oxygen saturation monitoring, using continuous pulse oximety and arterial blood gas estimations from time to time, is of the utmost importance; suboptimal brain oxygenation contributes significantly to poor outcome. Though the use of ICP monitoring carries small but established risks of infection (2–8 per cent), intracranial haemorrhage and epilepsy (1 per cent each), it is strongly advisable in the setting of severe head injury. The use of ICP monitoring makes the management of ICH and the regulation of CPP easier and more logical.

The frequency of raised ICP is as much as 80 per cent in comatose, head injured persons and is strongly associated with mortality and morbidity (10). Empirical and prophylactic therapy with steroids and barbiturates has proved unsuccessful. Ideally, therapy should be targeted at the *predominant* cause of the increase in ICP. In head injury these may be (i) an increase in cerebral blood volume best treated by hyperventilation and hypnotic drugs; (ii) an increase in brain water content best treated by osmotherapy and (iii) increased CSF outflow resistance best treated by CSF drainage. This last cause seldom predominates in head injury. We cannot rely on purely clinical indicators of raised ICP in the severely brain-injured, intubated and ventilated person. Moreover, the absence of conventional imaging signs of ICH are no guarantee of ICP being normal. Thus, it is advantageous to monitor ICP for at least three days post-injury, to cover the expected period for establishment of brain swelling. Monitoring should be continued for as long as ICH persists and may be discontinued after 48 hours of normal pressure trace. ICP should preferably be held under 20 mm Hg. Assuming that an intraventricular drain is in place, ICP should never be allowed to fall to zero or go negative, since this impedes pressure measurement and predisposes to catheter blockage.

In the supine patient, CPP is derived from the difference between mean arterial pressure and mean intracranial pressure (arterial and intracranial pressure transducers *must* be commonly *zero*-referenced at the level of the tragus). It is a helpful guide to the adequacy of cerebral circulation. In normal humans, CPP is in the range of 70 to 100 mm Hg; it should be maintained at the lower end of this range in the trauma setting. Conventionally, if CPP drops to 60 mm Hg for > 5 minutes, any elevation of ICP requires treatment. In the setting of suspected vasospasm, the CPP may be required to be maintained at the upper limit of the normal range.

Much valuable information may be obtained by monitoring cerebral metabolism and oxygenation (11). One such method is to continuously or intermittently monitor jugular venous oxygen saturation ($J\bar{v}SO_2$), which is normally 55 to 85 per cent. Values higher than normal are an index of generalized cerebral hyperaemia or brain death and values lower than normal indicate that cerebral blood flow (CBF) is reduced; the latter may herald impending ischaemia. More recent methods, of monitoring promise, are cerebral microdialysis for the measurement of brain oxygenation as well as for obtaining trends of brain lactate, aspartate, glutamate, adenosine and free radicals. Velocity of intracranial blood flow, notably in the middle cerebral artery, may be measured intermittently by using transcranial Doppler sonography. This again yields information on CPP and may indicate isolated major vessel spasm.

In the paralyzed and ventilated patient, monitoring EEG waveform with a method such as compressed spectral array may provide reassuring information of neurological function. It would also indicate seizures, which have been masked by muscle relaxants, but which may nonetheless cause bewildering haemodynamic swings.

Surgical Considerations

In cases where CT scan indicates an extra cerebral haematoma associated with > 5 mm of midline shift or an estimated volume of > 25 ml or both, urgent evacuation should be obtained. The patient's level of arousal is an appropriate guide to the urgency of evacuation: a sizeable haematoma in a person with rapidly sinking arousal or coma requires urgent evacuation. In such situations, minutes may count and a large bolus dose of mannitol (1mg/kg) should be administered *interim*.

The role of early operative treatment in the management of intracerebral haematomas and haemorrhagic contusions is controversial. While a school of thought favours early surgery, the increasing trend is to manage such persons conservatively at first, relying upon the level of arousal as well as continuous arterial and ICP monitoring. These parameters, clinical deterioration and repeat CT scan to demonstrate an increase in mass effect may then prompt operative evacuation. It is advisable to obtain a neurosurgical consultation earlier rather than later.

The other situation in which early neurosurgical intervention may be necessary is for complex head wounds such as compound, depressed skull fractures. This type of trauma may be associated with a dural tear in up to 50 per cent of cases. It is important that debridement, removal of contaminant materials and haematoma, as well as secure wound closure be attained as early as possible but preferably within six hours. It is advisable to bid for optimal operating conditions and to minimize brain swelling so that brain extrusions be avoided through such compound, infected wounds.

Medical Considerations

Persons are usually nursed in the supine position with a 20° to 30° head-high and with the head usually maintained neutral, so as to avoid jugular venous flow impediment. Tapes around the neck should be avoided on similar grounds. In persons who are artificially ventilated, arterial PCO_2 is kept between 25 and 30 mm Hg, and SaO_2 maintained as close to 100 per cent as possible, employing an increase in FIO_2 and positive end expiratory pressure (PEEP), if necessary. The latter may require to be *individualized*, since not all persons with intracranial hypertension (ICH) tolerate it without sustaining *detrimental* alterations in cardiac output or ICP. In fact, an increase in ICP is an important adverse effect of

PEEP; its effect on CPP is variable though significantly less disturbing (12).

Arterial pressure should not be allowed to fall. The commoner causes of hypotension are hypovolaemia (due either to inadequate fluid replacement or misplaced 'keeping dry') and the use of sedative drugs such as barbiturates. ICP should ideally be held below 20 mm Hg. Moderate increases up to even 30 mm Hg may be tolerated, so long as arterial pressure is sufficient to support a CPP of 70 mm Hg or more. On occasion, it may be necessary to support arterial pressure to support CPP; there is no consensus as yet on the pressor agent of choice though some observations favour norepinephrine over dopamine (13), particularly in terms of the effect these agents may have on ICP. If ICP rises above 25 mm Hg, simple extracranial causes must first be checked: is neck position neutral and unrotated? Is the airway obstructed? Is the effect of relaxants wearing off and leading to the person 'bucking' the ventilator? Is there an elevation in arterial PCO_2 or a fall in PO_2? Is there fever or occult seizure activity? On relaxants, the latter may be difficult to detect; bilateral pupillary dilatation, mild arterial pressure elevation and substantial ICP elevation is sometimes a useful diagnostic triad. EEG monitoring readily answers the question. Free-water overloading and resultant dilutional hyponatraemia is another important cause of ICH. An important factor leading to unexplained, delayed deterioration and ICH is delayed haemorrhage; this may manifest anywhere from 8 hours to 13 days, post injury.

When ICP rises above 25 mm Hg within the first 48 hours of injury, or above 30 mm Hg thereafter, CPP stands jeopardized; if simple measures fail to control ICH, specific therapy may be required. It is therapeutically useful to consider ICH as being due to *vascular* and *non-vascular* causes. Underlying vascular ICH is due to vasodilatation, with a resultant increase in venous and capillary intravascular volume leading to increased intracranial pressure. A logical step to counter the situation is purposeful hyperventilation with a reduction in $PaCO_2$ to 25 mm Hg. This leads to cerebral vasoconstriction with a resultant fall in intracranial pressure. The effects of this measure are relatively short-lived, since there is the very real risk of precipitating irreversible ischaemic change. If $J\bar{v}SO_2$ is being monitored, a fall to 45 per cent or less will clearly be an indicator of critical reduction of blood flow and impending brain ischaemia. Moreover, the more enduring forms of treatment are ineffective if cerebrovascular CO_2 reactivity is dampened. Longer term therapy of vascular ICH may be attempted with the continuous infusion of hypnotics (e.g. midazolam), thiopentone sodium, propofol and perhaps, indomethacin. Again, hypotension and impending ischaemia must be guarded against when using these drugs over some duration. Monitoring cerebral oxygenation with $J\bar{v}SO_2$ or with one of the methods mentioned above would be prudent.

In treating ICH of non-vascular origin, intravenous mannitol is appropriate. The lowest effective dose is administered as a *rapid* bolus; it is wise to start with 0.25 g/kg and optimize, as determined by the ICP response. Monitoring ICP makes this an easier and more logical exercise, minimizing the dangers of mannitol overuse.

The effect of this therapy may be enhanced by co-administering furosemide (1 mg/kg) and following mannitol by albumin infusion. A serum osmolality of > 320 mOsm/l *contraindicates* further osmotherapy, which would probably be ineffective as well as harmful to renal function.

Problems related to pulmonary care, deep venous thrombosis and pulmonary embolism, coagulopathies, fluid and electrolyte balance and nutrition are considered elsewhere.

Controversial Areas

Evidence-based medical practice does not, currently, support the use of *steroids* in the treatment of acute brain injury or acute post-traumatic brain oedema. Several studies have shown either variable or inconclusive results; moreover, existing trials are either too small or lack the statistical power to significantly demonstrate or to refute the possibility of a moderate but clinically important benefit. At this point in time, therefore, we desist from using them routinely. The Corticosteroid Randomization After Significant Head Injury (CRASH) trial is a large-scale, randomized, controlled trial, among adults with head injury and impaired consciousness, to evaluate the effects of a short-term infusion of corticosteroids on death and on neurological disability (14). The study will only be completed c. 2005. The use of steroids in the setting of unexpectedly delayed recovery is also controversial and open to study.

On closer review, *phenytoin prophylaxis* has been found to significantly lower the risk of *early* post-traumatic seizures (those occurring within 7 days after injury) as compared to controls (15). Anti-epileptic drug prophylaxis is probably not effective in decreasing the risk of *late* post-traumatic seizures; this is still an area of controversy, however. Thus, post-traumatic epilepsy occurring a week or more after head injury ought to be managed by conventional anti-epileptic drugs.

Opinions are sharply divided on the use of *prophylactic antimicrobials* in patients with intracranial air, CSF rhinorrhoea or CSF otorrhoea. They are clearly at increased risk of developing meningitis. Prophylactic antimicrobial use may encourage the development of antibiotic-resistant strains. While we do not advocate their prophylactic use, we remain watchful for the earliest indicators of meningitis and advise *early CSF examination*.

In Sweden, there exists a treatment protocol which is widely employed and which is based upon *the Lund concept*. At the heart of the Lund hypothesis are the following: the reduction of cerebral oedema by normalizing a high hydrostatic capillary pressure, using colloids to achieve normovolaemia, simultaneously normalizing colloid osmotic absorption pressure; and reducing filtration by antihypertensive therapy. Hyperventilation and mannitol osmotherapy are very sparingly used; barbiturate therapy is also handled differently. Though promising, some degree of controversy surrounds this treatment protocol, even among its proponents in Sweden (16).

The use of *neuroprotective agents*, largely targeted at free radicals, excitatory metabolites and their receptors, is still under evaluation and therefore is not common practice.

Outcome

The outcome of head injury must be viewed in terms of both *survival* and *disability*; and we learn, increasingly, that early and appropriate critical care has an impact on both these factors. When considering the use of the *initial* GCS for prognosis, the two most important problems are the reliability of the initial measurement, and its lack of precision for prediction of a good outcome if the initial GCS is low. If the initial GCS is reliably obtained and not tainted by prehospital medications or intubation, approximately 20 per cent of the patients with the worst initial GCS will survive and 8–10 per cent will have a functional survival (Glasgow Outcome Scale 4–5) **(17)**. Recent figures, based on a large series and a 20-year meta-analysis, indicate that mortality rate (at 6 months) and unfavorable outcome (assessed on the Glasgow Outcome Scale) *increased with age*: 21 and 39 per cent, respectively, for patients younger than 35 years and 52 and 74 per cent, respectively, for patients older than 55 years **(18)**.

Secondary events such as persistent ICH, low CPP and impaired cerebral metabolism appear to contribute significantly to poorer survival rates and greater disability figures. The critical care unit provides the basis for the early recognition and rapid attempted reversal of secondary insult. Neither should we forget the ongoing contribution of the critical care unit to the better understanding of the pathophysiology of traumatic brain insult and to its more appropriate management. The impact of the latter in mitigating disability and thus enhancing the quality of life in survivors and their families, must surely be *the* justification for our endeavours in the critical care of head injury.

REFERENCES

1. Murray C, Lopez A. (1996). Global Health Statistics. Boston, MA. Harvard University Press.

2. Sternbach GL. (2000). The Glasgow coma scale. J Emerg Med. 19, 67–71.

3. Lewén A, Matz P, Chan PH. (2000). Free radical pathways in CNS injury. J Neurotrauma. 17, 871–890.

4. Wilson JX, Gelb AW. (2002). Free radicals, antioxidants, and neurologic injury: possible relationship to cerebral protection by anesthetics. J Neurosurg Anesthesiol. 14, 66–79.

5. Hattori N, Huang SC, Wu HM et al. (2003). Correlation of regional metabolic rates of glucose with glasgow coma scale after traumatic brain injury. J Nucl Med. 44, 1709–1716.

6. Healey C, Osler TM, Rogers FB et al. (2003). Improving the Glasgow Coma Scale score: motor score alone is a better predictor. J Trauma. 54, 671–678; discussion 678–680.

7. Marshall LF, Bowers Marshall S, Klauber MR et al. (1991). A new classification of head injury based on computerized tomography. J Neurosurg. 75 (suppl), S14–20

8. Vos PE, van Voskuilen AC, Beems T et al. (2001). Evaluation of the traumatic coma data bank computed tomography classification for severe head injury. J Neurotrauma. 18, 649–655.

9. Firsching R, Woischneck D, Klein S et al. (2001). Classification of severe head injury based on magnetic resonance imaging. Acta Neurochir (Wien). 143, 263–271.

10. Miller JD, Piper IR, Dearden NM. (1993). Management of intracranial hypertension in head injury: matching treatment with cause. Acta Neurochir Suppl (Wien). 57, 152–159.

11. Sarrafzadeh AS, Kiening KL, Unterberg AW. (2003). Neuromonitoring: brain oxygenation and microdialysis. Curr Neurol Neurosci Rep. 3, 517–523.

12. Videtta W, Villarejo F, Cohen M, et al. (2002). Effects of positive end-expiratory pressure on intracranial pressure and cerebral perfusion pressure. Acta Neurochir Suppl. 81, 93–97.

13. Ract C, Vigué B. (2001). Comparison of the cerebral effects of dopamine and norepinephrine in severely head-injured patients. Intensive Care Med. 27, 101–106.

14. Roberts I. CRASH Trial Management Group. (2001). The CRASH trial: the first large-scale, randomised, controlled trial in head injury. Critical Care. 5, 292–293 www.crash.lshtm.ac.uk

15. Chang BS, Lowenstein DH; Quality Standards Subcommittee of the American Academy of Neurology. (2003). Practice parameter: antiepileptic drug prophylaxis in severe traumatic brain injury: report of the Quality Standards Subcommittee of the American Academy of Neurology. Neurology. 60, 10–16.

16. Naredi S, Koskinen LO, Grande PO et al. (2003). Treatment of traumatic head injury—US/European Guidelines or the Lund Concept. Crit Care Med. 31, 2713–2714

17. The Brain Trauma Foundation. The American Association of Neurological Surgeons. The Joint Section on Neurotrauma and Critical Care. (2000). Glasgow coma scale score. J Neurotrauma. 17, 563–571.

18. Hukkelhoven CW, Steyerberg EW, Rampen AJ et al. (2003). Patient age and outcome following severe traumatic brain injury: an analysis of 5600 patients. J Neurosurg. 99, 666–673.

C. ACUTE STROKE

Dr Sarosh M. Katrak & Dr Noshir H. Wadia

General Considerations

Strokes are one of the major causes of admission and death in any large general hospital. In the last 20 years the mortality of strokes has considerably reduced because of the recognition and treatment of the various risk factors. However, even today, a large ischaemic infarct carries a mortality of about 15 per cent and this increases to 30–50 per cent for large intracerebral haemorrhages, the final common terminal events being due to a rise of intracranial pressure. The other common causes of death following strokes are aspiration pneumonia, pulmonary embolism, cardiac arrhythmias and myocardial infarction.

A patient presenting with a stroke constitutes an emergency, and often requires critical care. Recent advances in basic and clinical research have shown potential for improvement in stroke patients, the main thrust being in the field of reperfusion and neuronal protection. All these newer therapies have to be administered within a time frame which constitutes the 'therapeutic window'. Patients with strokes should, therefore, be admitted as soon as possible into centres capable of treating stroke patients. Intensive stroke care units have had an impact in reducing the mortality and morbidity (1). The guidelines for a proper evaluation and treatment of strokes are given here in order to form a rational basis of therapy based on the recent advances in stroke management.

Classification of Strokes

The term 'stroke' usually applies to any form of cerebrovascular disease with either permanent or transient focal symptoms. These may be either ischaemic or haemorrhagic, the latter being further subdivided into parenchymatous bleed or subarachnoid haemorrhage (SAH). In Western centres, approximately 10 per cent of such patients would present with a transient attack (TIA). Unfortunately in India, patients usually present with a completed stroke and in an emergency setting this may constitute a large infarct or cerebral haemorrhage. The differentiation between a haemorrhagic and ischaemic stroke is important, as therapy is different for these two subtypes. Clinical indicators for an intracerebral haemorrhage may be a rapid deterioration in the level of consciousness, headache, vomiting and an elevated blood pressure. This differentiation is not always clear, and a CT scan should be done in all stroke patients as soon as possible as this is the most reliable way to differentiate between a haemorrhage and an infarct.

A SAH usually presents with a severe *de novo* headache with hardly any focal neurological weakness in the initial phases. Again, a CT scan with thin cuts through the basal cistern should be performed to confirm the diagnosis. Occasionally, the CT scan does not confirm the diagnosis when there is a small bleed or if the scan is performed after a delay of a few days. Under these circumstances, it is important to perform a lumbar puncture and examine the CSF for blood or xanthochromia.

The subclassification of ischaemic strokes is difficult but from a clinical and emergency unit setting may be divided into the following subgroups:

1. TIA/Residual ischaemic neurological deficit (RIND).
2. Large artery atherosclerotic infarcts due to stenosis or occlusion.
3. Embolic infarcts: the embolus most commonly arises from the heart or thoracic aorta.
4. Arteritis.
5. Dissection of carotid or vertebral arteries in the neck.
6. Infarct with unknown cause—source of embolus not found.

The basic pathology underlying these clinical subtypes is thrombosis or embolism or a combination of both. It is again important to make this distinction as aetiologies producing either thrombosis or embolism are different and further treatment for stroke prevention are likewise different. Patients with thrombosis usually have multiple risk factors producing atherosclerosis, whereas patients with embolism may have a history suggestive of arrhythmias or valvular disease. Embolic infarcts tend to be more cortical whereas thrombotic infarcts involve major vascular territories.

Arteritis is usually suspected in patients who are relatively young and without the usual risk factors. These patients may also have multifocal symptoms and signs. Dissection should be suspected in any patient with a stroke following physical exertion or trivial trauma and in patients with ischaemic strokes preceded by severe pain in the anterior (carotid dissection) or posterior (vertebral dissection) part of the neck. Haematological disorders can also underlie strokes. Sickle cell disease, polycythaemia, thrombocytosis, hypercoagulable states and excessive leucocytosis (leukaemia) are some of the conditions associated with strokes.

Diagnostic Evaluation

The purpose of diagnostic studies after a stroke is to establish the type of stroke, the probable aetiology and the systemic complications.

The most common and reliable method of differentiating the type of stroke is the CT scan. It is highly reliable in distinguishing a cerebral haemorrhage from an infarct. This distinction helps in the decision of whether to control the blood pressure actively in haemorrhage or to avoid precipitous drop of blood pressure in ischaemic strokes. It also helps in deciding whether to employ anticoagulant therapy. Once this decision has been made, further evaluation is needed to determine the probable aetiology. In an atypical intracerebral haemorrhage, an MRI scan increases the likelihood of detecting an arteriovenous malformation (AVM). If SAH has been detected on the CT scan, an arteriogram should be performed within the first 24–48 hours to detect an aneurysm or malformation. Surgery for clipping of the aneurysm or coiling through an endovascular route within the first 72 hours may reduce the mortality and morbidity from rebleeding. Angiography may also be required to detect arterial vasospasm following SAH, but transcranial Doppler ultrasound has largely replaced angiography for this purpose.

Patients with infarct in whom clinical examination suggests a cardio-embolic source, should have a 2-D echocardiogram and Holter monitoring for arrhythmias. If a cardiac source is strongly suspected and a 2-D echocardiogram is negative, a transoesophageal echocardiogram should be done and may detect abnormalities in the artial appendage or thoracic aorta in a large percentage of patients. Carotid ultrasound or MR angiography are commonly ordered in acute ischaemic stokes with clinical evidence of moderate or severe occlusive disease of the arteries. Recently, carotid endarterectomy has been proven to be effective for prevention of subsequent strokes in patients with TIAs or minor strokes associated with 70–99 per cent carotid stenosis (2). Hence careful evaluation of the extracranial carotid arteries is indicated in all patients with a carotid artery distribution of stroke and who are left with either mild or no neurological deficit. Such cases stress the importance of carotid Doppler ultrasound and MR angiography. Digital substraction angiography (DSA) should be carried out in all patients with severe carotid artery stenosis on Doppler or MR angiography, who are considered candidates for endarterectomy. DSA should also be performed in patients with a clinical syndrome suggestive of arterial dissection, vasculitis and cerebral venous occlusion.

Certain haematological and biochemical studies should be carried out in all stroke patients. These include a complete haemogram, platelet count, prothrombin time, partial thromboplastin time, blood urea nitrogen, creatinine, electrolytes, blood sugar and lipid profile. Other studies may be done in atypical strokes, strokes in the young or in patients with no risk factors and a stroke. These include studies for collagen vascular disease, anti-cardiolipin and anti-phospholipin antibodies, protein C and S, anti-thrombin III levels, serology for luetic infection and for HIV infection. An ECG and baseline chest X-ray should also be done for all patients. A lumbar puncture for CSF examination should be performed to detect SAH if this is suspected but not confirmed on CT scan, or in any patients in whom meningitis or vasculitis is suspected as an underlying pathology.

Thus the early clinical evaluation and diagnostic studies will basically divide the patients into three major categories of stroke, viz. acute ischaemic strokes, intracerebral haemorrhages and subarachnoid haemorrhage. The specific management differs in each subgroup, but certain principles of general management remain the same in all three groups.

General Management

In patients with completed stroke, careful attention to certain general measures helps in reducing mortality and morbidity. These 'vital signs' in stroke patients include blood pressure, temperature, seizure activity, oxygenation, intravascular volume and blood sugar.

Blood Pressure

Maintenance of adequate blood pressure is the single most important variable in the emergency care of the stroke patient. With a fluctuating basilar or carotid artery syndrome, most neurologists have the experience that rapid lowering of the blood pressure results in further deterioration. The problem is what should be the therapeutic approach in a patient with a static completed stroke and hypertension. Normally the cerebral blood flow (CBF) is autoregulated, i.e. the CBF remains fairly constant over a wide fluctuation of blood pressure. However, in the injured brain, autoregulation is often lost, so that CBF passively follows mean arterial blood pressure. Secondly, in hypertensive patients the auto-regulatory curve is further shifted to the right so that the CBF begins to fall at a higher mean arterial blood pressure. Hence, in patients with acute cerebral infarction the blood pressure should be lowered cautiously. Active reduction of blood pressure with parenteral drugs is only indicated in acute cerebral haemorrhage or in cases of cerebral infarction where there is evidence of angina or myocardial damage, hypertensive encephalopathy, acute renal damage, or when thrombolytic therapy is indicated. If the blood pressure has to be reduced, the best drug is either a parenteral beta-blocker such as labetalol or an infusion of nitroprusside. The advantage of nitroprusside is that the dose can be titrated to maintain the blood pressure at a desired level. However, nitroprusside is a cerebral vasodilator and can result in further rise of ICP in patients who already have a mass effect due to a large cerebral haematoma or infarct. In patients with cerebral infarct and moderate hypertension (systolic BP 170–200 mm and a diastolic BP of 90–110 mm of Hg) the recommendation is to withhold antihypertensive therapy in the acute stage as this is a reactive hypertension and the blood pressure spontaneously lowers over the next few days. Wallace and Levy (3), found that 84 per cent of 334 consecutive stroke patients had elevated blood pressure whereas only 50 per cent had a preceding history of hypertension. The blood pressure spontaneously declined on an average by 20 mm of Hg systolic and 10 mm of Hg diastolic in the first ten days following the stroke. This has been confirmed by other studies (4–6). Hence aggressive lowering of the blood pressure is detrimental to acute stroke patients. If the blood pressure remains elevated, it should be gradually lowered using oral therapy with an ACE inhibitor or a calcium antagonist. Sublingual use of a calcium antagonist should be avoided as it can produce a precipitous decline in the blood pressure. If antihypertensive therapy is used, the blood pressure should be carefully monitored and the dosage reduced as the blood pressure drops in the subsequent weeks after a stroke.

Temperature

It is now well recognized that hypothermia substantially reduces infarct size whereas hyperthermia increases cerebral damage by increasing the metabolic rate. For each degree celsius rise of body temperature the cerebral metabolic rate increases by 5–7 per cent. Many patients with strokes have aspiration pneumonia or pulmonary embolism complicating their stroke. Hence fever and the cause of infection should be scrupulously sought out and treated with appropriate antipyretics and antibiotics.

Seizure Activity

Seizure activity increases the cerebral metabolic requirements and if prolonged causes neuronal death even under normal circumstances and more so in the injured brain.

Oxygenation

Hypoxia will produce anaerobic metabolism increasing the levels of lactates and hydrogen ions in the brain thereby producing further brain damage. The most common causes of hypoxia in a stroke patient are aspiration pneumonia, pulmonary embolism or congestive heart failure. Aspiration usually results from premature oral feeding. In the early phases of a stroke, the patient's nutrition should be maintained by nasogastric tube feeding.

Blood Sugar Levels

Both hyperglycaemia and hypoglycaemia damage the injured brain. In experimental animals blood glucose levels greater than 155 mg/dl increase infarct size and worsen prognosis (7). Hence the patient must be maintained in a euglycaemic state.

All these simple but vital signs must be paid the utmost attention. The most important consideration is that the nurses and other paramedical personnel should be trained to observe the patient carefully so that fluctuations in the neurological status can be recognized and corrected appropriately, thus maximizing standard medical management. These are the benefits of a team in a dedicated stroke unit (1).

Acute Ischaemic Infarct

The three main strategies for treating acute cerebral infarction are (1) antithrombotic therapy, (2) reperfusion therapy and (3) neuronal protection.

1. Antithrombotic Therapy

Antithrombotic therapy is done with anticoagulants such as heparin followed by warfarin and with anti-platelet drugs. The indications for anticoagulant therapy have been clearly delineated and include (a) progressive stroke—unstable or progressive neurological deficit, (b) TIA/RIND associated with severe internal carotid artery stenosis, (c) embolic stroke due to a cardiogenic source, particularly non-valvular atrial fibrillation in the elderly, (d) cortical venous thrombosis and (e) dissection of the carotid or vertebral artery with thrombus formation. Most neurologists would use anticoagulants in the above situations. In the acute stage, intravenous infusion of heparin is started at the rate of 800–1000 IU/hour keeping the partial thromboplastin time and clotting time at 1.5 to 2.0 times the control value. In TIA/RIND associated with severe ICA stenosis, anticoagulation is usually employed prior to carotid endarterectomy. In cardiogenic embolization, anticoagulation has been proven to reduce recurrent embolization (8). However, with a large haemorrhagic infarct, anticoagulant therapy would be hazardous. Routine anticoagulation therapy after an ischaemic stroke, which does not fit into the above categories, cannot be justified as the risk of haemorrhagic complications is high.

The use of low molecular weight heparin has been shown to be effective and is associated with low rates of haemorrhagic complications.

Aspirin is the most commonly used anti-platelet drug and has been shown to reduce the incidence of subsequent TIAs and strokes in patients who are at risk. The recent IST and CAST studies involving approximately 40,000 patients have shown the value of aspirin in the acute stage of ischaemic strokes (9, 10).

2. Reperfusion Therapy

Reperfusion therapy is basically aimed at increasing cerebral blood flow and limiting the size of the infarct. Initially, vasodilators were tried for this purpose but have proven ineffective as the blood vessels in the ischaemic area are already maximally dilated. Subsequently, urgent thrombectomy was tried but went into disrepute because of excessive haemorrhagic complications and deterioration in the clinical state. Because thrombosis or embolic arterial occlusion are the leading causes of infarct, pharmacological therapy for arterial recanalization through thrombolysis is now gaining widespread attention and has replaced the above two methods for reperfusion. Intra-arterial streptokinase and urokinase as well as intra-venous tissue plasminogen activator (tPA) have been tried. The benefits of thrombolytic therapy are that it re-establishes blood flow, improves the ischaemic penumbra and thereby limits the size of the infarct. The risks involve rethrombosis, distal embolization, reperfusion tissue damage mainly haemorrhagic complications, and cerebral oedema. Early experience with urokinase and streptokinase were not very encouraging as they carried a high risk of haemorrhage, but therapy was started late—after 24–48 hours—and was done prior to the CT scan etc. Hence, small lobar haematomas could have been missed with deterioration in the patient's condition.

Recently, more 'clot specific' thrombolytic agents have been developed and the maximum experience is with tPA which is produced by a recombinant DNA technique. The advantages of tPA are that its functional half-life is approximately 5 minutes compared to about 16 minutes for urokinase and 23 minutes for streptokinase. Thus the thrombolytic action of the drug disappears shortly after the infusion is discontinued. Secondly, it is very 'clot specific' because of its high affinity for plasminogen in the presence of fibrin. This allows efficient activation of plasminogen in the clot but very little activation in the plasma. Hence, the systemic effects are modest. Lastly, it is non-antigenic and has practically no adverse reaction other than bleeding. In the mid 1990s, many double blind placebo controlled clinical trials were conducted to assess the clinical efficacy of tPA. The studies had negative results. The National Institute of Neurological Disorders and Strokes (NINDS) tPA stroke study (11) was the first and only clinical trial that showed beneficial results of intravenous tPA. There were several reasons for this success. The 'door to needle' time in the NINDS study was less than 3 hours with a median time of 90 minutes and the investigators used a lower dose compared to the other investigators who used larger 'coronary' doses. Patients included in the study were required to meet strict entry criteria (see **Table 15.10.3**).

Once the entry criteria were met, the patient was given

Table 15.10.3. Inclusion and exclusion criteria for the NINDS rt-PA Stroke Study

Inclusion

1. Ischaemic stroke with clearly defined symptom onset
2. Measurable deficit on NIH Stroke Scale
3. No evidence of intracranial blood on brain CT
4. 180 minutes or less from the time of symptom onset to initiation of rt-PA

Exclusion

1. Rapidly improving stroke symptoms
2. Stroke or serious head trauma within 3 months
3. Major surgery within 14 days
4. History of intracranial haemorrhage
5. Systolic BP > 185 mm Hg or diastolic > 110 mm Hg at the time of treatment initiation
6. Suspected SAH despite normal CT scan
7. Gastrointestinal or urinary haemorrhage within 21 days
8. Arterial puncture at a non-compressible site within 7 days
9. Seizure at onset of stroke
10. Use of heparin within 48 hours and elevated aPTT
11. PT > 15 seconds, platelet count < 100,000, glucose < 50 or > 400 mg/dl

NIH—National Institute of Health
aPTT—Activated Partial Thromboplastin Time
PT—Prothrombin Time

0.9 mg/kg body weight of tPA with a maximum dose of 90 mg. A 10 per cent bolus dose was given intravenously over one minute, with the remaining dose given over the following one hour. Antiplatelet and anticoagulants were prohibited over the next 24 hours, and the BP was monitored vigorously and treated with intravenous labetalol or sodium nitroprusside infusion when indicated. A favourable outcome was documented by three separate outcome scales. Although 6.4 per cent of patients in the tPA group had symptomatic intracerebral haemorrhage (compared to 0.6 per cent in the placebo group) the beneficial effect of tPA was well documented. A post-hoc analysis of cost effectiveness in the NINDS study found that therapy with tPA significantly reduces the cost of care (12). Since then, tPA has been used in several centres in the United States. In spite of protocol violations, varying from 32.6 to 54.5 per cent, the rate of symptomatic intracerebral haemorrhage was comparable to the NINDS study (13–15). The most common protocol violations were use of antiplatelet and anticoagulant drugs within the first 24 hours, inclusion of patients with an increased blood pressure and initiation of therapy after 3 hours. The rate of symptomatic intracerebral haemorrhage was much higher in these patients (11 per cent versus 4 per cent in non-violators) in one study (13). In India, very few centres have started thrombolytic therapy. The main constraints are the cost of tPA and more importantly very few patients come to the hospital within the 'therapeutic window' time. The latter is essentially due to a lack of awareness of the symptoms of stroke and difficulties in commuting to major hospitals in large cities like Mumbai.

In order to expand the 'therapeutic window' to 6 hours, the Prourokinase in Acute Thromboembolism trials, (PROACT-I and PROACT-II), were designed to assess safety, frequency of recanalization and clinical efficacy of recombinant prourokinase (r-proUK) directly into an occluded M1 or M2 segment of the middle cerebral artery (**16, 17**). Results from these studies showed that the frequency of recanalization was significantly more in the r-proUK group. The rate of symptomatic intracerebral haemorrhage was 15.4 per cent and was dependent upon the administered dose of heparin. The results of PROACT II show that there is a 15 per cent absolute increase in favourable outcome in the prourokinase treated group despite a frequency of symptomatic intracerebral haemorrhage of 10 per cent at 24 hours. Because r-proUK is not yet approved by the FDA in the United States, many clinicians use intra-arterial tPA.

3. Neuronal Protection

The list of neuroprotective drugs that have failed in acute ischaemic strokes is given in **Table 15.10.4**. The possible clinical explanation for failure may be long window of opportunity employed, the variable severity of the stroke studies and inappropriate drug delivery systems (the drug may not reach the target tissue).

Treatment of Cerebral Oedema after Infarction

Massive cerebral oedema with central or uncal herniation may complicate 10 per cent of large hemispheric infarcts. This oedema usually reaches a peak after 2–5 days. Initially the patient may be drowsy but with increasing oedema the level of consciousness deteriorates with an ipsilateral fixed dilated pupil and a positive Babinski's sign. When the level of consciousness deteriorates after cerebral infarction, the prime concern is reduction of intracranial pressure. The therapy for raised ICP after an ischaemic stroke is

Table 15.10.4. Overview of neuroprotection drug studies

Mechanism of action	Agent tested	Result
Anti-adhesion molecule	ICAM Ab, CD18 Ab	Study terminated: unsuccessful
Na+ channel antagonist	Fosphenytoin	Study terminated: unsuccessful
Ca+ channel blocker	Nimodipine	Negative results
	Flunarizine	Study terminated: unsuccessful
	Lubelozole	Study terminated: unsuccessful
Free radical scavengers	Tirilazad	Study terminated: unsuccessful
	Ebselen	Negative results
Glutamate antagonists	Selfotel	Negative results
	Eliprodil	Study terminated: unsuccessful
	Aptiganel	Study terminated: unsuccessful
Opioid antagonists	Nalmefene	Negative results
GABA agonists	Clomethiazole	Study terminated: unsuccessful
K+ channel modulation	BMS-204352	To be reported

the same in principle as outlined under increased intracranial pressure (ICP).

Since the mid 1990s, there is a resurgence of interest in decompressive hemicraniotomy (lateral-coronal skull bone removal) to relieve compression from acute grossly expanding cerebral hemisphere after a total occlusion of the middle cerebral artery (18, 19). In this situation, the mortality rates are as high as 80 per cent (18) and early i.e. within 24 hours decompressive hemicraniotomy improves both mortality and morbidity.

Intracerebral Haemorrhage

The management of intracerebral haemorrhage (ICH) is dependent upon the aetiology, location and size of the intracranial haematoma. Arterial hypertension is the presumed cause in 70–90 per cent of patients. It produces fibrinoid necrosis of the penetrating vessels of 80–300 μ diameter arising from the Circle of Willis or the basilar artery. Hence the characteristic location of hypertensive ICH is basal ganglia (35–45 per cent), subcortical white matter (25 per cent), thalamus (20 per cent), cerebellum (15 per cent), and pons (5 per cent). In about 10–30 per cent of patients with ICH, there is no evidence of hypertension and in patients over the age of 65 years, amyloid angiopathy is the most common cause after hypertension. The other aetiologies producing ICH are aneurysms, particularly during re-bleeding, AVMs, bleed into a tumour, abnormal coagulation, arteritis and haemorrhagic infarction from venous occlusion. Advances in therapy for ischaemic vascular disease have also been associated with increased incidence of brain haemorrhages, as mentioned earlier.

Clinical Syndromes

ICH presents abruptly with a rapid evolution of symptoms and signs. Headache and vomiting are often the initial symptoms soon followed by a change in the level of consciousness from stupor to coma. In a putamenal haemorrhage, there is conjugate deviation of the eyes towards the ipsilateral hemisphere, whereas the eyes are deviated downwards and medially, i.e. towards the nose, in a thalamic haemorrhage. The level of consciousness is closely associated with the degree of horizontal displacement of midline structures and is therefore more likely with haematomas in the temporal lobe. Pontine haemorrhage is most likely to lead to deep coma with pinpoint pupils. The light reflex in such pupils is often preserved if the pupils are observed with a magnifying glass. The eyes are conjugate in the primary position but oculocephalic and oculovestibular reflexes are absent. Progression of signs ultimately leads to cessation of respiration.

In the clinical setting of intracerebral haemorrhage, it is important to recognize intracerebellar haemorrhage because early surgical intervention has reduced the mortality and morbidity considerably. Intracerebellar haemorrhages usually present with repeated vomiting and vertigo and an inability to walk because of loss of balance. As the haematoma expands, it presses upon the brainstem and produces conjugate gaze deviation away from the side of the haemorrhage. Dysarthria and facial weakness may also develop. As the brainstem is further compressed, there is impairment of the level of consciousness and this can progress rapidly to pinpoint pupils and decerebration. Once these signs are elicited, it may be too late for surgical intervention. Hence, the need to recognize early clinical features of cerebellar haemorrhage.

Management
Initial Evaluation

As mentioned above, ICH produces a characteristic pattern and progression of signs and these help in identifying the location of the haemorrhage. The initial neurological examination must be brief but comprehensive and is essentially directed to assess the level of consciousness which is vital for prognosis as well as for further management decisions. Patients presenting to the ICU in coma or rapidly becoming comatose have a mortality rate of over 50 per cent (20). Once the initial clinical evaluation is complete, one should direct attention to 'vital signs' (mentioned earlier in general management) and start appropriate measures. If the patient requires intubation, it should be performed expertly by an anaesthesiologist using either a short-acting anaesthetic agent or local anaesthesia of the pharynx and larynx. If the patient strains during intubation, the intracranial pressure rises but more seriously there is a risk of re-bleeding with a precipitous rise of blood pressure. Hyperventilation when on ventilator support, and intravenous mannitol are recommended if there is evidence of increased intracranial pressure. Corticosteroids are not recommended in many units as they are not proven to be of use (21). However, some units continue to use dexamethasone 4 mg intravenously six-hourly in patients with raised intracranial pressure.

Hypertension is almost invariably seen after ICH. It should be reduced so that re-bleeding does not occur. For this purpose a systolic blood pressure of around 160 mm of Hg is ideal. Intravenous infusion of nitroprusside or a parenteral beta-blocker such as labetalol should be used for this purpose. However it is not prudent to reduce the systolic blood pressure in every patient of hypertensive intracerebral bleed. Patients with a large haemorrhage and a rise of ICP will require higher levels of systolic blood pressure in order to maintain adequate CPP. Once the patient has been clinically evaluated and emergency management initiated, the patient usually stabilizes to some extent and is then sent for CT scan evaluation.

Radiological Evaluation

The CT scan has revolutionized the diagnosis and management of ICH by allowing rapid anatomical diagnosis. It confirms the diagnosis reliably, assesses the size and location of the haematoma and also the extent of concomitant ventricular, subarachnoid and subdural blood. Hypertensive ICHs have a predilection for certain specific locations around the basal ganglia. Hence, if a haematoma is in an unusual location or has odd features, a contrast enhanced CT or MR scan must be performed to look for an underlying aneurysm, AVM or a neoplasm. With aneurysmal rupture the haematoma is either in the frontal or temporal lobe, largely within and around the Sylvian fissure. Digital subtraction angiography (DSA) is usually not part of the routine evaluation but if there is any doubt on a contrast enhanced CT scan, it should be performed as a DSA is the mainstay for identifying aneurysms. Re-bleeding from an aneurysm carries a high mortality; therefore an early DSA would give sufficient time to plan appropriate surgical clipping of an aneurysm. DSA also helps in identifying arteriovenous malformations and planning further management, i.e. either surgery or interventional radiology. Uncommonly, a malformation may be missed in an early DSA as the haemorrhage compresses and thereby 'masks' the malformation. If the suspicion of a malformation is high, then a DSA should be repeated after 2–3 weeks.

Specific Management

The specific management of an intracerebral haematoma varies with the size, location and aetiology of the haemorrhage. Small haemorrhages with mild to moderate deficits may only require close observation and conservative treatment for hypertension and oedema. Conversely, large haemorrhages with a comatose patient are unlikely to benefit from any therapy.

Therapy for Supratentorial Haematomas

Most clinicians agree that cerebellar and superficial lobar haematomas should be evacuated if the lesions are causing symptomatic mass effect. The value of surgery for deep-seated haematomas is controversial and has been evaluated in three prospective studies. In a Finnish study of 52 patients who were largely stuporous or comatose, emergency surgery was compared to conservative treatment (22). The mortality rate amongst the surgical group was lower. However, all these patients remained severely disabled and the study concluded that surgery did not offer any advantage over medical management. Similar findings were noted in an Austrian study (23) with putamenal and thalamic haemorrhages. However, surgical patients with sub-cortical haematomas showed a significantly lower mortality rate compared to medical therapy—30 vs 70 per cent. These patients also had a good outcome—40 per cent—than those in the medical group—25 per cent. Hence, it appears that surgical evacuation of a subcortical white matter clot is beneficial. In a small American study (24) evaluating 21 severely impaired patients, surgery proved of no help, but the small number of patients evaluated makes it difficult to draw any conclusion.

Cerebellar Haemorrhages

The outcome in patients with cerebellar haemorrhages is directly related to the level of consciousness at the time of admission as well as prior to surgery. As mentioned earlier, a high index of clinical suspicion and an early CT scan evaluation would go a long way in improving the outcome. Secondly, as the haematoma size increases, it compresses the brainstem and impairs consciousness. Hence the size of the haematoma and brainstem compression are also important in planning management. Haematomas of < 2 cm diameter can be managed medically provided the patient is alert (25). Haematomas larger than 3 cm should be operated on urgently even in patients who are alert or minimally drowsy. Haematomas between 2 and 3 cm can be managed medically if the patient is alert and CT scan does not demonstrate any evidence of brainstem compression (25). Patients presenting in deep coma with large cerebellar haematomas are not considered to be appropriate surgical candidates but should nevertheless be given an opportunity to survive through evacuation of the clot, even though the mortality is high. The patient's age, general medical condition and the length of time from ictus to surgery must also be considered in the decision to operate.

Brainstem Haemorrhage

Brainstem hemorrhages usually carry a poor prognosis and medical management for these lesions includes support of blood pressure and respiration. Occasionally hydrocephalus may develop and ventricular drainage may be required in some patients.

Lobar Haemorrhage

As in other areas of the brain, the size of the haemorrhage determines whether medical therapy alone or surgical evacuation is needed. The subcortical white matter is able to accommodate large haemorrhages but the location also determines the management decisions, e.g. a large haemorrhage may be accommodated in the occipital lobes with minimal change in the level of consciousness. A haemorrhage of a similar volume in the temporal lobe would produce a shift of the midline structures and brainstem compression, and would argue in favour of surgical evacuation. Hence, the size, location and clinical state would dictate management decisions.

In recent years, there has been an increasing application of minimally invasive stereotactic technique for evacuation of deep-seated intracerebral haematomas. The morbidity is limited as no general anaesthesia is required. The technique involves CT-guided stereotactic evacuation of the clot followed by insertion of a catheter into the haematoma cavity for serial clot lysis using fibrinolytic agents. The advantage of this minimally invasive surgical technique is that it can substantially decrease haematoma volume while avoiding the morbidity of major craniotomy, especially in the elderly and moribund patients. The results of two randomized controlled trials are promising with lower mortality rates and improved clinical outcome when compared to medical therapy (26, 27).

Subarachnoid Haemorrhage (SAH)

Rupture of an intracranial saccular aneurysm is the most common cause of subarachnoid haemorrhage which is a common and often devastating neurological emergency. About 25 per cent of the patients die within the first 24 hours from a re-rupture of the aneurysm. Arteriovenous malformation (AVMs) are also a common cause of SAH. Because aneurysms and AVMs have a high mortality and morbidity but are amenable to modern therapeutic techniques, such cases must be recognized early and referred to specialized centres with expertise to deal with these problems.

Clinical Presentation of Aneurysmal SAH

Prodromal symptoms may betray the localization of an unruptured aneurysm. Often the earliest suggestion of an expanding aneurysm of the junction of the internal carotid artery and posterior communicating artery is pain behind and above the medial aspect of the ipsilateral eye. This is soon followed by an ipsilateral third nerve palsy with pupillary involvement. An expanding cavernous sinus aneurysm may give rise to a sixth cranial nerve palsy. Compression of the optic chiasma by a supra-clinoid carotid aneurysm may give rise to bitemporal visual field defects or if anteriorly placed, monocular blindness. Pain in and around an eye with involvement of the temple is suggestive of an expanding middle cerebral artery aneurysm. Occipital or posterior cervical pain may indicate an aneurysm in the posterior cerebral circulation. *Any sudden unexplained severe headache in any location arouses the suspicion of SAH and requires an urgent CT scan.*

At the onset of any acute severe aneurysmal SAH, there may be a transient loss of consciousness in 45 per cent of cases. Most patients on regaining consciousness complain of severe headache associated with vomiting. Initially there may be an absence of focal neurological deficit or the cranial nerve palsies described above may persist after aneurysmal rupture. However, any aneurysm can rupture into the brain parenchyma, particularly during re-rupture, thereby producing focal deficits. The clinical picture is variable depending on the site of aneurysm and the extent of subarachnoid and parenchymatous haemorrhage.

Initial Radiological and Laboratory Evaluation

The CT scan is the mainstay in the diagnosis of SAH. If the scan is performed within 24 hours, SAH can be detected in 92 per cent of the cases (28). The CT scan is also useful in identifying the extent and location of subarachnoid blood and thereby locating the site of the aneurysm. This feature may also predict those patients likely to have cerebral vasospasm. If subarachnoid blood is more over the hemispheres rather than over the basal cisterns, an AVM or mycotic aneurysm should be suspected.

A selective DSA should be performed as soon as possible. The angiogram is extremely useful in localizing and characterizing the anatomy of the aneurysm and also in detecting the presence or absence of focal cerebral vasospasm. Subtle aneurysms in the anterior communicating artery or posterior circulation can be missed and it would be prudent to repeat the angiogram after 2–3 weeks.

Transcranial Doppler can be used for non-invasive diagnosis of aneurysms but is now mainly used for follow-up examination of cerebral vasospasm. It has a good correlation with the angiogram, particularly for vasospasms involving the middle cerebral artery stem. However, some centres still prefer angiography because of angioplasty therapy for vasospasm.

A baseline ECG is important because it may show changes simulating acute myocardial ischaemia. If so, CK-MB fraction should be done to exclude myocardial damage. Platelet count, bleeding time and other coagulation parameters should be documented. Because SAH can frequently precipitate inappropriate anti-diuretic hormone secretion and hence hyponatraemia, baseline electroyte levels should be documented.

Initial Management

Because of the risk of re-bleeding, all patients should be given bed rest and straining in any form (e.g. during defaecation) should be avoided. In heavy smokers, proper chest physiotherapy and nebulization should be instituted to avoid frequent coughing. Overhydration should be avoided because of the possibility of dilutional hyponatraemia. Some patients with SAH may have a rise of ICP. Dexamethasone and methylprednisolone have been used without any specific evidence of beneficial effect. However, they do reduce headache and neck pain. The blood pressure is invariably elevated immediately after an SAH. If the blood pressure remains elevated, treatment with antihypertensive agents remains controversial. Because of the risk of re-bleeding, it seems rational to reduce the blood pressure to around 150–160 mm Hg. However, randomized trials and observational studies have not shown any significant difference between treatment and conservative groups. Seizures are uncommon in SAH. If they do occur they should be promptly treated with an intravenous bolus of phenytoin sodium followed by oral therapy.

Surgical Therapy for Ruptured Aneurysm

The advent of the operating microscope in the late 1960s has made microsurgical clipping of a ruptured aneurysm a safe and effective method of preventing re-bleeding. In most series the re-bleeding rate has drastically reduced following direct surgical treatment of a ruptured aneurysm and can be as low as 1.2 per cent (29). There is still some controversy regarding the timing of surgery and recently there is a trend towards early surgical intervention, particularly in patients who are in a good clinical state. Surgery may be delayed in patients with a poor general medical condition in order to prepare them for the surgery. Hence the complexity of the aneurysm, the difficulty in surgical approach and the clinical state of the patient clearly influence the time of the surgery. More often than not, the timing of the surgery is tailored to the individual patient's requirement. Early surgical intervention also has the advantage of removing the clot around an artery, thereby eliminating the potential threat of vasospasm. Occasionally, aneurysms situated in a technically difficult location may require surgical wrapping or may benefit by endovascular coiling and total occlusion. This technique has been refined in recent years. Gugliemi detachable coils (GDC) can be delivered into the aneurysm via transfemoral angiography and spares the patient a major neurosurgical procedure. This technique is particularly useful in patients with a poor neurological or medical co-morbid condition. The recent ISAT trial enrolled 2143 patients with ruptured intracranial aneurysms and randomly assigned them to neurosurgical clipping (n=1070) or GDC coils (n=1073) (30). Because the interim analysis was significantly in favour of coiling, the trial was stopped short of its target of 2500 patients. At one year follow-up, the risk of death or significant disability was 30.6 per cent in the neurosurgical group compared to 23.7 per cent in the endovascular group— a 22.6 per cent relative risk reduction in favour of coiling. Because of the drawbacks of this study, the debate between 'clipping' and 'coiling' still continues. The development of newer catheters, coils and balloons continues to push the therapeutic decisions in favour of endovascular techniques.

Delayed Neurological Deficits

There are three major causes of delayed neurological deficits in patients with SAH: hydrocephalus, re-rupture and cerebral vasospasm.

Hydrocephalus

Hydrocephalus occurs in the acute, subacute or chronic form. The abrupt onset of stupor or the persistence of coma after the initial rupture would suggest acute hydrocephalus because of the presence of intraventricular and subarachnoid blood. This requires urgent ventriculostomy which may have to be bilateral because of the presence of thick clots in the third ventricle. In an occasional patient this manoeuvre will result in dramatic improvement but more often the improvement is gradual. A subacute form usually occurs within the first seven days after SAH. After an initial phase of improvement the patient may become progressively drowsy accompanied by upward gaze palsy. When this is suspected a CT scan should be repeated to confirm the diagnosis. Fortunately, in many patients this form of hydrocephalus gradually resolves and ventricular or lumbar drainage may not be required. Chronic (communicating hydrocephalus) is a frequent occurrence after SAH and usually presents with gait difficulty, precipitate micturition and a mild dementia. A ventriculoperitoneal shunt is required and there is a high rate of improvement in such cases.

Re-rupture

Re-rupture of an aneurysm is generally heralded by a sudden severe increase in headache, vomiting and new neurological deficits followed by rapid deterioration in consciousness. A repeat CT scan demonstrating an increase in the amount of blood in the subarachnoid space or a lumbar puncture showing fresh blood can confirm the diagnosis reliably. The incidence of re-rupture may be as high as 30 per cent and carries a significant morbidity and mortality. The highest incidence of re-bleeding is on the first day and is probably a major cause of mortality before hospitalization. Subsequently, the risk of re-bleeding is highest within the first three weeks and reduces considerably after the first month. The high rate of re-rupture and its significant mortality have prompted the trend towards early surgery for aneurysmal SAH.

The use of anti-fibrinolytic therapy—epsilon aminocaproic acid and tranexamic acid—has now largely fallen into disrepute because it is associated with a higher rate of cerebral ischaemic infarcts which offsets any beneficial effects of this therapy in preventing re-bleeding. It may be used in specific situations e.g. in a patient with a low risk of vasospasm and when general medical problems increase the risk of surgery.

Cerebral Vasospasm

Cerebral vasospasm is a major cause of delayed cerebral ischaemia or infarct leading to delayed morbidity and death. This occurs in about 30 per cent of patients with SAH. Most patients are stable after the initial ictus when signs appear between 4 and 14 days reaching a peak at 7 days. There is good evidence that the extent and location of clotted blood on CT scan in the basal cisterns and fissures can be used to predict the incidence, location and severity of vasospasm. Subarachnoid clots larger than 5 × 3 mm in the basal cisterns and a layer of blood 1 mm or more in the fissures predict vasospasm. The CT scan is thus a reliable method to pick up potential vasospasm in the anterior and middle cerebral artery territory. Unfortunately, the CT scan cannot detect clots in the posterior fossa and is therefore not reliable for the vertebro-basilar territory. Blood is usually 'washed out' after an SAH. Hence, time diminishes the sensitivity of the CT scan and in order to predict vasospasm reliably, the scan must be performed within the first three days. It is postulated, that once a clot encases the artery, haemoglobin breakdown products induce vasospasm. The clinical syndromes depend on the vessels involved and the extent of vasospasm. These can range from minor neurological deficits to completed infarcts producing aphasia, hemiparesis, dominant or non-dominant parietal lobe signs, abulic state, homonymous field defects and focal brainstem signs.

Therapy for vasospasm. Therapeutic efforts to prevent or treat symptomatic vasospasm have been generally disappointing. A number of prospective randomized trials for the oral calcium channel antagonist—nimodipine—have been initiated and the following conclusions have been reached. (1) Oral nimodipine consistently reduces poor outcome due to vasospasm in all grades of patients but the incidence of symptomatic vasospasm was not affected by nimodipine treatment. (2) Vessel caliber by angiography was not affected by nimodipine therapy. (3) The side effects and complications of this drug were minimal. Nimodipine 60 mg every 4 hours is therefore used routinely in SAH patients.

Induced hypertension, hypervolaemia with volume expanders and haemodilution—the triple H therapy—have been used in the past to 'break' the vasospasm. Only a small proportion of patients responded to this mode of therapy and stroke and death rate approached 15 per cent. The risks of this therapy include cardiac failure, cerebral oedema, bleeding abnormalities and rupture of an unclipped aneurysm.

Transluminal angioplasty (31) has been tried for patients with vasospasm refractory to other modes of therapy. Significant improvement in 60–80 per cent of patients was noted within hours after dilatation. Complications like rupture of the vessels or of an unclipped aneurysm occurred in 5 per cent of cases.

It must be remembered that patients with SAH are also prone to certain medical complications. Patients undergoing bed rest may develop deep vein thrombosis and pulmonary embolism. The ECG may suggest myocardial ischaemia or subendocardial infarction. This is very likely due to sympathetic overactivity mediated through alpha-adrenergic stimulation of the coronary arteries leading to coronary spasm. Such spasms can be treated by intravenous nitroglycerin or possibly by calcium-channel blockers. SIADH is also frequently noted in SAH and results in hyponatraemia. Restricting free water while maintaining adequate intravascular volume and cardiac output becomes important. Lastly, a rare patient with SAH may present with neurogenic pulmonary oedema.

REFERENCES

1. Indredavik B, Bakke F, Soleberg R et al. (1991). Benefit of a stroke unit: a randomized controlled trial. Stroke. 22, 1026–1031.
2. North American Symptomatic Carotid Endarterectomy Trial Collaborators. (1991). Beneficial effect of carotid endarterectomy in symptomatic patients with high-grade carotid stenosis. N Eng J Med. 325, 445–453.

3. Wallace JD, Levy LL. (1981). Blood pressure after stroke. JAMA, 246, 2177–2180.

4. Carlberb B, Apslund K, Haag E. (1991). Course of blood pressure in different subsets of patients after acute stroke. Cerebrovasc Dis. 1, 281–287.

5. Carlberg B, Apslune K. Haag E. (1991) Factors influencing admission blood pressure levels in patients with acute stroke. Stroke. 22, 527–530.

6. Loyke H. (1983). Lowering blood pressure after stroke. Am J Med Sci. 286, 2–11.

7. Kushner M. Nencini P, Reivich M et al. (1990). Relationship of hyperglycaemia early in ischaemic brain infarction to cerebral anatomy, metabolism and clinical outcome. Ann Neurol. 28, 129–135.

8. Cerebral Embolism Task Force. (1989). Cardiogenic brain embolism. Arch Neurol. 46, 727–743.

9. International Stroke Trial Collaborative Group. (1997). The International Stroke Trial (IST): A randomised trial of aspirin, subcutaneous heparin, both or neither among 19435 patients with acute ischaemic stroke. Lancet. 349, 1569–1581.

10. Chinese Acute Stroke Trial (CAST) Collaborative Group. (1997). CAST: A randomized placebo controlled trial of early aspirin use in 20000 patients with acute ischaemic strokes. Lancet. 349, 1641–1649.

11. The National Institute of Neurological Disorders and Stroke rt-PA Stroke Study Group. (1995). Tissue plasminogen activator for acute ischaemic strokes. N Engl J Med. 333, 1581–1587.

12. Fagan SC, Morgenstern LB, Petitta A et al. (1998). Cost-effectiveness of tissue plasminogen activator for acute ischaemic strokes: the NINDS rt-PA Stroke Study Group. Neurology. 50, 883–890.

13. Tanne D, Bates VE, Verro P et al. (1999). Initial clinical experiences with IV tissue plasminogen activator for acute ischaemic stroke: A multicentre survey. Neurology. 53, 424–427.

14. Albers GW, Bates VE, Clark WM et al. (2000). Intravenous tissue-type plasminogen activator for treatment of acute stroke: The Standard Treatment with Alteplase to Reverse Stroke (STARS) Study. JAMA, 283, 1189–1191.

15. Katzan IL, Furlan AJ, Lloyd LE et al. (2000). Use of tissue-type plasminogen activator for acute ischaemic stroke: the Cleveland area experience. JAMA. 283, 1151–1158.

16. del Zoppo GJ, Higashida RT, Furlan AJ et al. (1998). PROACT: a phase II randomized trial of recombinant pro-urokinase by direct arterial delivery in acute middle cerebral artery stroke. PROACT Investigators. Prolyse in Acute Cerebral Thromboembolism. Stroke. 29, 4–11.

17. Furlan AJ, Higashida RT, Wechsler L et al. (1999). Intra-arterial pro-urokinase for acute ischaemic stroke: The PROACT Study: a randomized controlled trial. Prolyse in acute cerebral embolism. JAMA. 2003–2011.

18. Schwab S, Steiner T, Aschoff A et al. (1998). Early hemicraniotomy in patients with complete middle cerebral artery infarction. Stroke. 29, 1888–1893.

19. Demchuk AM. (2000). Hemicraniotomy is a promising treatment in ischaemic stroke. Can J Neurol Sci. 27, 274–277.

20. Hier DB, Davis KR, Richardson EPJ et al. (1977). Hypertensive putamenal haemorrhage. Ann Neurol 1, 152–159.

21. Poungvatin N, Bhoopat W, Viriyavejakul A et al. (1987). Effects of dexamethasone in primary supratentorial intracerebral haemorrhage. N Engl J Med. 316, 1229–1233.

22. Juvela S, Heiskanen O, Poranen A et al. (1989). The treatment of spontaneous intracerebral haemorrhage. J Neurosurg. 70, 755–758.

23. Auer LM, Deinsherger W, Neiderkorn K et al. (1989) Endoscopic surgery versus medical treatment for spontaneous intracerebral haematoma: randomized study. J Neurosurg 70, 530–535.

24. Batjer HH, Reisch JS, Allen BC et al. (1990). Failure of surgery to improve outcome in hypertensive putamenal haemorrhage. Arch Neurol 47, 1103–1106.

25. Ito Z, Nakajima K. (1983). Surgical treatment of acute cerebellar haemorrhage. In: Hypertensive Intracerebral Haemorrhage (Ed. Mizukami, M), pp. 215–223. Raven Press, New York, NY.

26. Rohde V, Rohde I, Reinges MH et al. (2000). Frameless stereotactically guided catheter placement and fibrinolytic therapy for spontaneous intracerebral haematomas: technical aspects and initial clinical results. Mimin Invasive Neurosurg. 43, 9–17.

27. Mortes JM, Wong JH, Fayad PB et al. (2000). Stereotactic computed tomographic-guided aspiration and thrombolysis of intracranial haematoma: protocol and preliminary experience. Stroke. 31, 834–840.

28. Kassel NF, Torner JC, Haley EC Jr et al. (1990). The International Cooperative Study on the Timing of Aneurysm Surgery, I: Overall management resulrs. J Neurosurg 73, 18–36.

29. Sundt TM Jr, Kobayashi S, Fode NC et al. (1982). Results and complications of surgical management of 809 intracranial aneurysms in 722 cases: related and unrelated to grade of patient, type of aneurysm and timing of surgery. J Neurosurg. 56, 753–765.

30. ISAT Collaborative Group. (2002). International Subarachnoid Aneurysm Trial (ISAT) of neurosurgical clipping versus endovascular coiling in 2143 patients with ruptured intracranial aneurysms: a randomized trial. Lancet. 360, 1267–1274.

31. Barnwell SL, Higashida RT, Halbach VV, Dowd CF, Wilson CB, Heishima GB. (1989). Transluminal angioplasty of intracerebral vessels for cerebral arterial spasm: reversal of neurological deficits after delayed treatment. Neurosurgey 25, 424–429.

D. FULMINANT NEUROLOGICAL INFECTIONS

Dr Sohrab K. Bhabha

From time to time, the intensivist is faced with patients who appear to have life-threatening, rapidly progressing neurological disorders of suspected infectious aetiology. Such disorders may occur sporadically (e.g. herpes simplex encephalitis) or in an epidemic manner (e.g. arboviral encephalitis). They may be endemic to a region (e.g. cerebral malaria, cysticercal encephalitis), or related to an animal reservoir (e.g. rabies to dogs or bats, Kyasanur forest disease to ticks). All the same, these patients require preliminary *syndromic definition*, subsequent *differential diagnosis* and concurrent *critical care* to stem the tide of systemic and neurological deterioration. This chapter purports to provide such a working overview.

Syndromic Definition

A variety of syndromes may reach the critical care unit, in the setting of suspected fulminant neurological infection. They are essentially disorders related to the meninges and brain, rostral spinal cord or to the neuromuscular system. Formulating the *syndromic diagnosis* is the cornerstone to instituting appropriate management.

The *meningoencephalitis syndrome* is probably the commonest one to gain admission to the intensive care unit. It may begin as meningitis, with the constellation of fever, headache, drowsiness, photophobia, vomiting, signs of meningeal irritation and at times, delirium. Acute behavioural changes, amnesia, delirium, stupor, convulsions, patterns of central motor weakness, ataxia and involuntary movements in the presence of fever, all indicate an additional encephalitic component. The evolution of symptoms and signs is rapid; the nadir of clinical evolution is often noted within hours or at most, in a day or two.

Rapidly evolving focal neurodeficit (e.g. hemiplegia, ataxia) with or without seizures and the development of indicators of intracranial hypertension (ICH) point towards the *intracranial space-occupying lesion syndrome*. Among other factors, it is the alarming progress of seizures and ICH that require critical care, if secondary brain insult is to be prevented. Progressive obtundation leading to stupor or coma, vomiting, visual symptoms, evolving pupillary and extraocular movement impairment, bradycardia, widening pulse pressure and altered patterns of respiration all indicate the establishment of *intracranial hypertension*.

Asymmetric, painful, predominantly unilateral ophthalmoplegia, chemosis, proptosis, visual impairment, ophthalmic-trigeminal deficit and at times contralateral hemiparesis with preceding facial, nasal cutaneous or chronic paranasal sinus infection may indicate an evolving *cavernous sinus thrombosis*. Similarly, ear discharge and ataxia or hemideficit with ophthalmoparesis, with or without seizures, indicate petromastoid infection with secondary effects on the contents of the posterior and middle cranial fossae, respectively. Fulminant *polyneuritis cranialis* must always prompt

the consideration of *skull-base* and *cranial epidural space* infections, resulting from complicated paranasal sinusitis or petromastoiditis with pachymeningitis. Such infections are also termed *parameningeal*.

The *rostral (high) spinal cord syndrome* may present with quadriparesis (often acutely areflexic), retention, sensory impairment, catastrophic hypotension among other dysautonomic features and signs of low medullary dysfunction. The latter may include respiratory impairment and features of bulbar palsy such as dysphagia or dysphonia.

Acute generalized neuromuscular paralysis at once jeopardizes ventilation and leads to the tissue-damaging effects of respiratory failure (discussed elsewhere). This may evolve over hours and requires urgent ventilatory support if secondary brain insult and widespread systemic damage are to be prevented.

Lastly, we must be aware of fulminant neurological dysfunction (largely encephalopathic or meningoencephalitic) as part and parcel of vital organ disturbances (e.g. hepatic disorders) or severe systemic infections (e.g. salmonellosis) which culminate in overwhelming *sepsis*. *Infective endocarditis* may also lead to acute neurological disorders, though these are rarely infective in nature.

Differential Diagnosis

The Meningoencephalitis Syndrome

Fulminant meningitis is usually bacterial or aseptic in nature. The latter term refers to meningitides which are sterile on conventional culture. They are largely viral, though infections associated with fastidious atypical bacteria may share the same features. Aseptic meningitis may also be an indicator of a parameningeal source of infection. Organisms responsible for bacterial (pyogenic) meningitis vary according to a person's age. In adults, S. pneumoniae, N. meningitidis and H. influenzae predominate as the organisms causing community-acquired meningitis. Nosocomial meningitis is generally due to Gram-negative bacilli; following neurosurgery, Staphylococcus must be considered. Streptococci and Listeria preferentially infect immunocompromised persons, the elderly and puerperal women. Tuberculous meningitis and the early phase of various spirochaetal meningitides may on occasion assume a fulminant complexion, especially in the immunocompromised person.

Viral meningitis generally affects children and young adults. More than half of the infections are caused by enteroviruses such as coxsackie B or echovirus; less commonly, herpes simplex type 1 virus, mumps virus, lymphocytic choriomeningitis virus, varicella zoster virus or human immunodeficiency virus (HIV, all stages except late) may be implicated. These agents are not easy to culture; thus serology, including CSF serology is increasingly important. In the immunocompromised host, antibody responses are poor and contemporary methods, such as the polymerase chain reaction, may prove vital for the detection of antigenic moieties associated with the infective organism.

Reaching a definitive diagnosis of encephalitis is difficult, since a wide array of organisms may be responsible for this condition. As illustrated earlier, various clues may be obtained from predisposing and epidemiologic factors. Though viruses are by far the commonest cause of encephalitis, bacteria (e.g. Salmonella, Listeria, Borrelia, Leptospira), Mycobacteria, Rickettsiae, Mycoplasma, parasites (e.g. Amoebae, Pl. falciparum , Cysticercus, Toxoplasma) and fungi (e.g. Histoplasma, Cryptococcus, Coccidioides) may all induce the encephalitis syndrome. The toxic shock syndrome, associated with staphylococcal toxin elaboration, may present as a meningoencephalitis, as may the Vogt-Koyanagi-Harada syndrome, as well as sarcoidosis. Vasculitic disorders such as systemic lupus erythematosus and Behçet's disease may manifest as a febrile encephalitis.

It is *mandatory* to consider infection-induced exacerbation of underlying putative mitochondrial (e.g. respiratory chain disorders: MELAS, MERRF, Leigh; Reye syndromes) or other neurometabolic disorders (e.g. urea cycle enzymopathies: ornithine transcarbamylase defects), presenting as fulminant encephalopathy, before turning one's view to viruses.

Among epidemic encephalitides, arboviruses have the largest impact. Japanese encephalitis, dengue and Kyasanur Forest disease complex are some examples of these. Enteroviridae and influenza virus A and B may also cause epidemic encephalitis. Herpes simplex type 1 encephalitis (HSE) is the prototype of sporadic encephalitis. Other causes of this type of encephalitis are HIV (at all stages except late), mumps, measles, rubella, varicella-zoster virus (in the varicella phase), Epstein-Barr virus and adeno-viridae. Rabies is an example of a zoonotic encephalitis; lymphocytic choriomeningitis virus, associated with hamsters, also causes a meningoencephalitis.

The Intracranial Space-occupying Lesion Syndrome

This syndrome, with or without manifestations of intracranial hypertension (ICH), may be seen in a variety of infectious settings. Extraparenchymally, subdural empyema needs to be considered (streptococcal in 50 per cent, staphylococcal in 20 per cent, Gram-negative bacilli in 10 per cent of cases); the occasional mycobacterial granuloma may also exist in this location. Intraparenchymal infective space-occupying lesions include bacterial (polymicrobial), nocardial or aspergillus abscesses, mycobacterial (granulomas or abscesses, simple or complex), parasitic (cysticercal, toxoplasma, hydatid cysts, etc.) and fungal granulomas. The presence of primary brain abscess or of toxoplasma or fungal granulomas must prompt the further definition of underlying immune status, with special reference to acquired (e.g. HIV disease) or iatrogenic (post-transplant, post-chemotherapy, etc.) immunocompromise. In HIV or post-transplant settings, primary brain lymphoma and focal lymphoproliferative disorders may need consideration. When ICH co-exists, it may be due to brain oedema (generalized or compartmentalized) or as a result of associated hydrocephalus; this question must be suitably addressed.

The Intracranial Hypertension Syndrome

Briefly, this syndrome may be the result of different pathophysiological mechanisms. An infective intracranial space-occupying lesion usually evokes a considerable degree of perilesional inflammation. The resultant oedema may produce a marked elevation in intracranial pressure, compartmentalized or generalized, depending upon the topography of such lesions. If such lesions obstruct CSF pathways, hydrocephalus may result. Co-existent meningitis, such as may occur in tuberculosis, mycoses or cysticercosis, may also lead to the establishment of hydrocephalus. Intracranial infections may be associated with the development of fulminant cortical venous and venous sinus thrombophlebitis. This may lead to haemorrhagic infarction and precipitous brain swelling or, if the deep venous system is involved, to hydrocephalus. Pseudotumour cerebri may result if venous drainage is sufficiently impeded. Several mechanisms may thus lead to ICH, each one requiring a different therapeutic strategy.

Cavernous Sinus Thrombosis, Skull-base Infection, Polyneuritis Cranialis

Most often, cavernous sinus thrombosis is secondary to infections of the paranasal sinuses, rhinopharynx, deep orbit or facial soft tissues around the eye and nose. Staphylococci are the chief pathogens in the community-acquired form; fungi and anaerobes may complicate chronic paranasal sinusitis. Gram-negative organisms merit consideration in nosocomial cases. Petromastoid infections, usually the end-result of suppurative middle ear disease, must also be microbiologically defined if their brain complications are to be appropriately treated. At times, paranasal sinus infection of an indolent nature may spread across the skull-base to involve adjacent areas such as the temporal bone and lead to secondary petrositis. Focal suppuration may take the form of an intracranial epidural abscess. Fungal infections such as mucormycosis and aspergillosis must also be borne in mind, especially in the setting of immunodeficiency or poorly-controlled diabetes. Polyneuritis cranialis is *the* clinical indicator of the extent of skull-base and meningeal involvement; an occasional case of bulbar palsy due to lower cranial nerve palsy may present in the acute phase of faucial diptheria.

The Rostral Spinal Cord Syndrome

This syndrome, in the setting of infection, is usually due to mycobacterial, brucellar or fungal (blastomycotic) aetiology. The usual mechanism is compressive, due to extradural inflammatory tissue in the cervical spinal canal. At times, an abscess, usually epidural, may exist when prompt surgical aid may be required. The primary infective lesion usually arises in a discovertebral unit. As inflammation spreads, it may reach upwards towards the cervicomedullary region threatening bulbar and respiratory function. Spinal leptomeningitis ('arachnoiditis') and secondary vascular changes, resulting in spinal cord ischaemia at this level, though uncommon, are the most dreaded complications since they run a protracted course and carry a guarded prognosis.

Acute Generalized Neuromuscular Paralysis

In the post-poliomyelitis immunization era, this is thankfully an uncommon occurrence, though acute inflammatory demyelinating polyneuropathy of a parainfectious nature (the Guillain-Barré syndrome) is commonly encountered. Nonetheless, this situation brings enteroviral anterior horn cell diseases to mind, such as those caused by coxsackie and echoviruses. On occasion, infectious mononucleosis (Epstein-Barr virus) may present thus. *Campylobacter jejuni*-associated acute polyneuropathy may occasionally be encountered. Another infectious-toxic disorder which should be borne in mind is botulism; a history of envenomation (tic paralysis, snake, spider venoms) must be sought. Impending neuromuscular respiratory failure is the common denominator which brings all these conditions to the critical care unit. Infective disorders (in particular acute infective polyneuritis and acute poliomyelitis), causing generalized neuromuscular weakness or paralysis should be specifically differentiated from myasthenia gravis. Myasthenia frequently involves muscles supplied by the oculomotor and other motor cranial nerves. When myasthenia presents as acute respiratory failure, the differential diagnosis from other acute infective neuroparalytic conditions may be difficult. A careful history of easy fatiguability preceding acute neuromuscular weakness is of help. The diagnosis of myasthenia may be confirmed by an EMG; supramaximal stimulation of a motor nerve at 2–3 Hz, results in a 10 per cent or greater decrement of the amplitude of the evoked compound muscle action potential from the first to the fifth response. If this facility is not available in the critical care setting, the edrophonium (Tensilon) test (2 mg intravenous initially, followed by a further 8 mg if no adverse effects are noted), or the neostigmine test (1–1.5 mg intramuscular) are of diagnostic help. Either of these drugs results in dramatic improvement in myasthenic weakness.

Post-infective Demyelinating Disorders

One does well to bear in mind that infectious diseases may induce a process of immune-mediated post-infective demyelination, which may lead subsequently to a variety of neurological disorders. Among these are post-infective demyelinating encephalitis, acute disseminated encephalomyelitis, 'transverse' myelitis, cerebellitis, brainstem encephalitis, acute haemorrhagic leukoencephalitis, pseudotumour cerebri, acute inflammatory demyelinating polyneuropathy (the Guillain-Barré syndrome, above) and optic neuritis. Some of these may find their way to the critical care unit and may require to be differentiated from their infective counterparts (e.g. post-infective encephalitis vs. herpes simplex encephalitis).

Issues in Critical Care

The critical care of fulminant neurological infection is crucially dependent on a *working definition* of the disorder at hand. What follows is a selective consideration of critical care issues further to the syndromic and differential diagnostic considerations above. Invariably, such efforts require the seamless collaboration of the intensivist, the neurologist, the neurosurgeon, the microbiologist, the neuroradiologist and the neurophysiologist. Communication is of the utmost importance; documentation of observations, management and plans is mandatory.

Rapid *baseline evaluation* must include medical and neurological clinical surveys with fundoscopy, initial Glasgow Coma Scale Sumscore, accurate note of the pupillary light response and limb power with special reference to asymmetry. Routine critical monitoring is instituted, with intracranial pressure monitoring and EEG monitoring being performed when indicated. Laboratory investigations should include a haemogram, smear for malarial parasites, a broad biochemical profile, *serum ammonia, lactate, pyruvate,* blood gas analysis, coagulopathy profile (to include prothrombin time, activated partial thromboplastin time, platelet count, fibrinogen and fibrin degradation products, D-Dimer) and blood as well as body fluids for extended cultures, including viral culture. Acute phase serum should be sent for seroimmunology (to always include HIV, spirochaetal serology, clinically-prompted serology e.g. brucella, enterovirus, etc.) and *stored*, for subsequent immunological comparison with convalescent serum. A similar policy is adopted with CSF, which is invariably examined very early in the course of the illness and should be stored for immunological purposes. Obtaining brain imaging prior to CSF examination by lumbar puncture is not mandatory and is harmful if this delays early CSF examination. Clinical features of raised intracranial pressure must be sought (fundoscopy mandatory); these are enough to guide the safe performance of lumbar puncture with suitable precautions. The value of CSF examination cannot be overemphasized. This must include opening pressure *manometry*, a glucose *ratio* (this implies obtaining a concurrent blood glucose sample), cell count, smears for appropriate microbiological examination and immunostaining, cytohistopathology and serology as appropriate, including a treponemal test if TPHA or FTA Abs have not been requested on serum. CSF culture must be obtained on the best available and most appropriate media; short-changing this policy may prove extremely costly, since the *first* CSF examined is invariably the most revealing one. It is our practice to discuss appropriate culture methods, on a case-by-case basis, with our consultant microbiologist. Radiology should include a chest film and appropriate imaging. MR imaging with contrast enhancement is the imaging modality of choice. This may require supplementation with contrast enhanced CT imaging, particularly when contiguous skull or spine bone structure requires better visualization or when MR imaging is not feasible. The diagnostic EEG may provide fairly specific clues as in herpes simplex encephalitis; it invariably provides valuable data in the presence of specific *encephalopathies* and is usually diagnostic of the *rare* idiopathic epilepsy presenting in status, which may mimic an encephalitic illness. Bedside neurophysiology is invaluable for the elucidation of several myogenic and neuropathic disorders. Such an evaluation strategy should lead to the formulation of a *working diagnosis*, both anatomic and aetiologic.

The contemporary management of *acute meningoencephalitic*

disorders has been greatly facilitated by the improved monitoring and life support strategies available in the critical care setting, by standardized, specific seroimmunology, as well as by the development of antiviral drugs. Careful metabolic and haemodynamic monitoring, the readiness to institute ventilatory support and an aggressive seizure control policy (discussed elsewhere) are essential. The wider use of multimodal brain imaging, intracranial pressure monitoring, hyperventilation, high dose barbiturate therapy and selective decompressive surgery (CSF diversion, craniectomy) all help in reducing morbidity, mortality and in enhancing the quality of outcome. Meningoencephalitis can otherwise be anticipated to inexorably progress towards a state of unbridled inflammation with increasing intracranial pressure. Systemic infection control and prophylaxis for deep venous thrombosis and pulmonary embolism are part of routine management.

Specific drug therapy must be instituted, based on the most likely aetiology (e.g. cerebral malaria, herpes simplex encephalitis) or, sometimes unavoidably, based on a short-list of aetiologies (e.g. pyogenic vs acutely presenting TB meningitis). In the treatment of bacterial ('pyogenic') meningitis, there are now some grounds to consider the use of steroids (dexamethasone, 0.15 mg/kg six hourly for four days). This should be started 15 to 30 minutes before the first dose of antibiotic. Though this issue is not yet resolved, two facts emerge: first, such a short course of dexamethasone appears to have negligible, if any, ill-effects; second, there may be some reduction in the incidence of untoward neurologic sequelae (1–3). There appears to be a set of persons who clearly benefit by such treatment; current studies have not yet identified this set. Thus, there is an understandable trend towards such an abbreviated use of steroids. The institution of antimicrobial therapy, as indeed of all therapeutic efforts, must be swift. Lost time is extremely costly in terms of neurologic sequelae (4a, 4b, 5). The choice of antibiotic should be in accordance with the antibiotic policy of the hospital or critical care unit; this is especially important when empiric antibiotics are instituted. It is advisable to achieve CSF antibiotic levels 10 to 20 times higher than the minimum bactericidal concentration in vitro, for the organism in question. This usually implies using maximal doses parenterally. If treatment is instituted without delay, rapid improvement is expected. Failure to observe this within 48 to 72 hours should prompt a review of the working diagnosis. Though clinical improvement is apparent, it is justifiable to repeat CSF examination after 72 hours of treatment; at this juncture, improving trends in CSF are invariably observed in pyogenic and in most viral meningitides. The acute phase of chronic meningitis (e.g. TB meningitis) may show slower settling CSF trends. Septicaemic coagulopathies must always be watched for; severe meningococcaemia with its characteristic purpura is being currently treated with protein C concentrate on a trial basis (6). Most cases of viral (aseptic) meningitis are benign and self-limiting, requiring only adjunctive measures of treatment. The pitfall in management is to fail to exclude a specifically treatable cause; this should be diligently sought, keeping parameningeal infective sources (largely bacterial) in mind. The latter factor makes the free use of steroids

a reprehensible and potentially hazardous policy, in this setting. The true challenge in treating meningitis is not in completely eradicating the infection from the meninges alone; it is in locating the source of meningitis and once found, in eradicating this source so that the person is spared the hazards of recurrent meningitis.

The outcome of *viral encephalitis* largely depends upon the specific type of encephalitis, the quality of critical care received and the promptness with which specific drug treatment is instituted. This leads to the inevitable overuse of acyclovir, given the high suspicion of herpes simplex encephalitis in all sporadic cases. If subsequent viral studies indicate otherwise, treatment may be discontinued after 5 days.

Post-infective encephalitis is the result of an infection-related immune reaction, leading to myelin breakdown in various areas of the brain. This process is associated with an intense inflammatory response, during which brain swelling, seizures and a variety of focal deficits may occur. This form of demyelination is usually antigen-specific and thus is non-recurrent. Therapy aims at symptomatic and supportive measures of a similar nature to those employed in viral encephalitis. Steriods are used to stem the inflammatory response; they are usually administered in high doses for a short duration (e.g. intravenous methylprednisolone 500 to 1000 mg daily for 3 to 5 days).

Metabolic encephalopathy may present in a fulminant manner and this may be precipitated by systemic (non-neurological) infections. Such presentations are not uncommon in persons with *mitochondrial disorders* (7) and in those with a variety of *inherited enzymopathies* especially those related to the respiratory chain of mitochondrial enzymes and the urea cycle. Clinical clues must be sought for these disorders both in the person concerned and in family members. For this reason, every case of 'encephalitis' *must* have serum ammonia, lactate, pyruvate, thyroid hormones and autoantibodies estimated on admission (8). Such definition can dramatically change the management and outlook.

The *intracranial space-occupying lesion syndrome*, when suspected to be *infective*, can now be managed more logically largely due to contemporary imaging and neurosurgical methods. Seizure control and the management of intracranial hypertension are preliminary measures, which must be aggressively instituted. Various brain imaging patterns, themselves fairly definitive, prompt the clinician to seek further corroborative clinical and laboratory data, whether in other organ systems or by seroimmunology. At times however such data may not lead to satisfactory aetiologic management. It does well to bear in mind that timely, minimally-invasive, image-guided, neuronavigated aspiration or biopsy may provide vital definitive information with negligible risk. In the setting of a suspected infective space-occupying lesion, this approach may provide definitive diagnosis as well as valuable material for microbiological examination and provides the logical link to appropriate aetiologic management (9). Current literature emphasizes the polymicrobial nature of abscesses, the phenomenon of methicillin-resistant Staph. aureus and the collaborative imaging-medical-surgical approach to management (10).

Cerebral venous disorders can take many forms and present a host of regional and systemic challenges to the critical care team.

Seizures and intracranial hypertension require immediate attention. The thrombophilic state must be considered and extensively investigated. Venous sinus thrombosis and dural arterio-venous fistulae are often found to coexist; the reasons for this association are still not clearly understood though recent work indicates the operation of several thrombophilic phenomena such as heterozygote mutation of the prothrombin gene, factor V Leiden mutation, the presence of cardiolipin antibodies and dysfunctional protein C activity, among other abnormalities (11). In addition, regional and remote infective foci always require attention (12–14); metabolic factors such as underlying diabetes mellitus control and fluid balance must be optimized, normovolaemia being an important objective at all times. Occult neoplasms, immune-mediated disorders and immunocompromise require consideration. Observations have led to the wider use of anticoagulant therapy with variably aggressive thrombolysis (15,16). The status of the latter two therapies in the face of infective venous or sinus thrombosis is less clear (17). Infective cavernous sinus thrombosis is perhaps the most challenging situation (18). It calls for extreme care in data collection, beginning with baseline neurological and opthalmological assessment. Imaging must include multimodal MR, CT study of the brain, the skull-base, the orbits, the paranasal sinuses and the facial skeleton. At times, skull-base imaging may need to move across the floor of the middle cranial fossa to include the petromastoids. Non-invasive (at times invasive) imaging of vascular (venous and arterial) structures is mandatory. Ultrasound examination of the orbital contents may be required. Microbiology needs to extend across all these areas, too. Needless to say, collaboration with the microbiologist, opthalmologist, ENT surgeon, dental surgeon and neurosurgeon is vital. Fungi (mucorales, aspergillus) are the organisms most often implicated; amphotericin in combination with other antifungals invariably must be used, with repeated skillful debridement of necrotic tissue, as required. The contents of the orbit may require to be sacrificed. Periodically, and certainly at the outset, CSF examination is essential to assess to what extent dural-leptomeningeal barriers have been breached and a meningitic process established. Often, what begins as a focal fungal infection rapidly metamorphoses into a polymicrobial trans-compartmental head and neck infection with remote effects, including severe metabolic and coagulopathic features, requiring periodic intervention in the face of finely-balanced organ function (e.g. debridement procedures in a long-standing, poorly controlled diabetic with borderline renal function in the wake of amphotericin nephrotoxicity). The reduction in current mortality figures (earlier, close on 100 per cent; now, 20–30 per cent) is rewarding and is a reminder of the real impact of critical care on the management of such disorders (14).

Increasingly, we need to bring our attention to infections in *the immunocompromised host*. The background, in terms of both the underlying disorder(s) and the iatrogenic status, is of vital importance. HIV disease, post-chemotherapy immunosuppression and the post-transplant state are probably the commonest settings for the development of opportunistic infections in the immunocompromised. The privileged immune status of the nervous system makes it a sanctuary for the persistence of such infection. The muted immune response (both cell-mediated and humoral) detracts from the utility of most conventional immunodiagnostic methods, making us more dependent upon contemporary techniques for the amplification of antigenic moieties and gene sequencing, related to suspected organisms (19). Image-based patterns of nervous system pathology (largely with the help of contrast enhanced MR imaging of the neuraxis) are diagnostically invaluable. Still, we are learning of new presentations in this population (20); of new pathogenic mechanisms associated with old pathogens (21); of new pathogens (22, 23) and of new therapeutic strategies, often using old drugs (24,25). As we review successive epochs of antiretroviral drug therapy alone (26), we learn more about the immunobiology and novel behaviours of organisms such as toxoplasma, pneumocystis, measles virus, varicella-zoster virus, herpes simplex virus, cytomegalovirus, human polyomavirus, mycobacteria and cryptococci to name only a few old and heretofore 'well-known' organisms (27, 28). The presentations of such critically ill persons broadly conform to the syndromes discussed above; specific features, which ordinarily help in differential diagnosis, are invariably absent. The challenge of defining aetiology is multidisciplinary: it extends from the clinician even to the pathologist, who though armed with tissues, requires recourse to more refined ultrastructural, immunohistochemical, and molecular genetic tools to fulfill his task (29–31). The clinician must thus adopt an *initial* broad and 'inclusive' management strategy, pending narrower differential diagnosis aided by contemporaneous diagnostic modalities. Inclusive management demands frequent review of the syndromic diagnosis, which tends to alter over time. Collaboration and communication within the critical care team, meticulous attention to metabolic detail and documentation of observations and plans are never more crucial than in this setting. Symptomatic relief, whether concerning pain management, anxiety and sleep or other routines (e.g. bowel habit), is important. The pursuit of aetiologic diagnoses remains urgent and mandatory; *'judicious aggression'* best describes such a course of action. We must relentlessly obtain body fluids and tissues to prove our infective hypotheses and to record the adequacy of therapeutic responses. The successful treatment of infection is not enough in itself; surveillance and maintenance therapy (the consolidation phase) may be required lifelong. Decisions should, as far as possible be consensus ones in which the person and family members must participate; they require to be kept well informed of our endeavours. Overlooking these aspects of care can have unfortunate (litigant) implications.

Afterword

It is difficult to obtain data regarding the impact of critical care on the course and outcome of an inhomogeneous group of infective disorders. Nonetheless, it is illuminating to note that in the United States, the overall mortality rate for H. influenzae meningitis is less than 5 per cent. In the Gambia, 27 per cent of children hospitalized with culture-proven H influenzae meningitis, died in hospital despite receiving effective antibiotics. 38 per cent of the survivors had clinical sequelae, a quarter of whom had major disabilities (**32**). In herpes simplex encephalitis, the overall untreated mortality rate exceeds 70 per cent; delaying treatment until symptoms have been present for 4 days is associated with a mortality of 35 per cent and instituting treatment before a complete loss of consciousness reduces the mortality rate to 17 per cent. Similarly, it is our impression that critical care continues to contribute to a better outcome both in terms of survival rates and in the quality of life for survivors. Critical care has also afforded us the opportunity to observe the course of these disorders more closely and to explore new management strategies in the controlled environment of the critical care unit.

In memoriam, **Dr Prashant G Shetty MD, DNB, DMRD (1963–2001),** *Consultant Radiologist, The Hinduja Hospital and Medical Research Centre, Mumbai. Perceptive diagnostician, true student, human par excellence.*

REFERENCES

1. de Gans J, van de Beek D. (2002). Dexamethasone in adults with bacterial meningitis. N Engl J Med. 347, 1549–1556.

2. Tunkel AR, Scheld WM. (2002). Corticosteroids for everyone with meningitis? N Engl J Med. 347, 1613–1615.

3. van de Beek D, de Gans J, McIntyre P et al. (2003). Corticosteroids in acute bacterial meningitis. Cochrane Database Syst Rev. 3, CD004305.

4a. Begg N, Cartwright KAV, Cohen J et al. (1999). Consensus statement on diagnosis, investigation, treatment and prevention of acute bacterial meningitis in immunocompetent adults. J Infect. 39, 1–15.

4b. Heyderman RS, Lambert HP, O'Sullivan I et al. on behalf of The British Infection Society. (2003). Early management of suspected bacterial meningitis and meningococcal septicaemia in adults. J Infect. 46, 75–77.

5. Moller Kirsten Skinhoj P. (2000). Guidelines for managing acute bacterial meningitis. Speed in diagnosis and treatment is essential. BMJ. 320, 1290

6. Rintala E, Seppälä OP, Kotilainen P et al. (1998). Protein C in the treatment of coagulopathy in meningococcal disease. Crit Care Med. 26, 965–968.

7. Sharfstein SR, Gordon MF, Libman RB et al. (1999). Adult-onset MELAS presenting as herpes encephalitis. Arch Neurol. 56, 241–243.

8. Bernier FP, Boneh A, Dennett X et al. (2002). Diagnostic criteria for respiratory chain disorders in adults and children. Neurology. 12, 59, 1406–1411.

9. Le Moal G, Landron C, Grollier G et al. (2003). Characteristics of brain abscess with isolation of anaerobic bacteria. Scand J Infect Dis. 35, 318–321.

10. Roche M, Humphreys H, Smyth E et al. (2003). A twelve-year review of central nervous system bacterial abscesses; presentation and aetiology. Clin Microbiol Infect. 9, 803–809.

11. Gerlach R, Yahya H, Rohde S et al. (2003). Increased incidence of thrombophilic abnormalities in patients with cranial dural arteriovenous fistulae. Neurol Res. 25, 745–748.

12. Watkins LM, Pasternack MS, Banks M et al. (2003). Bilateral cavernous sinus thromboses and intraorbital abscesses secondary to Streptococcus milleri. Ophthalmology. 110, 569–574.

13. Colson AE, Daily JP. (1999). Orbital apex syndrome and cavernous sinus thrombosis due to infection with Staphylococcus aureus and Pseudomonas aeruginosa. Clin Infect Dis. 29, 701–702.

14. Ebright JR, Pace MT, Niazi AF. (2001). Septic thrombosis of the cavernous sinuses. Arch Intern Med. 10–24; 161, 2671–2676.

15. Stam J, De Bruijn SF, DeVeber G. (2002). Anticoagulation for cerebral sinus thrombosis. Cochrane Database Syst Rev. 4, CD002005.

16. Canhão P, Falcão F, Ferro JM. (2003). Thrombolytics for cerebral sinus thrombosis: a systematic review. Cerebrovasc Dis. 15, 159–166.

17. Bhatia K, Jones NS. (2002). Septic cavernous sinus thrombosis secondary to sinusitis: are anticoagulants indicated? A review of the literature. J Laryngol Otol. 116, 667–676.

18. Talmi YP, Goldschmied-Reouven A, Bakon M et al. (2002). Rhino-orbital and rhino-orbito-cerebral mucormycosis. Otolaryngol Head Neck Surg. 127, 22–31

19. Kupila L, Rantakokko-Jalava K, Jalava J et al. (2003). Aetiological diagnosis of brain abscesses and spinal infections: application of broad range bacterial polymerase chain reaction analysis. J Neurol Neurosurg Psychiatry. 74, 728–733.

20. Cone LA, Leung MM, Byrd RG et al. (2003). Multiple cerebral abscesses because of Listeria monocytogenes: three case reports and a literature review of supratentorial listerial brain abscess(es). Surg Neurol. 59, 320–328.

21. Speed B, Dunt D. (1995). Clinical and host differences between infections with the two varieties of Cryptococcus neoformans. Clin Infect Dis. 21, 28–34; discussion 35–36.

22. Bloch KC, Nadarajah R, Jacobs R. (1997). Chryseobacterium meningosepticum: an emerging pathogen among immunocompromised adults. Report of 6 cases and literature review. Medicine (Baltimore). 76, 30–41.

23. Guppy KH, Thomas C, Thomas K et al. (1998). Cerebral fungal infections in the immunocompromised host: a literature review and a new pathogen—Chaetomium atrobrunneum: case report. Neurosurgery. 43, 1463–1469.

24. Opravil M, Pechère M, Lazzarin A et al. (1995). Dapsone/pyrimethamine may prevent mycobacterial disease in immunosuppressed patients infected with the human immunodeficiency virus. Clin Infect Dis. 20, 244–249.

25. Knapp S, Turnherr M, Dekan G et al. (1999). A case of HIV-associated cerebral histoplasmosis successfully treated with fluconazole. Eur J Clin Microbiol Infect Dis. 18, 658–661.

26. Langford TD, Letendre SL, Larrea GJ et al. (2003). Changing patterns in the neuropathogenesis of HIV during the HAART era. Brain Pathol. 13, 195–210.

27. Makni F, Cheikrouhou F, Ayadi A. (2000). Parasitoses and immunodepression. Arch Inst Pasteur Tunis. 77, 51–54.

28. Gray F, Chrétien F, Vallat-Decouvelaere AV et al. (2003). The changing pattern of HIV neuropathology in the HAART era. J Neuropathol Exp Neurol. 62, 429–440.

29. Tattevin P, Schortgen F, de Broucker T et al. (2001). Varicella-zoster virus limbic encephalitis in an immunocompromised patient. Scand J Infect Dis. 33, 786–788.

30. Mustafa MM, Weitman SD, Winick NJ et al. (1993). Subacute measles encephalitis in the young immunocompromised host: report of two cases diagnosed by polymerase chain reaction and treated with ribavirin and review of the literature. Clin Infect Dis. 16, 654–660.

31. Di Patre PL, Radziszewski W, Martin NA et al. (2000). A meningioma-mimicking tumor caused by Mycobacterium avium complex in an immunocompromised patient. Am J Surg Pathol. 24, 136–139.

32. Goetghebuer T, West TE, Wermenbol V et al. (2000). Outcome of meningitis caused by Streptococcus pneumoniae and Haemophilus influenzae type b in children in the Gambia. Trop Med Int Health. 5, 207–213.

E. STATUS EPILEPTICUS

Dr Sarosh M. Katrak & Dr Noshir H. Wadia

Definition

Until recently status epilepticus (SE) was defined as a clinical state in which epileptic seizures occur so frequently that the patient does not recover from one seizure before getting another, or a condition in which an epileptic seizure is so prolonged as to create a fixed and lasting epileptic state (1). Since neuronal injury occurs as early as 30 minutes, there is a move to shorten the duration of the fixed and lasting epileptic state. In 1999, it was proposed that the duration of the epileptic state should be more than 5 minutes to fulfil the definition (2). This definition captures the essence of SE which is that the seizures are prolonged or repetitive because of a failure of seizure terminating mechanisms. This failure leads to certain pathophysiological changes and neurotransmitter defects which in turn lead to severe encephalopathy and more seizures.

Classification of SE

There are five major subtypes of SE:
1. Over-generalized convulsive SE (GCSE)
2. Subtle convulsive SE
3. Complex partial SE—also called non-convulsive SE
4. Absence SE—Petit mal status
5. Partial or focal SE—Epilepsy Partialis Continuum

All types of status may have serious consequences but GCSE is the most common and serious subtype of SE and constitutes a medical emergency. This chapter will only consider the various causes, pathophysiology and management of GCSE.

Causes of GCSE

The major causes of GCSE are:

1. Cerebral Trauma

Open head injuries tend to produce more status epilepticus than closed head injuries (3). Although the risks of epilepsy after neurosurgical procedures (a form of cerebral trauma), ranging from burr holes to open craniotomy, are known, the exact incidence of SE following surgery is not known but is believed to be negligible.

2. Cerebral infection

Any form of infection of the central nervous system can produce SE but the common ones are bacterial and tuberculous meningitis, abscesses, severe viral encephalitis especially herpes simplex encephalitis, cerebral malaria and more recently HIV infections.

3. Cerebral Tumours

Intra-axial tumours and rapidly growing tumours have a greater propensity to produce GCSE. Thus epilepsy and SE are more common in malignant gliomas as compared to oligodendrogliomas or meningiomas. The site is also important, GCSE being more common in the superficial tumours (closer to the cortex) and in the frontal area.

4. Cerebrovascular Disease

All forms of vascular insults to the brain can produce GCSE: these include intracerebral or subarachnoid haemorrhage, angiomatas or arteriovenous malformations (AVMs), cerebral infarcts and particularly haemorrhagic infarcts secondary to cortical venous thrombosis.

5. Metabolic Causes

Hypoglycaemia, hypocalcaemia and hypomagnesaemia are the most common metabolic causes of SE. SE is uncommon in acute hepatic coma unless associated with cerebral oedema. Hyperparathyroidism, porphyria, Wilson's disease and chronic disorders of calcium and magnesium can all produce SE.

6. Toxic Causes

Toxic exposure or withdrawal of drugs can produce SE. However in most studies this factor is grossly underrepresented. Drugs/toxins known to cause SE are (a) alcohol, abuse as well as sudden withdrawal (4), (b) isoniazid, (c) lidocaine and enflurane, (d) psychotropic drugs, (e) penicillin particularly if given intrathecally.

Most cases of GCSE do not occur as a result of a massive cerebral lesion. In fact there is usually a precipitating factor that causes the development of SE. The most frequent precipitating factors are sudden withdrawal of anti-epileptic drugs and fever (5, 6). Other causes include superadded metabolic defects—hypoglycaemia or hypocalcaemia, inadvertent withdrawal from sedative drugs, sleep deprivation and cerebral angiography. *Hence a precipitating factor for SE must be actively and vigorously sought and treated to facilitate seizure control.*

Clinical Presentation and EEG

GCSE generally follows a predictable course if untreated or refractory to therapy.

Motor events: The initial part—phase I—consists of a tonic phase followed by a clonic phase. Subsequently the tonic phase decreases in duration with continuing tonic/clonic seizures (7). The seizures may be bilateral and synchronous in 45 per cent of the patients; in the remainder, they may be adversive or focal in onset (8).

As tonic/clonic seizures continue they become shorter in duration and more restricted and focal. This does not necessarily imply a focal pathology. Later, the seizure activity may be reduced to a few myoclonic jerks and should not be mistaken for myoclonic SE. This phase is considered as phase II of GCSE and is what Treiman has aptly called 'Subtle GCSE' (8, 9).

The transition from phase I to II is determined by the extent of rostral to caudal transmission of neural impulses from the cerebral cortex to axial muscles. As GCSE progresses, certain pathophysiological events occur which dampen or impair the transmission of neural impulses resulting in more subtle restricted seizure activity.

Just as there is progression from clinically overt SE (phase I) to subtle SE (phase II), it is now recognized that the EEG also evolves over a period of time in SE. Treiman et al. (8) have shown a distinct 5 phase evolution of the EEG in GCSE:

1. Initially discrete EEG seizures separated by interictal slowing.
2. Merging seizure activity produces a waxing and waning character of amplitude and frequency of EEG rhythms.
3. Continuous ictal activity.
4. Continuous ictal activity punctuated by periods of relative flattening.
5. Periodic epileptiform discharges on a relatively flat background activity.

The time period for this evolution is not specified and these five phases may not be consistent in every patient.

Pathophysiological Changes in GCSE

The pathophysiological changes in both the phases of GCSE are summarized in **Table 15.10.5**.

Table 15.10.5. Pathophysiological changes during GCSE

	Early SE (Phase I)	Late SE (Phase II)
CBF/CPP	Elevated	Rapidly falls
ICP	Elevated	Remains elevated
Cerebral oedema	Mild	Severe
Systemic BP	Elevated	N or Hypotension
Blood glucose	Elevated	N or Hypoglycaemia
Arterial pH	Acidosis++	Acidosis+
Body temperature	Elevated	More elevated
Heart rate	Tachycardia	Tachycardia with arrhythmia
Respiratory rate	Tachyphnoea	Tachypnoea
Pulmonary oedema	Present	Worse
Catecholamines	Markedly elevated	Still elevated
Leucocytosis	Present	?

CBF = Cerebral Blood Flow; CCP = Cerebral Perfusion Pressure
ICP = Intracranial Pressure; N = Normal

Cerebral Blood Flow and Perfusion

In phase I, which is the compensated stage, cerebral metabolic rates are phenomenally raised. This is compensated by a marked increase in cerebral blood flow with increased delivery of oxygen and glucose. During transition from phase I to phase II (the decompensated phase) cerebral autoregulation fails. Hence, cerebral perfusion pressure becomes dependent on systemic blood pressure, hypotension develops and cerebral perfusion and blood flow decrease. This results in cellular hypoxia, particularly in epileptic tissues, where metabolic rates are high.

Systemic Blood Pressure

In phase I, systemic blood pressure is elevated because of an increase in plasma catecholamine levels. The heart rate is also increased (10). During phase II, the systemic blood pressure begins to fall with sustained hypotension. In prolonged SE, hypotension is common and secondary to cerebral and metabolic changes, drug therapy particularly if general anaesthetics are employed, and to desensitization of catecholamine receptors.

Blood Glucose Changes

At the onset of SE, because of the release of catecholamines, insulin and glucagon, there is moderate hyperglycaemia (11). Routine administration of dextrose to patients in SE who are not hypoglycaemic should be avoided as recent evidence shows that hyperglycaemia can produce cerebral neuronal damage by inducing cellular excitotoxicity (12). As SE becomes more prolonged and sustained, hypoglycaemia ensues because of exhaustion of glycogen stores, hepatic damage and rebound hyperinsulinaemia.

Acidosis

Acidosis is invariable in GCSE, because of neuronal and muscle activity, accelerated glycolysis, tissue hypoxia, and impaired respiration. Lactate levels are very high and serum potassium levels are low. An effective method of dealing with acidosis would be to control respiration and abolish seizure activity, the two major causes of lactic acidosis. Although acidosis is not an important cause of cerebral damage in adults, it is important in infants and children (13) and high levels of CSF lactate have been correlated with poor outcome (14).

Hyperpyrexia

An increase in the body temperature is common in SE because of muscle activity and massive catecholamine release. At times, hyperpyrexia can be severe and prolonged and is associated with neuronal damage particularly in the cerebellum (10). Hyperpyrexia is a strong determinant of poor outcome and is an independent risk factor for increased risk of death and neurological deficit (10).

Intracranial Pressure (ICP) and Cerebral Oedema

All epileptic seizures transiently elevate ICP. Hence, in GCSE, ICP is generally elevated but rapidly returns to normal with control of status. In phase II of GCSE, the combined effect of systemic hypotension and raised ICP results in decreased cerebral perfusion pressure, compromised cerebral circulation and cerebral oedema. In children, cerebral oedema is more severe with further impairment of circulation and infarcts in the watershed area (15). The development of cerebral oedema is more common in encephalitis and cerebral trauma than in SE due to drug withdrawal.

Pulmonary Oedema

Pulmonary hypertension and oedema commonly occur in phase II of GCSE probably as a result of seizure-related autonomic effects. The development of pulmonary oedema is a complication which worsens the outcome of SE (10).

Cardiac Arrhythmias

Seizure-induced autonomic effects, catecholamine release, hypoglycaemia, acidosis and cardiotoxic drugs all contribute to the development of cardiac arrhythmias in GCSE. Intravenous sedatives depress cardiac output and may precipitate congestive failure, if impaired cardiac function pre-existed.

Rhabdomyolysis and Myoglobinuria

Violent convulsive movements can produce rhabdomyolysis and occasionally this is severe enough to produce myoglobinuria and acute renal failure.

Disseminated Intravascular Coagulopathy (DIC)

DIC is a rare but serious complication of GCSE. The exact mechanism is not known.

Leucocytosis

Leucocytosis up to $20,000/mm^3$ is frequent in GSE. CSF leucocytosis can also occur in a smaller percentage of patients but is usually early and transient. If CSF leucocytosis is persistent an infective aetiology should be considered (16).

Electrolyte, Renal and Hepatic Dysfunction

Electrolyte disturbances do occur in GCSE, particularly hyperkalaemia in the presence of rhabdomyolysis. Similarly, acute renal failure with tubular necrosis may occur with myoglobinuria secondary to severe rhabdomyolysis. Hepatic failure may result from drug treatment, particularly with sodium valproate. Intractable status with acute hepatic failure leading to death should arouse the possibility of Alper's disease.

Pathological Consequences of SE

From experimental and human studies it is now well established that seizures per se produce neuronal damage (16, 17) and the severity of this damage is proportional to (a) the original aetiology producing SE, (b) the duration of the seizure activity, and (c) the time lapse between the onset of seizure activity and treatment. In human studies, persistent seizure activity for two or more hours before therapy is instituted, is usually associated with a poor outcome or morbidity (7, 16). In experimental models, the pathological changes are similar to the neuronal damage found in human beings, particularly in the selectively vulnerable areas such as the hippocampus (18). This damage does occur even if the systemic effects of SE are abolished by controlled ventilation and paralysis of the experimental animal (19) and occurs chiefly in phase II of GCSE.

The basic mechanisms by which neuronal damage occurs are not entirely clear but two types of basic mechanisms are postulated based on an experimental model of SE.

1. There is a reduction in blood flow in phase II of SE producing reduced cerebral perfusion pressure and neuronal injury especially hippocampal sclerosis. There is now substantial evidence that prolonged repetitive seizure activity causes hippocampal sclerosis and neuronal injury is similar to that seen in anoxia (20).

2. Repeated seizures cause the release of excitatory neurotransmitters particularly glutamate and related compounds. By their action on N-methyl D-aspartate (NMDA) receptors, they produce a number of cytotoxic effects, mediated through the entry of calcium intracellularly, producing neuronal damage. Other neurotoxic substances released during SE are aspartate, free fatty acids, arachidonic acid and free radicals (18, 21).

In survivors of SE the mechanism of neuronal injury is mainly inferred from animal data. In vivo markers could define subtypes of SE and serve as outcome measures for new treatments and interventions. Two such markers are neuronal specific enolase (NSE) and diffusion weighted images on magnetic resonance imaging (DW-MRI).

NSE is a key protein in glycolysis and is associated with neuronal injury in anoxia, stroke and SE. NSE leaks across the injured neuronal cell membrane and crosses the blood-brain barrier into the serum compartment (22). NSE levels correlate with the duration and outcome of SE (23).

Increased signal on DW-MRI is a highly reliable marker of acute ischaemic neuronal injury. These changes occur immediately after the ischaemia and persist for 2 weeks. Flacke et al. have shown that an increase in regional blood flow in the epileptic cortex of focal SE produces increased signal on DW-MRI (24).

Prognosis

The overall mortality in GCSE varies between 3 and 27 per cent (3, 7, 25). Death may be due to the original disease producing SE, medical complications, or overmedication. Unfortunately, there have been virtually no studies that have systematically evaluated the neurological and cognitive outcome following recovery from a prolonged GCSE. Hauser (25) states that epileptics who have had an episode of SE have a lower likelihood of remission from their fits. The methodological problem of assessing cognitive function in the post SE period are many but some studies have shown a slight deleterious effect on cognition following SE (26).

Principles of Management of Status Epilepticus

The main principles of management of SE are:

1. Maintain vital functions

The patient's position should be such as to avoid aspiration, suffocation or a fall. Tight clothing should be loosened. An ECG should be recorded and cardiac function monitored. Insert a soft *plastic* airway and tape it in place. Intubate the patient to secure the airway, prevent aspiration and allow mechanical ventilatory support. A fast-acting paralytic drug may be essential prior to intubating a convulsing patient. The role of hypoglycaemia is now debatable in an unconscious patient (12) but it is prudent to give 50 ml of 50 per cent dextrose as a bolus via a *large* intravenous catheter as hypoglycaemia may subsequently evolve with prolonged convulsions. Thiamine 100 mg intravenously may be given if alcohol withdrawal or chronic alcoholism is suspected.

2. Identify and treat the cause and precipitating factors

All the causes and precipitating factors have been outlined earlier and appropriate measures should be taken to treat or correct them.

3. Treat or prevent medical complications

The common pathophysiological changes have been listed in **Table 15.10.5**. Of these the ones requiring close attention are blood glucose, arterial pH and arterial blood gases, and body temperature.

4. Rapid control of seizure activity

This requires not only pharmacological therapy but also close attention to the above three principles of therapy.

Pharmacological Therapy

Pharmacological Principles

The ideal drug for status epilepticus should have the following properties:

1. Rapid entry into the brain.
2. Immediate anticonvulsant activity.
3. No significant depression of consciousness or respiration.
4. Long duration of action (**27, 28**).

As fast drug action is essential in SE, all drugs are administered parenterally, preferably intravenously. Highly lipid soluble drugs—diazepam, midazolam, chlormethiazole—have a very rapid onset of action but tend to redistribute from cerebral tissue to larger peripheral lipid tissue. Hence their action is usually short lived and repeated dosage may be necessary. With repeated doses, the peripheral fat tissue becomes saturated and redistribution does not occur rapidly from the cerebral tissue. Therefore subsequent intravenous doses may achieve high cerebral levels and precipitate hypotension, sedation and cardiorespiratory failure. Less lipid soluble drugs (phenytoin, phenobarbitone, lorazepam) have a relatively slower onset of action, but have a longer lasting effect without undue sedation or depression of cardiorespiratory function. Thus, although there is no single ideal anticonvulsant drug, a combination of intravenous diazepam followed by an intravenous bolus of phenytoin seems to be the ideal combination for the treatment of GCSE.

Phenytoin

Phenytoin is the drug of choice for established SE. Its pharmacological and clinical effects are well established and there is extensive experience of its use in adults and children. However a few points require clarification. In status epilepticus, the loading dose should be high—15–20 mg/kg—as optimal serum concentration for control of SE may be 25–30 µg/ml as against the normal therapeutic range of 10–20 µg/ml. Thus the initial loading dose in an adult is around 1000 mg. Regrettably, lower doses are often given and this is one of the most common reasons for uncontrolled SE. As phenytoin has to be infused at a rate of 50 mg/min and even slower (2–30 mg/min) in the elderly, this large dose would take 20–30 minutes for infusion. Based on the pharmacokinetics of intravenous

phenytoin, peak cerebral and CSF concentrations will be reached 1 hour later (**29**). Hence there is usually a delay of approximately 90 minutes before the peak effect of phenytoin is seen, even if therapy is instituted rapidly. It is for this reason that it is given in conjunction with a short but rapidly acting drug like diazepam.

The usual parenteral phenytoin solution has a pH of 12 and if added to intravenous fluids with a pH lower than the physiological pH (5 per cent dextrose), there is a danger of precipitation in the bottle or along with tubing. Use of normal (0.9 per cent) saline is safer. Being highly alkaline, phenytoin can produce chemical phlebitis. After an infusion the vein should be flushed with normal saline. Phenytoin should not be given rectally or intramuscularly. Constant monitoring of blood pressure and ECG is essential during high dose infusion of phenytoin particularly in the elderly. The toxicity of intravenous phenytoin is more dependent on the rate of infusion rather than on the total dose. Hence, it is prudent to infuse it at a slower rate (20–30 mg/min) in the elderly and in those with conduction defects. Known complications include hypotension, atrial and ventricular conduction depression, ventricular fibrillation and cardiovascular collapse with respiratory arrest (**29**).

Fosphenytoin

This is a prodrug of phenytoin and is significantly more soluble than phenytoin. It also has a significantly lower pH and as a result does not cause the same degree of pain when infused nor tissue necrosis when it extravasates into subcutaneous spaces. Fosphenytoin is expressed in phenytoin equivalents (PEs). It is given at a dose of 18–20 mg/kg PEs and infused at a rate of 50–150 mg/minute. It can produce therapeutic concentrations of phenytoin very rapidly (up to 10 minutes) and produces significantly less hypotension. Hence, it can be administered more rapidly than phenytoin. However, it is more expensive than phenytoin and rate reductions in the speed of infusion are still recommended in patients with cardiac or liver disease, in the elderly and in the critically ill (**30**).

Phenobarbitone

Phenobarbitone is indicated for the treatment of GCSE in patients who are allergic to phenytoin, have evidence of impaired cardiac conductivity, or in whom phenytoin has failed to control established SE. It is highly effective, has a rapid onset of action, a prolonged anticonvulsant effect and may be preferentially concentrated in metabolically active neurons like an epileptic focus. The main disadvantages of phenobarbitone are that it produces sedation, respiratory depression and hypotension. In practice, these effects are slight, particularly if the patient is already intubated and on a ventilator.

The recommended loading dose is 10 mg/kg given at a rate of 60–100 mg/min to a total of 700 mg in 7–12 minutes. This may be followed by daily maintenance doses of 1–4 mg/kg. Phenobarbitone should not be given intramuscularly to a patient in SE because peak serum levels are not reached quickly and seizures continue until the level rises into the therapeutic range.

Diazepam

Although diazepam is not considered as a primary drug for GCSE, it has a time-honoured place in the therapy of the early stages of SE. Because intravenous diazepam produces high serum and brain levels, it is a helpful adjunct to phenytoin therapy in SE. Peak levels are achieved in 1 minute of a standard bolus of diazepam. However being lipid soluble, it is redistributed amongst peripheral lipid stores and hence its action, though rapid, is very transient. The adult bolus intravenous dose is 1–20 mg given at a rate of 2–5 mg/min. Additional 10 mg can be given at 15 minute intervals to a total of 40 mg. Probably the most common and dangerous error is to treat repeated seizures with repeated boluses of diazepam without administering a long acting anti-epileptic drug or treating the precipitating cause.

The use of intravenous diazepam to control generalized tonic/clonic seizures after a full loading dose of phenytoin or phenobarbitone requires experience and judgement. This is usually necessary in refractory SE due to a structural lesion—large brain tumour, encephalitis or cortical venous thrombosis. In such cases, the smallest effective dose of diazepam is indicated if seizures compromise vital function.

Intramuscular and rectal diazepam are absorbed relatively slowly and should not be employed for SE. The most serious complication of diazepam is respiratory depression and hypotension. This occurs in about 6–12 per cent of cases of SE treated with diazepam and is common when there are repeated boluses or when diazepam is used in combination with other sedatives.

Lorazepam

A less lipid soluble benzodiazepine than diazepam, lorazepam can also be used in the early stages of SE as an adjunct to phenytoin. Its long duration of action (up to 12 hours) and strong cerebral binding are very significant advantages over diazepam. However a double blind study comparing lorazepam and diazepam in SE found no significant difference between the two drugs in seizure control, latency of action or toxicity in adults (31). In adults a bolus dose of 0.07 mg/kg (usually 4 mg) is given initially.

Midazolam

Midazolam has been recently introduced for SE. It is unique among the drugs used for SE in that it can be given intramuscularly, per rectum or intravenously. Bioavailability after an intramuscular injection is 80–100 per cent and peak levels are achieved in 25 minutes. Hence in early SE, if facilities for intravenous medication are not available, intramuscular midazolam has a great advantage. Its toxicity is similar to diazepam.

Intravenous Valproate

Rapid loading with intravenous valproate 25 mg/kg at a rate of 3–6 mg/kg/min produces effective blood levels with minimal hypotension or respiratory depression. Valproate appears safe in SE especially in the elderly with cardiovascular instability and hypotension. Unfortunately, no randomized trial of valproate in SE has been performed to date (32).

Refractory GCSE

If therapy is instituted rapidly, full loading doses of anti-convulsants (phenytoin and diazepam) are given and the precipitating factor is treated, most cases of GCSE come under control. If seizures do *not* respond to full doses of phenytoin and diazepam, a loading dose of phenobarbitone should be added. There are a small number of patients who do not respond to this therapy. These patients usually have a structural lesion—brain tumour, encephalitis, cortical venous thrombosis. These patients present difficult therapeutic problems and as seizures recur, they become more difficult to treat. Soon the decompensated phase II sets in with permanent brain damage (8, 18). Such refractory patients should be treated by general anaesthesia pentobarbital or thiopental or propofol. The advantages of general anesthesia are (1) it prevents tonic/clonic movements and also controls cerebral seizure activity, (2) it reduces cerebral metabolic needs, (3) it allows control of respiration.

All these factors also help in reducing the ICP which in this situation is invariably elevated. The use of short-acting barbiturates—pentobarbital, thiopental or propofol—has recently gained popularity because of their ease of administration, as compared to inhalation anaesthesia, and readily reversible effect.

Pentobarbital

The loading dose is 2–20 mg/kg by bolus or infusion pump at a rate of 25–100 mg/min. A loading dose of 200–400 mg over several minutes is a typical procedure. The maintenance dose ranges from 0.5 to 5 mg/kg/hr. The effectiveness of therapy is judged by abolition of clinical seizures and a 'burst suppression' pattern on EEG monitoring. Once effective, the patient is maintained in this state for 12–24 hours and then gradually reversed out (9, 33, 34).

Thiopental

The loading dose of thiopental is 0.5–30 mg/kg and maintenance doses of 2–55 mg/kg/hr have been used to maintain a burst suppression pattern in the EEG.

Propofol

This is a general anaesthetic. It is a highly water soluble lipid emulsion that is primarily metabolized in the liver. Single boluses or infusions of up to 24 hours have a short elimination half-life with rapid awakening within 10–15 minutes after cessation of the drip. Prolonged infusion over several days may result in slower clearance and a delay in awakening. Propofol can cause bradycardia and severe hypotension as a result of peripheral vasodilatation. Doses used for SE have been a bolus of 1–2 mg/kg followed by 2–10 mg/kg/hour. The experience with propofol in SE is limited and not yet defined. The advantages are a rapid awakening after short-term infusion which can be delayed with prolonged infusions (35, 36).

The use of anaesthetic-induced coma is associated with many risks:

1. The patient requires intubation and controlled ventilation as respiratory and cardiac depression may occur.

2. Hypotension may occur. Hence blood pressure and central venous pressure should be monitored. Hypotension may need to be treated with volume expanders or fluid challenge. Inotropic support may be necessary.

3. Other complications are poikilothermia and increased risk of nosocomial pneumonia.

Under barbiturate coma, a neurologic assessment is not possible. The average mortality in such cases is about 35 per cent and is usually due to the underlying disease and rarely due to the therapy *per se*.

Protocol for therapy of GCSE

A protocol for the treatment of acute GCSE is outlined in **Table 15.10.6**. The treating physician and his support team must be familiar with the treatment protocol, and as many good protocols are available they should adopt one for consistency (**9, 28, 34**).

Table 15.10.6. Protocol for treatment of acute GCSE

0–5 minutes

(i) Assess cardiorespiratory function. (ii) Simultaneously confirm diagnosis of SE by observing one tonic/clonic seizure activity. (iii) Insert oral airway and administer oxygen if necessary. (iv) Insert IV catheter. Draw blood for CBC, glucose, electrolytes, calcium, magnesium, BUN/creatinine. Collect arterial blood for ABG. (v) If airway is compromised intubate and secure airway.

6–9 minutes

Administer either IV diazepam 10–20 mg bolus at a rate of 2–5 mg/minute OR IV lorazepam 4 mg bolus at a rate of 1–2 mg/minute. Both can be repeated if seizures do not stop in 5 minutes.

10–30 minutes

If SE persists, administer IV phenytoin 15–20 mg/kg slow infusion at a rate of 50 mg/minute or 20–30 mg/minute in the elderly or when cardiac function is compromised. Fosphenytoin 18–20 mg/kg PEs infused at a rate of 50–150 mg/min is preferable in the elderly with compromised cardiac function. Phenytoin is incompatible with dextrose containing solutions. Hence, flush the IV line with normal saline before the infusion.

30–60 minutes

If SE is not controlled then give additional phenytoin 5 mg/kg OR infuse phenobarbitone 10 mg/kg at a rate of 60–100 mg/min IV. When phenobarbitone is given after diazepam/lorazepam, there is a great risk of apnoea. Hence pass an endotracheal tube (if this has not already been done), and initiate ventilator support. If SE persists, an additional 10 mg/kg of phenobarbitone may be given at 60–100 mg/min.

60–120 minutes

If SE persists, induce general anaesthesia with either pentobarbital, thiopental or propofol. EEG monitoring is essential. The loading dose of pentobarbital is 15 mg/kg given at a rate of 1–2 mg/kg/hr until seizures stop or EEG shows a burst suppression pattern. The loading dose of thiopental is 5–10 mg/kg followed by 2 mg/min via a micro-drip set for 30–60 minutes. Reduce the dose to 0.5 mg/min when SE is controlled. A bolus dose of propofol of 1–2 mg/kg followed by 2–10 mg/kg/hour infusion until SE is controlled adequately. The patient regains consciousness rapidly after cessation of infusion.

Note: Ventilator support should be promptly offered if seizures render ventilation inadequate or if the PaO_2 is lowered to < 70 mm Hg on supplemental oxygen. *It is best to anticipate ventilatory failure or hypoxia and use early ventilatory support.*

REFERENCES

1. Gastaut H. (1970). Clinical and electroencephalographical classification of epileptic seizures. Epilepsia. 11, 102–113.
2. Lowenstein D, Bleck T, MacDonald RL. (1999). It's time to revise the definition of status epilepticus. Epilepsia. 40, 752–758.
3. Oxbury JM and Whitty CWM. (1971). Causes and consequences of status epilepticus in adults: A study of 86 cases. Brain 94, 733–744.
4. Simon RP and Aminoff MJ. (1980). Clinical aspects of status epilepticus in an unselected urban population. Transactions of the American Neurological Association. 105, 46–49.
5. Jans D. (1962). Conditions and causes of status epilepticus. Epilepsia. 2, 170–177.
6. Kas S, Orszagh J. (1976). Clinical study of status epilepticus: Review of 11 statuses, Acta Univ Carol (Med) Praha. 22, 133–178.
7. Rowan AJ, Scot DG. (1970). Major status epilepticus: A series of 42 patients, Acta Neurol Scand. 46, 573–584.
8. Treiman DM, Waldrom NY, Kendrick CW. (1990). A progressive sequence of electroencephalographic changes during generalized convulsive status epilepticus. Epilepsy Res. 5, 49–60.
9. Teriman DM. (1990). The role of benzodiazepines in the management of status epilepticus. Neurology. 40 (suppl 2), 32–42.
10. Simon RP. (1985). Physiologic consequences of status epilepticus. Epilepsia. 26 (suppl 1), S58–S66.
11. Kreisman NR, Lamanna JC, Rosenthal M et al. (1981). Oxidative metabolic responses with recurrent seizures in rat and cerebral cortex: Role of systemic factors. Brain Res. 218, 175–188.
12. Pulsinelli WA, Levy DE, Sigabee B et al. (1983). Increased damage after ischaemic stroke in patients with hyperglycaemia with or without established diabetes. Am J Med. 74, 540–544.
13. Simpson H, Habel AH and George EL. (1977). Cerebrospinal fluid acid base status and lactate and pyruvate concentrations after convulsions of varied duration and aetiology in children. Arch Dis Child. 42, 844–849.
14. Calabrese VP, Gruemer HD, James K et al. (1991). Cerebrospinal fluid lactate levels and prognosis in status epilepticus. Epilepsia. 32, 816–821.
15. Brown JK and Hussin IHMI. (1991). Status epilepticus I, Pathogenis Dev Med Child Neurol. 33, 3–17.
16. Aminoff MJ, Simon RP (1980), Status epilepticus: causes, clinical features and consequences in 98 patients. Am J Med. 69, 657–666.
17. Meldrum BS and Brierley JB. (1973). Prolonged epileptic seizures in primates: ischaemic cell change and its relation to ictal physiological events. Arch Neurol. 28, 10–17.
18. Lothman E. (1990). The biochemical basis and pathophysiology of status epilepticus. Neurology. 40 (suppl 2), 13–23.
19. Meldrum BS, Vigoroux RA, Brierley JB. (1973). Systemic factors and epileptic brain damage: prolonged seizures in paralysed, artificially ventilated baboons. Arch Neurol. 28, 82–87.
20. Meldrum BS. (1983). Metabolic factors during prolonged seizures and their relation to nerve cell death. In: Advances in Neurology, Status Epilepticus (Eds Delgado-Escueta AV, Wasterlain CG, Treiman DM et al.). Vol 34, Raven Press, New York. pp. 261–275.
21. Siesjo BJ, Ingvar M, Folbergrova et al. (1983). Local cerebral circulation and metabolism in bicuculline induced status epilepticus: Relevance for development of cell change. In: Advances in Neurology, Status Epilepticus (Eds Delgado-Escueta AV, Wasterlain CG, Treiman DM et al.). Vol 34, Raven Press, New York. pp. 217–230.
22. Correale J, Rabinowicz AL, Heck CN et al. (1998). Status epilepticus increases CSF level of neurone specific enolase and alters the blood brain barrier. Neurology. 50, 1388–1391.

23. DeGiorgio CM, Heck CN, Rabinowicz AL et al. (1999). Serum neurone specific enolase in the major subtypes of status epilepticus. Neurology. 52, 746–749.

24. Flacke S, Wullner U, Keller E et al. (2000). Reversible changes in echo planar perfusion—and diffusion-weighted MRI in status epilepticus. Neuroradiology. 42, 92–95.

25. Hauser WA. (1990). Status epilepticus: Epidemiologic considerations. Neurology. 40 (suppl 2), 9–13.

26. Dodrill CB, Wilensky AJ. (1990). Intellectual impairment as an outcome of status epilepticus. Neurology. 40 (supple 2), S23–S27.

27. Browne TR. (1990). The pharmacokinetics of agents used to treat status epilepticus. Neurology. 40 (suppl 2), S28–S32.

28. Leppik IE. (1990). Status epilepticus: the next decade. Neurology. 40 (suppl 2), S4–S9.

29. Cranford RE, Leppik IE, Patrick BK et al. (1978). Intravenous phenytoin: Clinical and pharmacokinetic aspects. Neurology. 28, 874–880.

30. Physicians Desk Reference. (2001). Medical Economics Company, Montvale, New Jersey.

31. Leppik IE, Derivan AT, Homan RV et al. (1983). Double blind study of lorazepam, and diazepam in status epilepticus. JAMA. 249, 1452–1454.

32. Wheless JW, Venkataraman V. (1998). Safety of high IV loading dose of valproate. Epilepsia. 39 (suppl 6), S50 (abstract).

33. Osorio I, Reed RC. (1989). Treatment of refractory generalized tonic-clonic status epilepticus with phenobarbital anaesthesia after high dose phenytoin. Epilepsia. 30, 464–471.

34. Van Ness PC. (1990). Phenobarbital and EEG burst suppression in the treatment of status epilepticus refractory to benzodiazepines and phenytoin. Epilepsia. 31, 61–67.

35. Stecker MM, Cramer TH, Raps EC et al. (1998). Treatment of refractory status epilepticus with propofol. Clinical and pharmacologic findings. Epilepsia. 39, 18–26.

36. Treiman DM. (1997). Generalized convulsive status epilepticus. In: Epilepsy—A comprehensive textbook (Eds Engel J Jr, Pedley TA). pp. 669–680. Lippincott-Raven, Philadelphia.

F. PERI-OPERATIVE NEUROLOGICAL CARE

Dr Sohrab K. Bhabha

General Considerations

The demands of contemporary neurosurgery on critical care resources can be considerable. A good working rapport between intensivist, neuroanesthesiologist, neurologist and neurosurgeon does much to facilitate and simplify critical care. The practice of the neurologist or neurosurgeon *alone* assuming charge of critical care, while sometimes unavoidable, is to be strongly discouraged. Experience indicates that the *intensivist* should be the team leader during this crucial phase. It is also appropriate that the intensivist be involved in the pre-operative care of the person whom she or he will continue to manage through critical peri-operative and post-operative phases. It need hardly be stated that the results of painstaking neurosurgery can all too easily be undone, in more than one sense, by unskilled post-operative management. The scope of this chapter is to outline the critical care of the neurosurgical candidate.

Pre-operative Care

Intracranial Hypertension

The management of intracranial hypertension (ICH) in a variety of settings is discussed elsewhere. In the present setting, tumours and intracranial haemorrhage are possibly the commonest causes of ICH. As always, the structural and functional bases for ICH require consideration. The operative mechanism of ICH may then be best addressed. If an intracranial drain is in position, extreme caution must be exercised in venting pressure, since intracranial compartmental shifts may pre-exist and any acute change may be disastrous. Glucocorticoids are usually effective in the management of persons with peritumoural oedema. Dexamethasone (16–32 mg/day), or an alternative steroid, may be started as soon as the diagnosis is made (*excepting* in suspected cerebral lymphomas) and preferably at least 48 hours prior to surgery. If the response is poor, the daily dose may be elevated to 100 mg/day. For acutely decompensating situations, e.g. impending herniation, a bolus of 100 mg may be followed by a similar daily maintenance dose. This measure, sometimes combined with an intravenous mannitol bolus (at times preceded by furosemide), hyperventilation, or both, will salvage most situations.

Seizures

Seizures, generalized or partial, are most often tumour or bleed-associated phenomena in this setting. The incidence of seizures is higher in primary brain tumours than in secondary ones, with the exception of metastatic melanoma, which is frequently associated with seizures. Uncontrolled seizures lead to aggravation of an already decompensated intracranial pressure balance. Seizures may be anticipated in several supratentorial epileptogenic condi-

tions, when prophylactic anticonvulsant drug (ACD) therapy should be considered. The evidence-base for such prophylactic ACD use is slim, however (**1, 2**). It must also be added that contemporary literature seems to point to the underlying pathology, rather than the procedure, as the provocative factor. The presence of a seizure-provoking lesion should not prevent a search for co-existent metabolic derangements which lower seizure threshold, such as hypocalcaemia, hyponatraemia, hypoglycaemia, alcohol-withdrawal and hepatorenal compromise. Patients with primary or secondary brain tumours who receive iodinated radiologic contrast media are at an increased risk for seizures; pretreatment with 5–10 mg oral dose of diazepam, 1 hour prior to contrast injection, reduces the incidence of such seizures (**3**).

For most purposes, phenytoin is a satisfactory acute-care ACD which is available in several dosage forms. In previously untreated persons, a loading dose *must* be administered orally (15–18 mg/kg over 24 hours) *or* intravenously (rate not exceeding 50 mg/min), preferably while monitoring heart rate and blood pressure. We prefer oral loading. Subsequently, a daily dose of 5 mg/kg will usually maintain therapeutic serum levels. Stable serum levels should be ensured *pre-operatively*, as far as possible. A seizure on the operating table is an uncommon but dreaded event. The duration of continued prophylactic ACD use is contentious; current literature appears to indicate that their use must be based upon the epileptogenic potential of underlying pathology. The presence of pre-operative epilepsy or seizures requires altogether different considerations.

Peri-operative Critical Care

Head-Position and Airway

Appropriate head-positioning and fixation are vital steps, especially in the present era of microneurosurgery, image-guided techniques and neuronavigation, when head-position must be maintained over long periods of time. It is nonetheless important to ensure that the endotracheal tube is not compromised. Neck veins should not be obstructed in any way, since this will have an adverse effect on cranial venous return, haemostasis, brain oedema and operating time.

Air Embolism

Twenty five per cent or more of persons operated in the sitting position may suffer from air embolism. This occurs as a result of air entry through torn cortical or diploic veins or dural venous sinuses. Major air embolism causes right heart failure with catastrophic hypotension. Screening for a patent foramen ovale is pre-operatively mandatory for any neurosurgical procedure in the sitting or 'beach chair' position as well as in those procedures where one is likely to encounter prominent venous channels. Pre-operative contrast-enhanced transcranial Doppler ultrasonography (4) and monitoring with transoesophageal echocardiography as well as end-tidal PCO_2 (5) help to define the presence of a patent foramen ovale and establish significant air embolism. Aspiration of air from a right atrial or Swan-Ganz catheter is both diagnostic and therapeutic. Inspired gas should be switched to 100 per cent oxygen to decrease the volume expanding effect of nitrous oxide on the air embolus, and the person should be turned to the left lateral recumbent position. Vasopressors may be required to support arterial pressure. Air embolism can lead to acute pulmonary oedema (6), pulmonary infarction, and also to delayed gas-embolic stroke.

Reversal

The abrupt elevation of intrathoracic pressure commonly associated with *rapid reversal* and its transmitted effects on intracranial venous pressure prompts many neurosurgeons to desist from this method of reversal. Their prime concerns are early intracranial bleeding and intracranial pressure elevation. Therefore, such teams continue to ventilate persons post-operatively and permit them to '*emerge*' or '*float out*' of the effects of anaesthesia. If such a method is employed, it is *imperative* that the person be advised so pre-operatively, to allay his anxiety when he awakens. *This cannot be overemphasized.*

Prophylaxis for *gastrointestinal bleeding, deep venous thrombosis* and *pulmonary embolism* are important aspects of peri-operative neurosurgical care and are considered elsewhere.

Post-operative Critical Care

Effects of Anaesthesia vs. Immediate Neurologic Deterioration

Neurologically normal persons exhibit a variety of pyramidal signs as they emerge from general anaesthesia and up to an hour (or two) thereafter. These include hyperreflexia, ankle clonus and extensor plantar responses (7, 8). Similarly, a degree of confusion, mild worsening of previous hemiparesis, mild dysarthria and asterixis may all be residual anaesthetic effects. In addition, patients undergoing craniotomy for large intracranial mass lesions awaken more slowly than patients after spinal surgery or craniotomy for small brain tumours (9).

When confusion was not pre-operatively present, its presence in the post-operative phase must be viewed as representing a fresh brain event; brain swelling or an evolving intracranial haematoma should be considered. Other worrisome pointers are progressive headache, vomiting, drowsiness, evolving hemiparesis or pupillary changes and *de novo* bradycardia. Any progressive or fluctuating deterioration should be presumed to be of serious import. Additive anaesthetic and anticonvulsant toxicity may lead to toxic effects. Peri-operative phenytoin administration has been associated with post-operative hiccups and vomiting. Persistent ophthalmoplegia (beyond a few hours) may indicate fresh brainstem vascular insult or may unmask a rare case of myasthenia gravis. Brain imaging with CT or MRI is the mainstay of structural redefinition in such circumstances and ought to be used early and as often as may be

required. EEG and evoked response studies have a more limited role. At times, a substantial, transient change in post-operative neurological status may be anticipated, such as may occur in bulbar or ventilatory functions following some surgical procedures involving the brainstem, skull-base or craniovertebral region. This may necessitate anticipatory nutritional management (usually nasogastric intubation) or elective tracheostomy and short-term ventilation.

Haematomas

Haematomas can occur at the site of surgery or remotely, in established spaces such as the extradural or subdural space. Occasionally, they are seen distant to the operative site. Established systemic hypertension predisposes a person to this complication; tumour (typically meningioma) and arteriovenous malformation resection are the commonest settings. With gliomas, gross total resection is associated with a lower incidence of intraparenchymal haematoma development than subtotal resection (10). Extradural haematomas can sometimes be prevented by tenting sutures, especially where the dura has been drawn away from the inner table. Subdural haematomas may result from abrupt brain decompression, such as occasionally occurs when spinal or ventricular drainage is established or when brain swelling responds to bolus mannitol. Surgery in the seated position also predisposes to subdural haematoma, because of traction on bridging veins, particularly after posterior fossa surgery.

Blood Pressure Control

Established *systemic hypertension* should be kept well controlled both before and after craniotomy, since it has been associated with increased mortality in the critical care setting. The precise levels that represent a risk for cerebral oedema post-operatively are difficult to define and depend on the surgical pathology, surgical trauma and pre-operative control. In such persons, their regular antihypertensive treatment is started at approximately half to two-thirds the dose, as soon as possible post-operatively. Sedation often reduces antihypertensive requirements.

Hypertension after *carotid endarterectomy, angioplasty* and *arteriovenous malformation* surgery presents special problems. Malignant cerebral oedema and haemorrhage may occur. *Dysautoregulated hyperperfusion* is thought to underlie such developments. When mean arterial pressure exceeds 110–120 mm Hg, nitroprusside or labetalol may be the best choices to employ (see Chapter on Hypertensive Emergencies in the ICU). Trimetaphan is another agent, which has a negligible effect on intracranial pressure. Nitroglycerin and nifedipine are preferably avoided.

Aneurysmal subarachnoid haemorrhage poses several challenges to the intensivist. Among these are the management of *vasospasm* and *dysnatraemia*. The former may occur as early as a few days (2–4 days) of bleed or may set in as late as 2 weeks post-bleed. The result is variable ischaemic brain insult, even catastrophic infarction, which may significantly mar the quality of outcome. The currently favoured form of therapy is early intervention (either clipping via craniotomy or endovascular interventional obliteration) followed by a combination of induced hypertension, intentional hypervolaemia and haemodilution, also known as 'triple H therapy' (11). This form of therapy has never been subjected to controlled study, however (12). Sodium metabolic derangements related to subarachnoid haemorrhage are a complex of disorders, as yet not fully pathophysiologically understood. Generally, hypernatraemia carries a graver prognosis than hyponatraemia does (13). Bedside cerebral microdialysis is establishing itself as a useful tool for directly monitoring regional cerebral metabolic changes, some of which may help us to define impending neurological events (14).

Intracranial Hypertension

Intracranial hypertension (ICH) may be heralded by a failure to awaken as expected in the immediate post-operative period, a delayed change in the level of arousal ('consciousness') after initial recovery, or the development of an unexpected change or loss of neurological function. Its important causes include haematomas (discussed earlier), perilesional brain oedema, hydrocephalus, tension pneumocephalus and brain infarction (discussed later). Neuroimaging usually differentiates these and guides more specific treatment.

Post-operative *perilesional brain oedema* peaks at 36 to 72 hours. The tempo of evolving ICH is slower in oedema than in haematomas. Patients usually awaken as expected from anaesthesia, but between 6 and 36 hours post-operatively, they become lethargic or develop fresh neurologic deficits. Brain imaging is obtained to exclude a bleed; as soon as this is done, the steroid dose is increased and free water administration is decreased. Further measures to monitor and combat the resultant raised intracranial pressure, such as sedation and hyperventilation (discussed elsewhere), may be required.

Post-operative *hydrocephalus* is most often associated with posterior fossa or intraventricular neurosurgery, the latter carrying the greatest likelihood of introducing blood into the CSF pathways. Patients with symptomatic third ventricular tumours may abruptly develop hydrocephalus and decompensate to coma and sudden death. The latter phenomena are probably a result of *plateau waves*. A ventricular drainage procedure is most often indicated.

With the advent of skull base surgery, the incidence of *tension pneumocephalus* has increased. Continual efflux of CSF from the basal cisterns creates a negative pressure, which sucks in air intracranially. Operative measures to prevent this include dural closure, skull base reconstruction, re-expansion of the intracranial contents and the placement of an extradural drain. Clinical signs of tension pneumocephalus usually appear 2 to 4 days post-operatively, when the intracranial air, due to its mass effect, mimics a space occupying lesion. Persons at risk should be nursed in the head-low position, for 4 days post-operatively. A plain skull film or CT scan readily make the diagnosis clear. Once diagnosed, 100 per cent oxygen is administered and if rapid decompensation is encountered, needle aspiration or silastic catheter placement may be imperative. Water-seal drainage may be required to prevent reaccumulation. Definitive surgery may be the final corrective measure.

Post-operative Stroke

When encountered in the immediate post-operative setting, this event has invariably occurred intra-operatively. Precautions in this direction therefore must be adopted *before* and *at the time of surgery*. Rarely, brain infarction occurs as a post-operative event. Preventive measures include ensuring a normovolaemic state and normal arterial pressure. The post-operative, volume-depleted, hypotensive, hyponatraemic, altered haemorrhagic state predisposes to stroke. Careful fluid and electrolyte monitoring are therefore essential.

The goal of *fluid and electrolyte* management in the post-operative period is to keep the person normovolaemic and normo-to slightly hyper-osmolar, at the same time ensuring normal sodium balance. Several brain-related factors may cause fluid and electrolyte disturbances—e.g. SIADH and 'cerebral natriuresis'. These should be carefully considered and appropriately treated (see Section on Fluid and Electrolyte Disturbances in the Critically Ill).

Fever and Infection

Unsustained fever below 38.5°C can usually be attributed to atelectasis and the post-operative state. Higher temperatures or persistence beyond the first 6 hours require further investigations. Clinical examination, chest X-ray, sputum and urine cultures are the next step. *Central fever* is distinctly uncommon and should only be diagnosed when unremitting hyperthermia (> 40°C) occurs in patients with massive haemorrhage or basal brain lesions in proximity to the anterior hypothalamus. Fever may sometimes be due to a sinusitis, caused or exacerbated by nasogastric intubation over several days. Drug fever, usually associated with an antimicrobial or an anti-convulsant, must also be considered. When fever persists beyond 24 hours and is unexplained by the foregoing, spinal fluid must be examined. Bacterial meningitis must be differentiated from its aseptic counterpart (15). This is not always easy, since glucose ratios and cell counts are not so helpful. Fever, CSF leak, peripheral leucocytosis and culture postivity are better differentiators and favour bacterial meningitis. *S. aureus* and *Gram-negative bacilli* are the leading causes of post-operative bacterial meningitis. Even with satisfactory therapy, CSF cultures may still show Gram-negative bacilli for up to 2 weeks. CSF leaks require definitive management if treatment is to be lastingly effective. Other factors causing fever at this stage are craniotomy infections, subgaleal fluid collections or haematomas, salivary gland inflammation, deep venous thrombosis and acute adrenal insufficiency.

The use of prophylactic antimicrobials in *clean* neurosurgical procedures, whether monitoring ones (ICP monitoring, drains, microdialysis) or formal surgery, is undergoing a process of continual review and rationalization (16). The emerging trend is away from prophylactic use (particularly for monitoring ones) and increasingly towards extremely brief (single-dose, single-day, 3-day) use in formal ones.

REFERENCES

1. De Santis A, Villani R, Sinisi M et al. (2002). Add-on phenytoin fails to prevent early seizures after surgery for supratentorial brain tumors: a randomized controlled study. Epilepsia. 43, 175–182.

2. Baker CJ, Prestigiacomo CJ, Solomon RA. (1995). Short-term perioperative anticonvulsant prophylaxis for the surgical treatment of low-risk patients with intracranial aneurysms. Neurosurgery. 37, 863–870; discussion 870–871.

3. Pagain JJ, Hayman L A, Bigelow R H et al. (1983). Diazepam prophylaxid of contrast media induced seizures during computed tomography of patients with brain metastases. AJR. 140, 787–792.

4. Stendel R, Gramm HJ, Schröder K et al. (2000). Transcranial Doppler ultrasonography as a screening technique for detection of a patent foramen ovale before surgery in the sitting position. Anesthesiology. 93, 971–975.

5. Schmitt HJ, Hemmerling TM. (2002). Venous air emboli occur during release of positive end-expiratory pressure and repositioning after sitting position surgery. Anesth Analg. 94, 400–403.

6. Frim DM, Wollman L, Evans AB et al. (1996). Acute pulmonary edema after low-level air embolism during craniotomy. Case report. J Neurosurg. 85, 937–940.

7. Rosenberg H, Clofine R, Bialik. (1981). Neurologic changes during awakening from anesthesia. Anaesthesiology. 45, 125–130.

8. McCullock P R, Milne B. (1990). Neurological phenomena during emergence from enflurane or isoflurane anesthesia. Can J Anesth. 37, 139–142.

9. Schubert A, Mascha EJ, Bloomfield EL et al. (1996). Effect of cranial surgery and brain tumor size on emergence from anesthesia. Anesthesiology. 85, 513–521.

10. Fadul C E, Wood J, Thaler H et al. (1988). Morbidity and mortality of craniotomy for excision of supratentorial gliomas. Neurology. 38, 1374–1379.

11. Sen J, Belli A, Albon H et al. (2003). Triple-H therapy in the management of aneurysmal subarachnoid haemorrhage. Lancet Neurol. 2, 614–621.

12. Treggiari MM, Walder B, Suter PM et al. (2003). Systematic review of the prevention of delayed ischemic neurological deficits with hypertension, hypervolemia, and hemodilution therapy following subarachnoid hemorrhage. J Neurosurg. 98, 978–984.

13. Qureshi AI, Suri MF, Sung GY et al. (2002). Prognostic significance of hypernatremia and hyponatremia among patients with aneurysmal subarachnoid hemorrhage. Neurosurgery. 50, 749–755; discussion 755–756.

14. Sarrafzadeh AS, Sakowitz OW, Kiening KL et al. (2002). Bedside microdialysis: a tool to monitor cerebral metabolism in subarachnoid hemorrhage patients? Crit Care Med. 30, 1062–1070.

15. Ross D, Rosegay H, Dons V. (1988). Differentiation of aseptic and bacterial meningitis in postoperative neurosurgical patients. J Neurosurg. 69, 669–674

16. Cacciola F, Cioffi F, Anichini P et al. (2001). Antibiotic prophylaxis in clean neurosurgery. J Chemother. 13 Spec No 1, 119–122.

Critical Care After Open Heart Surgery

Critical Care After Open Heart Surgery

General Considerations

Open heart surgery has made great strides in India. The number of centres for open heart surgery in the large metropolitan cities of the country are increasing year by year. In our centre, 12–15 open heart surgeries are performed every week, and very often half the ICU beds are engaged at any one time, in the post-operative care of these patients. Coronary artery bypass grafting (CABG) is the most frequently performed open heart surgery, followed in order of frequency by valve replacements, and by repair of congenital defects in the heart.

The success of good surgical technique and good peri-operative care, can be easily ruined if critical care in the post-operative period is poor. In our unit, the mortality following CABG surgery is less than 1 per cent. In fact, in patients with good pre-operative left ventricular function, the mortality is almost nil. The surgeons are taking on more and more patients with poor left ventricular function (often with ejection fractions in the region of 15 per cent). Many of these poor-risk patients have associated problems in the form of aneurysmal dilatation of a part of the wall of the left ventricle, and blocked coronary arteries which not only need to be bypassed, but also require an endarterectomy. Patients who have a very poor pump function and have to be taken up for CABG surgery or some other open heart surgery, are often given dopamine support (5–7 µg/kg/min) as a pre-operative measure for 1–2 days immediately prior to surgery. In spite of the complexity of the surgical procedures, the mortality in what are really poor-risk cases, is < 5 per cent.

Till about three years ago, CABG surgery necessitated the use of cardiopulmonary bypass (CPB). Many centres in the world, including centres in India now prefer to perform CABG surgery on a beating heart without using CPB. This technique requires training, expertise and experience for good results. Cardiopulmonary bypass (CPB) is reserved for surgery on complicated coronary artery disease, for the surgical management of aneurysms of the aorta or ventricular wall, for valve replacement surgery and for surgery on congenital heart defects. Off-pump CABG surgery has been shown to decrease complications and shorten time for recovery. High-risk patients, unsuitable for CABG surgery using cardiopulmonary bypass, can now be successfully operated upon by this off-pump procedure. Though technically refined, CPB is still an abnormal state of perfusion. Anticoagulation, hypothermia, the absence of pulsatile perfusion, and trauma to the cellular elements of blood by exposure to air, tubings, filters and suction, are necessary but harmful features of this abnormal circulatory state. The effects of CPB are to an extent responsible for a number of management problems encountered during the post-operative phase. It is therefore necessary for the intensivist to be aware of the basic procedure and problems during CPB. This chapter will however confine itself to management problems after patients undergoing cardiac surgery have been transferred to the intensive care unit for post-operative critical care.

Monitoring on Transfer to the ICU

Before transfer to the ICU, the practice in our unit is to intravenously inject 500,000 units of aprotinin post-operatively, and then 500,000 units in an infusion over the next 12 hours, so that post-operative bleeding is reduced. Some units prefer to use the drug pre-operatively and if for any reason the risk of bleeding is increased, the post-operative dose can be suitably raised as well, up to 500,000 units/hour till the bleeding stops.

Patients are continuously monitored on arrival to the ICU. The arterial blood pressure is monitored through an arterial line, the central venous pressure through a central venous line, the urine output by an indwelling Foley's catheter, the ECG by a single lead ECG, and the oxygen saturation by a pulse oximeter. In addition, in selected instances, temporary epicardial atrial and ventricular pacing wires are left in situ for a few days, for the management of arrhythmias.

Some surgeons prefer to keep a left atrial line to measure the left atrial pressure, and thereby the left ventricular filling pressure. Others insert a Swan-Ganz catheter to measure the pulmonary capillary wedge pressure in the immediate post-operative period. We prefer to do without both these invasive monitoring lines. If difficulties arise in the management of a low cardiac output state, we may need to insert a Swan-Ganz catheter; however we do this only when absolutely necessary.

The mediastinum and the left pleural space have chest drains, and the drainage is measured every hour to determine if excessive bleeding is present. When both internal mammary arteries have been used as grafts, or if for any reason the right pleural space has been opened, a chest drain in the right pleural space becomes imperative as well. The rectal temperature, the heart rate and the respiratory rate are continuously monitored. The patient has an endotracheal tube in place, which is connected to a volume-cycled ventilator. The ventilator settings are noted—in particular the respiratory rate, the tidal volume, the minute ventilation, and the peak and pause inflation pressures.

A 12 lead ECG and a chest X-ray are taken immediately on arrival to the ICU. Blood is also collected for CBC, PCV, platelet count, serum electrolytes, urea, creatinine, glucose, arterial pH and blood gases. Relevant studies in relation to the blood chemistry, clotting parameters, and arterial pH and blood gas analysis are repeated as and when necessary.

Immediate Post-operative Management

Immediate post-operative goals include restoration of normal body temperature, monitoring of haemodynamic and respiratory functions with prompt correction of any abnormalities or complications that may arise, restoring and maintaining fluid, electrolyte and acid-base balance, and replacing blood loss which is estimated both clinically and by noting the volume of drainage through chest tube drains. Intravenous infusions should maintain adequate filling pressures within the ventricular chambers. The rate and quantity of intravenous infusions depend on the circulatory state after surgery, the ongoing blood loss and the urine output.

In our unit, patients undergoing CABG are often transferred from the operating theatre with an ongoing infusion of nitroglycerin at a rate of 5–10 μg/kg/min, to increase vascular capacitance in the immediate post-operative period, and to counter coronary artery vasoconstriction. They often are also on an infusion of dopamine (5–7 μg/kg/min), for immediate post-operative inotropic support. These infusions are tapered and stopped after the first 24 hours if the circulatory state is satisfactory, and the immediate post-operative period is uneventful. Aspirin (300 mg) is administered 8 hours after surgery and continued once daily throughout the post-operative period. After discharge the patient should continue 150 mg daily on an indefinite basis. Low molecular weight heparin is begun on the second or third day after surgery and continued for 7 days. Both aspirin and heparin may need to be omitted in the presence of excessive post-operative bleeding.

The following features are worthy of note in the immediate post-operative period.

(i) Serum K$^+$ levels during the early post-operative phase can fluctuate markedly. Serum K$^+$ should be maintained between 3.5–4.5 mEq/l.

(ii) Uncontrolled hyperglycaemia is frequent in diabetics and needs carefully titrated administration of insulin. In non-diabetics, blood sugar levels may also be high—between 250–350 mg/dl. Insulin is generally not required in these patients.

(iii) Significant acid-base disturbances e.g. metabolic acidosis or metabolic alkalosis may be present and need to be corrected.

(iv) Shivering is common, as the early period after CPB is characterized by a fall in the core temperature. Shivering commonly occurs during this phase, as patients begin to re-warm after the effects of the anaesthetic and muscle relaxant begin to wear off. Shivering interferes with effective mechanical ventilation, and causes an increase in the CO_2 production. It also increases oxygen consumption, and myocardial work, thereby making undue demands on a heart recovering from the effects of aortic cross-clamping and CPB. Minute ventilation should be appropriately increased to counter increased oxygen consumption and CO_2 production till such time as the patient's temperature slowly rises and remains stable. This may take 2–8 hours. Severe shivering, particularly when associated with haemodynamic instability, should be countered by the use of a muscle relaxant (pancuronium 2–4 mg intravenously). This controls the shivering, and allows the patient to rewarm slowly.

(v) Bleeding is one of the commonest problems encountered in the early post-operative period. Bleeding may be due to several causes—heparin rebound, acquired qualitative platelet defects due to CPB or drugs, thrombocytopaenia, clotting factor deficiencies, local or systemic fibrinolysis, and disseminated intravascular coagulopathy (1). The activated clotting time, bleeding time, prothrombin time, partial thromboplastin time, and platelet counts are routinely estimated and repeated as necessary. A full coagulation profile is often asked for, but results are generally available only after the lapse of some precious hours. Therefore, initial management of bleeding is more often than not empiric. Since heparin rebound is fairly common, protamine (50–100 mg) is given in an attempt to effectively neutralize heparin. Fresh frozen plasma should be given to replace a possible deficiency in the clotting factors. Desmopressin may be given in an infusion over 10 minutes, in a dose of 0.3 μg/kg, to increase levels of von Willebrand's factor and to restore platelet function (2). Thrombocytopaenia ($< 80,000/mm^3$) or a prolonged template bleeding time is managed by adequate platelet infusions. If the serum fibrinogen level is < 100 ng/dl, 8 U of cryoprecipitate are administered. If there is evidence of fibrinogenolysis with high levels of fibrin degradation products (FDP), epsilon aminocaproic acid may be given in a dose of 5–10 g intravenously in the first hour, followed by an infusion of 1 g/hr for 3–5 hours. Transfusions of red blood cells or whole blood should be guided by the rate of blood loss, the haematocrit and the existing haemoglobin values in blood. We prefer to maintain a haemoglobin concentration of between 11–12 g/dl.

The surgical decision to re-explore the chest for excessive bleeding through chest tube drains, is dependent on the volume and rate of blood loss, and the basic coagulation status. If this status (platelet count, CT, BT, PT, PTT, fibrinogen levels) is satisfactory, exploration is considered if the blood loss exceeds 1000 ml in the first 12 hours. Sudden increase in the blood loss to > 300 ml/hr for 2 hours, should prompt a possible re-exploration. Blood loss of 300 ml in the first hour, 250 ml in the second hour and 150 ml/hr subsequently, has been correlated with surgically correctable bleeding (3). Surgeons generally prefer to err on the safer side and risk a re-exploration, rather than await a possible haemodynamic collapse. Re-exploration may be rewarded by the presence of a discrete major source of bleeding which can be promptly controlled. Not uncommonly, a number of small bleeding points are present. Evacuation of a clot, and cauterization of these points generally suffice to stop the bleed. It is of critical importance to realize that a sudden cessation or sharp decrease in the chest tube drainage in a haemodynamically unstable patient, may be due to excessive bleeding within the chest, with clots blocking the drains. A chest X-ray in these patients shows a pleural opacity, and the presence of hypovolaemic shock should clarify the diagnosis. Urgent re-exploration with evacuation of the clots, with special attention to the bleeding points within the chest, is mandatory.

When bleeding from the chest drains is uneventful and within the normal range, the drains are generally removed by the second or third post-operative day. By this time, chest tube drainage is generally < 100 ml/day, and is chiefly serous in nature.

An infrequent but life-threatening reaction soon after cardiopulmonary surgery is a protamine reaction. Parillo describes three kinds of reactions (4). The first is caused by rapid administration of protamine; this leads to hypotension due to release of histamine from mast cells. The second is an anaphylactic reaction resulting in hypotension, bronchospasm, and vasodilatory shock. Anaphylaxis is more frequently observed in diabetics exposed to protamine insulin and in patients with a history of fish allergy. Also, patients who have undergone cardiac surgery in the past are at greater risk. The third kind of reaction is due to heparin-protamine complexes causing a release of thromboxane from the capillary bed. This results in acute pulmonary hypertension, right sided heart failure and a low output syndrome with hypotension. Treatment consists in the use of steroids, antihistaminics, inotropes, vasopressors and volume infusions. We are fortunate in not encountering serious life-threatening protamine reactions, or perhaps we have missed them attributing hypotension and low-output states to other common causes.

Cardiovascular Complications

With cross-clamping of the aorta during CPB, coronary blood flow ceases, and there is global myocardial ischaemia. Myocardial preservation is optimized by the use of potassium rich cold cardioplegia at 4°C, administered directly into the coronary arteries every 20–30 minutes. The shorter the cross-clamp time, the quicker the recovery of the myocardium after bypass. Crossclamp times of 120 minutes or even more are well tolerated, particularly by patients with good pre-operative left ventricular function. Even so, there is a significant degree of transient depression in myocardial function, which may last from 6–12 hours. This depression is often more marked and longer lasting if the cross-clamp time is excessive, particularly in patients who have poor left ventricular function to start with.

The important cardiovascular complications are discussed below.

A. Low-output Syndrome and Hypotension

This is one of the most frequently observed and important complications after open heart surgery. A persistent low cardiac output in the immediate post-operative period is associated with an increased frequency of multiple organ dysfunction, chiefly involving the renal, respiratory, hepatic and central nervous systems. It is clinically manifested by cold peripheries, low systolic arterial blood pressure (< 90 mm Hg), decreased urine output (< 30 ml/hour) and increasing acidosis. If haemodynamic measurements are made, these patients are noted to have a lowered cardiac index (often < 2.2. l/min) and a low mixed venous oxygen saturation.

There are two points worth noting in the recognition of low-output states.

(i) Low-output states can occur with a systolic arterial blood pressure > 90 mm Hg when a compensatory increase in peripheral vascular resistance helps to maintain arterial blood pressure.

(ii) It is important to distinguish hypotension caused by low-output states from hypotension due to vasodilatation.

Hypotension due to vasodilatation generally occurs in the first 24 hours after surgery. Vasodilatation results from decreased sympathetic tone leading to a reduced peripheral systemic vascular resistance (<1000 dynes-sec/cm⁵). It should be suspected when hypotension is associated with warm peripheries and a normal to low central venous pressure. Inhibition of sympathetic tone may be due to anaesthetic agents used during surgery, and to a marked increase in venous capacitance that occurs during the rewarming phase. Patients after CABG surgery are often transferred to the ICU with a nitroglycerine infusion to counter post-operative coronary vasoconstriction. The infusion may be too rapid, or the vessels may vasodilate due to marked sensitivity to the drug. At times vasodilatation is aggravated if the patient is on continuous dobutamine support. In the above instance, nitroglycerine infusions must be slowed or stopped and dobutamine replaced by dopamine. If both dopamine and dobutamine are being used for inotropic support, infusion rate of the former is increased and that of the latter reduced. Volume loading these patients further helps in restoring a satisfactory circulation.

Vasodilatation in the immediate post-operative period can occasionally also result from an adverse protamine reaction. Hypotensive vasodilatory shock after cardiac surgery has been recently attributed in some patients to a relative deficiency of vasopressin (5). Administration of arginine vasopressin corrects this form of hypotension.

Low-output states can be due to reduced preload, to poor myocardial contractility, to an increased afterload, to cardiac tamponade, cardiac arrhythmias, to metabolic derangements or to the adverse effects of antiarrhythmic drugs. Fulminating sepsis can also result in a low-output severely hypotensive shock (see **Table 16.1.1**).

It is important to consider each of these factors if appropriate treatment is to be administered. More than one factor is often present in a given patient.

(i) Reduced preload

The commonest cause of a low cardiac output and hypotension in the post-operative period is a reduced preload due to hypovolaemia. Hypovolaemia is due to excessive bleeding, loss of tissue fluids and/or excessive diuresis. Hypovolaemia immediately after transfer to the ICU can be due to insufficient return of fluids during cardiopulmonary bypass. It can also occur from leaking capillaries—

Table 16.1.1. Causes of a low-output syndrome and/or hypotension

1. Reduced preload
   * Hypovolaemia due to blood loss, fluid loss, excessive diuresis
2. Increased afterload
   * Vasoconstriction from increased endogenous catecholamine secretion
     – Painful stimuli
     – Hypothermia
     – Pre-existing hypertension
   * Vasoconstriction from excessive exogenously administered catecholamines
3. Poor pump function
   * Myocardial depression (impaired contractility)
     – Peri-operative infarction
     – Functional depression (< 24 hours)
     – Myocardial ischaemia
     – Inadequate myocardial preservation, intraoperatively
     – Pre-existing poor ejection fraction
     – Uncorrected mechanical lesions
        Incomplete vascularization
        Mechanical valve dysfunction
        Undetected or uncorrected valvular stenosis or insufficiency
   * Metabolic complications
     – Hypo and hyperkalaemia
     – Hypomagnesaemia
     – Hypercalcaemia
     – Hypoxia, acidosis
   * Arrhythmias and conduction defects
   * Antiarrhythmic drugs
4. Cardiac tamponade
5. Vasodilatation
   * Due to anaesthetic agents
   * Iatrogenic (e.g. nitroglycerine)
   * Poor sympathetic tone (e.g. diabetes, elderly)
   * Relative deficiency of vasopressin
   * Protamine reaction
   * Anaphylaxis to a drug
6. Fulminant septic shock

a feature of the post-pump syndrome. Cold peripheries, hypotension, tachycardia, a normal rectal temperature and a low CVP (< 5 cm H_2O) suggest hypovolaemia. Hypovolaemia is corrected by infusion of colloids, crystalloids, and by the transfusion of packed red blood cells if there is increased blood loss. In addition to a volume load the patient is often also put on inotropic support.

(ii) Poor Pump Function

Poor pump function may be due to left ventricular dysfunction and failure, to right ventricular dysfunction and failure, or may result from a global hypokinesia. When severe, pump dysfunction leads to cardiogenic shock. As mentioned earlier, poor pump function may not be related to an intrinsic abnormality within the myocardium but to metabolic disturbances, to arrhythmias, and to the effect of antiarrhythmic drugs.

Impaired ventricular function after CABG surgery can be due to peri-operative or post-operative myocardial infarction or severe ischaemia. Some degree of post-operative functional myocardial depression is at times observed, particularly after prolonged or difficult cardiac surgery. This generally lasts for not more than 24 to 36 hours. Myocardial oedema, ischaemia and even myocardial

necrosis can result from inadequate myocardial preservation during surgery. After valve replacement surgery, pump dysfunction with a low-output syndrome can result from mechanical valve dysfunction.

Severe left ventricular failure besides causing a low-output syndrome with hypotension also results in an increased pulmonary capillary wedge pressure and pulmonary oedema. This is recognized clinically, on a chest X-ray and by noting a progressive increase in the peak inflation pressures while on the ventilator without any change in the ventilator settings.

Severe right ventricular failure and global hypokinesia are characterized by a poor forward flow and poor tissue perfusion, but not necessarily by increased left ventricular filling pressures (i.e. increased pulmonary capillary wedge pressures).

The management of poor pump function is dealt with in a previous chapter, but is briefly recapitulated below for convenience.

1. Ensure that the left ventricular filling pressure is maintained between 15 to 18 mm Hg. Associated hypovolaemia is thus countered by a volume load.

2. If a low-output syndrome with hypotension is observed in the presence of high filling pressures, use inotropic support to an extent that ensures a satisfactory increase in the cardiac output and blood pressure. A continuous infusion of dopamine 5–20 µg/kg/min helps raise cardiac output and blood pressure. Dobutamine has little α-adrenergic activity but pronounced β_1 and β_2 adrenergic activity. It increases cardiac output by increasing cardiac contractility and rate and by its vasodilating effect. In patients with a low cardiac output and a marked increase in systemic vascular resistance, dobutamine is preferred to dopamine. Dobutamine is given in an infusion at 5–20 µg/kg/min. Dopamine and dobutamine can be given together but in separate infusions, the dosage of each being titrated to obtain an optimal circulatory effect.

When dopamine and/or dobutamine are ineffective an epinephrine infusion is used in a dose of 1 to 10 µg/minute. Epinephrine increases myocardial contractility and rate and in higher doses raises the blood pressure through its α mediated vasoconstrictor effect on peripheral vessels.

Norepinephrine which has both α and β adrenergic activity increases both myocardial contractility and blood pressure. It is given in an infusion at the rate of 4–10 µg/minute. Amrinone and milrinone are two inotropic drugs which increase cardiac output independent of adrenergic stimulation. Milrinone is an effective vasodilator as well, and should be tried in patients with low cardiac output who are severely vasoconstricted. The drug is given in a loading dose of 50 µg/kg over 10 minutes, followed by an infusion of 0.375 to 0.75 µg/kg/minute.

In difficult cases two or more inotropes and vasopressors may prove necessary to increase cardiac output and blood pressure.

3. Severe right ventricular failure can result in a markedly poor forward flow and a shock-like state. Though right atrial and central venous pressures are elevated, pulmonary capillary wedge pressures need not be high. Volume load and inotropic support as outlined earlier, form the mainstay of management.

4. Intravenous furosemide should be used in the presence of pulmonary oedema.

5. A low cardiac output with hypotension can result from a marked increase in the systemic vascular resistance (afterload). An increase in the afterload could be due to excessive endogenously produced catecholamines resulting from unrelieved pain, hypothermia, non-pulsatile flow during cardiopulmonary bypass, or pre-existing hypertension. An increased afterload can also be caused by exogenously administered vasopressors.

Factors contributing to an increased afterload should be corrected when possible. A titrated dose of intravenous nitroglycerine or intravenous nitroprusside also reduces afterload. Nitroprusside should preferably be avoided in patients with a systolic blood pressure < 90 mm Hg.

6. Hypoxia, metabolic acidosis and electrolyte imbalance, notably in relation to K^+, Mg^{++}, Ca^{++} can aggravate or cause myocardial dysfunction. These factors should be recognized and corrected. Antiarrhythmic drugs are myocardial depressants and may well contribute to myocardial dysfunction.

7. Shock-like syndromes after cardiac surgery may be due to rhythm disturbances and should be promptly rectified. These may be missed, as with supraventricular tachycardias with A-V block, or in A-V dissociation with a fast atrial and ventricular rate. Loss of effective atrial contraction may tilt the balance against the patient.

8. Bradycardia can lead to a low cardiac index and hypotension. This is because the cardiac output is a product of the stroke volume and heart rate. Intravenous atropine or atrial or atrioventricular pacing at 80–100/minute can restore a normal circulatory state.

9. Myocardial assist devices become necessary for cardiac support if poor pump function persists after optimizing rate, rhythm, preload, myocardial contractility, afterload, and if factors such as metabolic disturbances, arrhythmias and drug reactions are non-existent or stand corrected. Intra-aortic balloon pump support reduces the afterload of the left ventricle and helps to relieve myocardial ischaemia. Patients with very poor ejection fractions who undergo CABG surgery or those who suffer complications during surgery should best have a balloon pump inserted in the theatre before transfer to the ICU. Ventricular assist devices are more effective in increasing cardiac output as compared to the aortic balloon pump but we have no experience with these devices.

In summary, though a volume load and the use of inotropes is the usual response to a low output state and/or hypotension, it is important to tailor therapy appropriate to the cause. Thus for example, the steps detailed above would provide only temporary respite in a patient whose low cardiac output is due to tamponade or to graft closure.

(iii) Septic Shock

Hypotension with a shock-like state which to start with is associated with a normal or high cardiac output and a lowered systemic vascular resistance, characterizes septic shock. This condition has been dealt with at length in an earlier chapter. Sepsis may occur within the first 48 hours after surgery, or may occur later and interrupt an otherwise satisfactory progress. Sepsis may arise from a source in the operation theatre, or may be related to gadgetry used for invasive monitoring and treatment. Occasionally it results from a seeding into the blood from a source of infection within the body e.g. from the urinary tract, the lungs, an infected anal fistula, or an infected pilonidal sinus. It should be a dictum to avoid cardiac surgery till such time as a pre-existing infection is appropriately treated. Patients running even a low-grade fever should not be taken for elective cardiac surgery till the cause of the fever is discovered and eradicated.

In critically ill, low-output hypotensive patients management is significantly assisted by monitoring and measurement of circulatory haemodynamics through a Swan-Ganz catheter.

B. Cardiac Tamponade

This is an extremely important cause of a low-output shock-like state after open heart surgery. It is usually caused by a leak at the site of right atrial cannulation; the resulting haematoma compresses the right atrium and superior vena cava, restricting inflow of blood into the right atrium. There is a progressive elevation of right atrial and central venous pressures with a fall in cardiac output, tachycardia and hypotension. A rising right atrial pressure with an impaired filling of the right ventricle leads to a loss of the Y-descent in the right atrial pressure tracing. Equilibration of pressures in the right and left heart may not be observed when tamponade is due to a localized haematoma pressing upon the right atrium. Exploration to remove the haematoma is mandatory.

Cardiac tamponade due to pressure on both right and left ventricles can occur with mediastinal bleeding or from an extension of the right atrial haematoma over the front of the heart, or from a leak at the anastomotic site of a graft in CABG surgery. In addition to the clinical features of hypotension and raised central venous pressure there is invariably a widening of the mediastinal shadow. Cardiac tamponade should always be thought of when brisk bleeding and drainage through the chest tubes suddenly lessen or cease and the X-ray chest shows a widened mediastinum. Tamponade can well occur even in the presence of well-placed mediastinal drains. An increasing mediastinal shadow on chest X-ray, a diastolic collapse of the right atrium and right ventricle on echocardiography, coupled with the clinical findings stated above are diagnostic of cardiac tamponade. These patients would show equilibration of the right and left heart pressures on a haemodynamic study. A volume load and inotropic support should be given and the patient promptly taken up for surgery in order to remove clots and blood causing the tamponade.

C. Peri-operative Myocardial Infarction

The recent Bypass Angioplasty Revascularization Investigation study revealed that the incidence of Q wave infarction after bypass surgery was 4.6 per cent (6). Possible causes of infarction include incomplete revascularization, haemodynamic stress (in particular hypotension and arrhythmias) during surgery, or during intubation, diffuse atherosclerotic disease of distal vessels, formation and extension of a clot in an endarterectomized coronary vessel, coronary artery spasm, embolism or thrombosis of native coronary vessels or bypass grafts (7, 8).

The diagnosis of peri-operative myocardial infarction is based on the following:

(i) Appearance of new Q waves after surgery. ST-T changes occurring alone without Q waves are less specific.

(ii) CK-MB levels which are significantly or markedly elevated (>80 mg/dl) (9). A mild to moderate degree of rise in CK-MB is to be expected after cardiac surgery, without signifying a fresh infarction.

(iii) Peak troponin I levels greater than 3.7 µg/l and troponin T levels greater than 3.4 µg/l (10, 11).

(iv) The presence of a new regional wall abnormality on echocardiography. It is worth noting that the removal of the restraining effect of the pericardium consequent to surgery, may lead to a false positive reading of a new regional wall motion abnormality in the high anterior septal area.

Small peri-operative myocardial infarcts do well; larger infarcts have a high post-operative mortality which may be due to pump failure or to uncontrolled ventricular arrhythmias (12). Patients who are haemodynamically unstable or those with a large area of the myocardium in jeopardy should be taken to the catheterization laboratory, to determine if a graft is occluded. If so, the graft should be opened up through a balloon plasty.

D. Cardiac Arrhythmias

Post-operative cardiac arrhythmias are common. They should be promptly recognized and treated. Hypokalaemia, hyperkalaemia, acidosis, bleeding, poor pump function, ongoing myocardial ischaemia, or peri-operative myocardial infarction can all trigger arrhythmias in these patients. These precipitating factors should be looked for and if present promptly corrected. Excessive use of inotropics for cardiovascular support is an often forgotten cause of malignant ventricular arrhythmias. Nebulization of large doses of salbutamol in patients with airways obstruction can enhance supraventricular and ventricular arrhythmogenic activity in the post-operative phase of open heart surgery. Arrhythmias are commoner and more persistent in patients who have had an aneurysmorrhaphy or an aneurysmectomy performed during CABG surgery.

Arrhythmias may be supraventricular or ventricular. Premature atrial contractions may be ignored except when they trigger repeated episodes of atrial fibrillation, or compromise circulation in patients who depend on a synchronized atrial contraction for a proper stroke volume. Digoxin should be used to suppress ectopic activity in these patients.

Paroxysmal atrial fibrillation is frequently observed, generally occurring two to three days after open heart surgery. It often reverts to sinus rhythm spontaneously. In a multicentre study of patients undergoing CABG surgery, the incidence of atrial fibrillation was noted to be 27 per cent (13). The most common risk factor for peri- and post-operative atrial fibrillation is advanced age. If atrial fibrillation with a fast ventricular rate persists and compromises circulation, then the ventricular rate should be slowed with intravenous digoxin, followed if necessary by 5 mg increment doses of verapamil. An alternative is to administer a bolus of 300 mg amiodarone followed by an intravenous infusion of 700 mg to 1 g of amiodarone over 24 hours. Conversion to sinus rhythm is

frequently observed. The dose of amiodarone is gradually reduced over the next two days, oral amiodarone being finally substituted for the infusion as prophylaxis (see Section on Tachyarrhythmias in the ICU). Electrical cardioversion is unnecessary in most patients. It should only be used in the presence of acute decompensation caused by a very rapid ventricular rate, which is uncontrolled by intravenous digoxin. Repeated episodes of paroxysmal atrial fibrillation or persistent atrial fibrillation in the post-operative phase, may be due to pericarditis or pulmonary emboli. Intravenous dexamethasone 4–8 mg, offers dramatic relief and a return to sinus rhythm when the underlying cause is pericarditis. Supraventricular arrhythmias are perhaps more frequent in patients who have had an endarterectomy of the right coronary artery during CABG.

Transient second and third degree AV blocks are common after valve surgery. These are best treated with the aid of atrial and ventricular epicardial pacing wires placed during surgery. AV sequential pacing at a rate of 80–100/minute is preferred because of the contribution of atrial systole to cardiac output.

Ventricular arrhythmias are life-threatening. Ventricular tachycardia, not responding to a bolus dose of lidocaine, and which results in haemodynamic instability, should be converted to sinus rhythm by a synchronized DC shock of 200 J. Ventricular fibrillation needs prompt cardioversion. If 200 J is unsuccessful, a 300 J DC shock should be used. A bolus dose of lidocaine (1–2 mg/kg) is given after cardioversion in ventricular fibrillation; this is followed by a maintenance lidocaine drip at the rate of 1–3 mg/minute. Frequent ventricular ectopy is also treated with lidocaine as detailed above. If this drug fails to control multiple ventricular ectopics, or the patient has recurrent ventricular tachycardia or fibrillation, we prefer to use amiodarone 300 mg intravenously as a bolus dose followed by 1 g in an infusion over 24 hours. This is continued for 2–3 days, and followed by oral amiodarone (see Chapter on Tachyarrhythmias in the ICU). Rarely overdrive pacing may be required for control of persistent or recurrent ventricular tachycardia.

In patients who have received digitalis, digitalis toxicity should always be considered in the presence of multiple ventricular ectopics, atrial tachycardia with block, AV dissociation and ventricular tachycardias. Digitalis toxicity can occur even with serum digoxin levels within the therapeutic range. Details of management of various cardiac arrhythmias have been dealt with in an earlier chapter (see Chapter on Tachyarrhythmias in the ICU).

E. Pericarditis

Pericarditis is common in the first 3–7 days following CPB. A pericardial friction rub is always present, and may persist for over 5–7 days. In the asymptomatic patient, no treatment is required. Symptoms of the post-pericardiotomy syndrome generally occur 2 to 8 weeks after open heart surgery. Symptoms include fever, tachycardia, chest pain, a raised ESR (often close to 100 mm/hr), a left sided pleural effusion, occasionally a pericardial rub, and a tendency to supraventricular arrhythmias. The clinical condition improves with the use of nonsteroidal anti-inflammatory agents, particularly indomethacin. If the condition still persists we prefer a short course of corticosteroids; a small maintenance dose may be required for weeks or months. Rarely constrictive pericarditis is a sequel to the post-pericardiotomy syndrome.

F. Post-operative Hypertension

The incidence of post-operative hypertension with a systolic blood pressure > 140–150 mm Hg, occurs in over 40 per cent of patients (14). It is especially frequent after CABG and the surgical relief of left ventricular outflow tract obstruction (15).

The mechanisms of post-operative hypertension include (i) elevated circulating catecholamine levels with excessive sympathetic nervous system activity; (ii) rebound effect from withdrawal of pre-operatively given beta-blockers; (iii) pressor reflexes originating from the heart, coronary vessels and the aorta (16). Post-operative hypertension should be controlled promptly. Increase in systemic arterial blood pressure which is most often seen in the immediate post-operative period, can cause an increase in post-operative bleeding, disruption of suture lines of the grafts, aortic dissection, increase in afterload with ventricular dysfunction, and an increased incidence of strokes. A mild to moderate rise in blood pressure is best treated with a titrated dose of nitroglycerin in an intravenous infusion. A sharp marked rise in blood pressure is treated with a titrated intravenous infusion of sodium nitroprusside. Hypertension and tachycardia following beta-blocker withdrawal is treated with intravenous esmolol 50–250 µg/kg/min (17). The need for oral antihypertensives after the first 2 days, should be assessed for each patient. Oral beta-blockers should be restarted in patients who were on these drugs prior to surgery. They effectively control the hypertension and tachycardia in these patients.

Respiratory Care

Patients are generally weaned off ventilator support within 4 to 12 hours. Low risk, younger patients undergoing CABG surgery are often extubated in the recovery room before being transferred to the ICU. The indications for weaning are the same as those discussed in the Chapter on Mechanical Ventilation in the Critically Ill. The patient must be awake, haemodynamically stable with no significant abnormality on an X-ray chest. He should not be tachypnoeic on disconnecting the ventilator, and the blood gases after being kept on a T tube for 2 to 4 hours should show neither hypoxia nor hypercapnia. He could then be extubated. Pain relief is important to enable the patient to breathe freely. He should be given oxygen through nasal prongs so as to keep the O_2 saturation well over 90 per cent. We have always weaned patients by the T tube method and have never found the need to use SIMV. In patients who are difficult to wean because of atelectasis or oedema, we use CPAP before graduating to the T tube. CPAP or BiPAP through an orofacial mask can be continued after extubation. Patients with poor left ventricular function (LVEF < 20 per cent), those with respiratory complications, or serious complications involving other organ systems, are kept on ventilator support for 24–48 hours, or even longer. It is unwise to remove support prematurely in these

patients. The increased work of breathing in haemodynamically unstable patients can induce respiratory fatigue, hypoventilation and atelectasis with a progressive deterioration in the cardiorespiratory system.

More prolonged ventilator support is often necessary in those with chronic lung disease, particularly those patients with airways obstruction. If case selection has been correct, these patients can generally be weaned off support within 12 to 48 hours. Nebulization with salbutamol 4–6 hourly and ipratropium bromide 12 hourly is of help in keeping the airways open. A marked difference between the peak and pause inflation pressures, is a guide to the severity of airways resistance. Corticosteroids should be avoided except in patients who are steroid-dependent, or in patients with asthma who have a severe exacerbation of airways obstruction after surgery. The arrhythmogenic effects of beta-2 agonists and aminophylline in these patients should be borne in mind. The dangers of wound sepsis, other infections, and poor healing always accompany the use of corticosteroids.

Factors predisposing to prolonged ventilator support with difficulties in weaning are listed in **Table 16.1.2**.

Table 16.1.2. Factors predisposing to prolonged ventilator support with difficulties in weaning following open heart surgery

* Stormy post-operative period
* Re-exploration
* LV dysfunction
* Renal failure
* Infection (sepsis, pneumonia)
* Malnutrition
* Chronic airways obstruction
* Injury to phrenic nerve
* Aged, debilitated, poor-risk patients
* Multiple organ dysfunction/failure
* Stroke/encephalopathy

Pulmonary Complications

These include pulmonary oedema, atelectasis, nosocomial pneumonia, pleural effusion and diaphragmatic paralysis.

(a) Pulmonary oedema is generally due to raised left ventricular filling pressures consequent to left ventricular failure. Acute lung injury (ARDS) can occasionally result as a consequence of CPB even in the absence of infections or transfusion reactions. It is due to exposure of blood to foreign surfaces during prolonged CPB. Damage to the alveolar capillary membrane is induced by clumping of platelets, leucocyte sequestration and activation of the coagulation cascade, the complement and the fibrinolytic system. The mortality against the background of recent cardiac surgery is over 70 per cent (18). Risk factors include hypertension, smoking, emergency surgery and a low-output syndrome after surgery (18).

Patients on amiodarone before cardiac surgery are noted to be at greater risk for ARDS after surgery (19). ARDS develops 24 to 48 hours in the post-operative period and has a high mortality. We observed recently a severe rapidly progressive ARDS in a patient who had received amiodarone for over 4 days after surgery. No other explanation for ARDS was forthcoming in this patient. Management of ARDS involves prolonged ventilator support and the use of PEEP (see Chapter on ARDS).

(b) Pulmonary atelectasis invariably occurs because of poor respiratory care leading to retained respiratory secretions. Good physiotherapy, proper suction, and frequent change of posture are necessary, particularly in obese patients with short, thick chests. The use of PEEP during ventilator support is of help in opening up atelectatic areas.

The commonest cause of peri-operative respiratory failure (Type III failure) is atelectasis. Atelectasis may present with obvious atelectatic shadows in one or both lung fields. It however often presents with 'small volume' lungs on an X-ray chest, with high diaphragms. The small lung volumes on either side need not be symmetrically equal. Clinically the patient is tachypnoeic off the ventilator, breathes poorly, coughs poorly and ineffectively. This problem in our experience is commoner in females, particularly those with short 'stocky' chests. Ventilator support for a longer period with the use of PEEP helps keep the lungs open. Physiotherapy and pain relief help in breathing and clearing secretions. After extubation these patients should be given either CPAP or BiPAP through the night and for several hours during the day to keep the lung volumes from shrinking.

(c) Nosocomial pneumonias are infrequent in our set-up. Remarkably enough, the incidence is higher in those with poor left ventricular function (see Chapter on Fever and Acute Infections in a Critical Care Setting).

(d) Pleural effusion is common after cardiac surgery; it generally resolves spontaneously and should be tapped only if it produces symptoms. Rarely pleural effusion of moderate severity persists for weeks or months after CABG surgery. Infection, in particular tuberculosis should be excluded. When non-infective and persistent, a pleurodesis generally solves the issue.

(e) Diaphragmatic Paralysis. Partial paralysis is frequent on the left side and is due to phrenic nerve injury or to 'freezing' of the phrenic nerve because of the ice slush used for myocardial preservation. The raised left dome of the diaphragm is generally not associated with increased morbidity. In a very small number of these patients, total one-sided diaphragmatic palsy may be symptomatic, in that it can cause left lower lobe atelectasis and pose problems in weaning from ventilator support. A paradoxical movement of the dome of the diaphragm on 'sniffing' confirms diaphragmatic paralysis. Ventilator support may be required for as long as 6 weeks, as recovery of the phrenic nerve may take a long time. Bilateral phrenic nerve injury with diaphragmatic palsy occurs even more rarely. The patient becomes cyanosed on lying down and is promptly relieved on sitting up. We have had three patients with bilateral diaphragmatic paralysis following open heart surgery. Recovery occurred over a period of 6–10 weeks, during which time mechanical ventilator support was necessary.

If ventilator support is necessary for more than 14 days, we prefer to do an elective tracheostomy. The danger of sternal wound infection following a tracheostomy always exists, and this could involve the mediastinum to produce mediastinitis, mediastinal abscess, empyema, and a communication between the empyema and the mediastinal abscess. These complications are fraught with great danger and result in a very high morbidity and mortality. It is therefore unwise to do a tracheostomy when the sternal wound shows signs of infection. As far as possible, the operative wound must be clean and well healed before tracheostomy is advised for prolonged ventilator support.

Neurological Complications

Cerebrovascular accidents manifesting as transient ischaemic attacks or strokes, are an ever present danger of open heart surgery. Massive cerebral or brainstem infarction or a massive bleed must always be suspected if the patient does not recover from anaesthesia, and if the possibility of hypoxic brain damage is unlikely because of a smooth intra- and immediate post-operative course. If possible, patients who are unresponsive for 48 hours following surgery, are sent for CT scanning to determine the presence of organic disease or cerebral oedema. Mannitol 150 ml 8 hourly intravenously, dexamethasone 4 mg intravenously 6 hourly and hyperventilation to allow a $PaCO_2$ of 20–25 mm Hg, are tried to counter increased intracranial pressure. Unfortunately the patient with focal or global cerebral damage is diagnosed too late for any therapeutic measures to be effective. Risk factors for cerebrovascular accidents include the presence of pre-operative carotid bruits [20], previous history of a cardiovascular accident or a transient ischaemic episode [21], post-operative atrial fibrillation [21], and prolonged CPB [20]. Patients with symptomatic carotid bruits have successfully undergone carotid endarterectomy with their cardiac surgery in a single operative session.

Spinal ischaemia can occur after cross-clamping the thoracic aorta for repair of an aneurysm of the descending aorta. Encouraging results have been obtained by drainage of the cerebrospinal fluid and intrathecal injection of papaverine [22].

Rarely rib resection during a thoracotomy can produce a haematoma causing compression of the thoracic spinal cord. This may present with paraplegia or a Brown-Sequard syndrome. A CT scan or an MRI can prove the diagnosis; compression should be relieved by surgery.

Neuropathies in the upper limbs chiefly involving the ulnar nerve can occur following brachial plexus compression or traction

---

Table 16.1.3. Causes of cerebrovascular accident after cardiac surgery

* Embolism
  – Debridement or replacement of calcified aortic valve
  – Dislodgement of atherosclerotic plaque during aortic cannulation
  – Introduction of air into circulation during surgery
  – Atrial fibrillation
  – Thrombosis of mechanical prosthetic valve
  – Left ventricular thrombosis
  – Dislodgement of fragment of left atrial myxoma
* Haemorrhage
  – Peri-operative anticoagulation
  – Hypertension
* Infarction
  – Cerebral hypoperfusion while on CPB or during period of post-operative shock particularly when this occurs against a background of cerebral atherosclerosis or carotid or vertebral artery stenosis

injury (**23**). Recovery generally ensues in 2 months but may take as long as 9 months to a year. **Table 16.1.3** lists the causes of cerebrovascular accidents following bypass surgery.

Gastrointestinal Complications

These are rare but carry a high mortality. Ileus is often present for a few days if the gastroepiploic artery is used for revascularization. In patients with diffuse atherosclerotic disease, mesenteric ischaemia may lead to the picture of an acute abdomen. This is particularly seen in hypoperfusion states and in surgery on the abdominal aorta. Acute pancreatitis possibly related to hypoperfusion may occur suddenly and can lead to rapid deterioration in the clinical state. A high index of suspicion is necessary for a diagnosis. The diagnosis should not be solely based on high serum amylase levels as these are observed in over 30 per cent of patients undergoing cardiopulmonary bypass (**24**). Elevated serum lipase levels in conjunction with the clinical picture are of greater help in diagnosis. In patients with a low-output syndrome which is severe or long-lasting, liver cell dysfunction is observed with marked elevation of the enzymes and a rise in bilirubin. This 'shock-liver' syndrome improves if cardiac output, arterial blood pressure and tissue perfusion recover. Acute cholecystitis often attributed to visceral hypotension, is a rare but important complication within the first week after surgery. It is characterized by pain and tenderness in the right hypochondrium, increase in liver enzymes, and fever. The diagnosis can be confirmed by ultrasound examination. The overall mortality in these patients is over 30 per cent (**25**), the gall bladder being frequently gangrenous on explorative surgery. Gastointestinal bleeds from acute erosions or ulcers are common particularly in patients with a prolonged stormy post-operative course, in those who are septic, and following the use of corticosteroids. Most patients should receive sucralfate, H_2-antagonists or proton pump inhibitors prophylactically, the latter two being specifically indicated for high-risk patients. **Table 16.1.4** lists the causes of some common gastrointestinal complications seen after cardiac surgery.

Table 16.1.4. Common causes of gastrointestinal complications after cardiac surgery

Complication	Common Causes
1. Elevated Serum Bilirubin	
* Early (1–10 days)	– Haemolysis during CPB
	– 'Shock-Liver Syndrome'
	– Right sided heart failure
* Late (10–90 days)	– Infection (CMV or Hepatitis C virus)
	– Cholecystitis
2. GI Bleeds	– Stress gastric erosions or ulcerations
	– Peptic ulcer disease
3. Mesenteric Ischaemia	– Low cardiac output, embolic or due to thrombi, or vascular dissection by IABP
4. Pancreatitis	– Hypotension, thromboembolism of vascular supply, splanchnic vasoconstriction
5. Ileus	– Use of gastroepiploic artery for revascularization; related to mesenteric ischaemia.
6. Acute Noncalculous Cholecystitis	– probably related to hypoperfusion

Renal Complications

Acute oliguric failure after open heart surgery is rare (0.7 to 4.3 per cent) but carries a grave risk and a high mortality (**26, 27**) The incidence of a quickly rising creatinine, oliguria, anuria, the need for dialysis, and the occurrence of other complications is higher when pre-operative serum creatinine levels are beyond 1.7 mg/dl (**28**). The occurrence of oliguric renal failure after open heart surgery often precipitates fluid overload and pulmonary oedema. Early use of continuous arteriovenous haemofiltration to remove excess fluid is always indicated in these patients. Three patterns of renal failure are generally observed. The first occurs as a result of a renal insult, at or soon after surgery. It is characterized by a rise in serum creatinine from the second to the fifth post-operative days. Renal function then improves and serum creatinine levels return to normal over a week. During the phase of impaired renal function, it is important to omit as far as possible, all nephrotoxic drugs, in particular nonsteroidal anti-inflammatory agents and aminoglycosides. The second pattern is characterized by a more prolonged course of acute renal failure. It occurs in patients, who in addition to a peri-operative renal insult, have haemodynamic instability and poor tissue perfusion in the initial post-operative phase. Recovery of renal function occurs after 3–4 weeks. The last and the most serious pattern of renal failure is when complicating sepsis or a massive GI bleed is an added insult to early circulatory disturbances. This form of failure is often seen in patients who develop multiple organ failure, and carries a high mortality.

The principles of management of acute renal failure have been discussed in another chapter (see Chapter on Critical Care in Acute Renal Failure). We prefer to use continuous arteriovenous haemofiltration rather than haemodialysis in our patients of acute renal failure. We initiate haemofiltration early in the natural history of the disease.

Infectious Complications

These include wound infections, urinary tract infections, pneumonia and sepsis. Gram-negative and methicillin-resistant staphylococcal infections are most frequently encountered. A nasty nosocomial wound infection is indeed a dreaded complication of open heart surgery. Healing may be protracted and difficult. In the worst scenario, the sepsis syndrome with multiple organ failure results. At times local dehiscence may cause a total separation of the sternal wound with exposure of the mediastinum. Wound infections often necessitate prolonged ventilator support. Healing of infected wounds is doubly difficult in patients with poor pump function. The risk of nosocomial wound infection in the unit is significantly increased if there is even one patient with severe wound infection, who continues to need prolonged critical care within the unit.

Local attention to the wound should be left to the surgical team. Appropriate cultures of discharge from the wound should guide systemic antibiotic therapy. Mediastinitis, mediastinal abscess, pleural effusion (unilateral or bilateral), empyemas may all complicate a bad sternal wound infection. These need to be diagnosed and surgically treated. Wound infections are further discussed in a separate chapter (see Section on Surgical Infections).

Infective Endocarditis

Prosthetic valve endocarditis is a rare complication of cardiac surgery, occurring in 2–4 per cent of patients. Half of these are classified as early (< 60 days after surgery), and half as late cases (> 60 days following surgery). Early endocarditis is most often due to S. aureus (29, 30), and then in descending order of frequency, to the Gram-negative bacilli, diphtheroids and the fungi. Late endocarditis is more often due to the Streptococcus species, and the microbiologic spectrum causing infection is similar to that observed in native valve endocarditis. Mechanical valves typically show a ring abscess or a myocardial abscess, whereas infected porcine valves show stenosis or regurgitation. Antibiotic therapy depends on the organisms grown on blood culture. The regime against early endocarditis should include vancomycin to cover methicillin-resistant Staphylococci. Indications for surgery include prosthetic valve dysfunction, myocardial abscess, perivalvular infection and abscess, persistently positive blood cultures, relapse after antibiotic therapy, embolic episodes and cardiac dysfunction or failure (30, 31).

Peripheral Vascular Complications and Pulmonary Embolism

Embolic or thrombotic occlusion of vessels in the limbs, (particularly the lower limbs), may occasionally occur. Thrombectomy or revascularization surgery of the lower limbs, may be necessary to salvage the limb. Heparinization is indicated.

Deep vein thrombosis of the calves is a frequent complication. Rarely this may result in a massive embolism. Sudden hypotension with a shock-like state occurring after the sixth day of surgery, should suggest this complication. Major pulmonary embolism can be easily proven by an HRCT pulmonary angiography. Heparin in full doses—5000 units intravenously to start with, followed by 1000 units/hour, to keep the PTT to 2–2.5 times normal should be given. Streptokinase is avoided in view of major surgery in the very recent past.

Multiple Organ Dysfunction

This is a rare but dreaded complication of open heart surgery. It can occur very rarely because of a systemic inflammatory response syndrome initiated during CPB. In these cases, it manifests initially with mild to moderate degree of acute lung injury (ARDS). Progressive multiple organ dysfunction is more likely to occur if the patient has suffered a myocardial insult resulting in a prolonged period of poor perfusion, during or after surgery. Provided there is scope for recovery of myocardial function, and there is no complicating sepsis, multiple organ failure in this situation does not carry the grim prognosis forecast by many workers in the West.

We have had 3 patients who suffered an insult causing severe hypoperfusion before, during and after bypass surgery. They developed severe multiple organ failure involving all organ systems for more than 2 weeks, but still made a complete recovery. If severe sepsis complicates the above picture, then the prognosis is extremely grim, and death invariably results.

REFERENCES

1. Bick RL. (1985). Hemostasis defects associated with cardiac surgery, prosthetic devices and other extracorporeal circuits. Semin Thromb Hemost. 11, 249.

2. Salzman ED, Weinstein MJ, Weintraub RM et al. (1986). Treatment with desmopressin acetate to reduce blood loss after cardiac surgery: A double-blind randomized trial. N Engl J Med. 314(22), 1402.

3. Michelson EL, Torosian M, Morganroth J et al. (1980). Early recognition of surgically correctable causes of excessive mediastinal bleeding after coronary artery bypass graft surgery. Am J Surg. 139, 313.

4. Khan SS, Denton TA, Czer LSC. (2001). Management of the Patient after Cardiac Surgery. In: Critical Care Medicine (Eds Parillo JE, Dellinger RP). pp. 684–701. Mosby, USA.

5. Argenziano M, Chen JM, Choudhry AF et al. (1998). Management of vasodilatory shock after cardiac surgery: identification of predisposing factors and use of a novel pressor agent. J Thoracic Cardiovasc Surg. 116, 973.

6. BARI Investigators. (1996). Comparison of coronary bypass surgery with angioplasty in patients with multivessel disease. N Engl J Med. 335, 217.

7. Lemmer JH Jr, Krish MM. (1988). Coronary artery spasm following coronary artery surgery. Ann Thorac Surg. 46, 108.

8. Obarski TP, Loop FD, Cosgrove DM et al. (1990). Frequency of acute myocardial infarction in valve repairs versus valve replacement for pure mitral regurgitation. Am J Cardiol. 65, 887.

9. Gray RJ, Matloff JM, Conklin CM et al. (1982). Perioperative myocardial infarction: late clinical course after coronary bypass surgery. Circulation. 66, 1185.

10. Maire J, Larue C, Mair P et al. (1994). Use of cardiac troponin I to diagnose perioperative myocardial infarction in coronary artery bypass grafting. Clin Chem. 40 (11, Pt 1), 2066.

11. Carrier M, Pellerin M, Perrault LP et al. (2000). Troponin levels in patients with myocardial infarction after coronary artery bypass grafting. Ann Thorac Surg. 69, 435.

12. Bateman TM, Matloff JM, Gray RJ. (1984). Myocardial infarction during coronary artery bypass surgery—benign event or prognostic omen? Int J Cardiol. 6, 259.

13. Mathew JP, Parks R, Savio JS et al. (1996). Atrial fibrillation following coronary artery bypass graft surgery. JAMA. 276, 300.

14. Estafanous FG, Tarazi RC. (1980). Systemic arterial hypertension associated with cardiac surgery. Am J Cardiol. 46, 685.

15. Rocchini AP, Rosenthal A, Barger AC et al. (1976). Pathogenesis of paradoxical hypertension after coarctation resection. Circulation. 54, 382.

16. James TN, Hageman GR, Urthaler F. (1979). Anatomic and physiologic considerations of a cardiogenic hypertensive reflex. Am J Cardiol. 44, 852.

17. Gray RJ, Bateman TM, Czer LS et al. (1987). Comparison of esmolol and nitroprusside for acute post-cardiac surgical hypertension. Am J Cardiol. 59, 887.

18. Christenson JT, Aeberahrd JM, Badel P et al. (1996). Adult respiratory distress syndrome after cardiac surgery. Cardiovasc Surg. 4, 15.

19. Nalos P, Kass R, Gang E et al. (1987). Life-threatening postoperative pulmonary complications in patients with previous amiodarone pulmonary toxicity undergoing cardiothoracic operations. J Thorac Cardiovasc Surg. 93, 904.

20. Reed GL, Singer DE, Pilard EH. (1988). Stroke following coronary artery bypass surgery. A case control estimate of the risk of carotid bruits. N Engl J Med. 319, 1246.

21. Taylor GJ, Malik SA, Colliver JA et al. (1987). Usefulness of atrial fibrillation as a predictor of stroke after isolated coronary artery bypass grafting. Am J Cardiol. 60, 905.

22. Svensson LG, Steward RW, Cosgrove DM et al. (1988). Intrathecal papaverine for the prevention of paraplegia after operation on the thoracic or thoracoabdominal aorta. J Thorac Cardiovasc Surg. 96, 823.

23. Seyfer AE, Grammer NY, Bogumill GP et al. (1985). Upper extremity neuropathies after cardiac surgery. J Hand Surg (Am). 10, 16.

24. Missavage A, Weaver D, Bouwnan D et al. (1984). Hyperamylasaemia after cardiopulmonary bypass. Am Surg. 50, 297.

25. Sessions SC, Scoma RS, Sheikh FA et al. (1993). Acute acalculous cholecystitis following open heart surgery. Am Surg. 59, 74–77.

26. Bhat JG, Gluck MC, Lowenstein J, Baldwin DS. (1976). Renal failure after open heart surgery. Ann Intern Med. 84, 677.

27. Hilberman M, Myers BD, Carrie BJ et al. (1979). Acute renal failure following cardiac surgery. J Thorac Cardiovasc Surg. 77, 880.

28. Higgins TL, Paganini EP, Noor FA et al. (1990). Postoperative course of patients undergoing coronary artery bypass grafting (CABG) with elevated preoperative serum creatinine. Abstract presented at the Society of Cardiovascular Anesthesiologists Annual Meeting (Manuscript in preparation).

29. Wilson WR, Danielson GK, Giuliani ER et al. (1982). Prosthetic valve endocarditis. Mayo Clin Proc. 57, 155.

30. Cowgill LD, Addonizio VP, Hopeman AG et al. (1987). A practical approach to prosthetic valve endocarditis. Ann Thorac Surg. 43, 450.

31. Dinubile MJ. (1982). Surgery in active endocarditis. Ann Intern Med. 96, 650.

The Immunocompromised Patient

The Immunocompromised Patient

Immunocompromised patients who get infections, and are seriously ill under intensive care, are under grave risk and have a far greater mortality as compared to patients with a normal immune status. It is almost certain that in years to come intensive care units will be populated by an increasing number of immunosuppressed or immunocompromised patients. The occurrence of infection in compromised patients reflects the interaction between these patients' immune defence system and their endogenous and exogenous microbial environment. It is impossible to discuss in detail the normal immune defence mechanisms in this chapter, but a brief outline of immune responses that help fight infection, is of basic importance to doctors working in ICUs. This is because specific defects in the immune defence system predispose the immunocompromised patients to certain specific infections. Unfortunately in acutely ill patients it is not always possible to quickly identify these specific deficits, nor is it advisable to perform elaborate tests to do so.

Basic Host Defence Mechanisms

Host defence mechanisms are complex interacting systems. These mechanisms chiefly include:

(i) The Inflammatory Response

Circulating phagocytes, and in particular the neutrophils form the most important part of this inflammatory response. A wide variety of bacteria as well as fungi are capable of being ingested, digested and killed by neutrophils. Severe neutropaenia strongly predisposes a patient to infection by Gram-negative and Gram-positive bacteria, especially Pseudomonas aeruginosa, Klebsiella and Enterobacter species, E. coli, and Staphylococci aureus. Fungal infections, notably of the Aspergillus, Candida and Mucor species are also observed in neutropaenic patients.

(ii) The Complement System

The complement cascade especially C3a and C5a together with other mediators promote and direct phagocytes to the areas of inflammation. If the organisms within the area of infection have been opsonized by complement or antibodies, phagocytosis and destruction of the organism is facilitated. A complement deficiency therefore also predisposes to bacterial infection, particularly of the Neisseria species.

(iii) The Reticuloendothelial System

Circulating microorganisms are cleared from the blood stream by tissue phagocytes derived from circulating monocytes. The most important tissue phagocytes include the Kupffer cells in the liver, phagocytes in the spleen, lymph nodes, lung (alveolar macrophages), kidney (mesangial cells) and brain (microglial cells). Suppression or poor function of the reticuloendothelial system can lead to bacteraemia and sepsis from exogenous and/or endogenous microbial flora.

Immune Response

The B cell lymphocyte response to infection is the production of antibodies (IgG, IgA, IgM, IgE), and the T cell lymphocyte response leads to a cell-mediated immune defence. Humoral defence through antibody production and cell-mediated immunity are closely interrelated, inter-reactive and interdependent.

Humoral deficiency exposes the patient at times to overwhelming infection, particularly to Streptococcus and H. influenzae pneumonias.

Cell-mediated immune deficiency often renders the patient susceptible to protozoal, fungal, viral and rarer bacterial infections. Infections with Pneumocystis carinii, Toxoplasma gondii, Cryptococcus neoformans, Mycobacterial infections (tuberculosis and Mycobacterium avium-complex infections), infections by the Legionella species, and by Listeria monocytogenes are observed in these patients. Viral infections include infections due to Cytomegalovirus (CMV), Herpes simplex and Herpes zoster virus.

The following groups of immunocompromised patients are often seen in ICUs (1):

(i) Solid Organ Transplant Recipients

Most common in this group are patients who have received a kidney transplant. In Western countries, patients with heart, liver, lung, and pancreas transplants are also seen. These patients are all immunosuppressed, as they must have a lymphocyte depletion so that the transplants survive. They demonstrate an increase in suppressor T lymphocytes and limited T cell cytotoxic activity. In addition, they suffer from the effects of prolonged corticosteroid administration and the use of cyclosporine A. Infection, sometimes sudden and overwhelming, is an important and dreaded complication in all organ transplant recipients. Different infections generally occur in different time frames (early or late after transplant) and this serves as a rough aid in diagnosis (see Chapter on Critical Care of the Transplant Patient).

(ii) The Haemopoeitic Stem-cell Transplant Recipients

Haemopoeitic stem-cell transplants are increasingly used as therapy for various haematological malignancies, haemoglobinopathies, immunodeficiency disorders and even for solid tumours. Autologous stem-cell transplant is associated with neutropaenia as the primary immune defect. Allogenic transplants lead to a broader range of immune defects with more wide-ranging complications.

(iii) Patients with Malignant Disease

Advanced malignancy leads to immunosuppression; lymphomas, and in particular Hodgkin's lymphoma are also associated with immunosuppression of the cellular immune reaction.

(iv) Patients on Corticosteroid Therapy

Corticosteroids are amongst the most frequently used drugs in medicine, and the doctor in a critical care unit may be unaware of the history of corticosteroid ingestion by an acutely ill patient admitted as an emergency. Corticosteroids suppress the immune response and mask the underlying pathology and inflammation. Patients on maintenance steroid therapy for long periods of time may easily go into an acute adrenal crisis in the presence of overwhelming infection, if the attending doctor is unaware of the history of steroid ingestion, and if the dose of corticosteroids is not suitably increased during such a crisis.

(v) Patients on Antimitotic Drugs

All antimitotic drugs are immunosuppressive and therefore predispose to infection. Cyclophosphamide and nitrogen mustard affect cell replication and bone marrow function. Antimetabolites affect and interfere with purine and pyrimidine metabolism, and prevent an adequate cellular immune response to infection.

(vi) Splenectomised Patients

These patients have an altered immune function. IgM production in response to bacterial antigen is markedly slow, and patients are particularly prone to fulminant infections by pneumococcus and other encapsulated organisms.

(vii) Immune Suppression in Chronic Disease

This is one of the most important groups encountered in our ICUs, and includes patients with liver cirrhosis and liver cell failure, chronic renal failure and patients on chronic haemodialysis, severe diabetics, alcoholics and those with myeloproliferative disorders. In our country as well as in other third world countries, poor nutrition is a frequent background factor against which many acute infections evolve. These patients are prone to acute infections, and are more likely to die of these infections in critical care units.

(viii) Immune Suppression in HIV Infection

According to a WHO report, about 42 million people worldwide are infected with the human immunodeficiency virus (HIV), with nearly 90 per cent of the infected persons residing in developing countries (**2, 3**). Though the Indian national adult HIV prevalence is estimated at less than 1 per cent, India had the second highest HIV-prevalence with an estimated 3.97 million HIV-positive people by the end of 2001 (**2**).

The HIV virus causes a depletion in T4 lymphocytes with a marked deterioration in cell-mediated immunity. The most serious feature of AIDS is the occurrence of infectious complications, particularly by opportunistic organisms.

Approach to the Acutely Ill Immunocompromised Patient

The following features are worthy of note:

(i) Acute infections in immunocompromised individuals can be sudden, overwhelming and rapidly fatal.

(ii) The clinical manifestations of such infections are not usually of the same intensity and degree as compared to those in patients with normal immune mechanisms. Diagnosis is doubly difficult because of the paucity of signs and the short time available between the onset of symptoms and possible death.

(iii) Complications due to non-infective causes are also observed in immunocompromised patients. It may be difficult to distinguish them from actual infections.

(iv) The clinician must recognize that the immunosuppressed patient is exposed to, and is likely to be infected by two groups of microbial pathogens—(a) the usual pathogens which can also afflict immunocompetent patients; (b) opportunistic organisms which invariably affect immunosuppressed patients only.

(v) Treatment of acute infections in immunocompromised individuals in ICUs should be prompt. It is often empirical and tailored to counter more than one possible infection depending on the clinical picture, and on the background against which this picture evolves. Therapy for immunosuppressed patients often involves the use of drugs directed against opportunistic organisms, and is often different from therapy in acute infections afflicting patients with normal immunological responses.

Acute or Critical Infections in Immunocompromised Patients

In a critical care setting, infections in immunocompromised individuals generally present in the following manner:

    A. Fever with Neutropaenia

    B. Sepsis and Septic Shock

    C. Pneumonias

    D. Disseminated Tuberculosis

    E. Meningitis and CNS Infections

A. Pyrexia of Unknown Origin (PUO) with Neutropaenia

This is generally observed in patients with myeloproliferative disease, lymphoma and cancers after aggressive chemotherapy. Severe neutropaenia results in a loss of phagocytic function leading to infectious complications. Associated B cell and T cell dysfunction further contributes to these complications. The risk of infection depends on the degree and duration of neutropaenia. The infection rate is significantly increased if the neutrophil count is $< 1.0 \times 10^9/l$ and is highly probable if it further falls to $0.5 \times 10^9/l$. In our experience infection invariably results if the duration of severe neutropaenia is > 10 days. Many infections result from the patients' own endogenous flora (i.e. from the skin, gut, lungs); approximately half the infections are nosocomial in origin. In our unit, the organisms most frequently involved are the Gram-negative organisms, such as the Pseudomonas aeruginosa, Klebsiella, Enterobacter, Serratia, and Gram-positive organisms notably Staphylococcus aureus (including the methicillin resistant Staph) and Staph epidermidis. Invasive fungal infections due to Candida, Aspergillus and Mucor species are increasingly observed.

The organism causing fever in patients with severe neutropaenia is microbiologically identified in less than a quarter of cases. In another quarter, the clinical symptomatology suggests an infection, though the nature and site of infection again remains unproven and in half or more patients the fever remains of unknown origin. Thus in many such patients, a complete physical examination, basic radiological and ultrasound tests, blood tests including cultures of blood, urine, body secretions are all negative. It is therefore imperative that in patients with severe neutropaenia (to the extent described above), with fever (defined as a single oral temperature of 38.3°C or 38°C for at least one hour), empiric antibiotic therapy should be promptly commenced after relevant blood tests, culture of blood, urine, other body secretions and a chest X-ray have been done. One should never await results. We generally prefer to cover Gram-negative organisms (in particular Pseudomonas) with a third generation cephalosporin or a piperacillin derivative, plus an aminoglycoside. Gram-positive cover is provided with intravenous augmentin. If there is a strong suspicion of methicillin resistant Staphylococcus causing infection, vancomycin is substituted for augmentin. Further modification in antibiotic coverage depends on results of tests, and on response to therapy. We also administer the granulocyte stimulation factor daily to help increase the leucocyte and neutrophil count to safe levels.

Patients with a PUO and neutropaenia who fail to respond within three or four days of a broad-spectrum antibiotic cover should in addition be given amphotericin B to cover a possible fungal infection. Amphotericin B is used even earlier if the patient deteriorates quickly, if there is a background known to significantly increase fungal superinfection (as in patients on prolonged corticosteroid therapy) or if pleuritic pain, cough, haemoptysis point to infection in the chest and an HRCT of the chest is suggestive of a possible fungal infection.

Fibreoptic bronchoscopy with BAL and transbronchial biopsy should be performed only if the patient fails to respond to the above management protocol. This is because opportunistic infections such as Pneumocystis carinii pneumonia are rare in patients with fever and neutropaenia, except in patients with underlying lymphoma or in those on long-standing corticosteroid therapy.

Surgical biopsy is very rarely indicated—when for example, infiltrates in the lung persist in spite of therapy and the patient is deemed fit to withstand the surgical procedure.

The mortality of patients with fever and severe neutropaenia is significantly reduced with the empirical therapy described above. Afebrile neutopaenic patients should be watched closely, should avoid external contact with other individuals, and preferably be given prophylactic antibiotics—augmentin 650 mg twice daily, ciprofloxacin 750 mg twice daily.

B. Sepsis and Septic Shock

Sepsis or septic shock is probably the most dreaded complication in immunocompromised individuals. The source and nature of sepsis is at times obvious, and at times remains undetermined in spite of all investigations. The important sources of sepsis are:

(i) An abscess or infected haematoma anywhere within the body for which the patient requires critical care.

(ii) Intra-abdominal sepsis—the most frequent cause of this is a perforated gut due to any aetiology, with peritonitis. A delayed diagnosis and late surgery are sure pointers to a very high mortality in spite of excellent surgical techniques and good post-operative care. If the source of infection within the peritoneal cavity cannot be completely eradicated, death is inevitable.

(iii) Sepsis is sometimes related to a community-acquired bacterial infection—chiefly a pneumonia.

(iv) Sepsis also follows upon opportunistic infections—in particular viral and fungal infections.

(v) An immunocompromised patient may be admitted to an ICU for trauma or following surgery. These patients are extremely prone to nosocomial infections. Nosocomial pneumonias, and nosocomial sepsis through central lines, catheters, ventilator tubings and nebulization equipment are frequent, and carry a forbidding mortality. Sepsis may arise from the overgrowth of pathogenic bacteria in the gut and their translocation into the systemic circulation.

(vi) As mentioned earlier, the source and nature of sepsis at times remains undetermined.

The diagnosis of sepsis and septic shock has been discussed in an earlier chapter. In immunocompromised patients fever and leucocytosis may not be as high as in patients with a normal immune system. In fulminant cases, hypothermia and leucopaenia may be observed. Physical signs are subtle, and may be easily missed or ignored. Deterioration is often rapid, with a quick onset of multiple organ dysfunction and failure.

The principles of management discussed under Septic Shock are applicable to immunocompromised patients. It needs to be restressed that however ill the patient, a localized source of infection if accessible, should be promptly dealt with surgically. An abscess simply must be drained, and abdominal sepsis must be surgically tackled. The choice between aspirating a localized abscess under ultrasound or CT guidance, or incising and draining it should be left to the surgeon.

It is always necessary to start appropriate empiric antibiotic therapy promptly, after collection of secretions and of blood for culture has been done. We generally start with augmentin 1.2 g 8 hourly intravenously to counter possible coccal infections, a third generation cephalosporin like ceftazidime 2 g intravenously 8 hourly or cefoperazone 2 g 12 hourly intravenously daily, which acts against Gram-negative infections including Pseudomonas pyocyaneus, and an aminoglycoside, which also acts against Gram-negative infections. Any antibacterial regime against Gram-negative infections should include a combination of two antibiotics.

In nosocomial infections the choice of antibiotics is governed by the nosocomial organisms most frequently encountered in a particular intensive care setting. In our unit, Pseudomonas aeruginosa, Klebsiella and Enterobacter are the common organisms responsible for nosocomial infections. An alternative regime empirically followed comprises ticarcillin in combination with clavulanic acid, or a piperacillin derivative, together with an aminoglycoside. When there is a possibility of a staphylococcal infection, or in very ill patients, or in those who show no response within 36 hours of starting the above standard regime, we add vancomycin 500 mg 6 hourly intravenously to the management protocol.

In certain clinical settings the standard regime may need to be modified:

(i) If culture reports suggest that the patient is colonized and probably infected by an organism resistant to the regime chosen, or if the patient is admitted to a unit where an uncommon, resistant organism is known to be responsible for frequent infections, a drug acting against such an organism is added or substituted in the regime.

(ii) If the clinical situation suggests an associated anaerobic infection (as in abdominal sepsis, perianal or perirectal sepsis, or in sepsis following aspiration of gastric contents), the addition of metronidazole 500–750 mg intravenously every 8 hours, or clindamycin 600 mg intravenously 6 hourly, or penicillin 2 mega units intravenously 4–6 hourly, is warranted.

(iii) If sepsis is thought to be related to central lines, intravenous vancomycin 500 mg 6 hourly should always be included in the regime.

(iv) If Haemophilus influenzae is likely to be the incriminating organism, it is best to include a third generation cephalosporin (if not used), or use cefuroxime acetate 1.5 g intravenously every 8 hours.

(v) Ordinarily antifungal therapy is not included initially in the standard regime except when there is strong clinical evidence, right from the outset, of a fungal infection. However if an immuno-compromised patient with sepsis or septic shock fails to improve within 48 hours on an antibacterial regime outlined above, antifungal treatment with amphotericin B is added to the therapy. In patients with cancer, in those immunosuppressed by antimitotic drugs, or in those immunosuppressed patients who have received broad-spectrum antibiotics for prolonged periods of time and who suddenly deteriorate, many would prefer to initiate antifungal therapy promptly. In patients with sepsis and severe granulocytopaenia who fail to improve on antibacterial broad-spectrum antibiotics, or those who improve initially but then suddenly dete-

riorate, a fungal infection is strongly suspect, and amphotericin B should be added empirically to the therapeutic regime (see Section on PUO with neutropaenia).

(vi) In patients with cellular immune defects, antimicrobial therapy must consider coverage of Listeria monocytogenes (ampicillin 2 g every 4 hours and gentamicin 1 mg/kg every 8 hours). Fungal infections (chiefly Candida and Cryptococcus neoformans) and viral infections (Cytomegalovirus and Herpes virus) are also to be suspected in this situation.

There are no firm or objective guidelines regarding the duration of antibiotic treatment of sepsis in immunocompromised patients. Antibiotics should be continued till sepsis is well controlled—generally treatment lasts for at least 10–14 days, and often for much longer periods of time. If possible, the serum antibiotic concentrations of all patients with sepsis, and in particular septic shock, should be monitored. There are only a few hospitals in our city and in our country that have facilities to monitor antibiotic levels. Dose modifications may therefore be necessary, particularly in the presence of hepatic or renal dysfunction induced by the disease, by shock, or by previous treatment. Fortunately, at least in Mumbai, it is possible to monitor levels of a few important antibiotics, including the aminoglycosides gentamicin and amikacin. When using the former, it is advisable to aim for peak concentrations of 4–10 µg/ml and trough concentrations of 1–2 µg/ml; when amikacin is used, the peak concentrations should be 20–35 µg/ml and the trough concentrations 5–10 µg/ml.

The role of corticosteroids in sepsis has been discussed in the Chapter on Sepsis and Septic Shock. Immunoglobulin infusions or infusions of complement or transfer factor to augment the immune response, are of dubious clinical efficacy. However the use of granulocyte colony stimulating factor (5–10 µg/kg/day) in such patients is often rewarded by an increase in the granulocyte count after 2–5 days. A satisfactory granulocyte response may well turn the tide in the patient's favour.

C. Pneumonias

Infections in immunocompromised patients frequently take the form of pneumonias. In these patients, pneumonia very frequently results from the usual bacterial flora prevailing within the community. The commonest community-acquired pneumonia in India (as in other countries) is due to the Streptococcus pneumoniae. In older, particularly immunocompromised individuals, Gram-negative infections are frequent. In our country, as well as in all third world countries where tuberculosis is common, a flare-up of this disease always needs to be considered. The diagnosis may not be easy as many of these patients produce little or no sputum for examination.

Immunocompromised patients, in contrast to patients who are immunocompetent, are however increasingly prone to opportunistic infections. In the acquired immune deficiency syndrome (AIDS), pneumonia due to Pneumocystis carinii is frequently observed when the CD4 lymphocyte count is < 200/mm^3. Pneumocystis carinii infection can also occur in lymphomas, leukaemias, myeloproliferative disorders, organ transplant recipients, in patients on corticosteroid therapy and rarely in patients with rheumatoid disease on methotrexate therapy. Other opportunistic organisms causing pneumonia include the Cytomegalovirus, and the Herpes virus, Mycobacterium avium intracellulare, protozoa, helminths (Strongyloidosis), and fungi. Not uncommonly, more than one opportunistic organism is present in the same individual.

Finally, immunocompromised patients admitted to a critical care unit for non-infectious conditions (trauma, surgery) are specially prone to nosocomial pneumonia.

There are some noteworthy features in relation to pneumonia in immunocompromised patients:

(i) Pneumonias constitute a major cause of morbidity and mortality in diverse immunosuppressed populations, and therefore pose a problem of enormous magnitude. In one large reported study of renal transplant patients, pneumonia occurred in 20 per cent of patients, and accounted for 50 per cent of deaths (4). Similarly in patients with lymphomas, pneumonia is the commonest infection causing death (5). Interstitial pneumonia is reported to occur in 55 per cent of bone marrow transplant recipients who survive for 30 days after transplantation, and carries a mortality of 60 per cent (6).

(ii) In many patients the symptoms are few, and there is a paucity of physical signs. In neutropaenic patients, physical signs are virtually absent. An increase in the respiratory rate is probably the only important sign which may be observed. Radiological shadowing in neutropaenic patients is barely noticeable and may even be absent due to the total lack of neutrophilic response in such patients.

(iii) Pneumonias due to bacterial infections can be multilobar. Acute lung injury (ARDS) is more often observed in immunocompromised patients under the above circumstances. Similarly multiple organ dysfunction, failure and death are more frequently observed.

(iv) A quick diagnosis allows specific therapy to be promptly instituted and improves patient survival. In renal transplant patients, a mortality of 21 per cent was noted in those patients where a specific diagnosis was made within 5 days of the illness. In contrast, the mortality rate was 65 per cent in patients who were diagnosed after 5 days of illness (4).

(v) Each ICU must have a protocol or a plan of approach for dealing with an immunocompromised patient admitted with fever and pulmonary infiltrates. Good patient care in these patients necessitates a team approach which should however be orchestrated by a single individual in charge of patient care. It is unfortunate and sad that many microbiological and pathological laboratories in our country are ill-equipped to diagnose opportunistic infections, particularly Pneumocystis carinii, viral infections, and infections caused by rarer microbes—chiefly Legionella, Mycoplasma and Nocardia. Management protocols in third world countries should therefore take into account the facilities available for investigations.

(vi) *Fever with pulmonary infiltrates in an immunocompromised individual is not always related to infection.* It is vital to be aware of this fact. Non-infective causes of pulmonary 'shadows' or infiltrates include pulmonary oedema, pulmonary haemorrhage, pulmonary embolism, drug-induced pulmonary disease, ARDS, opportunistic neoplasms (lymphoproliferative disorders, Kaposi's sarcoma). Other non-infective lesions include recurrence of underlying tumour, lymphoma, leukaemia within the lungs, immune-mediated disorders (acute rejection after lung transplant, obliterative bronchiolitis after lung transplant or after an allogenic stem-cell transplant), and non-specific focal inflammation (See **Table 17.1.1**).

Table 17.1.1. Non-infective pulmonary infiltrates or 'shadows' in the immunocompromised host

* Pulmonary oedema
* Pulmonary haemorrhage
* ARDS
* Pulmonary embolism
* Drug-induced pulmonary disease
* Leukoagglutinin reaction
* Opportunistic neoplasms (lymphoproliferative disorders, Kaposi's sarcoma)
* Recurrence of a tumour of a lymphoma or a leukaemia in the lungs
* Immune-mediated disorders
    Acute rejection after lung transplant
    Obliterative bronchiolitis
* Non-specific inflammation

Clinical Approach to Diagnosis of Fever with Pulmonary Infiltrates in Immunocompromised Patients

(a) **Knowledge of the Background Disease.** Patients with cell-mediated immune deficiency e.g. HIV infection, prolonged corticosteroid therapy, Hodgkin's or other lymphomas, and those with organ transplants, are prone to infections by Mycobacterium tuberculosis, Pneumocystis carinii, Cytomegalovirus and other Herpes viruses, Cryptococcus, Nocardia and Legionella. On the other hand, patients whose main defect is a severe granulocytopaenia are prone to Gram-negative infections, staphylococcal and fungal infections (Aspergillus, Mucor, Candida).

In organ transplant patients the time of onset after transplantation, may be of diagnostic assistance. Cytomegalovirus pneumonias occur from 1–4 months after renal transplantation, but are relatively rare prior to or after this period (4). Pneumonias occurring within the first 3–4 weeks after a transplant are almost never due to an opportunistic organism, but result from the usual bacterial pathogens causing post-operative pneumonias in surgical patients. Between 1–4 months after the transplant, besides the Cytomegalovirus, infections due to Nocardia, Pneumocystis and fungi should be kept in mind. After 4 months, patients who have normally functioning grafts, and who are on minimal immunosuppression, are prone to the usual community-acquired infections. Those with poorly functioning grafts who require intensive immunosuppression, remain susceptible to the opportunistic infections stated above.

In the early part of the natural history of lymphomas, the patient is at greater risk for community-acquired pneumonias. As the disease progresses and particularly with repeated therapy, the patient is at greater risk for opportunistic pathogens.

Epidemiological clues should always be sought. In our country and in other third world countries, depressed cell-mediated immunity is most likely to exacerbate or result in infection with Mycobacterium tuberculosis. However, residence and exposure in areas endemic to fungi such as Histoplasma capsulatum or Coccidioides immitis, could predispose to histoplasmosis or coccidioidomycosis.

Infiltrates due to non-infectious causes also have a predictable time for making their appearance. Patients treated for acute myeloblastic leukaemia may develop interstitial pulmonary infiltrates. When these infiltrates occur within 4 days of a fall in the white blood cell count, they are suggestive of a leukaemic cell lysis pneumopathy (7). The mechanism of infiltrates and alveolar damage in this syndrome is perhaps related to the lysis of interstitial and alveolar blast cells. A pattern of pulmonary oedema developing within minutes to hours of transfusion of blood or other blood products, raises the possibility of a leukoagglutinin reaction (7). On the other hand, pulmonary shadows (sometimes localized), may be related to pulmonary oedema produced by overhydration, poor left ventricular function, or to a capillary leak as in early acute lung injury (ARDS).

Bleomycin is the commonest drug responsible for interstitial infiltrates after the patient has received a cumulative dose of 150 mg of the drug. However idiosyncratic reactions may occur with much smaller doses. Other antimitotic drugs, particularly methotrexate and busulphan, can also result in interstitial infiltrates.

(b) The Mode of Onset and the Tempo of Progression. These often provide crucial clues in the diagnosis. Their value is enhanced if the above features are considered in association with radiological findings (**Table 17.1.2**). An acute onset over 24–48 hours is suggestive of a conventional bacterial infection, or certain non-infectious causes such as pulmonary oedema, pulmonary haemorrhage, pulmonary embolism or a leukoagglutinin reaction. A subacute onset over a few days or weeks suggests tuberculosis, pneumocystis, viral, fungal or nocardial infections. The same presentation may however also be observed with certain non-infectious causes such as drug-induced pneumonitis, radiation pneumonitis, or the recurrence of a tumour against the background of a mitotic disease.

Table 17.1.2. Differential diagnosis of fever and pulmonary infiltrates in the immunocompromised patient, based on radiological signs and onset of symptoms

Chest X-ray	Symptoms	
	Acute Onset	Subacute or Chronic Onset
1. Consolidation	* Bacterial * Thromboembolic * Haemorrhage	* Fungal * Nocardial * Tuberculous
2. Peribroncho-vascular (interstitial) infiltrate	* Pulmonary oedema * Leukoagglutinin reaction	* Viral * Pneumocystis carinii * Radiation * Drug induced
3. Nodular infiltrates	* Bacterial * Pulmonary oedema	* Tumour * Fungal * Nocardial * Tuberculous

(c) Physical Examination. Physical examination may occasionally provide valuable clues. In sophisticated ICUs with high technology equipments, physical examination tends to be perfunctory; this should never be so. Repeated clinical examination might reveal clues which machines and elaborate investigations fail to detect. The features enumerated below are merely illustrative of the importance of a careful physical examination.

(i) Tachypnoea in an immunocompromised patient particularly in the absence of high fever is indicative of sepsis, pneumonia or acidosis. Physical signs in the chest may or may not be evident; an absence of signs on percussion or auscultation is often observed in these patients.

(ii) Skin lesions are occasionally present in cryptococcal, nocardial and candidal infections. They take the form of minimally painful or asymptomatic macules, papules or nodules, which on biopsy provide the correct diagnosis, thereby obviating the need for invasive diagnostic procedures. Erythema gangrenosum is occasionally observed in infections with Pseudomonas aeruginosa, and very rarely with other Gram-negative infections.

(iii) A careful search for enlarged lymph glands can be rewarding. Lymphadenopathy strongly suggests a tuberculous infection in our country, either due to Mycobacterium tuberculosis or in AIDS patients to a possible infection with Mycobacterium avium-intracellulare. An underlying lymphoma, presenting with an obscure pneumonia, has been occasionally diagnosed following the biopsy of a nondescript clinically palpable lymph node.

(iv) Ocular examination is important as ocular findings are common with disseminated Cytomegalovirus infection. The retina shows haemorrhages and yellowish-white exudates. Similar ocular findings have been noted in toxoplasmosis, and occasionally in candidiasis and aspergillosis.

(v) Examination of other systems is of crucial importance. Hepatosplenomegaly with lymphadenopathy may point to an underlying lymphoma or a myeloproliferative disorder. It is also commonly observed in disseminated haematogenous tuberculosis and toxoplasmosis.

Neurological examination may reveal subtle symptoms and signs suggesting meningitis or a focal neurological lesion. Brain abscess is common in nocardial infection, cryptococcal infection, and in disseminated disease due to Mycobacterium tuberculosis (see Chapter on Neurological Problems requiring Critical Care).

(vi) Radiological Investigations. Pulmonary infiltrates are never so specific on a chest X-ray to allow a definitive aetiological diagnosis to be made. Nevertheless, a study of serial chest X-rays when combined with an analysis of the mode of onset and the progress of the disease often helps in limiting the diagnostic possibilities.

Focal or multifocal consolidation of short duration (< 48 hours) seen on a chest X-ray, is invariably due to an acute bacterial infection. Slowly progressive consolidation with a subacute or chronic history favours tuberculosis, nocardial or fungal infections.

Interstitial infiltrates spreading outwards from the hilar area and evolving in a subacute or chronic manner, suggest Pneumocystis, viral or drug-induced infiltration, or may be due to lymphangitis carcinomatosis. Acutely evolving interstitial infiltrates suggest pulmonary oedema or a leukoagglutinin reaction.

Acute nodular localized alveolar consolidation, or localized nodular infiltrates suggest pulmonary oedema or bacterial bronchopneumonia. Nodular infiltrates which are subacute or chronic and slow in evolving could be tuberculous, fungal or nocardial in aetiology. Such infiltrates could also be due to the recurrence or spread of an original tumour.

These radiological observations are not sacrosanct, and as mentioned at the outset, an exact diagnosis can never be made by the mere description of shadows on a chest radiograph. The overall picture has to be considered.

Management Protocol (Fig. 17.1.1)

This should be organized and planned depending on the facilities present in an ICU, and the degree of sophistication of the pathology and microbiology departments of the hospital. Routine investigations include a blood count, blood chemistry, blood culture, sputum examination (Gram's stain, acid-fast stain), sputum culture, X-ray chest and often an HRCT chest. A Gram's stain of the sputum at times provides a direction to appropriate therapy. In some patients, nebulization with hypertonic saline helps to obtain a satisfactory sputum sample.

Empiric therapy should be started without awaiting results of blood and sputum tests. Therapy could be changed later if the results so necessitate. The protocol we use in an acutely ill immunocompromised patient is as follows:

1. If the patient presents with a focal alveolar infiltrate or consolidation, we use intravenous augmentin + a third generation cephalosporin like ceftazidime + an aminoglycoside, or alternatively use other broad-spectrum antibiotics that counter Gram-positive and Gram-negative infections, as outlined in the Section on Sepsis. The choice of the antibiotic regime depends on the possible nature of the organisms suspected in a given individual. Nosocomial pneumonias in immunocompromised patients should include vancomycin in the initial therapy to cover severe methicillin-resistant staphylococcal infection. In pneumonia associated with severe neutropaenia, particularly in those who have pleuritic pain, cough, haemoptysis and whose HRCT is compatible with an Aspergillus infection, we would add amphotericin B to the regime of broad-spectrum antibiotics on an empiric basis. If the patient responds to the above treatment, the antibiotic course is continued for a period of 2 weeks or even longer.

If the patient does not respond within 48 to 72 hours, or if the disease progresses, we would opt to do a bronchoalveolar lavage with a careful examination and culture of the lavage fluid. Whenever possible we recommend brush biopsies of the involved areas done by standard accepted techniques. A transbronchial biopsy of the lesion if thought appropriate, can be done during the same procedure. The biopsy material is processed promptly for staining of the organisms, histopathology, and for cultures.

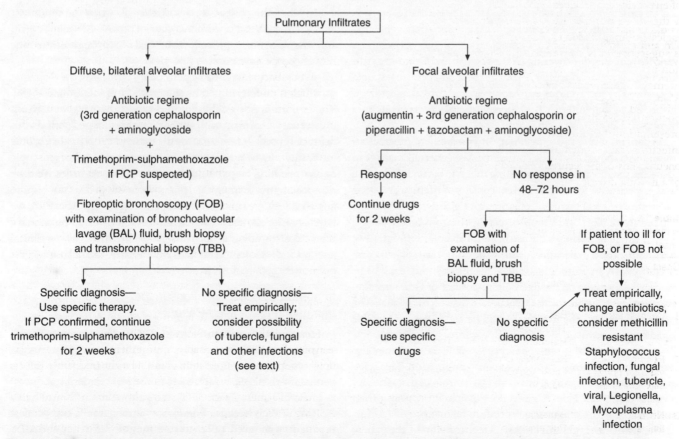

Fig. 17.1.1. Management protocol in acutely ill immunocompromised patients with fever and pulmonary infiltrates (see text for role of open lung biopsy and for details of management protocol).

The following aetiological agents are diagnosed by these techniques:

(i) Gram-negative or Gram-positive infections.

(ii) Mycobacterium tuberculosis. It is amazing how often this diagnosis would have been missed or would not have been seriously entertained if the above diagnostic procedure was not performed.

(iii) Other rare infections e.g. nocardial infections.

(iv) Pneumocystis carinii infection—the organism can be identified in lavage and in biopsy material by suitable staining.

(v) Cytomegalovirus infection can be diagnosed by the presence of inclusion bodies in cells normally observed in this infection.

(vi) Fungal infection, particularly aspergillus infection. Aspergilli in the BAL fluid of an immunocompromised patient with 'pneumonia', strongly suggests Aspergillus infection. It is unfortunate that very few laboratories in our country have the facilities to diagnose Legionella and other viral infections.

(vii) Opportunistic cryptococcal infection and toxoplasmosis may be occasionally diagnosed on a transbronchial biopsy.

If a specific aetiology is found by this procedure, the drugs used are, by and large, solely directed towards the eradication of the aetiological agent.

If the patient is too ill for a bronchoalveolar lavage or a transbronchial fibreoptic bronchoscopy, or if the ICU cannot organize these procedures, or if the pathological and microbiological backup is poor, further management should proceed on an empiric basis. For example, if augmentin, a third generation cephalosporin, and an aminoglycoside have been used initially with no effect, one could switch to ticarcillin-clavulanic acid combination, vancomycin and ciprofloxacin or to a combination of meropenem and vancomycin. Besides covering Gram-positive and Gram-negative infections, atypical organisms (e.g. Legionella, Mycoplasma) should be covered by intravenous erythromycin and fungal infection, if suspected, by amphotericin B. Opportunistic infection may at times be impossibly difficult to diagnose.

In patients with a subacute onset, the possibility of tuberculous pneumonia should always be considered. We generally manage to prove the diagnosis by demonstrating tubercle bacilli in bronchial lavage specimens. Specific treatment consists of rifampicin 600 mg daily, isoniazid 300 mg daily, ethambutol 1 g daily, pyrazinamide 750 mg twice daily and streptomycin 1 g intramuscularly daily.

2. If the patient shows diffuse bilateral alveolar infiltrates, we start with a third generation cephalosporin or ticarcillin in combination with an aminoglycoside. This regime may need to be modified depending on the likely Gram-positive or Gram-negative organism responsible for the infection in a given individual. The sicker the patient, the greater should be the cover for possible invading organisms. If the X-ray appearances and clinical background are compatible with pneumocystis infection, we may also start a trimethoprim-sulfamethoxazole combination. This is followed by bronchial lavage, brush and transbronchial biopsies for possible diagnostic help. If this is not possible for reasons earlier outlined, or if the diagnostic procedure fails to provide a clue, further treatment remains empiric. Deterioration of the patient should prompt the use of amphotericin B for cryptococcal, aspergillus or other rare fungal infections. If Legionnaires' disease is a clinical possibility, erythromycin is added. Disseminated tuberculosis should generally be evident by the demonstration of acid-fast bacilli in the samples obtained through a bronchial lavage.

3. If the patient has bilateral pulmonary parahilar interstitial infiltrates strongly suggestive of Pneumocystis infection, we start a trimethoprim-sulfamethoxazole combination, and follow this up with bronchial lavage, bronchial brush biopsy and rarely a transbronchial biopsy to prove the presence of Pneumocystis carinii. If the diagnosis is confirmed, specific treatment is continued for 2 weeks. If unconfirmed, the above-mentioned treatment should still be continued, and ganciclovir added for a possible cytomegalovirus infection.

4. The possibility that the 'shadows' or lung infiltrates in the lung could be non-infective in nature should be kept in mind, particularly if investigations, for an infective agent are persistently negative and the shadows persist in spite of antibiotic therapy.

The Role of an Open Lung Biopsy

Many units in the West are aggressive in their approach, and perform an open lung biopsy within 24 hours if the patient deteriorates, to obtain a specific diagnosis of the aetiology of the pneumonia. We rarely perform open lung biopsies on our patients as we feel that most of them are too ill to tolerate the procedure. Thoracoscopic lung biopsies are less traumatic than open lung biopsies. Lung biopsy is recommended under the following circumstances.

(i) When the patient is not critically ill, when the treatment directed towards the 'pneumonia' has not provided definite benefit, and when diagnostic procedures carried out through a fibreoptic bronchoscope have provided no yield.

(ii) In subacute or chronic pulmonary infiltrates, the diagnosis of which is undetermined by the procedures mentioned above. The importance of establishing a diagnosis here is that it avoids unnecessary treatment with antibiotics for prolonged periods, this being definitely detrimental for the patient. Subacute or chronic infiltrates may be non-infectious in nature, and a thoracoscopic or an open lung biopsy helps to confirm this. At times we have diagnosed chronic interstitial pneumonia which does not require any antibiotic treatment, on an open lung biopsy. Above all, we have occasionally diagnosed infiltrates to be due to pulmonary tuberculosis by doing an open lung biopsy in patients whose clinical features and radiological findings were bizarre, and did not suggest pulmonary tuberculosis in any way.

Important Specific Infections in the Immunocompromised Patient

Pneumocystis Carinii Pneumonia (PCP). Pneumocystis carinii is a protozoal parasite, and is an important cause of pneumonias in immunocompromised individuals. It most frequently infects patients with AIDS; in fact, early in the HIV epidemic about 80 per cent of patients with AIDS and pulmonary infiltrates had a PCP (8). This is because Pneumocystis infection is commonest in patients with severe cell-mediated immune deficiency, and AIDS is an example of the severest form of cellular immunity depression. However with the widespread use of antiretroviral therapy and chemoprophylaxis against P carinii, the incidence has fallen, and in 1991 only 46 per cent of pneumonias in AIDS were due to P carinii. In a recent Indian autopsy study on 143 patients with AIDS, only 5 per cent of lung pathologies were caused by P carinii (9). This is because AIDS patients in India die of pulmonary tuberculosis before they get a chance to acquire Pneumocystis infection (see Section on Pneumonia in AIDS). P carinii is also seen in other diseases with depressed cell-mediated immunity, e.g. lymphomas, in children with acute lymphoblastic leukaemia, patients on high doses of corticosteroids, organ transplant recipients and allogenic stem cell transplant patients.

In AIDS the disease is often subacute or insidious in onset (10), generally presenting with cough and bilateral perihilar infiltrates which slowly and progressively fan out into the periphery. As the disease progresses, it produces increasing breathlessness, but few physical signs. Hypoxia progressively increases so that the patient finally develops hypoxaemic respiratory failure, and at this stage the patient usually gets admitted to an ICU. If the background of AIDS is known, the diagnosis is generally obvious; if AIDS has not been diagnosed, the diagnosis may be missed if the clinician is unaware of its clinical and radiological features.

In diseases other than AIDS, pneumocystis pneumonia is more often an acute opportunistic infection, producing fever, increasing breathlessness and progressive interstitial infiltration fanning from the hilum to the periphery, and soon involving the greater part of both lungs. Death results from acute respiratory failure.

In the subacutely ill patient, nebulization of hypertonic saline (11) can give a yield of sputum positive for Pneumocystis carinii in more than 50–60 per cent of patients. In the acutely ill patient in an intensive care setting, the diagnosis can be proven by bronchial lavage, brush biopsies or transbronchial biopsy, as outlined earlier. Open lung biopsies are hardly ever necessary to establish a diagnosis.

Treatment. The drug of choice is a trimethoprim-sulpha-methoxazole (TMP/SMX) combination, the intravenous dose being trimethoprim 5 mg/kg and sulfamethoxazole 25 mg/kg given 6 hourly. The TMP/SMX combination can alternatively be given orally in the form of Bactrim Forte 2 tablets four times a day. Adverse reactions are frequent (12, 13) and over 50 per cent of patients treated with this combination exhibit rashes, liver cell and renal dysfunction, leucopaenia and thrombocytopaenia. A recent study reported that TMP/SMX had an amiloride-like effect, thus partly accounting for the hyponatraemia, which is frequently associated with the use of these drugs (14).

Pentamidine is also used in pneumocystis infections, particularly if the patient cannot tolerate the trimethoprim-sulphamethoxazole combination. The dose is 4 mg/kg given once daily, intravenously, over 60–90 minutes. Pentamidine is often more toxic than the trimethoprim-sulphamethoxazole combination, and can produce leucopaenia, thrombocytopaenia, hypotension, pancreatic islet cell dysfunction with either hypo- or hyperglycaemia, diabetes mellitus, renal dysfunction, gastrointestinal upset, elevated liver function enzymes, and repolarization abnormalities within the heart (15).

No convincing data are available to support the use of other alternative drugs in patients who fail to respond to either the trimethoprim-sulphamethoxazole combination, or to pentamidine.

Alternative therapies include the use of trimetrexate, dapsone, clindamycin-primaquine, or alpha-difluoromethyl ornithine (DFMO). We have used a combination of clindamycin-primaquine in patients who cannot tolerate trimethoprim-sulphamethoxazole or pentamidine. Studies suggest that corticosteroids are beneficial as adjunctive therapy in patients with hypoxaemic respiratory failure ($PaO_2 < 65$ mm Hg) (16). Methyl prednisolone 40–60 mg administered two to four times a day in tapering doses over 21 days appears beneficial.

The prognosis for the first episode of pneumocystis pneumonia if adequately treated, is good. Recovery occurs in 80–90 per cent of patients (17). Subsequent attacks carry a poorer prognosis (18). We have ventilated AIDS patients with pneumocystis pneumonia in the ICU in the past. We do not now do so if the patient is severely ill with other opportunistic infections, or if he is terminally ill.

Acute Viral Pneumonias Requiring Critical Care. The major viral pulmonary infection of concern in immunocompromised patients is the cytomegalovirus (CMV) infection. It can occur in any immunocompromised patient but is particularly common in certain patient populations. It is most common after allogenic bone marrow transplantation (19), in organ transplant recipients and in patients with AIDS.

The clinical features are characterized by fever, nonproductive cough, and increasing dyspnoea leading to a quickly progressive hypoxaemic respiratory failure. A chest X-ray shows progressive interstitial pulmonary infiltrates often indistinguishable from pneumocystis pneumonia. A miliary pattern on the chest X-ray is rarely observed in fulminant infections, leading to a quickly evolving arterial hypoxaemia and death.

Multisystem involvement is often observed in fulminant infections, and when present serves in most instances to distinguish CMV from pneumocystis infection. Thus, liver cell dysfunction, leucopaenia with atypical peripheral lymphocytes, lymphadenopathy, renal dysfunction probably due to virus-induced glomerulopathy and ocular changes may be observed. The frequency of CMV infection is undoubtedly underestimated, as diagnosis in critical care settings of developing countries is difficult. An important and rather peculiar feature of CMV infection is the ability of the CMV to further suppress cell-mediated immune responses in the host, thereby predisposing to further opportunistic infections. It is therefore not surprising that in AIDS, CMV infection often co-exists with mycobacterial and also with pneumocystis infections (20).

A quick diagnosis of CMV pneumonia in a critically ill patient can be only suspected by the presence of inclusion bodies within the cytoplasm of host cells in lung tissue obtained through transbronchial or open lung biopsies (21). CMV specific monoclonal antibodies are being studied to allow the diagnosis of CMV pneumonitis in tissues obtained from lung biopsies.

Therapy for CMV infection is unsatisfactory. Ganciclovir in a dose of 5 mg/kg, 12 hourly is reported to be of use; its main toxic effect is myelosuppression.

Other Acute Viral Pneumonias in Immunocompromised Patients. Several other viral infections can produce acute life-threatening pulmonary infections in immunocompromised patients. Measles and Varicella zoster viruses may present as disseminated infections with a fulminant fatal pneumonia. Generally, there is no diagnostic difficulty in either case because of the characteristic skin rash in each disease.

Herpes simplex virus rarely produces a haemorrhagic tracheo-bronchitis with a patchy pneumonia. The pathogen in most cases is due to an extension or aspiration of oral herpes simplex lesions, though in some cases there is a haematogenous spread. Bronchoscopy shows haemorrhagic ulcerating lesions within the bronchi covered with a white membrane. Material for specific cytological and virological studies may help establish a definite diagnosis. Therapy with intravenous acyclovir (5 mg/kg, 8 hourly) should be given in these patients. In the West, the incidence of herpes simplex viral infections in immunocompromised patients appears to be on the increase (22).

Nocardiosis. This is a rare infection produced chiefly by Nocardia asteroides in immunocompromised patients. It does not produce respiratory failure but presents in an intensive care setting as a pulmonary shadow of unknown aetiology in an immunosuppressed patient admitted for an unrelated problem. The X-ray picture shows one or more shadows often circumscribed and sometimes cavitating. A review of nocardial infection in 160 patients who had undergone heart transplant, provides a useful outline of the clinical profile of this disease (23). Fever and dry cough are presenting features but as mentioned above, an asymptomatic pulmonary shadow may be the first manifestation in 40 per cent of patients (23). Though generally subacute in its natural history, in some instances nocardial pulmonary infection in an immuno-suppressed host may resemble an acute bacterial pneumonia.

Nocardial infection can disseminate particularly to the CNS. One or more abscess-like cavities in the lungs and the brain in an immunocompromised patient should always suggest this diagnosis. Skin lesions occur in the form of nodules which on biopsy show the presence of Nocardia asteroides.

Diagnosis is difficult as nocardia is rarely present in sputum samples and cultures are frequently negative. This is one condition where a thoracoscopic or an open lung biopsy is indicated to establish a diagnosis. In two recent patients with nocardiosis, the diagnosis was arrived at by performing a CT-guided biopsy of the lesion in one patient, and by culture of material obtained through bronchial lavage in the other.

Treatment of nocardiosis is with sulfisoxazole (6–12 g/day) for a period of 3–6 months, extending to as long as a year in serious infections. Several authors have suggested that a trimethoprim-sulfamethoxazole combination maybe the treatment of choice in nocardial infections (24). This recommendation is based on a retrospective analysis of a small number of patients. We now use doxycycline 200 mg/day to start with, followed by 100 mg/day for 6 months to a year. Antibiotic sensitivity tests may be of help if the organism is grown on culture. Anecdotal reports claim success with a number of other drugs—minocycline, cycloserine, erythromycin and ampicillin.

Acute Fungal Pulmonary Infections. Fungal infections are being increasingly recognized in immunocompromised patients, and invasive fatal pulmonary infections due to Aspergillus are probably the commonest of these fungal infections. In AIDS patients however, cryptococcal lung disease appears to be significantly more common, but rarely leads to respiratory failure. Although disseminated candidiasis is a frequent opportunistic infection in immunocompromised patients in an intensive care setting, isolated or primary candida pneumonia is rare (25). Infection caused by the Mucor species (mucormycosis) should be kept in mind in immunocompromised patients (particularly in diabetics or those on corticosteroids) who have a maxillary sinusitis, or who have necrotic eschars over the sinuses, or within the nasal cavity, with orbital swelling and conjunctival oedema. Mucor tends to invade vessels leading to ischaemic necrosis of tissue supplied by these vessels.

Invasive rapidly spreading Aspergillus pneumonia almost exclusively occurs in severely immunocompromised and myelo-suppressed patients (26). Severe leucopaenia, and in particular marked granulocytopaenia, is a major risk factor in the evolution of invasive pulmonary aspergillosis. Patients with acute leukaemia develop invasive aspergillosis as a complication 20 times more frequently than patients with lymphomas or recipients of organ transplants (27, 28). In renal transplant patients the risk of invasive pulmonary aspergillosis increases with the use of high doses of corticosteroids.

Reports from the West continue to stress the importance of acute critical illnesses produced by invasive aspergillosis in patients with neoplastic disease and in heart transplant patients (23, 29). The spectrum of background diseases predisposing to invasive aspergillosis now includes patients with subacute hepatic necrosis treated with corticosteroids and intravenous antibiotics (30). We are fortunate in that the incidence of invasive pulmonary aspergillosis is low as compared to the West. Perhaps the frequency and the epidemiology of aspergillus infections is governed to an extent by the presence of airborne aspergillus in a particular eco-environment. Outbreaks of this infection have thus been related to the increased presence of this organism in the air, related to construction or to inadequate airconditioning systems (31–35).

Fever, nonproductive cough, haemoptysis, pleuritic chest pain, and a quick deterioration in the general condition of the patient is observed with invasive pulmonary aspergillosis. The X-ray pattern is of a patchy bronchopneumonia; occasionally a lobar involvement may occur. Pulmonary infarction due to vascular invasion by the Aspergillus produces peripheral shadows. Conventional chest X-rays are however not sensitive in the diagnosis of early invasive pulmonary aspergillosis. An HRCT of the chest is far more sensitive. The presence of single or multiple nodules surrounded by a 'ground glass' halo, or patchy areas of consolidation showing an air crescent is almost pathognomic of invasive aspergillosis. The clinical presentation at times resembles that of multiple pulmonary infarction. Necrosis of consolidated or infarcted areas may result in areas of cavitation. Chronic necrotizing pulmonary aspergillosis (24) producing a critical illness requiring intensive care has been reported in insulin-dependent diabetics, in patients on a modest dose of corticosteroids, or in cases following radiation therapy to the lungs.

Diagnosis of invasive aspergillosis is difficult. Sputum is rarely present and if present is rarely positive. Sputum cultures take a long time for growth of Aspergillus and in critically ill patients it is wrong to await reports when clinical suspicion is strong. Presence of Aspergilli in the BAL fluid in an immunocompromised patient is indicative of aspergillosis. An HRCT of the chest is far more sensitive in the diagnosis of invasive pulmonary aspergillosis than an X-ray chest, a sputum examination, or a bronchoscopic examination. A transbronchial biopsy is positive for Aspergillus in only 50 per cent of patients with invasive disease (36). An open lung biopsy is diagnostic but is not performed often, because of the poor condition of the patient. Empiric treatment is both indicated and justified in such situations.

Research in the detection of specific antibodies to Aspergillus or the detection of Aspergillus antigen continues. These are esoteric tests unavailable in our country; their sensitivity and specificity are undetermined, and it is wiser to err on the safer side and treat empirically whenever there is a strong clinical suspicion of invasive aspergillosis. Treatment is with amphotericin B (details in Chapter on Treatment of Fungal Infections in Critically Ill Patients).

Pneumonia in AIDS. The principles enunciated above in relation to pneumonia in immunosuppressed individuals apply to patients with AIDS as well.

A few points however need to be stressed in relation to these patients:

(i) There are some differences in the frequency of opportunistic pathogens in this syndrome. We are convinced that acute disseminated tuberculosis (including lung involvement), is the major opportunistic infection complicating the HIV epidemic worldwide (37–39). A study by Selwyn et al. showed a 7.6 per cent incidence of tuberculosis among anergic high-risk HIV-seropositive individuals (40). It is a general belief that Pneumocystis infection is uncommon in India. This is not so; it occurs later than tuberculosis in the natural history of HIV infection. The apparent infrequency of Pneumocystis carinii infection in patients with AIDS in India is because these patients are killed by the tubercle bacillus before the CD4 lymphocyte count drops to a level ($< 200/mm^3$) which predisposes them to P. carinii infection. Also, the latter infection is difficult to prove in units where microbiological and bronchoscopy facilities are inadequate.

An autopsy study of 143 patients with AIDS from Mumbai in 2001 (9) revealed a pulmonary pathology in 88 per cent of cases. The lesions identified were tuberculosis in 59 per cent, bacterial pneumonias in 18 per cent, CMV infection in 7 per cent, cryptococcal infection in 6 per cent, pneumocystis infection in 5 per cent, aspergillosis in 3 per cent, toxoplasmosis in 1 per cent, Kaposi's sarcoma in 1 per cent and squamous cell carcinoma in 1 per cent. Two or more infections were found in 13 per cent.

(ii) The clinical features of pulmonary infections in AIDS may be even more subtle than in other immunocompromised patients. This is so with all infections but is particularly observed with pneumocystis infection (which is generally subacute), disseminated tuberculosis and fungal infections.

(iii) Diagnostic procedures like examination of bronchoalveolar lavage fluid or the use of transbronchial biopsy, yield better or more definite results in diagnosing the aetiology of acute pulmonary infiltrates in AIDS as compared to other immunocompromised populations (28).

A plan for diagnostic evaluation of pulmonary infiltrates follows the same principles as in other immunocompromised patients and is briefly illustrated below in **Fig. 17.1.2.**

Specific antibiotic therapy (with the dose and duration of treatment) for organisms commonly encountered in immunocompromised patients, is listed in **Table 17.1.3.**

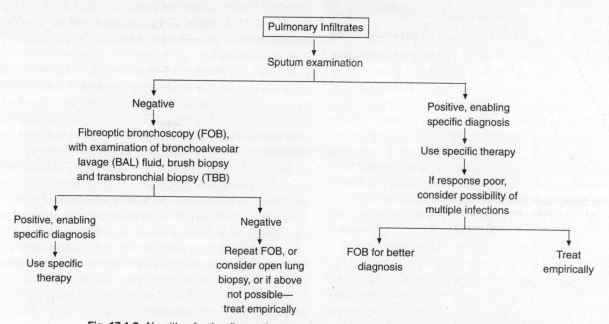

Fig. 17.1.2. Algorithm for the diagnostic evaluation of pulmonary infiltrates in patients with AIDS.

Table 17.1.3. Specific antibiotic therapy for commonly encountered organisms in immunocompromised patients

Organism	Drug and Dose	Average Duration of Treatment
1. Viruses		
* Herpes Simplex	Acyclovir 5 mg/kg 8 hrly IV	7–14 days
* Herpes Zoster	Acyclovir 10 mg/kg 8 hrly IV	7–14 days
* CMV	Ganciclovir 5 mg/kg 12 hrly IV	14 days
2. Bacteria		
* S. aureus	Cefazolin 2 gm 6 hrly IV	
	or	
	Cloxacillin 500 mg 6 hrly IV	
If MRSA suspected add	Vancomycin 500 mg 6 hrly IV	
* S. epidermidis	Vancomycin 500 mg 6 hrly IV	
* Ps. aeruginosa	Aminoglycoside (Gentamicin 60–80 mg 8 hrly IV or Amikacin 7.5 mg/kg 12 hrly IV) + Ticarcillin 1–3 g 4–6 hrly IV or Piperacillin 3–4 g 4 hrly IV	10–14 days
* Klebsiella/ Enterobacter	Gentamicin 1.5 mg/kg, 6 hrly IV + Cefazolin 2 gm 6 hrly IV	
* H. influenzae	Cefamandole 1.5 gm 4 hrly IV or third generation cephalosporine	
3. Protozoa		
* P. carinii	Trimethoprim 5 mg/kg 6 hrly IV + Sulphamethoxazole 25 mg/kg 6 hrly IV	14 days
* Toxoplasma gondii	Pyrimethamine 25 mg/day + Sulfadiazine 1 gm 6 hrly	orally for 4–6 weeks
4. Fungi		
* Candida species	Amphotericin B 0.6 mg/kg/day IV + Flucytosine 150 mg/day orally	till total of 1–2 g of amphotericin given
* Aspergillus species	Same as above	
* Cryptococcus neoformans	Amphotericin B 0.3–0.6 mg/kg/day IV + Flucytosine 150 mg/day orally	6 weeks

D. Disseminated Tuberculosis

This is an extremely important cause of a critical illness demanding intensive care in our country, and probably in all developing countries where tuberculosis is rampant. It occurs chiefly in patients whose cell-mediated immune response is suppressed or compromised. We have observed its frequent occurrence in AIDS, and in patients on chemotherapy or corticosteroids. The combination of chemotherapy and corticosteroids in high doses, given over a prolonged period, is a potent risk factor for haematogenous disseminated tuberculosis.

The clinical features, diagnostic methods, complications, and management are described in detail in the Section on Fever and Acute Infections in a Critical Care Setting.

E. Central Nervous System Infections

Immunosuppressed patients have an increased incidence of CNS infections necessitating critical care in an ICU.

Meningitis and brain abscesses are both important complications, and their diagnosis should be quick. Meningeal signs are almost never as florid as in patients with a normal immune status. In fact, they may be subtle and it is important to examine the CSF through a lumbar puncture even on a mere suspicion of a possible meningitis. If a brain abscess is suspected because of focal signs or because of evidence of increased intracranial pressure, a CT scan of the head with contrast study should be done prior to a spinal tap. Generally however, in such patients a spinal tap is best avoided particularly if the lesion is subtentorial, or there is increased intracranial pressure.

The choice of therapy in pyogenic meningitis depends on the organisms seen on Gram's staining of the CSF. Treatment should start promptly, the choice of empiric therapy being based on an evaluation of the clinical background of the individual patient. If the nature of the immunologic defect is known, therapy is easier to plan. For neutropaenic patients in whom Gram-negative bacillary infection is a strong possibility, a combination of ceftazidime 2 g intravenously 6 hourly together with gentamicin 1–1.5 mg/kg intravenously every 8 hours, is used. An alternative regime used, as in patients with Gram-negative sepsis, is a combination of ticarcillin or piperacillin with an aminoglycoside. If a coccal infection is suspect, ampicillin 2 g 4 hourly should be added to the above regime. On the other hand, if these patients have intracranial foreign bodies such as an Ommaya reservoir or a shunt, or have undergone a recent neurosurgical procedure, vancomycin 500 mg intravenously 6 hourly should be added.

Meningitis related to humoral or complement deficiencies is often due to S. pneumoniae or H. influenzae. Therapeutic regimes should include chloramphenicol 1 g intravenously every 6 hours, or cefotaxime 2 g intravenously every 6 hours.

Listeria monocytogenes is a rare cause of acute meningitis in patients with cell-mediated immune deficiencies. Therapy for this should include ampicillin 2 g intravenously 4 hourly and gentamicin 1–1.5 g intravenously 8 hourly. An alternative regime includes erythromycin 1g intravenously 6 hourly, and chloramphenicol 1g intravenously 6 hourly.

Tuberculous meningitis may occur in immunocompromised patients either by itself, or as a part of disseminated haematogenous disease. The clinical picture may be subacute, or may take the form of a fulminating meningo-encephalitis. Increase in CSF lymphocytes, raised proteins and a lowered CSF sugar level suggest the diagnosis. Acid-fast bacilli are almost never found in the CSF in our pathological laboratories.

Therapy of inflammatory space-occupying lesions must necessarily be empiric before a definitive diagnosis (by an invasive procedure) is made. Pyogenic abscesses are best treated with massive doses of penicillin or ampicillin. Vancomycin should be added to cover a staphylococcal infection. In leucopaenic patients, possible Gram-negative infections should be covered by ceftazidime and an aminoglycoside, or piperacillin together with vancomycin and amikacin.

Tuberculomas and tuberculous abscesses, sometimes multiple, are common in our country and in all third world countries where the incidence of tuberculosis is high. The CT findings with contrast studies are often distinctive enough to suggest a strong possibility of a tuberculous abscess. Specific treatment includes the use of rifampicin, isoniazid, pyrazinamide, ethambutol and streptomycin in the doses outlined earlier. Treatment should continue from 9 months to a year.

In patients with a cellular immune defect, a mass lesion may be due to toxoplasma infection. This requires the use of pyrimethamine 25–75 mg orally daily and sulphadiazine 1–2 g orally every 6 hours, with leucovorin calcium 10 mg intravenously daily. If toxoplasmosis is proven to be the cause of a mass lesion, all the three drugs mentioned above should be continued for at least 6 weeks, and a maintenance regime with a lower dose of these drugs should be continued life-long in patients with AIDS. Dexamethasone 4 mg 6 hourly intravenously should be used only when mass lesions are associated with cerebral oedema and with increased intracranial pressure.

Mass lesions may be due to other disseminated fungal infections. Definitive diagnosis can only be made by invasive procedures like a brain biopsy.

In patients with AIDS, inflammatory mass lesions described above need to be distinguished from tumours—particularly lymphomas, and viral infections viz. the mass lesions produced by the herpes simplex virus. The clinical background, the natural history of the disease and the CT findings help in the diagnosis. Definitive diagnosis more often than not, can only be made by a brain biopsy.

Table 17.1.4. Common opportunistic infections associated with HIV infection

| Organism | Clinical Manifestations | |
	Common	Infrequent
1. Protozoa		
* P. carinii	Pneumonia	Otitis, dissemination
* Toxoplasma	Encephalitis, retino-choroiditis	Pneumonia, dissemination
* Cryptosporidium	Enteritis	Cholangitis, bronchopleural lesions
* Isospora belli	Enteritis	
2. Fungi		
* Candida sp.	Stomatitis, oesophagitis	Proctitis, vaginitis, dissemination
* Cryptococcus neoformans	Meningitis, dissemination	Pneumonitis
* Histoplasma	Dissemination	
3. Nocardia	Dissemination	
4. Bacteria		
* M. tuberculosis	Pneumonia, dissemination	Meningitis
* Atypical mycobacteria	Dissemination	Pneumonia, diarrhoea
* Salmonella	Diarrhoea, sepsis	
* H. influenzae	Upper respiratory infection pneumonia, sepsis	
5. Viruses		
* Cytomegalovirus	Retino-choroiditis, pneumonia, colitis	Adrenal necrosis, hepatitis, encephalitis, myelitis
*Herpes simplex	Mucocutaneous (mouth, digit, rectum)	Pneumonia, encephalitis
* Herpes zoster	Dermatomal skin lesions	Encephalitis, disseminated skin lesions
* Epstein-Barr	Hairy leukoplakia ? neoplasia	
6. Helminth		
* Strongyloides	Bronchopneumonia	Dissemination

Infections in Patients with AIDS

These patients form a subset of the most severely immunocompromised patients. The principles in relation to infective complications and their management outlined earlier, are obviously applicable to these patients as well. The features characterizing pulmonary infiltrates in AIDS have already been briefly dealt with. Sepsis however can originate from almost any other site. The oral cavity, CNS, GI system, urinary system and breached surfaces of skin or mucosa are other important sites of infection in these patients. Great care should be taken to evaluate every possible source of infection; sepsis arising from indwelling catheters or central venous lines assume special importance.

Fungal oesophagitis, fungal (candidal) ulcers involving the lower oesophagus and stomach, bleeding from the GI tract, perianal abscesses, peforated diverticulitis or other acute abdominal catastrophies may pose problems in diagnosis and management. Symptoms may be even more insidious than in other subsets of immunocompromised patients. In our country, tuberculosis, salmonella infections, and overwhelming parasitic infections, head the list of infectious complications in this group of patients. Patients with AIDS form the only group of patients in our country in whom disseminated fungal infections (particularly cryptococcal and candidal infections) are quite common. All these infections should be assiduously searched for, investigated and treated. Not uncommonly, fungal, viral and parasitic infections in AIDS may be controlled during the acute stage but cannot be cured. Long-term suppressive therapy is needed to keep them under control, as they often flare up and cause acute illness if suppressive therapy is omitted, or if further deterioration occurs in the immune status of the patient. Infections in AIDS are usually multiple, often recurrent, with multiple organisms involving different sites. They are more severe, more disseminated, and elicit an even poorer tissue and body response as compared to patients immunocompromised due to other causes. They are often characterized by a very high density of organisms, a factor responsible for the poor results of therapy (41).

Finally, as already stressed earlier, any critical illness in a patient with AIDS may be due to tumours—in our country, lymphomas are probably observed with the same frequency as in the West; Kaposi's sarcoma however is rare.

Table 17.1.4 lists the common opportunistic infections recognized to be associated with HIV infection.

REFERENCES

1. Wilson RE. (1990). Management of the Critically Ill Immunodeficient Patient. In: Handbook of Critical Care, 3rd edn (Eds Berk JL, Sampliner JE). pp. 711–728. Little Brown and Company, Boston, Toronto, London.

2. Joint United Nations Programme on HIV/AIDS (UNAIDS) and World Health Organization (WHO). 2002. AIDS epidemic update.

3. Dayton JM, Merosn MH. (2000). Global dimensions of the AIDS epidemic: Implications for preventive Care. Infect Dis Clin North Am. 791–808.

4. Ramsey PG, Rubin RH, Tolkoff-Rubin NE et al. (1980). The renal transplant patient with fever and pulmonary infiltrates: Aetiology, clinical manifestations and management. Medicine (NY). 59, 206.

5. Bishop JF, Schimpff SC, Diggs CH et al. (1981). Infections during intensive chemotherapy for non-Hodgkin's lymphoma. Ann Intern Med. 95, 549.

6. Winston DJ, Gale RP, Meyer DV et al. (1979). Infectious complications of human bone marrow transplantation. Medicine (NY). 58, 1.

7. Fanta CH, Pennington JE. (1983). Pneumonia in the immunocompromised host. In: Respiratory Infections: Diagnosis and Management (Ed. Pennington JE). pp. 171–185. Raven Press, New York.

8. Centres for Disease Control. (1989). Guidelines for prophylaxis against Pneumocystis carinii pneumonia for persons with human immunodeficiency virus infection. MMWR. 38, 1–8.

9. Lanjewar DN, Duggal R. (2001). Pulmonary pathology in patients with AIDS: an autopsy study from Mumbai. HIV Med. 2(4), 266–271.

10. Kovacs J, Hiemenz J, Macher A et al. (1984). Pneumocystis carinii pneumonia: A comparison between patients with the acquired immunodeficiency syndrome and patients with other immunodeficiencies. Ann Intern Med. 100, 663–671.

11. Bigby T, Margolskee D, Curtis J et al. (1986). The usefulness of induced sputum in the diagnosis of Pneumocystis carinii pneumonia in patients with the acquired immunodeficiency syndrome. Am Rev Respir Dis. 133, 515–518.

12. Masur H, Lane C, Kovacs J et al. (1989). Pneumocystis pneumonia: From bench to bedside. Ann Intern Med. 111, 8813–8826.

13. Gordin F, Simon G, Wofsy et al. (1984). Adverse reactions to trimethoprim-sulfamethoxazole in patients with the acquired immunodeficiency syndrome. Ann Intern Med. 100, 495.

14. Weber R, Kustu H, Keller R et al. (1992). Pulmonary and intestinal microsporidiosis in a patient with the acquired immunodeficiency syndrome. Am Rev Respir Dis. 146, 1603–1605.

15. Stansell JD, Murray JF. (1994). Pulmonary complications of human immunodeficiency virus infection. In: Textbook of Respiratory Medicine, 2nd edn (Eds Murray JF, Nadel JA). pp. 2333–2367. WB Saunders Company, Philadelphia, London, Toronto, Montreal, Sydney, Tokyo.

16. National Institutes of Health—University of California Expert Panel. (1990). Consensus statement on the use of corticosteroids as adjunctive therapy for Pneumocystis pneumonia in the acquired immunodeficiency syndrome. N Engl J Med. 323, 1500–1504.

17. Mitchell DM, Johnson MA. (1989). Treatment of lung disease in patients with the acquired immunodeficiency syndrome. Thorax. 44, 219–224.

18. Garay SM. (1988). The Acquired Immunodeficiency Syndrome. In: Pulmonary Diseases and Disorders, 2nd edn (Ed. Fishman AP). pp. 1683–1705. MacGraw-Hill Book Company, New York, London, Montreal, Paris.

19. Meyers JD, Flournoy N, Thomas ED. (1982). Nonbacterial pneumonia after allogeneic marrow transplantation: A review of ten years' experience. Rev Infect Dis. 4, 1119.

20. Golden JA. (1989). Pulmonary complications of AIDS. In: AIDS—Pathogenesis and Treatment (Ed. Levy JA). pp. 403–447. Marcel Dekker Inc., New York and Basel.

21. Millar A, Patou G, Miller R et al. (1990). Cytomegalovirus in the lungs of patients with AIDS. Respiratory pathogen or passenger? Am Rev Respir Dis. 141, 1474–1477.

22. Graham BS, Snell JD. (1983). Herpes simplex virus infection of the adult lower respiratory tract. Medicine (NY). 62, 384.

23. Simpson GL et al. (1981). Nocardial infections in the immunocompromised host: A detailed study in a defined population. Rev Infect Dis. 3, 492.

24. Smego RA, Moeller MB, Gallis HA. (1983). Trimethoprim-sulfamethoxazole therapy for Nocardia infections. Arch Intern Med. 143, 711.

25. Masur H, Rosen PP, Armstrong D. (1977). Pulmonary disease caused by Candida species. Am J Med. 63, 914.

26. Rinaldi MG. (1983). Invasive aspergillosis. Rev Infect Dis. 5, 1061.

27. Gerson SL, Talbot GH, Hurwitz S et al. (1984). Prolonged granulocytopenia: The major risk factor for invasive pulmonary aspergillosis in patients with acute leukaemia. Ann Intern Med. 100, 345–351.

28. Worthington M. (1987). Viral, Opportunistic, and Fungal Infections in the Lung in the Intensive Care Unit. In: Respiratory Intensive Care (Eds Macdonnell KF, Fahey PJ, Segal MS). pp. 283–311. Little, Brown and Company, Boston, Toronto.

29. Meyer RD, Young LS, Armstrong D et al. (1973). Aspergillosis complicating neoplastic disease. Am J Med. 54, 6–15.

30. Binder RE, Faling LJ, Pugatch RD et al. (1982). Chronic necrotizing pulmonary aspergillosis: Discrete clinical entity. Medicine (NY). 61,109–124.

31. Rhame FS, Streifel AJ, Kersey JH Jr et al. (1984). Extrinsic risk factors for pneumonia in the patient at high risk of infection. Am J Med. 76, 42–52.

32. Kyriakides GK, Zinneman HH, Hall WH et al. (1976). Immunologic monitoring and aspergillosis in renal transplant patients. Am J Surg. 131, 246–252.

33. Aisner J, Schimpff SC, Bennett JE et al. (1976). Aspergillus infections in cancer patients: Association with fireproofing materials in a new hospital. JAMA. 235, 411–412.

34. Arnow PM, Anderson RL, Mainous PD et al. (1978). Pulmonary aspergillosis during hospital renovation. Am Rev Respir Dis. 118, 49–53.

35. Mahoney DH Jr, Steuber CP, Starling KA et al. (1979). An outbreak of aspergillosis in children with acute leukaemia. J Pediatr. 95, 70–72.

36. Albelda SM, Talbot GH, Gerson SL et al. (1984). Role of fiberoptic bronchoscopy in the diagnosis of invasive pulmonary aspergillosis in patients with acute leukemia. Am J Med. 76, 1027–1034.

37. Murray JF. (1989). The J Burns Amberson Lecture. The white plague: Down and out or up and coming? Am Rev Respir Dis. 140, 1788–1806.

38. Centres for Disease Control. (1989). Tuberculosis and human immunodeficiency virus infection: Recommendations of the Advisory Committee for the Elimination of Tuberculosis (ACET). MMWR. 39, 236–250.

39. Murray JF. (1991). Tuberculosis and human immunodeficiency virus infection during the 1990s. Bull Intern Union Tuberc Lung Dis. 66, 21–25.

40. Selwyn P, Sckell B, Alcabes P et al. (1992). High risk of active tuberculosis in HIV-infected drug users with cutaneous anergy. JAMA. 268, 504–509.

41. Glatt AE, Chirgwin K, Landesman SH. (1988). Treatment of infections associated with human immunodeficiency virus. N Engl J Med. 318, 1439.

Physical Injuries Requiring Critical Care

18.1 Intensive Care Management of Polytrauma

18.2 Management of Critically Ill Burns Patients

18.3 Critical Care in Poisonings

18.4 Critical Care in Envenomation

Intensive Care Management of Polytrauma

Contributed by Dr N.S. Laud, MS (Orth), Retired Professor and Head, Department of Orthopaedic Surgery and Chief Traumatology, LTM Medical College and LTMG Hospital, Mumbai, Consultant Orthopaedic Surgeon, Breach Candy Hospital, Mumbai

General Considerations

Polytrauma is a symptom complex with profound pathometabolic changes. Individual components may not be life-threatening but the cumulative effect can lead to a high early or late mortality. The incidence is on the rise due to rapid industrialization and urbanization and the need for mechanized transport. Even in rural areas its impact is seen due to the increased use of motorized equipment. International data indicate high early mortality in polytrauma. With adequate pre-hospital care with special regard to transportation, maintenance of a patent airway, breathing and circulation by paramedics, the mortality reduces drastically. In the United States, trauma management poses a special challenge because though mortality has been reduced by proper pre-hospital care, trauma victims occupy 22 million hospital beds. Hence the concept of a systems approach based on protocols is being implemented.

India is one of the ten most industrialized nations in the world. While India's vehicle population is less than 5 per cent of the world's, it accounts for the highest incidence of accidents in the world. More than 80,000 people lose their lives in accidents every year and it is estimated that about ten times that number are admitted in hospitals with injuries. The analysis from one of the 'A' level trauma centres indicates a mortality between 19 to 23 per cent. At the LTMG Hospital, which is one of the leading trauma centres, early intensive care with the participation of multispeciality residents, adequate monitoring and treatment based on protocols reduced the mortality of polytrauma from 23 per cent to 16 per cent. Further analysis of the patients salvaged indicated that mortality was highest in those arriving at the hospital after 24 hours and in those with with multiple injuries brought to the hospital without adequate transportation in the first six hours.

These observations indicate that pre-hospital care has a significant role in the management of polytrauma. In most developing countries pre-hospital care is non-existent. Patients are almost always transferred without any treatment, resulting in asphyxia, haemorrhage and shock.

Polytrauma is an endemic disease in the urban population and at times assumes epidemic proportions. While considering intensive trauma care, the following need to be analysed:

1. What constitutes intensive care for a trauma victim?
2. Where should it be made available?
3. When does it need to be instituted?
4. How should it be delivered?
5. How should it be organized?

Pathophysiology of Trauma Victims

The human body is a superbly balanced mechanism having multiple self-restoring safeguards which are activated when an injury occurs. It is vital to understand the pathophysiology of the human response to trauma, if we wish to reduce the morbidity and mortality of the victim.

Fig. 18.1.1 summarizes the various changes, and gives an idea of various levels at which one can intervene to interrupt the natural progression leading to death/permanent disability.

Injury to body
(soft tissue and/or bony architecture)
↓
Mechanical derangement
↓
Physiological changes
(↓ BP, ↑ HR, ↑ RR, ↓ urine output)
↓
Biochemical changes
leading to SIRS or MODS*
(Electrolyte abnormalities, ↓ PaO_2
↑ $PaCO_2$, ↓ pH, cardiac abnormalities)
↓
Permanent disability/death if not
adequately managed

*SIRS—Systemic Inflammatory Response Syndrome
MODS—Multiple Organ Dysfunction Syndrome

Fig. 18.1.1. Pathophysiology of trauma.

Physiological Response of the Body

The 'fight or flight' sympathetic response is activated as a result of any trauma. It helps to counter blood loss, altered pulmonary/cardiac functions, and maintains viability of vital organs.

Tachycardia, tachypnoea, peripheral vasoconstriction and selective shutdown of skeletal muscle microcirculation, help in keeping the kidneys, brain and heart adequately supplied with oxygenated blood. The reduced blood supply to skeletal muscle induces anaerobic metabolism and causes metabolic acidosis, which in turn stimulates the respiratory centres leading to hyperventilation.

Increased catecholamines, products of the activated complement system, and the liberation of cytokines and other inflammatory mediators by host cells, results in widespread damage to the endothelial lining of the microcirculation in various organ systems. There is also probably widespread impairment of cell function in various organs. The end result is multiple organ system failure. Involvement of the lungs is frequent and results in acute lung injury (ARDS). Renal and other systems also show progressive dysfunction. The lipid content of blood has a greater tendency to result in microfat embolism in patients with polytrauma. This tendency is augmented by associated skeletal fractures e.g. long bone/pelvic fractures. The above factors can worsen organ dysfunction, with particular reference to the lungs. The presence of an associated head injury or chest injury, can depress the respiratory drive, physically impair ventilation, and worsen the problems in relation to breathing and gas exchange.

The effect of altered oxygenation, altered acid-base balance and electrolytes, can lead to cardiac function abnormalities. Associated chest trauma or direct injury to thoracic viscera results in an added insult to the already stressed circulatory system; this may further lead to hypotension with reduced cerebral and renal perfusion.

Reduced renal perfusion results in electrolyte imbalance; if renal perfusion is significantly low for a prolonged period, it can cause acute tubular necrosis. This situation can develop quite early in an acutely injured person, even though there is no direct renal injury to begin with. Crushing of muscles, development of the compartment syndrome and myonecrosis, severe infection and sepsis are other concomitant causes which can lead to acute renal shutdown. Unless rapid and early precautions are taken in these situations, it is easy to lose an otherwise stable patient.

Presence of major bone fractures causing severe pain, limited mobility and other complications like fat embolism, injury to vessels or viscera, are important factors which contribute to increased mortality and morbidity.

The overall response of the human body to major stress is catabolic. The effect of this becomes more apparent if the time lag between severe injury and active intervention progressively increases. Absence of prompt critical care in severe trauma, results in the human body being trapped in a self-propagating vicious cycle of an increasingly severe systemic inflammatory response, that finally culminates in death. Hence as a provider of trauma care, our actions must be *urgent and on all fronts*. This is the precise reason why the patient with polytrauma warrants *intensive trauma care* (1).

T_1-T_2-T_3 Concept of Trauma Care (Fig. 18.1.2)

The events from the time of accident to recovery can be chronologically divided into 3 time spans, denoted as T_1, T_2 and T_3.

T_1 is the time of accident which is very short, and at the end of which the mechanical damage to the body is complete. Conse-

quently, no further mechanical damage can occur till the point of intervention. The physiological and biological changes are often minimal during this period. A small percentage of patients having injuries incompatible with life (e.g. cerebral lacerations, open or penetrating cardiac injuries, multiple injuries or fractures with severe internal/external bleeding) die during this period. These constitute the *First Peak* of trauma deaths. There is no way of salvaging these patients; the only way to reduce or eliminate this first peak is by preventive safety measures taken in industries or on roads to reduce the incidence of accidents.

T_2 is the period from the point of accident to the point of intervention. This is the time when the patient is literally left to nature for achieving homeostasis. The longer this period, the lesser the chances of a successful outcome. The aim of the *Golden Hour Project* which was started in cities like Mumbai, was to reduce this T_2 period to a minimum. Intervention within the first 60 minutes of an accident significantly improved the survival rate. A net of co-ordinated ambulances stationed at strategic points and working in unison with the local general practitioners and health workers, transported any trauma victim to the hospital within 1 hour of the accident. A central office which regulated the flow of patients to various trauma care centres helped in avoiding bottlenecks in the traffic. Many deaths are thus prevented by institution of prompt intervention.

T_3 is the intervention-recovery period. The duration of T_3 depends on the efficiency of the trauma care system. Delayed morbidity and mortality can occur in this period.

The best treatment can be offered to the patients if the modular concept of trauma care is adopted (**Fig. 18.1.3**). This includes Types A, B and C level trauma centres, with Type A being the most advanced with specialized units involving neurosurgery, reconstructive surgery, plastic surgery etc. Type C is the most basic or core unit which can provide the basic trauma intensive care for initial stabilization and emergency primary intervention. After stabilization, the patient can then be shifted to a more advanced unit for specialized treatment and/or rehabilitation (**1, 2**).

What Constitutes Intensive Trauma Care

Aim: To reduce mortality and long-term morbidity.

Conceptually it is basically divided into two: (1) Pre-hospital care and (2) Hospital care.

Pre-hospital Care

The previous concept of pick and run or stabilize and transport has now been replaced by a new concept of evacuation and salvage by paramedics. It essentially consists of (a) maintaining airway and circulation, (b) stabilizing neck with a cervical collar, (c) splinting of fractures, (d) transportation of patients on a supine flat board anticipating spinal injury, (e) covering the open wounds with sterile dressings with gentle manual pressure to prevent blood loss, and elevation of extremities. The new trauma ambulances are manned by emergency medical officers and emergency technicians whose job is to initiate resuscitation and maintain the patient's basic life support and communication during transportation to the

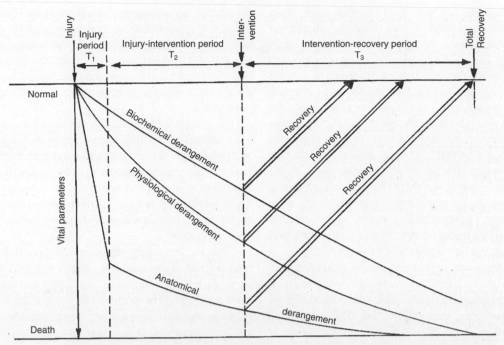

Fig. 18.1.2. The injury-intervention-recovery graph (a qualitative representation).

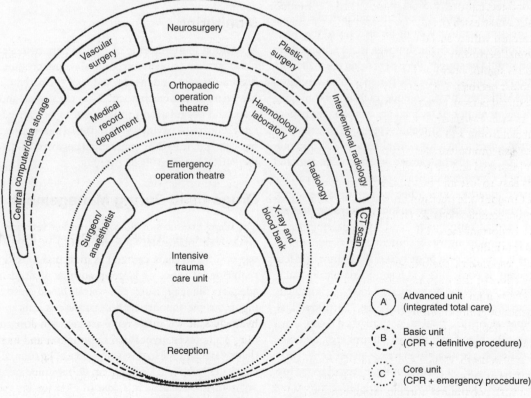

Fig. 18.1.3. Modular system of trauma units.

hospital care units. These paramedics assess the severity of injury and transport the patients to the specific centre for initial and further management. This concept reduces the initiation time of T_2 and load on A level trauma centres and redistributes the patients properly.

Management in Hospital and Further Care

Basic life support

The first 60 minutes are considered as the Golden Hour for trauma victims. Hence basic life support consisting of airway patency, and cardiorespiratory support must be instituted immediately. Primary assessment of injury and resuscitation should be carried out simultaneously. Snoring or gurgling sounds indicate an upper airways obstruction due to falling back of the tongue, or blood or vomitus in the oral cavity. The mouth should be cleared of all debris and secretions, and an oropharyngeal airway should be inserted. Endotracheal intubation with a cuffed tube not only keeps the airway patent, but also guards the tracheobronchial tree against aspiration of blood or vomitus in unconscious patients. *One should always bear in mind the possibility of upper cervical spine fracture, and the neck should be kept in the neutral position to avoid injury to the spinal cord.* The neck should not therefore be extended during endotracheal intubation in a suspected, or possible cervical spine dislocation or fracture. A nasotracheal intubation may be necessary in these patients. Rarely a tracheostomy may be required in patients with facio-maxillary injuries or fracture of the cervical spine.

Adequate ventilation must be promptly assured and maintained, particularly in patients with head injury, intoxication or with cardiopulmonary arrest following shock. Life-threatening conditions e.g. tension pneumothorax, haemothorax, flail chest, are detected by unequal expansion of the chest (together with evidence of external injury), poor air entry on auscultation, and a hypoxic, restless struggling patient. A tension pneumothorax is best treated with underwater intercostal drainage, or insertion of a 14–16 gauge needle in the second intercostal space in the midclavicular line as an emergency measure, without waiting for an X-ray of the chest. In cases of haemothorax where the drainage is > 1 l, immediate surgical opinion should be sought. Persistent drainage > 200 ml/hr is an indication for thoracotomy. The patient can be ventilated with mask and AMBU bag, or via an endotracheal tube and bag with oxygen supplementation. If facilities are available, the patient can be then put on mechanical ventilator support. In patients with absent peripheral pulses, check for central femoral, carotid pulsations; if these are also absent, cardiac arrest is suspected and without checking for presence of heart sounds, external cardiac massage is started together with other resuscitative measures. Distended neck veins, with tachycardia and hypotension, suggest a diagnosis of cardiac tamponade, and warrant emergency pericardiocentesis. Following establishment of an airway and institution of ventilation, the next priority is maintenance of circulation. If the patient is conscious and haemodynamically stable with a normal pulse and blood pressure, the blood loss is unlikely to be > 15 per cent of estimated blood volume (i.e. 750 ml in adults). However, a comatose restless patient, with marked tachycardia, hypotension (systolic blood pressure 60–90 mm Hg), and cold clammy extremities, suggests a blood loss > 30 per cent (1.5 l). This requires management on a war footing. External blood loss is managed by manual compression, splinting of fractures, and suturing of open wounds. Two intravenous lines (using large bore cannulae) are secured, one above and the other below the diaphragm. 1–2 l of Ringers lactate solution are administered promptly, and this usually restores the normal pulse and blood pressure if the blood loss is < 15 per cent, and there is no persistent bleeding. If 2 l of Ringers lactate solution fail to restore blood loss, and the patient remains haemodynamically unstable, 2 more litres

are infused and arrangements are made for blood transfusion. Bilateral intercostal drainage may be required to rule out the possibility of tension pneumothorax. If hypotension persists despite infusion of 4 l Ringers lactate and blood, the blood loss is likely to be > 40 per cent, and four-quadrant abdominal tapping is done. If the patient needs surgery, resuscitation is continued in the operation theatre.

The occurrence of ventricular tachycardia (causing haemodynamic instability), or fibrillation at any point in time after trauma will require DC defibrillation, starting with a DC shock of 100 Joules, and increasing if necessary to 360 Joules. Cardiopulmonary resuscitation is unquestionably of prime importance and of immediate priority in trauma patients who so require it (for details see Section on Cardiopulmonary Resuscitation and Cerebral Preservation in Adults).

After circulation and respiration have been stabilized, a careful neurological examination is carried out for localizing signs, particularly with reference to head injury and spinal cord injury. The fundus should be examined for papilloedema. Depending on the neurological findings, other neurological investigations like a CT scan, may well be necessary. A careful examination of the abdomen and other systems is warranted, with special attention to the musculoskeletal system.

Monitoring

In addition to monitoring of clinical parameters e.g. pulse rate, blood pressure, temperature, central venous pressure, urine output, respiratory rate, and mental status of the patient, investigations like haemoglobin, haematocrit, X-ray chest, renal and liver function tests, and coagulation profile need to be carried out. Oxygen saturation (pulse oxymetry) and arterial blood gases are monitored frequently. The PaO_2 is maintained between 75–100 mm Hg, and the $PaCO_2$ between 30–35 mm Hg.

Drugs Used During Management

The filling pressures of the right and left ventricle should be adequately maintained (CVP + 10 cm H_2O, PCWP 15 mm Hg). The use of a Swan-Ganz catheter is indicated in difficult problems requiring infusions of large quantities of fluids. If in spite of adequate filling pressures the systolic blood pressure is < 90 mm Hg, inotropic support with dopamine is indicated. Dopamine hydrochloride will dilate renal arterioles in doses of 2–5 µg/kg/min; it improves myocardial contraction and increases sympathetic vascular tone in doses of 5–15 µg/kg/min. If urine output continues to be < 0.5 ml/kg/hr, dobutamine can be added in a separate infusion drip, in a dose of 5–15 µg/kg/min.

Sodium bicarbonate should not be given routinely in large quantities at the start, as is often done. Metabolic acidosis gets corrected once tissue perfusion is restored. In fact excessive bicarbonate may lead to metabolic alkalosis (pH > 7.55) which is associated with an increased mortality rate. Arterial blood gas analysis should be done to estimate the pH and base deficit, and any abnormalities in pH should be corrected as per planned protocol (see Section on Acid-Base Disturbances in the Critically Ill).

The role of corticosteroids in the management of severe trauma victims, is controversial. Hydrocortisone 100 mg 6 hourly intravenously, or methyl prednisolone given in a pulsed dose of 1 g daily for 3 days, is believed by some workers to improve resistance to acute trauma, perhaps by causing vasodilatation and improving tissue blood flow. Dexamethasone 8 mg 8 hourly, may be used in patients with head injury.

Mechanical Ventilation

Indications (2)

Once the patient is stabilized with basic life support, advanced life support is instituted for vital organs like the lungs, heart, and kidneys. Ventilatory support ensures adequate arterial oxygenation. Proper oxygen delivery or oxygen transport to tissues is however only possible if cardiac output is well maintained. Normal, and at times supranormal levels of oxygen delivery are necessary to meet increased tissue demands for oxygen. Adequate tissue perfusion and increased oxygen delivery, reduce the incidence of late mortality due to multiple organ system failure. Ventilator support is mandatory for patients with head injury, chest injury (flail chest with pulmonary contusion), high cervical cord injury, acute lung injury (ARDS), sepsis syndrome, severe pneumonia. Elective mechanical ventilation is also indicated (i) in patients with blood loss > 40 per cent of estimated blood volume, haematocrit < 30 per cent and haemodynamic instability (low blood pressure, tachycardia, reduced urine output, temperature); (ii) in patients with an injury severity score > 30; (iii) in patients with multiple fractures (polytrauma); (iv) in some patients with head injury to control intra-cranial pressure, and thereby reduce mortality and morbidity.

Ventilator support should not be delayed till a point in time when the patient is in severe respiratory distress, or is obviously cyanosed. The indications for initiating ventilatory support are based on clinical assessment and results of arterial blood gases. Indications, together with details on management of ventilatory support have been dealt with in the Section on Mechanical Ventilation in the Critically Ill.

Weaning from Mechanical Ventilation (3)

Every effort should be made to discontinue ventilatory support as soon as the patient is haemodynamically stable and is able to resume and sustain spontaneous ventilation. Weaning criteria have been discussed in the Section on Mechanical Ventilation in the Critically Ill.

Re-evaluation and Continuous Re-assessment

The stabilized and/or primarily operated patient needs to be frequently re-assessed. This is necessary to detect certain complications of severe trauma e.g. acute lung injury, sepsis, continued bleeding etc. At times re-surgery or reconstructive procedures are necessary within 48–72 hours of the primary treatment. Delayed deaths or complications due to lack of adequate or infrequent follow-up will lead to loss of human life, and will negate the effort and expenditure spent on initial pick-up and stabilization.

Concept of Damage Control in Polytrauma

P. V. Giannoudis has described the concept of damage control in polytrauma (4–6). Initially it was thought that early stabilization of fractures had a grave risk related to pulmonary embolism and the fractures were treated essentially by prolonged rest and traction, leading to complications like bed sores, urinary tract problems, disuse atrophy, joint stiffness and pulmonary problems. Severely injured patients were at risk of multiple organ dysfunction. However, better understanding of the pathophysiology of polytrauma, availability of implants, and instrumentation to carry out stabilization of fractures by minimally invasive techniques (like intramedullary rod fixation described by AO Group in 1960s) brought about a revolutionary change in the concept (7).

The literature review in 1970 suggested that early skeletal stabilization of fractures helped to further maintain cardiopulmonary stabilization in patients with visceral injuries. It was believed to reduce the incidence of acute respiratory failure and post-operative complications. The skeletal fixation was carried out in the first 24 hours. Bone et al. in 1980 published a seminal study on the benefits of early stabilization of fractures on mortality and length of hospital stay (8). They introduced the terminology Early Total Care (ETC). ETC was an aggressive approach to management of polytrauma in patients suffering from visceral and skeletal injuries. However, by 1990, unexpected complications as a result of medullary reaming of femoral fractures to obtain rigid fixation by intramedullary nailing were reported (4, 9). A study by the American Orthopaedic Foundation confirmed that this method of stabilization through early surgery played a major role in the development of such complications. The ETC concept resulted in an increased incidence of ARDS and MODS and this higher incidence was noticed in patients with chest injuries or in patients with severe shock. A new concept states that early surgery constitutes a 'second hit phenomenon', the 'first hit phenomenon' being the injury itself. The type and severity of injury constituting the 'first hit phenomenon' could predispose an injured patient to deteriorate after surgery. The 'second hit phenomenon' imposes various burdens on the biological reserves of the patient, that could result in an adverse biological response and an adverse outcome. It is thus essential that the trauma teams understand that inappropriate clinical decisions may have a detrimental effect on the well-being of the patient. The treating physician faces a dilemma as to the proper time and need for skeletal stabilization to augment cardiopulmonary stabilization. Recent research indicates that it is difficult to quantify the biological impact caused after the initial injury and the additional effect of the surgical procedure. Clinical parameters are not useful in indicating the influence of surgical stress on the inflammatory system (10). A number of studies have highlighted the importance of inflammatory mediators viz. IL_6, IL_{10}, interferon-γ in response to trauma (9, 11, 12). These studies indicate that surgery causes several changes in patients with inflammation which could become clinically relevant with cumulative effect after the addition of several 'insults'. The concept of damage control orthopaedics for management of a polytraumatized patient was thus developed. The approach envisages the need for damage limitation and the need to reduce the magnitude of the adverse inflammatory response of the body following the 'second hit phenomenon'—i.e. after the surgical procedure.

Damage Control Orthopaedics

Benefit of early fixation of fracture has been well established; however, such early surgery in patients with severe chest trauma, pelvic fractures or cranial trauma may carry the risk of further deterioration, specially if surgery is prolonged (**5, 6, 8, 13**). The concept of damage control has an important role in the early total care of polytraumatized patients with severe skeletal injury. The patients are essentially categorized in four groups:

I. Stable patients after initial resuscitation, stabilized visceral injury with maintenance of basic parameters.

II. Borderline patients well resuscitated after major chest or abdominal injury and major skeletal fractures.

III. Unstable patients with major skeletal injury and visceral injury after initial management.

IV. Severely ill polytraumatized patients who are extremely unstable.

Trauma management regarding musculoskeletal injury is discussed in four different distinguished periods (**5**).

1. Acute or resuscitation period: 0–3 hours.
2. Primary or stabilization period: 3–72 hours.
3. Secondary or regeneration period: Days 3–8.
4. Tertiary or rehabilitation period: After Day 8.

For the management during the acute period, a trauma algorithm for trauma teams is described. It is a guide for diagnostic and therapeutic measures and consists of four different steps, viz. (1) first look, (2) shock treatment, (3) check up, (4) control and diagnosis.

The damage control operations indicate a different approach. In Groups I and II early skeletal fixation can be advocated. The operation should be done as early as possible and the preference is for minimally invasive surgery e.g. use of external skeletal stabilization in injury to the pelvis and closed intra medullary nailing using unreamed nail in proximal fractures. However, in Groups III & IV, the damage control operation concept envisages a stage wise approach.

Stage I—Management in emergency room and life saving operations like exploration of visceral injury to control haemorrhage and external skeletal stabilization of pelvic or proximal fractures.

Stage II—Shift to intensive care unit for intensive monitoring and further stabilization till the metabolic response to trauma is assessed and the patient's parameters return to normal, indicating a reduction in pro-inflammatory response. Urgent surgery for head and brain injuries, fractures with severe soft tissue injuries, visceral injuries, spinal cord injuries.

Stage III—Definitive reconstruction of chest or abdominal trauma or definitive osteosynthesis using plate, intra medul-

lary nail or screws is usually carried out between 7 to 10 days.

The incidence of infection following temporary external skeletal fixation, with conversion to internal fixation within one to two weeks is the same as that observed with primary intra medullary nailing (**12**). Damage control orthopaedic surgery has helped in early total stabilization of the patient, reduction in the need for ventilatory support, better pain relief, prevention of ARDS. Pain relief following definitive skeletal stabilization and very early mobilization of the injured limb or limbs reduce the chances of post immobilization muscle atrophy and help the patient attain a positive nitrogen balance. There is also a dramatic improvement in the functional and psychosomatic state of the patient. The advent of minimally invasive surgery and new implants has dramatically reduced the duration of hospital stay, has enabled early ambulation and has resulted in a reduction in secondary complications.

Prevention of Infection

Traumatized patients have a reduced capacity to fight infection, as the immune system is depressed under these conditions. The body is in a catabolic state following injury and subsequent surgical intervention. The use of steroids further reduces the capacity of the body to fight infection. Blood transfusions, presence of intravenous lines, central catheters, urinary catheters, endotracheal/tracheostomy tubes are all potential sources of sepsis (**12**).

The bedridden patient is also more prone to develop bedsores and basal hypostatic pneumonia. All these factors predispose to the development of overt or occult infection in polytraumatized patients. Open fractures and compound injuries further aggravate the problem. If infection occurs in these critically ill patients, it can rapidly push them downhill; prophylactic antibiotics are thus preferable. They should cover both Gram-positive as well as Gram-negative organisms, and also anaerobes. A combination of ampicillin with an aminoglycoside and metronidazole is usually used. Use of more specific antibiotics after culture and specific testing for antibiotic sensitivity is preferable, and can be instituted at a later date. If a specific infection is identified (e.g. urinary tract infection, or bone infection), a more specific antibiotic having better penetration in these systems can be used. General aseptic measures and limiting of traffic in the intensive care trauma unit (ITU) will help in reducing the incidence of these infections. Early mobilization of the patient by fixing bony injuries surgically, will go a long way in improving the general condition of the patient, and will thereby reduce the incidence of deep vein thrombosis, basal atelectasis, pneumonia and bed sores.

Nutritional Support

It cannot be overstressed that good nutrition is essential for survival in severe trauma victims. The importance of this is sadly ignored in many units in our country, resulting in a high morbidity and mortality. Enteral feeding is the best way of ensuring proper nutrition to a patient. However many situations preclude the use of the enteral route, and force the physician to resort to the parenteral route (see Section on Nutritional Support in the Critically Ill).

Pain Relief in the Trauma Victim (9)

This is an important feature in the care of critically ill trauma patients. Various methods are used for pain relief.

(i) Patient controlled analgesia (PCA) (14): A pump containing a maximally allowed total dose of an analgesic (usually narcotics like morphine or pethidine) is set up. The patient has a push button which when pressed will inject a small amount of the drug intravenously. A lag time is adjusted between 2 successive injections, to prevent a patient from overdosing himself by repeated use of the device. This is a very good system as the patient can himself decide when he requires relief from pain (9, 15).

(ii) Continuous analgesic intravenous infusion of small doses of morphine (0.1 mg/min) provides effective pain relief in most cases. Alternatively, 30 mg pentazocine together with 50 mg pethidine is added to 500 ml of 5 per cent dextrose/N saline and given intravenously as a slow infusion over 5–6 hours. This drip can be repeated after 12 hours depending on the patient's needs.

(iii) Oral analgesics can be given if the patient can tolerate them.

(iv) Regional blocks to anaesthetize the painful area (e.g. intercostal blocks in rib fractures where breathing is impaired due to pain), are also used to relieve pain.

(v) The placement of an epidural catheter with continuous patient-controlled/physician-controlled epidural injections of appropriate analgesics are being increasingly used in the ICU. In our set-up we commonly use buprenorphine 150 µg, diluted in 10–20 ml of N saline administered slowly. This provides highly effective pain relief, the analgesic effect lasting for approximately 12–16 hours. Morphine or pethidine may also be used via the epidural route. In acute cases, pain relief should consist of a combination of analgesics. Non-narcotics like diclofenac sodium can be combined with narcotics like morphine, pethidine or their derivatives. In cases of head injury, where the level of consciousness needs to be assessed, narcotic analgesics should be avoided. Effective pain relief reduces the patient's anxiety, and helps in controlling excessive sympathetic outflow.

Splinting of fractures, use of pinless fixators to stabilize broken limbs, and subsequent early stabilization, all go a long way in effective pain relief (9, 15).

General Nursing Care and Physiotherapy

Specific care to prevent bedsores is necessary in debilitated patients. Special foam mattresses, alternately inflating-deflating air beds and waterbeds are various ways of solving dependent skin pressure problems. Log rolling of the patient, active movements, and keeping the dependent pressure-bearing skin points dry, are also important. Deep breathing exercises and chest physiotherapy are essential in most patients. Passive mobilization of all joints, splinting of joints in their functional position in order to prevent contractures, and active movements to prevent muscle wasting, are also necessary. Care of the eyes and mouth (specially in unconscious patients) also constitutes an important aspect of general nursing in a severely traumatized victim.

Long-term Rehabilitation

This should be planned and discussed with the patient, keeping in mind his realistic functional outcome as soon as possible. This will allow the patient to mentally accept his disability, and will give him a psychological boost to try for maximum possible recovery.

REFERENCES

1. Taylor R, Shoemaker WC (Eds). (1991). Critical Care: State of the Art. Volume 12.
2. Tobin MJ (Ed.). (1990). Mechanical Ventilation. Critical Care Clinics. WB Saunders Co., London.
3. Netk LM, Morganroth M, Petty TL. (1984). Weaning from mechanical ventilation: A perspective and review of techniques. In: Critical Care: A Comprehensive Approach (Ed. Bone RC). pp. 171–188. American College of Chest Physicians, Park Ridge II.
4. Giannoudis PV, Abbott C, Stone M et al. (1998). Fatal systemic inflammatory response syndrome following early bilateral femoral nailing. Intensive Care Medicine. 24, 641–642.
5. Krettek C, Simon RG, Tscherne H. (1998). Management priorities in patients with polytrauma. Langenbeck's Arch Surg. 383, 220–227.
6. Pape HC, Giannoudis P. Krettek C. (2002). The timing of fracture treatment in polytrauma patients: relevance of damage control orthopedic surgery. American Journal of Surgery. 183 (6), June.
7. Mueller ME, Allgower M, Schneider R et al. (1970). Manual of osteosynthesis. Berling Etc. Springer Verlag.
8. Bone LB, Johnson KD, Weigelt J et al. (1989). Early versusu delayed stabilization of fractures: a prospective randomized study. J Bone Joint Surg (Am). 71–A, 336–340.
9. Giannoudis PV, Smith RM, Ramsden CW et al. (1996). Molecular mediators and trauma: effects of accidental trauma on the production of plasma elastase IL-6, sICAM-1 and sE-selectin. Injury. 27, 372.
10. Bone RC. (1996). Toward a theory regarding the pathogenesis of the systemic inflammatory response syndrome: what we do and do not know about cytokine regulation. Crit Care Med. 24, 162–172.
11. Giannoudis PV, Smith RM, Bellamy MC et al. (1999). Stimulation of the inflammatory system by reamed and unreamed nailing of femoral fractures; an analysis of the second hit. J Bone Joint Surg (Br). 81–B: 356–361.
12. Giannoudis PV, Smith RM, Perry SL et al. (2000). Immediate IL-10 expression following major orthopaedic trauma: relationship to anti-inflammatory response and subsequent development of sepsis. Intensive Care Med. 26, 1076–1081.
13. Pape HC, Auf'm'Kolk, Paffrath T et al. (1993). Primary intramedullary femur fixation in multiple trauma patients with associated lung contusion: a cause of post-traumatic ARDS? J Trauma. 34, 540–548.
14. Tawrsen A, Hartvig P, Eagerlund C et al. (1982). Patient controlled analgesic therapy: Clinical experience. Acta Anaesth Scand. 74(suppl), 157.
15. Bonica JJ (Ed.). (1990). The Management of Pain. Lea and Febiger, Philadelphia.

Management of Critically Ill Burns Patients

by Dr S.M. Keswani, Consultant Plastic and Cosmetic Surgeon, Breach Candy Hospital, Mumbai, with Dr F.E. Udwadia

General Considerations

Contrary to common belief, burns are essentially a medical problem, at least in the initial stages. The alterations in circulatory haemodynamics, renal function, cardiorespiratory physiology, the gastrointestinal and the haematopoietic systems, all require the attention of a team of specialists.

In India, burns are the second most common cause of injury after road accidents. Women and children are involved in 80 per cent of burn accidents; the majority of women who get burnt are between the ages of 15–20 years. 75 per cent of burns occur at home (1). Burn accidents occur throughout the year, but are commoner during the cold season. This is largely because the cold season is generally windy; it is the wind which fans a fire causing more extensive burns. During the festive season of Divali (the festival of lights) when firecrackers are widely used, burn accidents tend to increase in number. Suicidal and homicidal burns account for approximately 5 per cent of all burn accidents, particularly in young women. The majority of burns occur in the homes of the poor, which are usually small and at ground level. Here it is easy for the victim to rush out and seek help, and respiratory injury is uncommon. The loosely wrapped saree is ideal for burning; the thighs and legs which are the best skin donor areas get damaged in saree burns. It is an oft repeated myth that the Indian burn patient is anaemic and hypoproteinaemic. They become so after the burns, due to inadequate management.

Burns involving 70–80 per cent of body surface area had a 100 per cent mortality. In good burns centres the mortality rate is now < 50 per cent (2). There have been two major advances responsible for the sharp reduction in the mortality of severe burns. The first is the quick removal of burnt tissue prior to the onset of infection, and covering of the wound with available autoskin grafts and skin substitutes. Unfortunately in poor developing countries like India, facilities and infrastructure for prompt surgery in severe burns exist only in very few centres—mortality in extensive burns thus continues to be forbiddingly high. The second is the improvement in the critical care of burns patients, which enables the prevention of multiple organ failure during the period of resuscitation, surgical excision of the burns, and the healing process (2). Multiple organ

failure once it occurs, has a forbiddingly high mortality (> 80–90 per cent with severe three organ failure) and its treatment in the presence of burnt tissue is impossibly difficult, chiefly because the presence of remaining burnt tissue perpetuates and worsens organ system dysfunction. Though the critical care of burns patients has improved in the large centres of India, much more needs to be done in the country for better care. The leading cause of death in burns in poor countries, is still sepsis and its complications, whereas in the West the leading cause of death is now respiratory failure.

Pathophysiology of the Burn Wound

Skin is damaged by the total quantity of heat applied to it i.e. the intensity of the heat and the duration of time the heat is in contact with the tissue.

Jackson described three concentric zones of burn injury (3, 4). These zones are illustrated in **Fig. 18.2.1.**

The central 'Zone of Coagulation' represents the area of maximum damage, and consists of protein coagulation of the tissues including the blood vessels. Blood flow through the affected arte-

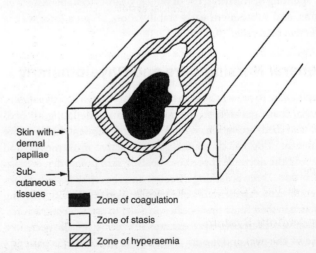

Skin with dermal papillae

Subcutaneous tissues

■ Zone of coagulation

□ Zone of stasis

▨ Zone of hyperaemia

Fig. 18.2.1. The 3 concentric zones of burn injury as described by Jackson (modified from Zawacki BE, 1974. Ann Surg. 180, 98, JB Lippincott Co., PA).

rial and venous channels ceases, resulting in a state of irreversible tissue death.

This central zone is surrounded by a zone of less damaged tissue, known as the 'Zone of Stasis'. The blood flow through this zone is completely slowed down, and tissues are starved of oxygen and nutrients. If left unprotected as with exposure treatment, this zone becomes dried up, dessicated, infected and the cells become irreversibly dead. If managed properly, the damage may be reversed and the 'Zone of Stasis' comes back to life. The aim of modern burn management is to prevent this 'Zone of Stasis' from getting dried up or infected. This can be achieved by the application of autografts, homografts, xenografts (other animal skin), synthetic skins, cultured skins or potato peel bandages (5). The burn wound must be kept moist, and should not become infected. Wound healing must not be disturbed by traumatic dressings.

Surrounding both these zones is the zone of least damage, the 'Zone of Hyperaemia'. In this zone the cells are hyperaemic, and heal spontaneously if provided with adequate care.

The Systemic Response to Burn Injury (6)

Cardiovascular System

The initial response to burn injury is decreased cardiac output and increased systemic vascular resistance (**Fig. 18.2.2**). This is proportionate to the size of the burn and the severity of hypovolaemia that may be allowed to occur. If corrected rapidly, the process may be reversed, the cardiac output increases and the peripheral vascular resistance decreases. During the second 24 hours post-burn period, the post-burn capillary hyperpermeability decreases, the extravasated fluid from the interstitial compartment returns to the vascular compartment, the volume deficit is corrected, and the cardiac output increases to above normal levels. It has been shown that the increase in blood flow is more in the burnt tissue than elsewhere, thus optimizing wound healing.

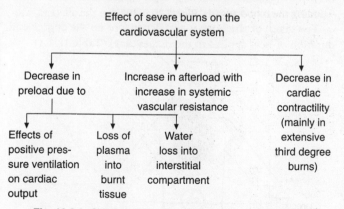

Fig. 18.2.2. Cardiovascular response to severe burn injury.

Respiratory System

Pulmonary complications are an important cause of morbidity and mortality, particularly in the West. Thermal injury in a closed environment causes pulmonary inhalation injury that can seriously damage the upper airways, larynx, trachea, bronchial tree, and the

pulmonary parenchyma. In addition, intoxication can result from inhalation of combustion products; the most important of these are carbon monoxide and cyanide. The physiopathology of pulmonary changes in severe burns is due to many factors. These include thermal inhalation injury, chemical irritation by smoke and other chemicals, secondary infection, the occurrence of acute lung injury (ARDS), fluid overloading and pulmonary embolism.

Physiological changes occur in the respiratory tract after every major burn injury. The respiratory rate and tidal volume increase in direct proportion to the size of the burn. With the large volume of resuscitation fluids infused, the chest wall oedema increases considerably, and if treated by exposure any burn on the thorax forms a tough constrictive eschar, which restricts movements of the thoracic cage. This requires correction with urgent escharotomy. However, it may be mentioned at this stage that the use of potato peel bandages keeps the burn wound supple, and has obviated the need for escharotomy in any patient, except when the patient reaches the burn centre late with already established, constricting eschars.

By the third to the fifth day post-burn, the extravascular fluid gets re-absorbed, and if the patient has been overinfused, pulmonary oedema progressing to acute lung injury (ARDS) may result. Hence, infusion of fluids during the initial resuscitation period has to be carefully calculated so as to maintain a normal blood volume, as also adequate tissue perfusion and renal perfusion.

Arterial hypoxia (a fall in PaO_2) may occur at the very start in severe burns. In other cases, arterial hypoxaemia and hypercapnia become manifest 8–14 days following the burns. Ventilation-perfusion inequalities, increase in the right to left shunt within the lungs, and inadequate ventilation in relation to metabolic needs, are responsible for these blood gas changes.

Renal System

With the onset of hypovolaemia following burns, the renal blood flow and glomerular filtration rate are both considerably reduced. If not corrected early, this may result in acute tubular necrosis and renal shutdown. Early and adequate correction of hypovolaemia is hence essential in the treatment of burns. Forty-eight hours following burns, when resorption of the extravasated fluid takes place, diuresis occurs.

Gastrointestinal System

Acute ulceration of the stomach or duodenum (Curling's ulcer) occurs in about 11 per cent of burns population. Multiple acute erosions may also occur and can cause severe GI bleeds. Post-burn hypovolaemia is also accompanied by reduction of gastrointestinal tract blood flow which manifests as ileus. If hypovolaemia is not allowed to supervene, this is rapidly corrected and ileus does not occur. Ileus causes gastric and intestinal distension and stasis with an increasing likelihood of translocation of intestinal bacteria. Contrary to earlier practice, early post-burn feeding is now encouraged, not only to provide nutrition through the natural pathway, but to preserve the integrity of the gut and to offset the complications which may ensue from bacterial translocation.

Central Nervous System

Specific neurologic changes following burn injury have not been described. Restlessness, disorientation and fits are observed and indicate cerebral hypoxia, cerebral oedema, fluid and electrolyte imbalance or sepsis. These should be investigated and corrected early.

Haematopoietic System

The red cells circulating in the burnt area are promptly coagulated. But many more are significantly damaged and become nonviable soon afterwards. In major burns this is often masked by the loss of fluid from the intravascular compartment, which results in severe haemoconcentration and an increased packed cell volume. It is only after the resorption of the extravasated fluid that the reduction in red cell mass becomes manifest. The loss of red cells may be as high as ten per cent of the total red cell mass per day, in major burns. Constant and regular monitoring of the blood count is therefore essential in all burns.

Changes in white cell count occur according to the level of infection in the body.

A reduction in platelet count is one of the earliest signs of impending sepsis. Transfusion of platelet concentrates and the use of appropriate antibiotics is indicated.

Coagulopathies may occur in the resuscitation phase. Disseminated intravascular coagulopathy is associated with reduction of various clotting factors including prothrombin, Factors V, VIII and IX. Thrombocytopaenia and thrombocytopathy necessitating platelet transfusions, may be observed. A hypercoagulable state may occur 2–4 weeks after a severe burn injury.

Immunologic Effects

The host immune response is suppressed in severe burn injuries. Complement and immunoglobulin levels are initially depressed, and chemotaxis is inhibited by the presence of a plasma inhibitor. Patients with burns are excessively prone to nosocomial infection, and in spite of the use of topical and systemic antibiotics, sepsis remains a major killer, particularly in poor developing countries.

Metabolic Effects

Increase in the metabolic rate with a markedly negative nitrogen balance, is greater than that in any other form of trauma. There is an increase in oxygen consumption and in carbon dioxide production. The stress response is mediated by catecholamines, other anti-insulin hormones, and is often associated with glucose intolerance in the early post-burn period. 'Insulin resistance' may be observed over a prolonged period of time. Hypermetabolism increases with sepsis, cooling, pain, and control of the above-mentioned factors plays an important role in management.

First Aid

Burn injury is caused by heat. Even after the flames are extinguished, the residual heat trapped in the skin continues to damage the tissues. A burning sensation indicates the presence of heat in the tissues. Cold water (not ice cold) should be poured over the burnt area till the burning sensation has subsided. This may take up to 6 hours. Cooling the burnt area reduces both the area and depth of burn. It is the easiest way to reduce the burn damage to the tissues, and to reduce the pain. Analgesics and sedatives should be avoided, as the restlessness seen after burn injury is often due to cerebral hypoxia; sedation may actually accentuate the cerebral hypoxia thereby increasing the restlessness. In chemical burns, the chemicals over the body should be washed away with copious amounts of water.

Transport

Loss of blood volume starts immediately following burn injury. It is most severe during the first 8 hours. In burns > 30 per cent of total body surface area, the leakage of plasma occurs all over the body. This fluid volume deficit must be replaced as early as possible. While in transport, fluid replacement should be actively undertaken if the time taken to reach a burn centre will take more than one hour.

Assessment of Burn Severity

The area of burns is estimated by the simple Wallace's 'Rule of Nine' (**Fig. 18.2.3**). A more accurate and better method is the estimation by Lund and Browder's chart (**Fig. 18.2.4**) **(7)**. Burns of over 10 per cent body surface area in a child, and over 15 per cent area in an adult can cause hypovolaemic shock and hence should not to be taken lightly. Burns of over 30 per cent of the body surface area are very serious.

Burn severity also varies with the depth of burn (**Fig. 18.2.5**). Burns which damage the full thickness of the skin are considered full thickness burns. When the depth of the burn is not complete, it is known as a partial thickness burn. Partial thickness burns heal by regeneration from the residual skin elements, if managed properly. Full thickness burns always require a skin graft to heal. They are therefore more difficult to manage.

The depth of the burn is also dependent on the degree and duration of heat applied to the tissues **(8, 9)** (**Table 18.2.1**).

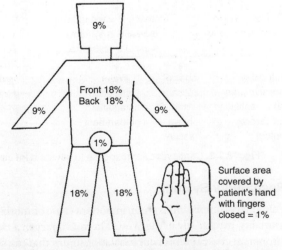

Fig. 18.2.3. Estimation of surface area by the Wallace's Rule of Nine.

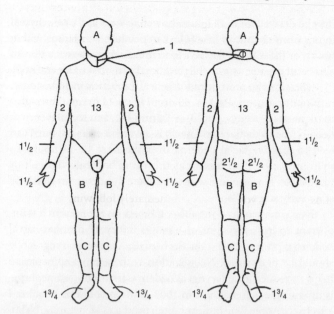

Area	Age	0	1	5	10	15	Adult
A = 1/2 of head		$9\frac{1}{2}$	$8\frac{1}{2}$	$6\frac{1}{2}$	$5\frac{1}{2}$	$4\frac{1}{2}$	$3\frac{1}{2}$
B = 1/2 of one thigh		$2\frac{3}{4}$	$3\frac{1}{4}$	4	$4\frac{1}{2}$	$4\frac{1}{2}$	$4\frac{3}{4}$
C = 1/2 of one leg		$2\frac{1}{2}$	$2\frac{1}{2}$	$2\frac{3}{4}$	3	$3\frac{1}{4}$	$3\frac{1}{2}$

Fig. 18.2.4. Estimation of extent of burns (per cent) by Lund and Browder's Chart (reference **7**).

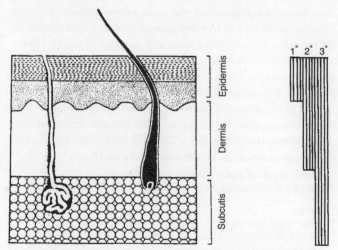

Fig. 18.2.5. Classification of burns according to the depth of injury.

Table 18.2.1. Production of full thickness burns depends on degree and duration of heat applied to skin (references **8, 9**)

Temperature	Time
At 44°C	In 6 hours
At 59°C	In 60 secs
At 62°C	In 30 secs
At 65°C	In 20 secs
At 70°C	In 10 secs

Immediate Management

Haemodynamic changes outlined earlier, occur rapidly following burns. These have to be anticipated and managed appropriately. Burn patients have massive evaporative heat loss and hence need treatment in a room with increased temperature. Air conditioning, i.e. cooling of the atmospheric temperature, is contraindicated. The burnt skin exposes the underlying tissues to infection, and such patients need strict aseptic management. A well-equipped burn centre staffed by specially trained personnel is an essential requirement for the management of these critically ill patients.

Management is best considered during the resuscitation phase (0–36 to 48 hours), the post-resuscitation phase (36 to 48 hours– 5 days), and the phase of inflammation and infection (6 days to period of wound healing).

Resuscitative and Immediate Post-resuscitative Management

The principles of therapy are:

(a) Fluid replacement and cardiovascular support to ensure maximum haemodynamic stability.

(b) Care of the airways and pulmonary support, as and when this becomes necessary.

(c) Correction of electrolyte and acid-base disturbances.

(d) Nutritional support.

(e) Care of the burn wound.

(f) Symptomatic treatment of pain and the use of antacids.

(a) Fluid Resuscitation and Cardiovascular Support

Several formulae are available and have strong proponents. The Parkland formula of Baxter is simple, practical and efficacious, has been adopted in most burn centres, and is currently the standard against which new formulae must be compared (**10**).

First 24 hours—Ringers Lactate solution, 4 ml/kg body weight/per cent burn, is administered. The total burn area is used in the calculation. Half of the calculated amount is given in the first 8 hours. The urine output should be approximately 50 ml/hour.

Second 24 hours—5 per cent dextrose and Ringers Lactate 0.5 ml/kg/per cent burn are used. Colloids are administered after the first 24 hours by which time the capillary leak is generally sealed. Some units favour the earlier use of colloids, administering them after the first 6 hours (**11–13**). The amount of colloid administered depends on the degree of burns—0.25 to 0.5 ml/kg/per cent of burn, or 20–60 per cent of calculated plasma volume. Albumin is often preferred; the only drawback is that it is very expensive. Dextravan, haemaccel or lomodex may also be used. Colloids and crystalloids must be infused at a constant rate. The sodium requirement is about 0.5 mmol/kg/per cent burns.

As mentioned earlier, various formulae have been recommended for fluid resuscitation and the use of colloids in the first 48 hours post-burn resuscitation period. These should serve merely as rough guidelines, and fluid adjustments should be titrated against patient response. Fluid resuscitation can be considered appropriate if tissue perfusion is adequate. In a young patient, a pulse rate ≤ 120/minute, a systolic blood pressure ≥ 100 mm Hg, a mean arterial blood pressure of about 85 mm Hg, a urine output of at least 0.7–1 ml/kg, and absence of base deficit, are parameters generally associated with adequate perfusion.

Renal and splanchnic blood flow are often selectively decreased during the first 24–48 hours after burns, and there is an increase in the secretion of aldosterone and antidiuretic hormone. We often use low dose dopamine (2 μg/kg/min) to maintain the urine output, rather than pushing excessive intravenous fluids, when other parameters of adequate perfusion have been satisfied.

Fluid Replacement during the Post-resuscitative Phase (36–48 hours to 5 days) (**Table 18.2.2**). This period is characterized by major fluid shifts. In deep burns, there is a continued loss of plasma into the burn tissue. In superficial burns there is a leak of plasma from the wound surface. The higher the capillary filtration pressure, the greater this loss. In addition, there is significant evaporative water loss from the wound surface. 5 per cent dextrose, alternating with dextrose saline is used to replace both loss of fluid from the burns, and evaporative loss from the wound surface. Hourly losses can be estimated from the formula:

ml/hr loss = (25 + per cent body surface burn) × m^2 surface area

Albumin may need to be continued to replace loss of plasma protein via the wound surface. Packed red blood cells may need to be given in patients with haemolysis, and for correction of anaemia produced by impairment of red blood cell production in the bone marrow. Packed cells are preferred and it is advisable to keep the haematocrit ≥ 30 per cent.

Monitoring volume replacement by the same tissue perfusion parameters described in the immediate 24–36 hour resuscitation period may be misleading after the first three days (**14**). This is because wound inflammation may commence around this time, and this produces a hyperdynamic circulatory state with marked tachycardia. The latter, if present at this stage, may not necessarily be due to hypovolaemia. In addition, the solute products of damaged tissue cells often induce a well-marked osmotic diuresis, so that the urine output may be excellent. It is necessary to check the specific gravity of the urine during this phase. A high specific gravity in association with a high urine output, generally indicates the need for more fluid administration.

Table 18.2.2. Fluid replacement in the post-resuscitative phase of burn injury (36–48 hours to 5 days)

---

* Replace evaporative water losses from wound surface and plasma loss into burn tissue with 5 per cent dextrose alternating with dextrose saline
* Correct protein losses by albumin infusions, maintaining serum albumin > 2.5 g/dl
* Correct anaemia by packed cell infusions, maintaining haematocrit > 30

(b) Care of the Airways and Pulmonary Support

It is vital to ensure that the airway is patent. An upper airway obstruction can develop suddenly with catastrophic results. Problems within the lungs, and in the large or small airways are most frequent in patients who have suffered a smoke inhalation injury. Inhalation of smoke in a fire causing burns, can lead to severe hypoxia causing immediate symptoms due to this hypoxic injury. Smoke inhalation injury can also cause upper airways obstruction from heat and chemicals. Symptoms of airways obstruction

may be delayed for 6–24 hours. Lower airways and parenchymal injury from chemicals in smoke can produce symptoms within hours, or these may take days to manifest. Airway problems can also occur in patients with full thickness burns to the face and neck.

Indications for prompt endotracheal intubation include stridor, respiratory distress, PaO$_2$ < 60 mm Hg on 4 l oxygen through a mask or nasal prongs, PaCO$_2$ > 50 mm Hg, and the presence of deep burns to the face and neck. A severe deep facial burn can lead to massive facial oedema over the next 12–18 hours, so that intubation if necessary at this time, becomes difficult or impossible. It is therefore wise to intubate these patients electively at an early stage.

Even when none of the above indications are present it is important to look for signs of airways injury. If oropharyngeal oedema is present, or the voice is hoarse an indirect laryngoscopy should be performed. Nebulization with racemic epinephrine helps to reduce local laryngeal oedema. If racemic epinephrine is unavailable, adrenaline 1 in 1000 dilution could be nebulized effectively. Adrenaline however often produces tachycardia. Nebulization with budecort could also help reduce laryngeal swelling and oedema. Systemic steroids may also be used for a day or two; prolonged use is contraindicated as it predisposes to infection. If upper airway oedema persists and causes airway obstruction, the patient should be intubated. If erythema alone is present without much oedema, the patient will still need close observation. Any deterioration in respiratory status on a close follow-up, merits securing of the airway by intubation. If endotracheal intubation is impossible because of oedema and swelling of the airways, a tracheostomy needs to be done. A tracheostomy in severe burns is generally associated with high morbidity and mortality, but in some patients is the only available option.

Endotracheal intubation is also often necessary in patients with severe chemical burns that cause bronchoconstriction, bronchorrhoea, and acute lung injury. The indications for endotracheal intubation in severe burns are listed in **Table 18.2.3**.

Table 18.2.3. Indications for endotracheal intubation in severe burns

---

* Stridor
* Respiratory distress
* PaO$_2$ < 60 mm Hg on 4 l oxygen via mask/nasal prongs; PaCO$_2$ > 50 mm Hg
* Deep facial or neck burns resulting in massive facial oedema
* Upper airways oedema
* Presence of airways injury—oropharyngeal oedema/erythema, hoarseness of voice, changing respiratory status
* Severe chemical burns causing bronchoconstriction, bronchorrhoea, acute lung injury

---

Ventilator support should be offered in the presence of acute respiratory failure or in the presence of incipient respiratory failure. Acute lung injury (ARDS) may occur at any time but is generally observed after the first 5–6 days. When present, it requires the use of PEEP. The patient may need to be paralyzed with pancuronium to enable efficient ventilatory support to be given. It is advisable to adjust ventilatory support so that peak inflation pressures do not exceed 30 cm H$_2$O, as these patients are particularly sensitive to barotrauma, and pneumothorax may easily occur.

During the post-resuscitative phase (36–48 hours to 5 days) fluid present in the interstitial compartment due to tissue oedema, often shifts back into the vascular compartment. This can cause hypervolaemia and worsen the acute lung injury (ARDS).

Optimal pulmonary support should always be given during and after any surgical procedure on the burn wound. Surgical procedures as far as possible should be of short duration and preferably not exceed 2 hours.

Nosocomial infection with nosocomial pneumonia is an important complication of ventilator support. It can occur at any time but is more frequent after the first week. Appropriate antibiotics are imperative as soon as a diagnosis of nosocomial pneumonia is made.

Injury from burns, particularly smoke inhalation injury, is sometimes complicated by carbon monoxide (CO) poisoning and rarely by cyanide poisoning. These produce immediate symptoms. Carbon monoxide poisoning is associated with mental disturbances and obtundation. A high index of suspicion is necessary for a correct diagnosis. CO poisoning should be suspected if the measured oxygen saturation of Hb is less than that predicted by the PaO_2, and if the patient has metabolic acidosis with a wide anion gap. The diagnosis can be confirmed by a carboxyhaemoglobin level > 5 per cent. Continuous administration of 100 per cent oxygen decreases the half-life of carboxyhaemoglobin from 4 hours on air, to about 80 minutes [15]. Cyanide intoxication may often be impossible to detect. Acute metabolic acidosis in the presence of a normal PaO_2 and a normal oxygen saturation of Hb should suggest the diagnosis. Anticyanide therapy includes the use of sodium nitrate, sodium thiosulphate and hydroxocobalamine.

(c) Electrolyte Disturbances

These are generally observed in the post-resuscitative period (from 36–48 hours to 5 days). The following electrolyte disturbances are commonly seen:

(i) *Hypernatraemia.* This is due to inadequate replacement of insensible water loss and the use of N saline in intravenous infusions. Salt restriction and infusion of 5 per cent dextrose should correct hypernatraemia.

(ii) *Hyponatraemia and hypokalaemia* may result from frequent washing or bathing of the burns patient with water, instead of an isotonic solution. Intravenous infusions of N saline with potassium supplements will correct this situation. Severe hyponatremia may need a titrated infusion of 3 per cent saline. Hypertonic saline should be avoided or used with great circumspection in the presence of pulmonary congestion.

(iii) *Hyperkalaemia* may occur in the early stages due to tissue damage and red cell destruction. Dextrose-insulin infusions help to reduce serum potassium levels. After 3–5 days, renal losses of potassium may be excessive so that potassium supplements of 80–200 mEq/day may be necessary.

(iv) *Hypocalcaemia* is invariably due to hypoalbuminaemia. Intravenous albumin infusions, and correction of hypoproteinaemia are then required.

Acid-Base Disturbances (16)

Severe thermal injury causes rapid acidosis. A combination of metabolic and respiratory acidosis exists in severe burns associated with smoke injury to the lungs. The metabolic component is due to tissues damaged by acid metabolites, and to relative hypoxia. The respiratory component is related to smoke injury to the lungs, or to hypoventilation in some patients. These need prompt correction, as acidosis has an adverse effect on myocardial function and on the overall circulatory system.

(d) Nutritional Support (17)

Early oral feeding is now the preferred method of nourishing a burns patient. It should be commenced when resuscitation is complete i.e. within 48–72 hours. As the patient will find it difficult to chew and masticate the food, liquid food must be specially prepared and given orally or through a nasogastric tube. Small measured quantities given hourly, are preferable to infrequently administered large nutrient boluses. The buttermilk diet (BMD) is a well-tried and safe diet providing 1 kcal/ml. Hence it is easy to monitor the amount of supplementary nutrition received by the patient. The composition of the BMD is given in **Table 18.2.4**. Starting with 10 ml/hour through the nasogastric tube, the quantity administered is increased by 10 ml/hour every 6 hours to reach a maximum of 2 ml/kg/hour for adults and 3–5 ml/kg/hour for children. Each feed is preceded by nasogastric aspiration to rule out gastric stasis and to prevent gastric dilatation. Some units prefer to administer enteral feeds by a continuous drip through a nasogastric tube, over a period of 14–16 hours. Generally after a period of 96 hours after the injury, the patient can be started on full diet with discontinuation of intravenous fluids.

Table 18.2.4. Composition of the buttermilk diet (BMD)

Curds	1 litre
Eggs	4
Bananas	4
Sugar	10 tablespoons

Total volume—1760 ml
Calories provided—1760 kcals
Proteins—60 g
Carbohydrates—340 g

In the presence of impaired gastrointestinal function, parenteral nutrition is necessary. This may be total or partial. A daily protein intake of 2–2.5 g/kg/day generally suffices, with a total caloric intake of 2500–3000 calories/day, the energy requirements being provided by dextrose and lipids (see Section on Nutritional Support in the Critically Ill). Vitamin supplements are necessary; hyperglycaemia may require the use of insulin.

(e) Local Care of the Burn Wound

Contamination of the burn, and invasive wound infection is the most dreaded complication. The wound must be covered as early as possible with a clean sheet over which cool water is constantly poured, to lower the temperature and withdraw heat from the wound. This helps to reduce the thermal damage.

Blisters or bullae *should not* be excised. They are just punctured and the fluid drained. If the bullae have already ruptured, the loose non-viable skin should not be excised, but cleaned with saline and evenly spread out over the burn. This non-viable skin serves to protect the burnt tissues underneath, and prevents dessication of the wound.

Tetanus is an important complication of burns in poor countries. Tetanus toxoid should be given on admission. Patients who have not been previously immunized should be given 250 units of tetanus human immunoglobulin and active immunization with tetanus toxoid should be commenced.

Treatment of the Burn Wound (18)

The exposure method of treatment has now been abandoned in burn centres all over the world, and the closed method of treatment has been universally accepted and adopted. After adequate resuscitation, the patient is given a bath and is dressed in the operating theatre. The choice of the antiseptic used over the burn wound varies. A silver sulphadiazine cream 1–2 per cent is most frequently used. Mefenide acetats 10 per cent cream or 5 per cent solution is preferred in some units in the West as this is believed to penetrate the eschar. It is unavailable in India and the silver sulphadiazine cream probably does just as well. Povidone Iodine is a good antiseptic but it is wise not to use it over a wide area. It is cytotoxic to fibroblasts and on systemic absorption can cause renal insufficiency and metabolic acidosis.

The nature of the agent used to dress and cover the wound varies. The *potato peel dressing* has been found to be eminently suited for this purpose. It is smeared with an antiseptic ointment (silver sulphadiazine cream) and gently applied over the burnt area; it is held in position with a gauze bandage. To prevent it from slipping, a single wet layer of plaster-of-Paris is spread over the dressing and allowed to dry into a thin shell, almost as thin as an eggshell—hence called the 'Egg Shell Dressing'. These dressings are changed once a day. Many prefer to use a *'collagen' dressing* to cover the wound. A very frequently used collagen dressing is termed *Integra*. This is a totally artificial material which is acellular and composed of two layers. The upper layer is of silistic and the lower layer is a cross-linked co-precipitate of collagen that is bovine in origin, and chondroitin-6-sulphate which comes from shark cartilage. Once the burned tissue is excised the Integra is sutured in place. When the lower layer has been populated by host cells, the silistic layer can be removed to provide an excellent vascularized mesodermal base. A freshly harvested thin epidermal graft can be laid on top of this to complete wound cover.

Cultured Autologous Epidermis (CAE)

A recent skin resurfacing technique is the use of cultured autologous epidermis to assist the timely closure of burn wounds. This technique requires expertise and special facilities, and to the best of our knowledge is not as yet in use in India.

The technique consists of taking a full-thickness skin biopsy consisting of a few square centimetres. After an in vitro culture period of 3–4 weeks, the autologous population of keratinocytes expands to approximately 1 m² of keratinocytes that are available for wound coverage. CAE has to be combined with dermal replacement in the form of INTEGRA, ALLODERA or CELL-FREE PORCINE DERMIS.

There are however several shortcomings with this technique. These include: (a) a relatively low rate of engraftment or 'take' of each CAE application; (b) graft fragility resulting in delayed loss; (c) prolonged immobilization of extremities in order to facilitate engraftment, leading to loss of function; (d) a very high cost when purchased commercially—about $ 2000 for each percentage of wound closure. This fact makes the above technique an impractical proposition for the poor countries of the world.

Whatever the method used to cover the burn wound, the joints must be positioned in their optimal functional positions. Once healing has occurred completely, gentle active physiotherapy restores the full range of movement. The axiom to remember is 'Heal First—Move Next'.

Escharatomy

It is not always possible for burn wounds in developing countries to be managed by the ideal, closed method of treatment. Through lack of facilities, burns are sometimes treated by the exposure method, and the patient is referred subsequently to a unit with better facilities. By the time of referral, the burn tissues on the surface have already formed a hard inelastic eschar. The oedema which occurs in the underlying tissues following burn injury, exerts an excessive compression on the vascular network, and impairs the circulation. Dry gangrene results very often, as does anaerobic infection when the eschar is circumferential. Such an eschar around the chest wall restricts the respiratory excursions and impairs ventilation. Releasing incisions in the midlateral positions of the involved extremity or trunk, have been recommended. The incisions should be made only through the eschar and subjacent tissue, lest the larger blood vessels are cut, resulting in excessive blood loss.

With the use of the potato peel bandages smeared with antibiotic ointment over the burn wound, an inelastic burn eschar is prevented from forming. The need for escharotomies has in our experience, been thereby considerably reduced.

Escharotomy and Split Skin Grafting

When the eschar separates out and is replaced by healthy granulation tissue (usually at 2–3 weeks post-burn), the wound is debrided and covered with a very thin split skin graft, preferably meshed 1:3. Blood loss at the time of surgery is rapidly corrected, or better still is reduced by subcutaneous infiltration of normal saline with adrenaline 1:1,000,000. Post-grafting dressings are done every 2–3 days thereafter.

Early Excision and Grafting of the Burn Wound

When good facilities exist, i.e. trained surgical and nursing staff, facilities for good anaesthesia, adequate dressing material and equipment, adequate supply of blood and homograft skin, the ideal treatment today consists of excision of all full thickness and deep partial thickness skin burns, starting within a few hours after the burn injury is sustained (19, 20). However such conditions are unavailable in most of our hospitals, and hence early excision and over grafting of skin is unfortunately impractical at present, and can be done in just a few special units.

Fascial Excision and Skin Grafting

This is indicated in severely infected burns with invasive burn wound sepsis ($> 10^5$ bacteria/g of burnt tissue on burn wound biopsy).

(f) Symptomatic Treatment of Pain and the Use of Antacids

A partial thickness wound is very painful. Also, the surface of a burn wound dries up if kept exposed, and the process whereby an eschar forms can be extremely painful. The application of a semipermeable membrane relieves pain to a great extent. A small dose of pethidine or morphine, titrated against the patient's response is frequently used in a continuous intravenous infusion, to relieve the pain. Ketamine is a very useful analgesic and anaesthetic agent in burns patients. Following a burn injury, acute stress often leads to upper GI bleeds from acute mucosal erosions and from a Curling's ulcer. Blood loss may be significant and may need to be replaced. Sucralfate or antacids may help in preventing or reducing the incidence of GI bleeds. In burns > 40 per cent, an intravenous H_2-antagonist is routinely given during the first 2 weeks post-burn.

Management during the Period of Inflammation and Infection

The hypermetabolic response to injury takes the form of the systemic inflammatory response syndrome (SIRS) which starts around the fifth day of burns, and peaks at 8–10 days. This response is not necessarily associated with infection, though infection is a frequent and dreadful complication. It is extremely difficult, and in the initial stages often impossible to distinguish inflammation-induced hypermetabolism from an infection-induced process. This phase is the most dangerous and difficult to manage in severe burns.

Symptoms and Signs of Invasive Wound Infections

Systemic features include tachycardia, tachypnoea, hyperthermia or hypothermia. Disorientation, ileus, hypotension, oliguria, glucose intolerance and acidosis may be present. Leucocytosis is frequent, but sepsis may causes severe leucopaenia and thrombocytopaenia. These systemic features are indistinguishable from sepsis produced by central line sepsis, fulminant urinary infections or nosocomial pneumonia. Physical changes in the appearance of the burn wound are therefore more reliable signs of invasive burn wound infection than systemic features. Clinical signs of burn wound infection include (a) focal dark or black discolouration of the wound; (b) conversion of a second degree burn to full-thickness burn; (c) unexpected rapid eschar formation; (d) haemorrhagic discolouration of eschar fat; (e) oedematous, inflamed, violaceous wound edges; (f) extensive foul smelling slough over the wound, with a greenish discharge suggesting a

Ps. aeruginosa infection; (g) abscess formation and infected lesions outside the burn wound area.

Surface cultures of the wound do not necessarily distinguish colonization from invasive infection. Quantitative cultures also lack sufficient sensitivity, though colony counts of $< 10^5$ per gram of biopsy tissue correlates with absence of invasive burn wound infection. Histological examination of a biopsy of the wound *and* underlying viable tissue is the best method of establishing invasive infection. The presence of micro-organisms in viable tissue points to tissue infection.

Wound Management

Severe burn wound infection is treated by local and systemic antimicrobial therapy. Twice daily applications of silver sulphadiazine ointment covered by sterile gauze dressings are used. Systemic antibiotics should be promptly started in full doses to treat not only local and systemic sepsis, but to prevent the onset and progression of multiple organ dysfunction and failure. Organisms most frequently encountered in infected burns include Pseudomonas, Klebsiella, E. coli, Staphylococcus aureus and Group A Streptococci. We have generally found a combination of ticarcillin clavulanic acid + an aminoglycoside + metronidazole to be effective. A proven or strongly suspected Staphylococcal infection would necessitate the use of augmentin or vancomycin. An alternative antibiotic regime for severely infected burns (chiefly due to Gram-negative organisms) is the use of imipenem-cilastin 500 mg intravenously eight hourly or meropenem 1 g eight hourly given as an intravenous infusion. Either of these can be combined with vancomycin 500 mg six hourly or 1 g twice daily in an intravenous infusion to cover possible staphylococcal infection. Local or systemic fungal infection merits the use of fluconazole and/or amphotericin B (see later Section on Antifungal Treatment in this chapter).

Broad guidelines for antibiotic usage are outlined below (21).

(i) Colonization of a large burn wound surface is impossible to prevent and invariably occurs. The mere culture of organisms is no indication for antibiotic use, in the absence of clinical evidence of infection.

(ii) When clinical (and in particular histological) evidence of wound sepsis is associated with growth of organisms from an unhealthy infected wound, the choice of antibiotics should be guided by culture, sensitivity reports. Gram-negative infections are most frequently responsible for wound infection and need an appropriate antibiotic cover.

(iii) Antibiotics once chosen should be continued for at least 5 to 7 days to allow them to act properly. Yet prolonged use of the same antibiotics can cause the emergence of resistant organisms. Appropriate antibiotic change should again be guided by culture, sensitivity reports.

(iv) The pharmacokinetics of antibiotics in severe burns is considerably changed. If possible, drug dosage should be adjusted to ensure adequate bactericidal serum concentration levels. Unfortunately, the penetration of antibiotics into a burn eschar is unreliable in spite of adequate serum concentration of the drug.

(v) The prophylactic use of antibiotics in burns should be reserved for: (a) Pre- and peri-operative administration associated with excision, debridement and autografting. (b) Early phases of burns in children: prophylactic antibiotics are administered in some units. (c) Cases of infection: in poor developing countries transport of patients with severe burns to an intensive care unit or to a burns unit, is often done in an unhygienic fashion so that infection is almost certain to occur. When this is so, many units in the city administer prophylactic antibiotics from the day of admission. Till definitive swab culture and sensitivity reports are available, a combination of ampicillin and an aminoglycoside is administered intravenously. The wisdom of this is disputable, though most experienced specialists in burns in this country believe that under existing circumstances, morbidity is reduced.

It should be noted that the mere use of local and systemic antimicrobial therapy does not always suffice. Aggressive surgical debridement and resection of infected tissue may occasionally be imperative. Bacteraemia, severe systemic sepsis, and even septic shock may follow such a major surgical procedure, and should be anticipated. The importance of correct local treatment to the burn wound by tropical antibiotics and aggressive excision *prior* to this phase cannot be overemphasized.

Fluid Replacement and Cardiovascular Support

Adequate fluid replacement should take into consideration evaporative water loss, and loss of blood and plasma from debridement of necrotic tissue. The catabolic state results in high fever necessitating further increase in evaporative losses at a rate of 8–10 per cent per degree of rise in body temperature. The haematocrit should continue to be kept at 35 per cent by packed cell infusions, and the albumin concentration should be maintained at around 3 g/dl. The hyperkinetic circulatory state is associated with a marked increase in the cardiac output to meet the increased oxygen demands. Myocardial dysfunction often supervenes, and inotropic support with dopamine and other inotropes as also vasopressors may be frequently necessary. Cardiopulmonary failure in this phase of severe burns is most frequently observed in elderly patients. This is because the circulatory and respiratory systems in the aged have a comparatively limited reserve which is unable to cope with the excessive metabolic demands of the stress response induced by severe burns.

Respiratory Support

Nosocomial pneumonia is a frequent complication, and the increased metabolic rate leads to increased carbon dioxide production necessitating increase in ventilatory requirements. Respiratory muscle fatigue often supervenes, so that patients who were breathing spontaneously, may now require ventilator support. Acute lung injury (ARDS) may also complicate the picture at this stage, and this worsens the prognosis markedly as it is often the forerunner of multiple organ failure.

Metabolic Support

Maintenance of adequate nutrition is vital for survival during this phase, as the hypermetabolic state leads to a severe loss in lean muscle mass. The enteral route is always to be preferred, and this may be supplemented if necessary, by parenteral nutrition. Total parenteral nutrition may be required at times.

Care of the Eyes and Ears

For protection of the eyes from infection, antibiotic eyedrops during the day and antibiotic ointment at night may be used. Mydriatics may also be used.

Chondritis is a dangerous complication which may result in the whole ear falling off due to infective destruction. It is treated by providing adequate fluffy padding for burnt ears with adequate antibiotic cream cover to prevent pressure necrosis of the fragile infected cartilage.

Control of Infection

A combination of an immunosuppressed host and bacterial colonization of the burn wound, the oropharynx and the tracheobronchial tree, strongly predisposes to nosocomial infection. Nosocomial pneumonia, vascular catheter sepsis, urinary catheter sepsis, and above all deep severe infection of the burn wound are all too common, and can trigger multiple organ failure.

A diagnosis of nosocomial pneumonia should be based on clinical and radiological grounds. Leucocytosis, fever, purulent sputum, or purulent tracheal aspirate showing many organisms on Gram's stain, with an increase or change in pulmonary shadowing, suffice to make a clinical diagnosis. Empiric antibiotic treatment should not be delayed pending sputum culture sensitivity reports.

If possible, vascular catheter sepsis should be prevented by judicious change of the central lines (every 7 to 10 days), by prompt removal of the arterial lines, and by avoiding the use of a Swan-Ganz catheter, unless this is absolutely mandatory. Catheter tips should be sent for culture, and blood cultures should always be done in each and every patient with nosocomial infection, so as to enable a proper choice of antibiotic therapy.

Antifungal Treatment

Invasive fungal infection of the burn wound and/or systemic fungal sepsis are important complications, particularly in extensive severe burns. They carry a high morbidity and mortality. Candida species frequently colonize a burn wound but rarely cause an invasive wound infection. Aspergillus however can cause an invasive fungal wound infection which generally is limited to subcutaneous tissue and only rarely crosses fascial planes. Rarely fungal invasion of the wound by Mucor species may also occur. Colonization of a burn wound with Candida or Aspergillus can be countered by the local application of clotrimazole. However if there is histologic evidence of fungal invasion of the wound, treatment consists of wound debridement and excision, and the use of intravenous amphotericin.

Systemic fungal sepsis with positive blood culture for fungi, is either nosocomial through vascular catheters, or results as a superinfection due to prolonged use of broad-spectrum antibiotics, or results from invasive fungal wound sepsis. Fluconazole and/or amphotericin need to be given in an intravenous infusion.

Some units use fluconazole prophylactically in situations where fungal infection is strongly anticipated.

Treatment of Complications and Support of Multiple Organ Systems

All organ systems need to be carefully supported. Renal failure may require dialysis. A progressively increasing serum creatinine and a progressively increasing blood urea nitrogen may necessitate dialysis regardless of the volume of urine excreted (22). Bacterial infection is a frequent hazard and complication, and death often results from infection rather than from renal failure.

Prevention

Burns treatment is far more advanced now than it was fifty years ago. The mortality and morbidity are much lower, but the pain suffered and the dreams shattered are as real as before. The basic aim or objective is to prevent burns. A great deal of research needs to be done in this direction for this objective to be adequately realized.

Rehabilitation

Physiotherapy is very important to maintain function. Pressure garments may be used to prevent hypertrophic scar formation. Moisturizing agents to soften scars and steroid creams to decrease itching are also commonly used.

REFERENCES

1. Keswani MH. (1986). The prevention of burning injury. Burns. 12, 533–539.
2. Pruitt BA, Goodwin CW, Jr. (2001). Critical Care Management of the Severely Burned Patient. In: Current Therapy in Critical Care Medicine (Eds Parrillo JE, Dellinger RP). pp. 1475–1500. Mosby, USA.
3. Jackson D MacG. (1969). Second thoughts on the burn wound. J Trauma. 9, 839.
4. Jackson D MacG. (1983). The burn wound—Its character, closure and complications. The William Gissane Lecture 1982. Burns. 10, 1.
5. Keswani MH, Patil AR. (1985). The boiled potato peel as a burn wound dressing—a preliminary report. Burns. 11, 220–224.
6. Freebairn RC, Oh TE. (1997). Burns. In: Intensive Care Manual, 4th edn (Ed. Oh TE). pp. 622–629. Butterworths-Heinemann, Sydney, London, Toronto.
7. Lund CC, Browder NC. (1944). The estimation of areas of burns. Surg Gynecol Obstet. 79, 352–358.
8. Moritz AR, Henriques FC. (1947). Studies of thermal injury. II. The relative importance of time and surface temperature in the causation of cutaneous injuries. Amer F Path. 23, 695–720.
9. Sevitt S. (1954). Pathological sequelae of burns. Proc Roy Soc Med. 47, 225–228.
10. Curreri PW, Luterman A. (1989). Burns. In: Principles of Surgery, 5th edn (Eds Schwartz SI, Shires GT, Spencer FC). pp. 285–305. McGraw-Hill Book Company, New York, London, Toronto.
11. Settle JAD. (1982). Fluid therapy in burns. J Royal Soc Med. 75(suppl 1), 6–11.
12. Hutches N, Haynes BW. (1972). The Evans formula revisited. J Trauma. 12, 453–455.
13. Artz CP. (1971). The Brooke formula. In: Contemporary Burn Management (Eds Polk HC Jr, Stone HH). pp. 43–51. Little, Brown and Company, Boston.
14. Venkatesh B, Meacher R, Muller MJ et al. (2001). Monitoring tissue oxygenation during resuscitation of major burns. J Trauma. 50, 485–494.
15. Fein A, Leff A, Hopewell PC. (1980). Pathophysiology and management of the complications resulting from fire and the inhaled products of combustion. Review of the literature. Crit Care Med. 8, 94–98.
16. Davies JWL. (1982). Physiological responses to burning injury. Academic Press, London.
17. Pasulka PS, Wachtel TL. (1987). Nutritional considerations for the burned patient. Surg Clin North Am. 67, 109–131.
18. Hansbrough JF. (1990). Current status of skin replacements for coverage of extensive burn wounds. J Trauma 30 (12 Suppl), S155–S160.
19. Burke JF. (1981). Early excision of the burn wound. J Trauma. 21(suppl 8), 726–727.
20. Heimbach DM. (1987). Early burn excision and grafting. Surg Clin North Am. 67, 93–107.
21. Dacso CC, Luterman A, Curreri PW. (1987). Systemic antibiotic treatment in burned patients. Surg Clin North Am. 67, 57–68.
22. Bartlett RH, Gentille DE, Allyn PA et al. (1973). Hemodialysis in the management of massive burns. Trans Am Soc Artif Int Org. 19, 264–276.

Critical Care in Poisonings

General Considerations

The evaluation and management of a patient who intentionally or accidentally ingests or is exposed to a poison, is an important aspect of critical care medicine. There are a vast number of poisons; important poisons include drugs which in toxic doses produce dangerous and often life-threatening effects.

The diagnosis of acute poisoning though often obvious, is at times difficult. The possibility of poisoning should always be considered in any obscure illness, or in any patient in whom the cause of unconsciousness is not clearly apparent.

Critical care of patients acutely ill with poisoning as a matter of urgent priority necessitates life support to keep them alive. Prevention of absorption of poisons, their quick elimination, and the use of specific antidotes are of further help in a number of situations.

This chapter outlines the principles of approach to poisonings in patients admitted to a critical care unit. It then briefly outlines the clinical features and management of a few important and common poisonings—particularly those observed in our part of the world.

Approach to Poisonings (1–7)

I. Life Support to Keep the Patient Alive

A patient brought to the unit following acute poisoning may be unconscious with poor respiration and circulation. If this is so, the immediate priority is towards life support.

(a) Care of the Airway and Respiratory Care

The airways should be kept open—the neck should be extended and the jaw pushed forward and secretions sucked from the back of the throat. Endotracheal intubation is promptly done if (i) the patient is deeply obtunded or unconscious; (ii) swallowing is impaired; (iii) the cough reflex is poor or absent, the patient being unable to protect his airways; (iv) the patient requires ventilator support either because ventilation is poor or because of pulmonary oedema.

Oxygen should be given in 100 per cent concentration. It can never do harm as an initial life support measure. The only relative contraindication is in patients with paraquat poisoning. In the latter situation, very high concentrations of oxygen can promote pulmonary fibrosis.

Ventilator support is necessary in patients with acute respiratory failure i.e. in those with hypoxia and/or hypercapnia. Ventilator support should also be offered in those with incipient respiratory failure—i.e. in acute poisoning known to rapidly lead to acute respiratory failure. The use of prophylactic PEEP is unwise; PEEP should however be given in patients with poison induced pulmonary oedema resulting from increased capillary permeability.

(b) Care of the Circulation

The circulation should be assessed *pari passu* with respiration. A large peripheral vein is promptly secured; a central venous line is also invariably necessary in acutely ill patients to determine central venous pressure, and to thereby allow adjustments for volume load. A self-retaining Foley's catheter is passed to enable the urine output to be monitored hourly. Hypotension should be immediately corrected as this causes poor tissue perfusion, metabolic acidosis and worsens prognosis. Hypotension in acute poisoning may be due to a variety of causes acting singly or in combination. These include a decrease in systemic vascular resistance causing arteriolar dilatation, venous pooling, myocardial depression and hypovolaemia. The initial management (except in the presence of pulmonary oedema) is a fluid challenge of 200 ml of a crystalloid solution. Repeated challenges are given provided the central venous pressure (CVP) is not beyond 10 mm Hg, the arterial blood pressure rises and the urine output is close to 60 ml/hour. If a volume challenge fails to raise the blood pressure, and the CVP is at the upper limit of normal, the patient is given dopamine support so that the systolic blood pressure is kept over 100 mm Hg and preferably around 120 mm Hg. The principles of inotropic support in patients with severe myocardial depression are the same as in patients with cardiogenic shock.

(c) Control of Seizures

A few poisons can produce frequent or continuous seizures. These can be life-threatening and need to be controlled. Benzodiazepines should be used initially; phenytoin and barbiturates may be needed if diazepam is ineffective. In refractory cases intravenous thiopental or the use of paralytic curare-like agents may be necessary to allow efficient ventilator support. It is however important to note that control of seizures may occasionally require therapy specific to the poison involved.

(d) Use of Emergency Drugs

Two important causes of deep coma or of mental obtundation with or without hypotension, are severe hypoglycaemia and narcotic poisoning. For diagnostic and therapeutic purposes it would be justified in giving first 50 g of dextrose intravenously to reverse possible hypoglycaemia. Blood is collected for blood glucose estimation before dextrose is administered. This can do no harm and produces a magical response in patients whose coma is due to very low blood sugar levels. 100 mg of thiamine are generally administered to prevent Wernicke's encephalopathy, particularly in alcoholics who are admitted with severe hypoglycaemia.

If intravenous dextrose produces no response, many critical care units would give a diagnostic and therapeutic trial to naloxone, a specific antagonist to narcotics. The initial dose is 2 mg intravenously. Improvement in respiration occurs in 2 minutes. Repeated dosing may be necessary, as the half-life of naloxone is shorter than the half-life of the narcotic agent. Some synthetic opiates (meperidine or propoxyphene), may require higher initial doses (6–8 mg) for reversal.

II. Evaluation of Poisoning

(a) History

A history is impossible in an obtunded or comatose patient. Even otherwise it is often unreliable particularly when a drug is taken with suicidal intent. It is important to question relatives, friends and co-workers to obtain as much information as possible. Vital clues may be given by the presence of specific drugs or poisons found at the site of a patient's home or workplace.

(b) Physical Examination

A quick physical examination may give a clue as to the nature of the poison. Physical examination is initially toxidrome oriented— which means oriented towards detection of symptom complexes that are associated with different groups of poisons.

The following features are quickly evaluated:

(i) *Vital Signs.* Sympathomimetic drugs, anticholinergics often produce tachycardia, hypertension. Anticholinergics produce a dry hot skin; cocaine can also produce hyperthermia, but with diaphoresis. Sedative-hypnotics or narcotics can produce respiratory depression, bradycardia and hypotension.

(ii) *A brief neurological examination* should determine the level of consciousness, the presence and nature of hallucinations, pupillary and motor responses.

Level of Consciousness: In severe poisonings with narcotics, hypnotics, and sedatives the patient is obtunded or comatose. Confusion, agitation and coma can also occur with poisons with a cholinergic action (e.g. organophosphorus compounds), as also with drugs that have an anticholinergic action (tricyclic antidepressants).

Hallucinations: These are frequently seen in atropine and dhatura poisoning, in poisoning with cocaine, phencyclidine and LSD. With cocaine, hallucinatory objects appear in the periphery of vision; with atropine, hallucinatory objects are small; dhatura poisoning is associated with finger picking movements, as if the patient is pulling threads from his finger tip; complex hallucinations characterize poisoning due to phencyclidine; LSD poisoning is associated with visual and auditory hallucinations and illusions where the patient can 'hear colours' or 'see sounds'.

Pupillary Responses: Miosis can be caused by organophosphate insecticides and by narcotics. Though opium and morphine cause pin-point pupils, in almost all such patients a very strong focused light produces a small contraction of the pupil, demonstrating the integrity of the third nerve and that portion of the midbrain concerned with the pupillary reflex. Both atropine and cocaine can result in mydriasis, though in cocaine poisoning the pupil will react to light.

Nystagmus: Alcohol, sedatives-hypnotics, and anti-epileptics like phenytoin, primidone can all cause nystagmus. Lithium poisoning and poisoning with carbamazepine and solvents also produce nystagmus.

Motor Response: Seizures can be induced by a number of poisons. The only important poison which can produce recurrent seizures with the patient remaining alert, and with muscle tone being normal in between seizures, is strychnine. Drug induced seizures often respond poorly to conventional antiepileptic therapy. Thus isoniazid-induced seizures (invariably associated with mental obtundation or psychosis) will respond to pyridoxine, and seizures induced by tricyclic antidepressants will respond to physostigmine.

(iii) *Auscultation of the lungs for pulmonary oedema and bronchospasm.* A number of poisons can induce pulmonary oedema; cholinergic drugs can induce severe bronchospasm and an increase in bronchial secretions. This is important both from the diagnostic and therapeutic point of view.

(iv) *Auscultation of the abdomen for bowel sounds.* Bowel sounds are feeble in severe sedative or narcotic poisoning; hyperperistalsis and abdominal cramps (if the patient is conscious) are observed with cholinergic poisons.

(v) *Skin temperature and moisture.* Sweating is frequently observed with poisons having a cholinergic and sympathomimetic action. The skin is dry and hot in persons with an anticholinergic effect.

Important features in physical examination in relation to 'toxidromes' or symptom complexes produced by poisons which exert a sedative-hypnotic effect, a cholinergic effect, anticholinergic effect and sympathomimetic effect are charted in **Table 18.3.1**.

(c) Laboratory Investigations

A blood glucose estimation is important in any individual who is obtunded or comatose. Routine investigations should include a blood count, urine examination, serum electrolytes, urea, creatinine, determination of the degree of anion gap, serum osmolality, calculated osmolar gap, liver function tests, X-ray chest, ECG, arterial blood gas analysis. The patient needs to be continuously monitored if there are arrhythmias. The QT interval should be measured, as an increase in this interval produced by a number of

Table 18.3.1. Various 'Toxidromes' observed with common poisons

Poison Group	Vital Signs				CNS Exam			RS Exam —Lungs	GI Exam —Bowel Sound	Exam of Skin, Moisture
	Temp	RR	BP	HR	Level of Consciousness	Pupils	Motor Response			
1. Sedative-Hypnotics (Barbiturates, Benzodiazepines, Alcohols, Opioids)	N or –	N or – or – –	N or –	N or –	Normal, Obtunded, Comatose	Miosis	N or –	N	N or –	N
2. Cholinergic Drugs (Organophosphorus Compounds)	N	+ or –	+	+ or –	Normal, Confusion, Coma	Miosis	Weakness, Paralysis, Fasciculations	Broncho-spasm, Bronch-orrhea	+ +	Diaphoresis + +
3. Anticholinergic Drugs (Tricyclic Antidepressants, Phenothiazines, Antihistaminics)	N or +	N or –	N or +	+ or + +	Delirium, Coma	Mydria-sis	N	N	– –	Dry, hot
4. Sympathomimetic Drugs (Cocaine, Amphetamine, Ephedrine, Phencyclidine)	N, + or + +	+ or –	+ +	+ +	Normal, Agitated, Paranoid, delusional	Mydria-sis	N	N	N or–	Diaphoresis

N = normal; + = increased; ++ = markedly increased; – = decreased; – – = markedly decreased.

drugs can precipitate serious rhythm disturbances. Other laboratory tests depend on the specific poison suspected in a given patient. Cyanosed patients with a normal PaO₂ and a lowered oxygen saturation, should have tests done for methaemoglobin and carboxyhaemoglobin.

Specific drug levels for drug intoxication due to specific suspected drugs may need to be done if facilities are available. Drug levels of salicylates, barbiturates, ethanol, digoxin, iron, theophylline and lithium are done in our laboratories. Serum levels of any of these drugs in suspected poisoning, help management. Estimation of blood levels of most common poisons is now possible at one of the medical centres in Mumbai.

Imaging Studies. A plain X-ray of the abdomen may show the presence within the gut of radiopaque drugs—iron tablets or enteric-coated tablets. These films also visualize drug packets in patients who ingest the latter to smuggle drugs through Customs.

History, clinical examination and relevant investigations should help diagnosis. Differential diagnosis of acute poisoning includes acute infections, particularly those involving the neuraxis, and metabolic problems, in particular hypoglycaemia, hypercalcaemia, liver and renal cell dysfunction. Head injury (when no wound is visible) can also mimic poisoning, as can a cerebrovascular accident particularly when the latter involves the brainstem. The neurological features produced by cyanide poisoning which is not immediately fatal, resemble brainstem infarction or the effects of severe hypoxia.

III. Further Management (8)

Life support, with a quick clinical assessment, and laboratory help to determine the nature of the poison, are now followed or accompanied *pari passu* by measures to prevent absorption, use of a specific antidote when this is available, and measures for removal of absorbed poison.

(a) Measures to Prevent Absorption

Most poisons are ingested orally either accidentally or with suicidal intent. There are three methods to prevent or reduce absorption— (i) inducing emesis; (ii) gastric lavage; (iii) use of activated charcoal.

(i) *Inducing emesis.* A home remedy to induce emesis is tickling the pharynx or by making the patient drink a glass of salt water and tickling the pharynx. Drugs used to induce vomiting are now used very rarely. They include apomorphine 0.6 mg/kg intravenously, and syrup ipecac 30 ml in 16 oz water given orally in adults, and 15 ml in 8 oz water orally in children.

Apomorphine has now been relegated to medical history books and is no longer used. Ipecac which also induces vomiting within 30–60 minutes, is also now rarely used because at best not more than 40–50 per cent of the ingested drug can be removed in this fashion.

(ii) *Gastric lavage* (**9, 10**). Gastric lavage through a large bore tube has totally replaced induced emesis by drugs. Lavage should be done through a large bore tube passed orally. The patient should always be in the lateral position, semiprone, with the foot end of the bed elevated by 15 degrees. Lavage should never be done with the patient supine for fear of aspiration. In a comatose or obtunded patient it is important to first intubate the patient, and seal off the respiratory tract from the gastrointestinal tract so that aspiration during lavage is avoided. Once the lavage tube has been correctly passed into the stomach, the stomach contents are completely aspirated before lavage is commenced. Lavage is performed by running 150–300 ml N saline down the tube; the fluid is then allowed to efflux from the stomach. Runs of N saline as stated above, are repeated again and again till the effluent is perfectly clear. Activated charcoal and a cathartic may be administered through the lavage tube before withdrawal.

The indications for gastric lavage are many and have been listed below in **Table 18.3.2**. The prime indication is a patient who is admitted to a unit within one hour of ingesting a drug which is known to be rapidly absorbed from the gut, and which can cause life-threatening problems.

Table 18.3.2. Indications for gastric lavage

* Patient admitted within 1 hour of ingesting a potentially life-threatening poison
* If the ingested substance slows gastric emptying
* If the ingested poison/drug is not absorbed very rapidly from GI tract
* If activated charcoal is ineffective in binding ingested substance

Complications of lavage include aspiration pneumonia and inadvertent passage of the tube through the larynx into the trachea with instillation of fluid into the lungs. Laryngeal spasm, oesophageal perforation and arrhythmias have been reported in rare instances.

Both induced emesis and lavage are absolutely contraindicated in poisoning due to caustic ingestion (either acid or alkali). Vomiting in these circumstances can lead to a worsening of oesophageal and mouth burns. Passage of a thick tube in caustic poisoning can induce perforation of the oesophagus or stomach.

(iii) *Use of activated charcoal* (11). The use of activated charcoal is becoming increasingly popular in the management of acute poisoning. Activated charcoal is an inert non-toxic adsorbent which binds high molecular weight compounds due to intermolecular attractions. Although activated charcoal binds many compounds, there are several potential poisons that do not bind well. These include bromides, caustics, methanol, ethylene glycol, lithium, isopropyl alcohol. When activated charcoal is used in repeated doses it can interrupt enterohepatic circulation and hence enhance the elimination of drugs whose pharmacokinetics includes enterohepatic circulation.

Activated charcoal is administered in a dose of 1 g/kg mixed in lemon barley, or water or fruit juice, and is either drunk or given through a nasogastric tube or preferably through a large lavage tube used for gastric lavage. When used in repeated doses to interrupt enterohepatic circulation of a poison or drug, 25 g is given every 2–4 hours in adults. In children 0.25–1 g/kg is given every 2–4 hours. Constipation can result from the use of activated charcoal. A laxative like magnesium sulphate should be added to the first dose of activated charcoal to counter constipation. Drugs amenable to repeat dose charcoal therapy include carbamazepine, diazepam, digoxin, phenobarbitol, phenytoin, salicylates, theophylline, tricyclic antidepressants (12).

The use of whole bowel irrigation by the administration of 1–2 l of polyethylene glycol has been tried in some units for the evacuation of ingested poison (12). It is a taxing procedure for the patient, and is not recommended for routine use.

Toxins and poisons can also enter the body through the skin, and through the ocular, pulmonary and parenteral routes. In ocular exposure the eyes should be irrigated with N saline for 30–40 minutes. Contamination of the skin with poisons should be countered by removal of the poison with soap and water. This is specially important with reference to organophosphates, hydro-carbons and herbicides. Separate drainage areas should be provided to dispose off the contaminated water used for cleansing the skin.

(b) Use of Specific Antidotes

Comparatively very few poisons have specific antidotes. Important antidotes to specific poisons are listed below in **Table 18.3.3**.

Table 18.3.3. Common poisons and their antidotes (with dosages)

Common Poisons	Antidotes	Dosages
1. Opiates (morphine, heroin, codeine)	Naloxone	0.4–2 mg IV bolus; can repeat to maximum of 10 mg
2. Tricyclic Anti-depressants	Physostigmine	0.5–2 mg slow IV push
3. Organo-phosphorus Compounds	Atropine	2 mg IV; repeat dose every 5 mins till atropinized
	+ Pralidoxime	0.5–2 g IV over 5–15 mins; can be repeated every 6–12 hrs
4. Paracetamol (acetaminophen)	Acetylcysteine	Loading dose 140 mg/kg orally, followed by 70 mg/kg every 4 hrs × 3 days
5. Cyanide	Amyl Nitrate, then Sodium Nitrate, Sodium Thiosulfate	Immediate inhalation; 10–15 ml IV in 5 mins; 50 ml of 25 per cent solution IV 8 hrly
6. Methyl Alcohol (methanol)	Ethanol	2 mg/kg of 50 per cent ethanol orally, or 10 per cent ethanol IV, at a rate of 0.05–0.1 mg/kg/hr
7. Ferrous Sulphate (iron)	Deferoxamine (Desferal)	5–7 g orally in 100–200 ml water, followed by 2 g in 6 ml distilled H_2O IM, then 7–10mg/kg/hr IV slowly to maximum of 80 mg/kg/day
	or Calcium EDTA	35–40 mg/kg/day orally of IV

(c) Measures for Removal of Poisons

There are three methods to help in the elimination of absorbed poisons—the use of repeated doses of activated charcoal, forced diuresis in combination with alkalinization of the urine, and the use of dialysis or charcoal haemoperfusion.

Frequent doses of activated charcoal can be given to help absorb a poison or drug (12). This method is particularly useful to absorb drugs that re-enter the gastrointestinal tract through the entero-hepatic circulation, or drugs that diffuse from the systemic circulation into the gastrointestinal tract because of a concentration gradient. Poisons which have a low volume of distribution within the body, and those which have low protein-binding, are lipophilic, and undergo an enterohepatic circulation, are best suited for removal by this means. The dose of activated charcoal is 1 g/kg and the initial dose is followed by 0.5 g/kg every 2–4 hours. A cathartic should be administered only once daily. Substantial decreases in the half-life of various compounds and drugs have been observed following repeated dosing with activated charcoal. It is important to remember that chlorpropamide clearance is not increased. Clearance of phenytoin, salicylates and imipramine is equivocal; this is probably related to the high protein binding of these drugs.

Forced diuresis with alkalinization of the urine. In our opinion this is rarely if ever necessary. If this modality is used, it should only be reserved for specific poisons—fluoride, barbiturates, primidone. Fluid diuresis with alkalinization of urine should be avoided in older people as it can cause pulmonary oedema. Hyponatraemia and a rise in intracranial pressure are other complications.

Haemodialysis and haemoperfusion. These methods are increasingly used to enhance elimination of poisons and drugs. Indications include patients refractory to general supportive care, those with extremely high levels of the poison in the blood necessitating quick removal, those in whom other routes of elimination are impaired (e.g. patients with renal and hepatic insufficiency). It is of course important that haemodialysis and haemoperfusion are used when poisons are capable of being removed by this form of therapy.

A list of important poisons whose removal is enhanced by multiple dosing with activated charcoal, haemodialysis and haemoperfusion is given in **Table 18.3.4.**

Table 18.3.4. Methods to enhance elimination of some common drugs and poisons

Drug/Poison	Multiple Doses of Activated Charcoal	Haemo-dialysis	Haemo-perfusion
1. Benzodiazepines	+ (?)	–	–
2. Amphetamine	–	+	–
3. Amitriptyline	+	–	+
4. Chloral Hydrate	–	+	+
5. Carbamazepine	+	–	–
6. Digitalis	+	–	+
7. Ethanol	–	+	–
8. Ethylene Glycol	–	+	–
9. Meprobamate	+	–	–
10. Methanol	–	+	–
11. Phenobarbital	+	+	+
12. Salicylates	+	+	–
13. Strychnine	–	+	–
14. Theophylline	+	+	+

Management of Specific Poisonings

(a) Overdose of Hypnotics-Sedatives (2, 13)

This is a common poisoning particularly in the comparatively affluent strata of society in India. Barbiturates are frequently involved in overdosage, and are generally taken with suicidal intent. The poisonous effect of a large dose of barbiturates is often potentiated by alcohol, by the simultaneous use of narcotics like opium, or by the ingestion of tranquilizers and antidepressants.

Clinical Features

Clinical features are characterized by progressive depression of the central nervous system culminating in paralysis of the brainstem and medulla. In the early stages, or in cases with mild overdose of sedative-hypnotics, there is ataxia and dysarthria with an altered sensorium, the clinical picture resembling acute alcoholic intoxication. Progressive depression of the CNS leads to stupor, followed by deepening coma. By the time the patient is in coma, his deep reflexes are not elicitable. There is flaccidity of the limbs, corneal reflexes are lost, conjugate doll's eye movements are absent, the pupils are dilated, and the respiration is feeble, shallow and irregular. Hypotension may be a prominent feature. These features signify severe depression of the brainstem and medulla. It is important to note that quite often a slight reaction of the pupils to a very strong light can be observed even when the patient has all other features of medullary paralysis. Death occurs from respiratory failure, severe hypotension due to vasomotor failure. Noncardiogenic pulmonary oedema may be observed. Hypothermia aggravates shock and hastens the end. Oliguria with renal failure can also occur.

Lethal Dose

The lethal dose of barbiturates cannot be stated with certainty. Short-acting barbiturates on the whole are more dangerous than long-acting ones. Blood levels compatible with a fatal outcome have varied from 10 mg/100 ml in long-acting barbiturates to 3 mg/100 ml in short-acting barbiturates. However patients with much higher blood levels have recovered, so that the finding of a raised barbiturate level in the blood does not necessarily constitute a prima facie evidence of death from barbiturate poisoning.

Diagnosis

The intensivist must bear in mind the numerous other causes of coma. It is important to ascertain that coma is not due to structural damage or organic disease within the brain. It is equally important to exclude all metabolic problems that can cause an impaired conscious state. The usual routine tests required for proper care have already been detailed earlier. Arterial blood gas analysis and a chest X-ray are both mandatory. A blood sample should be sent for estimation of barbiturate, bromide, glutethimide and phenothiazine levels.

Ingestion of non-barbiturate sedatives, such as chloral hydrate, glutethimide, methaqualone should be given differential consideration. Co-ingestion of alcohol, benzodiazepines is not uncommon in barbiturate poisoning with suicidal intent.

Management

This is based on the principles outlined above.

Cardiorespiratory Support is imperative in severe poisonings. Coma calls for prompt intubation. It is in our opinion important not to wait for the PaO_2 to fall to 60 mm Hg before initiating ventilator support. Ventilatory support is given to a comatose patient in anticipation of impending, worsening respiratory failure. Many of these patients have a dramatic and fairly abrupt fall in the PaO_2

to dangerously low levels, as also an abrupt rise in the PaCO$_2$. This should be anticipated and not awaited. Early ventilator support is therefore strongly advocated.

Gastric lavage should be done once ventilation and circulation are stable, provided the patient is brought within 2–4 hours of ingestion of the poison. Lavage in an unconscious patient should always be performed after a cuffed endotracheal tube has been inserted.

Activated charcoal is given repeatedly as outlined earlier.

Intake-output charts should be carefully kept, and fluid, electrolyte and acid-base balance should be carefully maintained.

Barbiturate poisoning is an indication for *forced diuresis with alkalinization of the urine,* in the hope that elimination of the drug is increased via the kidneys. Forced diuresis is more useful in poisoning by long-acting barbiturates which are largely excreted by the kidneys, than in short-acting barbiturates which are mainly metabolized by the liver. We have stopped using forced diuresis with alkalinization of the urine, as cardiorespiratory support with critical care suffices in the successful management of these patients.

Haemodialysis and haemoperfusion. These procedures in our opinion are rarely necessary. Their chief indication is in patients who are comatose and who are oliguric and in renal failure. They may also be used in patients who are known to have ingested large quantities of sedative-hypnotics, and who have blood phenobarbitone levels close to 100 µg/ml (levels of other barbiturates around 50 µg/ml). We have however found equally satisfactory results in these patients with just cardiorespiratory support and good overall critical care, provided renal function remains adequate.

(b) Narcotic Poisoning (2, 14)

Narcotic poisoning is encountered in patients attempting suicide with narcotics, and perhaps more frequently in addicts as a result of an accidental overdose. Children and elderly patients often show a marked sensitivity to morphine and other narcotics, so that serious toxic effects can occur with average usual doses. Myxoedema, adrenocortical insufficiency, chronic liver disease, renal failure, head injuries, and increased intracranial tension from any cause are important medical problems where the use of opium, morphine or heroin can prove disastrous.

The clinical features are characterized by increasing paralysis of the central nervous system with severe involvement of the brainstem. Unconsciousness, with extraselective depression of the respiratory centre (causing a very slow respiratory rate), and pin-point pupils, form a triad observed in narcotic poisoning. Bradycardia, hypotension, hypothermia also occur. Non-cardiogenic pulmonary oedema can occur in 50 per cent of the patients, particularly in heroin poisoning.

Organic or structural damage to the brainstem and organophosphorus poisoning can cause both coma and miosis. The intravenous atropine test is of great diagnostic value in organophosphorus poisoning. Organic or structural damage to the brainstem is associated with focal signs and disturbances in cranial nerve function or conjugate gaze. Patients with brainstem lesions are frequently hyperexcitable or have irregular breathing, rather than the slow shallow respiration observed in narcotic poisoning.

In addition to the toxic effect of a narcotic, an addict is exposed to a variety of neurological and infectious complications resulting from the use of crude adulterants (lactose, quinine etc), and various infectious agents (due to non-sterile administration). CNS complications from injections of heroin mixtures include toxic amblyopia and acute transverse myelopathy involving the cervical or thoracic cord resulting in paraplegia. Infective complications include sepsis, pyaemic abscesses, bacterial endocarditis most often involving the tricuspid valve, septic thrombophlebitis, Hepatitis B infection and HIV infection. Acute toxic myopathy with myoglobinuria causing renal failure, can occur after injections with adulterated heroin.

Management

The principles of management remain unaltered. Cardiorespiratory support, and in particular ventilator support is life-saving. Gastric lavage (with due precautions) should be done if the drugs have been taken orally.

Specific Antidote. Naloxone is fortunately a specific antidote. 0.4 to 0.8 mg is administered intravenously. When overdose is related to codeine, pentazocine or propoxyphen, a larger dose of 2 mg is given intravenously. Naloxone causes a dramatic improvement in respiration and circulation, the effect on respiration being observed within 2 minutes. It has however no effect on the pupils or on the level of consciousness. The drug has a short half-life and may need to be repeated frequently to reverse the effects of the narcotic on vital centres (**10**). If naloxone produces no effect on the shallow, slow respiration, the diagnosis of narcotic poisoning is questionable.

Complications of narcotic poisoning include pneumonia, atelectasis, pulmonary oedema, and bacterial endocarditis chiefly involving the tricuspid valve. These need critical care.

(c) Overdose with Tricyclic Antidepressants (15–18)

Tricyclic antidepressants such as amitriptyline, doxepin block uptake of norepinephrine in adrenergic nerves. Toxic effects are due to alpha-adrenergic blockade, strong anticholinergic activity and myocardial depression. As they reduce intestinal motility due to their anticholinergic effect, absorption may be slow and prolonged, increasing the half-life of the drug to 3–4 days.

Clinical Features

Peripheral anticholinergic effects include tachycardia, mydriasis, urinary retention, ileus, dry, hot skin, altered mental state, seizures and occasionally respiratory depression.

Cardiovascular effects include tachycardia, arrhythmias, atrioventricular block, hypotension. Hypotension is due to alpha-adrenergic blockade as also to myocardial depression. Death generally results from arrhythmias coupled with hypotension.

Diagnosis

A combination of anticholinergic effects and cardiovascular abnormalities should suggest the diagnosis. Tachycardia, prolonged PR interval and a prolonged QT interval on the ECG are commonly seen. The QRS interval is prolonged in patients with marked overdose; the mean QRS axis in the frontal plane is often upwards and to the right, causing a prominent R in avR and a prominent S in lead I and avF.

Management

(i) *Gastric lavage, use of activated charcoal and cardiorespiratory support* should be given according to principles stated earlier.

(ii) *Bicarbonate therapy.* Alkalinization of the blood to a pH of 7.5 is of great help. This reverses the major adverse effects of the drug including hypotension, arrhythmias and AV conduction abnormalities. Alkalinization can be achieved by using intravenous sodium bicarbonate in an appropriate dose, or by hyperventilation during ventilator support.

(iii) *Supportive care.* Severe agitation and seizures may necessitate the use of diazepam. Dysrhythmias which persist in spite of alkalinization, may need the use of suitable anti-arrhythmic drugs or cardioversion. Persistent hypotension may respond to a fluid challenge, or to the use of alpha-agonists like phenylephrine. Tricyclic antidepressants are strongly protein bound; hence haemodialysis or charcoal haemoperfusion does not help in eliminating the drug from the blood.

(d) Cocaine Poisoning (19–21)

Cocaine addicts are on the increase. The drug can be sniffed, taken orally, injected intravenously, and can be smoked in a free base form, or mixed with baking soda and water and smoked as the 'crack' form. Absorption from all sites is rapid.

Clinical Effects

Cardiovascular effects are most prominent. These include hypertension and arrhythmias. Hypertension may be severe enough to cause intracranial bleeding or an aortic dissection. Both supraventricular and ventricular arrhythmias may occur. Myocarditis has followed cocaine use; this is associated with gross ST-T changes on the ECG, and a rise in the CK-MB fraction. Cocaine is a vasoconstrictor, and this may result in organ ischaemia. Myocardial infarction, bowel infarction, renal infarction and ischaemia involving a limb, have all been noted to occur.

The CNS manifestations of cocaine are important—they may be the presenting feature. These include seizures, cerebral infarction, subarachnoid and intracerebral haemorrhage (22). Intracerebral aneurysms and arteriovenous malformations are frequent on angiographic examination. Overdosage of cocaine, even in addicts, can lead to severe mental obtundation and coma. Cocaine abuse should always be considered in the differential diagnosis of a stroke in young patients. Strokes may occur 24 hours after the use of cocaine. Though commoner in chronic cocaine use, they may also occur after the drug is used for the first time.

Severe cocaine intoxication can cause non-cardiogenic pulmonary oedema. Rhabdomyolysis and hyperthermia may occur with excessive muscle activity, particularly in those presenting with repeated seizures. Investigations should include an ECG, X-ray chest, CK estimation, urine for myoglobin. Relevant imaging studies of the head are necessary when CNS manifestations, in particular a neurologic focal deficit is observed. A toxicological screen for cocaine is asked for, to help diagnosis.

Differential Diagnosis

Overdose of sympathomimetic drugs, anticholenergic drugs, theophylline can produce a similar picture. Cocaine intoxication could be confused with CNS infections. Cocaine overdose, as stated earlier, should always enter into differential diagnosis of the aetiology of a stroke, particularly in young patients.

Management

Supportive measures include gastric lavage and the use of activated charcoal in those who have ingested the drug. Cardiorespiratory support is essential in acute severe overdosage.

Seizures should be controlled with diazepam, eptoin, and barbiturates. If uncontrolled and very frequent, the patient is paralyzed with a neuroparalytic drug, and kept on ventilator support.

Hypertension requires the use of antihypertensive drugs. Acute crisis may necessitate a titrated infusion of sodium nitroprusside.

Tachyrhythms may require the use of beta-blockers like esmolol or metoprolol. The patient needs to be observed to determine whether unopposed alpha-stimulation following beta-blockade does not worsen the hypertension.

Hyperthermia. Increase in body temperature may be marked in patients having repeated seizures. Physical methods to reduce temperature (cold sponges, wrapping a wet sheet and using a fan to help evaporation and promote cooling), should be used.

Rhabdomyolysis, when present is treated with intravenous fluids and alkalinization

(e) Organophosphorus or Insecticide Poisoning (23)

Organophosphates are found in insecticides and herbicides. Drinking organophosphorus compounds (chiefly TIK 20 or Parathion) with suicidal intent has been for the last 30 years, the commonest form of poisoning in the lower socio-economic strata of society in this country. Organophosphates act by causing irreversible inactivation of acetylcholinesterase. This results in the accumulation of acetylcholine at cholinergic receptors. Excess acetylcholine has muscarinic effects, nicotinic effects and toxic effects on the central nervous system.

Organophosphorus poisoning can occur from accidental ingestion of an insecticide, as also due to accidental dermal exposure. Inhalation via the lungs can also cause poisoning. Food, including stored grain contaminated by a spray of these insecticides has also been known to lead to severe toxicity.

Clinical Features

Peripheral muscarinic effects include bronchospasm, vomiting, diarrhoea, miosis, blurred vision, salivation, diaphoresis, lacrimation and urinary incontinence. Tachypnoea with severe respiratory distress is observed in many patients.

Nicotinic effects are chiefly observed in skeletal muscles—fasciculation, weakness and even paralysis.

Patients may have bradycardia or tachycardia and may be hypertensive or hypotensive, depending on whether the muscarinic or nicotinic effects predominate.

Excess of acetylcholine also has a toxic effect on the CNS—

confusion, seizures and ultimately coma result. The terminal picture is one of flaccid paralysis, respiratory cum peripheral circulatory failure, pulmonary oedema and deep coma. Respiratory failure is related to a combination of central depression, muscle weakness, bronchospasm and pulmonary oedema. Severe organophosphorous poisoning is characterized by multiple organ dysfunction and failure, the organs chiefly involved being the lungs, the cardiovascular system, the central nervous system and the renal system. High SOFA scores (> 10) are observed in some of these critically ill patients.

The recently described 'Intermediate Syndrome' occurs 1–4 days after an apparently well-treated cholinergic crisis. Its main clinical features are sudden respiratory paralysis, cranial motor nerve palsies, neck flexor muscle and proximal limb muscle weakness and paralysis. It has been documented for fenthion, diazinon, malathion, trichlorfon, dimethoate and sumithion. Treatment is by providing respiratory support; atropine and pralidoxime are ineffective. Recovery begins 5–15 days after onset of weakness (24, 25).

In some patients brought in a comatose state, increased motor tone resembling decorticate or decerebrate rigidity may be observed.

Diagnosis

Coma with pinpoint pupils should bring to mind the possibility of organophosphorus poisoning. There is often a characteristic garlic odour to the breath. This diagnosis can be proved by estimating cholinesterase levels in the blood. Levels below 50 per cent indicate intoxication. Treatment in suspected poisoning should be immediate.

Management (26, 27)

Gastric lavage should be given only if the patient is brought within 1 to 2 hours after the poisoning. Activated charcoal should be administered after the lavage.

Intravenous atropine is both of diagnostic and therapeutic value. A patient brought into a unit nearly dead with respiratory paralysis, coma, pulmonary oedema following organophosphorus poisoning can still be resuscitated with prompt use of atropine and good cardiorespiratory support.

A 2 mg dose of atropine is given slowly intravenously every 5 minutes till the pupils start to dilate. As much as 50–100 mg may need to be used in some patients. Once the pupils dilate to a normal size, atropine is stopped; if over a period of hours the pupils again constrict, further atropine is necessary. The continued use of atropine after the pupils have returned to normal size, can lead to atropine intoxication. Atropine antagonizes the muscarinic effect of excess acetylcholine and reduces the effect of the poison on the CNS. It has no action on the nicotinic effects on skeletal muscles, nor does it restore acetylcholinesterase.

Atropine also has no effect on respiratory paralysis. Ventilator support is necessary. PEEP may be used in the presence of pulmonary oedema, once the circulation and the blood pressure have stabilized.

Pralidoxime restores cholinesterase activity. The drug reverses the nicotinic effects of muscle weakness, and also reverses some of the CNS effects. It is used in conjunction with atropine. The dose of pralidoxime is 0.5–2 g (25–50 mg/kg), given intravenously over 5–15 minutes. Increased muscle strength and control of fasciculations are generally observed in 15–60 minutes. The drug can be repeated in 1–2 hours if muscle weakness and fasciculations persist or recur. Further doses of pralidoxime can be given every 6–12 hours if necessary.

In severe poisoning atropine and pralidoxime may need to be given for several days. The drugs are discontinued when clinical improvement is persistent and satisfactory, and when clinical features of toxicity do not recur, on withholding the drugs.

In many hospitals in the country, pralidoxime is not easily available. In its absence fresh blood transfusions should be tried.

Cardiorespiratory support is vital for survival. *Early intubation, ventilator support* (if necessary with PEEP) and *inotropic support* with dobutamine, dopamine, or even adrenaline are all necessary in hypotensive patients with respiratory failure. Support to all other organ systems is important as organophosphorous poisoning leads to multiple organ dysfunction and failure.

Charcoal haemoperfusion significantly increases the clearance of organophosphorus compounds and is indicated in severe poisoning.

Seizures may need symptomatic control with diazepam (10–20 mg intravenously) and by phenytoin sodium.

(f) Antihypertensives
Beta-blockers

Beta-blockers are among the most frequently used drugs in hypertensive patients. Patients may take a larger dose than that prescribed, by sheer accident, and manifest signs of drug toxicity. Rarely beta-blockers are consumed in large doses with suicidal intent. Toxicity generally occurs within 6 to 8 hours. Ingestion of extended release preparations and sotalol may be associated with delayed toxicity, necessitating observation for 24 to 48 hours.

Clinical findings of beta-blocker toxicity are hypotension, bradycardia and atrioventricular conduction abnormalities. The latter may take the form of first, second or third degree AV block. SA block is also observed and the QRS interval is often prolonged. In severe poisoning, the blood pressure is unrecordable, the cardiac output very low due to the depressant action of the drug on the myocardium, and the patient goes into cardiogenic shock. Death is due to asystole (28, 29).

The more lipophilic beta-blockers like propranalol, metoprolol, timolol, for unclear reasons can cause CNS dysfunction in the form of delirium, seizures and coma, even in the absence of significant hypotension. Hypoglycaemia may be observed.

Treatment

Patients who present within 2 to 4 hours after ingestion should benefit by gastric lavage. Activated charcoal should be given and the dose can be repeated. Patients who appear stable should be closely monitored for 24 to 48 hours.

Bradycardia and hypotension are initially treated with intravenous atropine and a volume load with isotonic saline. If bradycardia and hypotension persist, the specific drug to use is glucagon 5 mg intravenously; the dose can be increased to 10 mg if the response is poor. If a response to glucagon is satisfactory, the drug is given in an intravenous infusion at the rate of 10 mg/hour.

Calcium chloride 10 per cent may be given intravenously slowly up to a maximum of 3 g. This improves cardiac contractility and helps to reverse hypotension.

Catecholamine infusions should also be started if hypotension is severe and persistent. Very often a combination of dopamine, dobutamine and epinephrine or norepinephrine is used; very large doses may be necessary to produce a satisfactory response. The danger of tachyarrhythmias due to large doses of inotropes should be kept in mind. If a marked bradyrhythm persists, ventricular pacing is given a try. Pacing may increase the heart rate without increasing blood pressure or cardiac output. At times the pacemaker fails to capture.

In critically ill patients, management is helped by haemodynamic measurements made through a Swan-Ganz catheter.

Calcium Channel Blockers (30)

Calcium channel blockers are also frequently used in the management of hypertension. The most commonly used calcium channel blockers are verapamil, diltiazem and nifedipine. These drugs are well absorbed from the gastrointestinal tract; they are metabolized in the liver.

Calcium channel blockers in an overdose have a marked negative inotropic effect on the heart and induce severe peripheral vasodilatation. Patients present with bradycardia, hypotension and various degrees of heart block that may result in death.

Treatment

Calcium is administered intravenously. More often than not the result is unsatisfactory, as the calcium channels are blocked, so that additional calcium has little or no effect.

Glucagon should be used in the manner outlined for beta-blocker overdose. Atropine, 1 mg intravenously may help to increase the heart rate in some patients. Hypotension should be further combated by a volume load and by catecholamine infusions. As in the treatment of beta-blocker overdose, a combination of dopamine, dobutamine, and epinephrine or norepinephrine may be necessary. Transvenous pacing should be done in patients with severe heart block.

(g) Sympathomimetic Drug Overdose (30)

Sympathomimetic drugs like amphetamine and methamphetamine are very popular drugs of abuse. However sympathomimetic drugs are also present in over the counter preparations for 'cold', for appetite control, and include stimulants such as caffeine, ephedrine and pseudoephedrine.

These drugs (amphetamine and methamphetamine are classic examples) in an overdose, cause an excessive release of catecholamines—epinephrine and norepinephrine, resulting in a sympathomimetic toxidrome. The latter is characterized by tachycardia, hypertension, agitation, restlessness, anxiety and mydriasis. Hallucinations, acute and often paranoid psychosis and seizures

may occur. The psychosis is indistinguishable from that observed in schizophrenia. It is temporary, but may take weeks or even months to disappear.

Other cardiovascular and CNS effects observed with severe overdose include myocardial ischaemia, arrhythmias, strokes, intracranial haemorrhage. Hyperthermia, rhabdomyolysis, renal failure and diarrhoea may also occur.

Methamphetamine is more frequently used than amphetamine as a drug of abuse. It is termed 'ice' or 'crank'; the drug can be ingested, smoked, inhaled or given intravenously. Another amphetamine-like drug increasingly used not only in the West but also in India and many countries of the world is 3-4 methylenedroxymethamphetamine. It is popularly called 'Ecstasy' and acts both as a stimulant and hallucinogen. It produces the serotonin syndrome by inducing a release of serotonin in the brain and inhibiting its re-uptake. Besides its hallucinogenic and stimulant effect, the drug induces continuous physical activity. Complications include hyperthermia, rhabdomyolysis, circulatory collapse, strokes, intracranial haemorrhage and multiple organ dysfunction syndrome.

Diagnosis

When no history is available the sympathomimetic toxic syndrome should be distinguished from thyrotoxicosis, alcohol or benzodiazepine withdrawal, from poisoning caused by tricyclic antidepressants, and from symptoms induced by the interaction of monoamine inhibitors with other drugs.

Treatment

Treatment is directed to countering the CVS and CNS effects. Acute hypertension is an emergency that should be promptly controlled. A titrated solution of sodium nitroprusside given in an intravenous infusion is the quickest method to control a sharp rise in the blood pressure. Labetalol is a good choice in patients who have marked tachycardia and hypertension. Other beta-blockers should be avoided as increasingly severe hypertension could result from beta 2 adrenergic block and unopposed alpha-adrenergic stimulation.

Antiarrhythmics like verapamil or adenosine are used to revert supraventricular arrhythmias.

Seizures should be treated with benzodiapines, phenytoin and phenobarbitol. Benzodiapines are probably the drugs of choice in the management of psychosis. Hyperthermia can be lethal. Abolishing seizures and restlessness with benzodiapine and physical cooling of the skin by appropriate methods are important.

Myocardial ischaemia requires close ECG monitoring and serial cardiac enzyme estimation. Tachycardia should be controlled; nitrates either orally or as an intravenous infusion of nitroglycerine should be administered.

(h) Aspirin (Salicylate) Poisoning (2, 31)

Aspirin is one of the most commonly and widely used drugs today. Remarkably enough, poisoning with aspirin is rarely encountered in our country. The drug is available and sold over the counter as an aspirin preparation *per se*, or in combination with other drugs. Methyl salicylate (Oil of Wintergreen) poisoning occurs at times in children who ingest it because of its pleasant smell. This formulation contains as much as 7 g of aspirin per teaspoon, compared to the usual 300–600 mg aspirin per tablet in the usual aspirin preparations.

Aspirin after oral ingestion, reaches a peak level in the blood after 2 hours. It is metabolized in the liver, is also excreted by the kidneys and has a half-life of 4–6 hours. When an overdose is taken, the hepatic enzymes become saturated and the drug's half-life increases to 18–36 hours. The drug can now only be eliminated via the kidneys. When blood levels are high (> 40–50 mg/dl), serious toxic effects can occur.

It is best to consider patients with aspirin or salicylate poisoning as falling into 2 groups—those who ingest the drug with suicidal intent, and those who take the drug on a long-term basis to counter pain. Overdose with aspirin in the latter group can have subtle manifestations which are easily missed and which contribute significantly to morbidity and mortality.

Clinical Features

Tinnitus, vertigo, vomiting and impairment of hearing are frequent. Mental confusion, restlessness, excitability may resemble alcoholic intoxication. Sweating, dehydration and hypotension are often observed. In severe cases hallucinations, seizures, coma and death occur.

Salicylates initially stimulate the respiratory centre and induce hyperventilation with a respiratory alkalosis. They also directly cause a metabolic acidosis with an increase in the anion gap. Thus a combination of respiratory alkalosis with metabolic acidosis should strongly suggest the possibility of salicylate or aspirin poisoning. In children, or following large doses in adults, there can be a depression of the respiratory centre so that a combination of respiratory plus metabolic acidosis results with a life-threatening fall in the arterial blood pH.

Large doses produce haemorrhage due to hypoprothombinaemia. Haematemesis and malaena may result from acute erosive gastritis and duodenitis. Cerebral oedema can occur and non-cardiogenic pulmonary oedema results from increased capillary permeability. Salicylates uncouple the phosphoregulation process; this leads to increased glucose utilization, an increased metabolic rate and increased oxygen consumption. The clinical effects of the above are hypoglycaemia and fever.

It is extremely important to note that features of hyperventilation, seizures, dehydration and even coma, can occur in patients with chronic poisoning, even when salicylate levels are not inordinately high (35–50 mg/dl).

Diagnosis

The diagnosis may be difficult in the absence of a relevant history. Chronic overdose in patients is very easily missed.

The occurrence of metabolic acidosis + respiratory alkalosis, in the absence of diabetes and renal failure should suggest the possibility of salicylate poisoning. The diagnosis can be proved by measuring salicylate levels in blood. This can be done at the bedside by doing the Phensitix test which detects salicylates in the plasma if the level is more than 20 mg/dl.

Common laboratory findings in salicylism include an elevated anion gap metabolic acidosis, increased prothrombin time, hypernatraemia, hypo- or hyperglycaemia, ketonaemia, hypokalaemia, and increased levels of liver transaminases.

The differential diagnosis is from poisoning by CNS stimulants which can also cause an altered mental state, confusion, diaphoresis. Alcoholic ketoacidosis and other causes of metabolic acidosis need to be distinguished from salicylate poisoning. Encephalitis may present with hyperventilation, mental confusion and respiratory alkalosis. Sepsis can also be characterized by respiratory alkalosis or a combination of respiratory alkalosis plus metabolic acidosis.

Management

Lavage and the repeated use of *activated charcoal* are important. Lavage may be helpful even 12–24 hours after ingestion of the drug.

Correction of dehydration and shock, and efficient cardiorespiratory support are of prime importance. *Maintenance of electrolyte and acid-base balance* is crucial for survival in severe poisoning. Severe metabolic acidosis should be promptly corrected with 75–150 ml of intravenous sodium bicarbonate (see Chapter on Acid-Base Disturbances in the Critically Ill).

Use of forced diuresis with alkalinization of the urine. In an alkaline medium, salicylates remain in the ionized form and do not diffuse into the tissues. Alkalinizing the urine facilitates excretion of salicylates. One should aim to maintain a urine pH of 7.5–8. Salicylism is one poisoning where forced diuresis with alkalinization should as far as possible be attempted. The simplest method of alkalinization is to use 1 l of half strength (0.45 per cent) saline, to which is added 2 ampoules of 7.5 per cent sodium bicarbonate and infuse this at the rate of 150–250 ml/hr. Potassium deficits are appropriately replaced. Intravenous mannitol 300 ml, as also furosemide 40 mg intravenously may be administered to increase diuresis. The intake should continue to keep pace with the output, and it is important to check serum electrolytes frequently so that electrolyte balance is well maintained. Hypernatraemia, cerebral and pulmonary oedema are complications that need to be carefully watched for.

Haemodialysis and haemoperfusion (**32**). These very effectively reduce salicylate levels in blood and are indicated under the following circumstances:

(i) Serum levels > 120 mg/dl in acute poisonings observed within 6 hours of ingestion, or >100 mg/dl if observed after 6 hours of ingestion of the poison.

(ii) Chronic toxicity when blood level exceeds 60 mg/dl.

(iii) In patients with renal failure and /or hepatic dysfunction.

(iv) In the presence of pulmonary oedema which prevents the use of forced diuresis and alkalinization.

(v) In the presence of severe neurological toxicity—coma or seizures.

(vi) In the presence of clinical deterioration in spite of conservative conventional management.

Symptomatic measures. Seizures may need the use of diazepam; blood transfusions may be necessary to replace blood lost in haematemesis. Vitamin K should be given to counter hypoprothrombinaemia. Hypovolaemia should be treated by fluid infusions.

Non-cardiogenic pulmonary oedema can result from the effect of salicylates on pulmonary capillaries. Intubation and ventilator support then become necessary.

(i) Paracetamol (Acetaminophen) Poisoning (12)

Paracetamol is an antipyretic and analgesic very frequently used in medical practice. Overdose with suicidal intent is one of the commonest poisonings in the West, but is uncommon in our country. Patients may suffer poisoning from the drug by inadvertently consuming excessive quantities in an attempt to treat their own pain and fever. It is important to bear in mind the fact that paracetamol is often present in combination with other drugs bearing different brand names.

The drug after ingestion is metabolized in the liver via the cytochrome P 450 oxidase system. Excessive quantities of paracetamol deplete glutathione stores. This leads to accumulation of toxic metabolites that are severely hepatotoxic and can result in massive hepatic necrosis. In adults doses of less than 125 mg/kg are rarely toxic except when patients have pre-existing liver disease. Doses of 125–250 mg/kg result in varying toxicity, some patients suffering severe liver damage. Doses > 250 mg/kg invariably give rise to liver cell damage and often to massive hepatic necrosis. Death occurs within 4–15 days after ingestion of the drug in these patients.

Clinical Features

Patients with an overdose of paracetamol are minimally symptomatic in the first 24 hours. Sweating, nausea, vomiting may be observed. Hepatotoxicity starts after 24–48 hours, and is characterized by deepening jaundice, mental confusion, asterixis. Drowsiness progresses to coma; hypoglycaemia and excessive bleeding are observed. Death occurs from acute hepatic failure. The serum transaminases and bilirubin show a progressive rise *pari passu* with the clinical deterioration. The prothrombin time is markedly elevated and the serum ammonia levels are high.

Acute tubular necrosis with renal failure can also occur. Pancreatitis, myocardial dysfunction and hypersensitivity reactions have been reported.

Laboratory Investigations

The most important test is the serum acetaminophen level. It should be done 4 hours after ingestion of the drug. If this is over 150 µg/ml, the patient is at risk for massive hepatic necrosis and should be promptly treated with N-acetylcysteine.

Liver function tests need to be done and followed-up at periodic intervals in patients who show hepatotoxicity.

Management (33, 34)

(i) *Gastric lavage* is essential and should be given if the patient is admitted within 6 hours of ingestion of the drug. Activated charcoal should also be given if the time lag between ingestion of the poison and admission to a unit is < 6 hours. Activated charcoal also absorbs the antidote N-acetylcysteine, but the dose of the latter can be suitably increased. Lavage and use of activated charcoal are not likely to help in late admissions to hospital or to a critical care unit.

(ii) *Use of N-acetylcysteine* (35). The antidote is indicated (a) in patients who have consumed excess quantities of the drug; (b) in those with toxic serum levels as indicated earlier; (c) in those showing evidence of impaired hepatic function.

The drug is most effective when given within the first 8 hours of ingestion. After this period, its efficacy decreases, but it should nevertheless be given. There is no benefit in giving acetylcysteine in the first 4 hours after ingestion. The drug acts by increasing depleted glutathione stores, and by providing a glutathione substitute to allow for degradation and detoxification of metabolites of paracetamol within the liver.

N-acetylcysteine is usually given orally in a loading dose of 140 mg/kg followed by 70 mg/kg every 4 hours for 3 days. This antidote may unfortunately cause vomiting. Prochlorperazine or metoclopramide may be used to counter the latter. The drug can also be used intravenously in the same dose as stated above in patients where severe vomiting precludes oral use. It is best given in 500 ml of a diluent over a period of 2 hours.

(iii) *Supportive care* for liver cell failure is important. This has been discussed in another chapter.

(j) Carbon Monoxide Poisoning (36)

Carbon monoxide (CO) has a 200 times greater affinity for Hb compared to oxygen. It therefore readily displaces oxygen from oxyhaemoglobin (HbO_2), which is converted to carboxyhaemoglobin (HbCO). Severe tissue hypoxia results and this can cause death. An exposure concentration of 0.4 per cent of CO is fatal within an hour. Carbon monoxide is solely eliminated via the lungs, the time taken to reach half the original concentration being about 4 hours breathing air, and about 80 minutes breathing 100 per cent oxygen.

Clinical Features

Tissue hypoxia results in a loss of consciousness followed by respiratory failure. Circulation may continue for some minutes after respiration has failed. There is a cherry pink colour to the skin, nails and mucosa.

Diagnosis

This is generally obvious in the circumstances in which a patient is found. At times carbon monoxide poisoning is insidious. A slow gas leak may not be evident, and the diagnosis in a patient found unconscious in such circumstances is easily missed. A diagnosis of a brainstem infarct is erroneously made. Hypoxia produces lactic acid acidosis and a common finding is low arterial blood pH, a normal PaO_2 with lactic acid acidosis. A low oxygen saturation in the presence of a normal or near normal PaO_2, should promptly arouse suspicion of carbon monoxide poisoning or methaemoglobinaemia.

For the estimation of carbon monoxide, 3 ml of heparinized blood is collected under liquid paraffin, and sent to the laboratory. Spectroscopic examination of the blood reveals the typical band of carboxyhaemoglobin (HbCO), and confirms the clinical diagnosis. A rough but simple bedside test for carboxyhaemoglobin is as follows—1 ml of patient's blood is added to 10 ml distilled water plus 1 ml of 5 per cent NaOH. Carboxyhaemoglobin is present if the solution turns straw yellow (HbCO < 20 per cent), or remains pink (HbCO > 20 per cent). An HbO_2 solution turns brown.

Management

This involves immediate cardiorespiratory support. The patient is quickly intubated and put on ventilator support with 100 per cent oxygen. When facilities are available, hyperbaric oxygen at 2 atmospheres pressure rapidly produces dissociation of carbon monoxide from haemoglobin, and this promptly corrects tissue hypoxia. Hyperbaric oxygen if available, can help resuscitate even moribund patients.

If resuscitation from carbon monoxide poisoning is delayed, serious neurological sequelae can result even after complete recovery of consciousness.

(k) Cyanide Poisoning (36)

This is the quickest acting poison. It affects the cytochrome oxidase system within the cells thus preventing the latter from utilizing oxygen. 'Strangulation' literally occurs at the cellular level. Death occurs within a few minutes following inhalation or ingestion. Oral ingestion of hydrocyanic acid acts more slowly, death occurring within an hour. An odour of bitter almonds and the sudden catastrophic episode, point to the diagnosis.

Clinical features include coma, rigidity, respiratory depression, bradycardia and hypotension. A patient brought alive to the ICU immediately after ingestion of cyanide showed deep coma, marked bradycardia, hypotension, absent brainstem reflexes, severe rigidity and extensor thrusts as in a decerebrate state. Plantars were unelicitable. A diagnosis of a brainstem infarct or haemorrhage was entertained. The correct diagnosis was made retrospectively after the patient miraculously recovered just on cardiorespiratory support after a period of 10 hours. He confessed to ingesting a powder, which on analysis contained cyanide.

Management

(i) Immediate inhalation of amyl nitrate pearls (one every 2 minutes), should be followed by an intravenous injection of 10–15 ml of 3 per cent solution of sodium nitrate given over 5 minutes. The above measures produce a methaemoglobinaemia, and the cyanide is bound as stable cyanmethaemoglobin.

(ii) The next step is the administration of 50 ml of a 25 per cent solution of sodium thiosulfate. This helps conversion of cyanide liberated from cyanmethaemoglobin to thiocyanate.

Cyanide is rapidly destroyed in the body, so that if the patient can be tided over a period of a few hours, recovery may well occur.

(l) Methyl Alcohol (Methanol) Poisoning (37, 38)

Poisoning occurs through ingestion of methylated spirit due to suicidal intent or as a substitute for ethyl alcohol. Adulteration of ethyl alcohol with methanol is very common in what is termed in India as 'country liquor'.

Clinical Features

Toxic effects may occur after a latent period of 12–24 hours. These effects are caused directly by methanol as also by formic acid, into which some of the methyl alcohol is oxidized. An increase in formaldehyde in the blood is observed, which is also responsible for toxic symptoms. These include epigastric pain, vomiting, features of intoxication as in alcohol intoxication, and visual symptoms. The latter are chiefly characterized by blurred vision that may progress to blindness due to optic atrophy. Severe metabolic acidosis is also observed. Death may occur in coma from respiratory failure.

Laboratory Investigations

Metabolic acidosis with an increase in the anion gap is observed. An elevated osmolar gap may also occur.

Management (39)

(i) *Counter acidosis.* Intravenous sodium bicarbonate is administered to counter severe acidosis. Large amounts may need to be given because toxic acid metabolites are produced in large quantities. *Hypernatraemia may result from large doses of sodium bicarbonate.*

(ii) *Block or reduce toxic metabolites.* This is achieved by the administration of ethanol orally or intravenously. The dose of ethanol in an adult is 2 ml/kg of 50 per cent ethanol orally or 10 per cent ethanol intravenously. Ethanol infusions if given intravenously should be at the rate of 0.05–0.1 mg/kg/hr to provide ethanol levels of 100–150 mg/dl. Alcohol dehydrogenase which metabolizes methanol has a higher affinity for ethyl alcohol, and preferentially metabolizes the latter. The methanol therefore remains unmetabolized with less resulting toxic effects.

(iii) *Haemodialysis.* After the above measures are instituted, haemodialysis is used to remove both methanol and its toxic metabolites from the blood.

(iv) *Supportive treatment.* Folic acid in large doses (50 mg 8 hrly) is given to these patients. Fluid and electrolyte balance needs to be carefully maintained.

(m) Ferrous Sulphate (Iron) Poisoning

Soluble iron when ingested in a marked overdose produces intense vomiting, circulatory collapse, and at times even perforation of the stomach. Jaundice, metabolic acidosis, coma and respiratory failure are observed.

The specific antidote is deferoxamine mesylate (Desferal). This antidote combines with iron to form a harmless compound which is excreted in the urine. After a gastric lavage with 10 per cent sodium bicarbonate, 5–7 g of desferal in 100–200 ml of water is given orally. 2 g of desferal in 6 ml distilled water is given intramuscularly, and the drug is then given in a slow intravenous drip at the rate of 7–10 mg/kg/hr. The maximum dose should not exceed 80 mg/kg in 24 hours.

Calcium EDTA has also been used in a dose of 35–40 mg/kg/day orally, and in the same dosage intravenously over 24 hours.

Haemodialysis is effective in severe poisoning.

REFERENCES

1. Zimmerman JL, Rudis M. (2001). Poisonings. In: Critical Care Medicine (Eds Parrillo JE, Dellinger RP). pp. 1501–1524. Mosby, USA.

2. Mokhlesi B, Leikin J, Murray P et al. (2003). Adult Toxicology in Critical Care. Part I: General Approach to the Intoxicated Patient. Chest. 123, 577–592.

3. Bryson PD (ed.). (1989). Comprehensive review in toxicology, 2nd edn. Aspen Publications, Rockville, MD.

4. Ellenhorn MJ, Barceloux DG (eds). (1988). Medical Toxicology: Diagnosis and Treatment of Human Poisoning. Elsevier, New York.

5. Noji EK, Kelen EK (eds). (1989). Manual of toxicologic emergencies. Year Book Medical Publishers, Chicago.

6. Litovitz TL et al. (1991). Annual Report of the American Association of Poison Control Centers National Data Collection System. Am J Emerg Med. 9, 461–509.

7. Kulling P, Persson H. (1986). Role of the intensive care unit in the management of the poisoned patient. Med Toxicol. 1, 375–386.

8. Vernon DD, Gleich MC. (1997). Poisoning and drug overdosage. Crit Care Clin. 13(3), 647–667.

9. Hall AH. (1991). Gastrointestinal decontaminations: Sifting through supportive therapeutic options. Emerg Med Reports. 12, 171–178.

10. Vale JA. (1997). American Academy of Clinical Toxicology, European Association of Poison Centres and Clinical Toxicologists. Position statement: Gastric Lavage. J Toxicol Clin Toxicol. 35, 711–719

11. Vale JA, Krenzelok EP, Barceloux GD et al. (1999). American Academy of Clinical Toxicology/European Association of Poisons Centres and Clinical Toxicologists; Position statement and practice guidelines on the use of multi-dose activated charcoal in the treatment of acute poisoning. J Toxicol Clin Toxicol. 37, 731–751

12. Birnbaumer D. (2002). Poisonings and Ingestions. In: Current Critical Care Diagnosis and Treatment (Eds Bongard FS, Sue DY). pp. 829–864. McGraw-Hill, USA.

13. Gaudreault P. (1981). Barbiturates. Clin Toxicol Rev. 3,1.

14. Ungar JR, Schwartz GR, Levine DG. (1992). Drug and substance abuse emergencies. In: Principles and Practice of Emergency Medicine. 3rd edn (Schwartz GR et al.). Lea and Febiger.

15. Frommer DA, Kulig KW, Mark JA et al. (1987). Tricyclic antidepressant overdose: A review. JAMA. 257, 521–526.

16. Smilkstein MJ. (1990). Reviewing cyclic antidepressant cardiotoxicity: Wheat and Chaff. J Emerg Med. 8, 645–648.

17. Marshall JB, Forker AD. (1982). Cardiovascular effects of tricyclic antidepressant drugs: Therapeutic usage, overdose, and management of complications. Am J Cardiol. 103, 401.

18. Kerr GW, Mcguffie AC, Wilkies. (2001). Tricyclic antidepressant overdose: A review. Emerg Med J. 18, 236–241.

19. Derlet RW, Albertson TE. (1989). Emergency department presentation of cocaine intoxication. Ann Emerg Med. 18, 182–186.

20. Jacobs IG, Rosziler MH, Kelly JK et al. (1989). Cocaine abuse: neurovascular complications. Radiology. 170, 223–227.

21. Muller PD, Benowitz NL, Olson KR. (1990). Cocaine. Emerg Med Clin North Am. 8, 481–493.

22. Lichtenfeld PJ, Rubin DB, Feldman RS. (1984). Subarachnoid haemorrhage precipitated by cocaine snorting. Arch Neurol. 411, 223.

23. Lee P, Jai DY. (2001). Clinical features of patients with organophosphorus poisoning requiring intensive care. Intensive Care Med. 27, 694–699.

24. De Bleecker JL, De Reuck JL, Willems JL. (1992). Neurological aspects of organophosphate poisoning. Clin Neurol Neurosurg. 94(2), 93–103.

25. Senanayake N, Karalliede L. (1987). Neurotoxic effects of organophosphorus insecticides. N Engl J Med. 316, 761–763.

26. Finelstein Y, Kushnir A, Raikhlin-Eisenkraft B, Taitelman U. (1989). Antidotal therapy of severe acute organophosphate poisoning: A multi-hospital study. Neurotoxicol Teratol. 11, 593.

27. Bardin PG, Van Edden SF, Joubert JR. (1987). Intensive care management of acute organophosphate poisoning: A 7 year experience in the Western Cape. S Afr Med J. 9, 593.

28. Kerns W, Kline, Ford MD. (1994). Beta blocker and calcium channel blocker toxicity. Emerg Med Clin North Am. 12, 365–390.

29. Love JN, Howell JM, Litovitz TL et al. (2000). Acute beta blocker overdose, factor associated with the development of cardiovascular morbidity. J Toxicol Clin Toxicol. 38, 275–281.

30. Mokhlesi B, Leikin J, Murray P et al. (2003). Adult Toxicology in Critical Care. Part II: Specific Poisonings. Chest. 123(3), 897–922.

31. Woolf A. (1990). Salicylates. Clin Tox Rev. 12, 1.

32. Jacobsen D, Wiik-Larsen E, Bredersen JE. (1988). Hemodialysis or hemoperfusion in severe salicylate poisoning. Hum Toxicol. 7, 161.

33. Clark J. (2001). Acetaminophen poisoning and the use of intravenous acetylcysteine. Am Med J. 20, 16–17.

34. Kozer E, Koren G. (2001). Management of paracetamol overdose. Drug Saf. 24, 503–512.

35. Smilkstein MJ, Knapp GL, Kulig KW et al. (1988). Efficacy of oral N-acetylcysteine in the treatment of acetaminophen overdose. N Engl J Med. 319, 1557.

36. Corbridge TC, Murray P. (1998). Toxicology in Adults. In: Principles of Critical Care (Eds Hall JB, Schmidt GA, Wood LDH). pp. 1473–1525. McGraw-Hill, USA.

37. McMartin K, Ambre JJ, Tephly TR. (1980). Methanol poisoning in human subjects. Role for formic acid accumulation in the metabolic acidosis. Am J Med. 68, 414.

38. Jacobsen D, McMartin KE. (1986). Methanol and ethylene glycol poisonings: Mechanism of toxicity, clinical course, diagnosis and treatment. Med Toxicol. 1, 309–334.

39. McCoy HG, Cipolle RJ, Ehlers SM et al. (1979). Severe methanol poisoning: Application of a pharmacokinetic model for ethanol therapy and hemodialysis. Am J Med. 67, 804–807.

CHAPTER 18.4

Envenomation in the ICU

General Considerations

Envenomation from snake bites is an important medical emergency in India, Bangladesh, Sri Lanka, Africa, South America and in the greater part of South East Asia. In the last two decades of the twentieth century the annual death rate from snake bites in Brazil was about 4 per 100,000, in Burma 15 per 100,000 and in the United States about 2000 per year. In Europe death from snake bite is rare, but in India and Bangladesh there must be probably about 100 deaths every day from snake bite. Snake bite is estimated to account for a tenth as much mortality as malaria. This would roughly amount to over 100,000 deaths per annum. Unfortunately there is no global strategy against snake bite as there is against malaria. There is a tremendous shortage in the availability of snake antivenin all over the world, particularly in India and Africa. Research, development and funding for antivenin appear to have sadly lost momentum.

There are over 3500 species or kinds of snakes in the world, of which about 375 are poisonous (1–4). The important poisonous families are:

(i) Elapidae (cobras, kraits, mambas, coral snakes), found all over the world except in Europe.

(ii) Viperidae (true vipers), and the Crotalidae (pit vipers and rattle snakes).

(iii) Colubridae, seen as a few species with rear fangs in Africa.

(iv) Hydrophiidae (sea snakes) found in the sea close to the coastline, and in large collections of fresh water.

The common varieties of poisonous snakes in India are cobras, the common krait, Russell's viper, the E. carinatus and sea snakes. The cobras include the common Indian cobra and the King cobra. The krait is a small but extremely poisonous snake and includes the common krait and the banded krait. The vipers include the pit vipers, so called because of a 'pit' below the eyes, and the true vipers. The heads of the cobra and the Russell's viper are illustrated in **Fig. 18.4.1**.

All poisonous snakes have two fangs attached in front to the upper jaw, through which snake venom is injected into the prey. Fangs are specially developed teeth, either grooved or tubular. Poison glands (secreting venom or poison) are present on either side of the upper jaw. A duct carries the poison from the gland to the base of the fang on either side. When the snake bites, the poison gland is squeezed through the ducts into the fangs, and enters the prey (**Fig. 18.4.2**).

Composition and Effects of Snake Venom (5, 6)

Snake venoms contain numerous toxic proteins and proteolytic enzymes. The Indian Cobra contains a neurotoxin, a haemolysin,

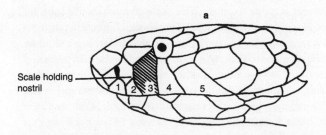
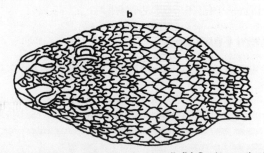

Scale holding nostril

Fig. 18.4.1. (a) A Cobra head showing the large third labial scale which touches the eye and the scale containing the nostril. **(b)** Scales on the head of a Russell's Viper. Note triangular head with small scales (from Vakil RJ, Udwadia FE. 1982. Diagnosis and Management of Medical Emergencies. OUP, Mumbai).

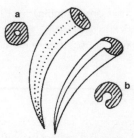

Fig. 18.4.2. (a) Canalized fang of a Russell's Viper. **(b)** Grooved fang of a Cobra (source as in Fig. 18.4.1).

a cardiotoxin, cholinesterases, phosphatases, phospholipase B, glycerophosphate, nucleotidase and an enzyme inhibiting cytochrome oxidase. The neurotoxins in cobra venom are polypeptide toxins. α-bungorotoxin and cobrotoxin are postsynaptic (α) neurotoxins that bind to acetylcholine receptors at the motor endplate. β- bungorotoxin is a presynaptic (β) neurotoxin that releases acetylcholine at the nerve endings and then damages the end-plate, so that further release of acetylcholine is arrested.

The viper venom besides containing digestive enzymes, hyaluronidase also contains a thrombin like factor X and a prothrombin activating factor.

Snake venom produces the following effects:

(i) Neurotoxic—This results in a curare-like paralysis of voluntary muscles, a paralysis of the muscles supplied by the cranial nerves, and terminally paralysis of the brainstem and medulla.

(ii) Necrotizing—the toxin causes severe inflammation and local necrosis.

(iii) Haemolytic and haemorrhagic—the toxin causes intravascular haemolysis and results in severe haemorrhage due to interference with and depletion of normal clotting factors.

(iv) Shock—which is produced by exudation of fluid into the bitten extremity, by vasodilatation with a generalized increase in capillary permeability, and by severe haemolysis and haemorrhage. In viperine bites, shock may occur before the local features are clinically marked, and before the occurence of haemorrhage or haemolysis.

The venom of elapids (cobra, kraits, coral snake) chiefly produces a neurotoxic effect, though some degree of haemolysis and local tissue necrosis may also occur.

The venom of viperidae (vipers) produces a severe local necrotizing lesion, haemolysis, disturbance in the coagulation mechanism with profuse haemorrhage and shock.

Clinical Features

Before discussing the clinical features the following points deserve notice.

(i) A bite from a poisonous snake does not necessarily cause envenomation. The patient might have been protected by clothing, or the snake may have emptied its poison on an earlier prey, so that very little or no venom may enter the patient.

(ii) A bite by any snake even if non-poisonous, can cause severe fright. A patient may faint from fright. Death has been known to occur from severe fright and acute panic. A history of the patient

turning violent and agitated soon after a bite is the result of a hysterical reaction induced by fright; it is not due to envenomation.

(iii) A bite from a poisonous snake leaves 2 prominent fang marks. Absence of clear fang marks in the wound points to a non-poisonous snake. The bite in the latter case takes the form of a inverted U (∩) without fang marks.

(iv) Envenomation is invariably far more serious in children than in adults.

(v) The presence of pathogenic bacteria in the mouth of the snake or on the skin of the victim, can lead to secondary infection of the wound. Tetanus and clostridial infections can complicate bites of poisonous and non-poisonous snakes.

(vi) If the victim is perfectly well 6–8 hours after a bite, the snake is generally non-poisonous. Exceptions are observed with some species of viperidae when acute haemolysis or a haemorrhagic tendency may manifest 24 hours or even later after a bite. However, even in these patients, some degree of local inflammation around the bite is invariably present.

Cobra Bite

A burning pain is felt over the bite in 5 minutes, often followed by a numbness around the wound which may spread a variable distance up the limb. A red inflamed ring is generally present around the fang marks, but the degree of inflammation is never as marked or necrotizing as with viperine bites.

The systemic effects are observed within 10 minutes to 2 hours of the bite. Early symptoms, before objective neurological features appear, include vomiting, vertigo, circumoral paraesthesia, excessive salivation, blurring of vision, and heaviness of the eyelids. This is followed by an increasing weakness and ataxia of the limbs so that the patient is unsteady and finds it difficult to walk. A progressive curare-like paralysis involves muscles supplied by the cranial nerves and skeletal muscles, so that muscle power is reduced and ultimately lost. Ptosis followed by a varying degree of ophthalmoplegia is generally the first paralytic sign to be observed. The pupils are increasingly dilated and fixed. Paralysis of the palate and pharynx make swallowing difficult, so that secretions collect in the back of the throat. The muscles of the tongue are often involved early; the tongue can be protruded with difficulty, and it feels heavy and stiff so that speech is indistinct. Salivation is often increased, and when associated with an inability to close the mouth and the lips, leads to continuous dribbling of saliva. Weakness of the muscles of the neck allows the head to fall forwards on the chest if the patient is made to sit up. The skeletal muscles are soon involved leading to a well-nigh total paralysis. Ultimately, paralysis involves the muscles of respiration, so that breathing is shallow and irregular. The patient hypoventilates and has both hypoxia and hypercapnia. Involvement of other vital centres in the brainstem particularly the vasomotor centre leads to hypotension and shock.

The patient is generally conscious to the end, perfectly aware and helpless against the relentless increase in the paralysis that ultimately kills him. Death generally occurs within 4–12 hours of the bite; it may however occur within an hour, or may be delayed for 72 hours. Some degree of haemolysis and a mild bleeding tendency may be observed in those who live more than 24 hours.

If the patient does not die, paralysis quickly recedes and recovery without any sequelae occurs.

Krait Bite

The symptoms are similar to cobra bite, with the addition of severe abdominal pain and cramps.

Sea Snake Bite

Headache, sweating, vomiting, thirst, heaviness of the tongue are first observed. Within $1/2$ to 4 hours, there is a painful stiffness of the muscles; trismus is frequent. This phase is followed by a generalized flaccid paralysis. Myoglobinuria following rhabdomyolysis occurs within 3 to 8 hours after the bite and may lead to renal failure. Hyperkalaemia often results due to the release of potassium from damaged muscles; it can lead to cardiac arrest.

Viperine Bites

Local Effects

These are marked and are observed very often within a few minutes of the bite. Severe pain, increasing redness, oedema, bulla formation are observed spreading outwards from the fang marks. A serosanguinous discharge oozes from the wound. The necrotizing inflammation involves the soft tissues, may even involve muscle, and may be severe enough to cause gangrene. It creeps up the limb if the bite is on an extremity.

Systemic Effects

(i) *Acute Circulatory Failure.* Shock with pallor, tachycardia, sweating, hypotension, restlessness and oliguria can occur within a few hours. Several factors contribute to shock. These include haemolysis, extravasation of fluid into the bitten limb, a generalized increase in capillary permeability and haemorrhage. In many patients shock occurs before all the above features are clinically apparent. It is probably due to specific factors within the venom that directly induce acute circulatory failure.

(ii) *Severe Intravascular Haemolysis.* Haemolysis causes a profound fall in haemoglobin, icterus, haemoglobinaemia, haemoglobinuria and acute tubular necrosis, resulting in renal failure.

(iii) *Disturbances in Clotting Mechanism with Haemorrhage.* Bleeding typically takes the form of epistaxis, haematuria, haematemesis, and rectal bleeding. Bleeding can also occur into various organs, such as the brain, lung, into the pleural space or into muscle and tissue. Disseminated intravascular coagulopathy can occur. Bleeding in some instances may only take place from one site e.g. a severe rectal bleed, or bleeding from the urinary tract. Though bleeding generally occurs within a few hours, it occasionally may occur 24 hours or even later after a bite. Bleeding from one or more sites may be the sole manifestation of a viperine bite.

(iv) *Fever* of 100°F to 104°F, with well marked leucocytosis (20,000–40,000/mm^3), is invariably present. Vomiting is early and frequent; rarely seizures may also occur.

(v) *Acute Renal Failure* is an important and frequent complication of viperine bites. It can result from acute circulatory failure and shock, from acute intravascular haemolysis, from disseminated intravascular coagulopathy or from a combination of factors. It is most often due to acute tubular necrosis.

Death when it occurs in viperine bites, generally occurs in 12–24 hours.

Management (7–10)

Unfortunately, envenomation from snake bite chiefly occurs in rural India and not in the large towns where critical care units or emergency departments are available. What is more, many patients after being bitten by a poisonous snake prefer to go to traditional healers rather than be treated by allopaths or be treated in hospitals.

Critical care or at least basic well-directed medical attention can however make a difference between life and death in patients suffering from severe envenomation following a snake bite. Critical or emergency care whenever possible, is mandatory under the following circumstances:

(i) Systemic effects of envenomation are present following a snake bite. The patient should be admitted to the intensive care unit even if systemic features are mild. Sudden clinical deterioration can occur, particularly in a krait or cobra bite.

(ii) Local inflammation around the bite is marked soon after a snake bite, even in the absence of systemic features. Bites causing acute inflammation within a matter of minutes or hours, are invariably due to poisonous snakes. Two tell-tale fang marks are generally visible. These are usually viperine bites, and sudden severe bleeds may occur within the first 24 hours.

Most patients with features of envenomation are admitted 2–4 hours after a bite or even much later. Slowing the absorption and spread of the venom by the application of a tourniquet proximal to the bite, though useful as an immediate emergency measure within 1–30 minutes of the bite, is not likely to help if admission is delayed beyond 30 minutes.

The continuous application of a tourniquet can lead to gangrene, increased fibrinolysis, bleeding distal to the tourniquet, compartmental ischaemia and increase in the local symptoms of envenomation. The current recommendation is to avoid the use of a tourniquet. Instead, the bitten limb is immobilized by bandaging it tightly with a crepe bandage, starting from the toes or fingers, and extending the bandage up to the knee or elbow. A splint is incorporated in this dressing for better immobilization. This method was developed by Struan Sutherland and his colleagues in Australia. It should be used only for cobra and krait bite, whose poison is chiefly neurotoxic. It should not be used for viperine bites as tight bandaging could worsen oedema and tissue necrosis of the limb.

Traditional first-aid measures of making cruciate incisions over the wound with attempts to suck the poison from the wound almost certainly do more harm than good, by introducing bacterial infection as an added complication. Similarly the use of ice packs to the wound are of dubious value. The important point is to immobilize the limb and discourage all movement.

During urgent transport to a hospital, emergency department or local dispensary, care is taken to avoid aspiration if the patient is vomiting. Oxygen is administered if there is cyanosis and adrenaline 0.5 ml subcutaneously administered for autonomic disturbances or hypotension. Cardiopulmonary resuscitation may be necessary during transport, in desperate situations.

The immediate priorities in severe envenomation after admission to the emergency department of a hospital or to a critical care unit are:

(i) Cardiorespiratory support, and also support to other organ systems.

(ii) Neutralization of the poison with antivenin.

Both these priorities should be addressed more or less simultaneously.

A large peripheral venous line is promptly secured and blood sent for a blood count, haematocrit, platelet count, bleeding time, clotting time, prothrombin time, electrolytes, urea and creatinine. In viperine bites presenting with bleeding, a coagulation profile is necessary. The reticulocyte count and tests for haemoglobinaemia, and haemoglobinuria should be done in patients with haemolysis. A urine examination is done and an intake-output carefully charted. A central venous line is secured for administration of fluid, drugs and for monitoring the central venous pressure. Arterial blood pH, and blood gases are estimated, and the patient's ECG monitored.

Neutralization of the Poison

The only effective treatment against venom that has entered the circulation is its neutralization by the use of antivenin. Ideally, to be most effective, antivenin should be given as soon as possible. It is however never too late to administer antivenin provided systemic signs of envenomation are present. It has thus been reported to be effective when given to patients who remain defibrinated weeks after a viperidae bite. In India, the Haffkine Institute in Mumbai prepares a polyvalent anti snake-venom serum. This is prepared by hyperimmunizing horses against the venoms of 4 common poisonous snakes—cobra, Russell's viper, common krait, and the Echus (saw-scaled viper). Each ml of the concentrated serum neutralizes the following quantities of dried venom when injected along with the venom in white mice; cobra 0.6 mg, Russell's viper 0.6 mg, common krait 0.45 mg, Echus 0.45 mg. The serum is lyophilized, and to be reconstituted has to be dissolved in distilled water.

Use of Antivenin

A sensitivity test is first performed. If the patient is not sensitive, 5 ml of the reconstituted polyvalent serum is injected locally around the wound. Local infiltration of antivenin should never be done into a finger or toe, as it can induce sloughing and gangrene.

The next step is the systemic use of antivenin. This is preferably preceded by the subcutaneous injection of 0.5 ml of 1 in 1000 adrenaline, as also by an injection of an antihistamine. Antivenin should as far as possible be administered intravenously, particularly in patients who are seriously ill or in shock. 100 ml of the polyvalent serum is added to 300–500 ml N saline, and given as a slow infusion over 1–2 hours. This dose may be repeated twice or even more frequently in serious life threatening situations.

In patients who are sensitive to the polyvalent serum, a rapid desensitization should be attempted. 0.05 ml subcutaneously is first given; this is followed by progressively increasing doses till 2 ml is given intramuscularly. A further gradual increase in intramuscular dosage to 10 ml and then to 40 ml is made. This may need to be done under cover of adrenaline, antihistamine and corticosteriods. If no reaction occurs to a large intramuscular dose then 10–20 ml of the polyvalent serum is diluted in 500 ml N saline, and given as a slow infusion over 2 hours. A careful watch should be kept for untoward reactions.

In small children in whom it may be impossible to quickly find a vein, polyvalent serum should be given intramuscularly. The dose in children is the same as in adults, since envenomation in children is always more serious than in adults. 60–100 ml (divided doses) is given intramuscularly with hyalase, to help absorption. If however a vein can be secured, the same dose is given as an infusion in normal saline over 2 hours. Intravenous administration whenever possible is to be preferred to the intramuscular use of the antivenin.

The use of antivenin is followed by a prompt reversal in the systemic features of envenomation. Spontaneous bleeding in viperidae bites stops within an hour and the coagulation profile reverts to normal within 6 to 12 hours. Systemic envenomation can however recur after hours or even days of initial good response. This is due to the continued absorption of the venom from the wound after it has been initially cleared from the blood stream by the antivenin. The dose of antivenin should then be repeated, and the patient observed closely for 3 to 5 days.

Cardiorespiratory Support

This is of vital importance in seriously ill patients. Immediate endotracheal intubation with ventilator support is necessary in cobra or krait bites that cause a curare-like paralysis. It is important to secure and protect the airway and anticipate respiratory failure in these patients. In bites of Elapidae causing a curare-like paralysis, prostigmine 2.5–5 mg intramuscularly has been tried (as in myasthenia gravis). Prostigmine generally produces little or no improvement. It should never be relied upon to prevent respiratory paralysis in these patients. Ventilatory support is also necessary in patients in severe shock, so often observed with viperine bites. Intensive respiratory care goes *pari passu* with ventilatory support.

A sufficient volume load should be given to ensure a left ventricular filling pressure of 15 mm Hg. This may require the use of a Swan-Ganz catheter. Inotropic support is also often necessary in these patients.

Support to Other Systems

(a) Acute haemolysis is treated by small packed cell transfusions of carefully matched blood.

(b) Severe haemorrhage due to deficiency of clotting factors is treated by infusions of fresh frozen plasma—8–10 units or more may be necessary. When fibrinolysis occurs following snake bite, the use of epsilon aminocaproic acid 0.1 g/kg in a slow intravenous infusion, is of help. Cryoprecipitate should be infused (8 to 10 units or even more), if fibrinogen levels are low.

(c) Renal function must be supported by care over fluid and

electrolyte balance, and avoiding the use of nephrotoxic drugs. Acute tubular necrosis with a mounting serum creatinine requires haemodialysis till such time as kidney function returns to normal.

(d) Metabolic acidosis if present, is countered by attempts to increase oxygen transport, and improve tissue perfusion. Intravenous sodium bicarbonate may be given so that the arterial pH is not < 7.3.

Care of the Wound and Surrounding Inflamed Area

Strict asepsis after admission to the unit is necessary. The wound should be washed with Condy's lotion or potassium permanganate, and suitably dressed with an antibiotic ointment. Tetanus toxoid should always be administered to prevent tetanus. Crystalline penicillin in a dose of 10 lac units, is given intravenously 6 hourly. If Gram-negative organisms are present on examination of the discharge from a wound, a third generation cephalosporin, like ceftadizime 1 g intravenously 8 hourly, may be given.

Pain in and around the wound is relieved by analgesics. Morphine is best avoided in cobra and krait bites.

Cryotherapy has been advocated locally in the treatment of viperine bites. It consists in packing the bitten extremity with fresh water ice in plastic bags, whilst keeping the rest of the body warm. The objective is to chill the tissues (and not freeze them) in order to retard the local proteolytic and enzymatic activity of the venom. It is important not to pack the bitten extremity in fresh water ice during administration of the antivenin, and for 12 hours after administration as reaction of the antivenin with the venom may otherwise be interfered with. Current experience however throws doubt on the efficacy of cryotherapy. It could do more harm by increasing tissue necrosis.

Use of Corticosteroids

Good results have been reported with the use of corticosteroids. In viperine bites both local and systemic effects of envenomation seem to be reduced. A correct and unbiased appraisal of the efficacy of corticosteroids in snake bites is however difficult. In severely ill patients, particularly those in shock, it is advisable to give hydrocortisone hemisuccinate 300 mg intravenously, followed by 300 mg in a slow infusion over 24 hours. 100 mg intravenously 8 hourly may then be given for the next 2–3 days.

Treatment of Late Complications

Late complications like renal shutdown, local gangrene, or severe tissue necrosis need expert specialized management. Haemodialysis is often necessary for the management of acute renal failure following viperine bites. In the southern part of our country, snake bites would constitute one of the most important causes of acute renal failure necessitating the use of haemodialysis. The management protocol used for snake bites has been summarized in **Table 18.4.1**.

Other Poisonous Bites

Scorpion Sting (11, 12)

Some species are deadly poisonous. The poisonous species encountered in Western Maharashtra is the Indian red scorpion

Table 18.4.1. Summary of management protocol in snake bites

1. Neutralization of poison promptly with antivenin
2. Cardiorespiratory support
   - Immediate endotracheal intubation with ventilator support in cobra/krait bites causing curare-like paralysis, and in patients in severe shock following viperine bites
   - Maintain left ventricular filling pressure around 15 mm Hg with use of sufficient volume load
   - Inotropic support may be required
3. Support to other organ systems
   - Treat haemolysis with transfusions of packed cells/whole blood
   - Deficiency of clotting factors treated by infusions of fresh frozen plasma. Epsilon aminocaproic acid may be useful for fibrinolysis
   - Support renal function by maintaining fluid and electrolyte balance, and avoiding use of nephrotoxic drugs
   - Counter metabolic acidosis
4. Care of the wound and surrounding inflamed area
5. Use of tetanus toxoid, antibiotics, analgesics
6. Use of corticosteroids
7. Treatment of late complications e.g. renal shutdown, local gangrene or severe tissue necrosis

Mesobuthus tamulus. In North Africa the yellow scorpion (genus Liturus) is chiefly responsible for lethal envenomation.

The venom from a scorpion sting deposited in the subcutaneous tissue may take as long as 6 to 8 hours for complete absorption. Elimination of the venom by the body is slower, with estimated half-life of 4.2–24 hours (13)

The local effects of envenomation following a scorpion bite are burning pain, inflammation, and ecchymosis. Scorpion venom stimulates the release of catecholamines and acetylcholine. Early symptoms include vomiting, sweating, abdominal colic, diarrhoea, salivation, piloerection and occasionally priapism. A tachy-brady rhythm may occur. Ultimately a shock like state with hypotension and tachycardia evolves. In a large study conducted over several years in a hospital in Mahad (situated on the outskirts of Mumbai), hypertension was observed in 27 per cent of patients and pulmonary oedema at times fulminant in 18 per cent (14, 15). The cause of hypertension in some patients is related to stimulation of the α-adrenergic receptors by the venom. The venom also has a toxic effect on both the left and right heart. Severe left ventricular dysfunction leads to a raised pulmonary capillary wedge pressure with resulting pulmonary oedema. (16). The cardiotoxic effect of the venom can also cause marked bradycardia and arrhythmias. The venom over a period of time can result in multiple organ dysfunction. Death generally results from acute circulatory failure or from fulminant pulmonary oedema.

Treatment

Mortality depends on the time lag between the scorpion sting and the start of medical treatment. It also depends to an extent on the quality of care offered. Death occurs in 5 to 35 per cent of patients.

If the patient is brought to the unit within 30 minutes of the bite, cryotherapy in the form of application of ice in plastic bags around the bitten area, may help to retard the local proteolytic effects of the poison.

Scorpion antivenin if available should be promptly administered intravenously. Experimental and clinical studies suggest that it could reverse the circulatory, metabolic and ECG changes caused by the venom. Unfortunately scorpion antivenin is even more scarce than snake antivenin.

Supportive treatment is imperative, particularly with regard to the cardiorespiratory system. Hypovolaemic shock is treated by a volume load. Severe pulmonary oedema particularly when associated with hypertension responds to an intravenous infusion of nitroprusside. Severe left ventricular dysfunction needs dobutamine support.

The study in Mahad referred to earlier suggests that prazosin (an alpha blocker) in a dose of 250 µg in children and 500 µg in adult given 3 hourly is of considerable use. It controls both hypertension and pulmonary oedema. Patients receiving prazosin early in this study did not develop pulmonary oedema (14, 15).

Centipede Bite

The clinical features are similar to a scorpion bite and may prove fatal, particularly in children. Local inflammation around the bite is followed by restlessness, salivation, diaphoresis with a shock-like state that may culminate in death.

Treatment is symptomatic; cardiorespiratory support with management of the shock-like state is important.

Bee and Wasp Stings

Multiple stings are observed particularly in hikers who unwittingly disturb a bee hive. The usual reaction to a sting is a sharp pain followed by a local wheal and severe oedema, particularly if the sting is on the face. A sting into a peripheral nerve leads to a temporary loss of function of the nerve. With multiple stings or in hypersensitive individuals, a picture of anaphylactic shock is observed—severe urticaria, bronchial spasm, and hypotension, followed at times by cardiac arrest.

If brought as an emergency to the intensive care unit, adrenaline in a dose of 0.75–1 ml is injected subcutaneously or intramuscularly. If hypotension and a state of anaphylaxis prevail, adrenaline may need to be given intravenously (see Chapter on Anaphylactic Shock), and emergency resuscitation with cardiorespiratory support should be promptly initiated. The airway should be quickly secured by endotracheal intubation in patients with increasing urticaria involving the skin and mucosa. Intravenous hydrocortisone and antihistamines are of help particularly in patients with severe urticaria.

REFERENCES

1. Dowling H, Minton SA Jr, Russell FE. (1968). Poisonous snakes of the world. US Government Printing Office, Washington DC.
2. Minton SA Jr, Minton MG. (1969). Venomous reptiles. Charles Scribner's Sons, New York.
3. Russell FE. (1983). Snake Venom Poisoning. Scholium International, Great Neck, NY.
4. Visser J, Chapman DS. (1978). Snakes and Snakebite. Purnell and Sons, Capetown.
5. Russell FE, Dart RC. (1990). Toxic effects of animal toxins. In: Casarett and Doull's Toxicology: The Basic Science of Poisons, 4th edn (Eds Doull J, Klassen CD, Amdur MO). Macmillan Publishing, New York.
6. Bieber AL. (1979). Metal and non-protein constituents in snake venoms. In: Snake Venoms (Ed. Lee CY). pp. 295–306. Springer-Verlag, New York.
7. Blackman JR, Dillon S. (1992). Venomous snake bite: Past, present and future treatment options. J Am Board Fam Prac. 5, 399–405.
8. Gold BS, Barish RA. (1992). Venomous snakebites: Current concepts in diagnosis, treatment, and management. Emerg Med Clin North Am. 10, 249–267.
9. Johnson CA. (1991). Management of snake bites. Am Fam Physician. 44, 174–180.
10. Warrel DA. (2003). Injuries, Envenoming, Poisoning and Allergic Reaction caused by Animals. In: Oxford Textbook of Medicine (Eds Warrel DA, Cox MD, Firth JD, Benz Jr EJ). pp. 923–936. Oxford University Press, London.
11. Macho JR, Schechter WP. (2002). Care of Patients with Environmental Injury—Envenomation. In: Current Critical Care Diagnosis and Treatment (Eds Bongard FS, Sue DY). pp. 875–879. McGraw-Hill, USA.
12. Rimza ME, Zimmerman DR, Bergeson DS. (1980). Scorpion envenomation. Pediatrics. 66, 298.
13. Ismail M. (1993). Serotherapy of the scorpion envenoming syndrome is irrationally convicted without trail. Toxicon. 31, 1077–1083
14. Bawaskar HS, Bawaskar PH. (1986). Prazosin in the management of cardiovascular manifestations of scorpion sting [letter]. Lancet 1, 510–511.
15. Bawaskar HS, Bawaskar PH. (1989). Stings by red scorpion (Buthotus tamulus) in Maharashtra State, India: A clinical study. Trans R Soc Trop Med Hyg. 83, 858–860.
16. Karnad DR (1998). Haemodynamic pattern in patients with scorpion envenomation. Heart. 79, 485–489.

SECTION 19
Critical Care of the Cancer Patient

Critical Care of the Cancer Patient

General Considerations

The cure rate in cancer has increased over the last 3 decades. Patients with common cancers like breast cancer, colorectal cancer, lung cancer, still defy a cure once these cancers have metastatized. There are however a number of cancers which can be cured even after metastasis. These include acute lymphatic or myeloid leukaemia, chronic myeloid leukaemia (after extensive radiation and allogenous bone marrow transplant), gestational choriocarcinoma, testicular tumours, Hodgkin's disease, aggressive non-Hodgkin's lymphomas, Wilm's tumour, Ewing's sarcoma, and in rare instances small cell lung carcinoma. Survival of patients with other forms of metastatic cancers can also be extended for varying periods of time.

As far as possible, particularly in poor countries with a serious financial resource crunch, patients with advanced cancer are best treated in the wards or at home. However an acute, life-threatening reversible pathology in cancer patients does need critical care. The priority for such care is obviously low if the basic disease process is so advanced as to sharply limit the expected life span. The priority increases if the patient has a cancer which is either potentially curable, or which if effectively treated can result in an extended period of survival. However, therapeutic considerations in the ICUs all over the world are being increasingly influenced by cost and outcome concerns. The intensivist, the treating physician or surgeon caring for a cancer patient faces the challenge in the ICU 'to decide not only what should or can be done but also to decide if and when to do it, or whether to do anything at all'.

Post-operative Critical Care

In surgical ICUs, ICU admissions are related chiefly to immediate post-operative care after major surgery, or to surgical and other complications arising soon after massive surgery. Principles of surgical care are exactly the same as after major surgery unassociated with cancer (1). The main post-operative support necessitating ICU stay is dependence on mechanical ventilation, especially over an extended period of time. Generally, the risks of untoward outcomes in the ICU correlate with the extent and magnitude of the surgical procedure. For example ovarian cancer surgery involving resection of the gut, ventilatory dependency and haemodynamic instability requiring the use of a Swan-Ganz catheter, carries a higher morbidity and longer stay in the ICU (2). Considering the recent advances in surgery, post-operative risks are determined to a lesser extent by the technical aspects of the surgical procedure, than by existing co-morbidity and general underlying factors that prevent an uncomplicated recovery.

Most surgical operations in cancer patients carry a procedure specific morbidity and mortality rate. Potentially lethal complications generally do not occur in the immediate or early post-operative phase, but later. Resurgery (for whatever reason) carries a high morbidity and mortality. Post-operative infection either in the surgical area or systemic infection is probably the greatest hazard, particularly in cancer patients who have received chemotherapy prior to surgery.

Critical care in cancer patients may be necessitated for several other reasons:

(i) Overwhelming or serious infection related to immunosuppression (see Section on The Immunocompromised Patient). Advanced malignancy is always associated with a reduction in immune response. Protein synthesis is abnormal, and continued rapid growth and spread of the tumour produces cachexia. Malnutrition worsens immunosuppression at this stage. A far more important cause of immunosuppression is related to severe neutropaenia observed as a feature of acute myeloproliferative disease, or related to the use of chemotherapy and/or radiation. The more dose-intensive the chemotherapy or radiation therapy regime, the greater the likelihood of damage to host cells, and of severe thrombocytopaenia and granulocytopaenia. Immunosuppression often leads to acute infection which may be due to the usual micro-organisms infecting immunocompetent patients, or to opportunistic organisms. This has been dealt with in the Section on The Immunocompromised Patient. Severe thrombocytopaenia following radiation or chemotherapy, may induce bleeding either within the skin and the mucosa, or in internal organs and other anatomical structures of the body.

(ii) Complications due to a mitotic lesion which can produce life-threatening emergencies. These complications can result directly from the tumour effects at the primary site, or from spread of the tumour. Non-metastatic complications of malignant diseases can also result in serious problems meriting critical care.

(iii) Complications directly related to the side effects of antimitotic drugs or radiation (other than immunosuppression already mentioned above).

Complications listed under (ii) and (iii) can best be considered in relation to different organ systems with specific reference to critical care requirements.

1. Metabolic Complications (2–5)

The main metabolic complications that may require critical care are the tumour lysis syndrome, hypercalcaemia, and fluid and electrolyte disturbances, notably the syndrome of inappropriate secretion of antidiuretic hormone (SIADH).

The Tumour Lysis Syndrome (6, 7)

This is particularly observed in rapidly proliferating tumours that are very sensitive to chemotherapy. The syndrome is classically associated with Burkitt's lymphoma (8), but in our part of the world is most frequently observed during treatment of other malignancies (9, 10). These include acute lymphoblastic leukaemia, chronic myeloid leukaemia in an acute blast crisis, non-Hodgkin's lymphoma, and occasionally in small cell cancer of the lung, and metastatic breast cancer.

The syndrome is caused by rapid lysis of malignant cells resulting in hyperuricaemia, hyperkalaemia, hyperphosphataemia, hypocalcaemia, and an increase in blood urea nitrogen. Though hyperuricaemia and increase in uric acid excretion typically occur following chemotherapy in malignancy, these abnormalities can also occasionally occur in untreated patients with rapidly growing tumours.

Life-threatening complications include acute renal failure from precipitation of uric acid in renal tubules with uric acid nephropathy, cardiac arrhythmias from hyperkalaemia and hypocalcaemia. Oliguria and azotaemia are warning features; hypocalcaemia can result in tetany, cramps and seizures.

Management

Prevention consists of hydrating patients before and during chemotherapy, and using allopurinol 500 mg/m^2/day for 3 days; this is reduced to 200 mg/m^2/day after 3 days of chemotherapy. Chemotherapy is best instituted 24–48 hours after proper hydration and use of allopurinol. During chemotherapy, relevant blood biochemistry should be done every 12–24 hours.

Treatment

If metabolic aberrations are observed in the form of increasing hyperuricaemia, oliguria and electrolyte abnormalities, as stated above, chemotherapy is either postponed or stopped. Allopurinol is given as above; the dose is decreased in the presence of renal insufficiency or if serum uric acid levels are controlled. Patients should be carefully hydrated, but in the presence of increasing oliguria, fluid overload should be watched for. Furosemide is given in a dose that maintains urine flow at over 100 ml/hour. An increase in urine output should be matched by an increase in oral and intravenous fluid intake. The urine should be alkalinized to a urine pH ≥ 7 by the use of intravenous sodium bicarbonate. This is given in a dose of 75–100 mEq/l to start with, and subsequently the dose is adjusted to maintain an alkaline urine. Once the urine output increases, and the serum uric acid falls, alkalinization of urine is no longer necessary. In patients who develop an acute renal shutdown, intravenous fluids are avoided for the purpose of hydration, else pulmonary oedema occurs.

Hyperkalaemia

Hyperkalaemia needs urgent attention with 50 per cent dextrose-insulin given intravenously, the use of intravenous bicarbonate, and of an exchange resin—sodium polystyrene sulfonate (see Section on Fluid and Electrolyte Disturbances in the Critically Ill).

Hypocalcaemia (11)

Hypocalcaemia is corrected by the use of 10 per cent calcium gluconate intravenously, which can be repeated as and when necessary.

Hyperphosphataemia

Hyperphosphataemia is typically severe (serum levels ranging from 6–35 mg/dl), and is due both to tumour lysis and increasing renal failure. It is treated with 20 per cent dextrose-insulin till the phosphate levels are < 6 mg/dl. Aluminum hydroxide 30–60 ml 6 hourly is given orally to bind phosphates in the gut. Good hydration, both orally and intravenously, helps excretion of phosphates via the urine.

Some patients do not respond to the above therapy. They develop increasing oliguria and renal failure with hyperuricaemia and persistent hyperkalaemia and hyperphosphataemia. The criteria for starting dialysis are as follows: (a) Serum uric acid levels > 10 mg/dl; (b) serum K$^+$ > 6 mEq/l; (c) serum phosphates > 10 mg/dl; (d) fluid overload; (e) symptomatic uncorrected hypocalcaemia.

Other Metabolic Problems in Malignancy
SIADH (12, 13)

The syndrome of inappropriate secretion of antidiuretic hormone can cause mental obtundation, coma, seizures and even death. It occurs most frequently with a small cell lung cancer, but can occur with other malignant lesions as well. Besides being a non-metastatic complication of the tumour itself, SIADH can also result from chemotherapy, notably following the use of cyclophosphamide or vincristine. The treatment has been detailed in the Section on Fluid and Electrolyte Disturbances in the Critically Ill. It is important to raise serum sodium gradually in these patients, so as to minimize the risk of central pontine myelinolysis.

Hypophosphataemia

Serum phosphate levels < 3 mg/dl are occasionally observed with rapidly growing tumours, and in severely malnourished cancer patients. The clinical features of hypophosphataemia are characterized by increased weakness which could also involve the respiratory muscles, poor myocardial function, as also leucocyte and platelet dysfunction. Phosphate levels < 1 mg/dl can cause haemolysis and rhabdomyolysis. Treatment in an emergency consists of the administration of 30–40 mmol/l of a neutral sodium or potassium phosphate solution at the rate of 50–100 ml/hour.

Hypercalcaemia (14–20)

Hypercalcemia is the commonest metabolic complication of malignancies, and one that most often requires critical care. It occurs in 10 per cent of cancer patients (3) and in some instances constitutes a life-threatening emergency. It is most frequently associated with multiple myeloma, lung cancer, breast cancer, cancers involving the head and neck, T-cell lymphomas, renal carcinoma, as well as other solid tumours. A rapid onset hypercalcaemia can cause confusion, obtundation, psychosis, and even coma. Vigorous hydration with intravenous N saline combined with the use of furosemide, is the standard therapy, and has been outlined in the Section on Fluid and Electrolyte Disturbances in the Critically Ill. Corticosteroids, diphosphonates, mithramycin, and calcitonin can all reduce serum calcium levels by reducing bone resorption of calcium. A combination of calcitonin and corticosteroids has the quickest effect in reducing serum calcium. Mithramycin has a good, but poorly sustained effect. Diphosphonates act slowly, but the effect is more sustained. Methods to counter hypercalcaemia have been discussed in an earlier chapter, but for reasons of convenience, the dosage schedules of corticosteroids, calcitonin, diphosphonates and mithramycin are given in **Table 19.1.1**.

Table 19.1.1. Dosages of commonly used agents in the treatment of hypercalcaemia

Drug	Route of Administration	Dosage
1. Prednisolone	Oral	1–2 mg/kg/day
2. Salmon Calcitonin*	Subcutaneous	100–400 U/6–12 hrs
3. Mithramycin	Intravenous	25 µg/kg, once or twice/week
4. Diphosphonates (Allendronate disodium)	Intravenous	7.5 mg/kg/day for 7 days

Also used as a nasal spray.

Hypocalcaemia (11)

Hypocalcaemia in cancer can result from the following causes:

1. Osteoblastic metastatic deposits in the bone from a prostate cancer or from a breast cancer on hormone therapy. Prostate cancer is the commonest cause of hypocalcaemia. More than 30 per cent of patients with prostate cancer and extensive osteoblastic deposits develop hypocalcaemia.

2. The tumour lysis syndrome can result in hyperphosphataemia, with an increase in calcium phosphate product leading to deposition of calcium in various soft tissues. Hypocalcaemia followed by the development of secondary hyperparathyrodism results.

3. Low vitamin D_3 levels can also lead to hypocalcaemia.

4. Magnesium deficiency leads to hypocalcaemia. This occurs in cancer patients on prolonged hyperalimentation when magnesium is not adequately replaced. It can also occur in patients on diuretics, in chronic diarrhoea, in patients on cisplatin therapy and in those receiving intravenous phosphate. Both calcium and magnesium need to be given to correct hypocalcaemia in these patients.

Clinical features have been described in the Chapter on Fluid and Electrolyte Disturbances in the Critically Ill. They include tetany, muscle cramps, laryngeal spasm, headache, irritability and seizures. Chvostek's and Trousseau's signs are often positive and the ECG shows a prolonged QT interval.

Treatment

Treatment consists of the intravenous administration of 10 ml 10 per cent calcium gluconate repeated after 20 to 30 minutes or as and when necessary. Magnesium in a dose of 1 g over 12 to 24 hours is given intravenously if there is an associated hypomagnesaemia. (< 1.5 mg/dl).

Hyperglycaemia

Hyperglycaemia can occur in malignant disease without insulin deficiency. It has been reported in glucagonomas, somatostatinomas, and rarely in pheochromocytoma and ACTH secreting tumours. Nonketotic hyperosmolar hyperglycaemic coma can occasionally result as a complication of cyclophosphamide, vincristine or prednisolone therapy, in patients who are mildly diabetic and in patients who are on intravenous alimentation. Hyperglycaemia generally responds to treatment of the tumour either by resection, radiation therapy or chemotherapy.

Hypoglycaemia

Hypoglycaemia due to tumours is most frequently due to an insulinoma. However, an insulin like substance causing severe persistent hypoglycaemia can be secreted by some tumours. These include large retroperitoneal fibrosarcoma, mesotheliomas, and renal, adrenal and primary hepatocellular carcinoma. Extensive metastasis within the liver can also lead to hypoglycaemia. Associated liver cell disease, hypopituitarism from any cause (including tumours), and myxoedema may also be responsible for hypoglycaemia.

The immediate treatment is an intravenous infusion of 10–20 per cent glucose to keep the blood glucose level > 60 mg/dl. Removal of the tumour whenever possible grants relief from hypoglycaemia.

Hypokalaemia due to Ectopic ACTH Secretion

Besides adrenocortical tumours secreting cortisol and thereby producing Cushing's syndrome, a number of other tumours can secrete ectopic ACTH resulting in hypokalaemia and Cushingoid features. These chiefly include small cell lung cancer, carcinoid tumours of the bronchi, cancers of the ovary, thyroid, and prostate, haematological malignancies and sarcomas.

The differential diagnosis of hypokalaemia, and potassium replacement in hypokalaemia are both considered in the Chapter on Fluid and Electrolyte Disturbances in the Critically Ill. Ideally the effective treatment of hypokalaemia and the induced Cushing's Syndrome due to ectopic ACTH secretion is removal of the underlying tumour. If the tumour is unresectable, chemotherapy should be tried.

2. Haematological Complications (3)

The chief haematological complication requiring intensive care is bleeding. Bleeding may be directly related to a cancerous lesion in the GI tract, or it may result from thrombocytopaenia, or may be due to disseminated intravascular coagulopathy (DIC). Thrombocytopaenia may result from neoplastic disease chiefly through infiltration of the bone marrow, or could be drug-induced. DIC can occur with a variety of cancers, but especially with promyelocytic leukaemia, prostatic carcinoma, and cancer of the breast, lungs and the GI tract. Patients with DIC require transfusions with whole blood, packed cells, fresh frozen plasma, and platelet infusions. Fibrinogenaemia is countered by intravenous infusions of cryoprecipitate—2–3 bags/10 kg body weight is infused initially, followed by 1 bag/15 kg body weight daily (see Chapter on Transfusion [Blood Product] Therapy).

3. Pulmonary Complications (3)

Pulmonary complications in malignancies, meriting critical care include:

(a) Acute respiratory failure.

(b) Central airways obstruction from tumour involvement of the upper airways, or from pressure on the airway by mediastinal glands.

(c) Massive atelectasis of a lung due to endobronchial obstruction, or to extrinsic pressure.

(d) Acute infections.

(e) Massive haemoptysis.

(a) Acute Respiratory Failure

This most frequently results from lymphangitis carcinomatosis, or alveolar cell carcinoma, or widespread metastatic spread of cancer within the lungs. *These patients should be treated in the wards and not in critical care units.* They should not in our opinion, be ventilated; treatment is directed towards symptomatic relief. Acute respiratory failure could also result from complicating pneumonia, due to community acquired, or nosocomial, or opportunistic infection, or due to pulmonary embolism. These patients need expert critical care for survival.

Acute myeloblastic leukaemia or chronic myeloid leukaemia in a blast crisis can cause leukostasis with obstructed blood flow to small pulmonary blood vessels. This can lead to hypoxaemic respiratory failure.

Respiratory failure may also result from treatment given to cancer patients (2, 21). A number of chemotherapeutic agents, in particular bleomycin and mitomycin, can cause pneumonitis with progressive pulmonary fibrosis, and increasing hypoxaemia (22). Similarly radiation therapy can produce acute pneumonitis over a period of 6 or more weeks. Progressive fibrosis with respi-

ratory failure can result due to a chronic radiation effect, particularly if large areas of the lung are irradiated, or the patient has simultaneously received chemotherapy. It is believed that radiation injury to the lungs, with damage to the alveolar capillary wall produced by chemotherapy, is due to the formation of free oxygen radicals. The pathogenesis of lung injury in these patients is similar to oxygen toxicity produced by inhalation of very high oxygen concentrations (FIO_2), over a long period of time. Administering a high concentration of oxygen to these patients could conceivably increase the degree of lung injury, and may well produce irreversible lung damage. The lowest possible FIO_2 that can maintain an oxygen saturation of haemoglobin around 90 per cent, should therefore be used.

(b) Central Airways Obstruction

Central airways obstruction from tumour involvement of the upper airways, or by extrinsic pressure from mediastinal glands, can produce asphyxia, and needs urgent surgical attention.

(c) Massive Atelectasis

Massive atelectasis from endobronchial obstruction can cause acute respiratory failure. Temporary relief of the obstruction by therapeutic procedures performed via the bronchoscope may help.

(d) Acute Infections

Acute leukaemias, chronic myelogenous leukaemia in blast crisis, Hodgkin's disease, malignant lymphomas, and other malignant lesions are often treated with high dose chemotherapy. Radiation together with bone marrow transplants are also used in the treatment of leukaemias. Patients with advanced breast cancer are also at times treated with very aggressive regimes. This causes prolonged severe neutropaenia and thrombocytopaenia. Bacterial, viral (particularly cytomegaloviral) and fungal infections can be fulminant and cause death in spite of vigorous antibiotic therapy and support. Cytomegaloviral pneumonia and diffuse interstitial pneumonia are dangerous complications following bone marrow transplants, and carry a high mortality (see Section on The Immunocompromised Patient).

(e) Massive Haemoptysis

Haemoptysis can be severe in some patients with non-small cell lung cancers, and is particularly severe in squamous cell lung cancer. Intrapulmonary haemorrhage with haemoptysis can also occur in patients with severe thrombocytopaenia; fluffy lung shadows with progressively increasing hypoxaemic respiratory failure result.

4. Cardiovascular Complications

Cardiac Tamponade (23)

Cardiac tamponade is an important complication that may necessitate critical care in patients with malignant disease. Tamponade is most frequently due to malignant pericardial effusion, but can be due to constrictive pericarditis arising from encasement of the heart by tumour tissue, or to irradiation fibrosis.

Pericardiocentesis is urgently required to reverse haemodynamic abnormalities in malignant pericardial effusions. Surgical procedures by experienced oncologists may be necessary for long-term benefit.

Congestive Cardiomyopathy (3)

An extremely important cardiovascular complication in patients with mitotic disease is congestive cardiomyopathy, induced by chemotherapeutic agents such as adriamycin, or high dose cyclophosphamide. Progressive cardiac enlargement, increasing breathlessness, pulmonary and systemic venous congestion can occur over a short period of 2–4 weeks, though in some patients the clinical features of heart failure may be delayed by a few months. A clinical follow-up, as also a follow-up by 2-D echocardiography with specific reference to the ejection fraction, is of value in early diagnosis. Management consists of strict bed rest, the use of digitalis, diuretics, and the use of angiotensin converting enzyme inhibitors to reduce the afterload. The incriminating drug should be avoided. Varying degrees of improvement in cardiac function may be observed with proper management.

Superior Mediastinal Syndrome (24–26)

The superior mediastinal syndrome most commonly results from a lymphoma or a metastatic carcinoma (chiefly from a carcinoma within the lung). However the possibility of a benign cause for a superior mediastinal syndrome should always be kept in mind. For this reason it is wrong in principle to give chemotherapy or radiation to such a patient without a tissue diagnosis. In our part of the world, massive mediastinal adenopathy with a superior mediastinal pressure syndrome can result from tuberculous adenitis, particularly in the younger age group.

Patients with cancer who have central venous catheters in situ, may develop superior vena caval thrombosis. This results in engorged neck veins, and resembles a superior mediastinal pressure syndrome. An infusion of urokinase, through a catheter placed directly above the clot in the superior vena cava, often dissolves the clot and gives excellent relief. This is preferably followed by an intravenous infusion of heparin at a rate of 1000 units/hour for 3–4 days. Long-term oral anticoagulation may be necessary in some patients.

Severe tracheal obstruction from a metastatic adenopathy due to cancer or lymphoma may need urgent relief. Stenting with a self-expanding metal endoprosthesis provides successful relief in 90 per cent of patients. Chemotherapy is used in patients with small cell lung cancer, lymphoma and germ cell tumours. Radiation therapy is the only alternative for other cancers. It may temporarily increase upper airway obstruction, or further obstruct the superior vena cava, necessitating the insertion of a stent within the trachea and the superior vena cava.

5. Gastrointestinal Complications (3)

Perforation of the gut may be a direct complication of a malignant lesion involving the GI tract. Perforation can also result from enterocolitis in neutropaenic patients. Fever, diarrhoea, abdominal pain and tenderness are present. The classical signs of acute abdomen after perforation may not be present in a severely neutropaenic patient. Surgery is imperative, but the morbidity and mortality are high.

Severe GI bleeds, or localized intra-abdominal abscesses may also be serious enough to merit critical care in some patients.

Obstruction to the gut may be due to the disease process itself. Surgery, radiation therapy, or intraperitoneal therapeutic interventions may however cause adhesions or damage to the gut, with resulting obstruction. It is often difficult to distinguish whether problems involving the gut are related to the malignancy per se, or to therapy used against the disease. Expert surgical advice is imperative.

6. Neurological Complications (2, 3, 27)

Acute complications requiring critical care include increase in intracranial tension because of a primary tumour within the brain, or due to metastasis within the brain.

Early diagnosis and prompt treatment of acute spinal cord compression due to metastatic disease or a primary neoplasm are of utmost importance. This requires a good clinical examination plus imaging studies. Cord compression diagnosed after myelopathy has already set in has the most unfortunate consequences on what remains of the patient's life—often a bedridden existence, with an indwelling catheter and with an increased risk of bed-sores, pneumonia and urinary infection.

Once a clinical diagnosis of chord compression is made, the patient should be given pulsed doses of 1 g methylprednisolone for 3 days, as this helps reduce cord oedema. Definitive neurosurgical treatment to decompress the cord should be prompt so as to avoid a permanent myelopathy.

Severe metabolic encephalopathy in a patient with malignant disease can be due to hyponatraemia, or hypercalcaemia. Antimitotic drugs like cytarabine, etoposide, methotrexate, ifosfamide can also cause metabolic encephalopathy. Interleukin-2 and interferon-α can also cause somnolence and confusion. Paranoid psychosis, seizures and coma have been reported with interleukin-2. Management is chiefly symptomatic and supportive, and the offending drug should be promptly stopped.

Anti-cancer Therapy Requiring Intensive Care

It is hardly ever necessary to give chemotherapy in an ICU setting. Recently however biological therapy chiefly with interleukin-2 (IL-2), is being increasingly administered under critical care conditions (3). IL-2 therapy is particularly useful in patients with renal cell carcinoma and melanoma, the results being superior to other modalities of treatment. Other biological factors being used are the tumour necrosis factor (TNF) and interleukin-1 (IL-1). IL-2 is presumed to have a lymphokine-activated killer (LAK) cell activity (3). An IL-2 regime however produces a predictable range of toxic effects which require management in a critical care setting (28–30).

IL-2 infusions can produce (a) severe hypotension due to an increased vascular capacitance with a lowered systemic vascular resistance; (b) non-cardiogenic pulmonary oedema (3).

The hypotension is similar to that observed in septic shock, and is associated with a warm skin, and a good pulse volume. Poor perfusion of organ systems results if the blood pressure is not raised. It is inadvisable to raise the blood pressure by a volume load, as this increases the tendency to produce non-cardiogenic pulmonary oedema. It is best to raise the blood pressure by an infusion of phenylephrine 50 mg in 250 ml of 5 per cent dextrose, the infusion being given at a rate of 20–40 µg/minute. If hypotension persists despite increasing doses of phenylephrine, the patient is given inotropic support either with dopamine or dobutamine. These patients invariably have a fair degree of left ventricular dysfunction. The deleterious cardiovascular effects of IL-2 are reversed within hours if the drug is discontinued. The drug can be restarted with a 25 per cent reduction in dose, after the patient is haemodynamically stable.

The danger of non-cardiogenic pulmonary oedema is minimized by restricting fluids and avoiding volume load. Hypoxia if present, is corrected by an appropriate increase in the FIO_2. If hypoxia persists with a haemoglobin oxygen saturation < 90 per cent, IL-2 is best omitted. It should be noted that the respiratory toxicity of IL-2 is not as easily reversed as the cardiovascular effects.

When LAK cells are infused together with IL-2, further complications include an additive effect on declining respiratory function, due to sludging of cells in the capillary bed. Bronchospasm and acute pulmonary oedema have also been observed. Continuous positive pressure breathing, or intubation with ventilatory support, may be necessary at times.

It is possible that in the decades to come, biological agents will be used with increasing frequency. The intensive care physician will therefore need to be aware of the potential grave complications, so that he can handle them successfully.

REFERENCES

1. Udwadia FE. (2003). Critical Care in Surgery. Indian J Surg. 65(3), 228–231.

2. Harrington DW, Tabbarah HJ. (2002). Critical Care of the Oncology Patient. In: Current Critical Care Diagnosis and Treatment (Eds Bongard FS, Sue DY). pp. 487–502. McGraw-Hill, USA.

3. Curti BD, Longo L. (2001). Intensive Care of the Cancer Patient. In: Current Therapy in Critical Care Medicine (Eds Parrillo JE, Dellinger RP). pp. 1439–1457. Mosby, USA.

4. Gradishar WJ, Hoffman PC. (1998). The Oncologic Emergencies. In: Principles of Critical Care (Eds Hall JB, Schmidt GA, Wood LDH). pp. 1075–1090. McGraw-Hill, USA.

5. Odell WD (1997). Endocrine / Metabolic Syndrome of Cancer. Semin Oncol. 24, 299–317.

6. Altman A. (2001). Acute tumor lysis syndrome. Semin Oncol. 28 (suppl 5), 3–12.

7. Lorigan PC, Woodings PL, Morgenstern GR et al. (1996). Tumor lysis syndrome: Care report and review of the literature. Ann Oncol. 7, 631–639

8. Cohen LF, Balow JE, Magrath IT et al. (1980). Acute tumor lysis syndrome: A review of 37 patients with Burkitt's lymphoma. Am J Med. 68, 486–491.

9. Tsokos G, Balow J, Spiegel R et al. (1981). Renal and metabolic complications of undifferentiated and lymphoblastic lymphoma. 60, 218.

10. Boccia R, Longo D, Licher M et al. (1985). Multiple recurrences of acute tumor lysis syndrome in an indolent non-Hodgkin's lymphoma. Cancer. 56, 2295.

11. Zaloga GP. (1992). Hypocalcemia in critically ill patients. Crit Care Med. 20, 251–262.

12. Robinson AG. (1985). Disorders of antidiuretic hormone secretion. Clin Endocrinol Metab. 14, 55.

13. Adrogue HJ, Madias NE. (2000). Hyponatremia. New Eng J of Med. 342, 1581–1589.

14. Bajournas DR. (1990). Manifestations of cancer-related hypercalcemia. Semin Oncol. 17, 16–25.

15. Bilezikian JP. (1992). Management of acute hypercalcemia. N Engl J Med. 326, 1196–1203.

16. Muggia FM. (1990). Overview of cancer related hypercalcemia: Epidemiology and etiology. Semin Oncol. 17, 3–9.

17. Ralston SH, Gallacher SJ, Patel U et al. (1990). Cancer associated hypercalcemia, morbidity and mortality: Clinical experience in 126 treated patients. Ann Intern Med. 112, 499–504.

18. Strewler GJ, Nissenson RA. (1990). Hypercalcemia in malignancy. West J Med. 153, 635–640.

19. Cooper JAD, White DA, Mathay RA. (1986). Drug-induced pulmonary disease. Part I: Cytotoxic drugs. Am Rev Respir Dis. 133, 321.

20. Mandy GR, Giuse TA. (1997). Hypercalcemia of malignancy. Am J Med. 103, 134–145.

21. Ginsberg SJ, Coomis RL. (1982). The pulmonary toxicity of antineoplastic agents. Semin Oncol. 9, 34.

22. White DA, Stover DE. (1984). Severe bleomycin-induced pneumonitis: Clinical features and response to corticosteroids. Chest. 86, 723.

23. Theologides A. (1978). Neoplastic cardiac tamponade. Semin Oncol. 5, 181.

24. Ahmann FR. (1984). A reassessment of the clinical implications of superior vena caval syndrome. J Clin Oncol. 2, 961–967.

25. Nieto A, Doty D. (1986). Superior vena cava obstruction: Clinical syndrome, etiology and treatment. Curr Prob Cancer. 10, 442.

26. Walker DI, Casciano DA (2000). Thoracic complications. In: Manual of Clinical Oncology, 4th edn (Eds Casciano DA, Lowitz BB), Lippincott Williams and Wilkins.

27. Sawaya R. (2001). Considerations in the diagnosis and management of brain metastasis. Oncology. 15, 1144–1148.

28. Lee RE, Lotze MT, Skibber JM et al. (1989). Cardiorespiratory effects of immunotherapy with interleukin-2. J Clin Oncol. 7, 7–20.

29. Margolin KA, Rayner AA, Hawkins MJ et al. (1989). Interleukin-2 and lymphokine-activated killer cell therapy of solid tumours: analysis of toxicity and management guidelines. J Clin Oncol. 7, 486–498.

30. Nora R, Abrams JS, Tait NS et al. (1989). Myocardial toxic effects during recombinant interleukin-2 therapy. J Natl Cancer Int. 81, 59.

Control of Pain and Anxiety and the Use of Muscle Relaxants in the Critically Ill

Control of Pain and Anxiety and the Use of Muscle Relaxants in the Critically Ill

Pain is an important symptom of disease, and indiscriminate suppression of pain may delay diagnosis and prevent correct management. Once a diagnosis is made and effective treatment planned, pain must necessarily be relieved. Post-operative and post-traumatic pain also needs effective relief, as it serves no useful purpose, and may prove detrimental to the patient in many ways (1).

The Anatomy of Pain (2)

Nociceptive stimuli are perceived by nerve endings throughout the body, and are conveyed by unmyelinated and small myelinated sensory axons to the posterior root ganglion in the spinal cord. A neuronal relay transmits the pain to the posterior horn cells. Many of the afferents terminating in the region of the spinal cord contain neuropeptides, including Substance P, cholecystokinin and somatostatin. These peptides probably play an important role in sensory transmission. The spinal dorsal horn is divided into a series of layers. Neurones processing noxious or nociceptive stimuli are found in a number of these layers. Unmyelinated afferents terminate in substantia gelatinosa (Layer II), while the myelinated afferents end in Layers I and V. The axons of neurones arising from the dorsal horn cross to the opposite side to ascend upwards as the ventrolateral spinothalamic tract. The spinothalamic tract can be conceptually divided into two systems based on its connections—a direct tract ending in the ventrolateral nucleus of the thalamus, and a phylogenetically older, spinoreticulothalamic tract that terminates at several levels within the reticular formation of the brainstem. This indirect tract is part of a polysynaptic system terminating in the medial thalamic nuclei.

Descending Analgesic Fibres (2)

In addition to this major ascending spinothalamic system, the nervous system contains descending nerve fibres that suppress nociceptive inputs. These descending fibres (at least in animals), originate in the periaqueductal grey matter, synapse in the nucleus raphe magnus in the medulla, and then project downwards into the spinal cord to the dorsal horns. The descending pathways can to an extent, gate or restrict the initial nociceptive stimuli received in the dorsal horns. The descending analgesic pathways described above, contain endogenous opiate peptides and opiate receptors. Opiate receptors are also present in the thalamus and the limbic system. These structures may therefore play an important role in the analgesic response to systemically administered narcotics.

Biogenic amines like serotinin and norepinephrine, are other neurotransmitters also present in the fine terminals of the descending analgesic pathways. A major descending analgesic pathway originates in the nucleus locus coeruleus of the pons. This pathway contains norepinephrine and inhibits nociceptive responses within the posterior horns through an alpha-adrenergic mechanism.

Physiopathology of Pain (2)

Perception of pain within the neuraxis excites segmental and central responses. Segmental response is characterized chiefly by increase in muscle tension, which intensifies pain. The central response consists of an increase in sympathetic tone resulting in tachycardia, and a rise in both blood pressure and cardiac output. The metabolic rate and both oxygen demand and oxygen consumption may increase. Pain also excites a neuroendocrine response. There is an increased secretion of catecholamines, cortisol, ACTH, aldosterone, antidiuretic hormone and glucagon. Insulin secretion can decrease. Severe unrelieved pain increases the catabolic state, and may cause a negative nitrogen balance; this could result in decreased immune function and delay wound healing (3). Nociceptive stimuli if unrelieved, can result in insomnia, nausea, vomiting, ileus, prolonged immobility and a feeling of increasing anxiety distress and frustration in the patient. Unabated chest pain as after cardiothoracic surgery can also contribute to poor respiration, through restriction of movements of the chest wall and diaphragm. This increases the chances of post-operative atelectasis. Management of pain and anxiety are therefore vital aspects of critical care.

The following section first describes the use of both narcotic and non-narcotic drugs for analgesia in a critical care setting. It then discusses the use of anxiolytic agents in critically ill individuals, and ends with a brief description of muscle relaxants in the intensive care unit.

The Use of Opioids or Narcotic Analgesics for Pain Relief (4)

Opioid or narcotic analgesics are the drugs most frequently used to relieve pain in critical care units. They may be used alone or in combination with non-steroidal anti-inflammatory agents. Remarkably enough, analgesics are often overused or underused. Their administration should be guided by the background disease, the immediate cause, and the severity of pain. The dose should always be individualized and titrated as needed. Pain relief must always be balanced against potential side effects of narcotics (chiefly respiratory depression, hypotension), and the effect these side effects could produce on the overall clinical outcome in a gravely ill individual.

Opioids (narcotic analgesics) can be given orally, intramuscularly or intravenously. Over the last 15 years new delivery systems have been developed, so that opioids can also be administered by the epidural, intrathecal, transdermal and transmucosal route. Opioids produce both analgesia and sedation through their action on the opioid receptors of the central nervous system

The intramuscular route of administering narcotic drugs is universally accepted for pain relief. We prefer to administer the drug as and when needed; the drug could also be given at fixed intervals (at 4 to 6 hours), provided the patient is carefully monitored. The major advantage of the intramuscular use of opioids is a lesser incidence of respiratory depression and hypotension, when compared to intravenous use. The disadvantage is a comparatively erratic absorption, erratic blood levels and slower action (4)

Relief of severe pain in a critical care setting is quicker and easier with a titrated intravenous administration of narcotic analgesic.

Intravenous Narcotic Analgesics (5)

The intravenous administration of narcotics brings prompt relief of pain and anxiety in an ICU setting. The dosage and the exact method of intravenous administration (either by bolus injections or by a continuous intravenous infusion) need to be individualized for each patient. 5 mg morphine or 0.1–0.3 mg buprenorphine given in a very slow intravenous bolus dose affords quick relief from pain. If intravenous morphine is given at intermittent intervals, the dose is 0.01–0.15 mg/kg every 2 hours, care being taken to ensure that respiration is not unduly depressed, and hypotension does not occur. Naloxone can reverse the respiratory depressant effect of morphine. A smaller dose of 2 mg morphine or 0.1 mg of buprenorphine should be initially given in elderly or frail patients so as to note the effect on respiration and circulation. Unfortunately morphine is generally unavailable except through a special permit and our ICUs make do with buprenorphine in its place.

Morphine or buprenorphine can also be given in a continuous intravenous infusion. An infusion rate of 0.07–0.5 mg/kg/hour of morphine, or 0.01 mg/kg/hour of buprenorphine, allows a steady level of the narcotic within the blood, and offers good relief. Alternatively, 30 mg pentazocine together with 50 mg promethazine is added to 500 ml of 5 per cent dextrose saline, and given intravenously in a slow infusion over 5–6 hours. The infusion can be repeated if necessary after 12 hours. Here again respiratory depressant and hypotensive side effects of the narcotic should be watched for. The patient should ideally remain sedated and free of pain, but yet easily arousable.

Hydromorphone (Dilaudid) is frequently used in the West for its potent analgesic effect. It is unavailable in our country, except through a special permit. When used intermittently the recommended dose is 10–30 µg/kg intravenously at 2 hourly intervals. The infusion dose ranges from 7–15 µg/kg/hour.

Other Synthetic Narcotic-Analgesics

Pentazocine

Pentazocine belongs to the benzmorphan group of synthetic compounds. It is indicated in the treatment of pain of intermediate severity. 30 mg of pentazocine is equivalent to 10 mg of morphine. The drug can be given intramuscularly, by intermittent intravenous injection, or in an intravenous infusion in the dose stated earlier. Its main advantage is that it does not cause dependence unless used in high doses for prolonged periods. Unlike pure narcotic agonists, its effects cannot be reversed by nalorphine. Intravenous naloxone is an effective antidote.

Pethidine (Meperidine)

Pethidine is similar to morphine, but has a shorter duration of action, and is less potent in relieving pain. It is usually administered in a dose of 1 mg/kg intravenously. Its use is contraindicated in patients who are on MAO inhibitors. Pethidine is metabolized by the liver; a principal product of metabolism is norpethidine, which can cause tremors, apprehension, delirium and seizures, and may interact with antidepressants.

Fentanyl is a recent synthetic opioid which is 50 to 100 times more potent for pain relief compared to morphine. The intravenous dose for a 60–70 kg adult is 0.1 mg. The drug has a short duration of action and has no significant effect on the circulatory system. It is increasingly used both in general anaesthesia and as a potent analgesic. Though fentanyl is the quickest and shortest acting analgesic, repeated doses may cause accumulation and prolonged effects. When administered as an intravenous infusion, the dose is 0.1 µg/kg/hour.

In patients with lesser degree of pain, fentanyl can be applied transdermally as a patch. The subdermis acts as a reservoir from which a slow and steady absorption of the drug occurs. Patches can deliver 25, 50, 75, 100 µg/hour. Peak analgesic levels occur after a time lag of 10–12 hours. A careful watch on possible respiratory depression and hypotension should be kept. Transdermal fentanyl should not be used for severe pain where need for urgent analgesic relief is important.

Remifentanil is even quicker and shorter acting than fentanyl, as it has a half-life of 3 to 10 minutes. It is given in an infusion in a dose of 0.6 to 15 µg/kg/hour. The short action and quick arousal after discontinuing the drug is useful when frequent clinical and in particular neurological assessment is called for.

Butorphanol tartarate is a recent opioid analgesic now available in India. It has a short half-life and is seven times more potent than morphine. When given intravenously its peak action is within 0.5 to 1 hour and its duration 3 to 4 hours. The intravenous dose is 1 mg repeated every 3 to 4 hours. Depressant effects on respiration and circulation need to be carefully watched for.

Ketamine is a potent synthetic opioid analgesic and anaesthetic. It is chiefly used in the ICU for bedside procedures and has been discussed in a later section of this chapter.

Patient Controlled Analgesia (PCA) (4, 6, 7)

PCA permits self-administration of a preset quantity of a narcotic intravenously, as and when needed. PCA enables a patient to control his own analgesic requirements. A lock-out device is incorporated into the system to prevent overdosage with the narcotic. This method provides effective analgesia, effective control over pain and anxiety, improves pulmonary function in post-operative patients, reduces sleep disturbances, and is shown to reduce the overall drug requirement, when compared to other methods of narcotic administration. The dosage in PCA needs to be individualized. An example of a prescribed dosage schedule with morphine is as follows—2–5 mg as a loading dose over 15–30 minutes, followed by a patient triggered bolus of 1–2 mg via the PCA pump, programmed with a lock-out interval of 15 minutes. This schedule may be changed according to the patient's response.

A similar schedule for norphine is as follows: 0.3–0.5 mg as a loading dose, followed by 0.1–0.2 mg of a patient triggered bolus via the PCA pump, with a lock-out interval of 15 minutes.

The PCA method of pain control can be combined with a slow infusion of a narcotic which allows a steady blood level of the drug to exert a continuous analgesic effect. It is essential to check the respiration, basic circulatory parameters, and the level of mental obtundation when using this combined approach to the relief of pain.

Recommendations for Analgesia in ICU Patients

It is important that the intensivist familiarizes himself with just a few opioid (narcotic) analgesics. The clinical practice guidelines on the use of analgesics in the critically ill adult have the following recommendations to make on analgesia (5):

(i) A therapeutic plan and goal of analgesia should be established for each patient.

(ii) If intravenous doses of an opioid analgesic are required, fentanyl and morphine are recommended agents. In our country where morphine is difficult to obtain, buprenorphine could substitute for morphine.

(iii) Scheduled opioid doses or a continuous infusion is preferred over an 'as needed' regime for consistent analgesia. In our opinion this may hold for a certain group or category of patients; an 'as needed' approach is safer and almost as effective.

(iv) Fentanyl is preferred for a rapid onset of analgesia in acutely distressed patients.

(v) Fentanyl or hydromorphone (not available in India) is preferred for patients with haemodynamic instability or renal failure.

(vi) Morphine (buprenorphine is the substitute we use) is pre-

ferred in intermittent therapy because of its longer duration of effect.

Adverse Effects of Opioids

The following are the adverse effects seen with the use of opioids:

(i) Depression of respiration. This needs to be carefully watched, particularly in the old and feeble.

(ii) Hypotension, due to a sympatholytic effect and a vagally mediated bradycardia.

(iii) Marked depression of the conscious level, which interferes with clinical assessment.

(iv) Rarely hallucinations and agitation are observed.

(v) Gastric hypomotility, ileus, urinary retention, constipation occur particularly with prolonged or frequent administration; these require symptomatic treatment.

(vi) Increase in intracranial pressure has been reported in patients with head injury.

Epidural and Intrathecal Opioids (8, 9)

Epidural and intrathecal administration of opioids relieves pain by acting on spinal pain receptors. Epidural administration of a narcotic is much more frequently used. It produces good relief with a relatively small quantity of the drug, without blocking motor and sympathetic nerves. It requires the placement of a catheter in the epidural space. Morphine or buprenorphine are the most frequently used analgesic narcotics. Since buprenorphine is more easily available, 150 µg of the drug diluted in 10–20 ml of N saline is administered slowly. This provides pain relief that may last for 12–16 hours, after which the dose can be repeated. Pethidine can also be used epidurally in a similar fashion, for pain relief.

Morphine and buprenorphine have been shown to spread in a cephalic direction to reach the fourth ventricle, after epidural administration. Two phases of respiratory depression may be observed. The first phase occurs within 30–45 minutes, and reflects absorption of the drug into the blood via the epidural veins. The second phase of depression occurs after 6–8 hours, and is due to rostral spread of the drug into the fourth ventricle, causing a direct depressant effect on the respiratory centre. It is best to avoid the systemic administration of narcotics if the epidural route is being used, as the danger of serious respiratory depression significantly increases.

Fentanyl, like morphine is a lipophilic agent which travels rostrally when given intrathecally, or through a catheter placed in the lumbar epidural space. It however travels in a cephalad direction less slowly than morphine, and is not as effective as the latter for relief of thoracic pain, but has fewer side effects (10, 11).

Epidural administration of narcotic analgesics can be given in the bolus form, as a continuous infusion (using an infusion pump), or can be administered as an infusion that can be controlled by the patient, as per his/her requirements (PCA).

Regional Anaesthesia (4)

Regional blocks to relieve pain are also of considerable use in certain circumstances. A typical example is the use of a regional intercostal block to relieve pain and ease breathing in a patient with rib fractures. Brachial plexus blocks can relieve severe pain in the upper limb, and local infiltration of a wound area in suitable cases can relieve pain arising from a serious wound. Regional anaesthesia blocks both afferent and efferent pathways of the reflex arc, and minimizes metabolic and neuroendocrine responses to painful stimuli. However, when local anaesthetics are used intrathecally, care must be taken to minimize side effects. These include hypotension and limb weakness or even paralysis secondary to sympathetic and somatic nerve block.

Lidocaine 0.5–1.5 per cent is the most commonly used local anaesthetic in the ICU, because of its rapid action lasting for a significant period of time, and its low incidence of side effects. It is used locally prior to the insertion of central lines and the pulmonary artery catheter. It is also used topically (in 4 per cent strength) in the nose, mouth, throat, tracheobronchial tree, oesophagus and urethra. An uncommon but important side effect following the local use of lidocaine, is a hypersensitivity reaction that rarely can cause anaphylaxis. Lidocaine is also used to provide pain control in spinal, epidural, caudal, nerve and field blocks

Bupivacaine is used in obstetric anaesthesia. It is slow-acting, but produces marked analgesia for a prolonged duration of time. It is often used for epidural anaesthesia and for intercostal nerve blocks. We have no experience with its use in a critical care setting.

Non-steroidal Anti-inflammatory Drugs (4)

These drugs probably act by exerting an inhibitory effect on prostaglandin synthesis. Non-steroidal anti-inflammatory drugs include diclofenac sodium (50 mg 8 hourly intramuscularly or

orally), and piroxicam (40 mg daily intramuscularly or orally). These drugs can relieve mild to moderate pain, but do not have the same efficacy observed with the narcotic group of drugs, in the relief of severe pain. They often cause gastritis, acute upper GI erosions which can bleed profusely, platelet dysfunction, and interstitial nephritis leading to renal dysfunction. Elderly patients, patients with hypovolaemia or hypoperfusion, and those with pre-existing renal insufficiency are more prone to NSAID-induced renal failure.

A number of oral NSAIDs are available—they include ibuprofen and naproxen. More selective COX-2 inhibitors are also available for oral administration. They are believed to produce less gastric irritation on long-term use. Acetaminophen is also useful to relieve mild pain. NSAIDs can on occasions be combined with the use of opioids for pain relief, so that the dose requirement of opioids is reduced.

A valuable addition to the non-steroidal anti-inflammatory drugs is ketorolac tromethamine, which can be given intramuscularly or intravenously for pain relief (4). This drug has no direct effect on opiate receptors. It is a potent analgesic—30–90 mg given intramuscularly has an efficacy comparable to 10 mg of morphine. Ketorolac can also be given intravenously in a dose of 15–30 mg repeated 6 to 8 hourly if necessary. The dose should be halved in elderly patients and the drug should preferably not be used for more than 5 days for fear of inducing renal insufficiency. Ketorolac is non-addicting and does not depress respiration. Its side effects are similar to those of other non-steroidal anti-inflammatory drugs. It should be avoided in patients with renal dysfunction, or in patients with a bleeding tendency. **Table 20.1.1** lists commonly used opioid and non-opioid analgesic drugs in a critical care setting.

Table 20.1.1. Common analgesics used in the ICU

Drug	Equianalgesic dose (IV)	Intermittent dose	Infusion dose	Main adverse effects
Morphine (special license needed for drug)	10 mg	0.01–0.15 mg/kg IV 2 hourly	0.07–0.5 mg/kg/hour	Depressed respiration, hypotension
Buprenorphine	0.3 mg	3 µg/kg	0.01 mg/kg/hour	Same as above
Fentanyl	200 µg	0.35–1.5 µg/kg IV at 0.5 to 1 hour	0.7–10 µg/kg/hour	Same as above, rigidity with high doses
Pentazocine	50 mg	0.5–1 mg/kg		Depressed respiration, hypotension
Pethidine (Meperidine)	75–100 mg	not recommended	not recommended	Same as above, occasionally, excitability, tremors, delirium, seizures
Hydromorphone (Not available in India)	1.5 mg	10–30 µg/kg/hour	7–15 µg/kg/hr	Depressed respiration, hypotension
Ketorolac		15–30 mg IV 6 hourly. Decreased in elderly patients. Avoid in renal insufficiency. Do not use > 5 days		Platelet dysfunction, GI bleed, renal dysfunction

Analgesics and Anaesthesia for Bedside Procedures (4, 12)

Cardioversion

5–10 mg of diazepam or 2–3 mg midazolam given intravenously is a safe and effective premedication prior to cardioversion, provided of course that there is sufficient time to use the premedication. Diazepam offers sedation, hypnosis and a period of amnesia.

Bedside Debridement of Wounds, Other Minor Surgical Procedures in the ICU, or Excision of Eschar in Burns Patients

Ketamine is a phencyclidine anaesthetic which produces dissociative anaesthesia, hypnosis and analgesia. When given intravenously in a dose of 2 mg/kg, it acts within 30–60 seconds. Its effect is short-lasting, and it has a plasma half-life of 2–3 hours (13). This excellent anaesthetic allows minor bedside surgical procedures like debridement of painful wounds, to be performed in the ICU. The drug when used intravenously as a short acting anaesthetic, is also extremely useful in the care of burns patients, particularly for the excision of eschars. Ketamine can also be given intramuscularly in a dose of 5–10 mg/kg, its onset of action then being 3–8 minutes. Ketamine in a dose of 1–2 mg/kg produces analgesia, with little change in the level of consciousness; the degree of analgesia is equivalent to that obtained with opioids. In the ICU, ketamine can be given before intubation, prior to changing surgical dressing, prior to orthopaedic manipulations and for other surgical procedures, such as incision, drainage of an abscess or a tracheostomy.

The short anaesthesia induced by intravenously administered ketamine (provided it is given slowly over 1 minute), is associated with preserved gag and laryngeal reflexes, and a slightly increased skeletal muscle tone. Ventilation is generally not depressed, and the patient does not require to be intubated. Emergence from anaesthesia may be associated with excitement and hallucinations, which can be easily controlled by diazepam, hyoscine or droperidol. Stimulation of the cardiovascular system may result in tachycardia and mild hypertension. Ketamine may induce profuse salivation, and hence an anti-sialogogue should be administered prophylactically.

Sedatives in the Critically Ill (14–17)

The intensive care unit is to an extent a hostile environment for critically ill patients. Noxious stimuli include pain, noise, suctioning of oropharyngeal and tracheal secretions, or tragedy involving other patients in the unit. Added to this is the sense of isolation, the difficulty encountered in communication (particularly in patients with an artificial airway), physical restraints associated with immobilization, other distressing sensory inputs, fear, anxiety, and often deprivation of sleep. All these features can lead to a stressful situation, eliciting a mental response that ranges from anxiety and depression, to anger, hostility, agitation or even psychosis.

Sedative-hypnotic medications are often necessary to calm the patient and dull the edge of anxiety and fear. The agents most frequently used are the benzodiazepines. Occasionally, propofol and barbiturates are also used; narcotics should preferably be given only for pain, or when pain and anxiety co-exist. The present discussion is restricted to the use of benzodiazepines. Ideally, a sedative and anxiolytic agent used in the ICU should have the following features—rapid onset of action, effective response, predictable duration of action, no adverse effects on vital functions, in particular on the respiratory and cardiovascular functions, and ease of administration. The drug should have a good therapeutic index, and if possible, a specific antagonist should be available in case of overdosage. Benzodiazepines satisfy many of the above requirements. They have sedative and anxiolytic effects, produce muscle relaxation, and have anticonvulsant properties.

The ideal level of sedation is one where the patient sleeps, yet is easily arousable. Severely hypoxic patients on mechanical ventilation or those on neuromuscular paralytic agents may require a higher degree of sedation.

Monitoring Sedation

No subjective or objective method or technique is ideal on monitoring sedation. Several monitoring protocols have been devised. The Ricker Sedation-Agitation Scale (SAS) has proved satisfactory for ICU patients (18, 19). The Vancouver Interaction and Calmness Scale is also used, and in children a widely used scale is the COMFORT scale (20, 21). A monitoring scale used in the ICU should be simple, yet should document the degree of anxiety present and the degree of sedation achieved with accuracy.

Diazepam

Diazepam is the most commonly used drug. It binds to specific receptors in the hypothalamic, thalamic and limbic areas of the brain (responsible for sedative effect), and to spinal receptors in the spinal cord, enhancing the inhibitory effects of gamma aminobutyric acid (GABA) and other inhibitory neurotransmitters (responsible for muscle relaxant effect). An intravenous dose acts within one minute, the maximum effect being observed in 2–5 minutes, and the duration of sedative action lasts for 4–6 hours. The drug is metabolized in the liver by microsomal oxidation and demethylation, its active ingredients being excreted by the kidneys. The drug should preferably not be given intramuscularly as its absorption is then erratic.

Diazepam is chiefly used as an anxiolytic agent which produces sedation and anterograde amnesia for stressful events. It is also used as a muscle relaxant (as in tetanus), and as an anticonvulsant (as in tetanus and in status epilepticus). It is the premedication of choice for cardioversion and for endoscopic procedures, and is also used in the management of addictive drug or alcohol withdrawal.

It is usually given slowly intravenously as a 2–10 mg bolus, and repeated after 6–8 hours if necessary. For cardioversion, 5–10 mg is given intravenously 5 minutes before the procedure. Status epilepticus is managed by 10 mg bolus doses of intravenous diazepam, or by an infusion of 30–50 mg of the drug in 500 ml of N saline. It is important to remember that individual response to the drug varies greatly, so that the dose should always be titrated to the response, particularly in feeble patients, or in the elderly.

Diazepam can produce prolonged drowsiness, and impairment of intellectual and psychomotor functions. Respiratory depression and even apnoea may occur, particularly if given rapidly. Bradycardia, hypotension, and even cardiac arrest have occurred in patients who are exquisitely sensitive to the drug, or when a large rapid bolus injection is used. The drug should be used with great caution, and as far as possible avoided altogether in patients with liver or renal dysfunction. Milder forms of anxiety are best treated by the oral use of the drug, 5–10 mg thrice daily.

Lorazepam

Lorazepam is a benzodiazepine with no specific advantage over diazepam. It acts on the benzodiazepine receptors in the central nervous system and spinal cord, enhancing the function of the inhibitory neurotransmitter GABA, by promoting the binding of this neurotransmitter to its receptors. It has the same sedative, anxiolytic, muscle relaxant and anticonvulsant properties as diazepam. The duration of action is 6–10 hours, and is longer than that observed with diazepam. The usual intravenous dose is 0.04 mg/kg. The maximum dose that can be administered is 2 mg intravenously and 4 mg intramuscularly. The bioavailability on intramuscular injection is better and more predictable than with diazepam. The dose however as with diazepam, needs to be titrated and individualized depending on the response. In status epilepticus, the drug is given in a 0.5–2 mg dose intravenously every 15 minutes, till seizures stop.

The side effects are exactly similar to those observed with diazepam. However venous thrombosis is infrequent with the use of lorazepam.

Midazolam (22)

The main advantage of this drug over diazepam is its very short duration of action. It is also two to three times more potent than diazepam. On intravenous use its action starts within one minute, peaks in 5 minutes, and lasts for 30–120 minutes. The drug has a short plasma half-life of 1.5–3 hours. Its metabolism is through mitochondrial oxidation in the liver, and its half-life (as with the other benzodiazepines) is significantly prolonged in liver cell dysfunction.

It is effective both intravenously and intramuscularly in a dose of 0.1 mg/kg, to a maximum of 2.5 mg/kg. Intermittent doses of 2.5–5 mg can be given every 3–4 hours. The drug in some instances can also be given as a slow intravenous infusion at the rate of 0.5–5 µg/kg/minute. The drug is freely available for use and it appears to have become the benzodiazepine of choice in many ICUs in the West. Its indications are exactly the same as for diazepam, and it has the same side effects. Apnoea and severe respiratory depression may occur, particularly in old, feeble patients. Myocardial depression and hypotension are also observed particularly in hypovolaemic patients who have received narcotics. A careful watch should be kept on cardiovascular and respiratory function, following its use.

Clinical features of overdosage with benzodiazepines are not uncommon in critical care units. This effect is either due to extreme sensitivity to the drug, or to overuse of the drug. Respiratory depression and hypotension can be life-threatening in some critically ill patients. *Flumazenil is the specific antidote for benzodiazepines*, and may be given slowly intravenously in a dose of 1mg. The dose can be repeated up to a total dose of 3 mg (23).

Propofol (Dipropylphenol)

Propofol is both an intravenous sedative and anaesthetic. It is short-acting and rapidly metabolized. When used as sedation, an initial intravenous dose of 0.5 to 1 mg/kg is given, followed by an infusion of 25 to 70 µg/kg/minute. The infusion rate is titrated to the level of sedation required. Patients become awake within 20 minutes of discontinuation of the drug. The shortness of action and quick arousal after stopping the drug is very similar to that of midazolam.

Propofol comes as a lipid emulsion and strict aseptic technique in administration should be followed for fear of nosocomial infection.

Side effects include hypotension and vasodilation. Sudden death has been reported from metabolic acidosis, particularly in children (24). Myoclonic jerks have been observed in some patients after drug withdrawal

Butyrephenones

These drugs inhibit dopamine-mediated neurotransmission in the cerebrum and basal ganglia, resulting in an improvement in abnormal thought patterns; a detachment of the patient from the environment is observed. Haloperidol (the most commonly used butyrephenone) is a useful drug to calm agitated patients. The drug is given parenterally in a dose of 0.5 mg to 5 mg; it takes 30 minutes for a full response to be evident. The drug could be repeated if agitation is uncontrolled or recurs. A small maintenance dose at night for 5 to 7 days may prevent night-time delirium or hallucinations.

Side effects include extrapyramidal signs, dyskinesia and very rarely the neuroleptic malignant syndrome. The drug also causes a prolongation of the QT interval; the ECG should therefore be monitored, particularly in cardiac patients.

Droperidol

Droperidol is similar to haloperidol but has a greater antiemetic and sedative effect than the latter. It can be combined with opioids to enhance sedation without causing further respiratory depression.

Barbiturates

They are one of the oldest of sedative hypnotic drugs. We use them chiefly as sedative hypnotics and as anticonvulsants in patients with seizures.

Table 20.1.2 lists the intravenous dose, onset of action, peak action, and duration of action of the commonly used sedatives.

Muscle Relaxants in Intensive Care (25)

Neuromuscular blocking agents are often used in critical care units. They are absolutely indispensable in the management of severe tetanus, and following major neurosurgery, or a head injury where restlessness, agitation and straining are to be controlled,

Table 20.1.2. Intravenous dosages, onset of action, peak action and duration of action of commonly used sedatives in the ICU

Drug	IV Dose	Onset of Action	Peak Action	Duration of Action
1. Diazepam	2–10 mg	1–2 mins	2–5 mins	4–6 hrs
2. Lorazepam	0.04 mg/kg	1–5 mins	60–90 mins	6–10 hrs
3. Midazolam	0.1 mg/kg	1–2 mins	2–5 mins	0.5–2 hrs
4. Propofol	1–2.5 mg/kg (maintenance dose 50–150 µg/kg/min)	< 1 min	1–2 mins	5–10 mins
5. Halopendol	0.15 mg/kg*	1–5 mins	60–90 mins	4–8 hrs

*IM dose

and where sedation is contraindicated for various reasons. Neuroparalytic agents are also indicated in status epilepticus which is uncontrolled or poorly controlled with the usual sedatives and antiepileptics. Mechanical ventilator support is mandatory in patients receiving neuroparalytic agents.

Perhaps the most frequent use of neuroparalytic agents in the ICU is to help in mechanical ventilator support in patients who continue to clash severely with the machine. In such instances, effective ventilation becomes impossible. Neuroparalytic agents should however only be used if all obvious correctable causes of a clash between the patient and the machine, are carefully excluded. These causes have been discussed in the Section on Mechanical Ventilation in the Critically Ill, and include incorrect ventilator settings, hypoxia, alveolar hypoventilation, a blocked airway, pneumothorax, airways obstruction, and a decreased compliance of the lungs due to oedema, pneumonia or atelectasis. There are however a number of patients where asynchrony between the patient and the ventilator is due to either uncontrolled agitation, or to a strong respiratory drive. The latter is most frequently observed in severe intrinsic lung disease (as in acute lung injury), and can only be abolished by the use of muscle relaxants. The use of inverse ratio mechanical ventilation in acute lung injury also often necessitates the use of muscle relaxants for proper ventilator support. Sedation, and relief of discomfort, pain and agitation with diazepam or narcotics, often enables the physician to offer ventilator support, without ultimately resorting to neuroparalytic drugs.

A patient paralyzed by a neuroparalytic agent has a feeling of extreme helplessness and dependency which leads to fear and anxiety. The use of benzodiazepines as sedatives, and anxiolytic agents is mandatory in all such patients, as also the use of analgesics for pain relief.

Table 20.1.3 lists the common indications for the use of muscle relaxants in the ICU.

Table 20.1.3. Indications for the use of muscle relaxants in the ICU

1. To facilitate mechanical ventilation
   – Facilitate endotracheal intubation
   – Machine-patient clash unrelieved by other methods
   – Severe ARDS, when using inverse-ratio pressure-controlled mode
2. Tetanus
3. Status epilepticus
4. To reduce work of breathing and oxygen consumption in critically ill patients
5. Hyperventilation in patients with increased intracranial pressure

Depolarizing Agents

Succinylcholine

This is the only clinically available depolarizing neuromuscular blocking agent. On intravenous administration it acts within 30 seconds, and has a short duration of action (5–10 minutes). It acts by binding to post-synaptic cholinergic receptors causing persistent depolarization and muscle paralysis. The drug however stimulates all cholinergic receptors, including autonomic ganglia, post-cholinergic nerve endings, and cholinergic receptors in the vessel walls.

The following side effects can be observed with succinylcholine:

(i) Bradycardia sometimes leading to sinus arrest. This is usually seen after administration of a single large bolus dose, or following a second dose of the drug.

(ii) Persistent muscle fasciculation. This can cause a hyperkalaemia which at times can lead to arrhythmias. Hyperkalaemia is enhanced in burns, following trauma, crush injuries, and following cerebrovascular accidents. Succinylcholine is therefore best avoided in these conditions.

(iii) Malignant hyperthermia can be triggered following its use.

(iv) A rise in intragastric pressure, which could cause regurgitation of gastric contents, and aspiration pneumonia.

The main use of succinylcholine in a critical care setting is to permit endotracheal intubation, when clenching of the jaw or increased muscle tone makes laryngoscopy impossible. The dose used is 1–2 mg/kg intravenously.

Non-depolarizing Neuromuscular Blocking Agents

These agents bind competitively to the post-synaptic cholinergic receptors at the neuromuscular junction, and prevent depolarization of the muscle by acetylcholine. They thereby induce a paralytic state in all voluntary muscles. The drugs in use are pancuronium, atracurium, and vecuronium.

Pancuronium

This is the main neuroparalytic agent easily available in poor countries. It is a long-acting water-soluble, non-depolarizing agent which is excreted mainly by the kidneys (90 per cent). Its renal clearance depends on the glomerular filtration rate. The drug is also metabolized and broken down into less active metabolites in the liver (10 per cent).

It is administered in a bolus dose of 2–6 mg intravenously (0.06–0.08 mg/kg). Muscle relaxation is observed in 2 minutes, and lasts for 30–40 minutes. Besides its neuroparalytic effect, pancuronium causes histamine release and has a mild vagolytic effect. It is unnecessary to aim for complete or total paralysis with this drug. The dosage should be titrated in such a manner as to enable the physician to achieve his objective. This does not always necessitate total paralysis. The drug can also be given as a continuous infusion through an infusion pump. We prefer the bolus method because it allows constant easy assessment of the patient, and in our opinion, a better titration of the dosage and frequency of administration of the drug, particularly when used over a long period of time.

Pancuronium in clinical practice, has little effect on the cardiovascular system. However after prolonged use (as in severe tetanus), each bolus dose may be followed by a transient drop in blood pressure due to histamine release. The elimination half-life of the drug is 90–160 minutes, and this is significantly prolonged in patients with hepatic or renal dysfunction. The dosage should be suitably reduced and carefully titrated in these conditions, else it can result in prolonged paralysis.

We have used this drug in patients with severe tetanus for as long as 6–8 weeks, with comparatively few or no side effects.

Atracurium

Atracurium is a non-depolarizing neuromuscular blocking agent which has an intermediate duration of action. Renal or hepatic dysfunction does not prolong its half-life; the drug is therefore safer to use when compared to pancuronium in renal or hepatic disease.

The intravenous dose in adults is 0.5 mg/kg. The onset of action is within 2 minutes, peak action occurs in 5 minutes, and the total duration of action is 20–60 minutes. Intravenous administration should be slow; a rapid bolus can cause significant histamine release and hypotension. It can be given by continuous infusion at a rate of 0.3–0.6 mg/kg/hour; in most instances recovery is rapid once the infusion is stopped. It is recommended for prolonged neuromuscular paralysis as in tetanus. It is however more expensive than pancuronium.

Vecuronium

Vecuronium is a shorter-acting monoquarternary analogue of pancuronium. Its great advantage is that it provokes no histamine release, has no vagolytic effects, and its use is therefore associated with a very stable cardiovascular system. The drug is chiefly metabolized by the liver, and is partially excreted by the kidneys.

In adults the drug is administered intravenously in a dose of 0.1 mg/kg. Its action starts within 2 minutes, peaks in 3–5 minutes, and duration of action lasts for 20–30 minutes. A continuous infusion of the drug is recommended in patients needing prolonged paralysis. The dose needs to be suitably reduced in patients with hepatic or renal dysfunction. Patients with cardiac disease do not require any adjustment in dosage. In patients with hepatic or renal disease, the duration of its effect may be variable and unpredictable. The drug is expensive.

Other Non-depolarizing Neuroparalytic Agents (4)

These include doxacurium, pipecuronium and mivacurium. Doxacurium and pipecuronium resemble pancuronium, but do not affect the cardiovascular system. Mivacurium has the shortest duration of action, its effect lasting for just 15–20 minutes. We have no experience with these drugs.

Complications Following the Use of Muscle Relaxants

Total or near total paralysis can induce fright and panic—hence the imperative need to use sedatives and anxiolytic agents in patients who are given muscle relaxants.

Pulmonary Complications

Paralyzed patients cannot cough. Secretions need to be carefully aspirated through the endotracheal tube or tracheostomy. Suction is often used in conjunction with expert physiotherapy to prevent atelectasis from retained secretions.

Neuromuscular Dysfunction

Delayed recovery from induced paralysis and neuromuscular dysfunction can occur after prolonged use of muscle relaxants (**26**). The following clinical syndromes are observed.

The first is a myopathy producing the clinical picture of flaccid quadriparesis. It is typically observed in severe asthmatics receiving high dose corticosteroids and who have been given muscle relaxants during ventilator support. Flaccid paralysis, increased creatinine kinase levels in blood, myonecrosis and slow recovery that can take several months characterize the clinical picture. Pancuronium, atracurium, vecuronium have all been reported to produce this syndrome. Steroid dose, and the dose of muscle relaxants should be kept to a minimum. The creatinine kinase level in the blood should be monitored and if the concentration increases, the muscle relaxant should as far as possible be stopped. The incidence of myopathy in asthmatics on both steroids and muscle relaxants, in our experience is between 10 to 20 per cent; the higher the dose of these drugs the greater the risk.

The second syndrome is a motor neuropathy without myopathy, following the long-term use of vecuronium and pancuronium. The neuropathy involves both upper and lower limbs, producing weakness, wasting of muscles and absent tendon reflexes. Weaning from mechanical ventilation is delayed and recovery may take weeks or even months.

A third syndrome observed following prolonged use of pancuronium or vecuronium is motor weakness of the limbs which on an EMG is related to failed neuromuscular transmission. Recovery occurs over several months.

Finally, a mixed neuropathic-myopathic syndrome may be observed. Notwithstanding the above description, we have been singularly fortunate in using pancuronium for prolonged periods of time in severe tetanus, without significant side effects.

Many sophisticated ICUs find it helpful to titrate the requirement and dose of muscle relaxants by the use of a peripheral nerve stimulator, with assessment of train-of-four (TOF) responses (**27**). This is a luxury we have dispensed with. Clinical judgment invariably suffices in adjusting both the dose and the frequency of administration.

Table 20.1.4 lists the common complications associated with the use of muscle relaxants in the ICU.

Reversal of Neuromuscular Blockade

Depolarizing agents have no specific antagonists. Neuromuscular block caused by non-depolarizing drugs can be reversed by anticholinesterase drugs. The drugs commonly used are neostigmine (0.06 mg/kg), pyridostigmine (0.2 mg/kg), and edrophonium (0.5 mg/kg). Atropine (0.01 mg/kg) is given simultaneously to counter the muscarinic side effects of these anticholinesterase drugs.

Table 20.1.4. Complications associated with the use of muscle relaxants

1. Ventilator failure or circuit disconnection can cause disaster if not promptly recognized
2. Pulmonary complications
   - Inability to cough—atelectasis
   - Pulmonary infection
   - Retained secretions—atelectasis
3. Prolonged paralysis after stopping muscle relaxant
   - Persistent neuromuscular blockade
   - Steroid-associated myopathy
   - Motor neuropathy
   - Neuromuscular dysfunction
   - A combination of the above
4. Immobility
   - Pressure sore
   - Peripheral nerve injuries
   - Deep venous thrombosis
   - Pulmonary embolism

REFERENCES

1. Drasner K, Katz JA, Schapera A. (1992). Control of Pain and Anxiety. In: Principles of Critical Care (Eds Hall JB, Schmidt GA, Wood LDH). pp. 958–973. McGraw-Hill International Inc., New York, London, Tokyo.

2. Maciewicz R, Martin JB. (1991). Pain: Pathophysiology and Management. In: Harrison's Principles of Internal Medicine, 12th edn (Eds Braunwald E, Isselbacher KJ, Petersdorf RG, Wilson JD, Martin JB, Fauci AS). pp. 93–97. McGraw-Hill Inc., New York, London, Tokyo.

3. Cuthbertson DP. (1980). Alterations in metabolism following injury: part I. Injury. 11, 175.

4. Lee Tai-Shion. (2002). Intensive Care Anesthesia and Analgesia. In: Current Critical Care Diagnosis and Treatment (Eds Bongard FS, Sue DY). pp. 104–125. McGraw-Hill, USA.

5. Pharm JJ, Fraser GL, Coursin DB et al. (2002). Clinical practice guidelines for the sustained use of sedatives and analgesics in the critically ill adult. Crit Care Med. 30(1), 119–141.

6. Eisenach JC, Grice SC, Dewan DM. (1988). Patient-controlled analgesia following Cesarean section: A comparison with epidural and intramuscular narcotics. Anesthesiology. 68, 444–448.

7. Tamsen A, Hartvig P, Fagerlund B et al. (1982). Patient-controlled analgesic therapy. Acta Anaesth Scand. 74, 157.

8. Crews JC. (1990). Epidural opioid analgesia. Crit Care Clin. 6, 315–342.

9. Stenseth R, Sellevoid O, Breivik H. (1985). Epidural morphine for post-operative pain: Experience with 1085 patients. Acta Anaesthiol Scand. 29, 148–156.

10. Hoffmann P. (1987). Continuous infusions of fentanyl and alfentanil in intensive care. Eur J Anesth. 1(Suppl), 71.

11. King MJ, Bowden MI, Cooper GM. (1990). Epidural fentanyl and 0.5 per cent bupivacaine for elective cesarean section. Anesthesia. 45, 285–288.

12. Ornato JP, Gonzalez ER. (1990). Drug Therapy in Emergency Medicine. Churchill Livingstone.

13. White PF, Way WL, Trevor AJ. (1982). Ketamine—Its pharmacology and therapeutic uses. Anesthesiology. 56, 119.

14. Ritz R, Spoendin M, Haefeli W. (1990). Long-term sedation in the critically ill. Update Intensive Care Emerg Med. 10, 723.

15. Bion JF. (1988). Sedation and analgesia in the intensive care unit. Hosp Update. 14, 1272.

16. Veselis RA. (1988). Sedation and pain management for the critically ill. Crit Care Clin. 4, 167–181.

17. Stone DJ. (1990). Sedation in the intensive care unit. Semin Anesth. 9, 162–168.

18. Riker RR, Fraser GL, Cox PM. (1994). Continuous infusion of halo-peridol controls agitation in critically ill patients. Crit Care Med. 22, 433.

19. Riker RR, Picard JT, Fraser GL et al. (1999). Prospective evaluation of the sedation-agitation scale for adult critically ill patients. Crit Care Med. 27, 1271.

20. de Lemos J, Tweeddale M, Chittock DR. (2000). Measuring quality of sedation in adult mechanically ventilated critically ill patients: the Vancouver Interaction and Calmness Scale. J Clin Epidemiol. 53 (9), 908.

21. Ambuel B, Hamlett KW, Marx CM et al. (1992). Assessing distress in pediatric intensive care environments: the COMFORT scale. J Pediatr Psychol. 17, 95.

22. Oldenhot H et al. (1988). Clinical pharmacokinetics of midazolam in intensive care patients: A wide interpatient variability. Clin Pharmacol Ther. 43, 263–269.

23. Bodenham A, Park GR. (1989). Reversal of prolonged sedation using flumazenil in critically ill patients. Anesthesia. 44, 603.

24. Parke TJ, Stevens JE, Rice ASC et al. (1992). Metabolic acidosis and fatal myocardial failure after propofol infusion in children: five case reports. Br Med J. 305, 613.

25. Durbin CG Jr. (1991). Neuromuscular blocking agents and sedative drugs: Clinical uses and toxic effects in critical care. Crit Care Clin. 7, 489–505.

26. Segredo V, Matthay MA, Sharma ML et al. (1990). Prolonged neuromuscular blockade after long-term administration of vecuronium in two critically ill patients. Anesthesiology. 72, 566–570.

27. Barnette RE, Fish DJ. (1995). Monitoring neuromuscular blockade in the critically ill. Crit Care Med. 23, 1790.

Critical Care of the Transplant Patient

CHAPTER 21.1

Critical Care of the Transplant Patient

Organ transplantation is an increasingly prevalent form of management in end-organ disease. Renal transplant, heart transplant, lung transplant, heart and lung transplant, liver transplant and pancreas transplant, are the solid organ transplants being practised in large centres in all Western countries, as also in a few countries in the East. In India, many centres have been carrying out renal transplants for several years. Stem-cell transplantation is in a way slightly different from solid organ transplants, and is also being done in a few centres in this country. Liver transplants have begun to be performed at centres in Mumbai, Delhi, Hyderabad and Chennai, and there have been a few successful heart transplants at centres in Delhi and Chennai. The reason for organ transplant surgery not keeping pace with countries in the West, is that the law in our country till recently did not legally recognize brain death, thereby excluding the donation of heart, lungs, liver, pancreas for transplant purposes. Fortunately, good sense has dawned on our lawmakers, and by an act of parliament, brain death has been accepted as a legal definition of death. This act has become law in most states of this country, which means that the era of organ transplantation in India is now about to begin. A social awareness of the need to donate organs under the right circumstances to save lives has unfortunately yet to be cultivated in our country. The infrastructure and organization necessary for the use of cadaver transplants in India is now being organized. It is to be ardently hoped that ethical safeguards for donor organs are strictly formulated and followed.

This section does not deal with the details of critical care of each individual organ transplant. There are however basic problems common to all transplant surgery. These are briefly dealt with below.

There are 3 major groups of complications in organ transplantation that determine outcome (1). These complications are common to all solid organ transplants. They include:

(i) Technical complications resulting from the surgical procedure of the graft implant.

(ii) Complications due to the effect of immunosuppressive therapy, and to rejection of the graft.

(iii) Complications due to infection (2).

Technical problems are generally observed in the early post-operative period, within the first 10–12 days. Rejection primarily occurs later in 10–60 days. Side effects of immunosuppressive drugs can occur early or late. Infectious complications can occur anytime after transplant surgery, due to active suppression of the immune system. However the pattern of infection in these patients in the early post-operative period (1–30 days), is different from the pattern observed in the period from 1–4 months, or even later.

Not all patients with organ transplantation require critical care. Renal transplants are not routinely managed in the ICU, unless age, background disease, or complications discussed below, necessitate close monitoring or critical care management. On the other hand, heart transplant, heart and lung transplant, lung transplant, liver transplant, pancreas transplant, all need critical care for a varying period of time after surgery. Many patients may also require critical care in the pre-transplant period for a varying length of time. A pre-operative assessment in all potential transplant recipients begins with a proper history, physical examination, ECG, X-ray chest, a full biochemical and blood profile, as also blood and tissue typing. Patients with evidence of coronary artery disease, undergo a more thorough cardiac evaluation, which includes a 2-D echocardiography, and when indicated a coronary angiography. Critical lesions in the coronaries should be preferably corrected before performing, for example, a renal transplant. Similarly endoscopy is indicated if there is a history suggestive of peptic ulcer, and transplant surgery is delayed till the ulcer has healed. The assessment of compliance is an important pre-operative feature of organ transplant surgery. A work-up prior to transplant surgery includes a study of Hepatitis B and C viral markers, other viral titers which should include antibodies for the cytomegalovirus (CMV), tests for HIV I and HIV II, urine culture, and cultures of a throat swab.

General contraindications for transplant surgery include malignancy, sepsis, manifest HIV infection, history of drug abuse, hepatitis, non-compliance, and advanced disease in an organ system, other than the one being considered for transplant.

Immediate Post-operative Care

The post-operative management of a transplant patient follows the general principles of post-operative care, with special reference to monitoring function of the organ transplanted. Heart, lung, liver transplants will require mechanical ventilation for at least 24 hours. Nasogastric suction through a nasogastric tube is required for intra-abdominal transplants, and in patients on ventilator support. Enteral feeds are started as soon as gut function returns.

The emphasis on laboratory data or on other investigational procedures, will depend on the organ transplant that has been done. Serial chest X-rays are important in the early post-operative period to assess the lung fields, and to check the placement of various lines and tubes. Common prophylactic measures include the use of antacids or sucralfate to protect against stress ulcers and the ulcerogenic effect of corticosteroids. Parenteral antibiotics in very good units are chiefly used peri-operatively for adequate antibacterial cover. Many units in the West use antifungal agents for oral candida prophylaxis, trimethoprim-sulfamethoxazole for prophylaxis against P. carinii (3), and gancyclovir for the first 3 months to prevent cytomegalovirus infection in solid organ transplants. Immunosuppressive therapy is a mandatory post-operative feature of all organ transplant regimes.

Complications in the Immediate Post-operative Period (0–10 days)

A. Technical Complications Related to Surgery

(i) *Vascular Thrombosis.* A major post-operative disaster is vascular thrombosis. This is rare in heart, or heart lung transplants, and is most common in liver transplants. The incidence of hepatic artery thrombosis following a liver transplant in adults, is 3 per cent. Vascular thrombosis is also observed after pancreatic transplants, though its incidence is on the decline. Thrombotic complications are relatively rare with renal transplants.

Recognition of vascular thrombosis is difficult because most patients are asymptomatic. Irreversible loss of the organ graft therefore results. Special ultrasonographic procedures can detect patency of the hepatic artery. Early diagnosis of hepatic artery thrombosis can be treated by thrombectomy, with a possible salvage of the transplanted liver. Biliary strictures however occur frequently, even when the transplant has been saved.

(ii) *Bleeding.* The management of post-operative bleeding in transplant patients is similar to that in other post-operative patients. A surgical cause for bleeding may need re-exploration. In liver transplant, severe bleeding may result from dysfunction of the graft leading to a coagulopathy. Replacement of clotting factors, and transfusions of packed red blood cells must be given till such time as graft function improves. Bleeding in the presence of good graft function, warrants early re-exploration.

B. Complications due to Immunosuppression

Immunosuppression protocols by and large are the same for all solid organ transplants. The complications related to immuno-suppression are also therefore similar. At times the occurrence of dysfunction of the transplanted organ causes difficulty in the evaluation of complications produced by the immunosuppressive drugs. The early side effects of immunosuppressive drugs are renal and neurologic dysfunction due to cyclosporine, hyperglycaemia, mental changes and acute gastroduodenal erosions due to corticosteroids, and leucopaenia and thrombocytopaenia from anti-lymphocyte preparations.

C. Infectious Complications

Infections in the immediate post-operative period are bacterial, and are similar in nature to those observed following other major surgery. Wound infection, nosocomial pneumonia, urinary sepsis related to urinary catheters, or infection introduced through central lines, are all observed. Gram-negative and staphylococcal infections are most frequently observed in our unit following renal transplant surgery.

Bacterial infections are treated with appropriate antibiotics, and by removal of lines that may have triggered the infection. Many units in our part of the world use prophylactic antibiotics after renal transplant surgery. The danger of superinfection with resistant organisms must always be kept in mind following unnecessary and wrong use of powerful antibiotics.

Complications in the Intermediate Post-operative Period (10 days to 1 month)

A. Technical Complications

Complications during this phase are generally related to break-down or leaks from anastomotic sites—ureterovesical anastomosis in renal transplant, tracheal or bronchial anastomosis in lung transplant, duodenovesical anastomosis in pancreatic transplant, and the bile duct anastomosis in liver transplant. The cause of anastomotic leaks is generally a poor blood supply to the anastomotic area. Treatment lies in immediate re-exploration. Re-exploration can be avoided in liver and kidney transplants, by drainage of bile or urine proximal to the leak. Ultrasound examination helps in the percutaneous drainage of localized fluid collections.

B. Rejection

Rejection is the major complication in this period. It leads to graft dysfunction; there are however other important causes of graft dysfunction, and it is vital to ascertain whether the dysfunction is related to rejection or to other causes. Thus oliguria following a renal transplant can be due to different aetiologies. A careful and quick diagnostic evaluation should distinguish between rejection and the other causes, so that correct management can be promptly instituted. A diagnostic work-up of oliguria after renal transplant surgery is given below in **Fig. 2.1.1a** and **b**.

A confirmed diagnosis of rejection is best made on histological grounds. In both heart and lung transplantation, a histological diagnosis of rejection can be made at a point in time when clinical and other functional parameters are barely, or only slightly altered. An early histological diagnosis of rejection can therefore lead to a suitable modification of immunosuppressive therapy, and result in improved graft survival. Graft surveillance by weekly biopsies of heart, lung and liver transplants, is an accepted feature of management. Early diagnosis of rejection allows of easier reversal, with less damage to the graft. Pancreatic biopsies to detect rejection are however best avoided because of the possible risk of pancreatitis. In renal transplants, some centres do not perform a diagnostic biopsy before the first treatment for rejection with corticosteroids. Most centres however do a diagnostic biopsy before a second course of treatment, or before using antilymphocytic preparations. In

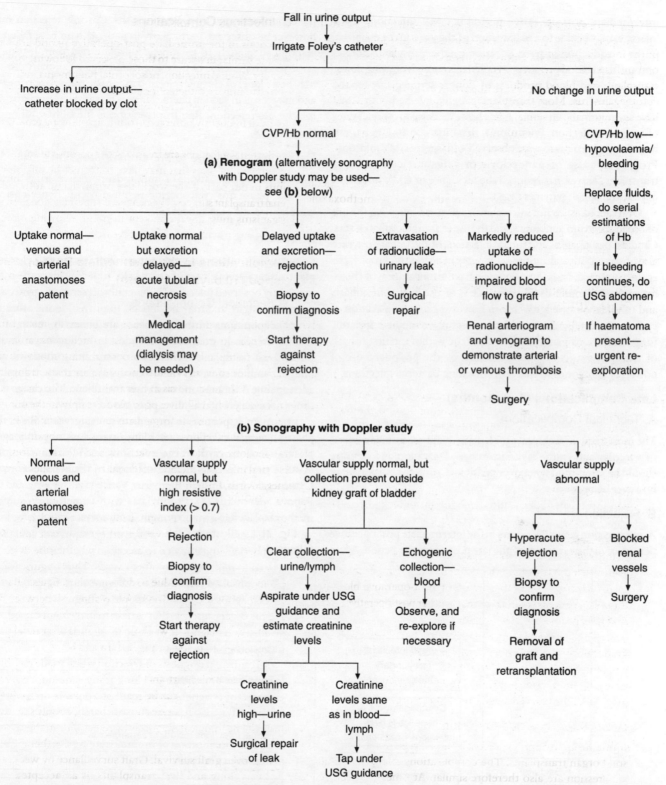

Fig. 21.1.1. Approach to post-operative oliguria in a patient with renal transplant: **(a)** using a renogram, and **(b)** using sonography with Doppler study.

renal transplant patients, cyclosporine therapy can unfortunately cause renal dysfunction, indistinguishable from renal dysfunction induced by rejection. The need for a biopsy and its correct interpretation, may help to distinguish between these two important causes of poor function of a renal graft.

C. Infection

Bacterial infections mentioned in the immediate post-operative period can continue to cause problems up to 1 month following transplant surgery. An important cause of morbidity in the intermediate post-operative period is CMV infection. CMV infection may be due to a reactivation of the virus in the recipient, or the introduction of fresh infection via the transplanted organ or transfused blood products. Prophylaxis consists of using donor transplants and blood products of donors seronegative for the cytomegalovirus. Most transplant patients infected with CMV have asymptomatic viraemia. A few however develop overt features of systemic infection. Pneumonia, hepatitis, chorioretinitis, and haemorrhagic colitis may be observed with severe CMV infection. Prophylactic use of gancyclovir or valgancyclovir in many transplant centres, has reduced the incidence of CMV infections in post-transplant patients (4, 5).

Oral candidiasis is not infrequently observed following the use of broad-spectrum antibiotics, and the use of immunosuppressants. Candidal oesophagitis and fungal infections of the urinary tract are also observed. Topical antifungal agents can be used for prophylaxis against oral candidiasis. Amphotericin B is the fungal agent of choice for systemic moniliasis. Fluconazole is of use in oral moniliasis and candidal oesophagitis. It can however cause an elevation of cyclosporine levels, which need to be carefully monitored. Systemic fungal infections generally do not occur within the first month of transplant surgery, unless induced by the prolonged use of powerful antibiotics to treat complicating bacterial infections.

Late Complications (1–6 months)

A. Technical Complications

The most frequent technical problems in this phase include stenosis of vascular and epithelial anastomosis. Dilatation and stenting should be attempted whenever possible. Corrective surgery may however be necessary.

B. Rejection

Acute rejection generally occurs in the intermediate post-operative period, or in the early part of the late post-operative period. Acute rejection is uncommon after 6 months. Chronic rejection may however be observed, particularly in patients who have failed to respond adequately to treatment for acute rejection. It usually presents as dysfunction of the transplanted organ. Coronary disease may be a sequel of chronic rejection in cardiac transplant patients, and may result in sudden death. There is no satisfactory treatment for chronic rejection. Retransplantation is the only solution to the problem.

C. Complications due to Immunosuppression

The chronic complications of immunosuppressive drugs during this late phase are cyclosporine nephrotoxicity, hypertension, lymphomas and skin cancer (6).

D. Infection

Opportunistic infections predominate after one month of transplant surgery. In our part of the world, tuberculosis is the most frequently observed infection. It generally presents as a pyrexia of unknown origin, and may be difficult to prove. Pleural effusion, lymphadenopathy within the chest or abdomen, are most often due to tubercle. Investigations include a bronchoalveolar lavage for acid-fast bacilli in patients with obscure lung shadows, and imaging studies to detect mediastinal, hilar or intra-abdominal adenopathy. A therapeutic trial with antituberculous drugs is at times necessary when all investigations have drawn a blank.

Important opportunistic organisms causing infections in this phase are fungal infections (including aspergillus), nocardia, toxoplasma infections, cryptococcal infections, and P. carinii infections. Possible viral infections include infections by the hepatitis C virus, Cytomegalovirus, Epstein-Barr virus, Varicella zoster virus and the Papova adenovirus (7). Prophylaxis with trimethoprin-sulphamethoxazol is often given to prevent Pneumocystis carinii infections.

Fig. 21.1.2 illustrates the time span for different infections following transplant surgery.

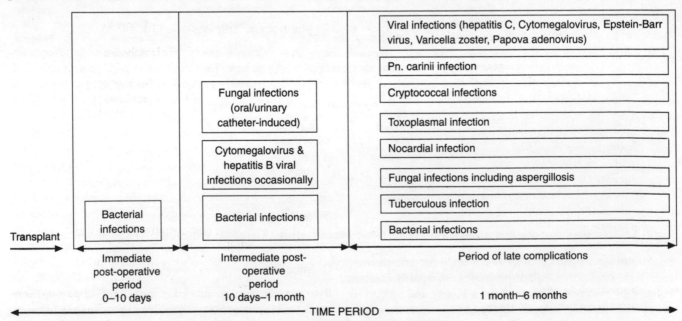

Fig. 21.1.2. Time span for occurrence of common infections in the organ transplant recipient.

Immunosuppression Therapy in Organ Transplants (8, 9)

Immunosuppressive drug regimes have been responsible for the great success of transplant surgery, and for the long-term survival of transplants. The critical care physician must be aware of the side effects of these drugs for two reasons—firstly they may be serious enough to necessitate critical care, secondly they need to be distinguished from other complications that follow transplant surgery.

The most important immunosuppressive drug in use today is cyclosporine. The drug is almost always used in combination with prednisolone. Some centres also add azathioprine to this immunosuppressive combination. A triple drug regime is often used in the hope that side effects from any one drug are lessened, and the combination may have an additive or even synergistic immunosuppresive effect.

Cyclosporine (10, 11)

Cyclosporine is the chief immuno-suppressant in use today. It prevents rejection, but is of little use in treating rejection once this has occurred. It is used intravenously in the immediate post-operative period, but after gut function returns the drug is given orally. Intravenous administration carries a greater risk of nephrotoxicity than the oral use of the drug. The drug inhibits the production of intrarenal prostaglandins, and thereby induces renal vasoconstriction. The intravenous drug dosage can be profitably reduced by the use of antilymphocytic preparations in the early post-transplant period. This schedule prevents rejection, and will allow the kidneys to recover function after surgery.

Sandimmune is the original oil-based cyclosporine preparation. Many units use the newer microemulsified preparation, neoral. Sandimmune requires the presence of bile salts for absorption. Neoral is less dependent on bile salts for absorption. Absorption of cyclosporine from the gut may prove a problem after liver transplantation, as bile is diverted from the gut by a T-tube. The drained bile should be re-fed through the nasogastric tube, thereby allowing absorption of the orally administered drug.

Drugs such as phenobarbitone, warfarin, phenytoin, rifampicin, which increase the activity of the P450 system, lead to increased metabolism of cyclosporine, with inadequate blood levels of the drug. On the other hand, ketoconazole, fluconazole, and erythromycin lead to increased blood levels of the drug.

Cyclosporine levels should be ideally estimated in the blood either by immunoassay or by the high performance liquid chromatography method. The immunoassay method is generally adequate, though it overestimates blood levels of the drug in the presence of cholestasis and jaundice. Unfortunately, very few centres in our country estimate cyclosporine levels by either of the above techniques.

The most important side effect of cyclosporine is renal dysfunction. It can occur early in the post-transplant period, and needs to be distinguished from renal dysfunction due to rejection of the graft. A biopsy of the renal graft is generally necessary for this purpose. Other side effects include headache, seizures, myoclonus, and hypertension. Gingival hyperplasia, hirsutism and hypercholesterolaemia may also be observed. Hyperkalaemia is an important side effect, and is related to hypoaldosteronism.

Tacrolimus (12)

Tacrolimus like cyclosporine is used to prevent acute rejection. It is protein bound, does not require bile salts for absorption and is given orally. Dose adjustments in patients with renal insufficiency are not necessary. As with cyclosporine, drug interactions between tacrolimus and other drugs can occur, thereby altering the blood level of tacrolimus. Side effects include hypertension, nephrotoxicity, tremors, abdominal pain and hyperglycaemia.

Corticosteroids (1)

Corticosteroids are useful both for prevention and treatment of rejection. At surgery a large dose of methylprednisolone 15–20 mg/kg is given. This is progressively tapered to a maintenance dose of 0.1–0.2 mg/kg within 2 months.

The important immediate side effects of corticosteroids are hyperglycaemia and mental changes severe enough to cause a psychosis. The hyperglycaemia lessens once the steroid dose is reduced; it may however need a titrated dose of insulin for its control. The long-term side effects of corticosteroids are numerous—obesity, cushingoid features, hypertension, osteoporosis, peptic ulcer, premature cataracts, and growth retardation in children.

Azathioprine (1)

This is useful in the prevention of rejection, but has no effect once rejection has occurred. Some units use azathioprine in their protocol from the outset; others use it after one episode of rejection has occurred. The major side effects are depression of the bone marrow and liver toxicity. The WBC count is best kept > 3500/ mm^3, and the liver functions should be monitored at periodic intervals.

Antilymphocytic Preparations (13, 14)

These preparations are antibodies to lymphocytes, whose functions are thereby inhibited. They are used to both prevent and treat rejection. The two preparations available are OKT3, a monoclonal preparation, and ATG (antithymocytic globulin), a polyclonal preparation.

In the immediate post-operative period, these drugs are given in sequential regimens with the purpose of delaying the initiation of cyclosporine therapy. Sequential therapy consists of an initial use of an antilymphocyte preparation, enabling renal function to improve and stabilize after surgery. Cyclosporine is added subsequently. The risk of renal dysfunction due to cyclosporine toxicity in the immediate post-operative period is thereby reduced (15). This regime was initially used in kidney transplants, but its use has now been extended in some centres to include other solid organ transplants, where renal dysfunction is a possibility due to intra-operative insults, or to pre-existing renal disease. ATG is initially used in preference to OKT3. This is because OKT3 appears to be more effective in treating rejection, and can be given via a peripheral vein on an outpatient basis. The early use of OKT3 may lead to sensitization that may hinder the future efficacy of the drug in treating rejection, if and when rejection occurs.

Antilymphocytic preparations, besides preventing rejection, are used to treat rejection in patients who have not responded to prior steroid therapy. ATG and OKT3 are associated with significant side effects related to cytokine release from lymphocyte activation. These include fever, hypotension, bronchospasm, and respiratory failure. The side effects can be controlled by the prior administration of methylprednisolone in a dose of 15–20 mg/kg. The antibodies in ATG can cross react with leucocytes (other than lymphocytes) and platelets, causing leucopaenia and thrombocytopaenia. A late hazard of antilymphocytic preparations is the development of lymphomas.

Newer Immunosuppressive Drugs

Several newer drugs are under trial and will probably come into use for post-transplant immunosuppressive therapy. The newest and most promising drug in clinical use is sirolimus. Further experience should decide whether sirolimus should be used as a first line drug together with other immunosuppressants, or whether it should only be reserved for patients who are at high risk for renal dysfunction, or for those who have developed nephrotoxicity following the use of cyclosporine and tacrolimus. The drug is administered orally, and has a half-life of 60 hours. It is metabolized in the liver; dose adjustments need to be made in patients with hepatic dysfunction but not in patients with renal dysfunction. Like cyclosporine and tacrolimus, sirolimus is metabolized by P450 enzyme systems. Drug interaction may occur with the use of drugs that interfere with this system. The main advantage is its comparative lack of nephrotoxicity. Side effects include hypercholesterolaemia, hypertrigyleridaemia. Anaemia, leucopaenia and thrombocytopaenia have also been observed (16).

REFERENCES

1. Barba L. (2002). Organ Transplantation. In: Current Critical Care Diagnosis and Treatment (Eds Bongard FS, Sue DY). pp. 777–798. McGraw-Hill, USA.

2. Rubin RH, Tolkoff-Rubin NE. (1991). The impact of infection on the outcome of transplantation. Transplant Proc. 23, 2068–2074.

3. Hughes WT, Rivera GK, Schell MJ et al. (1987). Successful chemoprophylaxis for Pneumocystis carinii pneumonitis. N Engl J Med. 316, 1627–1632.

4. Merigan TC, Renlund DG, Keay S et al. (1992). A controlled trial of ganciclovir to prevent cytomegalovirus disease after heart transplantation. N Engl J Med. 326, 1182–1186.

5. Pescovitz MD. (1999). Oral gangcyclovir and pharmacokinetics of volgancyclovir in liver transplant recipients. Transpl Infect Dis. (Suppl 1), 31–34.

6. Penn I. (1986). Collective Review—Cancer is a complication of severe immunosuppression. Surg Gynecol Obstet. 162, 603.

7. Smith SR, Butterly DW, Alexander BD et al. (2001). Vital infections after renal transplantation. Am J Kidney Dis. 37, 659–676.

8. Barry JM. (1992). Immunosuppressive drugs in renal transplantation: A review of the regimens. Drugs. 44, 554–566.

9. Bruce DS, Thistlewaithe JR. (1998). The Transplant Patient. In: Principles of Critical Care (Eds. Hall JB, Schmidt GA, Wood LDH). pp. 1325–1343. McGraw-Hill Inc., New York, London, Tokyo.

10. Kramer NC, Peters TG, Rohr MS et al. (1990). Beneficial effect of cyclosporine on renal transplantation. Transplantation. 49, 343.

11. Kahan BD. (1989). Cyclosporine. N Engl J Med. 321, 1725.

12. Testa G, Klintalm GB. (1997). Cyclosporine and Tacrolimus—The mainstay of immunosuppressive therapy in solid organ transplantation. Clin Liv Dis. 1(2), 417–437.

13. Thistlewaithe JR, Haag BW, Gaber AO et al. (1987). The use of OKT3 to treat steroid-resistant renal allograft rejection in patients receiving cyclosporine. Transplant Proc. 19, 1901.

14. Benvenisty AI, Cohen D, Stegall MD, Hardy MA. (1990). Improved results using OKT3 as induction immunosuppression in renal allograft recepients with delayed graft function. Transplantation. 49, 321.

15. Stock PG, Ascher NL, Osorio RW et al. (1993). Standard sequential immunosuppression with Minnesota antilymphoblast globulin and cyclosporine vs FK 506: A comparison of early nephrotoxicity. Transplant Proc. 25(1 Part 1), 675–676.

16. Chang J, Mahanty HD, Quan D et al. (2000). Experience with the use of sirolimus in liver transplantation—use in patients for whom calcineurin inhibitors are contraindicated. Liver Transpl. 6, 734–740.

Critical Care in Pregnancy

22.1 Introduction

22.2 Critical Illness Not Specific to Pregnancy

22.3 Critical Illness Specific to Pregnancy

Introduction

The critical care aspects of a pregnant patient have four differentiating features compared to the critical care of one who is not pregnant. First, there are specific differences in the physiology between the gravid and non-gravid patient. The physician or the intensivist has to be aware of these changes if he is to distinguish the 'normal' from the 'abnormal'. Second, critical care of the pregnant patient includes care not only for the woman but also of the foetus. Third, diagnostic procedures, interventions and drug therapy that may be optimal for the patient may pose actual or potential hazards to the foetus. Finally pregnant patients in critical care units could present with emergencies observed in non-pregnant women, and also with grave problems peculiar to the pregnant state.

This section first gives a very brief overview of the relevant physiological changes in pregnancy followed by relevant observations on critical illnesses in the obstetric patient not specific to pregnancy. It then goes on to describe the major critical illnesses requiring critical care that are specifically related to the pregnant state. These illnesses are (i) pre-eclampsia—eclampsia and their variants—the HELLP syndrome and the haemolytic uraemic syndrome (HUS); (ii) the acute fatty liver of pregnancy; (iii) amniotic fluid embolism; (iv) septic abortion.

Physiological Changes in Pregnancy (1)

Physiological changes in pregnancy should be looked upon as an adaptive process which provides maximum support for the foetus and minimizes the stress on the mother. Support to the foetus consists of ensuring an adequate placental blood flow, thereby providing enough oxygen and nutrients to the foetus. Reduction in maternal stress is chiefly through an expanded maternal blood volume, which acts as a buffer to compensate for substantial blood loss that always accompanies even a normal delivery. This expanded blood volume is responsible both for an increased cardiac output and an increased flow through the placental vessels (2).

Changes in the Cardiovascular System (1, 3)

A rise in the diaphragm that accompanies advancing pregnancy causes the heart to be more horizontally placed so that the apex is shifted to the left. The cardiac silhouette often appears larger than normal on an X-ray of the chest.

Haemodynamic changes are characterized chiefly by an increase in cardiac output by 30–50 per cent, most of which occurs by the first trimester. The increase in cardiac output is due to both an increase in stroke volume and cardiac rate. After about 6 months of pregnancy the cardiac output may decrease by over 20 per cent in the supine position because of pressure of the gravid uterus on the inferior vena cava; this results in a reduced venous return and a fall in cardiac output.

Peripheral vascular resistance as also pulmonary vascular resistance decrease during pregnancy. The hyperdynamic circulatory state in pregnancy is characterized by tachycardia, an increased cardiac output, and an increased pulse pressure with warm peripheries. There is a prominent third heart sound at the apex and a systolic flow murmur which is generally best heard over the pulmonary area. There is also to start with, a decrease in systemic blood pressure which reaches its nadir by the sixth month; the pressure then gradually increases but should not be greater than non-pregnant levels at any time during pregnancy.

Labour and delivery are associated with even greater stress. Cardiac output increases by over 40 per cent; there is an additional 15 per cent increase in cardiac output with each uterine contraction. Delivery of the foetus is associated with an even further increase in cardiac output, presumably because of autotransfusion of blood contained in the uterus. This extra cardiac stress can lead to decompensation in patients with background heart disease, or could induce a sharp rise in left atrial pressure, resulting in acute pulmonary oedema in patients with mitral stenosis.

Changes in the Respiratory System

Several aspects of pulmonary function change during pregnancy. There is an increase in tidal volume by about 40 per cent and a fall in residual volume by 20 per cent, as also a fall in the expiratory reserve volume. The forced vital capacity is unaltered.

The total oxygen uptake is increased by 30–40 ml/minute and there is a disproportionate increase in minute ventilation by about 50 per cent at full-term. This hyperventilation in pregnancy is probably hormonally mediated and results in a $PaCO_2 < 30$ mm Hg.

Changes in Renal Physiology

There is an increase in glomerular filtration rate, an increase in the creatinine clearance and lowered serum creatinine values

(< 0.9 mg/dl). A serum creatinine of say 1.4 mg/dl which would be considered normal in a non-pregnant female would indicate significant renal impairment in a pregnant female. As pregnancy progresses, there is a reduced sensitivity to endogenous vasopressors; this is responsible for decrease in the systolic and diastolic arterial pressures and the widened pulse pressure.

Changes in Gastrointestinal Physiology

Most of the changes in the GI tract are caused by progesterone related alteration of smooth muscle relaxation. Decreased lower oesophageal sphincter tone leads to gastro-oesophageal reflux. There is also a hormone-related generalized hypomotility of the gastrointestinal tract.

The abdominal viscera are pushed laterally, upwards and posteriorly by the enlarging uterus. The displacement of viscera may lead to problems in the interpretation of physical signs associated with common inflammatory abdominal pathologies. Thus as pregnancy advances, Mcburney's point and Murphy's sign do not have the same relevance as in non-pregnant patients.

Haematological Changes

These include an increase in plasma volume by 40–60 per cent and an increase in red blood cell mass by 25 per cent. There is therefore often a dilutional anaemia with a Hb concentration of 11 g/dl at 24 weeks of pregnancy. Biochemical changes include a fall in serum osmolarity and a slight decreased concentration in the serum levels of sodium, potassium, calcium and magnesium. The total proteins and serum albumin level are lowered in proportion to the degree of volume expansion. The levels of cholesterol and triglycerides may double in pregnancy.

The levels of clotting factors are altered. The fibrinogen level is as high as 600 mg/dl. Fibrin degradation products can be detected in traces. The risk of thromboembolism increases with a relative risk of 1.8 in gestation and 5.5 during puerperium. Increased venous stasis may contribute to the increased risk of thromboembolism.

Immune System

Pregnant women are at risk for certain infections. Reactivation of viral diseases and of tuberculosis appears more common in pregnancy. Varicella, pyelonephritis occurring in pregnancy are associated with more severe complications. The reason for this immune dysfunction has not been elucidated.

REFERENCES

1. Naylor DF, Olson MM. (2003). Critical care obstetric and gynecology. Crit Care Clin. 19, 127–149.

2. Martin C, Varner MW. (1994). Physiological changes in pregnancy: surgical implications. Clin Obstet Gynecol. 37, 241–255.

3. Beall M, Cedars LA, Fortson W. (2002). Critical care issues in pregnancy. In: Current Critical Care Diagnosis and Treatment (Eds Bongard FS, Sue DY), pp. 883–885. Mcgraw-Hill, USA.

Critical Illness Not Specific to Pregnancy

Serious illnesses necessitating critical care afflict pregnant and non-pregnant females equally. However the pregnant state can at times influence the incidence, occurrence and clinical manifestations of both medical and surgical problems that require intensive care. The intensivist needs to focus attention not only on the pregnant patient but also on the unborn foetus. Emergencies characterized by hypoxia or fulminant infections increase foetal mortality and morbidity. Foetal monitoring in critical illness is therefore mandatory, particularly in conditions which affect maternal pulmonary or cardiovascular function. Auscultation of the foetal heart rate is an easy method to monitor the presence and degree of foetal distress. Continuous foetal heart monitoring by an electronic monitor is indicated in the viable or near viable foetus (beyond 23 weeks) during crisis situations or during surgical procedures when hypotension, anaesthesia can lead to foetal compromise.

A very brief account of the possible influence of pregnancy on important critical illnesses (1) (not specific to pregnancy) is given below.

Respiratory Disease (2)

The important causes of acute respiratory failure in pregnancy are acute severe asthma, community acquired pneumonia, aspiration pneumonia, pulmonary oedema, and occasionally acute lung injury and ARDS.

In our experience acute severe asthma is the commonest medical emergency encountered in pregnancy. In asthmatic patients pregnancy causes a worsening of the asthmatic state in about one-third of patients. The asthma remains unchanged in another third and may improve in the remaining third. Other than the influence of high dose corticosteroids on the foetus, there is no evidence that the use of beta-agonists or theophylline increases the morbidity or mortality of the foetus. Management of acute severe asthma in pregnant patients should be no different from that in the non-pregnant patient.

Community acquired pneumonia is caused by the usual organisms, but treatment of pneumonia in the pregnant patient should include an awareness of the potential toxic effects of antibiotics on the foetus. Consideration should also be given to the harmful effects of diagnostic imaging involving the use of X-rays. Hypoxia caused by severe pneumonia or acute severe asthma should be corrected adequately and promptly; close monitoring for foetal distress is mandatory. The arterial oxygen saturation should be kept > 90 per cent to avoid foetal compromise.

Aspiration as a cause of pneumonia is frequent in the pregnant patient because of the hormonally induced reduced tone of the lower oesophageal sphincter and the increased transdiaphragmatic pressure due to the gravid uterus.

The causes of non-cardiogenic pulmonary oedema are the same as in the non-pregnant woman. However the use of tocolytic agents to retard the progression of labour is associated with an increased incidence of pulmonary oedema. Also, pulmonary oedema induced by tocolytic agents is observed to be at times more resistant to conventional therapy (1).

Ventilator management of pregnant patients is no different from that of the non-pregnant patient. Attention should be directed to the use of the lowest possible oxygen concentration, and the avoidance of both high inflation pressures and of respiratory alkalosis. The objective is to prevent hypoxia in the mother and the foetus; yet a high maternal PaO_2 (> 100 mm Hg) may lead to oxygen toxicity in the foetus. Higher than usual inflation pressure may however be necessary in late pregnancy to allow an adequate minute ventilation. We have found management of ARDS in late pregnancy distinctly more difficult than in the non-pregnant woman.

Cardiovascular Disease

The commonest cardiovascular disease in pregnancy necessitating intensive care is rheumatic heart disease with cardiac failure. Mitral stenosis is the most frequent cardiovascular problem meriting intensive care. Acute pulmonary oedema in mitral stenosis is often related to the tachycardia and high output state which is the normal physiology of the pregnant patient. Pulmonary oedema is worsened in the presence of atrial fibrillation with a fast ventricular rate. Digitalis and diuretics are safe during all stages of pregnancy.

Pulmonary embolism is an important hazard in pregnancy and the puerperium. Warfarin is contraindicated because of the danger of possible intracerebral bleed in the foetus and because of proven teratogenicity. Heparin is the preferred drug for anticoagulation. In patients with extensive venous thrombosis of the leg veins or in those with repeated embolic episodes, consideration should be given to the insertion of an inferior vena caval filter.

Major cardiac surgery is best avoided during pregnancy unless absolutely necessary. The surgical procedure that may be life-saving is a valvular commisurotomy for a tight mitral stenosis. However, coronary artery bypass surgery, valve replacement, repair of great vessels have all been performed at good centres with excellent results. Acute cardiomyopathy, though rare, is a recognized complication during the post-partum period. The cause is unknown and the treatment is as for any acute congestive cardiomyopathy.

Renal Disease (3)

Pregnant patients are particularly prone to acute pyelonephritis. The latter may take a fulminant course, causing overwhelming sepsis, acute renal failure and multiple organ dysfunction syndrome.

The specific causes of acute renal failure related to pregnancy are dealt with later.

Neurological Disease

Serious neurological problems are common to both pregnant and non-pregnant patients. However cortical venous thrombosis with thrombosis of the intracranial venous sinuses is more frequent in the pregnant state and the puerperium. It often presents with seizures and is often wrongly diagnosed as epilepsy, or stroke or meningitis.

Myasthenia gravis may undergo remission or exacerbation during pregnancy. It may also be associated with transient neonatal myasthenia from transplacental passage of acetylcholine antibodies.

Autoimmune Diseases

Autoimmune diseases may remit or exacerbate during pregnancy. The two important autoimmune diseases which may need critical care during pregnancy are systemic lupus erythematosus and the antiphospholipid syndrome (APS). The latter syndrome is associated with an increased rate of abortion, foetal loss and maternal mortality (4). Thrombocytopaenia and the propensity to arterial and venous thrombi characterize this syndrome. Aspirin and the use of heparin are advocated in the management of APS presenting as an emergency meriting critical care.

Endocrine Disease (1)

Control of insulin-dependent diabetes is more difficult in the pregnant state, yet ketoacidosis is uncommon. Gestational diabetes is characterized by reduced glucose tolerance initially diagnosed during pregnancy. Early gestational diabetes (before 20 weeks) often necessitates the use of insulin for proper control. There is also an increased risk of overt diabetes after pregnancy in these patients.

The features of thyrotoxicosis occurring in pregnancy may be wrongly attributed to the altered physiology in pregnancy. Tachycardia, palpitation, heat intolerance, are common both to

hyperthyroidism and to the pregnant state. Antithyroid drugs readily cross the placental barrier; they should be used with caution to prevent foetal hypothyroidism.

Surgical Emergencies

Surgical emergencies occur with the same frequency as in the non-pregnant woman and include in the main acute appendicitis, acute cholecystitis, biliary colic, peptic ulcer disease, intestinal obstruction and inflammatory bowel disease.

Acute appendicitis is the most frequent surgical emergency requiring operative intervention. The risk of conservative management clearly outweighs the risk of surgery at all stages of pregnancy. Progressive enlargement of the uterus may displace the caecum upwards, so that maximal tenderness may not be elicited over Mcburney's point. Ultrasound examination is of great help in atypical presentations. Laparoscopic appendicectomy is perhaps best confined to the first trimester; laparoscopic identification is difficult at full term.

Acute cholecystitis, particularly in the first and last trimesters is treated conservatively unless there are clinical features suggesting impending gangrene of the gall bladder. Surgical emergencies like intestinal obstruction, volvulus are difficult to diagnose particularly in advanced pregnancy. Surgery is indicated only after failure of medical management.

A surgical emergency that can be missed for a time is peritonitis due to accidental bowel perforation during the performance of a caesarian section. Abdominal guarding and rigidity are markedly reduced in these patients because of the stretching and laxity of the abdominal musculature caused by a fully gravid uterus. Persistent pain, free fluid within the abdomen and fever are warning signs that should not be ignored.

Drugs Used During Pregnancy

Drugs used for the mother can produce dangerous effects on the unborn foetus. The clinician must therefore be aware of the teratogenicity and toxic effects of drugs on the foetus. Though the mother's safety and life come first, the intensivist must consider possible alternative therapies which may be less dangerous to the foetus. Yet the principle underlying the choice of a drug or therapeutic modality is that the anticipated advantage to maternal health and recovery far outweighs the theoretical risk to the foetus. Thus the use of a life-saving drug for which there is no alternative is indicated in spite of its potential teratogenicity or toxicity to the foetus.

Cardiopulmonary Resuscitation in the Pregnant Woman

If cardiac arrest occurs in a pregnant woman, resuscitative measures are exactly as routinely recommended. Closed chest compression, defibrillation, use of adrenaline, vasopressors and other drugs should be carried out exactly as one would in a non-pregnant patient. It is often necessary to displace the uterus from the large abdominal vessels by a right hip wedge. If cardiopulmonary resuscitation is unsuccessful, the performance of perimortem caesarian section may be performed under appropriate circumstances, in the hope of extracting a live foetus.

REFERENCES

1. Naylor DF, Olson MM. (2003). Critical care obstetric and gynecology. Crit Care Clin. 19, 127–149.

2. Rizk NW, Kalassian KG, Gilligan T et al. (1996). Obstetric complications in pulmonary and critical care medicine. Chest. 110, 791–809.

3. Wing DA. (1998). Pyelonephritis. Clin Obstet Gynecol. 41, 515–526.

4. Breuster JA, Shaw NJ, Farquharson RG. (1999). Neonatal and pediatric outcome of infants born to mothers with antiphospholipid syndrome. J Perinat Med. 27, 183–187.

Critical Illness Specific to Pregnancy

Pre-eclampsia–Eclampsia

General Considerations

Pre-eclampsia is an important, common complication of pregnancy. It generally becomes evident in the second half of pregnancy, during labour, or for the first time in the immediate puerperium, without there being preceding evidence of the disease. The disease is typically characterized by hypertension (BP > 140/90 mm Hg), significant albuminuria ($\geq$ 300 mg / day) and generalized oedema, which however may be more apparent on dependent areas, such as the feet. The disease always resolves over a period of time after delivery. The aetiology of pre-eclampsia is obscure. The disease can be mild, moderate or severe, or graduate from mild to severe. The moderately severe and severe forms constitute a grave hazard to both mother and foetus and necessitate critical care.

Eclampsia is characterized by generalized seizures (for which there is no other cause) in a woman with pre-eclampsia. However eclampsia may strike suddenly in a pregnant woman who may often have no complaints or who exhibits mild to moderate hypertension very briefly before the onset of seizures.

It is best to consider pre-eclampsia–eclampsia as belonging to one clinico-pathological spectrum extending from the milder forms of pre-eclampsia to the severe form of eclampsia.

Incidence and Predisposing Factors

The incidence is probably about 1 in 20 or 30 pregnancies. It is more frequent in primigravidas than in multigravidas. Increasing maternal age, obesity, a history of previous pre-eclampsia and a family of history of pre-eclampsia are also additional risk factors. Medical disorders that add to the risk of pre-eclampsia are pre-existing chronic hypertension, chronic renal disease, diabetes, antiphospholipid antibody syndrome, background connective tissue disease and severe migraine.

Placental / foetal factors contributing to an increased risk of pre-eclampsia include advanced gestational age, multiple pregnancy, poor placentation, hydatiform mole, placental hydrops, trisomy 13, tripoidy (**Table 22.3.1**).

Physiopathology (1)

The physiopathology remains obscure. The presence of the placenta is crucial to the development of pre-eclampsia. There

Table 22.3.1. Factors predisposing to pre-eclampsia

Maternal Factors
* Primigravida
* Increased maternal age
* Obesity
* History of previous pre-eclampsia
* Pre-existing hypertension
* Chronic renal disease
* Diabetes
* Anti-phospholipid antibody syndrome
* Connective tissue disease

Placental Factors
* Advanced gestational age
* Multiple pregnancy
* Poor placentation
* Hydatiform mole
* Placental hydrops
* Trisomy 13
* Triploidy

appears to be a relative ischaemia due to changes in the uteroplacental circulation. The changes are two-fold. There is a partial lack of significant dilatation of the spiral arteries supplying the intervillous spaces; this dilation is necessary to accommodate the expanded uteroplacental flow in the second half of pregnancy. There is also an obstruction of these spiral arteries by fibrin, platelets and lipid-laden macrophages. Whether this impoverished uteroplacental circulation due to changes in the spiral arteries are primary features or merely associated features of pre-eclampsia is not clear.

The pathology in the maternal circulation has excited a great deal of interest. The full picture of pre-eclampsia–eclampsia is not just a primary hypertension problem, but is the consequence of diffuse endothelial dysfunction which results in disturbed function of various organ systems, widespread changes in the walls and lumen of arteries and arterioles, and coagulation abnormalities. The current belief goes a step further in postulating that the endothelial dysfunction is merely one aspect of a generalized systemic inflammatory response that also involves leucocytes, clotting factors and other components of the inflammatory system. This systemic inflammatory response in a very mild asymptomatic form is believed to be present in the last trimester of normal pregnancy. Pre-eclampsia results when this pregnancy induced inflammatory response for any reason accelerates and leads to decompensation of one or more organ systems (2). In other words, if this concept is indeed proven true, pre-eclampsia is merely an exaggeration or an aberration of a phenomenon present in every normal pregnancy (2). It is the decompensation of various organ systems in severe pre-eclampsia that is responsible for complications that could easily lead to death.

Clinical Features

The minimum criteria for the diagnosis of pre-eclampsia are: (a) sustained blood pressure elevation of 140 mm Hg systolic or 90 mm Hg diastolic in a previously normotensive woman after 20 weeks of pregnancy; (b) proteinuria of at least 300 mg in a 24 hour urine collection. Oedema is frequent but is not included as an essential feature because some degree of pitting oedema is often observed in the last trimester of a normal pregnancy. However a sudden increase in body weight and oedema often presages the occurrence of pre-eclampsia.

Hypertension is the essential feature and is caused by increased peripheral vascular resistance due to generalized endothelial dysfunction. The blood pressure is typically unstable. The circadian rhythm is often altered, with initially a loss of the normal fall of blood pressure at night, and later a paradoxical marked increase in blood pressure during sleep.

Severe pre-eclampsia is associated with dysfunction of various organ systems (3). It is of utmost importance to realize that changes in organ function do not necessarily correspond with the degree of rise in blood pressure.

Generalized oedema can occur but is inconsistent. Renal dysfunction could progress to acute tubular necrosis. CNS dysfunction takes the form of cortical blindness, cerebral haemorrhage and/or seizures (eclampsia). Involvement of the respiratory system can result in laryngeal oedema and acute lung injury/ARDS. Disturbances in the coagulation profile can lead to varying degree of disseminated intravascular coagulopathy. Hepatic dysfunction is characterized by right hypochondrial pain, tenderness, elevated liver enzymes, and rarely by hepatic infarction or even hepatic rupture. Left heart failure with pulmonary oedema is also observed.

Foetal crises are frequently observed. They include foetal distress, foetal asphyxia, abruptio placenta and intrauterine foetal death.

Complications associated with severe pre-eclampsia–eclampsia are listed in **Table 22.3.2**.

Pre-eclampsia is best classified as mild to moderate or severe. Severe pre-eclampsia is characterized by at least one of the following additional criteria: (i) blood pressure > 160 mm Hg systolic or > 110 mm Hg diastolic; (ii) proteinuria > 5 g in 24 hours; (iii) serum creatinine > 2 mg/dl; (iv) non-cardiogenic pulmonary oedema (ARDS); (v) oliguria < 500 ml/24 hours; (vi) microangiopathic haemolytic anaemia; (vii) thrombocytopaenia; (viii) hepatocellular dysfunction; (ix) symptoms of end-organ involvement (cortical blindness, severe headache, severe abdominal pain); (x) foetal growth restriction; (xi) eclampsia (seizures in a pregnant woman for which there is no other cause).

Table 22.3.2. Organ system involvement in severe pre-eclampsia–eclampsia

Maternal
* CNS—Cortical blindness, cerebral haemorrhage, grand mal seizures
* Acute renal tubular necrosis
* Acute cortical necrosis
* Generalized oedema, laryngeal oedema
* Acute left ventricular failure
* Acute lung injury, ARDS
* Disseminated intravascular coagulopathy
* Hepatic infarction, intrahepatic haemorrhage, hepatic rupture

Foetal
* Intrauterine death
* Intrauterine asphyxia
* Placental abruption

Eclampsia

Eclampsia is merely the severe end of the spectrum of pre-eclampsia. The term is applied to grand mal seizures in a patient with pre-eclampsia, in whom the seizures cannot be attributed to any other cause. As mentioned earlier, it can strike suddenly with the patient being unaware of having pre-eclampsia. Also the features of pre-eclampsia may antedate eclampsia by a very short period of time (less than a day or two). Seizures are often preceded by severe persistent headache. The occurrence of seizures is not necessarily related to the degree of hypertension, but is related to microangiopathic changes in cerebral vessels. Visual disturbances are frequent and often include cortical blindness. Cerebral oedema, cerebral haemorrhage, disseminated intravascular coagulopathy and ARDS are in our experience more often observed with eclampsia than in non-eclamptic patients.

There are two other syndromes which are currently considered complications or variants of the pre-eclampsia–eclampsia state. These are the syndromes characterized by haemolytic anaemia, elevated liver enzymes and lowered platelets (HELLP syndrome) and the other characterized by haemolysis and uraemia (the haemolytic uraemic syndrome—HUS).

HELLP Syndrome (2)

There is still controversy as to whether this syndrome is a separate entity or falls within the spectrum of pre-eclampsia. The haemolytic anaemia is due to a microangiopathic haemolytic process and rarely requires packed cell infusion. Thrombocytopaenia is moderate and platelet counts < 30,000/mm³ are only rarely observed. The elevated liver enzymes that characterize the HELLP syndrome are due to hepatocellular injury, perhaps caused by vasospasm and microangiopathic changes involving vessels supplying the liver cells. The rise in hepatic serum enzymes may be associated with hepatic infarction, intrahepatic haemorrhage, subcapsular haemorrhage and in rare instances hepatic rupture. The latter is an acute emergency needing prompt surgery. The maternal mortality in the HELLP syndrome is estimated to be 1–2 per cent.

Haemolytic Uraemic Syndrome (HUS)

This syndrome is believed to be a variant of thrombotic thrombocytopaenic purpura (TTP) without the presence of neurological features which typify TTP (2). It is rare in pregnancy and though considered to fall within the spectrum of pre-eclampsia may well be in our opinion, a separate rare entity. The HUS is characterized by renal dysfunction with high creatinine levels, an increase in the serum lactate dehydrogenase levels (> 1000 U/l), and decreased haptoglobin levels. The direct Coombs test is negative. Coagulation studies are within normal limits.

Differential Diagnosis

Hypertension occurring in the second half of pregnancy may be due to causes other than pre-eclampsia. These include chronic hypertension (pre-existing hypertension antedating pregnancy), gestational hypertension (pregnancy-induced hypertension with proteinuria), and elevated blood pressure seen in pregnant patients with acute fatty liver. Acute glomerulonephritis or pyelonephritis complicating pregnancy can also cause hypertension.

Coagulation abnormalities can be caused by conditions other than pre-eclampsia. These include amniotic fluid embolism and acute fatty liver of pregnancy.

A combination of elevated liver enzymes and thrombocytopaenia may occur with viral infections such as dengue, falciparum malaria and by other causes of hepatitis

Management (4)

Severe pre-eclampsia merits critical care. The patient should be closely monitored with regard to vital signs and with regard to laboratory tests to evaluate functions of different organ systems. A central venous line is inserted before any serious disturbance in the coagulation profile occurs. A careful monitoring of the arterial blood pressure is imperative. Arterial pH and blood gases are done and repeated as and when necessary. A close intake-output chart is vital and if possible the patient should be weighed daily.

Delivery. The definitive treatment of pre-eclampsia is delivery of the foetus. In severe pre-eclampsia this should be undertaken promptly. The features of severe pre-eclampsia are then relieved and subside over a period of time. If however, the mother's condition has stabilized and there is little or no organ dysfunction, conservative management with anti-hypertensives and support to all organ systems may be tentatively continued, only if the foetus is very immature. This is however controversial and should be entertained only when the anticipated benefit to the foetus is far greater than the risk to the mother or to both the mother and the foetus.

Control of Hypertension. The blood pressure should be kept below 140/90 mm Hg. We use a combination of hydralazine, alphamethyldopa and nifedipine to control blood pressure. When systolic blood pressure is > 180 mm Hg or diastolic > 110 mm Hg hydralazine in a dose of 5–20 mg is given intravenously. An alternative is the use of labetalol, 20 mg intravenously given as a bolus. The drug is repeated if necessary at a higher dose of 30–40 mg every 15 minutes till a suitable fall in blood pressure results.

Oral or sublingual nifedipine has been reported to produce a sharp fall in blood pressure, but we have used this drug safely without untoward effect. A carefully titrated and closely monitored infusion of nitroglycerine or sodium nitroprusside can also be used to control severe hypertension. Both drugs however cross the placental barrier and could exert toxic effects on the foetus.

It is debatable whether control of hypertension can reverse or delay maternal organ damage or increase foetal salvage rates. Hence the dictum that prompt delivery is the treatment of choice in patients with severe pre-eclampsia.

Support to All Organ Systems. Oliguria (< 30 ml urine/hour) can be due to a depleted intravascular volume, to cardiac failure or to isolated renal arteriolar spasm. Each of these requires appropriate treatment. Low dose dopamine infusion at 2–4 µg/kg/min may help improve urine output, particularly in the presence of renal arteriolar spasm.

Pulmonary Oedema. Pulmonary oedema may be precipitated by volume overload, by left heart failure or by damage to the alveolar capillary membrane (acute lung injury). Hypoalbuminaemia may contribute further to pulmonary oedema. Diuretics, use of oxygen, use of digitalis for heart failure and ventilator support for acute lung injury become necessary.

All other organs deserve efficient support—cerebral oedema is countered by the use of mannitol and coagulation disorders by the proper replacement of coagulation factors. Patients with severe pre-eclampsia should be given seizure prophylaxis with intravenous magnesium (see below).

Management of Eclampsia (5)

Management consists of control of seizures, control of hypertension with drugs and prompt delivery.

Seizures are controlled best by administering a 4 g intravenous bolus of magnesium sulphate over 10 minutes, followed by a continuous infusion of 2 g/hour. The infusion rate is titrated so as to keep the serum magnesium level between 4.5–8 mg/dl. If the patient has already been on intravenous magnesium as a prophylaxis (in severe pre-eclampsia), or if a recurrent seizure occurs after the initial seizure, a further 2 g bolus is administered.

Magnesium sulphate is undoubtedly the drug of choice for eclamptic seizures. If the latter are difficult to control in spite of the use of intravenous magnesium, a titrated infusion of diazepam (20–50 mg in 500 ml glucose) and intravenous dilantin sodium in an appropriate dose should be added to the therapy.

All organ functions need support, in particular the central nervous system, renal and haematological systems. Close monitoring of all vital parameters and of organ functions is imperative. Arterial pH and blood gases need to be frequently monitored; oxygen is almost always indicated. In patients with severe or recurrent seizures, or in obtunded patients, the airway should be promptly secured by endotracheal intubation. Mechanical ventilator support is indicated in the presence of hypoxia, recurrent or prolonged seizures, in the presence of pulmonary oedema, and when the patient is heavily sedated to suppress seizure activity.

Nosocomial infection should be quickly diagnosed and treated with appropriate antibiotics.

Management of HELLP Syndrome (6)

The haemolytic anaemia in this syndrome rarely needs packed cell infusions. The thrombocytopaenia is also generally not so marked as to require platelet infusions. Liver cell function should be supported by the use of intravenous glucose, vitamins and adequate nutrition. The latter may be difficult to achieve in the presence of right hypochondrial pain and vomiting. Symptomatic treatment for vomiting includes the use of phenergan, prochlorperazine (stemetil) and ondansetron (emeset).

Dexamethosone 10 mg intravenously 12 hourly usually results in clinical improvement and in a reversal of laboratory abnormalities. This therapy may permit some delay in delivery, if the foetus is far too premature. Dexamethasone also promotes lung maturation in the foetus. The abnormalities however all return when dexamethasone is discontinued.

Management of the Haemolytic Uremic Syndrome

The current treatment is the administration of plasma transfusions. Initially 30–40 ml/kg of plasma is infused, followed by a reduction to 15–20 ml/kg once stabilization occurs. If improvement is not seen, plasmapheresis should be promptly used. Corticosteroids (100–200 mg hydrocortisone intravenously 8 hourly), dipyridamole, immunoglobulins, and immunosuppressants have all been tried with limited success. Platelet infusion should be avoided except perhaps when there is marked thrombocytopaenia with severe bleeding, as platelets tend to promote further intravascular thrombosis.

REFERENCES

1. Redman CWG. (2003). Hypertension in Pregnancy In: Oxford Textbook of Medicine (Eds Warell DA, Cox TM, Firth JD, Benz EJ Jr.). pp. 396–402. Oxford University Press, Oxford, New York.

2. Redman CWG, Sacks GP, Sargent IL. (1999). Pre-eclampsia: an excessive maternal inflammatory response to pregnancy. American Journal of Obstetrics and Gynecology. 180, 499–506

3. Barton JR, Sibai BM. (1992). Acute life-threatening emergencies in pre-eclampsia–eclampsia. Clin Obst Gynecol. 35, 402–413.

4. Redman CWG, Robert JM. (1993). Management of pre-eclampsia. Lancet 341, 1451–1454.

5. The Eclampsia Trail Collaboration Group. (1995). Which anticonvulsant for women with eclampsia? Evidence from collaborative eclampsia trail. Lancet 345, 1455–1463.

6. Sibai BM, Ramadan MK, Usta I et al. (1993). Maternal morbidity and mortality in 442 pregnancies with hemolysis, Elevated liver enzymes and low platelets (HELLP syndrome). Am J Obst Gynecol. 169,1000–1006.

Acute Fatty Liver of Pregnancy

General Considerations

This is a very rare but catastrophic complication of pregnancy. Its incidence is believed to be 1 in 10,000 to 1 in 20,000 deliveries. It is characterized by severe hepatic dysfunction with massive fatty infiltration within the hepatocytes occurring either during the last trimester of pregnancy or in the immediate post-partum period (1). There are many who believe that this entity is a variant of pre-eclampsia, as the disease is frequently associated with hypertension and is more prone to occur in first pregnancies and with twin gestation (2). Earlier, the mortality in acute fatty liver of pregnancy was reported to be over 70 per cent. Currently the mortality is close to 20–30 per cent partly because less severe forms of the disease are recognized and partly because of early diagnosis and treatment.

The aetiology of acute fatty liver in pregnancy is unknown. It is possible that the disease is more likely to occur in mothers who carry foetuses which have a genetic defect in the oxidation of fatty acids (3).

Clinical Features (1)

The clinical features are characterized by nausea, vomiting and increasing anorexia for 4 to 7 days. This is followed by jaundice and a tender enlarged liver. The serum bilirubin is raised to a varying extent; liver enzymes and alkaline phosphate are raised. Hypertension is frequently present and may be associated with albuminuria and oedema.

In severe cases there is progressive deterioration of liver cell function characterized by hypoalbuminuria, ascites, hepatic encephalopathy and a progressive worsening coagulopathy. Hypoglycaemia due to worsening liver cell function, hepatorenal failure and metabolic acidosis are observed. Death when it occurs is due to severe multiple organ failure.

Pancreatitis is a noted complication and is associated with worsening abdominal pain and with elevation of serum amylase and lipase. Diabetes insipidus is a reported association; it may result in hypernatraemia.

Improvement in the patient's condition generally occurs following delivery of the foetus. There is an increased incidence of foetal deaths from uteroplacental insufficiency, if delivery is delayed.

The *differential diagnosis* is from other causes of acute or fulminant hepatitis, in particular viral hepatitis and drug-induced hepatitis. The diagnosis can be confirmed by a liver biopsy which demonstrates microvesicular fat within the hepatocytes. A USG of the abdomen demonstrates increased echogenicity of the liver; a CT or MRI reveals decreased attenuation of the liver parenchyma.

Management

Critical care is required for patients with acute fatty degeneration of the liver.

Monitoring. Close monitoring of the patient and the foetus is imperative. Foetal heart sounds should be continuously monitored to detect foetal distress or compromise. Liver functions, blood chemistry, blood glucose and functions of all organ systems need careful monitoring, in particular the renal and coagulation profiles. A central line should be inserted to help measure central venous pressure and guide fluid replacement early in the natural history of the disease.

Stabilization. Critically ill patients should be urgently stabilized. Hepatic encephalopathy should be treated on the usual lines (see Chapter on Fulminant Hepatic Failure). Hypoglycaemia poses a danger to both mother and foetus. Fluid and electrolyte disturbances are common and need to be restored to normal. Alteration of the coagulation profile should be countered by appropriate infusions of fresh frozen plasma, platelets and cryoprecipitate as indicated. Renal dysfunction is present in critically ill patients, necessitating fluid restriction and occasionally renal replacement therapy. Hypertension is frequently present and may require the use of hydralazine and other antihypertensives indicated earlier. If acute fatty degeneration of the liver is associated with other features of severe pre-eclampsia, magnesium sulphate should be used prophylactically (in the dose indicated earlier) to prevent seizures.

Delivery. Once the patient is stabilized, delivery is done preferably through a caesarian section. Spinal or epidural anaesthesia should only be risked if the coagulation profile and platelets have returned to normal. General anaesthesia is otherwise used, taking care to avoid agents which are hepatotoxic.

Following delivery. Management involves meticulous multi-organ support, particularly to the liver. Proteins are avoided or sharply reduced in planning nutritional support. Calories should consist chiefly in the form of carbohydrates given as intravenous glucose or through a nasogastric tube. Branched-chain aminoacids intravenously help supply proteins (see Chapter on Nutrition in the Critically Ill). Lactulose 30 ml thrice or four times a day helps to reduce ammonia production and absorption from the large bowel. A bowel wash using metrogyl is also of help.

Fluid and electrolyte balance is important. Vitamin K should be administered daily and the coagulation profile is kept normal through proper blood product replacement therapy. Nosocomial infection is frequent, particularly in ventilated patients; it needs the use of appropriate antibiotics.

REFERENCES

1. Bacq Y. (1998). Acute fatty liver of pregnancy. Semin Perinatol. 22, 134–140.
2. Naylor DF, Olson MM. (2003). Critical care obstetrics and gynecology. Crit Care Clin. 19, 127–149.
3. Ibdah JA, Bennett MJ, Rinaldo P et al. (1999). A foetal fatty acid oxidation disorder as a cause of liver disease in pregnant women. N Engl J Med. 340, 1723–1731.

Amniotic Fluid Embolism

General Considerations

Pulmonary embolism is a dreaded complication during pregnancy, at labour or in the puerperium. The source of embolism is generally the deep veins of the lower limbs, occasionally the pelvic veins or the large uterine venous sinuses. Women particularly at risk are those confined to bed because of pre-eclampsia or eclampsia, or those who have had a caesarian section. Venous thromboembolism is considered an important cause of death in the above situations.

In contrast, amniotic fluid embolism is rare, but catastrophic. It was first described in 1926. The overall incidence is unknown, but is believed to be 1 in 8000 to 1 in 80,000 deliveries (1). The maternal mortality can be as high as 85 per cent; the foetal mortality is less, about 20 per cent. Although very rare, it remains the third leading cause of maternal deaths in the United Kingdom after thromboembolism and hypertensive disorders of pregnancy (1).

This catastrophic emergency is associated with increased maternal age, multiparity, protracted difficult labour, placental disruption and signs of foetal distress as evinced by meconium-stained amniotic fluid. It has been reported as a complication of termination of pregnancy in the first or second trimester, during normal pregnancy and the puerperium. The greatest risk is during labour. The emergency is caused by the escape and release of amniotic fluid into the maternal pulmonary circulation, blocking the pulmonary vasculature and triggering an inflammatory host response mediated by leukotrienes and other arachidonic acid metabolites. Activation of the coagulation pathways leads to disseminated intravascular coagulopathy.

Clinical Features (2)

Massive amniotic fluid embolism is characterized by a sudden progressive deterioration in the clinical condition of the mother, characterized by hypotension, dyspnoea, hypoxia, cyanosis, culminating in cardiac arrest.

If the patient survives the immediate catastrophe, the clinical features are those of the acute respiratory distress syndrome. Hypoxia, tachypnoea, crackles over both lungs with bilateral shadowing on the X-ray of the chest are observed. Tachycardia and hypotension are generally present.

A third presentation, generally associated with ARDS, is the occurrence of disseminated intravascular coagulopathy (DIC) probably triggered by the inflammatory response induced by the contents of amniotic fluid. DIC may occur in 40–50 per cent of patients.

Diagnosis

The diagnosis is suspected from the clinical presentation. There is no confirmatory diagnostic test during life. The classic autopsy finding is the presence of foetal squamous cells in the maternal pulmonary circulation.

Management

Treatment is supportive. It includes cardiopulmonary resuscitation, and circulatory support through volume infusions plus the use of inotropes and vasopressors. Intubation with mechanical ventilator support is mandatory. ARDS is managed on conventional lines as discussed in an earlier chapter (see Chapter on Acute Respiratory Distress Syndrome). Coagulopathy should be treated with infusion of appropriate blood products. Prompt delivery of the foetus through a caesarian section should be considered if there is a cardiopulmonary arrest, which does not respond to resuscitative efforts.

REFERENCES

1. Naylor DF, Olson MM. (2003). Critical care obstetric and gynecology. Crit Care Clin. 19, 127–149.
2. Locksmith GJ. (1999). Amniotic fluid embolism. Obs Gynecol Clin North Am. 26, 435–444.

Sepsis in Obstetrics

Conditions leading to sepsis in the non-pregnant female can also produce sepsis in the pregnant female. Diagnosis is rendered difficult in the presence of a gravid uterus and by constraints on imaging techniques that could be potential hazards to the foetus. Management of sepsis unrelated to pregnancy and delivery is the same as in the non-pregnant female. Surgery is technically more difficult in the presence of a gravid uterus and surgical interference can pose a danger to the foetus.

The most important condition causing sepsis directly related to pregnancy is septic abortion; this section briefly deals with this entity.

Septic abortion is sepsis associated with the spontaneous or induced termination of a recent pregnancy. Septic abortion is much more frequent in poor, developing countries where abortion is often performed by quacks in filthy conditions and by crude and dangerous methods. The chances of complications are greater when abortions are attempted in later pregnancy and when dilatation of the cervix and evacuation procedures are performed.

Maternal sepsis can also occur after the delivery of a child at full-term, particularly if labour is conducted improperly with unsterile instruments. Maternal sepsis is also a feature of a dead, retained, macerated foetus within the uterus.

Clinical Features (1)

In a patient with a recent history of instrumentation to end pregnancy, the cardinal features of sepsis are fever, lower abdominal and pelvic tenderness, tenderness of the uterus on vaginal examination and a serosanguinous or purulent vaginal discharge. Vaginal bleeding, sometimes exsanguinating, may at times be the presenting symptom.

Fever and tachycardia are invariably present. Tachypnoea, hypotension and the features of increasing septic shock can evolve with frightening rapidity. Disturbances in organ function become manifest early. Elevated liver enzymes, a modest rise in serum creatinine and a slight prolongation of the prothrombin time are forerunners of multiple organ failure. In severe cases, disseminated intravascular coagulopathy sets in with bleeding from various sites, in particular from the uterus. Death occurs from hypotensive shock and/or multiple organ failure.

Laboratory Examination

Blood, urine, cervical secretions should be sent for routine examination and culture. Leucocytosis is frequent but severe leucopaenia often accompanied by thrombocytopaenia is also an indication of sepsis. Gram's stain of cervical secretions may guide initial therapy before culture reports are available. This is of utmost importance in the early diagnosis of infection with Clostridia

perfigens. The latter appear as Gram-positive rods on Gram's stain of cervical secretions or of curetted material. Imaging studies may reveal gas in the myometrium and in fulminant cases a crepitus can be felt in the soft tissues of the vagina and vulva.

X-ray of the abdomen may also detect perforation of the uterus or bowel which may complicate the use of dangerous procedures to achieve abortion.

An ultrasound of the abdomen may reveal the presence of retained products of conception as also inflammatory pathologies and abscesses within the pelvis and in the adnexa. A CT of the abdomen and pelvis would help to define and localize an abscess even better than an ultrasound. It would also clearly reveal the presence of gas in the myometrium and soft tissues of the pelvis in clostridial infection

Laboratory investigation should include determination of function of various organ systems; these parameters should be repeated as and when necessary. A coagulation profile is imperative as is the estimation of arterial pH and blood gases. An X-ray of the chest may reveal acute lung injury or even ARDS.

Management

Principles of management have already been outlined in the Chapter on Sepsis and Septic Shock.

Immediate intravenous use of appropriate antibiotics which cover Gram-negative, Gram-positive organisms and also anaerobes is mandatory. Antibiotic therapy may subsequently be tailored according to culture sensitivity reports. Clostridial infections are treated with 2 million units of penicillin G four hourly, intravenously. Hysterectomy may be life-saving in serious clostridial infection.

All organ systems need support; the coagulation profile should be restored by infusion of appropriate blood products. Cardio-respiratory support is vital and seriously ill patients need to be intubated and kept on mechanical ventilation. Details of management have been discussed in the Chapter on Sepsis and Septic Shock.

Pelvic surgery may be necessary to drain abscesses or collections of infected blood. Retained products of conception should be removed by careful curettage as they contribute to further infection. Close co-operation between the intensivist and the obstetrician is mandatory for patient survival.

REFERENCE

1. Stubblefield PG, Grimes DA. (1994). Septic abortion. N Engl J Med. 331, 310–314.

SECTION 23

The Critically Ill Child

23.1 Cardiopulmonary Resuscitation in Infants and Children

23.2 Respiratory and Haemodynamic Monitoring of the Critically Ill Child

23.3 Approach to Shock in the Paediatric Intensive Care Unit

23.4 Hypertensive Emergencies in Paediatrics

23.5 Heart Failure in Neonates and Children

23.6 Acute Respiratory Failure in Children and Hyaline Membrane Disease

23.7 Fluid and Electrolyte Disturbances in the Critically Ill Child

23.8 Nutritional Support in the Paediatric Intensive Care Unit

23.9 Paediatric Life-threatening Infections Requiring Critical Care

23.10 Acute Renal Failure in Infants and Children

CHAPTER 23.1

Cardiopulmonary Resuscitation in Infants and Children

Contributed by Dr Y.K. Amdekar, MD, DCH, Consultant Paediatrician, Breach Candy Hospital and Jaslok Hospital, Retired Honorary Professor of Paediatrics, Grant Medical College and the JJ Group of Hospitals, Mumbai.

A systematic approach to CPR in children is rarely emphasized during the training of medical graduates, and hence there exists a general lack of skill even in hospital settings, whereas pre-hospital CPR in children is almost non-existent. This is true even in Western countries.

Unlike in adults, cardiopulmonary arrest in children is often gradual in onset, and results from deterioration of respiratory and/or circulatory function. Hence an arrest can often be anticipated and prevented by early recognition of respiratory failure and/or shock. Although respiratory failure and shock may begin as clinically distinct entities, they ultimately deteriorate to a state of cardiorespiratory failure, before culminating in an arrest.

Rapid cardiopulmonary assessment may prompt initiation of proper therapy to prevent an arrest (1). It consists of an evaluation of respiratory function by noting the respiratory rate, increased work of breathing and cyanosis; the circulatory status is evaluated by monitoring the pulse rate, blood pressure, peripheral circulation and end-organ perfusion as evidenced by capillary refill, mental state and urine output. Primary response to hypoxaemia in neonates is bradycardia, unlike in older children, in whom tachycardia is the first response. Also bradycardia in a distressed child is an ominous sign of impending arrest. Besides respiratory failure and shock, children with severe trauma, burns, seizures and critically ill children on the ventilator as well as with tracheostomy, are potential candidates for arrest. In neonates, besides birth hypoxic injury, hypothermia, metabolic derangements like hypoglycaemia and hypokalaemia also predispose to arrest.

Sudden Infant Death Syndrome (SIDS) leads to arrest without warning. The exact aetiology of SIDS is not known, though interplay of various factors is incriminated; these include prematurity, babies who have recovered from the respiratory distress syndrome, abnormality in thermoregulation and the respiratory centre, and chronic hypoxia due to elevated foetal haemoglobin. Of late, the prone position during sleep has also been blamed (2). Besides a foreign body in the airway, SIDS is the only condition that may cause a sudden cardiac arrest, without any prior warning.

The sequence of CPR in children is essentially similar to that in adults with a few differences (3). Rescue breathing in older children and adults is carried out by mouth to mouth breathing, whereas in infants it is both mouth to nose, and mouth to mouth. Often in infants, this leads to gastric distension, especially if the airway is partially blocked. Gastric distension hampers adequate ventilation and hence should be prevented by limiting ventilation volume and if necessary by insertion of a nasogastric tube. Pressure over the abdomen is dangerous as it may lead to aspiration of stomach contents into the lungs. Circulation is assessed by palpation of the brachial artery in infants, as the carotid pulse is often difficult to palpate due to a short neck.

As the heart lies higher in the chest in infants and children, and also due to differences in heart rate and respiratory rate at various ages, chest compression will vary in site, rate and also depth. In an infant, the chest is compressed by two fingers placed below the intermammary line to a depth of 0.5"–1" at the rate of 100–120/min. In toddlers, chest compression is carried out by the heel of one hand placed just above the notch between the sternum and the rib-cage to a depth of 1"–1.5" at the rate of 80–100/min. Older children may need chest compression by two hands like in adults. The ratio of chest compression to breathing is 5:1 at all ages.

In case of airway obstruction due to a foreign body, the child should be encouraged to cough. Relief of obstruction is attempted only if coughing is ineffective or respiratory difficulty worsens with increasing stridor. In children, the Heimlich manoeuvre consisting of subdiaphragmatic abdominal thrusts is tried, while in infants, back blows and chest thrusts are attempted, so as to avoid injury to abdominal organs. Following such manoeuvres, rescue breathing is attempted, and if this is found to be unsuccessful, the procedure is repeated.

If breathing cannot be initiated and mantained by rescue breathing, bag and mask ventilation with oxygenation is necessary. Well-fitting masks of proper size, with a good seal around the nose and mouth are necessary. Smaller bags of 250–750 ml volume are used in children to deliver small tidal volumes. The pressure applied has to be just sufficient to inflate the chest. In neonates, 2–3 fingers are used to squeeze the bag, while in bigger children, the bag is squeezed by one hand. Gentle pressure is sufficient, and care should be taken to avoid a pneumothorax.

In most situations, basic life support is enough to resuscitate infants and children. In newborns, before initiating CPR, drying of the skin surface and providing optimal warmth, as also gentle tactile stimulation by rubbing the back or sole, are necessary to establish breathing. Suction of the nostrils and the oral cavity generally clears the airway. If breathing is not established, oxygen delivered by a catheter placed 1 cm from the nostrils is often adequate. In a majority of cases, breathing is established by such manouevres; if not, CPR is begun.

If breathing cannot be adequately maintained by bag and mask ventilation, endotracheal intubation (using an uncuffed tube), may become necessary. A laryngoscope with a straight blade is preferred in infants and small children. A proper sized tube is selected as per the baby's size—this varies from 2.5 in premature babies to 3–3.5 in full term neonates, and proportionately larger sizes subsequently. Tube size as depicted by the internal diameter (ID), may be approximated by the formula:

$$ID \ (mm) = \frac{16 + Age \ in \ Years}{4}$$

Proper-sized suction catheters varying in size from French 5 upwards, are used. Various oxygen delivery systems may be used, including an oxygen hood. Oxygen is toxic especially in preterm neonates, and may lead to retrolental fibroplasia and bronchopulmonary dysplasia; hence it should be used judiciously.

Vascular access is often difficult in infants and children. In newborns, the umbilical vein may be used for a short period, till a peripheral vein can be secured. In infants and children, intraosseous infusions of fluids may be tried in the tibial bone, and as soon as the circulatory state improves, a peripheral vein is secured. Emergency drugs may be administered through the endotracheal tube, though such an access may pose special problems. The amount infused through the endotracheal tube must be limited to 5 ml to prevent atelectasis due to altered or destroyed surfactant. Any drug that is administered through an endotracheal tube may form an intrapulmonary depot of the drug as it is not washed off quickly, and hence the drug may have a prolonged effect.

Fluids may have to be infused to maintain an adequate circulatory volume. A bolus of 20 ml/kg body weight of isotonic fluids like Ringer Lactate or normal saline are administered as the first step in resuscitation of volume. Further infusions are decided by the circulatory status.

Certain medications may be required in the last step of CPR. As endotracheal intubation is often planned in children, premedication with atropine is ideal. A minimum dose of 0.1mgm of atropine is used at any age; the actual dose works out to be 0.02 mg/kg body weight. This is to avoid smaller doses which often cause a paradoxical CNS-mediated bradycardia. Other medications required are similar to those used in adults, and include sodium bicarbonate to counter acidosis, and inotropes for circulatory support. Thus dopamine, dobutamine, isoproterenol or epinephrine infusions may be necessary. The paediatric dosages of inotropes are as follows—dopamine infusion at 2–20 µg/kg/min; dobutamine infusion at 5–20 µg/kg/min; epinephrine 0.01 mg/kg (0.1 ml/kg of 1:10,000 solution) stat, followed by an infusion at the rate of 0.1–1 µg/kg/min; isoproterenol infusion at 0.1–1 µg/kg/min. Ventricular extrasystolies and rhythm disturbances are often due to hypoxia, and are thus abolished by oxygen administration. Lidocaine in the dose of 1 mg/kg stat, followed by an infusion at a rate of 20–50 µg/kg/min may however be necessary. Fluid and electrolyte abnormalities are common in the paediatric age group, and the use of dextrose, dextrose saline and Ringer Lactate infusions should be carefully monitored.

REFERENCES

1. Leon Chameides (Ed.). (1988). Textbook of Pediatric Advanced Life Support. American Heart Association.
2. Willenger M, Hoffman HJ, Hartford RB. (1994). Infant sleep position and risk of sudden infant death syndrome. Pediatrics. 93(5), 814–820.
3. Von Seggern K, Egar M, Fuhrman BB. (1986). Cardiopulmonary resuscitation in pediatric ICU. Crit Care Med. 14, 275.

Respiratory and Haemodynamic Monitoring of the Critically Ill Child

Contributed by: *Dr Joseph Britto, MD, Consultant Paediatric Intensivist and Clinical Director, ISABEL Clinical Decision Support Systems www.isabel.org.uk.*

Dr P. Ramnarayan, MRCP(UK), Paediatric Intensive Care, Great Ormond Street Hospital for Children, London, UK.

Over the past few decades, advances in medical technology have enabled the intensive care clinician to use an amazing array of devices and systems to monitor critically ill children. Ironically, although advances in monitoring have enabled the measurement of a range of hitherto unmeasured physiological parameters, frequently led by the belief that more is always better, they may often lead to information overload, and make the intensivist's job more demanding (1). Furthermore, there is no hard evidence to support the assumption that monitoring a wide range of parameters, invasively or otherwise, in the critical care unit, leads to better patient care (2). Therefore, if the intensivist is to decide which biological parameter needs to be monitored and by what method, to be able to reliably interpret the values obtained, and then respond appropriately, it is vital that he/she possesses a firm understanding of the physiological principles on which each monitoring system is based, as well as the benefits and limitations of each method. Despite the attraction, it is also crucial that time-tested clinical skills and knowledge are retained, and not simply replaced by relatively untested new technology.

In general, when interpreting data presented on monitors, it is wise to take into consideration changes in the trend of a parameter, rather than reacting in knee-jerk fashion to a single abnormal value; and to interpret data in the context of the 'whole clinical picture', rather than in isolation.

Respiratory Monitoring

Physical Examination

History taking and detailed bedside clinical examination have an important role in the early diagnosis of impending respiratory failure and in deciding the need for tracheal intubation and/or respiratory support (**Table 23.2.1**). Various parameters can be assessed non-invasively: these are especially relevant in non-muscle relaxed, unsedated, unintubated patients.

Respiratory Rate

Other than visual inspection, the technique used most commonly for measuring respiratory movements is impedance pneumography (3). The method requires placement of at least three leads over the chest, one over the heart and one each on the opposite sides of the lower lateral thorax. Displacement of the leads, poor contact, and

Table 23.2.1. Signs indicative of respiratory failure

General
Fatigue
Sweating
Hypoxia
Cyanosis
Abnormal respiratory pattern

Respiratory
Tachypnoea, bradypnoea and apnoea
Nasal flaring
Retractions
Accessory muscle use
Grunting
Poor air entry
Crackles (rales)

Upper/Lower airway
Steator (obstruction above level of vocal cords)
Stridor (obstruction below level of vocal cords)
Wheeze/Ronchi

Cardiac
Bradycardia or tachycardia
Hypotension or hypertension
Palpable pulsus paradoxus

Cerebral
Restlessness or irritability
Headache
Reversal of sleep pattern
Altered level of consciousness
Seizures

excessive movement may all lead to false alarms (4). Like many other physiological parameters, respiratory rate varies with age (**Table 23.2.2**).

Table 23.2.2. Respiratory rate as function of age

Age (years)	Mean breaths/min	± SD
2	25	17–33
4	23	18–28
6	21	17–27
8	20	15–26
10	18	15–25
12	18	14–26
14	17	15–23
16	17	12–22

From: Iliff A, Lee V. (1952). Pulse rate, respiratory rate and body temperature in children between two months and eighteen years of age. Child Development. 23, 237.

Worsening tachypnoea in a sick child is a highly specific indicator of respiratory deterioration, although not the most sensitive (5). However, in children with neuromuscular weakness, impending respiratory failure may not manifest as tachypnoea, and respiratory pattern may be more informative.

Respiratory pattern

Clinical signs of respiratory distress include the use of accessory muscles, subcostal and intercostal retractions, and changes in respiratory pattern. Respiratory pauses may occur in children less than 3 months of age and are usually less than 15 seconds in duration. Pauses occur in groups of 3 or more, are separated by less than 20 seconds, and are resolved by 6 months of age (6). Infantile apnoea is defined as cessation of breathing for greater than 20 seconds or *any* respiratory pause associated with bradycardia, pallor or cyanosis (7). While respiratory pauses or apnoeas may be a physiological finding in early infancy, they indicate respiratory fatigue and impending respiratory arrest in older children.

Central Neurogenic Hyperventilation and Cheyne-Stokes pattern of breathing may be seen in children with worrying intracranial pathology; the characteristic Cushing triad of hypertension, bradycardia and bradypnoea is indicative of impending brain herniation, and constitutes a medical emergency; deep, sighing breathing (Kussmaul's breathing) may indicate a child with metabolic acidosis (e.g. diabetic ketoacidosis, salicylate toxicity).

Pulse Oximetry

Pulse oximetry is the most convenient non-invasive method of continuous monitoring of arterial oxygen saturation. Visual detection of cyanosis is subject to considerable observer bias, and depends on the haemoglobin concentration. Cyanosis is detected in only 95 per cent of patients by experienced observers when the arterial saturation falls to 89 per cent. In anaemic patients, cyanosis may be difficult to detect, while in contrast, plethoric or polycythaemic patients may appear cyanosed despite adequate arterial oxygen tensions (8).

Pulse oximetry is based on the spectrophotometric characteristics of pulsatile arterial blood, and the principle that reduced haemoglobin and oxyhaemoglobin have different light absorption characteristics (9). Light at wavelengths of 660 nm (red) and 940 nm (infrared) are used because the absorption characteristics of the two haemoglobins are different at these two wavelengths. A microprocessor programmed with experimentally derived data calculates the amount of reduced haemoglobin and oxyhaemoglobin and thus the oxygen saturation. These devices are typically calibrated against results of a carbon monoxide oximeter. A miniaturized light source is applied to any area of the body that is thin enough so that light can traverse a pulsating capillary bed and be sensed by a photo detector. In children, fingers and toes, as well as earlobes have been used as recommended sites; in infants, the palm has been used; and the whole foot may be used in newborns.

In a well-perfused, normothermic individual, the oxygen saturation of normal haemoglobin determined by the pulse oximeter correlates very closely to the oxygen saturation determined by the co-oximeter (correlation coefficient of 0.98), especially when the saturation is between 65 and 100 per cent (10). This has been recently borne out in a European multi-centre trial (11).

Conventional pulse oximetry can be an invaluable tool in patients at risk of hypoxaemia, if the following limitations are borne in mind:

1. *Low perfusion states:* Pulse oximeters require pulsatile, arterial blood flow at the site of measurement in order to render accurate results. In the presence of shock, concurrent use of vasopressors, severe tissue oedema or peripheral vascular disease, the photodetector may not detect a reliable signal. In these cases, the earlobe or the nasal septum may be tried as alternate sites (the anterior ethomoidal artery flow may be maintained even in low-perfusion states). Conversely, the presence of an arterial waveform is only a very crude indication of peripheral perfusion, and does not guarantee adequacy of cardiac output, arterial blood pressure, or cardiac rhythm. A waveform may also be displayed in the absence of a genuine arterial pulse.

2. *Ambient light:* False signals can be produced by ambient light. Covering the limb bearing the probe may prevent this.

3. *Motion artefacts:* A considerable number of false alarms are generated by pulse oximeters when the measurement site is not held still, a requirement that is often violated in paediatric and neonatal critical care (12). Newer technology to correct this problem, called Masimo signal extraction, has been shown to reduce the incidence of false alarms in the neonatal population (13).

4. *Dyshaemoglobinaemias:* A persistent shortcoming of pulse oximetry has been the failure to detect reduction in oxyhaemoglobin resulting from methaemoglobinaemia and carbon monoxide poisoning. Carboxyhaemoglobin and oxyhaemologin have similar absorbencies at 660 nm. Thus, carboxyhaemoglobin is interpreted as oxyhaemoglobin by the photodetector of the pulse oximeter, and this causes the pulse oximeter to overestimate oxyhaemoglobin concentrations in carbon monoxide poisoning (smoke inhalation or coma of uncertain cause). It is vital that pulse oximetry is not relied upon when either of these two dyshaemoglobinaemias is suspected; co-oximetry must be used to determine oxygen saturation.

5. *Oxygen saturation and PaO$_2$:* Oxygen saturation becomes a useful indicator of PaO$_2$ only when it has fallen below 90 per cent (a PaO$_2$ of about 60 mm Hg)—'the steep portion of the oxygen dissociation curve', due to the nature of the oxygen dissociation curve (**Fig. 23.2.1**). Pulse oximetry cannot be used to monitor hyperoxaemia in situations where exact knowledge of the upper level of PaO$_2$ is critical (e.g. in neonates)—'the flat portion of the oxygen dissociation curve'. However, in a recent study, newer pulse oximeters have been shown to be more reliable for this purpose (14).

6. *Oxygen saturation and hypoventilation:* (A = alveolar, a = arterial) Stable oxygen saturations may lull clinicians into a false sense of security, if the patient has hypoventilation (raised PaCO$_2$), but is breathing supplemental oxygen e.g. a child with upper airway obstruction on 100 per cent FIO$_2$. If the patient were on room air, oxygen saturation would fall early and point to hypoventilation. However, if the patient is on supplemental oxygen, PAO$_2$ (and PaO$_2$) are maintained much higher, and increasing alveolar PACO$_2$

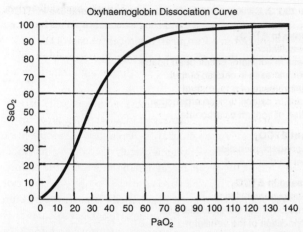

Fig. 23.2.1. Schematic of oxygen dissociation curve. It is clear from the diagram that a rise in oxygen saturation from 95% to 96% may be accompanied by significant rise in PaO_2, leading to oxygen toxicity.

(and $PaCO_2$) will have to progress before hypoxaemia sufficient to produce measurable desaturation occurs. *A normal oxygen saturation, in the presence of an increased inspired oxygen concentration, gives no information about the adequacy of ventilation ($PaCO_2$).* Accurate assessment of alveolar hypoventilation in this situation is only possible by measuring the $PaCO_2$ by arterial blood gas analysis.

Blood Gas Analysis

Blood gas analysis is indispensable for the assessment of oxygenation status, adequacy of alveolar ventilation and the acid-base status of the critically ill child **(15)**. In the analysis of patients with respiratory failure, the setting up and adjustment of mechanical ventilators and oscillators and in interpreting blood gases the authors strongly advocate the approach of *decoupling* oxygenation (O_2) from ventilation (CO_2). For clinical interpretation of blood gas reports, the reader is referred to other sections of this book.

Measurement of Oxygen Status (Also See Chapter on Basic Cardiopulmonary Physiology in the Intensive Care Unit)

FIO$_2$ is the fraction of inspired oxygen. Room air has FIO_2 of 0.21.

PaO_2 is the oxygen tension in arterial blood and *PAO_2* is the oxygen tension in the alveoli. A lowered PaO_2 can be due to a fall in ambient pressure (as at high altitudes), a fall in FIO_2 and in patients with alveolar hypoventilation. In all the above situations the alveolar oxygen tension (PAO_2) is also lowered. A low PaO_2 is frequently observed in patients who have ventilation/perfusion inequality. Unequal ventilation perfusion ratios constitute the commonest cause of hypoxia in clinical medicine. Right to left shunts either within the lungs (as with perfusion of atelectatic alveoli) or in the heart (as with congenital cyanotic heart disease) also markedly reduce the PaO_2. Finally, a significant fall in diffusion capacity also reduces the PaO_2. It is to be noted that a fall in the diffusion capacity is invariably associated with ventilation perfusion inequality in clinical medicine.

CaO_2. The oxygen content of arterial blood is the oxygen content in 1 dl of arterial blood. It is dependent on the total haemoglobin concentration, arterial oxygen saturation—SaO_2 (which in turn is dependent on the PaO_2) and the fraction of Hb capable/incapable of transporting oxygen. It is given by the formula:

$$O_2 \text{ content} = 1.39 \times \frac{\% \text{ saturation}}{100} + 0.003 \times PO_2$$

Oxygen Transport or Oxygen Delivery ($\dot{D}O_2$) is equivalent to the cardiac output × arterial oxygen content. A satisfactory oxygen transport is vital to prevent tissue hypoxia.

p50 is the capability of blood to release oxygen. It is related to position of the oxygen disassociation curve, arterial and end-capillary PO_2 values and the affinity of oxygen for haemoglobin.

Alveolar-arterial oxygen gradient *(A-a O_2 gradient).* The alveolar-arterial oxygen gradient is the difference in the PAO_2 and the PaO_2. The normal A-a O_2 gradient in a child is < 10 mm Hg, in an adult around 15 mm Hg and in the elderly around 20 mm Hg and not more than 25–30 mm Hg. An increase in the A-a O_2 gradient above normal denotes a problem in oxygenation and the larger the gradient the greater the problem. The A-a O_2 gradient is unaltered in patients with alveolar hypoventilation. It is increased in patients with ventilation perfusion inequality, in true right to left shunts within the lungs (i.e. perfusion of atelectatic alveoli), in right to left shunts within the heart, and in diffusion defects. The hypoxia caused by ventilation-perfusion inequalities or abnormalities in diffusion is abolished significantly by increasing the FIO_2. However hypoxia caused by true pulmonary right to left shunts (i.e. by perfusion of atelectatic alveoli) is not significantly altered by increasing FIO_2.

The A-a O_2 gradient is a measure of the above listed factors that can result in impaired oxygenation of arterial blood and is subtly different from the PaO_2 / FIO_2 ratio and the oxygenation index. The A-a O_2 gradient is influenced by changes in positive pressure, but it is important to remember that the numerical value of changes in mean airway pressure (e.g. during a recruitment manoeuvre) are not reflected in the calculation of the A-a O_2 gradient.

$$\begin{aligned}
\text{A-a } O_2 \text{ gradient} &= PAO_2 - PaO_2 \\
&= PIO_2 - (PACO_2 \times 1/R) - PaO_2 \\
&= 716 \times FIO_2 - (PACO_2 \times 1/R) - PaO_2 \\
&= 716 \times FIO_2 - (PaCO_2 \times 1/R) - PaO_2
\end{aligned}$$

(Also see Chapter on Basic Cardiorespiratory Physiology in the Intensive Care unit.)

Oxygenation index *(OI).* OI is another useful marker of oxygenation but differs from PaO_2/FIO_2 and A-a gradient. OI is particularly for mechanically ventilated or patients on HFOV with high mean airway pressures (MAP). It is useful to track the impact of increasing MAP (e.g. using recruitment strategies) on oxygenation as the latter is taken account of in the calculation of OI. In this respect OI is more useful than the A-a gradient.

$$OI = \frac{MAP \times FIO_2 \times 100}{PaO_2}$$

For example a patient with a MAP of 5 cm H_2O, an FIO_2 of 0.21 and PaO_2 of 100 mm Hg has an OI of 1. As the formula above indicates the higher the OI the worse the oxygenation problem.

Capnometry and Capnography

Capnometry is the measurement of expired CO_2. Its value is enhanced by capnography, which is defined as the graphic representation of expired CO_2 over time. Capnogram is the waveform produced by variations in CO_2 concentration throughout the respiratory cycle. A capnogram can form a sensitive indicator of alterations in metabolic rate, tissue perfusion, various aspects of pulmonary ventilation/perfusion relationships, and of the mechanics of ventilation (16). At the bedside, CO_2 concentration in respiratory gases is conveniently measured by infrared spectroscopy. The latter is based on the principle that each gas has unique absorption characteristics that can be used to quantify its amount in a mixture of gases. Infrared spectroscopy requires three components: an infrared light source, a detector and a gas chamber.

Sampling is easiest if the trachea is intubated or if there is a tight fitting face mask. There are two main methods by which gas is sampled: mainstream, in which the measurement chamber in which respiratory gases are sampled is attached inline to the endotracheal tube; and sidestream, where the sensor is remote from the patient. In the latter, a small amount of gas is aspirated from a T-piece inline with the circuit into the sensor. In the former, the infrared source and the detector are placed on either side of the sampling chamber. Sidestream capnometers are more prone to being blocked by secretions or water, and may not yield accurate waveforms in neonates who have low tidal volumes. In mainstream capnometers, secretions can be prevented from occluding the light source and detector by placing a humidifying filter in the circuit. However, this method also adds some dead space to the system, which can cause traction on the ventilator tubing and cause ventilation problems in small children (17). Microstream capnometers have been recently described, which use the sidestream method, but require minimal sample flow rate (50 ml/min) and cell volume (15 ml), enabling use in the neonatal population (18).

$ETCO_2$ is defined as the highest CO_2 value during the expiratory phase of respiration (**Figure 23.2.1**). This approximates $PaCO_2$, when ventilation and perfusion are well matched, and when CO_2 production is stable. Clinical conditions associated with alterations in $ETCO_2$ are given in **Table 23.2.3**.

The uses of $ETCO_2$ in the paediatric intensive care unit include the following:

Table 23.2.3. Clinical conditions associated with alterations in $ETCO_2$

Increase in $ETCO_2$
Hypoventilation
Increase in ventilator circuit dead space
Sudden increase in cardiac output
Sudden release of a tourniquet
Increase in carbon dioxide production
Injection of sodium bicarbonate

Absent $ETCO_2$
Oesophageal intubation
Absent cardiac output

Decrease in $ETCO_2$
Sudden hyperventilation
Obstruction of the endotracheal tube
Disconnection of the ventilator
Leakage around endotracheal tube
Leakage in the ventilator circuit
Sudden decrease in cardiac output
Decrease in pulmonary perfusion
Massive pulmonary embolism
Air embolism
Decrease in oxygen consumption

1. Non-invasive estimation of $PaCO_2$

Capnometry usually reveals the $ETCO_2$ value to be less than the $PaCO_2$ by about 2–5 mm Hg, if there is no leak around the endotracheal tube. In pre-pubertal children (where the use of cuffed endotracheal tubes is not common), the difference between $ETCO_2$ and $PaCO_2$ is greater than 5 mm Hg. In such cases, the $ETCO_2$ can only be used as a trend to monitor the adequacy of CO_2 removal.

2. Evaluation of Respiratory Rate and Pattern

Analysis of the capnogram can detect mechanical failure in a ventilated patient; mechanical breaths can be distinguished from spontaneous breaths; and inspiratory efforts generated by a partially paralysed diaphragm can be diagnosed (curare cleft).

3. Analysis of End-inspiratory CO_2 ($EICO_2$)

$EICO_2$ should always be near zero. If $EICO_2 > 0$, it implies that the patient is inhaling previously exhaled gas containing CO_2. This could be due to inadequate fresh gas flow rate or from spontaneous breath occurring during mechanical expiration with

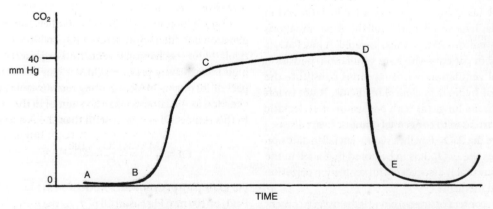

Fig. 23.2.2. Representation of exhaled CO_2 as a function of time. Point D is End Tidal CO_2.

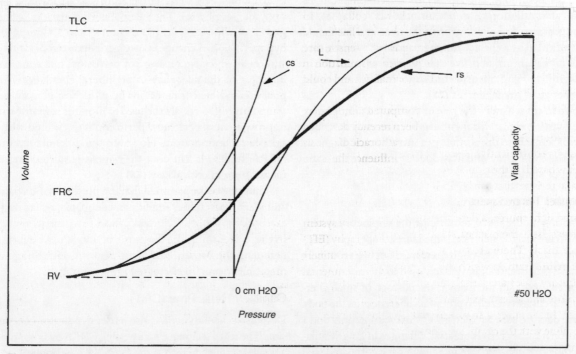

Fig. 23.2.3. Pressure volume curve. The curve is shifted to the right with a steeper slope in conditions of decreased lung compliance such as ARDS (reproduced from Caples SM, Hubmayr RD. Respiratory monitoring tools in the intensive care unit. Curr Opin Crit Care. 2003 Jun; 9(3), 230–235). Lippincott Williams and Wilkins.

the expiratory valve open, thus allowing the patient to inhale CO_2 rich gas.

4. Confirmation of Intubation

The new Paediatric Advanced Life Support guidelines stipulate that all intubations must be confirmed by some form of $ETCO_2$ measurement. A steady capnogram is considered the gold standard for tracheal intubation. In cases of oesophageal intubation, the capnogram would either be absent, or rapidly decline within 15 sec (if carbonated drinks have been ingested previously, or a prolonged period of exhaled gas ventilation had been carried out).

5. During cardiopulmonary circulation

In children who are being resuscitated from a cardiorespiratory arrest, initially $ETCO_2$ values are initially very high, reflecting accumulation of CO_2 in the lungs during the respiratory arrest phase. This then falls to a low level and then rises with adequate CPR, indicating cardiac output, returning to normal levels with return of spontaneous circulation. In addition, a recent study suggested that an $ETCO_2$ value of < 10 mm Hg for 20 minutes after initiation of CPR predicted death, indicating that CPR could be terminated in those patients (19).

Transcutaneous Blood Gas Determination

This technique involves the placement of skin electrodes to measure transcutaneous values of PO_2 and PCO_2. If the skin is 'arterialized' by warming to 41–44°C, the values obtained are close to that of arterial blood. However, this technique requires frequent calibration and change of location of the heated electrode to prevent skin burns. Other factors that affect the correlation between transcutaneous and arterial concentration of O_2 and CO_2 are the thickness and temperature of the skin, the arterial pressure, and other factors such as acidosis and drugs that affect peripheral perfusion. The technique can be used in neonatal units on normotensive, normothermic and normovolaemic ill infants. As a result of the limitations described above, and the development of pulse oximeter and capnography technology, very few paediatric intensive care units use this technology routinely (20).

Pressure-volume and Flow Curves

The pressure-volume curves reflect the mechanical properties of the respiratory system (chest wall plus lungs), and can be used to calculate the compliance (change in volume per unit change in pressure) and elastance (reciprocal of compliance) of the system (**Figure 23.2.3**). In ventilated patients, numerous techniques are used to measure these values, including the interrupter and multiple occlusion methods. Serial analysis of the pressure-volume and flow curves of a mechanically ventilated patient provides invaluable information about: a) setting the optimum length of the inspiratory time (Ti) for given pressure / volume settings; b) achieving lung recruitment by determining upper and lower deflection points; c) the value of set PEEP, measurement and visualization of intrinsic PEEP (PEEPi); d) compliance of the lungs. These values and measurements are indispensible in any recruitment strategy and in prevention of de-recruitment, overdistension and ventilator induced lung injury.

Imaging of the Lungs

Chest X-ray is the most commonly used modality for lung imaging. This allows the intensivist to monitor changes in lung parenchyma, assess distension of the lung, and identify associated complications of mechanical ventilation (e.g. pneumothorax, collapse). In addition, the position of an endotracheal tube or central line should always be confirmed by a chest X-ray. In a paediatric intensive care unit chest X-rays are more sensitive than physical examination in detecting significant and unsuspected abnormalities and could result in a change of management (21).

In addition to chest X-rays, the role of computed tomography (CT) of the chest in ventilated patients has been recently described (22). Chest CT can add to the accuracy of intrathoracic diagnosis provided by the chest X-ray, and may directly influence the acute management of some children.

Experimental Techniques

Newer promising modalities of monitoring the respiratory system during critical care include electrical impedance tomography (EIT) and pulmonary acoustics. Although these have not been routinely used in clinical practice, they have been used in an experimental setting for many years. In the former, the passage of small alternating electrical currents result in potential differences on the body surface; these data are used to calculate electrical impedance and a two-dimensional tomogram is created. Changes in lung ventilation assessed by this non-invasive technique have correlated well with adjustments in ventilator settings and oxygenation (23).

Haemodynamic Monitoring

The most effective and sensitive monitoring of haemodynamic status in a critically ill child is repeated and careful physical examination.

Assessment of the Microcirculation and Peripheral Perfusion

Children have excellent compensatory homeostatic mechanisms. The first signs of haemodynamic compromise relate to the body's compensatory mechanisms. Changes in peripheral perfusion, heart rate, pulse characteristics and urine output invariably precede changes in blood pressure and central perfusion. In essence, the body's compensatory mechanism is to maintain vital organ perfusion at the expense of the peripheries. Therefore assessment of the microcirculation and the peripheral perfusion is crucial in the haemodynamic monitoring of critically ill children. This is easily done at the bedside by assessing the core-peripheral temperature gradient and the capillary refill time.

Core-Peripheral Temperature Gradient

Core and peripheral temperatures should be monitored in all seriously ill children. This is easily and continuously done by means of temperature probes. The rectum is the optimal site for measurement of core temperature, although the urinary bladder and the tympanic membrane have been recently shown to be adequate substitutes (24). Temperatures measured in the mouth or in the axillae are regarded as core temperatures, but are subject to ambient temperature and peripheral perfusion, and are therefore less

than optimal. Peripheral temperature can be measured on the skin over the peripheries. The normal core-peripheral temperature gap is usually < 2°C. A gap of more than 5°C implies marked hypoperfusion. A change in core-peripheral temperature gap constitutes an objective measure of perfusion, and a more sensitive indicator of the adequacy of peripheral circulation than blood pressure and heart rate (25). The reduction of core-peripheral temperature gap can also be used to monitor response to therapy; improvement in peripheral perfusion is associated with a rise in peripheral temperature. However, the diagnostic value of this reliable finding is lost once the patient is started on vasoactive medications in critical care (26).

Thus, it may be assumed that the presence of palpable pulses and warm extremities implies an adequate cardiac output. The exceptions to this are warm septic shock or a patient on vasodilators. In these situations, the diagnosis of shock can be facilitated by detecting the presence of lactic acidosis, indicating anaerobic metabolism and/or decreased urine output.

Capillary Refill Time (CRT)

Decreased capillary refill is also a useful indicator of tissue perfusion. The usual technique for assessing CRT is by firm pressure over a bony prominence such as the forehead, anterior tibia or sternum for 5 seconds. Normally, the blanched area disappears in less than 3 seconds. CRT greater than 5 seconds is clearly abnormal. CRT greater than 7–10 seconds implies marked haemodynamic compromise. The advantages of this simple measure are that it is easily measured, and can be followed over time to help gauge response to therapy. However, CRT is not a very specific or sensitive indicator of tissue perfusion and therefore needs to be correlated with other indices of perfusion (urine output and base deficit on blood gas analysis). CRT should not be used to titrate fluid resuscitation in a hospital setting. Ambient temperature is a major confounding factor in estimating a reliable CRT. In addition, the site of measurement has a major influence on the value (limb CRT > central CRT).

Heart Rate, Rhythm and Pulse Characteristics

Tachycardia is an early, compensatory response to shock in children. Young children have a small relatively fixed stroke volume; augmentation of cardiac output (product of heart rate and stroke volume) is much more dependent on tachycardia than an increase in stroke volume. All critically ill children should be continuously monitored with ECG for heart rate and rhythm. Persistent tachycardia despite correction of other causes (fever, anaemia and pain) and/or a low volume pulse are signs of inadequate perfusion. Palpable pulsus paradoxus in a spontaneously breathing child may indicate obstructive airway disease or myocardial dysfunction. An increase in pulse volume with mechanical ventilation may indicate impaired myocardial contractility; a decrease in pulse volume during a mechanical breath may indicate decreased preload.

Arterial Blood Pressure Monitoring

As discussed above, the earliest signs of shock are signs of the body's compensatory mechanisms, i.e. signs of poor peripheral perfusion, tachycardia and tachypnoea. It is important to remember that hypotension can be a very late sign in shock and a fall in blood pressure indicates severe haemodynamic compromise. Thus, blood pressure may still be normal in children, even when cardiovascular function and/or tissue perfusion are very abnormal (27). Despite these limitations in its use as an early marker of haemodynamic status, blood pressure monitoring (systolic, diastolic and mean pressures) provides crucial information in the subsequent management of the critically ill child.

Techniques for Continuous Intra-arterial Blood Pressure Monitoring

Intra-arterial measurement is considered the gold standard for continuous, beat-to-beat monitoring of blood pressure. It is imperative that all children being managed for haemodynamic compromise have their blood pressure measured, preferably in continuous fashion. Most children admitted to a paediatric intensive care unit will have invasive intra-arterial catheters for this purpose. This may be replaced with non-invasive measurements by the oscillometric technique or a sphygmomanometer in a few children (**Tables 23.2.4, 23.2.5, 23.2.6**). During continuous intra-arterial blood pressure monitoring, an indwelling arterial cannula is placed,

Table 23.2.4. Indications for intra-arterial blood pressure monitoring

Shock

Hypothermia

Cardiopulmonary resuscitation

Haemodynamic instability
  Surgery
  Blood loss
  Marked shifts of body fluid

Indirect blood pressure measurement difficult
  Extensive burns

Arterial blood sampling
  Blood gas analysis
  Severe metabolic derangement
  Anticoagulation

Table 23.2.5. Precautions and nursing management of an arterial line

Check distal perfusion at least once every 8 hours
  Capillary refill
  Skin temperature
  Skin colour
Remove catheter if
  Poor perfusion is detected
  Blood withdrawal is difficult
  Arterial tracing remains constantly damp

Table 23.2.6. Suggested arterial cannula size and gauge (G)

	< 3 kg	3–10 kg	10 kg
Radial artery	24 G	22 G	22 G
Dorsalis pedis/posterior tibial artery	24 G	22 G	22 G
Axillary artery	22 G	22/20 G	20 G
Femoral artery	22 G	22/20 G	20 G

and connected by a catheter to a pressure transducer to permit direct measurement of the blood pressure. Arterial cannulation also permits regular sampling of arterial blood without disturbing the steady state; and it allows analysis of the pressure waveform. Indirect blood pressure monitoring by sphygmomanometry is unreliable in critically ill children and may falsely read lower values especially in the presence of shock and hypothermia. The use of an oversized cuff could also lead to an underestimation of indirect blood pressure. Direct blood pressure measurements usually average 5–20 mm Hg higher than indirect measurements. If indirect measurements are higher than direct pressures, the discrepancies are almost always due to errors in zeroing of the pressure transducer, large air bubbles in the catheter system and small bore or excessively long catheters. It is worth remembering that in peripheral vascular disease, direct pressures recorded distally may be significantly lower than proximal cuff readings.

Sites of Arterial Cannulation

The artery chosen for cannulation should be large enough to reflect accurately the true systemic blood pressure. Prior to cannulation the adequacy of collateral blood flow must be tested using the modified Allen's test (28). In patients with a right-to-left extracardiac shunt through a patent ductus arterious, the effect of the anatomic site on the blood oxygenation values is an important consideration. Oxygen values from the right upper limb (pre-ductal) represent blood oxygen saturation which will be higher than that going to the other limbs, and reliance on the latter values will result in unnecessarily vigorous treatment. When the upper extremity is used, the non-dominant side is preferable, in the unlikely event of a complication.

Radial Artery: The radial artery usually has good collateral blood flow via the ulnar artery and is the preferred site in neonates and children. However, of 1000 consecutive adult hands studied prior to cardiac catheterization in a study, 27 per cent demonstrated a negative Allen's test suggesting lack of good collateral circulation (29). Therefore it is imperative to ascertain the presence of collateral flow by performing the modified Allen's test in every child. The risk of arterial thrombosis increases with prolonged cannulation, beyond the first 24–36 hours.

Dorsalis Pedis and Posterior Tibial Artery: These arteries are the second choice for arterial cannulation. Collateral blood flow should be tested in a manner analogous to the modified Allen's test. The incidence of thrombosis is about 7 per cent (30).

Axillary Artery: The use of the axillary artery is becoming increasingly popular. It has a rich collateral circulation; thrombosis and occlusion are seldom seen. Due to the artery's proximity to the circulation of the aortic arch, embolism remains a concern, and great care must be taken not to vigorously flush the system. Theoretical concerns of brachial plexus injury have not been seen in practice.

Femoral Artery: When attempts at the other sites mentioned above have been unsuccessful, the femoral artery can be used. Ease of access and complication rate have not been significantly different from other arterial sites (31). Although femoral access should be avoided in the presence of occlusive vascular disease of the leg, this is not a major concern in children. In infants, cannulation of the femoral vein and artery in the same leg may lead to venous and/or arterial obstruction and limb ischaemia. If the artery is punctured above the inguinal ligament, there is a risk of occult retroperitoneal haemorrhage.

Brachial and Temporal Arteries: These are the least desirable arteries for cannulation due to the paucity of adequate collateral circulation. Occlusion of the brachial artery can lead to loss of the entire distal arm.

Analysis of arterial waveform

There has been renewed interest in analysis of the arterial waveform to provide further information about haemodynamic status. Variation in both systolic and pulse pressures over the course of a respiratory cycle in mechanically ventilated patients has been used as a marker of preload responsiveness, i.e. to identify patients in whom a fluid bolus will augment cardiac output (32, 33). In normotensive sedated patients, the difference between the maximum and minimum values of systolic BP does not exceed 8–10 mm Hg. During hypovolaemia, this may rise up to 20 mm Hg, and decrease with fluid administration (**Figure 23.2.4**). These changes are not seen in spontaneously ventilating patients. In addition, as seen in the following section where estimation of cardiac output is discussed, analysis of the arterial pulse contour has been used to assess left ventricular stroke volume and stroke volume variation (SVV). These are also regarded as indicators of preload-responsiveness (34).

Central Venous Pressure (CVP)

CVP reflects right-sided filling pressure and is monitored in patients with septic shock, myocardial impairment or pulmonary disease. The major determinants of CVP are ventricular function and compliance, pulmonary vascular resistance (afterload) and intravascular blood volume. *Intravascular blood volume is only one contributing factor to right-sided filling pressure.*

The normal values are 1–5 mm Hg. CVP monitoring has been used as a measure to assess response during preload augmentation with fluid administration (if the CVP remains low, volume overload is not likely). A CVP greater than 7–10 mm Hg indicates myocardial dysfunction; increased right ventricular afterload; or volume overload. Further preload augmentation could be deleterious; inotropic support should be considered. However, many of the established beliefs about the utility of CVP in this context have been questioned in the past few years (35, 36).

The indications for insertion of a central venous catheter are listed in **Table 23.2.7**. There are several anatomic sites at which access to large central veins can be gained. The key advantages and problems with each site are summarized in **Tables 23.2.8** and **23.2.9**. Triple (and even quadruple) lumen central venous catheters are now available in several sizes and lengths for paediatric patients, enabling multiple infusions to be delivered easily through one venous access point (**Table 23.2.10**).

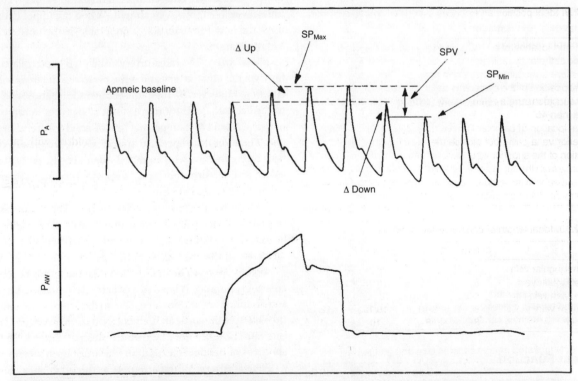

Figure 23.2.4. Stroke volume variation in ventilated patients.
Δ Down, the subsequent decrease in systolic pressure; Δ Up, the increase in systolic pressure immediately after the positive pressure breath; P$_A$, arterial pressure; P$_{AW}$, airway pressure; SP$_{Max}$, maximum systolic pressure after a positive pressure breath; SP$_{Min}$, minimum systolic pressure after a positive pressure breath; SPV, the difference between the SP$_{Max}$ and SP$_{Min}$ or the sum of Δ Up and Δ Down. From: Gunn. (2001). Current Opinion in Critical Care, 7(3), 212–217. Lippincott Williams and Wilkins.

Table 23.2.7. Indications for insertion of a central venous catheter

Measurement of CVP
Septic shock, hypovolaemia
High PEEP ventilation
Cardiac failure
Raised intracranial pressure

Other
Difficult peripheral venous access
Insertion of transvenous pacemaker

Secure, large-bore venous access
Cardio-pulmonary arrest
Rapid volume replacement e.g. shock states
Hypertonic infusions e.g potassium chloride, calcium gluconate, >10% dextrose, TPN, Inotrope administration

Table 23.2.8. Sites for insertion of a central venous catheter

Subclavian Vein
Anatomically most consistent central vein
Catheter not subject to movements of the neck
Less risk of infection with medium-term use
Risk of haemo/pneumothorax during insertion

Femoral vein
Least invasive
Does not reflect intrathoracic pressures

Internal Jugular Vein
Subject to anatomic variation (~8.5%)
Preferred central vein if clinical coagulopathy +/– thrombocytopaenia
To be avoided in raised intracranial pressure

Table 23.2.9. Ideal position and location of central venous catheters (CVC)

* Position and location of a CVC should always be confirmed before use of the catheter by radiography, blood gas analysis to check $S\bar{v}O_2$ and pressure transduction/waveform analysis

* The ideal position of the catheter is parallel to the vessel wall, failing which the incident angle of the catheter to the vessel wall should not be more than 40°

* The ideal location of catheter tip (internal jugular or subclavian) is in the superior vena cava, but outside the pericardium. An estimate of the junction of the superior vena cava with the right atrium is a third of the distance from the suprasternal notch to the xiphoid process. Internal jugular and subclavian venous catheters have demonstrated forward tip movement of 1–3 cm with neck and shoulder motion

Table 23.2.10. Ideal length of central venous catheters (in cm)

	0–8 kg	9–15 kg	16–30 kg	31–45 kg
Right internal jugular vein	5	8	8/10	10/12
Left internal jugular vein	8	8/10	10/12	12/15
Right subclavian vein	5	8	8/10	10/12
Left subclavian vein	8	8/10	10/12	12/15
Femoral vein	8	8	10	12

End-organ Function

In unsedated, sick children, the effects of impaired cardiovascular function can be easily assessed at the bedside by examining the end-organs: brain, kidneys and skin. In mechanically ventilated patients, the kidneys provide the most useful information about end-organ function. Oliguria usually occurs early in shock, even before the onset of tachycardia or changes in the blood pressure. A normal urine output (1–3 ml/kg/hour in children) is probably as good an indicator of adequate intravascular volume as cardiac filling pressures in a patient with normal renal function. Thus, measuring urine output on an hourly basis with a catheter in the bladder is perhaps more useful and efficient than a central venous or a pulmonary artery catheter. A urine output of less than 1 ml/kg/hour may indicate intravascular volume depletion or excessive antidiuretic hormone secretion. Recently, the effects of circulatory status on splanchnic perfusion have been assessed in children, by the use of gastric tonometry to measure gastric mucosal pH (37).

Measurement of Cardiac Output

Cardiac output (CO) is a product of heart rate and stroke volume. The gold standard technique for the measurement of CO has been the thermodilution technique using the pulmonary artery catheter (PAC). However, PAC insertion has never been standard practice in paediatric critical care due to technical difficulties and associated complication rate; for this reason, CO measurement was not commonly adopted. Recently, less invasive methods to measure CO have been described, and compare well with standard PAC-thermodilution techniques (38, 39). These techniques require the presence of an arterial and a central venous catheter, both of which are usually already present in children in critical care units. In one method, using lithium chloride dilution (LiDCO, London, UK) to calibrate a PulseCO™ monitor, cardiac output is measured continuously by examining the arterial waveform using pulse contour analysis. In another, a special arterial catheter tipped with a thermistor serves as a replacement for the PAC. In the latter case, a thermal fluid bolus injected into a central venous catheter (recent studies have shown that accurate results are possible even with peripheral intravenous injections) is sensed by the thermistor-tipped arterial catheter to calculate CO.

Both techniques, as with standard thermodilution, cannot be used to provide accurate results in children with intra-cardiac shunts.

Non-invasive Assessment of Haemodynamic Function

Echocardiography with Doppler is used extensively in paediatric intensive care units to assess myocardial contractility (stroke volume, shortening fraction and ejection fraction), pulmonary vascular resistance, abnormal cardiac structure and the presence of pericardial effusion, vegetations or intra-cardiac thrombus (40).

To Monitor or Not to Monitor

Monitoring will almost always provide more and interesting information. The key question an intensivist must ask is 'Is this additional information likely to change my management?' If the management is not going to change with the additional information provided by the monitoring then one must seriously consider the need for monitoring, especially invasive monitoring. 'The challenge is not so much contriving new things to do (there is enough for that) but figuring when to do them and understanding what was done' (41).

REFERENCES

1. McIntosh N. (2002). Intensive care monitoring: past, present and future. Clin Med. 2(4), 349–355.

2. Pinsky MR. (2003). Rationale for cardiovascular monitoring. Curr Opin Crit Care. 9(3), 222–224.

3. Mayotte MJ, Webster JG, Tompkins WJ. (1994). A comparison of electrodes for potential use in paediatric/infant apnoea monitoring. Physiol Meas. 15(4), 459–467.

4. Hamilton PS, Curley M, Aimi R. (2000). Effect of adaptive motion-artifact reduction on QRS detection. Biomed Instrum Technol. 34(3), 197–202.

5. Brooks AM, McBride JT, McConnochie KM et al. (1999). Predicting deterioration in previously healthy infants hospitalized with respiratory syncytial virus infection. Pediatrics. 104(3 Pt 1), 463–467.

6. Pasterkamp H. (1990). The history and physical examination. In: Kendig's disorders of the respiratory tract in children (Ed. Chernick V). p. 59. W B Saunders, Philadephia.

7. Little G (ed.). (1987). Infantile apnea and home monitoring: report of a consensus development conference. Bethesda, Maryland: National Institutes of Health, NIH 87–2905, 3.

8. Hutton P, Clutton-Brock T. (1993). The benefits and pitfalls of pulse oximetry. Brit Med J, 307, 457–458.

9. Caples SM, Hubmayr RD. (2003). Respiratory monitoring tools in the intensive care unit. Curr Opin Crit Care. 9(3), 230–235.

10. Yelderman M, New W. (1983). Evaluation of pulse oximetry. Anesthesiology, 59, 349.

11. Wouters PF, Gehring H, Meyfroidt G et al. (2002). Accuracy of pulse oximeters: the European multi-center trial. Anesth Analg. 94(1 Suppl), S13–S16.

12. Hay WW Jr, Rodden DJ, Collins SM et al. (2002). Reliability of conventional and new pulse oximetry in neonatal patients. J Perinatol. 22(5), 360–366.

13. Sahni R, Gupta A, Ohira-Kist K et al. (2003). Motion resistant pulse oximetry in neonates. Arch Dis Child Fetal Neonatal Ed. 88(6), F505–F508.

14. Bohnhorst B, Peter CS, Poets CF. (2002). Detection of hyperoxaemia in neonates: data from three new pulse oximeters. Arch Dis Child Fetal Neonatal Ed. 87(3), F217–F219.

15. Hayden W R, Greenberg RS, Nichols DG. (1992). Respiratory monitoring. In: Textbook of Pediatric Intensive Card (Ed. Rogers M C), pp. 204–228. Williams & Wilkins, Baltimore.

16. Snyder J, Elliot L, Grevnik A. (1982). Capnography. In: Clinics of critical care medicine (Ed. Spence A), pp. 100–121. Churchill Livingstone, Edinburgh.

17. Bhende MS. (2001). End-tidal carbon dioxide monitoring in pediatrics: concepts and technology. J Postgrad Med. 47, 153–156.

18. Singh S, Venkataraman ST, Saville A et al. (2001). NPB-75™: a portable quantitative microstream capnometer. Am J Emerg Med. 19, 208–210.

19. Levine RL, Wayne MA, Miller CC. (1997). End-tidal carbon dioxide and outcome of out-of-hospital cardiac arrest. N Engl J Med. 337, 301–306.

20. Fanconi S, Doherty P, Edmonds JF et al. (1985). Pulse oximetry in pediatric intensive care: comparison with measured saturations and transcutaneous oxygen tension. J Pediatr. 107(3), 362–366.

21. Hauser G, Pollock M, Sivit C et al. (1989). The routine chest radiographs in paediatric intesive care: a prospective study. Pediatrics 83, 465.

22. Thomas KE, Owens CM, Britto J et al. (2000). Efficacy of chest CT in a pediatric ICU: a prospective study. Chest. 117(6), 1697–1705.

23. Frerichs I, Schiffmann H, Hahn G et al. (2001). Non-invasive radiation-free monitoring of regional lung ventilation in critically ill infants. Intensive Care Med. 27(8), 1385–1394.

24. Lefrant JY, Muller L, de La Coussaye JE et al. (2003). Temperature measurement in intensive care patients: comparison of urinary bladder, oesophageal, rectal, axillary, and inguinal methods versus pulmonary artery core method. Intensive Care Med. 29(3), 414–418.

25. Wetzel R C, Tobin J R. (1992). Shock. In: Textbook of Pediatric Intensive Care (Ed. Roger MC). pp. 563–613. Williams & Wilkins, Baltimore.

26. Tibby SM, Hatherill M, Murdoch IA. (1999). Capillary refill and core-peripheral temperature gap as indicators of haemodynamic status in paediatric intensive care patients. Arch Dis Child. 80(2), 163–166.

27. Pollard AJ, Britto J, Nadel S et al. (1999). Emergency management of meningococcal disease. Arch Dis Child. 80(3), 290–296.

28. Kaye W. (1983). Invasive monitoring techniques: arterial cannulation, bedside pulmonary artery catheterization and arterial puncture. Heart Lung. 12, 400.

29. Benit E, Vranckx P, Jaspers L et al. (1996). Frequency of a positive modified Allen's test in 1,000 consecutive patients undergoing cardiac catheterization. Cathet Cardiovasc Diagn. 38(4), 352–354.

30. Wetzel RC, Tabata BK, Rogers MC (1992). Haemodynamic monitoring considerations in paediatric critical care. In: Textbook of Pediatric Intensive Care (Ed. Rogers MC). pp. 61–35. Williams & Wilkins, Baltimore.

31. Venkataraman ST, Thompson AE, Orr RA. (1997). Femoral vascular catheterization in critically ill infants and children. Clin Pediatr (Phila). 36(6), 311–319.

32. Tavernier B, Makhotine O, Lebuffe G et al. (1998). Systolic pressure variation as a guide to fluid therapy in patients with sepsis-induced hypotension. Anesthesiology. 89(6), 1313–1321.

33. Michard F, Boussat S, Chemla D et al. (2000). Relation between respiratory changes in arterial pulse pressure and fluid responsiveness in septic patients with acute circulatory failure. Am J Respir Crit Care Med. 162(1), 134–138.

34. Reuter DA, Felbinger TW, Schmidt C et al. (2002). Stroke volume variations for assessment of cardiac responsiveness to volume loading in mechanically ventilated patients after cardiac surgery. Intensive Care Med. 28(4), 392–398.

35. Nelson LD. (1997). The new pulmonary artery catheters: continuous venous oximetry, right ventricular ejection fraction, and continuous cardiac output. New Horiz. 5(3), 251–258.

36. Pinsky MR. (2002). Functional hemodynamic monitoring. Intensive Care Med. 28, 386–389.

37. Hamilton MA, Mythen MG. (2001). Gastric tonometry: where do we stand? Curr Opin Crit Care. 7(2), 122–127.

38. Linton NWF, Linton RAF. (2001). Estimation of changes in cardiac output from the arterial blood pressure waveform in the upper limb. Br J Anaesth, 86, 486–496.

39. Jonas MM, Tanser SJ. (2002). Lithium dilution measurement of cardiac output and arterial pulse waveform analysis: an indicator dilution calibrated beat-by-beat system for continuous estimation of cardiac output. Curr Opin Crit Care. 8(3), 257–261.

40. Mohan UR, Britto J, Habibi P et al. (2002). Noninvasive measurement of cardiac output in critically ill children. Pediatr Cardiol. 23(1), 58–61.

41. Brigham KL. (1987). A note from Nashville. Int. Care Med. 13, 428.

Approach to Shock in the Paediatric Intensive Care Unit

Contributed by Dr Y.K. Amdekar, MD, DCH, Consultant Paediatrician, Breach Candy Hospital and Jaslok Hospital, Retired Honorary Professor of Paediatrics, Grant Medical College and the JJ Group of Hospitals, Mumbai.

General Considerations

Shock is defined as a state of circulatory dysfunction that results in failure to provide adequate oxygen and other nutrients to meet the metabolic demands of the tissues. This is usually due to a reduction in cardiac output, maldistribution of regional blood flow, or a combination of both factors. Rarely it may occur due to increased metabolic requirements or impaired oxygen utilization at the cellular level. Such cellular oxygen deficiency leads to altered metabolism and decreased energy production, which if uncorrected, may result in death.

Ever-changing metabolic demands of tissues are met with primarily by adjustments in the cardiac output, which is the product of stroke volume and heart rate. In infants and young children, it is mainly the increase in the heart rate which tries to maintain the cardiac output, whereas in older children (as in adults), stroke volumes can be efficiently increased to improve cardiac output, without significant change in the heart rate. Thus infants and young children are at high risk of decompensation at an earlier stage as compared to older children. Besides suitable modification of cardiac output, the metabolic demands of a particular organ can be met by augmenting the regional blood flow by appropriate changes in the vasomotor tome mediated through neurohumoral mechanisms. When such physiological changes fail to meet the metabolic requirements, shock ensues. In paediatric practice, shock is a common accompaniment of many disease states; however the pathogenesis of shock varies depending upon the nature of disease. The different clinical forms of shock are briefly enumerated below.

(i) *Hypovolaemic Shock* results from decreased circulating blood volume commonly due to loss of fluids from the extravascular or intravascular compartment; it may also be due to third space fluid losses associated with the capillary leak syndromes.

(ii) *Distributive Shock* results from maldistribution of blood flow due to widespread abnormalities in vasomotor tone. Vasodilatation leads to venous pooling with decreased preload and shock ensues. Septic shock represents this type of shock. Other aetiologies like CNS injury, anaphylaxis and drug intoxication may also result in distributive shock.

(iii) *Cardiogenic Shock* results from decreased myocardial contractility. It may occur in patients with congenital heart defects,

in whom shock is preceded by congestive cardiac failure, or in children with previously normal hearts who have suffered hypoxic injury or metabolic derangements.

(iv) *Obstructive Shock* results from mechanical obstruction to venous inflow to the heart, as seen in cardiac tamponade, or to tight ventricular outflow as in pulmonary embolism.

(v) *Dissociative Shock* occurs in conditions like methaemoglobinaemia and carbon monoxide poisoning where oxygen is not released from haemoglobin to the tissues, in spite of normal tissue perfusion.

The first three types of shock are quite common while the last two varieties are rather rare.

Pathophysiology of Shock (1, 2)

Reduced cardiac output is the main factor in the evolution of shock. Hypovolaemic shock, results from a decrease in preload due to contraction of the intravascular volume as a result of blood or fluid loss. In septic shock, decrease in preload is the result of much more complex mechanisms. In sepsis, bacterial products interact with the reticulo-endothelial cells to produce a wide variety of mediators, which exert a potent effect on vascular tone and permeability leading to maldistribution of blood flow. Activated complement components promote leucocyte and platelet aggregation in capillaries, resulting in mechanical obstruction to blood flow. These changes in microcirculation which are the hallmark of septic shock also depress myocardial function, which further reduces cardiac output, as in cardiogenic shock. Thus, diminished cardiac output and resultant lowering of blood pressure trigger a series of changes that are characteristic of the clinical shock states.

Compensated Stage

With the onset of shock, the body tries to compensate for the reduced cardiac output by sympathetic discharge which leads to vasoconstriction, thereby increasing the heart rate and myocardial contractility. This results in improved cardiac output and blood pressure. However if the basic condition leading to shock is not controlled quickly, continued sympathetic overactivity beyond a certain limit proves detrimental to the patient, precipitating the decompensated stage of shock.

Decompensated Stage

Increasing heart rate leads to reduced myocardial perfusion and excessive oxygen consumption, which results in lowering of cardiac output. Hence the very mechanisms which are compensatory in the early stage of shock, prove to be detrimental at a later stage, perpetuating tissue ischaemia, impairing cell function and ultimately resulting in cell death. Tissue ischaemia releases biochemical mediators which exert potent effects on capillary endothelium and other cellular elements, thereby aggravating existing damage.

Cellular Response to Ischaemia

Tissue ischaemia with resultant lack of oxygen gives rise to anaerobic cell metabolism. Only 2 moles of ATP are produced per mole of glucose, instead of 38 moles produced by aerobic metabolism. Cellular ATP levels fall leading to failure of energy dependent processes. Anaerobic glycolysis with excess of lactate production and increased organic phosphates from ATP hydrolysis, results in extracellular and intracellular acidosis. This leads to influx of sodium, calcium and water into the cell, and efflux of potassium out of the cell; this damages the cell membrane and further impairs cell-ion regulation. Such changes impair energy production and promote release of acid hydrolases, which in turn cause tissue inflammation and injury.

Chemical Mediators in Shock

In all types of shock, but particularly in septic shock, mediators play an important role in initiating and sustaining impairment in tissue perfusion (2). These agents cause vasospasm, platelet aggregation and thrombus formation; they also increase capillary permeability, and promote maldistribution of blood flow.

A variety of arachidonic acid metabolites have been implicated as being modulators of shock. Thromoboxane A_2 is the most important of these compounds. It is mainly formed by the platelets and also by vascular smooth muscle, lung and the spleen. It is a potent vasoconstrictor and has platelet aggregating thrombogenic properties. These effects further reduce blood flow in an already compromised microcirculation, producing extension of tissue ischaemia and death. Vasoactive prostaglandin PGF alpha-2 is also formed by the platelets and is a potent vasoconstrictor. Prostacyclin is believed to neutralize the deleterious effect of thromboxane and is produced by healthy capillary endothelium. However as the capillaries are damaged, insufficient prostacyclin is produced and hence the shock state is perpetuated. Leukotrienes are produced by different types of cells like leucocytes, macrophages and mast cells. They enhance capillary permeability, produce intense vasoconstriction and have a myocardial depressant action. Intrinsic myocardial depression exists in all types of shock, mediated through several haemodynamic mechanisms. Irrespective of these factors, a small peptide released from pancreatic acinar cells due to ischaemia, is known to exert a negative inotropic effect, and is named the myocardial depressant factor. This mediator depresses myocardial function even in the presence of normal coronary flow, preload and afterload. This factor also causes pancreatic ischaemia, as well as depression of the reticulo-endothelial system. Endogenous opiates, most widely implicated in the pathogenesis of shock, are released from the pituitary in response to stress.

Clinical Approach

In vulnerable clinical settings, one must suspect and watch for early signs of shock. Much before clinical signs manifest clearly, there may be early clues, raising a suspicion of shock. Disproportionate tachycardia and tachypnoea indicates systemic inflammatory response and is a forerunner of impending sepsis. An increase in the difference between the core and skin temperatures, and postural hypotension may suggest impending shock. Subsequently typical clinical signs develop which consist of increasing tachycardia, increasing tachypnoea, low or normal blood pressure, cool and mottled extremities, poor colour and prolonged capillary refill, more than 2–3 seconds. In the early stage of distributive shock, patients may be febrile with a dry hot skin, and normal blood pressure often referred to as 'warm' shock. Urine output is an excellent indicator of renal perfusion and must be monitored on an hourly basis. A depressed neurological state may ensue later. All the above-mentioned clinical signs must be periodically assessed; however, they have to be supplemented by appropriate biophysical and biochemical parameters.

Septic shock is a clinical challenge for early diagnosis and prompt management. Though Gram-negative bacterial infections are more commonly the causative factors in the evolution of septic shock, Gram-positive bacterial infections as well as viral infections, parasitic infections (like malaria), and even myobacterial and fungal infections may lead to septic shock in children. In fact, any infection in a vulnerable setting, constitutes a potential threat to develop into septic shock. It is the sound knowledge of interactions between host factors and infections that guide a clinician to anticipate the outcome in a given infection. If an infection, instead of localizing, threatens to spread, a competent host develops a systemic inflammatory response syndrome (SIRS). SIRS is a measure of a counter-regulatory process, clinically evident by disproportionate tachycardia and tachypnoea. This stage represents early sepsis. If infection further worsens, the counter regulatory mechanisms fail to maintain the body's homeostasis. This corresponds to a stage of severe sepsis. On further deterioration, organ failure ensues and this heralds the development of septic shock. In unfavourable conditions, a patient may pass through these stages rapidly within 12–24 hours, giving little time for action. Hence clinical anticipation and early monitoring are key factors for successful management.

For the sake of understanding, three distinct phases (early sepsis, severe sepsis and septic shock) may be defined; each phase however overlaps the other, and there are no clinical or investigatory parameters for their precise diagnosis. It is the continuous monitoring of vital parameters together with periodic biochemical monitoring, that predicts the trend in a given disease state. A single record of any parameter is of much less significance than the trend observed over a period of time. Besides continuous display of heart rate, respiratory rate, core and skin temperatures, and non-invasive blood pressure readings, arterial oxygen saturation, and end-tidal PCO_2 monitoring help in optimum management. Central venous pressure (CVP) monitoring helps in the infusion of adequate amount of fluids especially in septic shock. Children with septic shock need very large amounts of fluid and are in constant danger of both under- or over-perfusion, in the absence of proper monitoring facilities. Sophisticated monitoring may entail the study of metabolism at cellular level, and assessing both oxygen delivery and consumption (3, 4).

Management

Early rapid infusion of fluids to replenish the intravascular volume, often decides the ultimate outcome of a patient in shock (5). In septic shock the source of sepsis should be promptly identified and eradicated. The earlier this is done, the better the prognosis. Empiric use of antibiotics in patients where the nature of infection cannot be immediately proven, is on the same principles as in adults.

Diagnosis of early shock should be followed by volume challenge of at least 20 ml/kg body weight of Ringer Lactate. If this produces improvement in vital prarameters, then appropriate infusions are continued and the patient is monitored clinically. However, if there is no adequate improvement on such a challenge, then further infusions should be planned by CVP monitoring. Crystalloids are commonly used; they may be safely infused to an amount equivalent to 50 per cent of circulating blood volume, beyond which point peripheral tissue and pulmonary oedema may develop. Colloids like plasma, blood or dextran are administered under close monitoring, as they are likely to expand the intravascular space by a volume greater than that infused, and may cause circulatory overload. Dextran solutions have an advantage of improving microcirculation by decreasing RBC aggregation and improving oxygen transport; however, their administration should not exceed 20 ml/kg/day. In hypotensive patients dopamine may be required to augment cardiac output, whereas in low cardiac output states with normal blood pressure, dobutamine may be the drug of choice. Vasodilators may be indicated in the late stages of shock where vasoconstriction is the prominent feature. Cardiac failure and rhythm disturbances may need appropriate therapy.

If in spite of adequate replacement, hypotension and hypoperfusion persist, CVP monitoring alone may not suffice, and further invasive monitoring is often required to assess the right and left atrial pressures and cardiac output; however, this is not routinely required. In case of renal hypoperfusion, diuretics should be used only after adequate volume expansion.

Metabolic status including oxygenation should be periodically evaluated and adequate steps are necessary to correct abnormalities. Hypoxia at the cellular level is the key factor in the pathogenesis of shock, and hence adequate oxygenation is mandatory in every patient. Blood gas determinations should guide timely interventions, including mechanical ventilator support.

The use of corticosteroids in the management of shock is controversial. Though theoretically steroids are supposed to exert a beneficial effect through various mechanisms, controlled studies have not found statistically significant benefits, and hence no definite recommendations can be made. Many other drugs have been tried, like the opiate antagonist naloxone, and thyrotropin, but as yet these cannot be recommended for routine use. Future drugs used in shock would essentially antagonize the actions of the numerous chemical mediators involved in shock. Till then, early recognition, maintenance of a satisfactory circulatory and metabolic state, and above all prompt eradication of the underlying pathology, remain the mainstays of management.

Table 23.3.1. Resuscitation in shock

Goal of therapy
* To maintain normal blood pressure and keep mixed venous O_2 saturation > 70 per cent.

Management
* Recognize poor perfusion—reduced urine output and blunted mental status
* Maintain airway and secure vascular access
* Aggressive volume replacement
  – Push 20 ml/kg body weight of isotonic saline in 20 minutes—if need be repeat two more pushes over next 40 minutes
  – If fluid refractory shock—establish CVP and start dopamine
  – If fluid refractory and dopamine resistant shock—epinephrine for cold shock and norepinephrine for warm shock
  – If catecholamine resistant shock—hydrocortisone

REFERENCES

1. Mouchawar A, Rosenthal M. (1993). A pathophysiological approach to the patient in shock. Int Anesth Clin. 31, 1–20.

2. Casteillo L, Sanchez M. (1993). Septic shock: Pathogenesis and treatment. Indian J. Pediatr. 60(3), 367–369.

3. Connor TA, Hall RT. (1994). Mixed venous oxygenation in critically ill neonates. Crit Care Med. 22(2), 343–346.

4. Sear M, Wensley D, Mocnab A. (1993). Oxygen consumption oxygen delivery relationship in children. J. Pediatr. 123(2), 208–214.

5. Carcillo JA, Davis AL, Zaritsky A. (1991). Role of early fluid resuscitation in pediatric septic shock. JAMA. 266(9), 1242–1245.

Hypertensive Emergencies in Paediatrics

Contributed by Dr Y.K. Amdekar, MD, DCH, Consultant Paediatrician, Breach Candy Hospital and Jaslok Hospital, Retired Honorary Professor of Paediatrics, Grant Medical College and the JJ Group of Hospitals, Mumbai.

In children, severe hypertension is almost always secondary. In fact, primary hypertension is mild and asymptomatic. About 80 per cent of children with hypertension have underlying kidney disease—two-thirds of them mesoparenchymal and one-third renovascular. Ten per cent of patients suffer from hypertension due to coarctation of aorta or aortoarteritis of various aetiologies. The remaining patients comprise endocrinal disorders and other miscellaneous causes.

Hypertensive emergencies may occur in patients with known kidney disease. However at times hypertension may be the only presenting feature, often manifesting with vague non-specific symptoms that may suggest primary CNS, cardiovascular or ocular disease. Hence in any seriously ill child who presents with ill-defined encephalopathy (headache, vomiting, irritability, change in sensorium), or cardiac failure, or visual disturbances of unknown aetiology, the blood pressure must be recorded. Accurate measurement of blood pressure is difficult in children and demands a proper size cuff, correct technique and patience on the part of the clinician. As the blood pressure is markedly elevated in hypertensive emergencies, a small error in the blood pressure recording does not change the interpretation or the management.

It is the sudden rise in the blood pressure that presents as an emergency, rather than chronically elevated blood pressure which has fewer symptoms. The child may present with convulsions and demonstrate various neurological abnormalities mimicking intracranial infection. Fundus examination may show evidence of papilloedema or retinal haemorrhages. Sudden onset of left ventricular failure, especially in the presence of overhydration may be a manifestation of acute glomerulonephritis and may be mistaken for myocarditis or bronchopneumonia.

Management (1–3)

The main aim of therapy is to reduce the blood pressure to a safe level, control various complications like seizures, cardiac failure and airways obstruction, and treat the primary cause as and when feasible. Reduction of blood pressure should be achieved over 3–4 days to a level of 95th percentile appropriate for the age. A sudden precipitous fall in blood pressure may be associated with development of neurological signs and impairment of cerebral and renal blood flow. Several drugs are available for prompt reduction of blood pressure. Diazoxide and labetalol are not easily available, and nifedipine is the drug most often used in our set-up. Though sublingual administration is known to lead to a sudden fall in blood pressure, in our experience it occurs rarely. Sodium nitroprusside is an excellent drug for continuous infusion; it is extremely potent and needs careful titration of the dose by constant monitoring. Hydralazine is another drug, but is rather slow in action. In case of accompanying fluid overload, diuretics like furosemide can be used; otherwise, diuretics may in fact be harmful as they may lead to volume depletion and hypotension. Dosage of drugs commonly employed in the treatment of hypertensive emergencies are given in **Table 23.4.1**.

Supportive measures include control of seizures by diazepam 0.3 mg/kg/dose, and antifailure treatment in case of cardiac failure. Surgical intervention may be necessary at times. Maintenance therapy for hypertension can be continued orally.

Table 23.4.1. Drugs commonly used (with route of administration and dosage) for treatment of hypertensive crisis in the paediatric age group

Drug	Route of Administration	Dosage
Nifedipine	Sublingual	0.5 mg/kg every 4–6 hrs
Sodium Nitroprusside	IV Infusion	0.5 µg/kg/min
Labetalol	IV	1–3 mg/kg
Diazoxide	IV	1–5 mg/kg every 4–6 hrs
Hydralazine	IV	0.2 mg/kg every 4–6 hrs
Furosemide	IV	2–5 mg/kg

REFERENCES

1. Deal JE, Barrat TM, Dillon MJ. (1992). Management of hypertensive emergencies. Arch Dis Child. 67, 1089–1092.

2. Calhoun DA. (1990). Current concepts—Treatment of hypertensive crisis. N Engl J Med. 323, 1177–1183.

3. Roy LP. (1988). Drug therapy in childhood hypertension. Ind J Pediatr. 55, 359–371.

CHAPTER 23.5

Heart Failure in Neonates and Children

Contributed by Dr Y.K. Amdekar, MD, DCH, Consultant Paediatrician, Breach Candy Hospital and Jaslok Hospital, Retired Honorary Professor of Paediatrics, Grant Medical College and the JJ Group of Hospitals, Mumbai.

Cardiac failure is a state in which the heart cannot maintain adequate output to sustain metabolic demands of the body. In the early stages, the heart tries to maintain optimum output by physiological adjustments; however after a certain point, compensatory mechanisms fail, and decompensated stage of cardiac failure ensues. Clinical manifestations vary a great deal between neonates and older children. No age is exempt from cardiac failure, but the aetiological factors are so diverse in the different age groups, that prompt recognition of cardiac failure and diagnosis of its aetiology, often pose a challenge to the clinician. Morever, the majority of these patients present as medical emergencies, with very rapid decompensation. This is due to the limitations of physiological compensatory mechanisms in children. Unlike adults, where stroke volume can be modified to a considerable extent by appropriate changes in myocardial contractility, preload, and afterload, in children it is mainly changes in the heart rate that try to maintain cardiac output, without much change in the stroke volume. However, increase in the heart rate beyond an optimum level, in fact results in poor coronary filling, and increased oxygen consumption leading to early decompensation. Thus early recognition of cardiac failure is far more important in young children.

In our experience, 10 per cent of patients in any paediatric ICU manifest with significant cardiac problems. Though congenital defects and acquired heart diseases presenting with cardiac failure are common to all age groups, certain conditions predominate in specific age groups. Besides congenital defects like hypoplastic left heart, transposition of the great vessels and large left to right shunts, birth asphyxia is an important cause of cardiac failure in newborns. Occasionally a baby is born with hydrops foetalis as a result of cardiac failure due to severe anaemia caused by isoimmune haemolytic disease. Severe anaemia in the newborn may also be caused by foetomaternal transfusion, haemorrhage due to birth injury or a bleeding diathesis. In infants and young children, cardiac failure may result from large left to right shunts, endocardial fibroelastosis, cardiomyopathy, viral myocarditis and hypertension, including coarctation of the aorta. In older children > 5 years of age, rheumatic heart disease is a major cause of cardiac failure in our country. Other important conditions include infective endocarditis, viral myocarditis, diphtheritic myocarditis, and

pericardial effusion due to tuberculosis or other infections. Acute hypertension often presents with cardiac failure in this age group. Cor pulmonale, thyrotoxicosis, and beriberi, are rare in children.

Clinical Features (1)

Newborns and infants present with varied and vague symptoms that are often unrelated to the cardiovascular system. Poor feeding, vomiting, diarrhoea may be initial symptoms while restlessness, excessive sweating and crying may offer clues to the diagnosis of cardiac failure. Tachypnoea, chest retractions and tachycardia are invariably present. Hepatomegaly is a constant feature, though tenderness and the hepatojugular reflux are difficult to elicit. Normally, the liver is palpable in newborns and young infants, and has a clearly defined edge. In case of cardiac failure, the liver edge becomes rounded and is a good clinical pointer to a pathological liver. Oedema of feet is often absent. Marked tachycardia, gallop rhythm and murmurs if present, are commonly observed clinical signs.

In older children, symptoms and signs are similar to those seen in adults, and hence easily detected. Breathlessness, oedema on dependent parts, right hypochondrial pain, and oliguria are the classical symptoms. Besides tachycardia and tachypnoea, a tender, enlarged liver with a positive hepatojugular reflux, cardiomegaly, basal crepitations in the lungs, soft heart sounds and murmurs if any, are the characteristic clinical signs. Signs of cardiogenic shock may ensue at any stage.

Investigations

In newborns and young infants, mild cardiomegaly is difficult to assess radiologically. ECG needs proper-sized chest leads, and interpretations are essentially age-dependent. 2D echocardiography with Doppler study is very useful in delineating anatomical defects, as well as assessing the functional state of various chambers and valves. Vegetations can be picked up easily in cases of active rheumatic carditis as well as in infective endocarditis. Other relevant investigations include serum electrolytes, acid-base balance, and oxygenation status.

Management (2–5)

Cardiac failure is an emergency which especially in infants and young children, needs prompt management. Non-pharmacological measures are as important as drug treatment. A proper position (ideally propped-up), is comfortable for older children, but infants may have to be managed even on the mother's lap. Humidified oxygen is given by a hood in an infant, at the rate of 8–10 l/min; this may be administered by mask or nasal prongs in older children. Adequate sedation maybe necessary at times in young children, either with chloral hydrate (20–25 mg/kg per dose orally), or in very sick infants with pulmonary oedema, even with morphine (0.1 mg/kg per dose subcutaneously). Adequate hydration and nutrition need to be maintained by suitable methods—either orally or intravenously. Salt restricted diet with sufficient calories, and appropriately restricted fluids may have to be planned to meet the increased energy requirements, without overloading the child with salt and water.

Cardiac output may be increased by using inotropic drugs combined with diuretics and vasodilators as and when necessary. Digoxin is an important drug in the control of cardiac failure (**2, 3**). In paediatric patients rapid digitalization (0.04–0.05 mg/kg) over 24 hrs is generally required; however in certain conditions in older children, slow digitalization over a week, may be ideal. Later, a maintenance dose of 0.01 mg/kg/day is administered. Other inotropes like dopamine and dobutamine are used in cardiogenic shock, asphyxia and post-surgical conditions. Diuretics like furosemide (1–2 mg/kg/day), thiazides (1–2 mg/kg/day) and spironolactone (1–2 mg/kg/day) are used judiciously in combination with digoxin, starting with a low dose and titrating the same as per the clinical state. Vasodilators like captopril (0.5–2 mg/kg/day) may be useful in cases of pulmonary oedema due to mitral or aortic regurgitant lesions, as well as in post-operative patients with cardiac failure. Precipitating factors like anaemia, electrolyte disturbances, arrhythmias, and infective endocarditis must be appropriately treated for successful management of cardiac failure.

REFERENCES

1. Behrman RE. (1992). The Cardiovascular System. In: Textbook of Paediatrics, 14th edn (Eds Behrman RE, Kliegman RM). pp. 1125–1228. WB Saunders Company, Philadelphia.

2. Young B. (1992). A prospective randomized study of ventricular failure and efficacy of digoxin. J Am Coll Cardiol. 19, 259A–262A.

3. Adam DT. (1989). A new look at digoxin in congestive heart failure and sinus rhythms. Postgrad Med J. 65, 715–717.

4. William F, Freidman HD, Boubal I. (1984). New concept sand drugs in the treatment of congestive heart failure. Pediatr Clin North Am. 31, 1197–1222.

5. Artam M, Graham T. (1987). Guidelines for vasodilator therapy of congestive heart failure in infants and children. Am Heart J. 113–121.

Acute Respiratory Failure in Children and Hyaline Membrane Disease

---

Contributed by Dr Y.K. Amdekar, MD, DCH, Consultant Paediatrician, Breach Candy Hospital and Jaslok Hospital, Retired Honorary Professor of Paediatrics, Grant Medical College and the JJ Group of Hospitals, Mumbai.

Acute Respiratory Failure in Children (1)

Respiratory failure, either impending or manifest, is a significant threat in many patients in paediatric practice. In our experience, 20 per cent of patients in a paediatric ICU are admitted for primary respiratory emergencies, though in many other conditions secondary respiratory problems ensue, needing prompt respiratory care. Such diseases include cardiac failure, peripheral nervous system disorders as in the Guillain-Barré syndrome, poliomyelitis, myopathies, CNS disorders, and shock states. Thus respiratory dysfunction is a common denominator in many paediatric ICU patients.

Common pulmonary diseases presenting with respiratory failure include pneumonia, severe asthma, acute bronchiolitis (2), pulmonary oedema, and the croup syndrome. Other problems causing acute respiratory failure include foreign body obstruction and hydrocarbon poisoning. Epiglotitis causing upper respiratory obstruction is rarely seen in our country. The important causes of acute respiratory failure in the paediatric age group are listed in **Table 23.6.1**.

Table 23.6.1. Important causes of acute respiratory failure in the paediatric age group

1. Pulmonary Causes
* Pneumonia
* Severe asthma
* Acute bronchiolitis
* Pulmonary oedema
* The croup syndrome
* Obstruction by foreign body
* Epiglotitis causing upper respiratory obstruction

2. Non-pulmonary Causes
* Cardiac failure
* Neuromuscular disorders e.g. Guillain-Barré syndrome, myopathies
* Central nervous system disorders e.g. poliomyelitis
* Shock states

Neonates may present with hyaline membrane disease, meconium aspiration, persistent pulmonary hypertension, congenital malformations like diaphragmatic hernia and lobar emphysema, as well as pneumonias, birth asphyxia and pulmonary haemorrhage. Extrapulmonary conditions include central nervous

Table 23.6.2. Important causes of acute respiratory failure in neonates

1. Pulmonary Causes
* Hyaline membrane disease
* Persistent pulmonary hypertension
* Congenital malformations e.g. diaphragmatic hernia, lobar emphysema
* Pneumonia
* Pulmonary haemorrhage
* Birth asphyxia

2. Extra-pulmonary Causes
* Central nervous system infections e.g. neonatal tetanus
* Cardiac diseases (generally congenital heart disease)

system infections, and cardiac diseases. The important causes of acute respiratory failure in neonates are given in **Table 23.6.2**.

Acute respiratory failure in terms of arterial blood gas estimation is defined as $PaCO_2 > 50$ mm Hg and/or $PaO_2 < 55$ mm Hg, while breathing room air. It may be clinically classified into pump failure (disorders of mechanics of respiration), and lung failure (diseases of airways and lung parenchyma). 'Pump failure' is characterized by an increase in $PaCO_2$ and a fall in PaO_2; whereas lung failure is characterized by a decreased PaO_2 with a normal or low $PaCO_2$. Later in the natural history of lung disease, the occurrence of alveolar hypoventilation or of respiratory muscle fatigue can cause a gradual rise in the $PaCO_2$. The above classification has an implication both in relation to aetiology and management. Thus an increase in $PaCO_2$ in pump failure may well be an indication for initiating mechanical ventilator support. On the other hand, a decrease in PaO_2 with a low $PaCO_2$ may respond to an increase in the FIO_2, if hypoxia is chiefly due to a ventilation-perfusion mismatch produced by lung disease. If however a decrease in PaO_2 is chiefly due to a right to left shunt within the lungs, increase in FIO_2 will not produce a significant increase in the PaO_2. Ventilator support will be required in these patients, as also in those who ultimately show a progressive increase in the $PaCO_2$.

In newborns and young children respiratory failure can develop rapidly due to various unfavourable anatomical and physiological factors, like poor compliance of the lungs, easy blockage of air passages, immaturity of the cough reflex and the higher centres, and poor respiratory reserve with early fatiguability of respiratory muscles.

Clinical Features

It is important to realize that respiratory distress may occur in the absence of respiratory disease or failure. Conversely, respiratory failure may be present without respiratory distress as in patients with muscular weakness or CNS depression. Diseases like encephalitis and Reye's syndrome, as well as diseases causing metabolic acidosis may present with hyperventilation, which may be mistaken for respiratory distress. Apnoea may be the manifestation of respiratory failure in neonates. Respiratory distress, with activity of accessory muscles of respiration, along with chest retractions, stridor, grunting or wheezing, are important clinical manifestations. Symptoms and signs of hypoxaemia manifested by restlessness, confusion, hypotonia and cyanosis may supervene. Muscle fatigue may be evident by paradoxical breathing and see-saw movements of the chest and upper abdomen. Convulsions, shock and cardiorespiratory failure ultimately supervene.

The clinical features of neonatal tetanus are characterized by difficulty in suckling and swallowing due to spasm and rigidity of the muscles of the face and of deglutition. Risus sardonicus with the characteristic tetanus facies is diagnostic of the disease. In neonatal tetanus, skeletal and truncal rigidity is quickly followed by convulsive seizures. Breathing is impaired, atelectasis is frequent and acute hypoxaemic respiratory failure results. Death generally results from cardiorespiratory failure (3).

Diagnosis

The clinical diagnosis of respiratory failure should be supplemented by relevant investigations. Arterial blood gas estimation defines the type and severity of respiratory failure. This can be further monitored by non-invasive parameters like SaO_2, transcutaneous PO_2, and capnography. These non-invasive methods certainly have limitations, but are very useful for defining the trends in progress. Chest X-ray is helpful in evaluating the cause, progress and complications of respiratory disease. Ultimately, cardiac, CNS, and other organ dysfunctions need to be monitored by appropriate tests.

Management

Pump failure is rather easy to manage. Mechanical ventilation is required with an increasing $PaCO_2$ due to ventilatory failure. In our experience, patients with ventilatory failure who to start with have normal lungs, tolerate prolonged mechanical ventilation for several weeks without any complications. We have had a newborn with congenital amyelinosis, and a six week old infant with severe poliomyelitis who despite being on mechanical ventilation for longer than 12 weeks, presented no problems in management. However lung failure is a challenge to the clinician (4). It is in this type of failure that skilful management may change the outcome, because in lung disease there exists a high risk of inflicting further damage by the use of both high inflation pressures and high concentrations of inspired oxygen. The aim of management is to maintain blood gases and acid-base status within the optimum range. This is primarily done by adequate oxygenation and ventilation. Humidified oxygen is administered at suitable flow rates depending on the method of delivery used—be it by oxygen hood, mask or nasal prongs. In paediatric practice, Venturi mask is rarely required as we do not encounter patients with chronic respiratory disease, dependent on the hypoxic central drive. Except in preterm neonates, where FIO_2 needs to be stringently monitored, short-term high oxygen concentrations are well tolerated.

In children, ventilatory settings depend on the age and body size. **Table 23.6.3** details the standard ventilator settings used in infants and children. However these may be modified depending on the disease and its pathophysiology. Pressure-limited time-cycled ventilation is ideal for newborns and infants, whereas older children require volume-control ventilation. The peak inspiratory pressure should not exceed 15–20 cm H_2O in neonates and infants, and 20–25 cm H_2O in older children. PEEP is often used in children to improve oxygenation, though too much PEEP is harmful. Square wave pressure generation with prolonged inspiration time may be ideal to improve oxygenation in acute lung disease.

Table 23.6.3. Standard ventilator settings in neonates and older children

Settings	Newborns and Infants	Older Children
Tidal Volume	10 ml/kg	10 ml/kg
Respiratory Rate	25–30/min	20/min
Peak Inspiratory Pressure	15–20 cm of H_2O	20–25 cm of H_2O
PEEP	2 cm of H_2O	2 cm of H_2O
I:E Ratio	1:2	1:2

CPAP is an intermediate method between mechanical ventilation and spontaneous breathing. It is normally delivered through an endotracheal tube, though it may also be employed to some extent through a nasopharyngeal tube, or even through a tight-fitting mask in small children. Specific treatment of the underlying disease and management of dysfunction of other organ systems are as important as the primary management of respiratory failure.

Orotracheal intubation with proper length and size of endotracheal tube is a prerequisite. Nasotracheal intubation is technically difficult in small children, and its long-term use is known to be associated with higher incidence of middle ear infections. In children, mechanical ventilation is required for a short time in most cases. The size of the endotracheal tube should be such as to allow a small leak under positive pressure. Tight fitting tubes with a tight seal, may lead to tracheal stenosis. At the same time, too large a leak may hamper adequate ventilation. The formula of (16 + age in years) ÷ 4 is a useful guide for determining the size of the endotracheal tube. An endotracheal tube of a small diameter in paediatric patients is prone to get blocked by thick secretions, and hence proper humidification of the respiratory tract is an important yet often neglected aspect of management. On the other hand, enthusiastic overhumidification may lead to absorption of a considerable amount of water. Frequent suction by sterile techniques is necessary in many ventilated children. Bag and tube ventilation with 100 per cent oxygen prior to suctioning, prevents hypoxaemia. Suction should be done whilst withdrawing the catheter gradually over 8–10 seconds. Between each suctioning, 100 per cent oxygen is administered by 'bagging'. An end-hole catheter is preferred to a side-hole one, to avoid trapping of respiratory mucosa. Development of bradycardia is indicative of hypoxaemia and suctioning must be immediately stopped, and the patient ventilated with 100 per cent oxygen. Infection must be prevented by proper asepsis including hand washing, use of disposables and proper sterilization of equipments including ventilators. Delicate parts of the ventilator circuits like transducers, are chemically sterilized in alcohol. Colonization of ventilators, humidifiers and endotracheal tubes by Gram-negative organisms, including pseudomonas infection, is a major problem in management. Scrupulous attention must be paid to prevent infections. Respiratory tubings must be changed every 2–3 days, or more frequently in the presence of colonization.

Patients needing mechanical ventilation often require some form of sedation or muscle relaxants. We use pancuronium bromide in the dose of 0.15 to 0.2 mg/kg intravenously, as an initial dose and repeat this every 2–4 hours as required. Paralyzing patients for prolonged periods may cause a gradual fall in the compliance of the lungs, and sudden accidental disconnection of the ventilator may be fatal in a paralyzed child.

Hyaline Membrane Disease (Respiratory Distress Syndrome)

Hyaline membrane disease occurs primarily in premature neonates. Its incidence is inversely proportional to the gestational age—60–80 per cent in infants less than 28 weeks of gestation, and rare in term babies. The incidence is also increased in infants born to diabetic mothers and in those delivered by caesarean section.

Absence of surfactant results in high surface tension and keeps the alveoli atelectatic. Along with atelectasis, formation of hyaline membrane and interstitial oedema make the lungs poorly compliant. High compliance of the chest wall in preterm infants offers less resistance against the tendency of the lungs to collapse. This results in poorly ventilated, though well perfused alveoli, leading to hypoxia. Poor lung compliance and alveolar hypoventilation, increased dead space, small tidal volumes and extra work of breathing, all contribute to hypercarbia. A combination of hypoxia, hypercarbia and acidosis results in pulmonary vasoconstriction leading to right to left shunting, reduced pulmonary flow and ischaemic injury to alveolar cells, thus worsening the vicious cycle.

Clinical presentation occurs early at birth, or within a few hours after birth, with tachypnoea, chest retraction and cyanosis. This may progress over the next 24–48 hours to cause severe hypoxic injury leading to shock, hypotension, myocardial failure and renal dysfunction. Persistent hypoxaemia in a typical setting, with diffuse lung infiltrates on chest X-ray, clinch the diagnosis of hyaline membrane disease. Pulmonary infections are difficult to exclude. Complications besides acute respiratory failure and shock, include air-leak syndromes and shunting through a patent ductus and foramen ovale.

Management is aimed at improving oxygenation and reducing hypercarbia and acidosis by proper oxygenation and ventilation. Artificial surfactant can be instilled into the air passages through the endotracheal tube, which helps in reverting early pathological changes (5). Other drugs may be necessary to deal with accompanying problems—tolazoline for persistent foetal circulation, aminophylline and doxapram to counter respiratory depression.

Prevention of hyaline membrane disease is possible by administering steroids to mothers 24–48 hours prior to delivery, especially before 32–34 weeks of gestation, trying to prevent preterm labour, and controlling maternal diabetes throughout pregnancy.

Surfactant Therapy

Exogenous surfactant therapy is widely used in preterm neonates with RDS and it is increasingly used in other respiratory conditions as well. There are two types of surfactants—natural and synthetic. The predominant and most efficient phospholipid in these products is DPPC (dipalmitoylphosphatidylcholine). However DPCC adsorbs very slowly to the air-liquid interface (6). Its adsorption is enhanced by other lipids and proteins contained in these products, including four major apoproteins—SP-A, SP-B, SP-C and SP-D (6). They provide defence against inhaled pathogens. Among them SP-A is most efficient in regulating lowering of surface tension. None of the presently available preparations contain SP-A. Synthetic surfactants lack many of the components of natural surfactant (7). Use of natural surfactants is preferred though it needs refrigeration for storage. Synthetic surfactant is available in lyophilized form, can be stored at room temperature and reconstituted with sterile water before use.

While use of surfactant in preterm neonates is well established, there used to be a debate over timing of its use and number of doses required. However, in recent times, such a controversy is settled. In a neonate at risk of developing RDS, prophylactic use of surfactant immediately after stabilization is preferred to 'rescue' therapy employed after development of RDS, even though such practice may result in the use of surfactant in a small number of neonates who may not have required it (8, 9). In those neonates who do not receive prophylactic surfactant therapy, early administration before 2 hours of age has better outcome than at a later age. In patients who demonstrate good response to the first dose but deteriorate after some time, multiple doses are administered—3–4 doses over the first 72 hours. Such a strategy has proved to be useful (8, 9).

Current evidence suggests that surfactant administered through double-lumen endotracheal tube or a catheter passed through a suction valve appears to be more effective and minimizes related adverse effects (including hypoxia) as compared to administration through the use of a simple catheter or side-port.

Adverse effects are few and not serious. Long-term follow-up of these neonates who receive surfactant is reassuring.

With the knowledge that surfactant deficiency occurs in many acquired disorders leading to acute lung injury, surfactant has been tried in such diseases with varying benefits (8). Evidence suggests that preterm neonates with bronchopulmonary dysplasia and prolonged mechanical ventilation also experience surfactant dysfunction; however, exogenous surfactant therapy beyond the first week of life has not been well studied. Surfactant replacement therapy has been studied for use in other respiratory disorders, including meconium aspiration syndrome and pneumonia (8). Commercial surfactant preparations currently available are not optimal, given the variability of surfactant protein content and their susceptibility to inhibition. Further progress in the treatment of neonatal respiratory disorders may include the development of 'designer' surfactant preparations.

Recently, natural exogenous surfactant replacement has been used in experimental models and clinical trials for the treatment of severe respiratory syncytial virus (RSV) disease. It has been shown that surfactant therapy improves gas exchange and respiratory mechanics and shortens the duration of ventilatory support and intensive care unit stay in infants with severe RSV-induced respiratory failure.

There is strong evidence that alterations in the pulmonary surfactant system play an important role in the pathophysiology of lung disease, including ARDS. Although it is still unclear whether mortality and morbidity of ARDS will be reduced, surfactant replacement therapy has been shown to improve oxygenation and improve lung compliance, and decrease need for ventilator support. Further studies will also be needed to elucidate the optimal timing and dosage regimen for different disease processes. Some evidence supports the measurements of surfactant protein levels as markers for predicting the onset and outcome of ARDS and perhaps providing a window for early treatment of patients at risk to develop ARDS. Continued investigation into the role of surfactant in the immune regulation of the lung may also provide additional information to support the efficacy of surfactant replacement in lung disease.

However meta-analysis of various trials has shown that exogenous surfactant administration has proven inconsistent as a therapeutic modality for patients with acute respiratory distress syndrome. This is because of the severity of the injury at the time of treatment and because of the variable surfactant preparations, dosing regimes, and delivery methods used in the different trials. Moreover, with the recognition that surfactant also plays an important role in host defence, the future for surfactant therapy is exciting.

In summary, the role of surfactant is well established in preterm neonates suffering from RDS and it is now a standard practice to institute prophylactic therapy. However, its use in other conditions has met with varying success and at present cannot be recommended as a standard form of treatment. Its benefit to improve host defence may find favourable indications in future.

High Frequency Ventilation (HFV)

High frequency ventilation is a form of mechanical ventilation that uses small tidal volumes, sometimes less than anatomical dead space and extremely rapid ventilatory rates. Inherent to many modes of HFV are the small pressure swings during the respiratory cycle, which allow for higher mean airway pressures than those safely achieved with CMV. This has the potential to reduce lung injury by limiting volutrauma, whereas maintaining bigger lung volumes at end-expiration may reduce atelectrauma. HFV has an ability to provide adequate gas exchange using lower proximal airway pressures in the lung already injured by barotraumas and volutrauma. It also enables preservation of normal lung architecture, even when high mean airways pressure are required. Normally efficient gas exchange depends upon adequate alveolar volumes ($V_A = V_T - V_D$). It is quite perplexing and intriguing that tidal volume as small as anatomical dead space used in HFV can provide effective gas exchange.

The increasing understanding of the pathogenesis of acute lung injury, including concepts such as volutrauma, barotraumas, oxytrauma and atelectrauma, has led to a renewed interest in the role of HFV in lung-protective ventilation strategies.

There are three types of HFV—high frequency positive pressure ventilation (HFPPV) produced by conventional or modified CMVs operating at rapid rates, high frequency jet ventilation (HFJV) ventilator that delivers high velocity jet of gas into airways and high frequency oscillatory ventilation (HFOV) produced by a device that moves gas back and forth through airway opening (10). HFJV and HFOV enhance both distribution and diffusion of gases. HFO is the only mode with an active expiration phase. This characteristic, combined with superior gas conditioning, may make HFO a promising ventilatory strategy for adults. Although a significant amount of data exists in the literature to support the application of HFO in infants and children who have acute respiratory failure, clinical data on the use of HFO in adults is only now emerging.

HFOV is a mode of ventilation that can achieve oxygenation and ventilation while maintaining maximal lung recruitment on the deflation limb of its pressure-volume curve (11). The primary theoretical advantages of HFOV over CMV in the management of acute lung injury are that HFOV allows adequate alveolar ventilation with minimal peak-trough pressure changes, provides lung recruitment, and avoids end-inspiratory overdistension of the relatively compliant nondependent lung. Taken together, the results of studies in animals, preterm and term neonates, and older paediatric patients reveal that an 'open-lung' strategy, with the goal of a high end-expiratory lung volume is safe and superior to CMV in both the short-term (rapidly improved oxygenation and/or ventilation) and longer-term (lower incidence of chronic lung disease) (11). The improved longer-term clinical outcomes on HFOV are presumably because of less ventilator-induced lung injury. As experience with HFOV in older patients grows, ventilator technology matures, and understanding of the pathophysiology of acute respiratory distress syndrome (RDS) deepens, it is likely that HFOV will find widespread use for the management of respiratory failure caused by acute lung injury in patients from preterm neonates to adults.

The full potential of HFV is yet to be realized in spite of 20 years of intensive studies. In airleak syndromes, including pulmonary interstitial emphysema and bronchopleural fistula, HFV improves outcome (11). In congenital diaphragmatic hernia or pulmonary hypoplasia, its benefits are not clear. In seemingly intractable respiratory failure, HFV can be an alternative to extra-corporeal membrane oxygenation and at least some patients would be able to avoid ECMO if HFV is first tried. In neonates with respiratory distress syndrome, earlier trials with HFV have been contradictory but later trials are encouraging, especially along with the use of surfactant (11).

Standard guidelines for use of HFV in neonates and older children are yet not available. Most clinical guidelines have been arbitrary and heavily depend upon experience, biases and at times idiosyncrasies of authors. Many different systems are in use all over the world and each HFV system is different in its functioning. There is no clear 'standard of practice'.

HFV has its own problems. As HFV is known to produce higher end-tidal volumes at lower proximal airway pressures, it can lead to an increasing auto PEEP. In many trials, pulmonary leaks increased in HFV as compared to CMV. Also, it is difficult to adjust the tidal volume so that there is neither underdistension and atelectasis of alveoli nor overdistension of alveoli (11). Close observation and repeated X-rays of the chest may be necessary to determine if the lungs are inflated to the right extent. Even so, it is difficult to monitor lung volumes at the bedside.

Due to economic constraints and select indications, we have had little experience with HFV. Outcome of preterm neonates with RDS has considerably improved with the use of surfactant. However, in our experience conventional ventilation in RDS generally suffices and the need for HFV is not commonly felt (12, 13, 14). In older children presenting with ARDS, who fail to improve on conventional ventilation strategies, the availability of HFV would perhaps make a difference.

In summary HFV looks to be an exciting and useful form of ventilation. However indication for its use is limited to a select few patients and is not yet standardized.

REFERENCES

1. Vidyasagar D, Sarnaik AP. (1985). Respiratory care in children. In: Neonatal and Pediatric Intensive Care. pp. 59–74. PSG Publishing Company Inc., Littletone, Massachusetts.
2. Cherian T, Simoes EAF, Steinhoff MC. (1990). Bronchiolitis in tropical South India. Am J Dis Child. 144, 1026–1030.
3. Udwadia FE.(1994). Tetanus. Oxford University Press, Bombay.
4. Stempel DA, Redding GJ. (1992). Management of Acute Asthma. Pediatr Clin N Am. 39, 1311–1325.
5. Vaucher YE, Harker L, Meritt TA et al. (1992). Randomized placebo-controlled trial of human surfactant. J Pediatr. 122, 125–132.
6. Poynter SE, LeVine AM. (2003). Surfactant biology and clinical application. Crit Care Clin. 19 (3), 459–472.
7. Lewis JF, Brackenbury (2003). A. Role of exogenous surfactant in acute lung injury. Crit Care Med. 31 (4 Suppl), S324–S328.
8. Merrill JD, Ballard RA. (2003). Pulmonary surfactant for neonatal respiratory disorders. Curr Opin Pediatr. 15(2), 149–154.
9. Soil RF. (2001). Use of surfactant in RDS (Cochrane review) in Cochrane library issue 2.
10. Priebe GP, Arnold JH. (2001). High-frequency oscillatory ventilation in pediatric patients. Resp Care Clin N Am.7(4), 633–645.
11. Sign JM, Stewart TE. (2002). High-frequency mechanical ventilation principles and practices in the era of lung-protective ventilation strategies. Resp Care Clin N Am. 8(2), 247–260.
12. Cools F, Offringa M. (1999). Meta-analysis of elective HFV in preterms with RDS Arch. Dis. Child Fetal Neonatal ed. 80. F15.
13. Henderson-Smart DJ, Bhuta T, Cools F, Offlinga M. (2000). Elective HFV versus conventional ventilation in acute pulmonary dysfunction in neonates. Cochrane Database Syst Rev. CD 000104.
14. Curtney SE, Durrand DJ, Asselin J et al. (2002). HFV versus conventional mechanical ventilation in low birth weight infants. N Engl J Med. 347, 643.

Fluid and Electrolyte Disturbances in the Critically Ill Child

Contributed by Dr Y.K. Amdekar, MD, DCH, Consultant Paediatrician, Breach Candy Hospital and Jaslok Hospital, Retired Honorary Professor of Paediatrics, Grant Medical College and the JJ Group of Hospitals, Mumbai.

Infants and children contain higher amounts of body water and electrolytes per kg body weight as compared to adults. Immaturity of renal function particularly in early infancy, and increased vulnerability to dehydration and electrolyte disturbances, make the management of fluid and electrolyte imbalance an integral part of paediatric intensive care.

Enteral vs Parenteral Therapy

Though the enteral route is most physiological and ideal, intravenous fluid and electrolyte administration is imperative in almost every PICU patient for a variety of reasons. In a normal preterm neonate, the GI tract needs to be rested for the first few days, till it stabilizes and starts functioning optimally. Also in every serious illness, the GI tract and the skin are always sacrificed in preference to more important vital organs, and hence the need for intravenous fluid therapy at least till the acuity of illness peaks off. Persistent vomiting, respiratory distress and risk of aspiration are additional factors necessitating intravenous therapy so as to prevent and rapidly treat significant dehydration and dyselectrolytaemia. With the advent of several devices like butterfly scalp-vein needles, intracaths, and infusion syringes and pumps, fluids can be infused in any desired composition and concentration at any given speed, at any age over any period of time. Though intravenous fluid therapy is no longer a difficult technique, it should never be taken lightly as it carries the risk of infection, thrombophlebitis, overloading and cardiac failure.

Normal Requirements (1–3)

On day one of life, a newborn needs 50 ml/kg body weight of fluids per day, increasing on every subsequent day by 10 ml/kg, to reach 100 ml/kg body weight/day by the fourth or fifth day. Till one year of age, or up to 10 kg of body weight, fluid requirements are constant at the rate of 100 ml/kg/day. Between 10 and 20 kg of weight, fluid requirements are computed at 100 ml + 50 ml/kg/day for each kg beyond 10 kg weight, and subsequently over 20 kg body weight as 1500 ml + 20 ml/kg/day for each kg body weight. Sodium and potassium are the two major electrolytes concerned with fluid therapy, though calcium and magnesium also play a role, especially in sick infants and children. A normal newborn is not able to handle electrolytes efficiently during the first 3–4 days, and should not be given supplements of sodium or potassium. Thereafter, 2–4 mEq/kg/day of both the electrolytes are sufficient as maintenance requirements, spread uniformly over 24 hours. Potassium should never be infused in a concentration > 40–60 mEq/l of fluid, even in the presence of normal renal function. Hyperosmolar solutions containing higher dextrose concentrations (> 10–12.5 per cent) are particularly harmful in small children. Similarly in neonates and young infants, the rate of the dextrose infusion should be maintained constant at 5–6 mg/kg/minute so as to avoid hypoglycaemia or hyperglycaemia.

Pathological States

Dehydration

Acute diarrhoea is the most common condition leading to dehydration in paediatric patients; other causes of dehydration include persistent vomiting, polyuria or a diminished intake. Depending on the severity of dehydration, the deficit to be replaced may amount to 50, 100 or even 150 ml/kg/day of total fluids during infancy; further ongoing losses may also have to be replenished. Based on the type of fluids lost as in diarrhoea or vomiting, the electrolyte composition of infusion fluids needs to be modified. Commercial preparations like Isolyte-P contain a balanced composition of electrolytes. If these are not available, combinations of dextrose saline with required amounts of potassium chloride and sodium bicarbonate may be administered according to the need. In the majority of infants with diarrhoea, dehydration is accompanied by hyponatraemia, hypokalaemia and metabolic acidosis, while in patients with vomiting, a hypochloremic metabolic alkalosis exists. In diabetic coma, dehydration may be accompanied by ketoacidosis, hyponatraemia and hyperkalaemia. In capillary leak syndromes as in septic shock, due to third space losses dehydration may co-exist with increased total body water.

Other Special Situations

Acute renal failure demands stringent balance between intake and output of fluids to maintain optimum fluid and electrolyte balance. In acute liver cell failure, constriction of the intravascular volume along with co-existent oedema may justify the simultaneous use of intravenous fluids and diuretics. In acute bronchiolitis, restriction of fluids due to fear of worsening the pulmonary oedema is no longer justified, as multiple variable factors are known to increase the fluid requirements in such cases. The same principle holds true in patients with acute brain cell oedema where better monitoring in individual patients should decide the actual fluid requirements, rather than routinely restricting fluids to two-thirds the normal maintenance levels. A case of burns is a special situation needing large amounts of fluid replacement, including colloids.

Significant electrolyte disturbances often accompany states of dehydration as well as oedema. Clinical judgement of dyselectrolytaemia is usually difficult and must be supplemented by biochemical and biophysical monitoring. Serum levels of sodium and potassium should be considered in conjunction with the acid-base status, total body electrolyte content, urinary electrolyte concentrations, electrocardiographic and neuropsychological states. As water and electrolytes are in dynamic equilibrium, correction of one element may precipitate changes in the other, and demands careful handling. Swings from undercorrection to overcorrection are difficult to assess and are harmful to the patient. Daily biochemical monitoring is the only guide in optimum management especially in complex situations.

REFERENCES

1. Singer GG, Brenner BM. (2001). Fluid and Electrolyte Disturbances. In: Harrison's Principles of Internal Medicine, 15th edn (Eds Braunwald E, Fauci AS, Kasper DL, Hauser SL, Longo DL, Jameson JL). pp. 271–283. McGraw-Hill, USA.

2. Schrier RW. (1992). Fluid and Electrolyte Disorders, 4th edn. Little, Brown and Company, Boston.

3. Narins RG. (1982). Diagnostic strategies in disorders of fluid and electrolyte hemostasis. Am J Med. 72, 496.

CHAPTER 23.8

Nutritional Support in the Paediatric Intensive Care Unit

Contributed by Dr Y.K. Amdekar, MD, DCH, Consultant Paediatrician, Breach Candy Hospital and Jaslok Hospital, Retired Honorary Professor of Paediatrics, Grant Medical College and the JJ Group of Hospitals, Mumbai.

Nutritional failure is a serious problem especially in patients suffering from subacute or chronic illnesses and also in acute conditions in the younger age group (1–3). Newborns or young infants may suffer from significant nutritional depletion within 4–7 days of lack of feeding, and ideally need nutritional support to avoid deleterious effects. Nutritional failure may lead to delayed recovery from infection, and wound healing is slow due to impaired immune mechanisms. Prolonged nutritional depletion results in malnutrition with decrease in muscle mass and easy fatiguability. This may interfere with normal respiratory effort and cause difficulty in weaning the patient off the ventilator. In addition to a lack of nutritional intake, critically ill children also have increased caloric needs due to catabolic stress. Thus the goal of nutritional support is to achieve a positive nitrogen balance. This is done by giving 100–120 calories/day and 2–3 g/kg/day of proteins.

The enteral route is always preferred because of ease of administration. It helps to maintain the normal physiological processes of digestion and absorption as it stimulates the gut hormones and enzymes. Also it is safe, cheap, effective, and does not need any monitoring. Milk enriched with oil (preferably coconut oil), egg-flips or commercial formulae may be administered through the nasogastric tube, or other semisolids may be fed with a spoon. Necessary supplements of vitamins and minerals as well as extra proteins can be easily supplied through available market preparations.

However, when enteral feeding is not possible or contraindicated, one has to resort to parenteral feeding (especially if enteral feeding is not possible for > 4–5 days). The main indications for parenteral alimentation include extremely premature babies (very low birth weight—VLBW), after major surgical procedures, in post-traumatic conditions, burns, severe gastrointestinal disorders, disseminated infections and multiorgan failure. Total parenteral nutrition (TPN) should be administered ideally by infusions through a central vein and should consist of adequate calories optimally derived from carbohydrates, proteins and fats. Minerals and vitamins should always be supplied. 55–60 per cent of calories must be supplied from carbohydrates, 30–35 per cent from fats and 5–10 per cent from proteins. Peripheral venous access can also be conveniently used, in which case a concentration of not more than 10–12.5 per cent dextrose solution can be given. In such a situation, fats may be infused in slightly higher amounts to make up for the calories. Proteins are supplied in the form of amino acid mixtures, while fats are provided as intralipids containing adequate essential fatty acids. Commercial solutions for parenteral nutritional are freely available, and are administered through a three-way connection so that infusions of amino acids, intralipids and dextrose are administered separately and get combined at the vein entrance. In infants and children, we preferably use a peripheral venous access. Routine protocol consists of dextrose infusions for the first 3–4 days, followed by additional amino-acid mixtures over the next 3–4 days; intralipids are added at a later stage if enteral feeding is still not possible.

Catheter-related complications are rare when a peripheral vein is used. However infection and sepsis are the most commonly encountered problems. Other complications include hepatic dysfunction and cholestasis, metabolic acidosis, disturbed glucose metabolism, hyperammonaemia and fat overload. Vitamin and mineral deficiencies are easily prevented by proper supplementation. Repeated biochemical monitoring is mandatory, and includes daily serum electrolyte estimations, blood glucose, acid-base status, urine examination, frequent liver function tests and other relevant haematological parameters.

Clinical experience with total parenteral nutrition has shown that when used in selected situations, it has improved survival rates in paediatric ICU patients. However TPN is costly, technically difficult and needs careful monitoring. The cost-risk-benefit ratio should always be considered before starting on this form of nutritional support.

REFERENCES

1. Pollack MM, Willey JS, Holbook DR. (1981). Early nutritional depletion in critically ill children. Crit Care Med. 9, 580.

2. Lee B Chang, Jacobs S. (1990). Intermittent nasogastric feeding. Intensive Care Med. 16, 100–103.

3. McLaren DS, David Burman (Eds). (1982). Textbook of Pediatric Nutrition, 2nd edn. Churchill Livingstone, London.

Paediatric Life-threatening Infections Requiring Critical Care

Contributed by Dr Y.K. Amdekar, MD, DCH, Consultant Paediatrician, Breach Candy Hospital and Jaslok Hospital, Retired Honorary Professor of Paediatrics, Grant Medical College and the JJ Group of Hospitals, Mumbai.

Infections are common in an ICU setting. It has been observed that 30–40 per cent of paediatric admissions to the ICU are related to community-acquired infections. A number of other admissions in the paediatric age group are likely to develop infections due to a variety of adverse background factors e.g. specific organ dysfunction, trauma or surgery. Infections pose a constant threat to life, despite proper treatment with antimicrobial drugs. Prevention, early diagnosis, and prompt treatment of existing infections, are important challenges faced in the management of paediatric ICU patients (1–2).

Several factors contribute to the increased vulnerability to life-threatening infections in the ICU. Younger age itself makes a paediatric patient more susceptible to serious infections, as newborns and infants are physiologically more deficient in natural defence mechanisms. Malnutrition (3), especially when induced by lactation failure, promotes easy access to infection, with quick dissemination of infection, with an increased morbidity and mortality. Developmental defects and anatomical malformations are additional risk factors. Immune deficiency disorders (4), either congenital or acquired (as in malignancy or in patients on steroid therapy), are also occasionally responsible for infection in the paediatric age group. Children with ventriculoperitoneal shunts or prosthetic valves, and patients with severe burns, are particularly vulnerable to serious infections. Nosocomial infections are difficult to prevent in an ICU setting, especially in patients on ventilators with central lines and other invasive interventions.

The site of infection and host responses to various types of microbial invasions, decide the outcome of infections. Intracranial infections like encephalitis and meningitis, fulminant pneumonias, endomyocarditis and necrotizing enterocolitis may lead to specific organ failure, endangering life. On the other hand, any infection may induce severe immune-mediated responses in the host and may threaten life, as is seen in septic shock, staphylococcal or streptococcal toxic shock syndrome and staphylococcal scalded skin syndrome.

Aetiology

A majority of serious infections are bacterial—both Gram-positive and Gram-negative. Staphylococcal infections and infections due to Ps. aeruginosa, Klebsiella and Proteus can often turn fulminant and life-threatening. Many other infections in the paediatric age group may require critical care, particularly in vulnerable situations. Tuberculous meningo-encephalitis and miliary tuberculosis pose a significant threat to life, especially in infants. It is feared that tuberculosis in HIV infected individuals will constitute a significant proportion of life-threatening infections in the near future.

Viruses also cause life-threatening infections—though not as commonly as bacterial infections. It is difficult to prove viral infections due to constraints of relevant laboratory facilities, though in clinical practice, some of the viral infections can be diagnosed by characteristic clinical findings. These include measles, poliomyelitis, and infections due to the herpes virus. Measles encephalitis or pneumonia, poliomyelitis affecting the brainstem or causing weakness of the respiratory muscles, herpes encephalitis, and viral myocarditis constitute life-threatening infections in children. Dengue fever and Japanese B viral encephalitis deserve special mention, as they occur in some parts of our country, and are associated with a significant morbidity and mortality.

Parasitic infections are rarely life-threatening though with a resurgence of malaria, cerebral malaria due to Pl. falciparum infections is a distinct threat to life. Fungal sepsis is being recognized in patients treated with prolonged antibiotic therapy. In immunocompromised patients, other opportunistic infections such as those due to Pneumocystis carinii, Toxoplasma and Cytomegalovirus may endanger life. Anaerobic bacterial infections may cause serious disease in certain situations.

Clinical Approach

It is the high index of suspicion based on clinical experience, evaluation of host factors, and knowledge of epidemiology, that may lead to an early diagnosis. Newborns and infants may demonstrate a wide spectrum of clinical presentations, some often vague without localization. Refusal of feeds, lethargy, temperature instability, behaviour disturbances, disproportionate tachypnoea and tachycardia, widened core skin temperature difference, mottling of skin, prolonged capillary refill, are some of the symptoms and signs suggesting serious infections. Localizing symptoms and signs of meningitis or pneumonia offer easy clues to the diagnosis and demand close monitoring of specific organ functions.

Investigations

Non-specific tests like the blood count, acute phase reactants like the erythrocyte sedimentation rate and C-Reactive Protein, routine urine analysis, spinal tap, chest X-ray may support a diagnosis of infections. Though any acute infection may present with neutrophilic leucocytosis with a shift to the left and eosinopaenia, newborns often react with leucopaenia. In fact a normal blood count does not rule out the possibility of infection. Anaemia and thrombocytopaenia may favour a diagnosis of malaria. Low platelet counts may suggest disseminated intravascular coagulopathy, which may be confirmed by raised levels of fibrin degradation products, and a decrease in coagulation factors. Abnormal CSF may denote intracranial infection, though at times in children, it is difficult to differentiate partially treated bacterial meningitis from tuberculous meningitis.

Specific diagnosis rests on demonstration of organisms on smear, or culture of blood, CSF, urine, stools, or any other body fluids. Pretreatment with antibiotics, and poor techniques including a risk of contamination, makes the diagnosis of bacterial infection difficult. Often, the clinician has to resort to a presumptive diagnosis of infection based on circumstantial evidence. Special techniques are required to culture viruses and other organisms. Detection of antigen by rapid immunological methods, as well as demonstration of antibodies, are suitable alternatives, though often not easily available. Interpretation of antibody levels against specific infections needs to be considered against the background of local epidemiology. Other tests are required to monitor specific organ functions, and include various non-invasive or invasive interventions.

Management

Specific treatment with chemotherapeutic agents or antibiotics whenever available, forms the mainstay of curative management. Obviously, the choice of such a therapy depends upon a precise diagnosis of the infection. As this is often not feasible, empirical treatment is started based on clinical judgment of specific situations. For example, newborns and young infants are covered with a broad-spectrum combination of penicillin and an aminoglycoside (ampicillin + gentamicin). Nosocomial infections may often need newer antibiotics so as to take care of resistant strains of Staphylococci, Pseudomonas, and other organisms. Immunocompromised hosts may justify antifungal, antiviral or antiparasitic drugs in addition to antibacterial agents.

Supportive management includes maintenance of fluid, electrolyte and acid-base balance, adequate ventilation and oxygenation, maintenance of optimum cardiac output and circulatory state, and homeostasis of other organ functions. In addition, newborns and sick children need an isothermal environment, specially in centrally airconditioned units, where special heating devices like radiant warmers are necessary. In special circumstances, even intravenous infusions and humidified oxygen may have to be warmed, as in newborns cold injury is often lethal. Adequate

nutrition and a positive nitrogen balance are desirable, and are important, particularly in the long-term management of such patients. Though enteral feeding is the first choice, in conditions where enteral feeds are contraindicated or not tolerated, one may have to resort to total or partial parenteral nutrition.

Having realized that outcome of infection is decided by immunological response of the host, induced by interactions with the organism, immune response modifiers have been tried. These include steroids, NSAIDS, interferons, growth factors, intravenous immunoglobulins, monoclonal antibodies, and naloxone. Transfusion of blood and its components, as well as exchange transfusions have also been tried. All these measures have given equivocal results and many of them are costly, rarely available in developing countries, and may produce considerable side effects. With the exception of a few agents, most of them cannot be advocated for routine use.

Prevention

Early diagnosis and prompt treatment of trivial infections often prevent life-threatening infections. Vaccine-preventable diseases are easily controlled by proper immunization. Hand-washing, proper asepsis and use of disposables go a long way in preventing nosocomial infections. ICUs should formulate specific policies regarding entry of staff and visitors, isolation of patients, disposal of patients' excreta and infected secretions, general cleanliness, fumigation, sterilization of equipments, bacteriological surveillance, and antibiotic usage. All such infection control measures should be monitored by specially designated staff guided by an infection control committee, comprising clinical and laboratory experts. Prophylactic antibiotics are best avoided in general, as they may often lead to infections by resistant strains of organisms. In certain situations, post-operative antibiotic prophylaxis may be used for one or two doses.

Special Infections

CNS Infections

Meningococcaemia with or without meningitis, is a life-threatening disease. Acute onset of fever followed by purpuric spots offers a clue to the probable aetiology. Meningococcaemia without meningitis carries a poor prognosis, death resulting from adrenal failure and shock. Development of meningitis denotes ability to localize the disease, and has a better prognosis. Early diagnosis and prompt treatment with penicillin is mandatory for survival.

Other bacteria causing meningitis have many features in common. Risk factors include younger age, marked change in sensorium, focal neurological abnormalities, persistent increase in intracranial tension, and gross CSF abnormalities. Besides proper antibiotic therapy (**Table 23.9.1**), control of increased intracranial tension and seizures is important. Early administration of steroids (5) before administration of the first dose of antibiotic, has been shown to be beneficial in minimizing the sequelae, specially in H. influenzae and pneumococcal meningitis. Cerebral oedema in tuberculous meningitis requires prompt control with mannitol (2 g/kg/day in 4–6 divided doses), and steroids (hydrocortisone 10 mg/kg/day). Hydrocephalus should be treated by a timely ventriculoperitoneal shunt. Ideally, patients suffering from meningitis should undergo continuous monitoring of intracranial pressure; this however is not possible in most of the institutions in our country.

Cerebral malaria is an immune-mediated disseminated vasculitis occurring as a result of Pl. falciparum infection. Diagnosis is difficult unless blood smears demonstrate parasites. In many situations clinical suspicion may justify therapy with quinine (25 mg/kg/day). Mortality is high unless promptly treated early in the course of the disease.

Herpes encephalitis may be considered in the presence of xanthochromic CSF and localized temporal lesions, as evidenced by an EEG or a CT scan. Early institution of therapy with acyclovir (25 mg/kg/day) is life-saving.

Toxic Shock Syndrome (TSS) (6)

Though most of the superficial infections of skin and soft tissue are benign, a few toxin-producing strains of Staphylococci and Streptococci may lead to a fulminant infection with the development of shock. Such infections often follow trauma or surgical procedures. If not recognized early, they may be fatal.

Staphylococcal Scalded Skin Syndrome (SSSS) (7)

This syndrome is seen primarily in younger children; at times epidemics in newborn nurseries have been reported. It is a toxin-mediated disease, characterized by skin lesions which vary from bullous impetigo to widespread exfoliative dermatitis. Early recognition and treatment are mandatory for survival.

Septic Shock (8)

Cardiac output is manipulated in children mainly by altering the heart rate, and not by significant changes in the stroke volume. There is therefore limited ability to maintain cardiac output in adverse situations, often resulting in early decompensation in shock. Thus progression from sepsis to severe sepsis, and thence to septic shock and multiple organ dysfunction, occurs rather rapidly in children. Recognition of early sepsis and of the reversible stage of shock, assumes added importance in proper management. Apart from this, the pathogenesis and management of septic shock in children is similar to that in adults.

Infections in the Immunocompromised and Critically Ill Children

These differ not only in aetiology but also in clinical presentation. Many of these children have serious infections without any fever. Clinical symptoms, signs, and progression vary a great deal, and aggressive treatment is mandatory in these individuals.

Any infection in newborns and infants must be viewed as a potentially life-threatening one; the distinction between mild or trivial and life-threatening infections however is not easy, and calls for sound clinical judgment.

Table 23.9.1 details the empiric treatment of acute fulminant paediatric infections, and lists the important drugs, their dosages, and the common organisms encountered in life-threatening paediatric infections.

Table 23.9.1. Empiric antibiotic therapy in paediatric life-threatening infections

Age	Suspected organism		Antibiotic	IV Dose
1. Bacterial Infections				
Birth to 3 months	Gram +ve	– Staphylococci – Streptococci	Ampicillin +	200 mg/kg/day
		– Listeria	Gentamicin or	7.5 mg/kg/day
	Gram –ve	– E. coli – Klebsiella	Ampicillin +	200 mg/kg/day
		– Pseudomonas	Ceftazidime	200 mg/kg/day
3 months to 5 years	Gram +ve	– Staphylococci – Streptococci	Ampicillin and/or	200 mg/kg/day
	Gram –ve	– H. influenzae	Chloramphenicol	100 mg/kg/day
		– Klebsiella – Pseudomonas	+ Ceftazidime	200 mg/kg/day
> 5 years	Gram +ve	– Staphylococci – Strep. pneumoniae	Ampicillin and/or	200 mg/kg/day
	Gram –ve	– H. influenzae – Meningococci	Chloramphenicol	100 mg/kg/day
			+ Ceftriaxone	200 mg/kg/day

Comments: Therapy is later modified as per bacteriological reports. Other antibiotics which can be used are amikacin 15 mg/kg/day, and vancomycin 30 mg/kg/day.

2. Other Organisms				
All Ages		Herpes virus	Acyclovir	25 mg/kg/day
		Pl. falciparum	Quinine	25 mg/kg/day
		Fungal infections	Fluconazole	5 mg/kg/day

REFERENCES

1. Miller MK, Pan JSC. (1989). Life-threatening infections in the newborn. In: Textbook of Critical Care, 2nd edn (Eds Shoemaker WC, Ayres S, Grenvik A, Holbrook PR, Leigh Thompson W). pp. 817–825. WB Saunders Company, Philadelphia, London, Sydney, Tokyo.

2. Kanter RK, Weiner LB. (1989). Pediatric life-threatening infections. In: Textbook of Critical Care, 2nd edn (Eds Shoemaker WC, Ayres S, Grenvik A, Holbrook PR, Leigh Thompson W). pp. 825–830. WB Saunders Company, Philadelphia, London, Sydney, Tokyo.

3. Aref GH, Osman MZ, Zaki A et al. (1992). Clinical and radiologic study of the frequency of presentation of chest infections in children with severe protein-energy malnutrition. J Egypt Public Health Assoc. 67(5–6), 655–673.

4. Hughes WT. (1993). Prevention of infections in patients with T-cell defects. Clin Infect Dis. Nov 17, suppl 2, 9368–9371.

5. Kennedy WA, Hout MJ, McCracken GH Jr. (1991). Role of corticosteroid therapy in children with pneumococcal meningitis. Am J Dis Child. 145(12), 1374–1378.

6. Strausbaugh LJ. (1993). Toxic Shock Syndrome—Are you recognising its changing presentation? Postgrad Med. 94(6), 107–108.

7. Resnick SD. (1992). Staphylococcal toxic shock syndromes in children. Intensive Care Med. 18(3), 175–176.

8. Hazinski MF, Iberti TJ, MacIntyre NR et al. (1993). Epidemiology, pathophysiology and clinical presentation of gram-negative sepsis. Am J Crit Care. 2(3), 224–235.

CHAPTER 23.10

Acute Renal Failure in Infants and Children

Dr B.V. Gandhi MBBS, Diplomate American Board of Medicine and Nephrology. Consultant Nephrologist, Breach Candy Hospital, Jaslok Hospital, Mumbai.

Acute renal failure (ARF) is defined as an abrupt decline in the renal regulation of water, electrolytes, and acid-base balance of sufficient magnitude to result in the retention of nitrogenous waste products. Acute renal failure is potentially fatal, but may be often reversible if promptly diagnosed and treated (1).

There are two types of ARF—(a) Oliguric Renal Failure and (b) Nonoliguric or High Output Renal Failure (2). Nowadays we see an increasing number of cases of nonoliguric renal failure. These are chiefly due to the use of nephrotoxic drugs (mainly aminoglycosides and non-steroidal anti-inflammatory drugs [NSAIDs]), loop diuretics and/or inotropes e.g. dopamine.

Oliguria is defined as urine output below 0.5 ml/kg/hr or less than 300 ml/m^2/day.

ARF in Newborns and Infants

All premature and full term infants void within the first 24 hrs after birth. If an infant does not void in 24 hours, a search should be initiated for underlying anatomic abnormalities. The common causes of ARF in infants are renal dysgenesis, obstructive uropathy, renovascular accidents, congenital heart disease, dehydration, sepsis, anoxia, and renal vein thrombosis. **Table 23.10.1** lists the main causes of ARF in infants.

The ultimate prognosis depends upon the cause and treatment available. Peritoneal dialysis can be done in infants; acute and even chronic renal failure (CRF) can be treated with CAPD catheters. This is however difficult, and chances of long-term survival are less in patients with CRF.

Table 23.10.1. Common causes of acute renal failure in infants

* Renal dysgenesis
* Obstructive uropathy
* Renovascular accidents
* Congenital heart disease
* Dehydration
* Sepsis, hypoxia
* Renal vein thrombosis

ARF in Paediatric Patients

Common causes of ARF in the paediatric population are vomiting, diarrhoea, sepsis, G6PD deficiency with haemolysis, malaria,

haemolytic uraemic syndrome, and certain types of nephritis. Obstructive uropathy is common in both infants and in the paediatric group of patients. Common causes of obstructive uropathy are posterior urethral valves, bilateral pelviureteric junction obstruction, and severe forms of vesicoureteric reflux. The main causes of acute renal failure in older children can be classified as prerenal, renal and postrenal and are listed in **Table 23.10.2**.

Table 23.10.2. Common causes of acute renal failure in children

1. Prerenal Causes
* Hypovolaemia
* Hypotension
* Hypoxia

2. Renal Causes
* Glomerulonephritis
* Renal vein thrombosis
* Acute tubular necrosis
* Acute interstitial nephritis
* Hereditary nephritis

3. Postrenal Causes
* Obstructive nephropathy
* Vesicoureteric reflux
* Calculi

In the majority of patients with ARF, the common causes are mainly extrarenal; renal causes are responsible for ARF in only a few patients.

Prerenal causes of ARF produce decreased renal circulation due to hypovolaemia. Diminished blood volume leads to a fall in cardiac output and decrease in glomerular filtration rate. If this condition is detected in time and treated promptly, the patient recovers quickly as kidney damage is not present in early stages. If hypotension persists for a longer time, damage to renal parenchyma occurs producing acute tubular necrosis.

Clinical Features

The clinical features are usually related to the precipitating disease. The signs and symptoms related to renal failure are oliguria, oedema, hypertension, pallor, nausea, vomiting and lethargy. At a later stage the patient may present with mental obtundation progressing to coma due to hypertensive encephalopathy or uraemia; gastrointestinal bleeding is often observed.

Diagnosis

A careful history will aid in the diagnosis in a majority of patients. Vomiting, diarrhoea and fever suggest dehydration. At times these symptoms may be present in a patient with HUS (Haemolytic Uraemic Syndrome) or renal vein thrombosis. A history of a throat or skin infection will suggest the diagnosis of post-streptococcal glomerulonephritis. History of exposure to drugs (antibiotics, analgesics or other forms of therapy) may suggest interstitial nephritis due to drugs. Presence of a mass in the renal area may suggest diagnosis of renal vein thrombosis or tumour. Presence of rash, purpuric spots, with history of arthralgia or fever may suggest the diagnosis of Henoch-Schonlein purpura or systemic lupus erythematosus (SLE).

Laboratory Investigations

Urine Examination is of utmost value in cases of renal failure. Presence of proteinuria and haematuria with red blood cell casts point to a glomerulonephritis, while urine with a large number of pus cells indicates urinary tract infection. The urine may be normal in acute tubular necrosis and in obstructive uropathy.

Urinary indices are of utmost importance in deciding whether renal failure is prerenal or renal in origin. A low urinary sodium (< 10 mEq/l), FE sodium (< 1), and a high urinary osmolality go in favour of prerenal failure. The urinary indices which help to distinguish between prerenal and renal causes of ARF are listed in **Table 23.10.3**.

Table 23.10.3. Urinary indices which distinguish between prerenal and renal causes of acute renal failure

	Prerenal	Renal
Urinary Na (mEq/l)	< 10	> 50
Fractional Excretion of Na (%)	< 1	> 2
Urine Osmolality (mOsm/kg H_2O)	> 500	< 300
Urine/Plasma Osmolality	> 1.5	< 1.2
BUN/Creatinine	> 20	20 or less

Other Tests. All patients with ARF usually have anaemia (mild to moderate) with a raised BUN and serum creatinine. Anaemia may be due to haemolysis, bone marrow depression due to lack of erythropoietin or blood loss. Presence of leucopaenia may be suggestive of SLE or severe septicaemia. Thrombocytopaenia may indicate diagnosis of septicaemia, HUS or SLE. Hyponatraemia (most likely dilutional) and hyperkalaemia with acidosis is common in patients with advanced renal failure. Positive ANA and anti-DNA tests with diminished complement levels will be present in cases of SLE. The ASO titer is raised in cases of post-streptococcal glomerulonephritis.

Radiology

Cardiomegaly may be noted on chest X-ray due to overhydration and hypertension.

Ultrasonography of the kidneys and bladder is of great help in establishing the aetiology in ARF. It is mandatory to do this investigation to rule out any correctable pathology. In selected patients, a micturating cystourethrogram may be done to rule out vesicoureteric reflux. Renal biopsy may be necessary in a few cases of non-resolving acute glomerulonephritis (to rule out rapidly proliferative glomerulonephritis [RPGN]).

Management

The treatment of ARF is as follows:

1. Assess the circulatory volume by careful physical examination—dry skin and mucus membranes with associated tachycardia suggest dehydration, while peripheral oedema with gallop rhythm, hepatomegaly, bilateral crepitations and hypertension, point to fluid overload. In doubtful cases it may be advisable to insert a central venous catheter for accurate assessment of central venous pressure.

2. In cases of suspected hypovolaemia, give a fluid challenge—10 to 20 ml/kg of normal saline.

3. Avoid use of diuretics and vasopressor agents till hypovolaemia is corrected.

4. If there is adequate response with fluid challenge continue fluid replacement under close medical supervision.

5. If response to fluid challenge is inadequate, as judged by the urine output, do not give more fluids as the patient may have developed acute tubular necrosis. Excess fluid may produce overhydration, hypertension and congestive cardiac failure.

6. A trial of diuretics is given after correction of hypovolaemia—furosemide 1 mg/kg is given intravenously and the response is noted. If the response is poor give a higher dose (up to 10 mg/kg), and this may be repeated every 6–8 hours.

7. A high dose of furosemide helps in converting oliguric renal failure to nonoliguric renal failure. This helps in clinical management as hyperkalaemia and hypervolaemia are less likely to occur in patients with nonoliguric renal failure.

8. Low dose of dopamine (1–2.5 µg/kg) also helps in improving the renal circulation and urine output.

9. Hyperkalaemia should be promptly corrected (3) (**Table 23.10.4**).

Table 23.10.4. Emergency treatment of hyperkalaemia

Drugs	Dose	Onset of Action	Duration of Action
* Calcium gluconate	0.5 ml/kg over 5–10 mins, slowly	Within minutes	30–60 mins
* Sodium bicarbonate	1–2 mEq/kg over 15–30 mins	Within minutes	1–2 hrs
* Dextrose with insulin	0.5–1 g/kg dextrose with 0.1–0.2 units insulin/kg slowly	Within minutes	2–4 hrs
* Kayexalate	1 g/kg in 70% sorbitol orally, or in 30% sorbitol as a retention enema	30 minutes	4–6 hrs

Management of Established Renal Failure

Management of acute tubular necrosis (a common and important pathology), is briefly described below. It aptly illustrates the basic principles of treatment in established acute renal failure.

Good conservative therapy will go a long way in preventing complications and avoiding or postponing the need for dialysis. Most of these patients have oliguric renal failure and usually do not respond to volume load and the use of furosemide as described above. These patients should then be treated as follows:

1. Thorough daily physical examination.

2. Maintenance of accurate intake and output charts (record output from all sources), with record of daily weight.

3. Daily laboratory investigations—HB, PCV, BUN, serum creatinine, serum electrolytes, arterial pH and arterial blood gases; chest X-ray for cardiac size and evidence of pulmonary congestion.

4. Intake to be restricted as per output + 400 ml/m^2/day.

5. Pay particular attention to serum potassium and avoid fruits, fruit juices, coconut water, dry fruits, chocolates, soups, and soft drinks to prevent hyperkalaemia.

The treatment of hyperkalaemia (3) is given in **Table 23.10.4**.

6. Replace sodium as needed.

7. Use diuretics and a dopamine drip (2 μg/kg) for its dopaminergic effect.

8. Avoid an indwelling catheter unless patient is unconscious, as a catheter is a potential source of infection.

9. Maintain nutrition giving sufficient calories with a high carbohydrate and low protein (0.5 to 0.7 g/kg) diet.

10. Antibiotics are administered if needed. Avoid nephrotoxic drugs as far as possible. If they have to be used, give in appropriate dosages, preferably monitoring blood levels.

11. Use sodium bicarbonate to counter acidosis.

12. Control hypertension. For severe hypertension administer diazoxide, hydralazine, or a calcium-channel blocker sublingually. In patients with mild to moderate hypertension use beta-blockers or alpha-methyldopa together with a diuretic.

Dialysis

Even with good conservative therapy some patients will require dialysis. Dialysis may be either peritoneal dialysis, haemodialysis or continuous arteriovenous haemofiltration (CAVH).

Peritoneal dialysis is safest but cannot be done in patients with recent abdominal surgery, hypercatabolic patients, or in patients with severe respiratory distress.

Haemodialysis requires vascular access and the availability of a dialysis machine with trained staff. It also requires use of heparin. Even minimal use of heparin can produce bleeding and hypotension in some patients. Patients with cardiac instability do not tolerate this form of dialysis.

Critically ill patients in a catabolic state or even severely overhydrated patients may be treated with CAVH (Continuous Arteriovenous Haemofiltration) or CAVHD (Continuous Arteriovenous Haemodiafiltration). This form of dialysis is life saving in critically ill patients and can be done in an ICU setting when it is difficult to transfer the patient to the dialysis unit. However it requires expert technical know-how and a good ICU set-up. Fluid removal to the extent of 100 to 300 ml or more per hour may be possible and may require large fluid replacement with close monitoring of patients. It also requires use of heparin in large dosages and may therefore produce bleeding. Patients with prolonged

oliguria, and those who require hyperalimentation are ideal candidates for CAVH or CAVHD.

Indications for dialysis are as follows:

1. Gross overhydration.

2. Intractable hyperkalaemia.

3. Severe acidosis.

4. Signs and symptoms of uraemia.

5. Severe prolonged oliguria during which period hyperalimentation is necessary to maintain an adequate caloric intake.

Renal Replacement Therapy (RRT)

In Neonates

RRT in neonates has a high morbidity and mortality during acute and chronic treatment phase.

In general RRT is only indicated if aggressive symptomatic treatment fails to manage life-threatening conditions such as hyperkalaemia, fluid overload, severe acidosis or hypertension. Peritoneal dialysis (PD) or continuous arteriovenous haemofiltration (CAVH) or venovenous haemofiltration (CVVH) have been done in small series of patients.

PD is the method of choice because of its simplicity, easy availability, effectiveness and relative safety in any age group including low birth weight neonates and infants. CAVHD and CVVHD is the treatment of choice in patients with very significant fluid overload and in refractory acidosis as well as severe catabolic renal failure. This mode of therapy requires an expensive machine with a special haemofiltration cartridge as well as tubing for neonates. The risk of hypotension and bleeding is very high. This should be done in very well experienced units only. However, many ethical and medical problems have to be considered in decision-making.

In Paediatric Patients

RRT becomes mandatory when conservative treatment fails and the child develops signs and symptoms of uraemia, fluid overload, hyperkalaemia, electrolyte imbalance or severe refractory acidosis.

Three modalities of therapy are available—peritoneal dialysis (PD), haemodialysis (HD) or continuous arteriovenous or venovenous haemofiltration (CAVH or CVVH).

Peritoneal Dialysis

It is relatively easy to perform and can be done with availability of paediatric size PD catheter and PD fluid. It is safe and easily tolerated by most patients including very small patients; hypovolaemia or hypotension are less likely to occur with this procedure compared to HD or CAVHD/CVVHD. However, fluid removal is limited in patients with hypotension; abdominal distension with respiratory embarrassment and a high risk of infection are likely.

Haemodialysis

HD is very effective in treating hyperkalaemia, acidosis and fluid overload. HD requires availability of HD machines along with special haemodialysis cartridges and very well trained staff as children tend to develop hypotension easily.

CAVH/CAVHD

Easy to do and does not require any special continuous renal replacement therapy (CRRT) machine. The main disadvantages are the need for good arterial access (femoral) and continuous anticoagulation with heparin. It is difficult in patients with hypotension.

CVVH/CVVHD

This is very good for catabolic patients and patients who require removal of large amounts of fluid. However, this modality requires access to a CRRT machine, special haemofiltration cartridge, patient immobilization and anticoagulation.

Recovering Phase of Renal Failure

A patient may remain in the oliguric phase for three days to three weeks, and at times even longer. After this the patient passes into the diuretic phase. In the diuretic phase, the patient starts passing large quantities of urine; close monitoring of fluids and electrolytes is mandatory as these patients may get dehydrated and/or have severe electrolyte imbalance. This phase lasts for a few days. The commonest error committed by the physician during the management of this phase, is chasing the urine output for a prolonged period. The urine output should be chased (intake increased as per urine output) for the first 2–3 days; subsequently the intake should be gradually decreased over the next 2–3 days. The electrolytes should be carefully monitored, as hyponatraemia and hypokalaemia are frequently observed.

ARF due to Other Aetiologies

(i) Post-Streptococcal Glomerulonephritis

Post-streptococcal glomerulonephritis causes oliguria with haematuria. These patients should be treated with fluid and salt restriction and a low protein diet. Potassium should be restricted (avoid coconut water and fruit juices), and hypertension controlled with either nifedipine or alpha-methyl dopa and furosemide. Steroids are contraindicated, and long-term penicillin therapy is not necessary. The majority of patients recover within 7 days; a few patients however may require dialysis. The common indications for dialysis are overhydration, acute left ventricular failure due to severe hypertension and/or overhydration, hyperkalaemia and uraemia.

(ii) Rapidly Proliferative Glomerulonephritis (RPGN)

These patients present with rising BUN and serum creatinine levels.

They may be wrongly diagnosed as acute post-streptococcal glomerulonephritis. However, as mentioned earlier, cases of post-streptococcal glomerulonephritis resolve within a few days time. In the event of such cases not resolving within this period, a renal biopsy is mandatory for arriving at a correct diagnosis and instituting early treatment.

Common causes of RPGN are Goodpasture's syndrome (kidney and lung involvement), systemic lupus erythematosus, and vasculitis. The following tests should be done prior to performing a renal biopsy—ANA, anti-DNA, anti-GBM antibodies, and anti-cytoplasmic antibody (ANCA), along with complement levels. The ultimate diagnosis however depends upon a renal biopsy; this shows crescentic glomerulonephritis—cellular crescents along with linear IGG antibodies along the capillary walls in Goodpasture's syndrome. Dialysis may be required before doing a renal biopsy.

Once a diagnosis of RPGN (crescentic glomerulonephritis) is established by a renal biopsy, patients require aggressive therapy with pulsed doses of methylprednisolone sodium succinate (15–20 mg/kg) for 3 days followed by oral prednisolone (1 mg/kg), along with immunosuppressive therapy (cyclophosphamide or azathioprine 2 to 3 mg/kg/day). The patient should be closely monitored, and the dose of the immunosuppressant adjusted weekly depending on the WBC count. In severe cases plasma exchange may be required.

The patient's diet and fluid intake should also be supervised; antihypertensive therapy as well as antibotic therapy may be necessary. Patients usually need to be treated for long periods; a few patients will however progress to end-stage renal failure despite all measures, and will need a renal transplant.

(iii) Systemic Lupus Erythematosus

This condition is relatively uncommon in very young patients. The patient may present with fever, arthralgia and skin rash along with renal involvement, which may progress from azotaemia to frank renal failure. Positive ANA and anti-DNA tests, together with diminished complement levels of C_3 and C_4 confirm the diagnosis. A renal biopsy may be indicated if the patient presents with renal failure or the nephrotic syndrome, in order to establish the type of nephropathy.

Treatment is with prednisolone (initially in high doses of 1–2 mg/kg/day), followed by a maintenance dose of 10–20 mg on alternate days for a few months. There may be an acute exacerbation even while the patient is on treatment. Acutely ill patients, and patients who require high doses of steroids for maintaining remissions, may require the addition of immunosuppressants.

(iv) Henoch-Schonlein Purpura

This disease is characterized by non-thrombocytopaenic purpura, arthralgia, abdominal pain and glomerulonephritis (haematuria and proteinuria). Henoch-Schonlein purpura may be mistaken for acute post-infection glomerulonephritis.

A renal biopsy shows variable features and IGA levels may be raised in 50 per cent of patients. The disease usually runs a benign course, though progressive renal failure may occur in a few patients. Treatment is symptomatic; there is no definite evidence that either steroids or immunosuppressive agents are beneficial.

REFERENCES

1. Maxiscalco MM. (1994). Acute Renal Failure. In: Principles and Practice of Pediatrics (Ed. Oski FA). pp. 1093–1096.

2. Bergstein JM. (1992). Renal Failure. In: Nelson's Textbook of Pediatrics (Ed. Behrman RE). pp. 1352–1355.

3. Gaudio KM, Siegel NJ. (1987). Pathogenesis and treatment of acute renal failure. Pediatric Clin of North Am. 34, 771–787.

Appendix

1. Normal Blood Gas and Respiratory Parameters, and Gas Transport Equations

Abbreviation	Parameters (full form)	Equations	Normal Values
pH			7.35–7.45
PAO_2	Partial pressure of oxygen in alveolus		104 mm Hg
$PACO_2$	Partial pressure of carbon dioxide in alveolus		40 mm Hg
PaO_2	Partial pressure of oxygen in arterial blood		75–100 mm Hg
$PaCO_2$	Partial pressure of carbon dioxide in arterial blood		35–45 mm Hg
$P\bar{v}O_2$	Partial pressure of oxygen in mixed venous blood		35–40 mm Hg
SaO_2	Arterial oxygen saturation		96–100%
$S\bar{v}O_2$	Mixed venous oxygen saturation		70–80%
RQ	Respiratory quotient	$\dot{V}CO_2/\dot{V}O_2$	0.8
CaO_2	Arterial oxygen content	$(1.39 \times SaO_2 \%/100 \times [Hb])$ $+ (0.0031 \times PaO_2)$	18–21 ml/dl
$C\bar{v}O_2$	Mixed venous oxygen content	$(1.39 \times S\bar{v}O_2 \%/100 \times [Hb])$ $+ (0.0031 \times P\bar{v}O_2)$	14–15 ml/dl
$C(a\text{-}\bar{v})O_2$	Arteriovenous oxygen difference	$CaO_2 - C\bar{v}O_2$	4–6 ml/dl
CcO_2	Pulmonary capillary oxygen content	$(1.39 \times [Hb])$ $+ (0.0031 \times PAO_2)$	20–23 ml/dl
$\dot{V}O_2$	Oxygen consumption	$C(a\text{-}\bar{v})O_2 \times CO \times 10$	195–285 ml/min
$\dot{D}O_2$	Oxygen delivery	$CaO_2 \times CO \times 10$	950–1150 ml/min
O_2ER	Oxygen extraction ratio	$C(a\text{-}\bar{v})O_2/CaO_2$	0.24–0.28
$(A\text{-}a)DO_2$	Alveolar-arterial oxygen gradient On $FIO_2 = 0.21$ On $FIO_2 = 1.0$	$PAO_2 - PaO_2$	 5–25 mm Hg 25–65 mm Hg
$\dot{Q}_S/\dot{Q}_T$	Shunt fraction	$(CcO_2 - CaO_2)/$ $(CcO_2 - C\bar{v}O_2)$	3–8%
V_D/V_T	Dead space fraction	$[PaCO_2 - P_ECO_2]/PaCO_2$	0.25–0.4

CO = Cardiac output; P_ECO_2 = Partial pressure of carbon dioxide in expired gas.

2. Arterial Blood Gases (at sea level) while Breathing Room Air at Different Ages

Age (years)	PaO_2 (mm Hg)	$PaCO_2$ (mm Hg)	$(A\text{-}a)PO_2$ (mm Hg)
20	84–95	33–45	4–17
30	85–94	34–45	7–21
40	80–90	34–45	10–24
50	75–90	34–45	14–27
60	75–88	34–47	17–31
70	70–86	34–47	21–34
80	67–80	34–47	25–38

3. Alveolar Oxygen Tension (PAO_2) in Non-acclimatized Subjects Breathing Air at Sea Level and at Varying Altitudes

(Modified from Cotes JE, Lung Function—Assessment and Application in Medicine. 1979. pp. 463. Blackwell Scientific Publications, Melbourne, London.)

Altitude		Barometric Pressure (mm Hg)	P_AO_2 (mm Hg)
metres	feet		
0	(sea level) 0	760	102
1500	5000	632	82
3000	10,000	523	61
4600	15,000	429	44
6100	20,000	349	35
7600	25,000	282	33

4. Normal Haemodynamic Parameters and Calculations

See Chapter on Cardiac Monitoring in Adults

5. Daily Requirements of Important Electrolytes in Critically Ill Patients

Electrolytes	Enteral Nutrition	Parenteral Nutrition
* Sodium	1.3–3.3 g 60–150 mEq	60–150 mEq
* Potassium	2–5.5 g 40–80 mEq	40–80 mEq
* Chloride	40–100 mEq	40–100 mEq
* Magnesium	350 mg 10–20 mEq	10–20 mEq
* Phosphorus	800 mg 10–60 mmol	10–60 mmol
* Calcium	800 mg 5–20 mEq	5–20 mEq

6. Daily Vitamin Requirements in Critically Ill Patients

Vitamins	Enteral Nutrition	Parenteral Nutrition
* Vitamin A	3300 IU	3300 IU
* Vitamin D	400 IU	200 IU
* Vitamin E	10–20 IU	10 IU
* Vitamin K		10 mg/week IM
* Vitamin C	50–60 IU	100 IU
* Thiamine	1.5 mg	3 mg
* Riboflavin	1.8 mg	3.6 mg
* Niacin	20 mg	40 mg
* Pyridoxine	2 mg	4 mg
* Pantothenic acid	7 mg	15 mg
* Folic acid	200 µg	400 µg
* Vitamin B_{12}	2 µg	5 µg
* Biotin	100 µg	60 µg

7. Daily Requirements of Important Trace Elements in Critically Ill Patients

Trace Element	Enteral Nutrition	Parenteral Nutrition
* Zinc	3 mg	2.5–4 mg
* Copper	1.5 mg	1–1.5 mg
* Iron		1–2 mg
* Manganese	150–800 µg	200–800 µg
* Molybdenum	75–250 µg	100–200 µg
* Selenium	40–120 µg	40–120 µg
* Chromium	10–15 µg	10–20 µg
* Cobalt	1.1 mg	
* Iodine		120 µg

8. Composition of Plasma Compared to Some Commonly Used Crystalloid Solutions

Solution	Na$^+$ (mEq/l)	Cl$^-$ (mEq/l)	K$^+$ (mEq/l)	Ca^{++}/Mg^{++} (mEq/l)	Buffer	pH	Osmolality (mOsm/kg)
Plasma	141	103	4–5	5/2	HCO_3^- (26)	7.4	289
0.9% Saline	154	154	–	–	–	4.5–7	308
Ringer Lactate	130	109	4	3/0	Lactate (28)	6–7.5	273
Dextrose-Saline	154	154	–	–	–	3.5–6.5	586

9. Important ICU Drugs with their IV Dosages and Infusion Rates

A. Dopamine

Preparation: 600 mg in 500 ml 5% dextrose
Concentration: 1200 µg/ml or 20 µg/microdrop

Desired Effect	Dose (µg/kg/min)	Weight (kg)						
		40	50	60	70	80	90	100
		Infusion Rate (microdrops/min)						
Renal vasodilatation	1	2	2.5	3	3.5	4	4.5	5
(1–5 µg/kg/min)	5	10	12.5	15	17.5	20	22.5	25
Increase in cardiac	6	12	15	18	21	24	27	30
output (6–10 µg/kg/min)	10	20	25	30	35	40	45	50
Vasoconstriction	11	22	27.5	33	38.5	44	49.5	55
(11–20 µg/kg/min)	20	40	50	60	70	80	90	100

B. Dobutamine

Preparation: 500 mg in 500 ml 5% dextrose
Concentration: 1000 µg/ml or 16.7 µg/microdrop
Usual Dose: 5–15 µg/kg/min

Dose (µg/kg/min)	Weight (kg)						
	40	50	60	70	80	90	100
	Infusion Rate (microdrops/min)						
5	12	15	18	21	24	27	30
10	24	30	36	42	48	54	60
15	36	45	54	63	72	81	90
20	48	60	72	84	96	108	120
40	96	120	144	168	192	216	240

C. Norepinephrine

Preparation: 4 mg in 500 ml saline
Concentration: 8 µg/ml
Administration: Beta dose 1–10 µg/min
    Alpha dose > 10 µg/min

Dose (µg/min)	Infusion Rate (ml/hr)
1	7.5
2	15
4	30
6	45
8	60
10	75
12	90
14	105
16	120
18	135
20	150

D. Nitroglycerin

Preparation: 100 mg in 500 ml 5% dextrose
Concentration: 200 µg/ml or 3.33 µg/microdrop
Dose: Venodilator Dose 1–50 µg/min
    Usual Dose 1–400 µg/min

Dose (µg/min)	Infusion Rate (microdrops/min)
5	1.5
10	3
25	7.5
50	15
100	30
150	45
200	60
250	75
300	90
350	105
400	120

E. Lidocaine and Procainamide

Preparation: 1 g in 250 ml 5% dextrose
Concentration: 4 mg/ml
Usual Dose: 1–4 mg/min

Dose (mg/min)	Infusion Rate (ml/hr)
1	15
2	30
3	45
4	60

F. Nitroprusside

Preparation: 50 mg in 500 ml 5% dextrose
Concentration: 100 µg/ml or 1.67 µg/microdrop
Usual Dose: In heart failure 0.5–2 µg/kg/min*
　　　　　　 In hypertension 2–5 µg/kg/min

Dose (µg/kg/min)	Weight (kg)						
	40	50	60	70	80	90	100
	Infusion Rate (microdrops/min)						
0.5	12	15	18	21	24	27	30
1.0	24	30	36	42	48	54	60
1.5	36	45	54	63	72	81	90
2.0	48	60	72	84	96	108	120
2.5	60	75	90	105	120	135	150
3.0	72	90	108	126	144	162	180
3.5	84	105	126	147	168	189	210
4.0	96	120	144	168	192	216	240
4.5	108	135	162	189	216	243	270
5.0	120	150	180	210	240	270	300

* In patients with heart failure, 50 mg of nitroprusside are added to 250 ml of 5% dextrose, and the infusion rate is halved.

10. Serum Levels of Commonly Used ICU Drugs

Drug	Serum Levels	
	Therapeutic Range	Toxic Range
* Paracetamol	10–30 µg/ml	> 200 4 hrs post-ingestion
* Amikacin	Peak: 25–35 µg/ml	> 35
	Trough:1–4 µg/ml	> 10
* Gentamicin	Peak: 5–10 µg/ml	> 10
	Trough: 1–2 µg/ml	> 2
* Vancomycin	Peak: 40–50 µg/ml	> 80
	Trough: 5–15 µg/ml	> 20
* Tobramycin	Peak: 8–10 µg/ml	> 10
	Trough: 1–2 µg/ml	> 2
* Barbiturates		
– Short-acting	1–2 µg/ml	> 5
– Intermediate acting	1–5 µg/ml	> 10
– Phenobarbitone	15–40 µg/ml	> 40–nystagmus; > 65–coma
* Lithium	0.6–1.2 mEq/l	> 2
* Amitryptyline	120–250 ng/ml	> 500
* Desimipramine	75–160 ng/ml	> 1000
* Imipramine	125–250 ng/ml	> 500
* Chlorpromazine	50–300 ng/ml	> 750
* Diazepam	100–1000 ng/ml	> 5000
* Pentazocine	0.1–1 mg/l	> 2
* Pethidine	600–650 µg/l	> 10 mg/l
* Phenytoin	10–20 µg/ml	> 20–nystagmus; > 40–mental status
* Disopyramide	3–7 µg/ml	> 7
* Lidocaine	1.5–6 µg/ml	> 6
* Quinidine	2–5 µg/ml	> 6
* Procainamide	4–10 µg/ml	> 10
* Theophylline	10–20 µg/ml	> 20
* Digoxin	0.8–2 ng/ml	> 2
* Acetylsalicylic acid	100–350 mg/l	> 350

11. Important Drug Interactions in the ICU

(From The ICU Book,1991. [Ed. Marino PL] Lea and Febiger, Philadelphia, London.)

IV Drug	Serum Level	
	Increased By	Decreased By
* Catecholamines	Agents which alkalinize the urine—diamox	Agents which acidify the urine—Vitamin C
* Lidocaine	Cimetidine, beta-blockers	
* Procainamide	H₂-antagonists—cimetidine, ranitidine	
* Beta-blockers		
– Metoprolol	Cimetidine	Rifampicin
– Propranolol	Cimetidine, furosemide	
* Aminophylline	Cimetidine, propranolol, erythromycin	Phenobarbital, rifampicin,
* Digoxin	Quinidine, amiodarone, verapamil, diazepam, erythromycin, spironolactone	Rifampicin
* Diazepam	Propranolol	Phenytoin
* Phenytoin	Cimetidine	Phenobarbital, rifampicin, diazepam
* Pancuronium	Verapamil, clindamycin	Theophylline
* Cimetidine		Rifampicin, phenobarbital

12. Compatibility Chart for Commonly Used Critical Care Drugs

(From Guglielmo J, 1994. Pharmocotherapy. In: Current Critical Care Diagnosis and Treatment, [Eds Bongard FS and Sue DY], pp. 191–198, McGraw Hill Companies, NY.)

Key: C-documented compatibility; M-mixed results; I-documented incompatibility; N-no documented information.

	Aminophylline	Amiodarone	Amrinone	Bretylium	Dobutamine	Dopamine	Heparin	Isoproterenol	Lidocaine	Norepinephrine	Nitroglycerin	Nitroprusside	Phenylephrine	Procainamide	Verapamil
Aminophylline	■	I	N	C	I	N	I	I	I	C	C	N	N	N	I
Amiodarone	I	■	N	C	C	C	N	C	C	C	C	N	C	C	C
Amrinone	N	N	■	N	N	N	N	N	N	N	N	N	N	N	N
Bretylium	C	C	N	■	C	C	N	N	NC	C	C	N	N	M¹	C
Dobutamine	I	C	N	C	■	C	I	C	C	C	C	C	N	C	C
Dopamine	N	C	N	C	C	■	C	N	N	C	C	N	C	N	C
Heparin	I	N	N	N	I	C	■	C	I	C	N	N	N	N	C
Isoproterenol	I	C	N	N	C	N	C	■	N	I	N	N	N	N	C
Lidocaine	C	C	N	C	C	C	C	I	■	I	C	N	C	C	C
Norepinephrine	I	C	N	N	C	N	I	N	I	■	N	N	N	N	C
Nitroglycerin	C	C	N	C	C	C	N	N	N	C	■	N	N	N	C
Nitroprusside	N	N	N	N	N	N	N	N	N	N	N	■	N	N	N
Phenylephrine	N	C	N	N	C	N	N	N	N	C	N	N	■	N	N
Procainamide	N	C	N	M¹	C	N	N	N	N	C	N	N	N	■	C
Verapamil	I	C	N	C	C	C	C	C	C	C	C	C	N	N	■

¹May be concentration dependent

Note:

(a) Administration should be done through y-sets. Most compatibilities are visual i.e. no visible precipitation.

(b) All compatibility data are for 24 hrs in D₅W or normal saline. Some combinations may be compatible for shorter durations or under specific conditions.

13. Glasgow Coma Score, Trauma Score, Revised Trauma Score, CRAMS Scale and APACHE II Score

See Chapter on Critical Care Scoring

14. Correlation between APACHE II score and Mortality

(From: Breach Candy Hospital ICU data 2001–2003.)

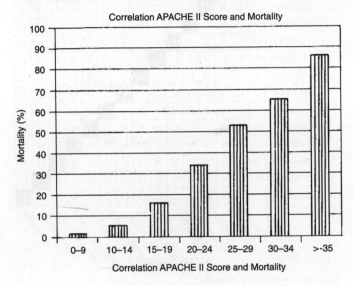

Correlation APACHE II Score and Mortality

15. Criteria for Diagnosis of Brain Death*

[From: ICU Book, 1991, [Ed. Marin PL]. Lea and Febiger, Philadelphia, London.)

Brain death has occurred if the following criteria are met on two consecutive occasions, at least two hours apart:
1. Does not localize in response to noxious stimuli (i)
2. Body temperature > 34°C
3. Serum levels of the following are negligible or subtherapeutic:
   (a) Ethanol; (b) CNS depressant drugs
4. The following movements are absent:
   (a) Decorticate posturing; (b) decerebrate posturing;
   (c) shivering; (d) spontaneous movements
5. The following reflexes are bilaterally absent (ii)
   (a) pupillary light reflex; (b) corneal reflex;
   (c) oculovestibular reflex; (d) oculocephalic reflex (doll's eyes)
6. EEG is isoelectric at maximal gain (iii)
7. Apnoea test is confirmatory (iv)
   (a) PaO_2 at end of test _____; (b) $PaCO_2$ at end of test _____

(i) Painful stimuli should be localized to cranial nerve areas because of the risk for spinal cord reflexes with peripheral stimuli. The favoured test is supraorbital pressure.

(ii) Pupillary light reflexes can also be absent after eye injury, neuromuscular blocking agents, atropine, mydriatics, scopolamine and opiates.

(iii) Isoelectric EEG does not exclude brainstem activity, and is not to be used in isolation to diagnose brain death.

(iv) The apnoea test is confirmatory if there is no evidence of spontaneous ventilatory efforts for at least 3 minutes, and the $PaCO_2$ is > 60 mm Hg at the end of the test. If history of chronic CO_2 retention is present, the PaO_2 should be < 55 mm Hg at the end of the test.

(Modified from the University of Pittsburgh criteria for brain death, with permission of BC Decker Inc., Philadelphia.)

Index

Acid-base disturbances, 361–71
 basic concepts in, 361
 kidneys in, 363
 metabolic acidosis, 367–8
 metabolic alkalosis, 369–70
 laboratory diagnosis in, 364
 respiratory acidosis, 370
 respiratory alkalosis, 370–71
 terminology in, 363–4
Acute coronary syndromes, 162–164, see also myocardial infarction, unstable angina
Activated Protein C, 151–2, 285–6
Acute disseminated haematogenous tuberculosis, 424–5
Acute left ventricular failure, see left ventricular failure
Acute lung injury, 274–87
 aetiology of, 275–7
 cardiopulmonary physiology in, 278–9
 clinical features of, 279
 definition and concept of, 274–5
 management of, 280–7
 imaging in, 89
 in multi-organ dysfunction, 279
 in nosocomial pneumonia, 279
 investigations in, 279–280
 O_2 uptake and utilization in, 278
 pathology of 277
 pathogenesis of 277–8
 prognosis of 280
Acute myocardial infarction, see myocardial infarction
Acute necrotizing pancreatitis, see pancreatitis, acute necrotizing
Acute renal failure, see renal failure, acute
Acute respiratory failure, see respiratory failure, acute
Acute respiratory crisis in COPD, see COPD
Acute severe asthma, see asthma, acute severe
Acute stroke, see stroke, acute
Acyclovir, 616
Adenosine, 206, 210
Adrenal crisis, 535–7
Adrenalin, see epinephrine

Advanced cardiac life support, 24–9
Airway management, 255–66
Amoebic infections, fulminant, 426–7
Aminoglycosides, 435
Amiodarone, 206–8
Amniotic fluid embolism, 698
Amphetamine poisoning, 648
Amphotericin B, 440–2
Anaphylactic shock, 159–60
Anaphylactoid reaction, 159
Anion gap, 367–8
Antibiotic-associated colitis, 409
Antibiotics in the ICU, 431–9
Anti-coagulant therapy,
 in myocardial infarction, 172, 179
 in stroke, 564
 in unstable angina, 166–8
Anti-platelet therapy,
 in myocardial infarction, 172, 179
 in stroke, 564
 in unstable angina, 166, 168
Antivenin, use of, 656–8
Aortic dissection, 217–9
 imaging of, 95, 101–2
APACHE scores, 15–6, 465–6
Artificial airways, 256
ARDS, see Acute lung injury
Aspiration pneumonia, 396–7
Aspirin,
 in DVT, 226
 in MI, 173
 toxicity of, 648–50
 in unstable angina, 168
Asthma, acute severe, 288–94
 clinical features of, 289
 investigations for, 289–90
 pathophysiology of, 288–89
 treatment of, 290–3
Asystole, 27–8
Atelectasis,
 imaging in, 91
 in mechanical ventilation, 331
 respiratory failure due to, 231
Atrial fibrillation, 193–5

Atrial flutter, 191–3
Atrioventricular block, 203–4
Automatic atrial tachycardia, 196
Auto-PEEP, 331–2
Aztreonam, 437–8

Barbiturate poisoning, 644–5
Basic life support, 22–4
 in polytrauma, 625–6
Beta-blockers,
 in hypertensive crisis, 215
 in myocardial infarction, 172, 174–5, 179
 in paediatrics, 718
 in tachycardias, 539
 in unstable angina, 166–7
 toxicity of, 647
Blood products, 530–2
Blood gas analysis, 79
 in children, 707
Body water, 341
Bradyrhythms, see heart blocks
Bretylium tosylate, 206, 209
Burns, 630–9
 assessment, 632–33
 management, 632–9
 physiopathology, 630–2

Café coronary, 22
Calcium-channel blockers
 in hypertensive crisis, 215
 in myocardial infarction, 172, 174, 179
 in paediatrics, 214–5
 in unstable angina, 166–7
 toxicity of, 648
Cancer patient, critical care in, 661–6
Candiduria, 408
Capsofungin, 440
Carbon monoxide poisoning, 650–1
Cardiac compressive shock, see cardiac tamponade
Cardiac monitoring in adults, 59–76
Cardiac output, 35
 measurement of, 71–3, 713
Cardiac tamponade, 155–8
 after open heart surgery, 595

clinical features and diagnosis, 155–7
management of, 157–8
physiopathology of, 155–6
Cardiac surgery, *see* open heart surgery, critical care after
Cardiogenic shock, 128–40
clinical features and diagnosis of, 129–30
haemodynamic changes and profiles in, 130–2
management of, 132–3, 138–40
physiopathology, 128–9
Cardiopulmonary resuscitation, 21–32
in infants and children, 703–4
Cardiopulmonary physiology in intensive care unit, 35–44
Catheter-related infections, 402–5
Cavernous sinus thrombosis, 572
Central venous catheterization, 50–2
Central venous pressure monitoring, 63–6
in children, 712–3
Cephalosporins, 436–7
Cervical spine trauma, airway management in, 265
Chest tube drainage, 53–5
Ciprofloxacin, 437
Clostridial myonecrosis, 451–2
Clotting factors, 532
Cocaine poisoning, 646
Coagulation disorders, 524–8
Combitube, 458
Community-acquired pneumonia, 295–300
aetiology of, 295
clinical features of, 296
complications of, 297
differential diagnosis of, 298
investigations in, 298–9
management of, 295, 299–300
pathogenesis of, 296
Complete heart block, 203–4
Compliance, pulmonary, 81–2
Continuous haemofiltration and diafiltration, 487
COPD, acute respiratory crisis in, 267–73
precipitating factors of, 267–8
diagnosis of, 268–9
management of, 269–73
complications during, 272–3
CRAMS scale, 15
Cranial trauma, 557–61
imaging in, 106–7
Cricothyroidotomy, 48–9
Cryoprecipitate, 530, 532
Cyanide poisoning, 651

Dalfopristin/ Quinopristin 438
Demyelinating disorders, 573
Dengue haemorrhagic fever, 427–9
Diabetic ketoacidosis, 543–8
Dialysis, 485–7, 489–90

Dieulafoy's ulcer, 514
Differential lung ventilation, 329–30
Difficult intubation in ICU, 258–60
Digitalis, *see* digoxin
Digoxin, 206, 210–1
arrhythmias induced by, 200–1
in atrial fibrillation, 193–5
in cardiogenic shock, 136
in left ventricular failure, 187
use of, 206, 210–1
Dissection of aorta, 217–9
Disseminated intravascular coagulopathy, 526–7
Dobutamine, use of, 27
in acute lung injury, 285
in left ventricular failure, 187–8
in paediatrics, 717
in pulmonary embolism, 226
in shock, 135, 150, 150
Dopamine, use of, 27
in acute lung injury, 285
in left ventricular failure, 187–8
in paediatrics, 717
in pulmonary embolism, 226
in shock, 135, 150, 150

ECG monitoring, 59–60
Echocardiography,
in cardiac tamponade, 157
in acute stroke, 563
Eclampsia, 694–5, 697
Emergency airways, 256–7
Endotracheal intubation, 47–8, 264–5
Empyema, imaging in, 91–2
Enteral nutrition, 380–3
Envenomation in the ICU, 653–8
Epilepsy, *see* status epilepticus
Epinephrine, 25, 27,
in acute severe asthma, 290
in anaphylactic shock, 160,
in shock, 137,
Esmolol, 206, 209, 216
Ethical issues in terminal illness, 6
Euthanasia, 7
Extracellular fluid, 341–2
Extracorporeal membrane oxygenation (ECMO), 330

Fever with neutropaenia, 607
Fever in the ICU, 391–3
non-infectious causes of, 392–3
physiopathology of, 391–2
Fick principle, 43–4
Fluconazole, 440–2
Flucytosine, 440–2
Fluid and electrolyte disturbances,
in the critically ill adult, 341–58
in the critically ill child, 626–7
Fresh frozen plasma, 530, 532

Fungal infection, treatment of, 440–3

Gas exchange, physiology of, 40
Gastric lavage, 642–3
Gastric tonometry, 75
Gastrointestinal bleeding, acute, 510–9
imaging in, 101
in hepatic failure, 498–501
lower, 514–9
upper, 510–4
Glasgow coma scale, 14
Glycoprotein IIb/IIIa receptor antagonists,
in myocardial infarction, 172, 178–9
in unstable angina, 166, 168
Gram-negative infection, 425–6

Haematemesis, 498–501
Haemodialysis, 486
Haemodynamic monitoring
in adults, 69–76
in children, 710–13
Haemofiltration
in metabolic alkalosis, 370
Haemolytic-uraemic syndrome, 695–7
Haemoptysis, massive, 301–7
causes of, 301–3
clinical features of, 302–3
diagnosis of, 303
management of, 303–6
Haemorrhagic disorders, 520–1
Haemorrhagic shock, *see* hypovolaemic and haemorrhagic shock
Head injury, 557–61
imaging in, 106–7
Heart blocks, 202–4
atrioventricular block, 203–4
complete heart block, 203–4
sinoatrial block, 202–3
Wenckibach block, 203
Heart failure,
in infants and children, 719–20
nutrition in, 387
physiopathology of, 38–9
with pulmonary oedema, 183–9
Heimlich manoeuvre, 22–3
HELP syndrome, 695
Henderson-Hesselbah equation, 362
Hepatic encephalopathy, 497–8
Hepatic failure, chronic, 497–502
coagulation defects in, 526
nutrition in, 386
Hepatitis, critical care in fulminant, 491–6
Aetiology of, 491
Definitions in, 491
clinical features and diagnosis of, 492–3
management of, 494–6
High dependency ward, 12
High frequency ventilation (HFV), 329
in paediatrics, 724–5

Hyperbaric oxygen, 250, 448, 452
Hypercapnia, 238 *see also* permissive hypercapnia
Hyperglycaemia, nutritional considerations, 543
Hyperglycaemic hyperosmolar non-ketotic coma, 548
Hypercalcaemia, 354
    in cancer patients, 663
Hyperkalaemia, 349
Hypermagnesaemia, 356
Hypernatraemia, 348
Hyperphosphataemia, 355
Hypertensive crisis
    in eclapmsia, 217, 695
    in paediatrics, 718
    in the ICU, 213–7
Hypochloric acid, use of, 370
Hypocalcaemia, 353–4
    in cancer patients, 662–3
Hypokalaemia, 349
    in cancer patients, 663–4
Hypomagnesaemia, 355–6
Hyponatraemia, 345
Hypophosphataemia, 354–5
    in cancer patients, 662
Hypovolaemic and haemorrhagic shock, 120–7
    blood transfusion in, 122–6
    clinical features of, 121–2
    differential diagnosis of, 123
    fluid resuscitation in, 122–6
    haemodynamic patterns in, 122–3
    in intra-abdominal sepsis, 457–8
    monitoring of, 122–3
    physiopathology of, 120–1
Hypoxaemic respiratory failure, 233–6
Hypoxia, 236–7

Imaging in intensive care, 87–111
    imaging techniques in the abdomen, 96–105
    imaging techniques in the chest, 88–95, 709–10
    neuroimaging techniques, 106–11
Imipenem, 437
Immunonutrition and immunity-enhancing formulas, 387
Immunocompromised patient, critical care in, 605–19
Infection, fulminant Gram-negative, 425–6
Injury severity score, 15
Intra-abdominal sepsis, 453–61
    aetiology of, 453–4
    clinical features and diagnosis of, 457–9
    investigations in, 459
    management of, 460
    physiopathology of, 454–6
Intra-aortic balloon pump (IABP), 56–7
    in unstable angina, 168–9
Intracellular fluid, 341

Intracerebral haemorrhage, 566–7
    imaging in, 107–8
Intracranial space occupying lesion syndrome, 572
Intracranial tension, increased,
    airway management in, 265–6
    monitoring, 57, 552–3
    physiopathology, 550–2
    syndrome, 572
Inverse ratio ventilation, 283
Iron poisoning, 651–2

Jugular venous pressure, 63–6

Lactic acid acidosis, 368–9
Laryngeal mask airway (LMA), 257–8
Lactic acid acidosis, 368–9
Left ventricular failure, acute, *see* pulmonary oedema
Leptospirosis, 429
Lidocaine, 205–7
Linezolid, 438
Lithium dilution technique for cardiac output monitoring, 73
Liver cell failure, chronic, 497–502
    coagulation defects in, 526

Malaria, *see* Plasmodium falciparum infection, fulminant
Malignant hypertension, 216–7
Mallory-Weiss syndrome, 510–4
Malaria, *see* Plasmodium falciparum infection, fulminant
Mechanical ventilation, 311–338
    complications of, 330–3
    criteria for initiating, 315–6
    guidelines in practical management of, 321–3
    indications for, 313–5
    in polytrauma, 627
    modes and strategies for, 323–5
    newer and less frequently used modes of, 328–30
    objectives of, 320–1
    physiological principles of, 311–3
    trouble-shooting in, 336–7
    types of ventilators in, 316–9
    use of PEEP in, 325–8
    ventilatory patterns in diseases requiring support, 321
    weaning from, 333–6
Meningoencephalitis syndrome, 571–2
Meropenem, 437
Metabolic acidosis, 367–8
Metabolic alkalosis, 369–70
Methanol poisoning, 651
Mixed venous oxygen saturation, 74–5
Morphine, 185–6
Multiple organ dysfunction score, 17

Multiple organ dysfunction syndrome (MODS), 465–78
    aetiology of, 467–9
    after open heart surgery, 600
    definition and concept of, 465–7
    epidemiology of, 469
    in pancreatitis, 504–5
    natural history and clinical features of, 469–71
    physiopathology of, 471–3
    prognosis of, 473–4
    prevention of, 474
    treatment of, 474–5
Muscle relaxants in the ICU, 674–7
Myocardial infarction, acute, 171–82
    complications in, 180–1
    diagnosis of, 171–2
    haemodynamic assessment in, 180
    management of, 172–80
    peri-operative, 595–6
Myxoedema coma, 540–2

Narcotic poisoning, 645
Necrotizing fasciitis, 450–1
Neuromuscular paralysis, acute generalized, 573
Neurological infections, fulminant, 571–6
Nitrates
    in hypertensive crisis, 214–5
    in left ventricular failure, 185, 187
    in myocardial infarction, 172, 174, 179
    in paediatrics, 718
    in unstable angina, 166–7
Non-paroxysmal AV junctional tachycardia, 197–9
Non-invasive ventilator support, 330
    in ARDS, 275–7
Norepinephrine, use of, 150
Nosocomial infection, 392–412
    epidemiology of, 394–5
    prevention and control of, 410–2
Nosocomial pneumonia, 396–402
    antibiotic therapy in, 400–1
    diagnosis of, 398–400
    pathogenesis of, 396–7
    predisposing factors for, 397–8
    prevention of, 401
    prognosis in, 401
Nutritional support, 375–88
    indications for, 376
    in special conditions, 385–7, 628–9, 728
    methods of, 380
    objectives of, 377
    requirements in, 378–9
    timing for, 376–7

Open heart surgery, critical care after, 591–601
    complications and their management, 593–600

immediate management, 592–3
in myocardial infarction, 179–80
monitoring and transfer to the ICU, 591–2
Open lung concept, 284–5, 328–9
Organization of intensive care unit, 9–12
Organophosphorus poisoning, 646–7
Osmolality, plasma, 342

Pain management, in the ICU, 669–73
Pancreatitis, acute necrotizing, 503–9
aetiology of, 503–4
clinical features and diagnostic evaluation of, 504–6
complications of, 504, 508–9
imaging in, 97–8
management of, 506–9
nutrition in, 387
physiopathology of, 504
Paracetamol poisoning, 650
Parenteral nutrition, 383–5
PEEP, 282, 325–8, 331–2
Penicillins, 433–5
Percutaneous dilatational tracheostomy, 49–50
Peri-operative neurological care, 584–7
Peritoneal dialysis, 486, 489
Permissive hypercapnia,
in ARDS, 284
Pericardiocentesis, 55–6, 157
Peritoneal dialysis, 486–7
Physiology in the ICU, cardiopulmonary, 35–44
Plasmodium falciparum infection, fulminant, 413–7
clinical features and complications in, 414–5
imaging in, 109–10
management in, 415–7
mortality in, 417
physiopathology of, 413–4
Platelet transfusions, 530–2
Pneumocystis carinii pneumonia, 612–3
Pneumonia
community-acquired, *see* community-acquired pneumonia
hospital-acquired, *see* nosocomial pneumonia
imaging in, 90–1
Pneumothorax,
imaging in, 92
Pneumomediastinum,
imaging in, 92
Polytrauma, 623–9
Poisonings, approach to, 640–4
Post-operative wound infection, 447–8
antibiotic prophylaxis in, 448
classification of, 447
clinical features of, 448
predisposing factors for, 448
treatment of, 448–9
Pre-eclampsia, 694–5

Pregnancy, critical care in, 689–99
Primary angioplasty, 172, 178
Procainamide, 206–7
Procedures in the ICU, 47–58
Prone position ventilation, 283–4
Proportional assist ventilation, 329
Pseudocyst of pancreas, 504–6, 508–9
Pulmonary artery pressure monitoring, 66–71
Pulmonary embolism, 220–7
after open heart surgery, 600
clinical presentation of, 221
diagnosis of, 221–224
management of, 225–6
physiopathology of, 220–1
peventive measures in, 226–7
Pulmonary oedema,
diagnosis of, 185
haemodynamic profiles in, 183–4
imaging in, 88–9
invasive monitoring in, 188–9
management of, 185
precipitating factors for in the ICU, 188
Pulse oximetry, 79
in children, 706–7

Quinidine, 206–7
Quinolones, 437–8
Quinopristin/Dalfopristin 438

Renal failure,
acute, 479–90
in infants and children, 733–6
nutrition in, 385–6
Respiratory acidosis, 370
Respiratory alkalosis, 370–1
Respiratory failure, acute, 231–44
clinical features of, 237–9
diagnostic assessment of, 239–41
failure of O_2 transport in, 236
failure of O_2 uptake in, 237
in children, 721–3
management of, 241–43
nutrition in, 386–7
respiratory muscle fatigue in, 236–7
types of, 231–6
Respiratory distress syndrome in neonates, 723–4
Respiratory monitoring,
in adults, 77–84
in children, 705–10
Rostral spinal cord syndrome, 572

Salicylate poisoning, 648–50
Salt balance, 343
SAPS score, 17
SARS (Severe Acute Respiratory Syndrome), 296–7
Scoring systems in critical care, 14–8
Scorpion sting, 657–8
Sedatives in the ICU, 673–4

Sengstaken-Blakemore tube, 500–1
Sepsis and septic shock, 141–54
clinical features of, 142–3
definitions, 141–2
haemodynamic effects of, 145
haemodynamic profiles in, 145–7
in immunocompromised patients, 607–8
in paediatrics, 731
laboratory features of, 143
management of, 147–52
physiopathology of, 143–4
Shock syndromes, 115–9
in paediatrics, 715–7
management of, 116–8
overview of, 115–6
SIADH, 345–7,
in cancer patients, 662
Sinoatrial block, 202–3
Sinus bradycardia, 202
Sinus tachycardia, 191
Snake bites, 653–7
SOFA score, 17
Subarachnoid haemorrhage, 567–70
Supraventricular tachycardia, 191–7
with delayed conduction, 195–6, 199
Status epilepticus, 577–83
Stress ulcers, 514
Stroke, acute, 562–7
classification of, 562
diagnostic evaluation of, 562–3
imaging in, 107–8
management of, 563–7
Swan-Ganz catheter, 66–71
Systemic Inflamatory Response Syndrome (SIRS), 469–73

Tachyrhythms, 190–201
Teicoplanin, 436
Tetanus, 417–24
altered haemodynamics in, 418
clinical features and diagnosis, 418–9
complications of, 419–21
diagnosis of, 421
management of, 421–3
mortality in, 423
physiopathology in, 418
prevention of, 423
Thoracic electrical bioimpedence, 72–3
Thrombocytopaenia, 522–4
Thrombolytic therapy,
in myocardial infarction, 172, 174–5
in stroke, 564–5
in unstable angina, 166, 168
Thyroid emergencies, 537–42
Torsade de Pointes, 199
Toxic shock syndrome, 152–3
in paediatrics, 731
Trauma care, 624–9
Tracheostomy, 260–4
Transfusion therapy, 530–4